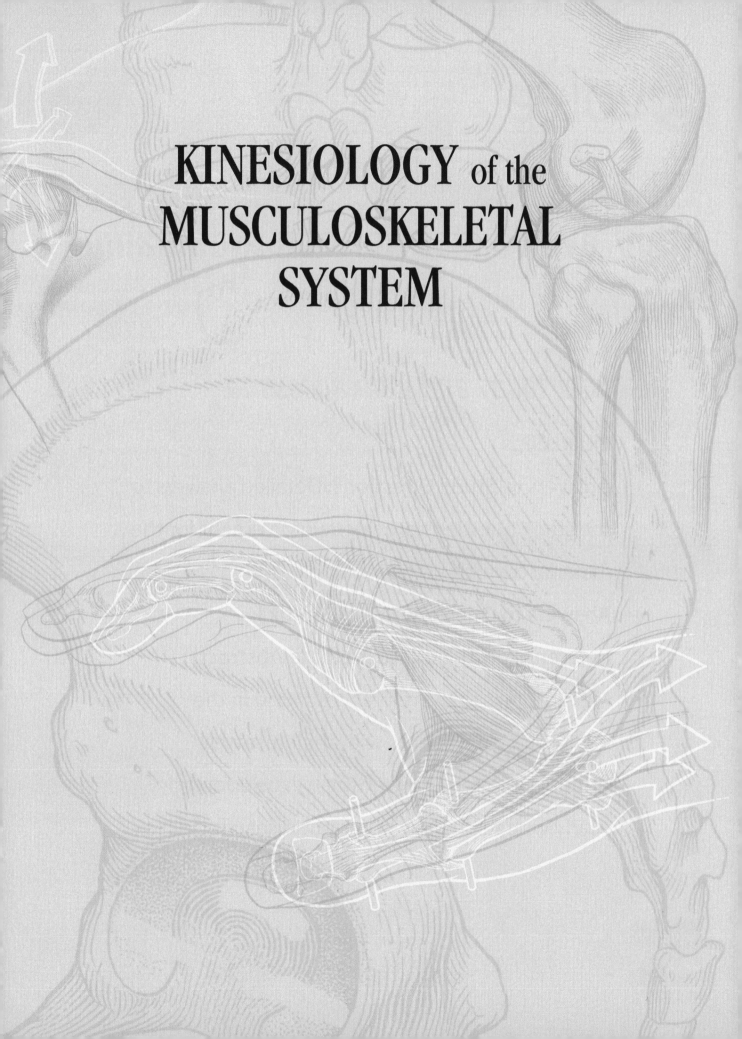

KINESIOLOGY of the
MUSCULOSKELETAL
SYSTEM

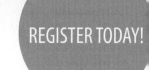

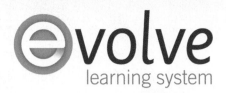

evolve
learning system

To access your Student Resources, visit:

http://evolve.elsevier.com/Neumann/

Register today and gain access to:

- **Video Clips**

- **Answers to Study Questions:** Detailed answers to the study questions provide reinforcement for the material covered in the textbook.

- **Answers to Questions in Appendix I**

- **References with links to Medline Abstracts:** Medline links to the references found in the textbook help students with their research.

- **Annual Updates:** The website will be updated yearly with references to current research.

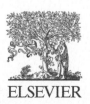

ELSEVIER

KINESIOLOGY of the MUSCULOSKELETAL SYSTEM

Foundations for Rehabilitation

Second Edition

DONALD A. NEUMANN, PT, PhD, FAPTA

Professor
Department of Physical Therapy and Exercise Science
Marquette University
Milwaukee, Wisconsin

Primary Artwork by

ELISABETH ROEN KELLY, BSc, BMC

CRAIG KIEFER, MAMS

KIMBERLY MARTENS, MAMS

CLAUDIA M. GROSZ, MFA, CMI

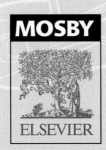

MOSBY

ELSEVIER

MOSBY
ELSEVIER

3251 Riverport Lane
St. Louis, Missouri 63043

KINESIOLOGY OF THE MUSCULOSKELETAL SYSTEM:
Foundations for Rehabilitation   978-0-323-03989-5

Artwork introducing the Additional Clinical Connections in Chapters 5-15 from
Barcsay J: *Anatomy for the Artist*, ed 2, London, 1958, Spring Books.

Library of Congress Cataloging-in-Publication Data
Neumann, Donald A.
  Kinesiology of the musculoskeletal system : foundations for rehabilitation / Donald A. Neumann ; artwork by Elisabeth R. Kelly, Craig Kiefer, Jeanne Robertson.—2nd ed.
      p. ; cm.
  Includes bibliographical references and index.
  ISBN 978-0-323-03989-5 (hardcover : alk. paper) 1. Kinesiology.   2. Human mechanics.
3. Musculoskeletal system—Diseases—Patients—Rehabilitation.   I. Title.
  [DNLM: 1. Kinesiology, Applied.   2. Biomechanics.   3. Movement.   4. Musculoskeletal Physiological Phenomena. WB 890 N492ka 2010]
  QP303.N465 2010
  613.7—dc22
                                                                   2009031123

Vice President and Publisher: Linda Duncan
Senior Editor: Kathy Falk
Senior Developmental Editor: Melissa Kuster Deutsch
Publishing Services Manager: Patricia Tannian
Senior Project Manager: Sarah Wunderly
Design Manager: Teresa McBryan
Art Assistance: Jeannie Robertson

Printed in the United States

Last digit is the print number: 9 8 7 6 5 4

To those whose lives have been strengthened
by the struggle and joy of learning

About the Author

Donald A. Neumann

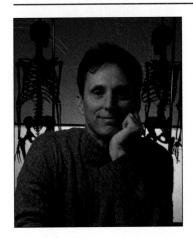

Don was born in New York City, the oldest of five siblings. He is the son of Charles J. Neumann, a meteorologist and world-renowned hurricane forecaster, who has lived for 60 years with the affects of polio, which he contracted flying as a "hurricane hunter" in the Caribbean Sea in the 1950s. Don grew up in Miami, Florida, the location of the United States Weather Bureau, where his mother (Betty) and father still live today.

Soon after graduating from high school, Don was involved in a serious motorcycle accident. After receiving extensive physical therapy, Don chose physical therapy as his lifelong career. In 1972, he started his study and practice of physical therapy by earning a 2-year degree from Miami Dade Community College as a physical therapist assistant. In 1976, Don graduated with a bachelor of science degree in physical therapy from the University of Florida. He went on to practice as a physical therapist at Woodrow Wilson Rehabilitation Center in Virginia, where he specialized in the rehabilitation of patients with spinal cord injury. In 1980, Don attended the University of Iowa, where he earned his master's degree in science education and a PhD in exercise science.

In 1986, Don started his academic career as a teacher, writer, and researcher in the Physical Therapy Department at Marquette University. His teaching efforts have concentrated on kinesiology as it relates to physical therapy, anatomy, and rehabilitation of people with spinal cord injury. Don remained clinically active as a physical therapist on a part-time basis until 2002, working primarily in the area of rehabilitation after spinal cord injury, outpatient orthopedics, and geriatrics. Today he continues his academic career as a full professor at Marquette University.

Dr. Neumann has received many awards for his scholarship in physical therapy (www. marquette.edu). In addition to receiving several prestigious teaching and research awards from the American Physical Therapy Association, Dr. Neumann received a Teacher of the Year Award at Marquette University in 1994, and in 2006 he was named by the Carnegie Foundation as Wisconsin's College Professor of the Year. In 2008, Donald was named a Fellow of the American Physical Therapy Association.

Over the years, Dr. Neumann's research and teaching projects have been funded by the National Arthritis Foundation and the Paralyzed Veterans of America. He has published extensively on methods to protect the arthritic or painful hip from damaging forces. Don has received multiple Fulbright Scholarships to teach kinesiology in Kaunas Medical University in Lithuania (2002), Semmelweis Medical University in Budapest, Hungary (2005 and 2006), and Shinshu University in Matsumoto, Japan (2009 and 2010). In 2007, Don received an honorary doctorate from the Lithuanian Academy of Physical Education, located in Kaunas, Lithuania. Donald also serves as an associate editor of the *Journal of Orthopaedic & Sports Physical Therapy.*

Don lives with his wife, Brenda, and two dogs in Wisconsin; his son Donald, Jr. ("Donnie") and family, and his stepdaughter, Megann, also live in Wisconsin. Outside of work, Donald enjoys photography, a wide range of music, mountaineering, and paying close attention to the weather.

About the Illustrations

The collection of art in this edition has undergone extensive transformation from the first edition. Some of the art is brand new, some of it has been extensively modified, and nearly all the illustrations have been fully colorized. Most of the more than 700 illustrations are original, produced over the course of compiling the first two editions of this text. The illustrations were first conceptualized by Dr. Neumann and then meticulously rendered to their pre-colored state through the unique talents of Elisabeth Roen Kelly. Dr. Neumann states, "The artwork really drove the direction of much of my writing. I needed to thoroughly understand a particular kinesiologic concept at its most essential level in order to effectively explain to Elisabeth what needed to be illustrated. In this way, the artwork kept me honest; I wrote only what I truly understood."

Dr. Neumann and Ms. Kelly produced three primary forms of artwork for this text. Elisabeth depicted the anatomy of bones, joints, and muscles by hand, creating very detailed pen-and-ink drawings (Figure 1). These drawings started with a series of pencil sketches, often based on anatomic specimens carefully dissected by Dr. Neumann. The pen-and-ink medium was chosen to give the material an organic, classic feeling. Color was added to these drawings in this edition by a talented and dedicated team of illustrators: Craig Kiefer, Kimberly Martens (from the art studio of Martens & Kiefer), and Claudia Grosz. Craig Kiefer, who led the colorization team, worked diligently with Dr. Neumann to develop a process of adding color that maintained the integrity of Ms. Kelly's original line art.

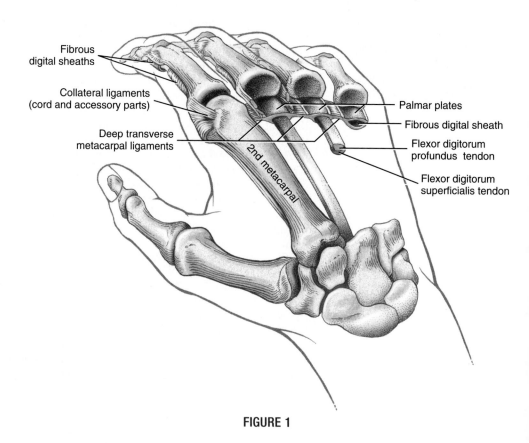

FIGURE 1

The second form of art used a layering of artistic media, integrated with the use of computer software (Figure 2). Neumann and Kelly often started with a photograph that was transformed into a simplified outline of a person performing a particular movement. Images of bones, joints, and muscles were then electronically embedded within the human outline. Overlaying various biomechanical images further enhanced the resultant illustration. The final design displayed specific and often complex biomechanical concepts in a relatively simple manner, while preserving human form and expression. Final coloring was skillfully provided primarily by the team of Kiefer, Martens, and Grosz.

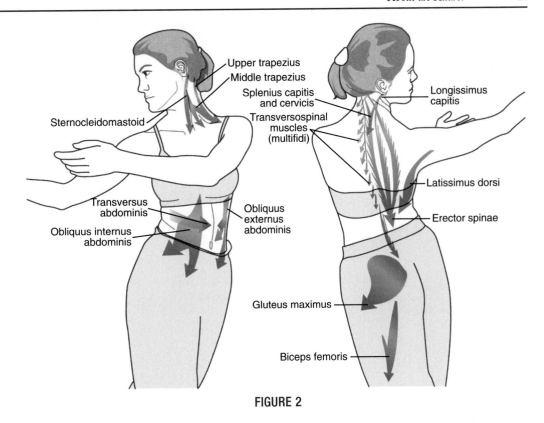

FIGURE 2

A third form of art was specifically developed by Neumann and Kelly for this edition (Figure 3). With the help of software, prepared anatomic specimens were rendered to a textured three-dimensional shape. The depth and anatomic precision of these images provides important insight into the associated kinesiology.

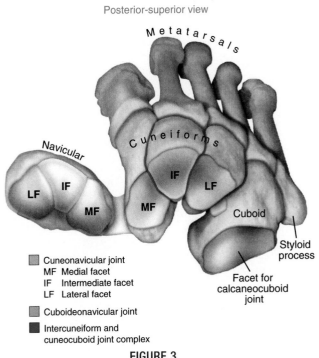

FIGURE 3

About the Contributors

Peter R. Blanpied, PT, PhD

Professor, Physical Therapy Department, University of Rhode Island, Kingston, Rhode Island

http://www.uri.edu/

Dr. Blanpied received his basic training at Ithaca College, graduating with a bachelor of science degree in physical therapy in 1979. After practicing clinically in acute, adult rehabilitation, and sports settings, he returned to school and completed an advanced master of science degree in physical therapy from the University of North Carolina in 1982, specializing in musculoskeletal therapeutics, and a PhD from the University of Iowa in 1989. Since then, he has been on faculty at the University of Rhode Island teaching in the areas of biomechanics, research, and musculoskeletal therapeutics. In addition to continuing clinical practice, he has also been active in funded and unfunded research and is the author of many peer-reviewed research articles, and national and international professional research presentations. He is an associate editor of the *Journal of Orthopaedic & Sports Physical Therapy,* and is active in the Research Section of the APTA. He lives in West Kingston with his wife Carol (also a physical therapist) and their two sons.

Sandra K. Hunter, PhD

Associate Professor, Exercise Science Program, Marquette University, Milwaukee, Wisconsin

http://www.marquette.edu/

Dr. Hunter received a bachelor of education degree in physical education and health from the University of Sydney, a Graduate Diploma in human movement science from Wollongong University, and a PhD in exercise and sport science (exercise physiology) from The University of Sydney where her research focused on neuromuscular function with aging and strength training. Dr. Hunter moved to Boulder, Colorado, in 1999 to take a position as a postdoctoral research associate in the Neurophysiology of Movement Laboratory directed by Dr. Roger Enoka. Her research focused on the mechanisms of neuromuscular fatigue during varying task conditions. She has been a faculty member in the Exercise Science Program in the Department of Physical Therapy at Marquette University since 2003 where her primary area of teaching is advanced exercise physiology and research methods. Dr. Hunter's current research program focuses on understanding the mechanisms of neuromuscular fatigue and impairment in muscle function in clinical populations under different task conditions. She is the author of several book chapters, many peer-reviewed research articles, and national and international research presentations. Dr. Hunter has received research funding from the National Institutes of Health (NIH), including the National Institute of Aging and National Institute of Occupational Safety and Health, as well as from many other funding sources. She is on the editorial board for the *Journal of Applied Physiology.* In her free time, Sandra enjoys traveling, camping, hiking, cycling, and the occasional triathlon. She lives in Wisconsin with her husband Jeff and her daughter Kennedy.

Guy G. Simoneau, PT, PhD

Professor, Department of Physical Therapy, Marquette University, Milwaukee, Wisconsin

http://www.marquette.edu/

Dr. Simoneau received a bachelor of science degree in physiotherapy from the Université de Montréal, Canada, a master of science degree in physical education (sports medicine) from the University of Illinois at Urbana-Champaign, Illinois, and a PhD in exercise and sport science (locomotion studies) from The Pennsylvania State University, State College, Pennsylvania, where he focused much of his work on the study of gait, running, and posture. Dr. Simoneau has been a faculty member in the Department of Physical Therapy at Marquette University since 1992. His primary area of teaching is orthopedic and sports physical therapy. He has also published several book chapters and research articles on topics related to orthopedic/sports physical therapy and biomechanics. Dr. Simoneau has received research funding from the National Institutes of Health (NIH), the National Institute of Occupational Safety and Health (NIOSH), the Arthritis Foundation, and the Foundation for Physical Therapy, among others. His research and teaching efforts have been recognized through several national awards from the American Physical Therapy Association. In 2007, Guy received an honorary doctorate from the Lithuanian Academy of Physical Education, located in Kaunas, Lithuania. Dr. Simoneau is currently the editor-in-chief of the *Journal of Orthopaedic & Sports Physical Therapy.* In his free time, Guy enjoys traveling and hiking.

Original Contributors

David A. Brown, PT, PhD

Associate Professor and Associate Chair for Post-Professional Education, Department of Physical Therapy & Human Movement Sciences, Feinberg School of Medicine, Northwestern University, Chicago, Illinois

http://www.feinberg.northwestern.edu/

Dr. Brown is the son of a physical therapist (Elliott). David graduated with a master's degree from Duke University in 1983 and received a PhD in exercise science from the University of Iowa in 1989. He is now the director of the NUPTHMS Locomotor Control Laboratory. His area of clinical expertise is in neurorehabilitation with an emphasis on locomotion following stroke. In his current role as an educator and scientist, Dr. Brown is a named inventor on four patents, including the KineAssist Walking and Balance System, and has authored many articles in peer-reviewed journals. He has received research funding from the National Institutes for Health, Department of Education, Department of Veterans Affairs, and Foundation for Physical Therapy. Dr. Brown is married, has one child, and enjoys hiking, biking, travel, classical music, theater, and reading American literature.

A. Joseph Threlkeld, PT, PhD

Associate Professor, Department of Physical Therapy, Creighton University, Omaha, Nebraska

http://spahp2.creighton.edu/

A 1976 physical therapy graduate of the University of Kentucky, Lexington, Kentucky, Dr. Threlkeld has been involved in the clinical management of musculoskeletal dysfunctions, particularly arthritis and related disorders. In 1984, he completed his doctoral work in anatomy with a focus on the remodeling of articular cartilage. He is currently Director of the Rehabilitation Science Research Laboratory at Creighton University. Dr. Threlkeld teaches courses on kinesiology and pathomechanics and co-teaches clinical electrophysiology and prosthetics to physical therapy students. His research pursuits include investigating the role of lower extremity loading in the generation, control, and rehabilitation of pathologic gait patterns. His hobbies include music, remodeling his house, and equine adventure.

Deborah A. Nawoczenski, PT, PhD

Professor, Program in Physical Therapy, School of Health Sciences and Human Performance, Ithaca College, Rochester, New York

http://faculty.ithaca.edu/

Dr. Nawoczenski has both a bachelor of science degree in physical therapy and a master of education degree from Temple University, Philadelphia. She also has a PhD in exercise science (biomechanics) from the University of Iowa, Iowa City. Dr. Nawoczenski is co-director of the Movement Analysis Laboratory at Ithaca College's Rochester Campus. She is engaged in research on the biomechanics of the foot and ankle. Dr. Nawoczenski also holds a position as an Adjunct Assistant Professor of Orthopaedics in the School of Medicine and Dentistry at the University of Rochester, Rochester, New York. She has served as an editorial board member for the *Journal of Orthopaedic & Sports Physical Therapy* and was co-editor of the two-part special issue on the foot and ankle. Dr. Nawoczenski has co-authored and co-edited two textbooks: Buchanan LE, Nawoczenski DA (eds): *Spinal Cord Injury: Concepts and Management Approaches*, and Nawoczenski DA, Epler ME (eds): *Orthotics in Functional Rehabilitation of the Lower Limb*.

Reviewers

Francisco Alencar, PhD, DDS
Marquette University College of Dentistry
Milwaukee, Wisconsin

Carlyn Alt, PT, PhD
Physical Therapy Program
University of Wisconsin-Milwaukee
Milwaukee, Wisconsin

Paul D. Andrew, PT, PhD
Department of Physical Therapy
School of Rehabilitation Sciences
Hyogo University of Health Sciences
Kobe, Japan

James W. Bellew, EdD, PT
Associate Professor
Krannert School of Physical Therapy
College of Health Sciences
University of Indianapolis
Indianapolis, Indiana

Teri Bielefeld, PT, CHT
Zablocki VA Medical Center
Milwaukee, Wisconsin

Paul-Neil Czujko, PT, DPT, OCS
Stony Brook University
Physical Therapy Program
Stony Brook, New York

Kevin Farrell, PT, OCS, FAAOMPT, PhD
Physical Therapy
Saint Ambrose University
Davenport, Iowa

McKenzie L. Fauth, DPT
Marquette University
Milwaukee, Wisconsin

Michael Karegeannes, PT, LAT, MHSc
Freedom Physical Therapy Services
Fox Point, Wisconsin

Jeremy Karman, PT
Physical Therapy Department
Aurora Sports Medicine Institute
Milwaukee, Wisconsin

Clare Kennedy, DPT
Chicago Rehabilitation Services
Chicago, Illinois

Rolandas Kesminas, MS, PT
Lithuanian Academy of Physical Education
Applied Physiology and Physiotherapy Department
Kaunas, Lithuania

Ted King, PhD, OTR
Occupational Therapy Program
University of Wisconsin—Milwaukee
Milwaukee, Wisconsin

Jon D. Marion, OTR, CHT
Marshfield Clinic
Marshfield, Wisconsin

Brenda L. Neumann, OTR, BCIAC
Center for Neurophysiologic Learning
Milwaukee, Wisconsin

Jessica Niles, DPT
Marquette University
Milwaukee, Wisconsin

Ann K. Porretto-Loehrke, DPT, CHT, COMT
Hand & Upper Extremity of Northeast Wisconsin, Ltd.
Appleton, Wisconsin

Christopher J. Simenz, PhD, CSCS
Department of Physical Therapy and Program in Exercise Science and
    Athletic Training
Marquette University
Milwaukee, Wisconsin

Guy Simoneau, PT, PhD
Department of Physical Therapy and Program in Exercise Science
Marquette University
Milwaukee, Wisconsin

Andrew Starsky, PT, PhD
Department of Physical Therapy and Program in Exercise Science
Marquette University
Milwaukee, Wisconsin

Carolyn Wadsworth, PT, MS, OCS, CHT
Advance, North Carolina

David Williams, MPT, ATC, PhD
Physical Therapy Program
University of Iowa
Iowa City, Iowa

Preface

I am pleased to introduce the second edition of *Kinesiology of the Musculoskeletal System: Foundations for Rehabilitation*. This edition is a natural offspring of the first, expanding upon many new concepts that have been fueled by a rapidly growing body of knowledge. Over 2000 references are cited in this second edition to support the science and clinical relevance behind the kinesiology. Any respected textbook must continue to grow and keep pace with the expanding knowledge base of the discipline and the professions it helps support.

The overwhelming popularity of the illustrations created in the first edition stimulated the efforts to take the art in the second edition to the next level. Every piece of art was revisited and thoroughly examined, and virtually every piece was revised. Through the full colorization of the existing work as well as the creation of many new or modified illustrations, the artwork in this edition has been significantly upgraded. As in the first edition, the art drives much of the teaching of this textbook.

Many new instructional elements have been added to the second edition, such as Study Questions and a section called Additional Clinical Connections. These clinical connections allow the students to apply their newly learned kinesiology to specific and often complex clinical situations. Furthermore, a more extensive website has been developed to extend the teaching effectiveness of this book.

Naturally, I used the first edition of the text to teach my classes on kinesiology to students at Marquette University. The close working relationship among the textbook, students, and I generated many practical ideas on ways to improve the writing, the organization or flow of topics, and clarity of images. Many improvements in both the text and illustrations are a result of the direct feedback I have received from my own students, as well as from other students and instructors around the United States and in other countries. As the second edition finds its way into the classrooms of universities and colleges, I look forward to receiving continued feedback and suggestions on improving this work.

Background

Kinesiology is the study of human movement, typically pursued within the context of sport, art, or medicine. To varying degrees, *Kinesiology of the Musculoskeletal System: Foundations for Rehabilitation* relates to all three areas. This textbook is intended, however, primarily to provide kinesiologic foundations for the practice of rehabilitation, which strives to optimize functional movements of the human body. Although worldwide the subject of kinesiology is presented from many different perspectives, I and my contributing authors have focused primarily on the mechanical and physiologic interactions between the muscles and joints of the body. These interactions are described for normal movement and, in the case of disease, trauma, or otherwise altered musculoskeletal tissues, for abnormal movement. I hope that this textbook provides a valuable educational resource for a wide range of health- and medical-related professions, both for students and clinicians.

Approach

This textbook places a major emphasis on the anatomic detail of the musculoskeletal system. By applying a few principles of physics and physiology to a good anatomical background, the reader should be able to mentally transform a static anatomic image into a dynamic, three-dimensional, and relatively predictable movement. The illustrations created for *Kinesiology of the Musculoskeletal System* are designed to encourage this mental transformation. This approach to kinesiology reduces the need for rote memorization and favors reasoning based on mechanical analysis, which can assist students and clinicians in developing proper evaluation, diagnosis, and treatment related to dysfunction of the musculoskeletal system.

This textbook represents the synthesis of nearly 35 years of experience as a physical therapist. This experience includes a rich blend of clinical, research, and teaching activities that are related, in one form or another, to kinesiology. Although I was unaware of it at the time, my work on this textbook began the day I prepared my first kinesiology lecture as a brand-new college professor at Marquette University in 1986. Since then, I have had the good fortune of being exposed to intelligent and motivated students. Their desire to learn has continually fueled my ambition and love for teaching. As a way to encourage my students to listen actively rather than to transcribe my lectures passively, I developed an extensive set of kinesiology lecture notes. Year after year, my notes evolved, forming the blueprints of the first edition of the text. Now, eight years later, I present the second edition of this text.

Organization

The organization of this textbook reflects of the overall plan of study used in my two-semester kinesiology course sequence as well as other courses in our curriculum. The textbook contains 15 chapters, divided into four major sections. *Section I* provides the essential topics of kinesiology, including an introduction to terminology and basic concepts, a review of basic structure and function of the musculoskeletal system, and an introduction to biomechanical and quantitative aspects of kinesiology. *Sections II* through *IV* present the specific anatomic details and kinesiology of the three major regions of the body. *Section II* focuses entirely on the upper extremity, from the shoulder to the hand. *Section III* covers the kinesiology of the axial skeleton, which includes the head, trunk, and spine. A special chapter is included within this section on the kinesiology of mastication and ventilation. *Section IV* presents the kinesiology of the lower extremity, from the hip to the foot. The final chapter in this section, "Kinesiology of Walking," functionally integrates and reinforces much of the kinesiology of the lower extremity.

This textbook is specifically designed for the purpose of *teaching*. To that end, concepts are presented in layers, starting with Section I, which lays much of the scientific foundation for chapters contained in Sections II through IV. The material covered in these chapters is also presented layer by layer, building both clarity and depth of knowledge. Most chapters begin with *osteology*–the study of the morphology and subsequent function of bones. This is followed by *arthrology*–the study of the anatomy and the function of the joints, including the associated periarticular connective tissues. Included in this study is a thorough description of regional kinematics, from both an arthrokinematic and osteokinematic perspective.

The most extensive component of most chapters in Sections II through IV highlights the *muscle and joint interactions*. This topic begins by describing the muscles within a region, including a summary of the innervations to both muscles and joint structures. Once the shape and physical orientation of the muscles are established, the mechanical interplay between the muscles and the joints is discussed. Topics presented include: strength and movement potential of muscles; muscular-produced forces imposed on joints; intermuscular and interjoint synergies; important functional roles of muscles in movement, posture, and stability; and the functional relationships that exist between the muscles and underlying joints. Multiple examples are provided throughout each chapter on how disease, trauma, or advanced age may cause reduced function or adaptations within the musculoskeletal system. This information sets the foundation for understanding many of the evaluations and treatments used in most clinical situations to treat persons with musculoskeletal as well as neuromuscular disorders.

Distinctive Features

Key features of the second edition include the following:
- Full-color illustrations
- Special Focus boxes
- Chapter at a Glance boxes
- Additional Clinical Connections boxes
- Study questions
- Evidence-based approach

Ancillary Materials

An Evolve website has been created specifically to accompany this textbook and can be accessed via the following link: http://evolve.elsevier.com/Neumann. A wealth of resources is provided to enhance both teaching and learning, as follows:

For the Instructor

- **Image Collection**: All of the textbook's artwork is reproduced online for download into PowerPoint or other presentations.
- **Lab Ideas**

For the Student and Instructor

- **Video Clips**: Video segments are provided to highlight kinesiologic concepts discussed in the text. These include videofluoroscopy of joint movements, demonstrations of persons with partial paralysis showing how to substitute for muscle weakness, and various methods of teaching concepts of kinesiology.
- **Answers to Study Questions**: Detailed answers to the study questions provide reinforcement for the material covered in the textbook.
- **Answers to Biomechanical Problems contained in Appendix I**
- **References with links to Medline Abstracts**: Medline links to the references found in the textbook help students with their research.
- **Yearly Citation Updates**: The website will be updated yearly by the author with references on current research related to kinesiology.

Acknowledgments

I welcome this opportunity to acknowledge a great number of people who have provided me with kind and thoughtful assistance throughout the evolution of this textbook to its second edition. I am sure that I have inadvertently overlooked some people and, for that, I apologize.

The best place to start with my offering of thanks is with my immediate family, especially my wife Brenda who, in her charming and unselfish style, supported me emotionally and physically during both editions. I thank my son, Donnie, and stepdaughter, Megann, for their patience and understanding. I also thank my caring parents, Betty and Charlie Neumann, for the many opportunities that they have provided me throughout my life.

Many persons significantly influenced the realization of *Kinesiology of the Musculoskeletal System: Foundations for Rehabilitation*. Foremost, I wish to thank Elisabeth Roen Kelly, the primary medical illustrator of the text, for her years of dedication, incredible talent, and uncompromisingly high standard of excellence. I also thank Craig Kiefer and his colleagues for their care and skill with transitioning the art into full color. I also extend a thank you to the Elsevier staff and affiliates for their patience, in particular Melissa Kuster Deutsch, Sarah Wunderly, and Jeannie Robertson.

I wish to express my sincere gratitude to Drs. Lawrence Pan and Richard Jensen, present and past directors, respectively, of the Department of Physical Therapy at Marquette University, as well as Drs. Jack Brooks and William Cullinan, past and present deans of the College of Health Sciences at Marquette University. These gentlemen unselfishly provided me with the opportunity and freedom to fulfill a dream.

I am also indebted to the following persons who contributed special chapters to this textbook: Peter R. Blanpied, Sandra K. Hunter, Guy G. Simoneau, David A. Brown, Deborah A. Nawoczenski, and A. Joseph Threlkeld. They provided an essential depth and breadth to this textbook. I am also grateful to the many persons who reviewed chapters, who did so without financial remuneration. These reviewers are listed elsewhere in previous sections.

Several people at Marquette University provided me with invaluable technical and research assistance. I thank Dan Johnson, Chief Photographer, for most of the photography contained in this book. I also wish to thank Ljudmila ("Milly") Mursec, Martha Gilmore Jermé, and other fine librarians at Raynor Library for their important help with my research.

Many persons affiliated directly or indirectly with Marquette University provided assistance with a wide range of activities throughout the evolution of this edition. This help included proofreading, listening, verifying references or concepts, posing for or supplying photographs, taking x-rays, and providing clerical or other technical assistance. For this help, I am grateful to Santana Deacon, Caress Dean, Kerry Donahue, Rebecca Eagleeye, Kevin Eckert, Kim Fowler, Jessica Fuentes, Gregg Fuhrman, Mary Beth Geiser, Barbara Haines, Douglas Heckenkamp, Lisa Hribar, Erika Jacobson, Davin Kimura, Stephanie Lamon, John Levene, Lorna Loughran, Christopher Melkovitz, Melissa Merriman, Preston Michelson, Alicia Nowack, Michael O'Brien, Ellen Perkins, Gregory Rajala, Janet Schuh, Robert Seeds, Elizabeth Shanahan, Bethany Shutko, Jeff Sischo, Pamela Swiderski, Michelle Treml, Stacy Weineke, Andy Weyer, Sidney White, and David Williams.

I am very fortunate to have this forum to acknowledge those who have made a significant, positive impact on my professional life. In a sense, the spirit of these persons is interwoven within this text. I acknowledge Shep Barish for first inspiring me to teach kinesiology; Martha Wroe for serving as a role model for my practice of physical therapy; Claudette Finley for providing me with a rich foundation in human anatomy; Patty Altland for emphasizing to Darrell Bennett and myself the importance of not limiting the functional potential of our patients; Gary Soderberg for his overall mentorship and firm dedication to principle; Thomas Cook for showing me that all this can be fun; Mary Pat Murray for setting such high standards for kinesiology education at Marquette University, and Guy Simoneau for constantly reminding me what an enduring work ethic can accomplish.

I wish to acknowledge several special people who have influenced this project in ways that are difficult to describe. These people include family, old and new friends, professional colleagues, and, in many cases, a combination thereof. I thank the following people for their sense of humor or adventure, their loyalty, and their intense dedication to their own goals and beliefs, and for their tolerance and understanding of mine. For this I thank my four siblings, Chip, Suzan, Nancy, and Barbara; as well as Brenda Neumann, Tad Hardee, David Eastwold, Darrell Bennett, Tony Hornung, Joseph Berman, Robert and Kim Morecraft, Guy Simoneau, and the Mehlos family, especially Harvey, for always asking "How's the book coming?" I wish to thank two special colleagues, Tony Hornung and Jeremy Karman, two physical therapists who have assisted me with teaching kinesiology at Marquette University for many years. They both help keep the class vibrant, fun, and clinically relevant.

Finally, I want to thank all my students, both past and present, for making my job so rewarding. Although I may often look too preoccupied to show it, you honestly make all of this worth it.

DAN

Contents

Section IV **Lower Extremity,** 463

KINESIOLOGY of the
MUSCULOSKELETAL
SYSTEM

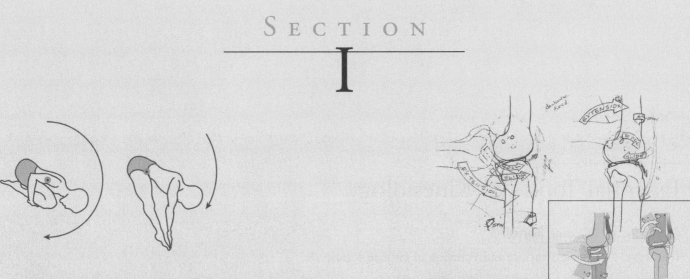

Essential Topics of Kinesiology

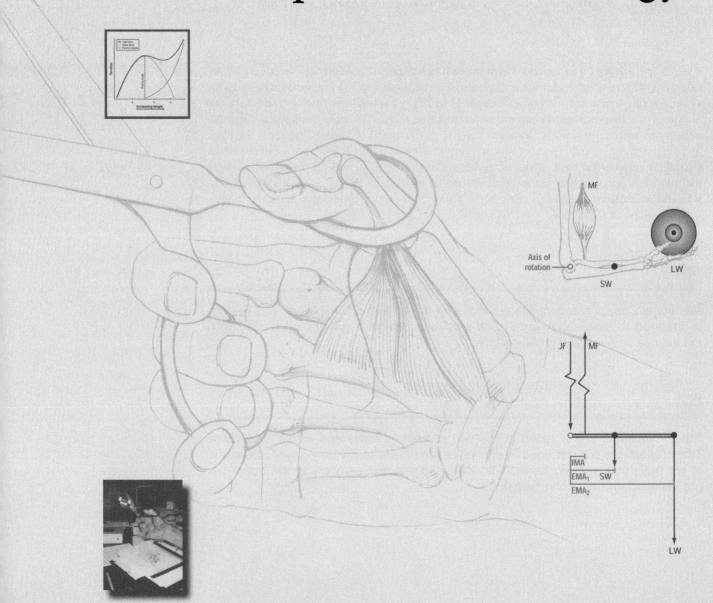

SECTION I

Essential Topics of Kinesiology

SECTION I is divided into four chapters, each describing a different topic related to kinesiology. This section provides the background for the more specific kinesiologic discussions of the various regions of the body (Sections II to IV). Chapter 1 provides introductory terminology and biomechanical concepts related to kinesiology. A glossary of important kinesiologic terms with definitions is located at the end of Chapter 1. Chapter 2 presents the basic anatomic and functional aspects of human joints–the pivot points for movement of the body. Chapter 3 reviews the basic anatomic and functional aspects of skeletal muscle–the source that produces active movement and stabilization of the skeletal system. More detailed discussion and quantitative analysis of many of the biomechanical principles introduced in Chapter 1 are provided in Chapter 4.

ADDITIONAL CLINICAL CONNECTIONS

Additional Clinical Connections are included at the end of Chapter 4. This feature is intended to highlight or expand on particular clinical concepts associated with the kinesiology covered in the chapter.

STUDY QUESTIONS

Study Questions are included at the end of each chapter and within Chapter 4. These questions are designed to challenge the reader to review or reinforce some of the main concepts contained within the chapter. The answers to the questions are included on the Evolve website. ⊖

Chapter 1

Getting Started

DONALD A. NEUMANN, PT, PhD, FAPTA

WHAT IS KINESIOLOGY?

The origins of the word *kinesiology* are from the Greek *kinesis*, to move, and *logy*, to study. *Kinesiology of the Musculoskeletal System: Foundations for Rehabilitation* serves as a guide to kinesiology by focusing on the anatomic and biomechanical interactions within the musculoskeletal system. The beauty and complexity of these interactions have been captured by many great artists, such as Michelangelo Buonarroti (1475-1564) and Leonardo da Vinci (1452-1519). Their work likely inspired the creation of the classic text *Tabulae Sceleti et Musculorum Corporis Humani,* published in 1747 by the anatomist Bernhard Siegfried Albinus (1697-1770). A sample of this work is presented in Figure 1-1.

The primary intent of this textbook is to provide students and clinicians with a firm foundation for the practice of physical rehabilitation. A detailed review of the anatomy of the musculoskeletal system, including its innervation, is presented as a background to the structural and functional aspects of movement and their clinical applications. Discussions are presented on both normal conditions and abnormal conditions that result from disease and trauma. A sound understanding of kinesiology allows for the development of a rational evaluation, a precise diagnosis, and an effective treatment of disorders that affect the musculoskeletal system. These abilities represent the hallmark of high quality for any health professional engaged in the practice of physical rehabilitation.

This text of kinesiology borrows heavily from three bodies of knowledge: anatomy, biomechanics, and physiology. *Anatomy* is the science of the shape and structure of the human body and its parts. *Biomechanics* is a discipline that uses principles of physics to quantitatively study how forces interact within a living body. *Physiology* is the biologic study of living organisms. This textbook interweaves an extensive review of musculoskeletal anatomy with selected principles of biomechanics and physiology. Such an approach allows the kinesiologic functions of the musculoskeletal system to be reasoned rather than purely memorized.

OVERALL PLAN OF THIS TEXTBOOK

This text is divided into four sections. *Section I: Essential Topics of Kinesiology* includes Chapters 1 to 4. To get the reader started, Chapter 1 provides many of the fundamental concepts and terminology related to kinesiology. A glossary is provided at the end of Chapter 1 with definitions of these fundamental concepts and terms. Chapters 2 to 4 describe the necessary background regarding the mechanics of joints, physiology of muscle, and review of applied biomechanics.

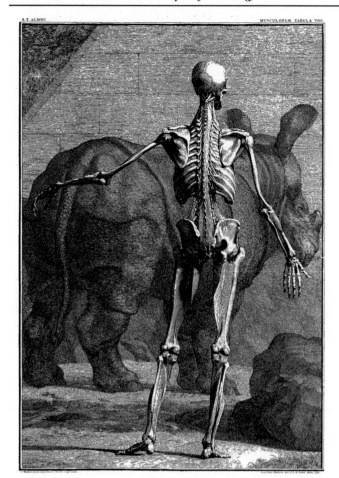

FIGURE 1-1. An illustration from the anatomy text *Tabulae Sceleti et Musculorum Corporis Humani* (1747) by Bernhard Siegfried Albinus.

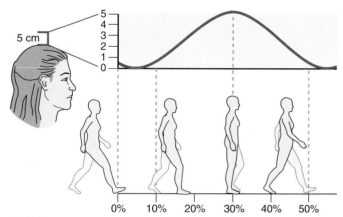

FIGURE 1-2. A point on the top of the head is shown translating upward and downward in a curvilinear fashion during walking. The horizontal axis of the graph shows the percentage of completion of one entire gait (walking) cycle.

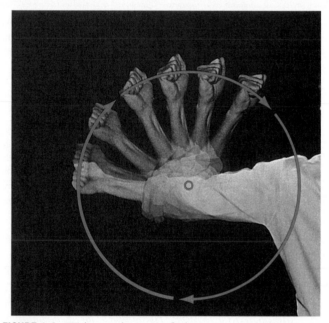

FIGURE 1-3. With a stroboscopic flash, a camera is able to capture the rotation of the forearm around the elbow. If not for the anatomic constraints of the elbow, the forearm could, in theory, rotate 360 degrees around an axis of rotation located at the elbow (open circle).

The material presented in Section I sets forth the kinesiologic foundation for the more anatomic- and regional-based chapters included in Sections II to IV. Section II (Chapters 5 to 8) describes the kinesiology related to the upper extremity; Section III (Chapters 9 to 11) covers the kinesiology involving primarily the axial skeleton and trunk; finally, Section IV (Chapters 12 to 15) presents the kinesiology of the lower extremity, including a closing chapter that focuses on walking.

KINEMATICS

Kinematics is a branch of mechanics that describes the *motion* of a body, without regard to the forces or torques that may produce the motion. In biomechanics the term *body* is used rather loosely to describe the entire body, or any of its parts or segments, such as individual bones or regions. In general, there are two types of motions: translation and rotation.

Translation Compared with Rotation

Translation describes a linear motion in which all parts of a rigid body move parallel to and in the same direction as every other part of the body. Translation can occur in either a straight line (*rectilinear*) or a *curved line (curvilinear)*. During walking, for example, a point on the head moves in a general curvilinear manner (Figure 1-2).

Rotation, in contrast to translation, describes a motion in which an assumed rigid body moves in a circular path around some pivot point. As a result, all points in the body simultaneously rotate in the same angular direction (e.g., clockwise and counterclockwise) across the same number of degrees.

Movement of the human body as a whole is often described as a translation of the body's *center of mass*, located generally just anterior to the sacrum. Although a person's center of mass translates through space, it is powered by muscles that *rotate* the limbs. The fact that limbs rotate can be appreciated

TABLE 1-1. **Common Conversions between Units of Kinematic Measurements**	
SI Units	**English Units**
1 meter (m) = 3.28 feet (ft)	1 ft = 0.305 m
1 m = 39.37 inches (in)	1 in = 0.0254 m
1 centimeter (cm) = 0.39 in	1 in = 2.54 cm
1 m = 1.09 yards (yd)	1 yd = 0.91 m
1 kilometer (km) = 0.62 miles (mi)	1 mi = 1.61 km
1 degree = 0.0174 radians (rad)	1 rad = 57.3 degrees

by watching the path created by a fist while the elbow is flexing (Figure 1-3). (It is customary in kinesiology to use the phrases "rotation of a joint" and "rotation of a bone" interchangeably.)

The pivot point for angular motion of the body or body parts is called the *axis of rotation*. The axis is at the point where motion of the rotating body is zero. For most movements of the limbs or trunk, the axis of rotation is located within or very near the structure of the joint.

Movement of the body, regardless of translation or rotation, can be described as active or passive. *Active movements* are caused by stimulated muscle, such as when lifting a glass of water toward the mouth. *Passive movements,* in contrast, are caused by sources other than active muscle contraction, such as a push from another person, the pull of gravity, tension in stretched connective tissues, and so forth.

The primary variables related to kinematics are position, velocity, and acceleration. Specific units of measurement are needed to indicate the quantity of these variables. Units of meters or feet are used for translation, and degrees or radians are used for rotation. In most situations, *Kinesiology of the Musculoskeletal System* uses the *International System of Units,* adopted in 1960. This system is abbreviated *SI,* for Système International d'Unités, the French name. This system of units is widely accepted in many journals related to kinesiology and rehabilitation. The kinematic conversions between the more common SI units and other measurement units are listed in Table 1-1. Additional units of measurements are described in Chapter 4.

Osteokinematics

PLANES OF MOTION

Osteokinematics describes the *motion of bones* relative to the three cardinal (principal) planes of the body: sagittal, frontal, and horizontal. These planes of motion are depicted in the context of a person standing in the *anatomic position* as in Figure 1-4. The *sagittal plane* runs parallel to the sagittal suture of the skull, dividing the body into right and left sections; the *frontal plane* runs parallel to the coronal suture of the skull, dividing the body into front and back sections. The *horizontal* (or *transverse*) *plane* courses parallel to the horizon and divides the body into upper and lower sections. A sample of the terms used to describe the different osteokinematics is shown in Table 1-2. More specific terms are defined in the chapters that describe the various regions of the body.

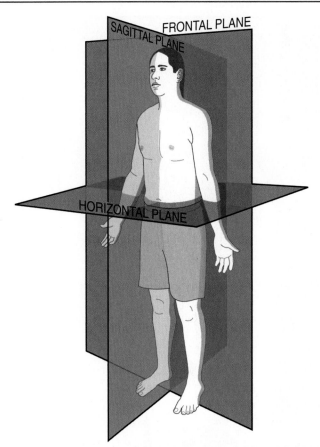

FIGURE 1-4. The three cardinal planes of the body are shown as a person is standing in the anatomic position.

TABLE 1-2. **A Sample of Common Osteokinematic Terms**	
Plane	**Common Terms**
Sagittal plane	Flexion and extension Dorsiflexion and plantar flexion Forward and backward bending
Frontal plane	Abduction and adduction Lateral flexion Ulnar and radial deviation Eversion and inversion
Horizontal plane	Internal (medial) and external (lateral) rotation Axial rotation

Many of the terms are specific to a particular region of the body. The thumb, for example, uses different terminology.

AXIS OF ROTATION

Bones rotate around a joint in a plane that is perpendicular to an *axis of rotation*. The axis is typically located through the convex member of the joint. The shoulder, for example, allows movement in all three planes and therefore has three axes of rotation (Figure 1-5). Although the three orthogonal axes are depicted as stationary, in reality, as in all joints, each axis shifts slightly throughout the range of motion. The axis of rotation would remain stationary only if the convex

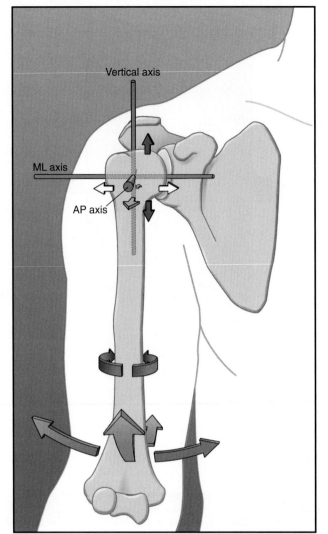

FIGURE 1-5. The right glenohumeral (shoulder) joint highlights three orthogonal axes of rotation and associated planes of angular motion: flexion and extension *(green curved arrows)* occur around a medial-lateral (ML) axis of rotation; abduction and adduction *(purple curved arrows)* occur around an anterior-posterior (AP) axis of rotation; and internal rotation and external rotation *(blue curved arrows)* occur around a vertical axis of rotation. Each axis of rotation is color-coded with its associated plane of movement. The short, straight arrows shown parallel to each axis represent the slight translation potential of the humerus relative to the scapula. This illustration shows both angular and translational degrees of freedom. (See text for further description.)

member of a joint were a perfect sphere, articulating with a perfectly reciprocally shaped concave member. The convex members of most joints, like the humeral head at the shoulder, are imperfect spheres with changing surface curvatures. The issue of a migrating axis of rotation is discussed further in Chapter 2.

DEGREES OF FREEDOM

Degrees of freedom are the number of independent directions of movements allowed at a joint. A joint can have up to three degrees of angular freedom, corresponding to the three car-

dinal planes. As depicted in Figure 1-5, for example, the shoulder has three degrees of angular freedom, one for each plane. The wrist allows only two degrees of freedom (rotation within sagittal and frontal planes), and the elbow allows just one (within the sagittal plane).

Unless specified differently throughout this text, the term *degrees of freedom* indicates the number of permitted *planes of angular motion* at a joint. From a strict engineering perspective, however, degrees of freedom apply to translational (linear) as well as angular movements. All synovial joints in the body possess at least some translation, driven actively by muscle or passively because of the natural laxity within the structure of the joint. The slight passive translations that occur in most joints are referred to as *accessory movements* (or joint "play") and are commonly defined in three linear directions. From the anatomic position, the spatial orientation and direction of accessory movements can be described relative to the three axes of rotation. In the relaxed glenohumeral joint, for example, the humerus can be passively translated slightly: anterior-posteriorly, medial-laterally, and superior-inferiorly (see short, straight arrows near proximal humerus in Figure 1-5). At many joints, the amount of translation is used clinically to test the health of the joint. Excessive translation of a bone relative to the joint may indicate ligamentous injury or abnormal laxity. In contrast, a significant reduction in translation (accessory movements) may indicate pathologic stiffness within the surrounding periarticular connective tissues. Abnormal translation within a joint typically affects the quality of the active movements, potentially causing increased intra-articular stress and microtrauma.

OSTEOKINEMATICS: A MATTER OF PERSPECTIVE

In general, the articulation of two or more bony or limb segments constitutes a joint. Movement at a joint can therefore be considered from two perspectives: (1) the proximal segment can rotate against the relatively fixed distal segment, and (2) the distal segment can rotate against the relatively fixed proximal segment. These two perspectives are shown for knee flexion in Figure 1-6. A term such as *knee flexion*, for example, describes only the *relative motion* between the thigh and leg. It does not describe which of the two segments is actually rotating. Often, to be clear, it is necessary to state the bone that is considered the primary rotating segment. As in Figure 1-6, for example, the terms *tibial-on-femoral movement* and *femoral-on-tibial movement* adequately describe the osteokinematics.

Most routine movements performed by the upper extremities involve distal-on-proximal segment kinematics. This reflects the need to bring objects held by the hand either toward or away from the body. The proximal segment of a joint in the upper extremity is usually stabilized by muscles, gravity, or its inertia, whereas the distal, relatively unconstrained, segment rotates.

Feeding oneself and throwing a ball are common examples of distal-on-proximal segment kinematics employed by the upper extremities. The upper extremities are certainly capable of performing proximal-on-distal segment kinematics, such as flexing and extending the elbows while one performs a pull-up.

The lower extremities routinely perform both proximal-on-distal and distal-on-proximal segment kinematics. These

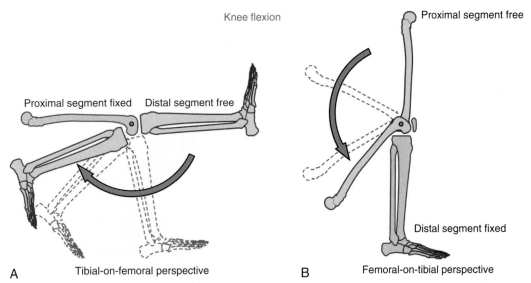

FIGURE 1-6. Sagittal plane osteokinematics at the knee show an example of **(A)** distal-on-proximal segment kinematics and **(B)** proximal-on-distal segment kinematics. The axis of rotation is shown as a circle at the knee.

kinematics reflect, in part, the two primary phases of walking: the *stance phase*, when the limb is planted on the ground under the load of body weight, and the *swing phase*, when the limb is advancing forward. Many other activities, in addition to walking, use both kinematic strategies. Flexing the knee in preparation to kick a ball, for example, is a type of distal-on-proximal segment kinematics (see Figure 1-6, *A*). Descending into a squat position, in contrast, is an example of proximal-on-distal segment kinematics (see Figure 1-6, *B*). In the latter example, a relatively large demand is placed on the quadriceps muscle of the knee to control the gradual descent of the body.

The terms *open* and *closed kinematic chains* are frequently used in the physical rehabilitation literature and clinics to describe the concept of relative segment kinematics.[9,20,25] A *kinematic chain* refers to a series of articulated segmented links, such as the connected pelvis, thigh, leg, and foot of the lower extremity. The terms "open" and "closed" are typically used to indicate whether the distal end of an extremity is fixed to the earth or some other immovable object. An *open kinematic chain* describes a situation in which the distal segment of a kinematic chain, such as the foot in the lower limb, is *not fixed* to the earth or other immovable object. The distal segment therefore is free to move (see Figure 1-6, *A*). A *closed kinematic chain* describes a situation in which the distal segment of the kinematic chain is *fixed* to the earth or another immovable object. In this case the proximal segment is free to move (see Figure 1-6, *B*). These terms are employed extensively to describe methods of applying resistive exercise to muscles, especially to the joints of the lower limb.

Although very convenient terminology, the terms *open* and *closed kinematic chains* are often ambiguous. From a strict engineering perspective, the terms apply more to the *kinematic interdependence* of a series of connected rigid links, which is not exactly the same as the previous definitions given here. From this engineering perspective, the chain is "closed" if *both ends* are fixed to a common object, much like a closed circuit.

In this case, movement of any one link requires a kinematic adjustment of one or more of the other links within the chain. "Opening" the chain by disconnecting one end from its fixed attachment interrupts this kinematic interdependence. This more precise terminology does not apply universally across all health-related and engineering disciplines. Performing a one-legged partial squat, for example, is often referred to clinically as the movement of a closed kinematic chain. It could be argued, however, that this is a movement of an open kinematic chain because the contralateral leg is not fixed to ground (i.e., the circuit formed by the total body is open). To avoid confusion, this text uses the terms *open* and *closed kinematic chains* sparingly, and the preference is to explicitly state which segment (proximal or distal) is considered fixed and which is considered free.

Arthrokinematics

TYPICAL JOINT MORPHOLOGY

Arthrokinematics describes the motion that occurs *between the articular surfaces* of joints. As described further in Chapter 2, the shapes of the articular surfaces of joints range from flat to curved. Most joint surfaces, however, are at least slightly curved, with one surface being relatively convex and one relatively concave (Figure 1-7). The convex-concave relationship of most articulations improves their congruency (fit), increases the surface area for dissipating contact forces, and helps guide the motion between the bones.

FUNDAMENTAL MOVEMENTS BETWEEN JOINT SURFACES

Three fundamental movements exist between curved joint surfaces: roll, slide, and, spin.[27] These movements occur as a convex surface moves on a concave surface, and vice versa (Figure 1-8). Although other terms are used, these are useful for visualizing the relative movements that occur within a joint. The terms are formally defined in Table 1-3.

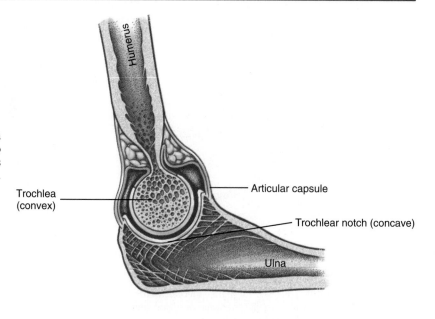

FIGURE 1-7. The humero-ulnar joint at the elbow is an example of a convex-concave relationship between two articular surfaces. The trochlea of the humerus is convex, and the trochlear notch of the ulna is concave.

Trochlea (convex)

Articular capsule

Trochlear notch (concave)

Ulna

TABLE 1-3.	Three Fundamental Arthrokinematics: Roll, Slide, and Spin	
Movement	**Definition**	**Analogy**
Roll*	*Multiple points* along one rotating articular surface contact *multiple points* on another articular surface.	A tire rotating across a stretch of pavement
Slide†	A *single point* on one articular surface contacts *multiple points* on another articular surface.	A non-rotating tire skidding across a stretch of icy pavement
Spin	A *single point* on one articular surface rotates on a *single point* on another articular surface.	A toy top rotating on one spot on the floor

*Also termed *rock*.
†Also termed *glide*.

Roll-and-Slide Movements

One primary way that a bone rotates through space is by a *rolling* of its articular surface against another bone's articular surface. The motion is shown for a convex-on-concave surface movement at the glenohumeral joint in Figure 1-9, *A*. The contracting supraspinatus muscle rolls the convex humeral head against the slight concavity of the glenoid fossa. In essence, the roll directs the osteokinematic path of the abducting shaft of the humerus.[22]

A rolling convex surface typically involves a concurrent, oppositely directed slide. As shown in Figure 1-9, *A*, the inferior-directed *slide* of the humeral head offsets most of the potential superior migration of the rolling humeral head. The offsetting roll-and-slide kinematics are analogous to a tire on a car that is spinning on a sheet of ice. The potential for the tire to rotate forward on the icy pavement is offset by a continuous sliding of the tire in the opposite direction to the intended rotation. A classic pathologic example of a convex surface rolling *without* an offsetting slide is shown in Figure 1-9, *B*. The humeral head translates upward and impinges on the delicate tissues in the subacromial space. The migration alters the relative location of the axis of rotation, which may alter the effectiveness of the muscles that cross the glenohumeral joint. As shown in Figure 1-9, *A*, the concurrent roll-and-slide motion maximizes the angular displacement of the abducting humerus and minimizes the net translation between joint surfaces. This mechanism is particularly important in joints in which the articular surface area of the convex member exceeds that of the concave member.

Spin

Another primary way that a bone rotates is by a *spinning* of its articular surface against the articular surface of another bone. This occurs as the radius of the forearm spins against the capitulum of the humerus during pronation of the forearm (Figure 1-10). Other examples include internal and external rotation of the 90-degree abducted glenohumeral joint, and flexion and extension of the hip. Spinning is the primary mechanism for joint rotation when the longitudinal axis of the long bone intersects the surface of its articular mate at right angles.

Motions That Combine Roll-and-Slide and Spin Arthrokinematics

Several joints throughout the body combine roll-and-slide with spin arthrokinematics. A classic example of this combination occurs during flexion and extension of the knee. As shown during femoral-on-tibial knee extension (Figure 1-11, *A*), the femur spins internally slightly as the femoral condyle rolls and slides relative to the fixed (stationary) tibia. These arthrokinematics are also shown as the tibia extends relative

Convex-on-concave arthrokinematics

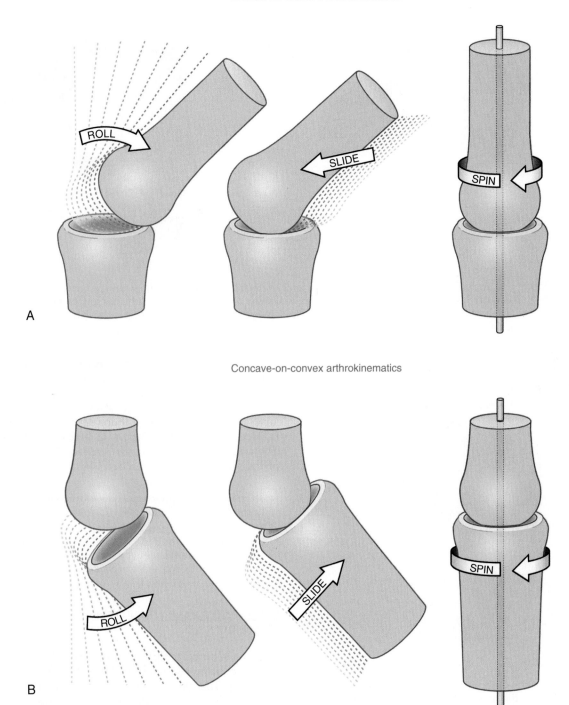

FIGURE 1-8. Three fundamental arthrokinematics that occur between curved joint surfaces: roll, slide, and spin. **A,** Convex-on-concave movement. **B,** Concave-on-convex movement.

to the fixed femur in Figure 1-11, *B.* In the knee the spinning motion that occurs with flexion and extension occurs automatically and is mechanically linked to the primary motion of extension. As described in Chapter 13, the obligatory spinning rotation is based on the shape of the articular surfaces at the knee. The conjunct rotation helps to securely lock the knee joint when fully extended.

PREDICTING AN ARTHROKINEMATIC PATTERN BASED ON JOINT MORPHOLOGY

As previously stated, most articular surfaces of bones are either convex or concave. Depending on which bone is moving, a convex surface may rotate on a concave surface or vice versa (compare Figure 1-11, *A* with Figure 1-11, *B).* Each

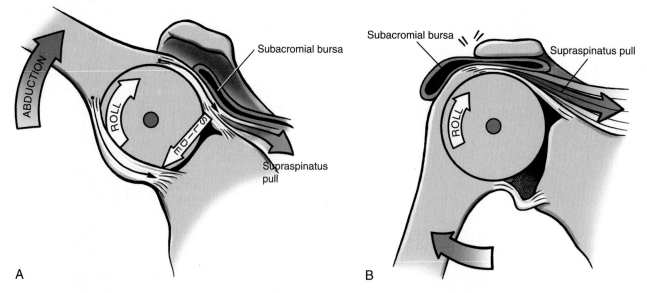

A   **B**

FIGURE 1-9. Arthrokinematics at the glenohumeral joint during abduction. The glenoid fossa is concave, and the humeral head is convex. **A,** Roll-and-slide arthrokinematics typical of a convex articular surface moving on a relatively stationary concave articular surface. **B,** Consequences of a roll occurring without a sufficient offsetting slide.

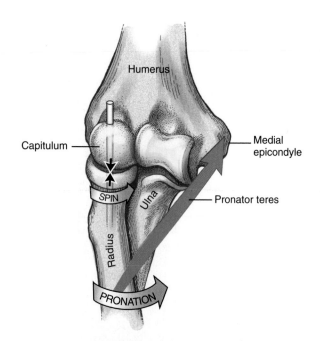

FIGURE 1-10. Pronation of the forearm shows an example of a spinning motion between the head of the radius and the capitulum of the humerus. The pair of opposed short black arrows indicates compression forces between the head of the radius and the capitulum.

scenario presents a different roll-and-slide arthrokinematic pattern. As depicted in Figures 1-11, *A* and 1-9, *A* for the shoulder, during a *convex-on-concave movement,* the convex surface rolls and slides in *opposite directions.* As previously described, the contradirectional slide offsets much of the translation tendency inherent to the rolling convex surface. During a *concave-on-convex movement,* as depicted in Figure 1-11, *B,* the concave surface rolls and slides in *similar directions.* These two principles are very useful for visualizing the arthrokinematics during a movement. In addition, the prin-

ciples serve as a basis for some manual therapy techniques. External forces may be applied by the clinician that assist or guide the natural arthrokinematics at the joint. For example, in certain circumstances, glenohumeral abduction can be facilitated by applying an inferior-directed force at the proximal humerus, simultaneously with an active-abduction effort. The arthrokinematic principles are based on the knowledge of the joint surface morphology.

Arthrokinematic Principles of Movement

- For a convex-on-concave surface movement, the convex member rolls and slides in *opposite* directions.
- For a *concave-on-convex* surface movement, the concave member rolls and slides in *similar* directions.

CLOSE-PACKED AND LOOSE-PACKED POSITIONS AT A JOINT

The pair of articular surfaces within most joints "fits" best in only one position, usually in or near the very end range of a motion. This position of maximal congruency is referred to as the joint's *close-packed position.*[27] In this position, most ligaments and parts of the capsule are pulled taut, providing an element of natural stability to the joint. Accessory movements are typically minimal in a joint's close-packed position.

For many joints in the lower extremity, the close-packed position is associated with a habitual function. At the knee, for example, the close-packed position is full extension—a position that is typically approached while standing. The combined effect of the maximum joint congruity and stretched ligaments helps to provide transarticular stability to the knee.

All positions other than a joint's close-packed position are referred to as the joint's *loose-packed positions.* In these posi-

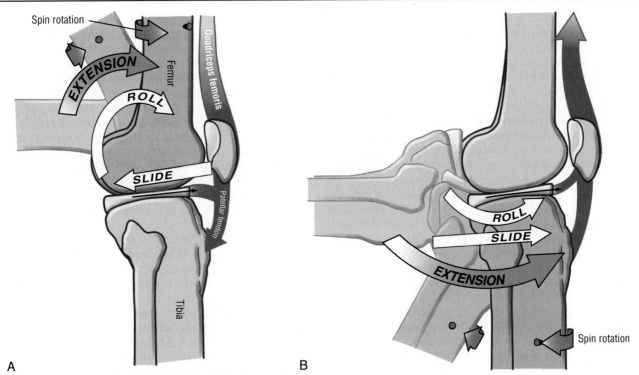

FIGURE 1-11. Extension of the knee demonstrates a combination of roll-and-slide with spin arthrokinematics. The femoral condyle is convex, and the tibial plateau is slightly concave. **A,** Femoral-on-tibial (knee) extension. **B,** Tibial-on-femoral (knee) extension.

tions, the ligaments and capsule are relatively slackened, allowing an increase in accessory movements. The joint is generally least congruent near its midrange. In the lower extremity, the loose-packed positions of the major joints are biased toward flexion. These positions are generally not used during standing, but frequently are preferred by the patient during long periods of immobilization, such as extended bed rest.

KINETICS

Kinetics is a branch of the study of mechanics that describes the effect of forces on the body. The topic of kinetics is introduced here as it applies to the musculoskeletal system. A more detailed and mathematic approach to this subject matter is provided in Chapter 4.

From a kinesiologic perspective, a *force* can be considered as a push or pull that can produce, arrest, or modify movement. Forces therefore provide the ultimate impetus for movement and stabilization of the body. As described by Newton's second law, the quantity of a force (F) can be measured by the product of the mass (m) that receives the push or pull, multiplied by the acceleration (a) of the mass. The formula $F = ma$ shows that, given a constant mass, a force is directly proportional to the acceleration of the mass: measuring the force yields the acceleration of the body, and vice versa. A net force is zero when the acceleration of the mass is zero.

The standard international unit of force is the *newton (N)*: $1\ N = 1\ kg \times 1\ m/sec^2$. The English equivalent of the newton is the pound (lb): $1\ lb = 1\ slug \times 1\ ft/sec^2$ ($4.448\ N = 1\ lb$).

Musculoskeletal Forces

IMPACT OF FORCES ON THE MUSCULOSKELETAL SYSTEM: INTRODUCTORY CONCEPTS AND TERMINOLOGY

A force that acts on the body is often referred to generically as a *load*.[23] Forces or loads that move, fixate, or otherwise stabilize the body also have the potential to deform and injure the body.[23,24] The loads most frequently applied to the musculoskeletal system are illustrated in Figure 1-12. (See the glossary at the end of this chapter for formal definitions.) Healthy tissues are typically able to partially resist changes in their structure and shape. The force that stretches a healthy ligament, for example, is met by an intrinsic tension generated within the elongated (stretched) tissue. Any tissue weakened by disease, trauma, or prolonged disuse may not be able to adequately resist the application of the loads depicted in Figure 1-12. The proximal femur weakened by osteoporosis, for example, may fracture from the impact of a fall secondary

to *compression or torsion (twisting), shearing,* or *bending* of the neck of the femur. Fracture may also occur in a severely osteoporotic hip after a very strong muscle contraction.

The ability of periarticular connective tissues to accept and disperse loads is an important topic of research within physical rehabilitation, manual therapy, and orthopedic medicine.[14,18] Clinicians are very interested in how variables such as aging, trauma, altered activity or weight-bearing levels, or prolonged immobilization affect the load-accepting functions of periarticular connective tissues. One method of measuring the ability of a connective tissue to tolerate a load is to plot the force required to deform an excised tissue.[8,22] This type of experiment is typically performed using animal or human cadaver specimens. Figure 1-13 shows a hypothetic graph of the tension generated by a generic ligament (or tendon) that has been stretched to a point of mechanical failure. The vertical (Y) axis of the graph is labeled *stress,* a term that denotes the internal resistance generated as the ligament resists deformation, divided by its cross-sectional area. (The units of stress are similar to pressure: N/mm^2). The horizontal (X) axis is labeled *strain,* which in this case is the percent increase in a tissue's stretched length relative to its original, preexperimental length.[24] (A similar procedure may be performed by *compressing* rather than stretching an excised slice of cartilage or bone, for example, and then plotting the amount of stress produced within the tissue.[29]) Note in Figure 1-13 that under a relatively slight strain (stretch), the ligament produces only a small amount of stress (tension). This *nonlinear* or "toe" region of the graph reflects the fact that the collagen fibers within the tissue are initially wavy or *crimped* and must be drawn taut before significant tension is measured.[18] Further elongation, however, shows a *linear relationship* between stress and strain. The ratio of the stress (Y) caused by an applied strain (X) in the ligament is a measure of its *stiffness* (often referred to as *Young's modulus*). All normal connective tissues within the musculoskeletal system exhibit some degree of stiffness. The clinical term "tightness" usually implies a pathologic condition of abnormally high stiffness.

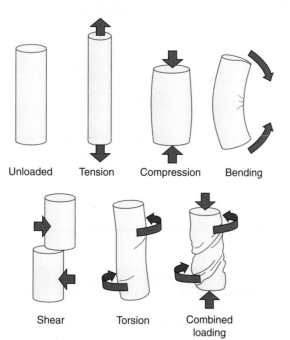

FIGURE 1-12. The manner by which forces or loads are most frequently applied to the musculoskeletal system is shown. The combined loading of torsion and compression is also illustrated.

FIGURE 1-13. The stress-strain relationship of an excised ligament that has been stretched to a point of mechanical failure (disruption).

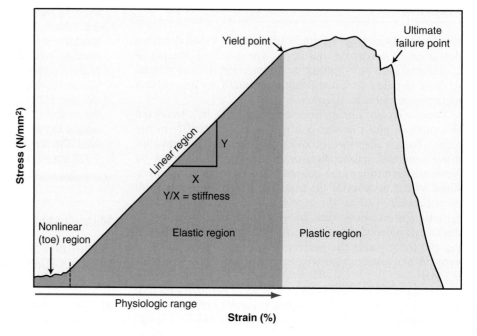

The initial nonlinear and subsequent linear regions of the curve shown in Figure 1-13 are often referred to as the *elastic region.* Ligaments, for example, are routinely strained within the lower limits of their elastic region. The anterior cruciate ligament, for example, is strained about 4% during an isometric contraction of the quadriceps with the knee flexed to 15 degrees.[3,4] It is important to note that a healthy and relatively young ligament that is strained within the elastic zone returns to its original length (or shape) once the deforming force is removed. The area under the curve (in darker blue) represents *elastic deformation energy.* Most of the energy used to deform the tissue is released when the force is removed. Even in a static sense, elastic energy can do useful work at the joints. When stretched even a moderate amount into the elastic zone, ligaments and other connective tissues perform important joint stabilization functions.

A tissue that is elongated beyond its physiologic range eventually reaches its *yield point.* At this point, increased strain results in only marginal increased stress (tension). This physical behavior of an overstretched (or overcompressed) tissue is known as *plasticity.* The overstrained tissue has experienced *plastic deformation.* At this point microscopic failure has occurred and the tissue remains permanently deformed. The area under this region of the curve (in lighter blue) represents *plastic deformation energy.* Unlike elastic deformation energy, plastic energy is not recoverable in its entirety even when the deforming force is removed. As elongation continues, the ligament eventually reaches its *ultimate failure point,* the point when the tissue partially or completely separates and loses its ability to hold any level of tension. Most healthy tendons fail at about 8% to 13% beyond their prestretched length.[31]

The graph in Figure 1-13 does not indicate the variable of *time* of load application. Tissues in which the physical properties associated with the stress-strain curve change as a function of time are considered *viscoelastic.* Most tissues within the musculoskeletal system demonstrate at least some degree of viscoelasticity. One phenomenon of a viscoelastic material is creep. As demonstrated by the tree branch in Figure 1-14, *creep* describes a progressive strain of a material when exposed to a constant load over time. Unlike plastic deformation, creep is reversible. The phenomenon of creep helps to explain why a person is taller in the morning than at night. The constant compression caused by body weight on the spine throughout the day literally squeezes a small amount of fluid out of the intervertebral discs. The fluid is reabsorbed at night while the sleeping person is in a non–weight-bearing position.

The stress-strain curve of a viscoelastic material is also sensitive to the *rate* of loading of the tissue. In general, the slope of a stress-strain relationship when placed under tension or compression increases throughout its elastic range as the rate of the loading increases.[24] The rate-sensitivity nature of viscoelastic connective tissues may protect surrounding structures within the musculoskeletal system. Articular cartilage in the knee, for example, becomes stiffer as the rate of compression increases,[23] such as during running. The increased stiffness affords greater protection to the underlying bone at a time when forces acting on the joint are greatest.

In summary, similar to building materials such as steel, concrete, and fiberglass, the periarticular connective tissues within the human body possess unique physical properties when loaded or strained. In engineering terms, these physical

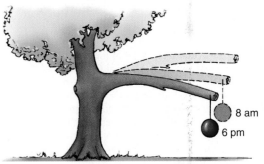

FIGURE 1-14. The branch of the tree is demonstrating a time-dependent property of creep associated with a *viscoelastic material.* Hanging a load on the branch at 8 AM creates an immediate deformation. By 6 PM, the load has caused additional deformation in the branch. (From Panjabi MM, White AA: *Biomechanics in the musculoskeletal system,* New York, Churchill Livingstone, 2001.)

properties are formally referred to as *material properties.* The topic of material properties of periarticular connective tissues (such as stress, strain, stiffness, plastic deformation, ultimate failure load, and creep) has a well-established literature base.* Although much of the data on this topic are from animal or cadaver research, they do provide insight into many aspects of patient care, including understanding mechanisms of injury, improving the design of orthopedic surgery, and judging the potential effectiveness of certain forms of physical therapy, such as prolonged stretching or application of heat to induce greater tissue extensibility.†

INTERNAL AND EXTERNAL FORCES

As a matter of convenience, the forces that act on the musculoskeletal system can be divided into two sets: internal and external. *Internal forces* are produced from structures located *within* the body. These forces may be "active" or "passive." Active forces are generated by stimulated muscle, generally but not necessarily under volitional control. Passive forces, in contrast, are typically generated by tension in stretched periarticular connective tissues, including the intramuscular connective tissues, ligaments, and joint capsules. Active forces produced by muscles are typically the largest of all internal forces.

External forces are produced by forces acting from *outside* the body. These forces usually originate from either *gravity* pulling on the mass of a body segment or an external load, such as that of luggage or "free" weights, or *physical contact,* such as that applied by a therapist against the limb of a patient. Figure 1-15, *A* shows an opposing pair of internal and external forces: an internal force (muscle) pulling the forearm, and an external (gravitational) force pulling on the center of mass of the forearm. Each force is depicted by an arrow that represents a vector. By definition, a *vector* is a quantity that is completely specified by its magnitude and its direction. (Quantities such as mass and speed are scalars, not vectors. A scalar is a quantity that is completely specified by its magnitude and has no direction.)

*References 1, 13, 15-17, 19, 28, 32.
†References 2, 7, 11, 14, 18, 21, 30.

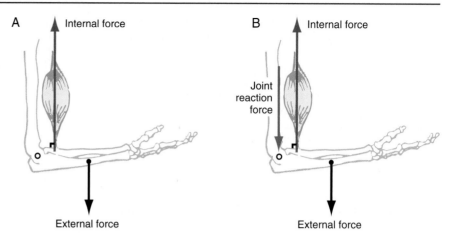

FIGURE 1-15. A sagittal plane view of the elbow joint and associated bones. **A,** Internal (muscle) and external (gravitational) forces are shown both acting vertically, but each in a different direction. The two vectors have different magnitudes and different points of attachment to the forearm. **B,** Joint reaction force is added to prevent the forearm from accelerating upward. (Vectors are drawn to relative scale.)

SPECIAL FOCUS 1-2

Productive Antagonism: the Body's Ability to Convert Passive Tension into Useful Work

A stretched or elongated tissue within the body generally produces tension (i.e., a resistance force that opposes the stretch). In pathologic cases this tension may be abnormally large, thereby interfering with functional mobility. This textbook presents several examples, however, illustrating how relatively low levels of tension produced by stretched connective tissues (including muscle) perform useful functions. This phenomenon is called *productive antagonism* and is demonstrated for a pair of muscles in the simplified model in Figure 1-16. As shown by the figure on the left, part of the energy produced by active contraction of muscle A is transferred and stored as elastic energy in the stretched connective tissues within muscle B. The elastic energy is released as muscle B actively contracts to drive the nail into the board (right illustration). Part of the contractile energy produced by muscle B is used to stretch muscle A, and the cycle is repeated.

This transfer and storage of energy between opposing muscles is useful in terms of overall metabolic efficiency. This phenomenon is often expressed in different ways by multi-articular muscles (i.e., muscles that cross several joints). Consider the rectus femoris, a muscle that flexes the hip and extends the knee. During the upward phase of jumping, for example, the rectus femoris contracts to extend the knee. At the same time, the extending hip stretches the active rectus femoris across the front of the hip. As a consequence, the overall shortening of the rectus femoris is minimized, which helps preserve useful passive tension within the muscle.

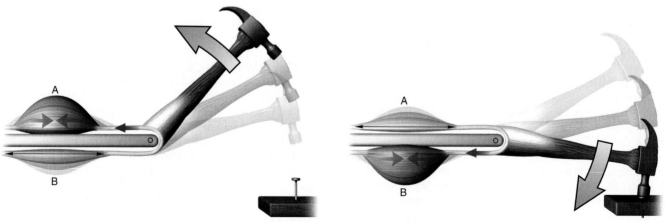

FIGURE 1-16. A simplified model showing a pair of opposed muscles surrounding a joint. In the left illustration, muscle A is contracting to provide the force needed to lift the hammer in preparation to strike the nail. In the right illustration, muscle B is contracting, driving the hammer against the nail while simultaneously stretching muscle A. (Redrawn from Brand PW: *Clinical biomechanics of the hand,* St Louis, Mosby, 1985.)

In order to completely describe a vector in a biomechanical analysis, its magnitude, spatial orientation, direction, and point of application must be known. The forces depicted in Figure 1-15 indicate these four factors.

1. The *magnitude* of the force vectors is indicated by the length of the shaft of the arrow.
2. The *spatial orientation* of the force vectors is indicated by the position of the shaft of the arrows. Both forces are oriented vertically, often referred to as the Y axis (further described in Chapter 4). The orientation of a force can also be described by the angle formed between the shaft of the arrow and a reference coordinate system.
3. The *direction* of the force vectors is indicated by the arrowhead. In the example depicted in Figure 1-15, *A,* the internal force acts upward, typically described in a *positive* Y sense; the external force acts downward in a *negative* Y sense. Throughout this text, the direction and spatial orientation of a muscle force and gravity are referred to as their *line of force* and *line of gravity,* respectively.
4. The *point of application* of the vectors is where the base of the vector arrow contacts the part of the body. The point of application of the muscle force is where the muscle inserts into the bone. The *angle-of-insertion* describes the angle formed between a tendon of a muscle and the long axis of the bone into which it inserts. In Figure 1-15, *A,* the angle-of-insertion is 90 degrees. The angle-of-insertion changes as the elbow rotates into flexion or extension. The point of application of the external force depends on whether the force is the result of gravity or the result of a resistance applied by physical contact. Gravity acts on the *center of mass* of the body segment (see Figure 1-15, *A,* dot at the forearm). The point of application of a resistance generated from physical contact can occur anywhere on the body.

Factors Required to Completely Describe a Vector in Most Simple Biomechanical Analyses
- Magnitude
- Spatial orientation
- Direction
- Point of application

As a push or a pull, all forces acting on the body cause a potential translation of the segment. The direction of the translation depends on the net effect of all the applied forces. In Figure 1-15, *A,* because the muscle force is three times greater than the weight of the forearm, the net effect of both forces would accelerate the forearm vertically upward. In reality, however, the forearm is typically prevented from accelerating upward by a *joint reaction force* produced between the surfaces of the joint. As depicted in Figure 1-15, *B,* the distal end of the humerus is pushing *down* with a reaction force (shown in blue) against the proximal end of the forearm. The magnitude of the joint reaction force is equal to the difference between the muscle force and external force. As a result, the sum of all vertical forces acting on the forearm is balanced, and net acceleration of the forearm in the vertical direction is zero. The system is therefore in *static linear equilibrium.*

Musculoskeletal Torques

Forces exerted on the body can have two outcomes. First, as depicted in Figure 1-15, *A,* forces can potentially *translate* a body segment. Second, the forces, if applied at some distance perpendicular to the axis of rotation, can also produce a potential *rotation* of the joint. The perpendicular distance between the axis of rotation of the joint and the force is called a *moment arm.* The product of a force and its moment arm produces a *torque* or a moment. A torque can be considered as a rotatory equivalent to a force. A force acting without a moment arm can push and pull an object generally in a linear fashion, whereas a torque rotates an object around an axis of rotation. This distinction is a fundamental concept in the study of kinesiology.

A torque is described as occurring around a joint in a plane perpendicular to a given axis of rotation. Figure 1-17 shows the torques produced within the sagittal plane by the internal and external forces introduced in Figure 1-15. The *internal torque* is defined as the product of the internal force (muscle) and the internal moment arm. The *internal moment arm* (see D in Figure 1-17) is the perpendicular distance between the axis of rotation and the internal force. As depicted in Figure 1-17, the internal torque has the potential to rotate the forearm around the elbow joint in a counterclockwise, or flexion, direction. (Other conventions for describing rotation direction are explored in Chapter 4.)

The *external torque* is defined as the product of the external force (such as gravity) and the external moment arm. The *external moment arm* (see D₁ in Figure 1-17) is the perpendicular distance between the axis of rotation and the external force. The external torque has the potential to rotate the forearm around the elbow joint in a clockwise, or extension, direction. Because the magnitude of the opposing internal and external torques is assumed to be equal in Figure 1-17,

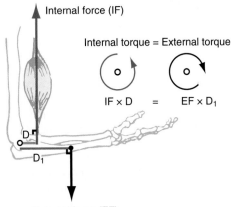

FIGURE 1-17. The balance of internal and external torques acting in the sagittal plane around the axis of rotation at the elbow *(small circle)* is shown. The *internal torque* is the product of the internal force multiplied by the internal moment arm (D). The internal torque has the potential to rotate the forearm in a counterclockwise direction. The *external torque* is the product of the external force (gravity) and the external moment arm (D₁). The external torque has the potential to rotate the forearm in a clockwise direction. The internal and external torques are equal, demonstrating a condition of static rotary equilibrium. (Vectors are drawn to relative scale.)

no rotation occurs around the joint. This condition is referred to as *static rotary equilibrium.*

The human body typically produces or receives torques repeatedly in one form or another. Muscles generate internal torques constantly throughout the day, to unscrew a cap from a jar, turn a wrench, or swing a baseball bat. Manual contact forces received from the environment in addition to gravity are constantly converted to external torques across joints. Internal and external torques are constantly "competing" for dominance across joints—the more dominant torque is reflected by the direction of movement or position of the joints at any given time throughout the body.

Torques are involved in most therapeutic situations with patients, especially when physical exercise or strength assessment is involved. A person's "strength" is the product of their muscles' force and, equally important, the internal moment arm: the perpendicular distance between the muscle's line of force and the axis of rotation. *Leverage* describes the relative moment arm length possessed by a particular force. As explained further in Chapter 4, the length of a muscle's moment arm, and hence leverage, changes constantly throughout a range of motion. This partially explains why a person is naturally stronger in certain parts of a joint's range of motion.

Clinicians frequently apply manual resistance against their patients as a means to assess, facilitate, and challenge a particular muscle activity.[12] The *force* applied against a patient's extremity is usually perceived as an external *torque* by the patient's musculoskeletal system. A clinician can challenge a particular muscle group by applying an external torque by way of a small manual force exerted a great distance from the joint, or a large manual force exerted close to the joint. Because torque is the product of a resistance force and its moment arm, either means can produce the same external torque against the patient. Modifying the force and external moment arm variables allows different strategies to be employed based on the strength and skill of the clinician.

SPECIAL FOCUS 1-3

Muscle-Produced Torques across a Joint: an Essential Concept in Kinesiology

How muscles produce torques across joints is one of the most important (and often difficult) concepts to understand in kinesiology. An understanding of this concept can be helped by considering a simple analogy between a muscle's potential to produce a torque (i.e., rotation) and the action of a force attempting to swing open a door. The essential mechanics in both scenarios are surprisingly similar. This analogy is described with the assistance of Figure 1-18, *A* and *B*.

Figure 1-18, *A* shows top and side views of a door mounted on a vertical hinge (depicted in blue). Horizontally applied forces (C to F) represent different attempts at manually pulling open the door. *Although all forces are assumed equal*, only forces C and E (applied at the doorknob) are actually capable of rotating the door. This holds true because only these forces meet the basic requirements of producing a torque: (1) each force is applied in a plane *perpendicular* to the given axis of rotation (hinge in this case), and (2) each force is associated with a *moment arm* distance (dark black line originating at the hinge). In this example the torque is the product of the pulling force times its moment arm. Force E will produce a greater torque than force C because it has the longer moment arm (or greater leverage). Nevertheless, forces C and E both satisfy the requirement to produce a torque in the horizontal plane.

Forces D and F, however, cannot produce a torque within the horizontal plane and therefore are not able to rotate the door, regardless of their magnitude. Although this may seem intuitively obvious based on everyone's experience closing or opening doors, the actual mechanical reasoning may not be so clear. Forces D and F are directed *through* the axis of rotation (the hinge in this case) and therefore have a zero moment arm distance. Any force multiplied by a zero moment arm produces zero torque, or zero rotation. Although these forces may compress or distract the hinge, they will not rotate the door.

Forces G and H shown at the right in Figure 1-18, *A* also cannot rotate the door. Any force that runs *parallel* with an axis of rotation cannot produce an associated torque. A torque can be generated only by a force that is applied *perpendicularly to a given axis of rotation.* Forces G and H therefore possess no ability to produce a torque in the horizontal plane.

To complete this analogy, Figure 1-18, *B* shows two views of the hip joint along with three selected muscles. In this example the muscles are depicted as producing forces in attempt to rotate the femur within the horizontal plane. (The muscle forces in these illustrations are analogous to the manually applied forces applied to the door.) The axis of rotation at the hip, like the hinge on the door, is in a vertical direction (shown in blue). As will be explained, even though all the muscles are assumed to produce an identical force, only one is capable of actually rotating the femur (i.e., producing a torque).

The force vectors illustrated on the left side of Figure 1-18, *B* represent the lines of force of two predominately horizontally aligned muscles at the hip (the piriformis and obturator externus). The piriformis is capable of producing an external rotation torque within the horizontal plane for the same reasons given for the analogous force C applied to the door (Figure 1-18, *A*). Both forces are applied in a plane perpendicular to the axis of rotation, and each possesses an associated moment arm distance (depicted as the dark line). In sharp contrast, however, the obturator externus muscle *cannot* produce a torque in the horizontal plane. This muscle force (as with the analogous force D acting on the door) passes directly *through* the vertical axis of rotation. Although the muscle force will compress the joint surfaces, it will not rotate the joint, at least not in the horizontal plane. As will be described in Chapter 12, which studies the hip, changing the rotational position of the joint often creates a moment arm distance for a muscle. In this case the obturator

Muscle-Produced Torques across a Joint: an Essential Concept in Kinesiology—cont'd

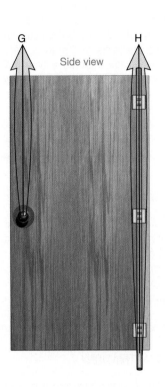

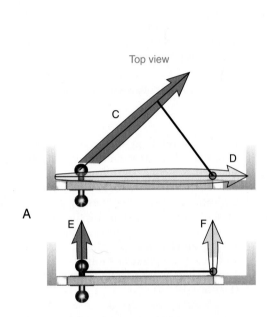

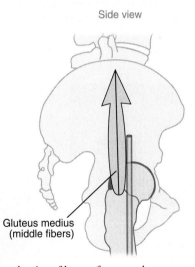

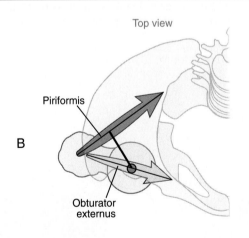

FIGURE 1-18. Mechanical analogy depicting the fundamental mechanics of how a force can be converted into a torque. **A,** Six manually applied forces are indicated *(colored arrows)*, each attempting to rotate the door in the horizontal plane. The vertical hinge of the door is shown in blue. The moment arms available to two of the forces (on the left) are indicated by dark black lines, originating at the hinge. **B,** Three muscle-produced forces are depicted *(colored arrows)*, each attempting to rotate the femur (hip) in the horizontal plane. The axes of rotation are shown in blue, and the moment arm as a dark black line. As described in the text, for similar reasons, only a selected number of forces is actually capable of generating a torque that can rotate either the door or the hip. For the sake of this analogy, the magnitude of all forces is assumed to be the same.

Continued

Muscle-Produced Torques across a Joint: an Essential Concept in Kinesiology—cont'd

externus may generate external rotation torque at the hip, although small.

The final component of this analogy is illustrated on the right of Figure 1-18, *B.* The middle fibers of the gluteus medius are shown attempting to rotate the femur in the horizontal plane around a vertical axis of rotation (depicted as a blue pin). Because the muscle force acts essentially *parallel* with the vertical axis of rotation (like forces G and H acting on the door), it is incapable of generating a torque in the horizontal plane. This same muscle, however, is very capable of generating torque in other planes, especially the frontal.

To summarize, a muscle is capable of producing a torque (or rotation) at a joint only provided it (1) produces a force in a plane perpendicular to the axis of rotation of interest, and (2) acts with an associated moment arm distance greater than zero. Stated from a different perspective, an active muscle is *incapable* of producing a torque if the force either *pierces or parallels* the associated axis of rotation. This applies to all axes of rotation that may exist at a joint: vertical, anterior-posterior (AP), or medial-lateral (ML). These principles will be revisited many times throughout this textbook.

Muscle and Joint Interaction

The term *muscle and joint interaction* refers to the overall effect that a muscle force may have on a joint. This topic is revisited repeatedly throughout this textbook. A force produced by a muscle that has a moment arm causes a torque, and a potential to rotate the joint. A force produced by a muscle that lacks a moment arm will not cause a torque or a rotation. The muscle force is still important, however, because it usually provides a source of stability to the joint.

TYPES OF MUSCLE ACTIVATION

A muscle is considered activated when it is stimulated by the nervous system. Once activated, a healthy muscle produces a force in one of three ways: isometric, concentric, and eccen-

tric. The physiology of the three types of muscle activation is described in greater detail in Chapter 3 and briefly summarized subsequently.

Isometric activation occurs when a muscle is producing a pulling force while maintaining a constant length. This type of activation is apparent by the origin of the word *isometric* (from the Greek *isos*, equal, and *metron*, measure or length). During an isometric activation, the internal torque produced within a given plane at a joint is equal to the external torque; hence, there is no muscle shortening or rotation at the joint (Figure 1-19, *A*).

Concentric activation occurs as a muscle produces a pulling force as it contracts (shortens) (see Figure 1-19, *B*). Literally, *concentric* means "coming to the center." During a concentric activation, the internal torque at the joint exceeds the oppos-

Three types of muscle activation

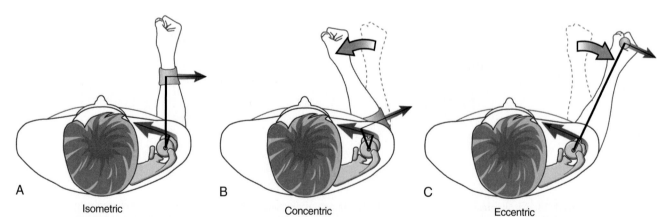

| A | B | C |
| Isometric | Concentric | Eccentric |

FIGURE 1-19. Three types of muscle activation are shown as the pectoralis major produces a maximal-effort force to internally rotate the shoulder (glenohumeral) joint. In each of the three illustrations, the internal torque is assumed to be the same: the product of the muscle force *(red)* times its internal moment arm. The external torque is the product of the external force applied throughout the arm *(gray)* and its external moment arm. Note that the external moment arm, and therefore the external torque, is different in each illustration. **A,** Isometric activation is shown as the internal torque matches the external torque. **B,** Concentric activation is shown as the internal torque exceeds the external torque. **C,** Eccentric activation is shown as the external torque exceeds the internal torque. The axis of rotation is vertical and depicted in blue through the humeral head. All moment arms are shown as thick black lines, originating at the axis of rotation piercing the glenohumeral joint. (Vectors are not drawn to scale.)

ing external torque. This is evident as the contracting muscle creates a rotation of the joint in the direction of the pull of the activated muscle.

Eccentric activation, in contrast, occurs as a muscle produces a pulling force as it is being elongated by another more dominant force. The word *eccentric* literally means "away from the center." During an eccentric activation, the external torque around the joint exceeds the internal torque. In this case the joint rotates in the direction dictated by the relatively larger external torque, such as that produced by the hand-held external force in Figure 1-19, *C.* Many common activities employ eccentric activations of muscle. Slowly lowering a cup of water to a table, for example, is caused by the pull of gravity on the forearm and water. The activated biceps slowly elongates in order to control the descent. The triceps muscle, although considered as an elbow "extensor," is most likely inactive during this particular process.

The term *contraction* is often used synonymously with *activation,* regardless of whether the muscle is actually shortening, lengthening, or remaining at a constant length. The term *contract* literally means to be *drawn together;* this term, however, can be confusing when describing either an isometric or eccentric activation. Technically, contraction of a muscle occurs during a concentric activation only.

MUSCLE ACTION AT A JOINT

A *muscle action* at a joint is defined as the potential for a muscle to cause a torque in a particular rotation direction and plane. The actual naming of a muscle's action is based on an established nomenclature, such as flexion or extension in the sagittal plane, abduction or adduction in the frontal plane, and so forth. The terms *muscle action* and *joint action* are used interchangeably throughout this text, depending on the context of the discussion. If the action is associated with a nonisometric muscle activation, the resulting osteokinematics may involve distal-on-proximal segment kinematics, or vice versa, depending on which of the segments comprising the joint is least constrained.

The study of kinesiology can allow one to determine the action of a muscle without relying purely on memory. Suppose the student desires to determine the actions of the *posterior deltoid* at the glenohumeral (shoulder) joint. In this particular analysis, two assumptions are made. First, it is assumed that the humerus is the freest segment of the joint, and that the scapula is fixed, although the reverse assumption could have been made. Second, it is assumed that the body is in the anatomic position at the time of the muscle activation.

The first step in the analysis is to determine the planes of rotary motion (degrees of freedom) allowed at the joint. In this case the glenohumeral joint allows rotation in all three planes (see Figure 1-5). Before further analysis is made, it is theoretically possible, therefore, that any muscle crossing the shoulder can express an action in up to three planes. Figure 1-20, *A* shows the potential for the posterior deltoid to rotate the humerus in the frontal plane. The axis of rotation passes in an anterior-posterior direction through the humeral head. In the anatomic position, the line of force of the posterior deltoid passes inferior to the axis of rotation. By assuming that the scapula is stable, a contracting posterior deltoid would rotate the humerus toward adduction, with strength equal to the product of the muscle force multiplied by its internal moment arm (shown as the dark line from the axis). This same logic is next applied to determine the muscle's action in the horizontal and sagittal planes. As depicted in Figure 1-20, *B* and *C,* it is apparent that the muscle is also an external (lateral) rotator and an extensor of the glenohumeral joint. As will be described throughout this text, it is common for a muscle that crosses a joint with at least two degrees of freedom to express multiple actions. A particular action may not be possible, however, if the muscle either lacks a moment arm or does not produce a force in the associated plane. Determining the potential action (or actions) of a muscle is a central theme in the study of kinesiology.

The logic just presented can be used to determine the action of *any* muscle in the body, at any joint. If available, an articulated skeleton model and a piece of string that

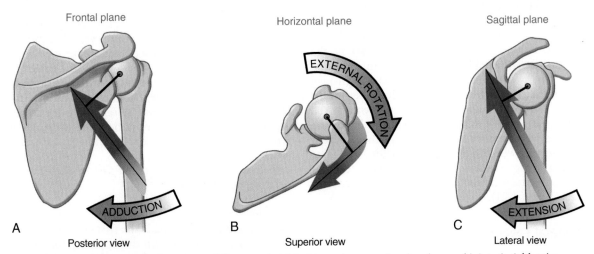

FIGURE 1-20. The multiple actions of the posterior deltoid are shown at the glenohumeral joint. **A,** Adduction in the frontal plane. **B,** External rotation in the horizontal plane. **C,** Extension in the sagittal plane. The internal moment arm is shown extending from the axis of rotation (small circle through humeral head) to a perpendicular intersection with the muscle's line of force.

mimics the line of force of a muscle are helpful in applying this logic. This exercise is particularly helpful when analyzing a muscle whose action switches depending on the position of the joint. One such muscle is the posterior deltoid. From the anatomic position the posterior deltoid is an *adductor* of the glenohumeral joint (previously depicted in Figure 1-20, *A*). If the arm is lifted (abducted) well overhead, however, the line of force of the muscle shifts just to the *superior* side of the axis of rotation. As a consequence the posterior deltoid actively abducts the shoulder. The example shows how one muscle can have opposite actions, depending on the position of the joint at the time of muscle activation. It is important, therefore, to establish a reference position for the joint when analyzing the actions of a muscle. One common reference position is the anatomic position (see Figure 1-4). Unless otherwise specified, the actions of muscles described throughout Sections II to IV in this text are based on the assumption that the joint is in the anatomic position.

Terminology Related to the Actions of Muscles

The following terms are often used when the actions of muscles are described:

- The *agonist* is the muscle or muscle group that is most directly related to the initiation and execution of a particular movement. For example, the tibialis anterior is the agonist for the motion of dorsiflexion of the ankle.
- The *antagonist* is the muscle or muscle group that is considered to have the opposite action of a particular agonist. For example, the gastrocnemius and soleus muscles are considered the antagonists to the tibialis anterior.
- Muscles are considered *synergists* when they cooperate during the execution of a particular movement. Actually, most meaningful movements of the body involve multiple muscles acting as synergists. Consider, for example, the flexor carpi ulnaris and flexor carpi radialis muscles during flexion of the wrist. The muscles act synergistically because they cooperate to flex the wrist. Each muscle, however, must neutralize the other's tendency to move the wrist in a side-to-side (radial and ulnar deviation) fashion. Paralysis of one of the muscles significantly affects the overall action of the other.

Another example of muscle synergy is described as a muscular force-couple. A muscular *force-couple* is formed when two or more muscles simultaneously produce forces in different linear directions, although the resulting torques act in the same rotary direction. A familiar analogy of a force-couple occurs between the two hands while turning a steering wheel of a car. Rotating the steering wheel to the right, for example, occurs by the action of the right hand pulling down and the left hand pulling up on the wheel. Although the hands are producing forces in different linear directions, they cause a torque on the steering wheel in the same rotary direction. The hip flexor and low back extensor muscles, for example, form a force-couple to rotate the pelvis in the sagittal plane around the hip joints (Figure 1-21).

Musculoskeletal Levers

THREE CLASSES OF LEVERS

Within the body, internal and external forces produce torques through a system of bony levers. Generically speaking, a lever

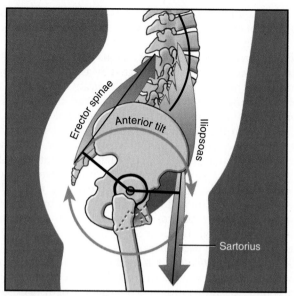

FIGURE 1-21. Side view of the force-couple formed between two representative hip flexor muscles (sartorius and iliopsoas) and back extensor muscles (erector spinae) as they contract to tilt the pelvis in an anterior direction. The internal moment arms used by the muscles are indicated by the black lines. The axis of rotation runs through both hip joints.

is a simple machine consisting of a rigid rod suspended across a pivot point. The seesaw is a classic example of a first-class lever (Figure 1-22). One function of a lever is to convert a linear force into a rotary torque. As shown in the seesaw in Figure 1-22, a 672-N (about 150-lb) man sitting 0.91 m (about 3 ft) from the pivot point produces a torque that balances a boy weighing half his weight who is sitting twice the distance from the pivot point. In Figure 1-22, the opposing torques are equal ($BW_m \times D = BW_b \times D_1$): the lever system therefore is balanced and in equilibrium. As indicated, the boy has the greatest leverage ($D_1 > D$). An important underlying concept of the lever is that with unequal moment arm lengths, the opposing torques can balance each other only if the opposing forces (or body weights in the preceding figure) are of different magnitudes.

Within the body, internal and external forces produce torques through a system of bony levers. The most important forces involved with musculoskeletal levers are those produced by muscle, gravity, and physical contact within the environment. The pivot point, or fulcrum, is located at the joint. As with the seesaw, the internal and external torques within the musculoskeletal system may be equal, such as during an isometric activation; or, more often, one of the two opposing torques dominates, resulting in movement at the joint.

Levers are classified as either *first, second,* or *third class* (see inset in Figure 1-22).

First-Class Lever

As depicted in Figure 1-22, the first-class lever has its axis of rotation positioned *between* the opposing forces. An example of a first-class lever in the human body is the head-and-neck extensor muscles that control the posture of the head in the sagittal plane (Figure 1-23, *A*). As in the seesaw example, the head is held in equilibrium when the product of the muscle

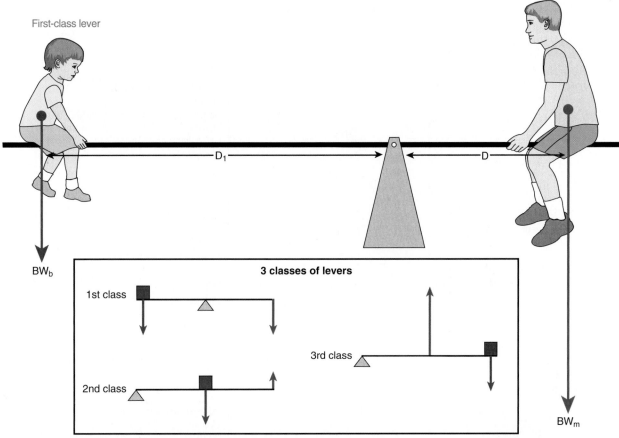

FIGURE 1-22. A seesaw is shown as a typical first-class lever. The body weight of the man (BW$_m$) is 672 N (about 150 lb). He is sitting 0.91 m (about 3 ft) from the pivot point (man's moment arm = D). The body weight of the boy (BW$_b$) is only 336 N (about 75 lb). He is sitting 1.82 m (about 6 ft) from the pivot point (boy's moment arm = D$_1$). The seesaw is balanced because the clockwise torque produced by the man is equal in magnitude to the counterclockwise torque produced by the boy: 672 N × 0.91 m = 336 N × 1.82 m. The inset compares the three classes of levers. In each lever the opposing forces may be considered as an internal force (such as a muscle pull depicted in red) and an external force or load (depicted in gray). The axis of rotation or pivot point is indicated as a wedge. (Force vectors are drawn to scale.)

force (MF) multiplied by the internal moment arm (IMA) equals the product of head weight (HW) multiplied by its external moment arm (EMA). In first-class levers, the internal and external forces typically act in similar linear directions, although they produce torques in opposing rotary directions.

Second-Class Lever

A second-class lever always has two features. First, its axis of rotation is located at one end of a bone. Second, the muscle, or internal force, possesses greater leverage than the external force. Second-class levers are very rare in the musculoskeletal system. The classic example is the calf muscles producing the torque needed to stand on tiptoes (see Figure 1-23, *B*). The axis of rotation for this action is assumed to act through the metatarsophalangeal joints. Based on this assumption, the internal moment arm used by the calf muscles greatly exceeds the external moment arm used by body weight.

Third-Class Lever

As in the second-class lever, the third-class lever has its axis of rotation located at one end of a bone. The elbow flexor muscles use a third-class lever to produce the flexion torque required to support a weight in the hand (see Figure 1-23, *C*). Unlike with the second-class lever, the external weight supported by a third-class lever always has greater leverage than the muscle force. The third-class lever is the most common lever used by the musculoskeletal system.

MECHANICAL ADVANTAGE

The *mechanical advantage* (MA) of a musculoskeletal lever can be defined as the ratio of the internal moment arm to the external moment arm. Depending on the location of the axis of rotation, the first-class lever can have an MA equal to, less than, or greater than one. Second-class levers always have an MA greater than one. As depicted in the boxes associated with Figure 1-23, *A* and *B*, lever systems with an MA greater than one are able to balance the torque equilibrium equation by an internal (muscle) force that is *less than* the external force. Third-class levers always have an MA less than one. As depicted in Figure 1-23, *C*, in order to balance the torque equilibrium equation, the muscle must produce a force much *greater than* the opposing external force.

First-class lever

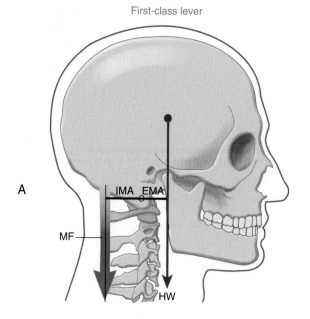

A

> **Data for first-class lever:**
> *Muscle force (MF) = unknown*
> *Head weight (HW) = 46.7 N (10.5 lbs)*
> *Internal moment arm (IMA) = 4 cm*
> *External moment arm (EMA) = 3.2 cm*
> *Mechanical advantage = 1.25*
>
> $MF \times IMA = HW \times EMA$
> $MF = \dfrac{HW \times EMA}{IMA}$
> $MF = \dfrac{46.7\ N \times 3.2\ cm}{4\ cm}$
> $MF = 37.4\ N\ (8.4\ lbs)$

Second-class lever

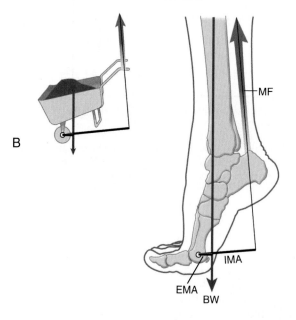

B

> **Data for second-class lever:**
> *Muscle force (MF) = unknown*
> *Body weight (BW) = 667 N (150 lbs)*
> *Internal moment arm (IMA) = 12 cm*
> *External moment arm (EMA) = 3 cm*
> *Mechanical advantage = 4*
>
> $MF \times IMA = BW \times EMA$
> $MF = \dfrac{BW \times EMA}{IMA}$
> $MF = \dfrac{667\ N \times 3\ cm}{12\ cm}$
> $MF = 166.8\ N\ (37.5\ lbs)$

Third-class lever

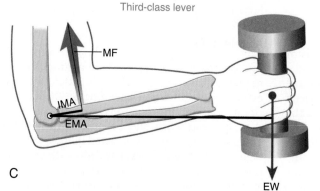

C

> **Data for third-class lever:**
> *Muscle force (MF) = unknown*
> *External weight (EW) = 66.7 N (15 lbs)*
> *Internal moment arm (IMA) = 5 cm*
> *External moment arm (EMA) = 35 cm*
> *Mechanical advantage = 0.143*
>
> $MF \times IMA = EW \times EMA$
> $MF = \dfrac{EW \times EMA}{IMA}$
> $MF = \dfrac{66.7\ N \times 35\ cm}{5\ cm}$
> $MF = 467\ N\ (105\ lbs)$

FIGURE 1-23. Anatomic examples are shown of first-class (**A**), second-class (**B**), and third-class (**C**) levers. (The vectors are not drawn to scale.) The data contained in the boxes to the right show how to calculate the muscle force required to maintain static rotary equilibrium. Note that the mechanical advantage is indicated in each box. The muscle activation (depicted in red) is isometric in each case, with no movement occurring at the joint.

The majority of muscles throughout the musculoskeletal system function with an MA of much *less than one*. Consider, for example, the biceps at the elbow, the quadriceps at the knee, and the supraspinatus and deltoid at the shoulder.[10,26] Each of these muscles attaches to bone relatively close to the joint's axis of rotation. The external forces that oppose the action of the muscles typically exert their influence considerably *distal* to the joint, such as at the hand or the foot. Consider the force demands placed on the supraspinatus and deltoid muscles to maintain the shoulder abducted to 90 degrees while an external weight of 35.6 N (8 lb) is held in the hand. For the sake of this example, assume that the muscles have an internal moment arm of 2.5 cm (about 1 inch) and that the center of mass of the external weight has an external moment arm of 50 cm (about 20 inches). (For simplicity, the weight of the limb is ignored.) In theory, the 1/20 MA requires that the muscle would have to produce 711.7 N (160 lb) of force, or *20 times* the weight of the external load! (Mathematically stated, the relationship between the muscle force and external load is based on the *inverse* of the MA.) As a general principle, most skeletal muscles produce forces several times larger than the external loads that oppose them. Depending on the shape of the muscle and configuration of the joint, a typically large percentage of the muscle force produces large compression or shear forces across the joint surfaces. These *myogenic* (muscular-produced) forces are most responsible for the amount and direction of the joint reaction force.

Dictating the Trade-off between Force and Distance

As previously described, most muscles are obligated to produce a force much greater than the resistance applied by the external load. At first thought, this design may appear flawed. The design is absolutely necessary, however, when considering the many functional movements that require large displacement and velocity of the more distal points of the extremities.

Work is the product of force times the distance through which it is applied. In addition to converting a force to a torque, a musculoskeletal lever converts the work of a contracting muscle to the work of a rotating bone and external load. The MA of a particular musculoskeletal lever dictates *how* the work is to be performed. Because work is the product of force and distance, it can be performed through *either* a relatively large force exerted over a short distance or a small force exerted over a large distance. Consider the small mechanical advantage of 1/20 described earlier for the supraspinatus and deltoid muscles. This MA implies that the muscle must produce a force 20 times greater than the weight of the external load. What must also be considered, however, is that the muscles need to contract only 5% (1/20) the distance that the center of mass of the load would be raised by the abduction action. A very short contraction distance (excursion) of the muscles produces a much larger vertical displacement of the load. When considering the element of *time* in this example, the muscles produce a relatively large force at a relatively slow contraction *velocity*. The mechanical benefit, however, is that a relatively light external load is lifted at a much faster velocity.

In summary, most muscle and joint systems in the body function with an MA of much less than one. This being the case, the distance and velocity of the load displacement will

---

Mechanical Advantage: a Closer Look at the Torque Equilibrium Equation

As stated, the mechanical advantage (MA) of a musculoskeletal lever can be defined as the ratio of its internal and external moment arms.

- First-class levers may have an MA less than 1, equal to 1, or greater than 1.
- Second-class levers always have an MA greater than 1.
- Third-class levers always have an MA less than 1.

The mathematic expression of MA is derived from the balance of torque equation:

$$MF \times IMA = EF \times EMA \qquad \text{(Equation 1-1)}$$

where
MF = Muscle force
EF = External force
IMA = Internal moment arm
EMA = External moment arm

Equation 1-1 can be rearranged as follows:

$$IMA/EMA = EF/MF \qquad \text{(Equation 1-2)}$$

- In some first-class levers, IMA/EMA = 1; the torque equation is balanced only when MF = EF.
- In some first-class and all second-class levers, IMA/EMA >1; the torque equation is balanced only when MF is less than EF.
- In some first-class and all third-class levers, IMA/EMA <1; the torque equation is balanced only when MF is greater than EF.

As indicated by Equation 1-2, MA can also be expressed by the ratio of external force to muscle force (EF/MF). Although this is correct, this text uses the convention of defining a muscle-and-joint's MA as the ratio of its internal-to-external moment arms (IMA/EMA).

---

always exceed that of the muscle contraction. Obtaining a high linear velocity of the distal end of the extremities is a necessity for generating large contact forces against the environment. These high forces can be used to rapidly accelerate objects held in the hand, such as a tennis racket, or to accelerate the limbs purely as an expression of art and athleticism, such as dance. Regardless of the nature of the movement, muscle-and-joint systems that operate with an MA of less than one must pay a force "penalty" by generating relative large internal forces, even for seemingly low-load activities. Periarticular tissues, such as articular cartilage, fat pads, and bursa, must partially absorb or dissipate these large myogenic forces. In the absence of such protection, joints may partially degenerate and become painful and chronically inflamed. This presentation is often the hallmark of osteoarthritis.

Surgically Altering a Muscle's Mechanical Advantage

A surgeon may perform a muscle-tendon transfer operation as a means to partially restore the loss of internal torque at a joint.[5] Consider, for example, complete paralysis of the elbow flexor muscles after poliomyelitis. Such a paralysis can have profound functional consequences, especially if it occurs bilaterally. One approach to restoring elbow flexion is to surgically reroute the fully innervated triceps tendon to the anterior side of the elbow (Figure 1-24). The triceps, now passing anteriorly to the medial-lateral axis of rotation at the elbow, becomes a flexor instead of an extensor. The length of the internal moment arm for the flexion action can be exaggerated, if desired, by increasing the perpendicular distance between the transferred tendon and the axis of rotation. By increasing the muscle's mechanical advantage (MA), the activated muscle produces a *greater torque per level of muscle force*. This may be a beneficial outcome, depending on the specific circumstances of the patient.

An important mechanical trade-off exists whenever a muscle's MA is surgically increased. Although a greater torque is produced per level of muscle force, a given amount of muscle shortening results in a *reduced angular displacement of the joint*. As a result, a full muscle contraction may produce an ample torque, but the joint may not complete its full range of motion.[6] In essence, the active range of motion "lags" behind the muscle contraction. The reduced displacement and velocity of the distal segment of the joint may have negative functional consequences. This mechanical trade-off needs to be considered before the muscle's internal moment arm is surgically enhanced. Often, the greater torque potential gained by increasing the moment arm functionally "outweighs" the loss of the speed and distance of the movement.

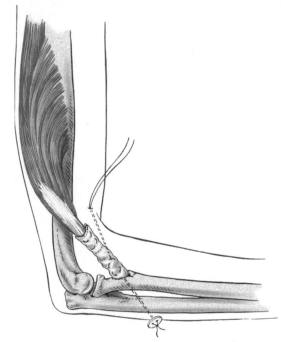

FIGURE 1-24. An anterior transfer of the triceps tendon after paralysis of the elbow flexor muscles. The triceps tendon is elongated by a graft of fascia. (From Bunnell S: Restoring flexion to the paralytic elbow, *J Bone Joint Surg Am* 33:566, 1951.)

SUMMARY

The human body moves primarily through rotations of its limbs and trunk. Two useful terms that describe these movements are osteokinematics and arthrokinematics. Osteokinematics describes movement of the limbs or trunk in one of the three cardinal planes, each occurring around an associated axis of rotation. Osteokinematic descriptors, such as internal rotation or extension, facilitate the study of these movements. Arthrokinematics are the movements that occur between the articular surfaces of joints. The wide acceptance of arthrokinematic descriptors such as roll, slide, and spin, for instance, has improved the ability of clinicians and students to conceptualize movements that occur at joints. This terminology is used extensively in manual-based therapy—treatment based largely on the specific movements that occur *between* joint surfaces. The strong association between arthrokinematics and articular morphology has stimulated the growth of the topic of arthrology: the study of the structure and function of joints and their surrounding connective tissues.

Whereas *kinematics* refers to the *motion* of bones and joints, *kinetics* refers to the *forces* that cause or arrest the motion. Muscles produce the forces that propel the body into motion. A fundamental concept presented in Chapter 1 is an appreciation of how a muscle force acting in a linear direction pro-

duces a torque around a joint. An internal torque is the angular expression of a muscle force, with a magnitude that equals the product of the muscle force times its moment arm; both variables are equally important when one considers the strength of a muscle action. Also important to the study of kinesiology is the understanding of how an external torque affects a joint. An external torque is defined as the product of an external force (such as gravity or physical contact) times its associated moment arm. Ultimately, movement and posture are based on the instantaneous interaction *between* internal and external torques—the prevailing direction and extent of which are determined by the more dominant torque.

Most muscles in the body act through a skeletal lever system with a mechanical advantage of much less than one. This design favors a relative high speed and displacement of the distal end of the extremities. This so-called biomechanical "advantage" is at the expense of a muscle force that is usually much *larger* than the combined weight of the limb and supported external load. The obligatory large muscle forces are usually directed across the surfaces of joints and on to bone and are most often described in terms of compression and shear. In order for these forces to be physiologically tolerated over a lifetime, the articular ends of most bones are relatively large, thereby increasing their surface area as a means to reduce peak contact pressure.

Additional protection is provided though the presence of a spongelike, relatively absorbent subchondral bone located just deep to articular cartilage. These features are essential for the dissipation of forces that would otherwise cause degeneration, possibly leading to osteoarthritis.

The study of kinesiology pays strict attention to the actions of individual muscles and their unique lines of force relative to the joint's axes of rotation. Once this is understood, the focus of study typically shifts to understanding how multiple muscles cooperate to control complex movements, often across multiple joints. Muscles act synergistically with one another for many reasons. Muscular interactions may serve to stabilize proximal attachment sites, neutralize unwanted secondary or tertiary actions, or simply augment the power, strength, or control of a particular movement. When muscle function is disrupted by disease or injury, the lack of such synergy is often responsible for the pathomechanics of a movement. Consider, for example, the consequences of paralysis or weakness of a selected few muscles within a functional muscle group. Even the healthy unaffected muscles (when acting in relative isolation) have a dominant role in an abnormal movement pattern. The resulting kinetic imbalance across the region can lead to certain compensatory movements or postures, possibly causing deformity and reduced function. Understanding how muscles interact normally is a prerequisite to comprehending the overall pathomechanics of the region. Such an understanding serves as the foundation for designing effective therapeutic interventions, aimed at restoring or maximizing function.

Kinesiology is the study of human motion, studied both in healthy, ideal conditions and those affected by trauma, disease, or disuse. To facilitate this study, this textbook focuses heavily on the structure and function of the musculoskeletal system. A strong emphasis is placed on the interaction among the forces and tensions created by muscles, gravity, and connective tissues that surround the joints. This chapter has helped to establish a foundation of many of the basic concepts and terminology used throughout this textbook.

GLOSSARY

Acceleration: change in velocity of a body over time, expressed in linear (m/sec^2) and angular ($degrees/sec^2$) terms.

Accessory movements: slight, passive, nonvolitional movements allowed in most joints (also called *joint play*).

Active force: push or pull generated by stimulated muscle.

Active movement: motion caused by stimulated muscle.

Agonist muscle: muscle or muscle group that is most directly related to the initiation and execution of a particular movement.

Anatomic position: the generally agreed on reference position of the body used to describe the location and movement of its parts. In this position, a person is standing fully upright and looking forward, with arms resting by the side, forearms fully supinated, and fingers extended.

Angle-of-insertion: angle formed between a tendon of a muscle and the long axis of the bone into which it inserts.

Antagonist muscle: muscle or muscle group that has the action opposite to a particular agonist muscle.

Arthrokinematics: motions of roll, slide, and spin that occur between curved articular surfaces of joints.

Axial rotation: angular motion of an object in a direction perpendicular to its longitudinal axis; often used to describe a motion in the horizontal plane.

Axis of rotation: an imaginary line extending through a joint around which rotation occurs (also called the *pivot point* or the *center of rotation*).

Bending: effect of a force that deforms a material at right angles to its long axis. A bent tissue is compressed on its concave side and placed under tension on its convex side. A bending moment is a quantitative measure of a bend. Similar to a torque, a bending moment is the product of the bending force and the perpendicular distance between the force and the axis of rotation of the bend.

Center of mass: point at the exact center of an object's mass (also referred to as *center of gravity* when considering the weight of the mass).

Close-packed position: unique position of most joints of the body where the articular surfaces are most congruent and the ligaments are maximally taut.

Compliance: the inverse of stiffness.

Compression: a force, applied perpendicularly to the contact surface, that pushes or pulls one object directly against another.

Concentric activation: activated muscle that shortens as it produces a pulling force.

Creep: a progressive strain of a material when exposed to a constant load over time.

Degrees of freedom: number of independent directions of movements allowed at a joint. A joint can have up to three degrees of translation and three degrees of rotation.

Displacement: change in the linear or angular position of an object.

Distal-on-proximal segment kinematics: type of movement in which the distal segment of a joint rotates relative to a fixed proximal segment (also called an *open kinematic chain*).

Distraction: a force, applied perpendicularly to the contact surface, that pushes or pulls one object directly away from another.

Eccentric activation: activated muscle that is producing a pulling force while being elongated by another more dominant force.

Elasticity: property of a material demonstrated by its ability to return to its original length after the removal of a deforming force.

External force: push or pull produced by sources located *outside* the body. These typically include gravity and physical contact applied against the body.

External moment arm: perpendicular distance between an axis of rotation and the external force.

External torque: product of an external force and its external moment arm (also called *external moment*).

Force: a push or a pull that produces, arrests, or modifies a motion.

Force-couple: two or more muscles acting in different linear directions, but producing a torque in the same rotary direction.

Force of gravity: potential acceleration of a body toward the center of the earth as a result of gravity.

Friction: resistance to movement between two contacting surfaces.

Internal force: push or pull produced by a structure located within the body. Most often, *internal force* refers to the force produced by an active muscle.

Internal moment arm: perpendicular distance between the axis of rotation and the internal (muscle) force.

Internal torque: product of an internal force and its internal moment arm.

Isometric activation: activated muscle that maintains a constant length as it produces a pulling force.

Joint reaction force: force that exists at a joint, developed in reaction to the net effect of internal and external forces. The joint reaction force includes contact forces between joint surfaces, as well as forces from any periarticular structure.

Kinematics: branch of mechanics that describes the motion of a body, without regard to the forces or torques that may produce the motion.

Kinematic chain: series of articulated segmented links, such as the connected pelvis, thigh, leg, and foot of the lower extremity.

Kinetics: branch of mechanics that describes the effect of forces and torques on the body.

Leverage: relative moment arm length possessed by a particular force.

Line of force: direction and orientation of a muscle's force.

Line of gravity: direction and orientation of the gravitational pull on a body.

Load: general term that describes the application of a force to a body.

Longitudinal axis: axis that extends within and parallel to a long bone or body segment.

Loose-packed positions: positions of most synovial joints of the body in which the articular surfaces are least congruent and the ligaments are slackened.

Mass: quantity of matter in an object.

Mechanical advantage: ratio of the internal moment arm to the external moment arm.

Moment arm: perpendicular distance between an axis of rotation and the line of force.

Muscle action: potential of a muscle to produce a torque within a particular plane of motion and rotation direction (also called *joint action* when referring specifically to a muscle's potential to rotate a joint). Terms that describe a muscle action are flexion, extension, pronation, supination, and so forth.

Osteokinematics: motion of bones relative to the three cardinal, or principal, planes.

Passive force: push or pull generated by sources other than stimulated muscle, such as tension in stretched periarticular connective tissues, physical contact, and so forth.

Passive movement: motion produced by a source other than activated muscle.

Plasticity: property of a material demonstrated by remaining permanently deformed after the removal of a force.

Pressure: force divided by a surface area (also called *stress*).

Productive antagonism: phenomenon in which relatively low-level tension within stretched connective tissues performs a useful function.

Proximal-on-distal segment kinematics: type of movement in which the proximal segment of a joint rotates relative to a fixed distal segment (also referred to as a *closed kinematic chain*).

Roll: arthrokinematic term that describes when multiple points on one rotating articular surface contact multiple points on another articular surface.

Rotation: angular motion in which a rigid body moves in a circular path around a pivot point or an axis of rotation.

Scalar: quantity, such as speed or temperature, that is completely specified by its magnitude and has no direction.

Segment: any part of a body or limb.

Shear: a force produced as two compressed objects slide past each other in opposite directions (like the action of two blades on a pair of scissors).

Shock absorption: the act of dissipating a force.

Slide: arthrokinematic term describing when a single point on one articular surface contacts multiple points on another articular surface (also called *glide*).

Spin: arthrokinematic term describing when a single point on one articular surface rotates on a single point on another articular surface (like a top).

Static linear equilibrium: state of a body at rest in which the sum of all forces is equal to zero.

Static rotary equilibrium: state of a body at rest in which the sum of all torques is equal to zero.

Stiffness: ratio of stress (force) to strain (elongation) within an elastic material, or N/m (also referred to as *Young's modulus* or *modulus of elasticity*).

Strain: ratio of a tissue's deformed length to its original length. May also be expressed in units of distance (m).

Stress: force generated as a tissue resists deformation, divided by its cross-sectional area (also called *pressure*).

Synergists: two or more muscles that cooperate to execute a particular movement.

Tension: application of one or more forces that pulls apart or separates a material (also called a *distraction force*). Used to denote the internal stress within a tissue as it resists being stretched.

Torque: a force multiplied by its moment arm; tends to rotate a body or segment around an axis of rotation.

Torsion: application of a force that twists a material around its longitudinal axis.

Translation: linear motion in which all parts of a rigid body move parallel to and in the same direction as every other point in the body.

Vector: quantity, such as velocity or force, that is completely specified by its magnitude and direction.

Velocity: change in position of a body over time, expressed in linear (m/sec) and angular (degrees/sec) terms.

Viscoelasticity: property of a material expressed by a changing stress-strain relationship over time.

Weight: gravitational force acting on a mass.

REFERENCES

1. Akeson WH, Amiel D, LaViolette D, et al: The connective tissue response to immobility: an accelerated ageing response? *Exp Gerontol* 3:289-301, 1968.
2. Belisle AL, Bicos J, Geaney L, et al: Strain pattern comparison of double- and single-bundle anterior cruciate ligament reconstruction techniques with the native anterior cruciate ligament, *Arthroscopy* 23:1210-1217, 2007.
3. Beynnon BD, Fleming BC: Anterior cruciate ligament strain in-vivo: A review of previous work, *J Biomech* 31:519-525, 1998.
4. Beynnon BD, Fleming BC, Johnson RJ, et al: Anterior cruciate ligament strain behavior during rehabilitation exercises in vivo, *Am J Sports Med* 23:24-34, 1995.
5. Brand PW: *Clinical biomechanics of the hand*, St Louis, 1985, Mosby.
6. Brand PW: The reconstruction of the hand in leprosy, *Clin Orthop Relat Res* 396:4-11, 2002.

7. Debski RE, Weiss JA, Newman WJ, et al: Stress and strain in the anterior band of the inferior glenohumeral ligament during a simulated clinical examination, *J Shoulder Elbow Surg* 14:24S-31S, 2005.

8. Dvir Z: *Clinical biomechanics*, Philadelphia, 2000, Churchill Livingstone.

9. Fleming BC, Oksendahl H, Beynnon BD: Open- or closed-kinetic chain exercises after anterior cruciate ligament reconstruction? *Exercise Sport Sci Rev* 33:134-140, 2005.

10. Graichen H, Englmeier KH, Reiser M, Eckstein F: An in vivo technique for determining 3D muscular moment arms in different joint positions and during muscular activation–application to the supraspinatus, *Clin Biomech (Bristol, Avon)* 16:389-394, 2001.

11. Hashemi J, Chandrashekar N, Mansouri H, et al: The human anterior cruciate ligament: Sex differences in ultrastructure and correlation with biomechanical properties, *J Orthop Res* 26:945-950, 2008.

12. Ireland ML, Willson JD, Ballantyne BT, Davis IM: Hip strength in females with and without patellofemoral pain, *J Orthop Sports Phys Ther* 33:671-676, 2003.

13. Keller TS, Spengler DM, Hansson TH: Mechanical behavior of the human lumbar spine. I. Creep analysis during static compressive loading, *J Orthop Res* 5:467-478, 1987.

14. Kolt SK, Snyder-Mackler L: *Physical therapies in sport and exercise*, Philadelphia, 2003, Churchill Livingston.

15. Ledoux WR, Blevins JJ: The compressive material properties of the plantar soft tissue, *J Biomech* 40:2975-2981, 2007.

16. Little JS, Khalsa PS: Material properties of the human lumbar facet joint capsule, *J Biomech Eng* 127:15-24, 2005.

17. Lu XL, Mow VC: Biomechanics of articular cartilage and determination of material properties, *Med Sci Sports Exerc* 40:193-199, 2008.

18. Lundon K: *Orthopaedic rehabilitation science: principles for clinical management of nonmineralized connective tissue*, St Louis, 2003, Butterworth-Heinemann.

19. McNamara LM, Prendergast PJ, Schaffler MB: Bone tissue material properties are altered during osteoporosis, *J Musculoskelet Neuronal Interact* 5:342-343, 2005.

20. Mellor R, Hodges PW: Motor unit synchronization of the vasti muscles in closed and open chain tasks, *Arch Phys Med Rehabil* 86:716-721, 2005.

21. Michlovitz SL: *Thermal agents in rehabilitation*, ed 3, Philadelphia, 1996, FA Davis.

22. Neumann DA: Arthrokinesiologic considerations for the aged adult. In Guccione AA, editor: *Geriatric Physical Therapy*, ed 2, Chicago, 2000, Mosby.

23. Nordin M, Frankel VH: *Basic biomechanics of the musculoskeletal system*, ed 2, Philadelphia, 1989, Lea & Febiger.

24. Panjabi MM, White AA: *Biomechanics in the musculoskeletal system*, New York, 2001, Churchill Livingstone.

25. Perry MC, Morrissey MC, King JB, et al: Effects of closed versus open kinetic chain knee extensor resistance training on knee laxity and leg function in patients during the 8- to 14-week post-operative period after anterior cruciate ligament reconstruction, *Knee Surg Sports Traumatol Arthrosc* 13:357-369, 2005.

26. Pigeon P, Yahia L, Feldman AG: Moment arms and lengths of human upper limb muscles as functions of joint angles, *J Biomech* 29:1365-1370, 1996

27. Standring S: *Gray's anatomy: the anatomical basis of clinical practice*, ed 40, St Louis, 2009, Elsevier.

28. Stromberg DD, Wiederhielm CA: Viscoelastic description of a collagenous tissue in simple elongation, *J Appl Physiol* 26:857-862, 1969.

29. Szerb I, Karpati Z, Hangody L: In vivo arthroscopic cartilage stiffness measurement in the knee, *Arthroscopy* 22:682, 2006.

30. Withrow TJ, Huston LJ, Wojtys EM, et al: Effect of varying hamstring tension on anterior cruciate ligament strain during in vitro impulsive knee flexion and compression loading, *J Bone Joint Surg Am* 90:815-823, 2008.

31. Woo SL, Gomez MA, Woo YK, et al: Mechanical properties of tendons and ligaments. II. The relationships of immobilization and exercise on tissue remodeling, *Biorheology* 19:397-408, 1982.

32. Woo SL, Matthews JV, Akeson WH, et al: Connective tissue response to immobility. Correlative study of biomechanical and biochemical measurements of normal and immobilized rabbit knees, *Arthritis Rheum* 18:257-264, 1975.

STUDY QUESTIONS

1 Contrast the fundamental difference between *kinematics* and *kinetics.*

2 Describe a particular movement of the body or body segment that incorporates both *translation* and *rotation* kinematics.

3 Note the accessory movements at the metacarpophalangeal joint of your index finger in full flexion and in full extension. Which is greater? Which position (flexion or extension) would you assume is the joint's close-packed position?

4 Figure 1-8 depicts the three fundamental movements between joint surfaces for both convex-on-concave and concave-on-convex arthrokinematics. Using a skeleton or an image of a skeleton, cite an example of a specific movement at a joint that matches each of these six situations. Examples may include *combinations* of roll and slide.

5 Provide examples of how the six forces depicted in Figure 1-12 could naturally occur at either the disc or spinal cord associated with the junction of the fifth and sixth cervical vertebrae.

6 Contrast the fundamental differences between *force* and *torque.* Use each term to describe a particular aspect of a muscle's contraction relative to a joint.

7 Define and contrast *internal torque* and *external torque.*

8 The elbow model in Figure 1-17 is assumed to be in static equilibrium. While maintaining this equilibrium, how would a change in the variables EF, D_1, or D independently affect the required amount of internal force (IF)? How can a change in these variables "protect" an arthritic joint from unnecessarily large joint reaction forces?

9 Slowly lowering a book to the table uses an eccentric activation of the elbow flexor muscles. Explain how changing the speed at which you lower the book can affect the type of activation (e.g., eccentric, concentric) and choice of muscle.

10 Assume a surgeon performs tendon transfer surgery to increase the internal moment arm of a particular muscle relative to a joint. Are there potential negative biomechanical consequences of increasing the muscle's moment arm (leverage) too far? If so, please explain.

11 Describe a possible pathologic situation in which the inferior-directed joint reaction force (JRF) depicted in Figure 1-15, *B* is *not* able to be generated by the distal humerus.

12 What is the difference between force and pressure? How could these differences apply to protecting the skin of a patient with a spinal cord injury and reduced sensation?

13 Describe the difference between mass and weight.

14 Most muscle and joint systems within the body function as *third-*class levers. Cite a biomechanic or physiologic reason for this design.

15 Assume a patient developed adhesions with marked increased stiffness in the posterior capsular ligaments of his knee. How would this change in tissue property affect full *passive* range of motion at the joint?

Answers to the study questions can be found on the Evolve website.

CHAPTER

2

Basic Structure and Function of Human Joints

DONALD A. NEUMANN PT, PhD, FAPTA
A. JOSEPH THRELKELD, PT, PhD

CHAPTER AT A GLANCE

A *joint* is the junction or pivot point between two or more bones. Movement of the body as a whole occurs primarily through rotation of bones about individual joints. Joints also transfer and dissipate forces produced by gravity and muscle activation.

Arthrology, the study of the classification, structure, and function of joints, is an important foundation for the overall study of kinesiology. Aging, long-term immobilization, trauma, and disease all affect the structure and ultimate function of joints. These factors also significantly influence the quality and quantity of human movement.

This chapter focuses on the general anatomic structure and function of joints. The chapters contained in Sections II to IV of this text describe the specific anatomy and detailed function of the individual joints throughout the body. This detailed information is a prerequisite for understanding impairments of joints as well as employing the most effective rehabilitation of persons with joint dysfunction.

CLASSIFICATION OF JOINTS BASED ON MOVEMENT POTENTIAL

One method to classify joints focuses primarily on their movement potential. Based on this scheme, two major types of joints exist within the body: *synarthroses* and *diarthroses* (Figure 2-1).

Synarthroses

A *synarthrosis* is a junction between bones that allows slight to essentially no movement. Based on the dominant type of periarticular connective tissue that reinforces the articulation, synarthrodial joints can be further classified as *fibrous* or *cartilaginous*.[63]

Fibrous joints are stabilized by specialized dense connective tissues, usually with a high concentration of collagen. Examples of fibrous joints include the sutures of the skull, the distal

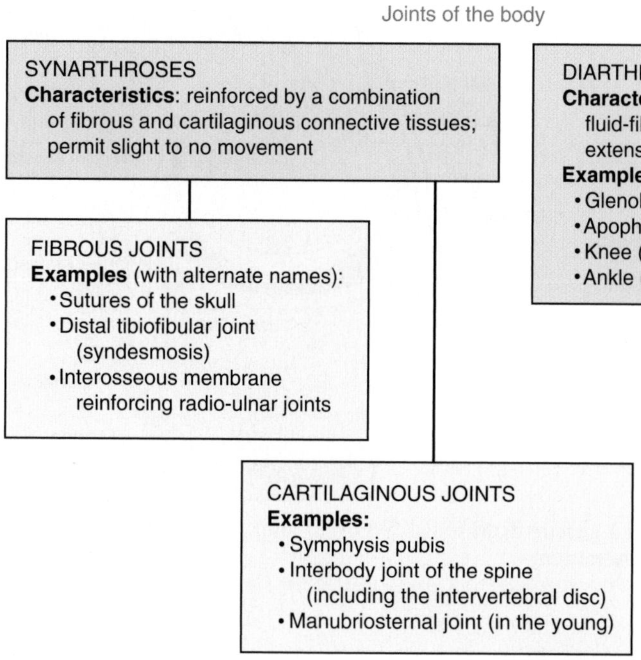

Joints of the body

```
┌─────────────────────────────────────┐          ┌─────────────────────────────────────┐
│ SYNARTHROSES                         │          │ DIARTHROSES                         │
│ Characteristics: reinforced by a     │          │ Characteristics: possess a synovial │
│  combination of fibrous and          │          │  fluid-filled cavity; permit        │
│  cartilaginous connective tissues;   │          │  moderate to extensive movement     │
│  permit slight to no movement        │          │ Examples:                           │
└─────────────────────────────────────┘          │  • Glenohumeral joint               │
                                                  │  • Apophyseal (facet) joint of      │
          ┌─────────────────────────────┐        │    the spine                        │
          │ FIBROUS JOINTS              │         │  • Knee (tibiofemoral joint)        │
          │ Examples (with alternate    │         │  • Ankle (talocrural joint)         │
          │  names):                    │         └─────────────────────────────────────┘
          │  • Sutures of the skull     │
          │  • Distal tibiofibular joint│
          │    (syndesmosis)            │
          │  • Interosseous membrane    │
          │    reinforcing radio-ulnar  │
          │    joints                   │
          └─────────────────────────────┘

              ┌─────────────────────────────────────┐
              │ CARTILAGINOUS JOINTS                │
              │ Examples:                           │
              │  • Symphysis pubis                  │
              │  • Interbody joint of the spine     │
              │    (including the intervertebral    │
              │    disc)                            │
              │  • Manubriosternal joint (in the    │
              │    young)                           │
              └─────────────────────────────────────┘
```

FIGURE 2-1. A classification scheme for describing two main types of articulations found in the musculo-skeletal system. Synarthrodial joints can be further classified as either fibrous or cartilaginous.

tibiofibular joint (often referred to as a *syndesmosis*), and other joints reinforced by an interosseous membrane. *Cartilaginous joints*, in contrast, are stabilized by varying forms of flexible fibrocartilage or hyaline cartilage, often mixed with collagen. Cartilaginous joints generally exist in the midline of the body, such as the symphysis pubis, the interbody joints of the spine, and the manubriosternal joint.[63]

The function of synarthrodial joints is to strongly bind and transfer forces between bones. These joints are typically well supported by periarticular connective tissues and, in general, allow very little movement.

Diarthroses: Synovial Joints

A *diarthrosis* is an articulation that allows moderate to extensive motion. These joints also possess a synovial fluid–filled cavity. Because of this feature, diarthrodial joints are frequently referred to as *synovial joints*. Synovial joints comprise the majority of the joints within the musculoskeletal system.

Diarthrodial or synovial joints are specialized for movement and always exhibit seven elements (Figure 2-2). *Articular cartilage* covers the ends and other articular surfaces of bones. The joint is enclosed by a peripheral curtain of connective tissue that forms the *joint* (or *articular*) *capsule*. The joint capsule is composed of two histologically distinct layers. The external, or fibrous, layer is composed of dense connective tissue. This part of the joint capsule provides support between the bones and containment of the joint contents. The internal layer of the joint capsule consists of a *synovial membrane*,

which averages 3 to 10 cell layers thick. The cells within this specialized connective tissue manufacture a *synovial fluid* that is usually clear or pale yellow, with a slightly viscous consistency.[63] The synovial fluid contains many of the proteins found in blood plasma, including hyaluronan and other lubricating glycoproteins.[63,75] The synovial fluid coats the articular surfaces of the joint. This fluid reduces the friction between the joint surfaces as well as providing some nourishment to the articular cartilage.

Ligaments are connective tissues that attach between bones, thereby protecting the joint from excessive movement. The thickness of ligaments differs considerably depending on the functional demands placed on the joint. Most ligaments can be described as either capsular or extracapsular. *Capsular ligaments* are usually thickenings of the articular capsule, such as the glenohumeral ligaments and deeper parts of the medial (tibial) collateral ligament of the knee. Capsular ligaments typically consist of a broad sheet of fibers that, when pulled taut, resist movements in two or often three planes. Most *extracapsular ligaments* are more cordlike and may be partially or completely separate from the joint capsule. Consider, for example, the lateral (fibular) collateral ligament of the knee or the alar ligament of the craniocervical region. These more discrete ligaments are usually oriented in a specific manner to optimally resist movement in usually one or two planes.

Small *blood vessels* with capillaries penetrate the joint capsule, usually as deep as the junction of the fibrous layer of the joint capsule and the adjacent synovial membrane. *Sensory nerves* also supply the external layer of the capsule and ligaments with receptors for pain and proprioception.

Elements ALWAYS associated with
diarthrodial (synovial) joints
- Synovial fluid
- Articular cartilage
- Joint capsule
- Synovial membrane
- Ligaments
- Blood vessels
- Sensory nerves

Elements SOMETIMES associated with
diarthrodial (synovial) joints
- Intra-articular discs or menisci
- Peripheral labrum
- Fat pads
- Bursa
- Synovial plicae

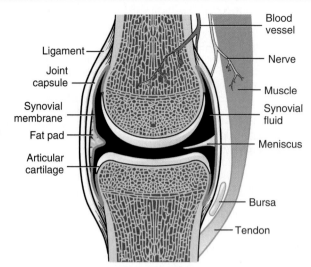

FIGURE 2-2. Elements associated with a generic diarthrodial (synovial) joint. Note that a peripheral labrum and plica are not represented in the illustration.

To accommodate the wide spectrum of joint shapes and functional demands, other elements may sometimes appear in synovial joints (see Figure 2-2). *Intra-articular discs,* or *menisci,* are pads of fibrocartilage imposed between articular surfaces. These structures increase articular congruency and improve force dispersion. Intra-articular discs and menisci are found in several joints of the body (see box).

Intra-articular Discs (Menisci) Found in Several Synovial Joints of the Body
- Tibiofemoral (knee)
- Distal radio-ulnar
- Sternoclavicular
- Acromioclavicular
- Temporomandibular
- Apophyseal (variable)

A *peripheral labrum* of fibrocartilage extends from the bony rims of the glenoid fossa of the shoulder and the acetabulum of the hip. These specialized structures deepen the concave member of these joints and support and thicken the attachment of the joint capsule. *Fat pads* are variable in size and positioned within the substance of the joint capsule, often interposed between the fibrous layer and the synovial membrane. Fat pads are most prominent in the elbow and the knee joints. They thicken the joint capsule, causing the inner surface of the capsule to fill nonarticulating joint spaces (i.e., recesses) formed by incongruent bony contours. In this sense, fat pads reduce the volume of synovial fluid necessary for proper joint function. If these pads become enlarged or inflamed, they may alter the mechanics of the joint.

Bursae often form adjacent to fat pads. A bursa is an extension or outpouching of the synovial membrane of a diarthrodial joint. Bursae are filled with synovial fluid and usually exist in areas of potential stress. Like fat pads, bursae help absorb force and protect periarticular connective tissues, including bone. The subacromial bursa in the shoulder, for example, is located between the undersurface of the acromion of the scapula and the head of the humerus. The bursa may become inflamed because of repetitive compression between the humerus and the acromion. This condition is frequently referred to as *subacromial bursitis.*

Synovial plicae (i.e., synovial folds, synovial redundancies, or synovial fringes) are slack, overlapped pleats of tissue composed of the innermost layers of the joint capsule. They occur normally in joints with large capsular surface areas such as the knee and elbow. Plicae increase synovial surface area and allow full joint motion without undue tension on the synovial lining. If these folds are too extensive or become thickened or adherent because of inflammation, they can produce pain and altered joint mechanics. The plicae of the knee are further described in Chapter 13.

CLASSIFICATION OF SYNOVIAL JOINTS BASED ON MECHANICAL ANALOGY

Thus far in this chapter, joints have been classified into two broad categories based primarily on movement potential. Because an in-depth understanding of synovial joints is so crucial to an understanding of the mechanics of movement, they are here further classified using an analogy to familiar mechanical objects or shapes (Table 2-1).

A *hinge joint* is generally analogous to the hinge of a door, formed by a central pin surrounded by a larger hollow cylinder (Figure 2-3, *A*). Angular motion at hinge joints occurs primarily in a plane located at right angles to the hinge, or axis of rotation. The humero-ulnar joint is a clear example of a hinge joint (see Figure 2-3, *B*). As in all synovial joints, slight translation (i.e., sliding) is allowed in addition to the rotation. Although the mechanical similarity is less complete, the interphalangeal joints of the digits are also classified as hinge joints.

TABLE 2-1. Classification of Synovial Joints Based on Mechanical Analogy

	Primary Angular Motions	Mechanical Analogy	Anatomic Examples
Hinge joint	Flexion and extension only	Door hinge	Humero-ulnar joint Interphalangeal joint
Pivot joint	Spinning of one member around a single axis of rotation	Doorknob	Humeroradial joint Atlanto-axial joint
Ellipsoid joint	Biplanar motion (flexion-extension and abduction-adduction)	Flattened convex ellipsoid paired with a concave trough	Radiocarpal joint
Ball-and-socket joint	Triplanar motion (flexion-extension, abduction-adduction, and internal-external rotation)	Spheric convex surface paired with a concave cup	Glenohumeral joint Coxofemoral (hip) joint
Plane joint	Typical motions include slide (translation) or combined slide and rotation	Relatively flat surfaces apposing each other, like a book on a table.	Carpometacarpal joints (digits II to IV) Intercarpal joints Intertarsal joints
Saddle joint	Biplanar motion; spin between bones is possible but may be limited by interlocking nature of joint	Each member has a reciprocally curved concave and convex surface oriented at right angles to the other, like a horse rider and a saddle	Carpometacarpal joint of the thumb Sternoclavicular joint
Condyloid joint	Biplanar motion; either flexion-extension and abduction-adduction, or flexion-extension and axial rotation (internal-external rotation)	Mostly spheric convex surface that is enlarged in one dimension like a knuckle; paired with a shallow concave cup	Metacarpophalangeal joint Tibiofemoral (knee) joint

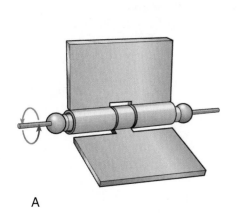

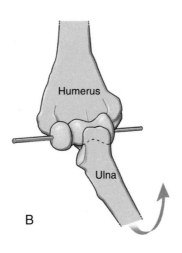

FIGURE 2-3. A hinge joint **(A)** is illustrated as analogous to the humero-ulnar joint **(B).** The axis of rotation (i.e., pivot point) is represented by the pin.

A

B

A *pivot joint* is formed by a central pin surrounded by a larger cylinder. Unlike a hinge, the mobile member of a pivot joint is oriented parallel to the axis of rotation. This mechanical orientation produces the primary angular motion of spin, similar to a doorknob's spin around a central axis (Figure 2-4, *A*). Two examples of pivot joints are the humeroradial joint, shown in Figure 2-4, *B*, and the atlanto-axial joint in the craniocervical region.

An *ellipsoid joint* has one partner with a convex elongated surface in one dimension that is mated with a similarly elongated concave surface on the second partner (Figure 2-5, *A*).

The elliptic mating surfaces severely restrict the spin between the two surfaces but allow biplanar motions, usually defined as flexion-extension and abduction-adduction. The radiocarpal joint is an example of an ellipsoid joint (see Figure 2-5, *B*). The flattened convex member of the joint (i.e., carpal bones) significantly limits the spin within the matching concavity (i.e., distal radius).

A *ball-and-socket joint* has a spheric convex surface that is paired with a cuplike socket (Figure 2-6, *A*). This joint provides motion in three planes. Unlike the ellipsoid joint, the symmetry of the curves of the two mating surfaces of the

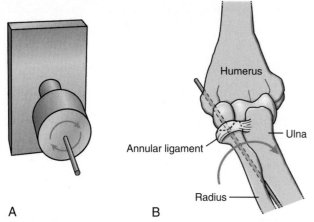

FIGURE 2-4. A pivot joint **(A)** is shown as analogous to the humeroradial joint **(B).** The axis of rotation is represented by the pin, extending through the capitulum of the humerus.

ball-and-socket joint allows spin without dislocation. Ball-and-socket joints within the body include the glenohumeral joint and the hip joint. As will be described further in Chapter 5, most of the concavity of the glenohumeral joint is formed not only by the glenoid fossa, but also by the surrounding muscle, labrum, joint capsule, and capsular ligaments.

A *plane joint* is the pairing of two flat or relatively flat surfaces. Movements combine sliding and some rotation of one partner with respect to the other, much as a book can slide or rotate across a tabletop (Figure 2-7, *A*). As depicted in Figure 2-7, *B*, the carpometacarpal joints within digits II to V are often considered as plane, or modified plane, joints. Most intercarpal and intertarsal joints are also considered plane joints. The forces that cause or restrict movement between the bones are supplied by tension in muscles or ligaments.

Each partner of a *saddle joint* has two surfaces: one surface is concave, and the other is convex. These surfaces are oriented at approximate right angles to each other and are reciprocally curved. The shape of a saddle joint is best visualized

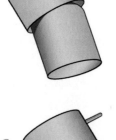
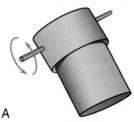
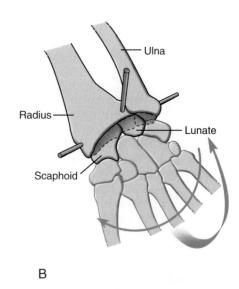

FIGURE 2-5. An ellipsoid joint **(A)** is shown as analogous to the radiocarpal joint (wrist) **(B).** The two axes of rotation are shown by the intersecting pins.

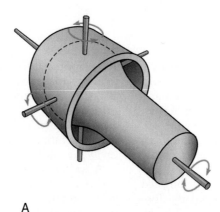
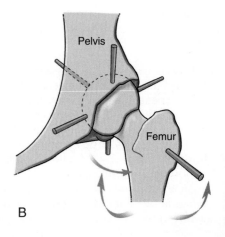

FIGURE 2-6. A ball-and-socket articulation **(A)** is drawn as analogous to the hip joint **(B).** The three axes of rotation are represented by the three intersecting pins.

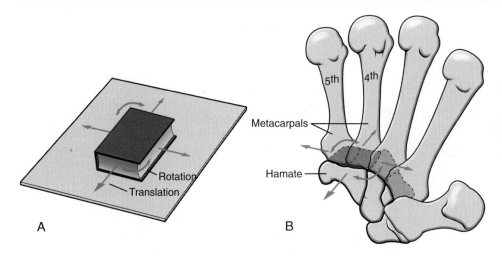

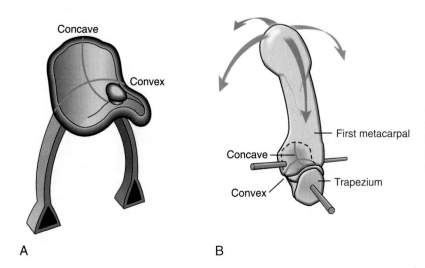

FIGURE 2-7. A plane joint is formed by opposition of two flat or nearly flat surfaces. The book moving on the tabletop **(A)** is depicted as analogous to the combined slide and rotation at the fourth and fifth carpometacarpal joints **(B).**

FIGURE 2-8. A saddle joint **(A)** is illustrated as analogous to the carpometacarpal joint of the thumb **(B).** The saddle in **A** represents the trapezium bone. The rider, if present, would represent the base of the thumb's metacarpal. The two axes of rotation are shown in **B.**

using the analogy of a horse's saddle and rider (Figure 2-8, *A*). From front to back, the saddle presents a concave surface reaching from the saddle pommel in front to the back of the saddle. From side to side, the saddle is convex, stretching from one stirrup across the back of the horse to the other stirrup. The rider has reciprocal convex and concave curves to complement the shape of the saddle. The carpometacarpal joint of the thumb is the clearest example of a saddle joint (see Figure 2-8, *B*). The reciprocal, interlocking nature of this joint allows ample motion in two planes but limited spin between the trapezium and the first metacarpal.

A *condyloid joint* is much like a ball-and-socket articulation except that the concave member of the joint is relatively shallow (Figure 2-9, *A*). Condyloid joints usually allow 2 degrees of freedom. Ligaments or bony incongruities often restrain the third degree. Condyloid joints often occur in pairs, such as the knees (see Figure 2-9, *B*) and the atlanto-occipital joints (i.e., articulation between the occipital condyles and the first cervical vertebra). The metacarpophalangeal joint of the finger is another example of a condyloid joint. The root of the word *condyle* actually means "knuckle."

The kinematics at condyloid joints vary based on joint structure. At the knee, for example, the femoral condyles

fit within the slight concavity provided by the tibial plateau and menisci. This articulation allows flexion-extension and axial rotation (i.e., spin). Abduction-adduction, however, is restricted primarily by ligaments.

Simplifying the Classification of Synovial Joints: Ovoid and Saddle Joints

It is often difficult to classify synovial joints based on an analogy to mechanics alone. The metacarpophalangeal joint (condyloid) and the glenohumeral joint (ball-and-socket), for example, have similar shapes but differ considerably in the relative magnitude of movement and overall function. Joints always display subtle variations that make simple mechanical descriptions less applicable. A good example of the difference between mechanical classification and true function is seen in the gentle undulations that characterize the intercarpal and intertarsal joints. Several of these joints produce complex multiplanar movements that are inconsistent with their simple "planar" mechanical classification. To circumvent this difficulty, a simplified classification scheme recognizes only two articular forms: the ovoid joint and the saddle joint (Figure 2-10). Essentially all synovial joints of the body with

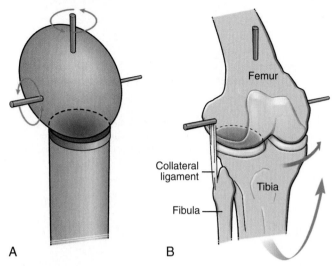

FIGURE 2-9. A condyloid joint **(A)** is analogous to the tibiofemoral (knee) joint **(B).** The two axes of rotation are shown by the pins. The potential frontal plane motion at the knee is blocked by tension in the collateral ligament.

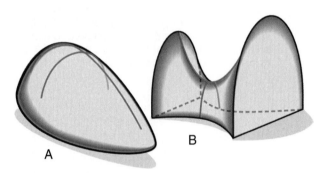

FIGURE 2-10. Two basic shapes of joint surfaces found in the body. **A,** The egg-shaped *ovoid surface* represents a characteristic of most synovial joints of the body (e.g., hip joint, radiocarpal joint, knee joint, metacarpophalangeal joint). The diagram shows only the convex member of the joint. A reciprocally shaped concave member would complete the pair of ovoid articulating surfaces. **B,** The *saddle surface* is the second basic type of joint surface, having one convex surface intersecting one concave surface. The paired articulating surface of the other half of the joint would be turned so that a concave surface is mated to a convex surface of the partner.

the notable exception of planar joints can be categorized under this scheme.

An *ovoid joint* has paired mating surfaces that are imperfectly spheric, or egg-shaped, with adjacent parts possessing a changing surface curvature. In each case the articular surface of one bone is convex and of the other is concave. Most joints in the body fit this scheme. A *saddle joint* has been previously described. Each member presents paired convex and concave surfaces oriented at approximately 90 degrees to each other. This simplified classification system is functionally associated with the arthrokinematics of roll, slide, or spin (see Chapter 1).

AXIS OF ROTATION

In the analogy of a door hinge (see Figure 2-3, *A*), the axis of rotation (i.e., the pin through the hinge) is *fixed* because it remains stationary as the hinge opens and closes. With the axis of rotation fixed, all points on the door experience equal arcs of rotation. In anatomic joints, however, the axis of rotation is rarely, if ever, fixed during bony rotation. Determining the exact position of the axis of rotation in anatomic joints is therefore not a simple task. A method of estimating the position of the axis of rotation in anatomic joints is shown in Figure 2-11, *A*. The intersection of the two perpendicular lines bisecting a to a' and b to b' defines the *instantaneous axis of rotation* for the 90-degree arc of knee flexion.[70] The word *instantaneous* indicates that the location of the axis holds true only for the specified arc of motion. The smaller the angular range used to calculate the instantaneous axis, the more accurate the estimate. If a series of line drawings is made for a sequence of small angular arcs of motion, the location of the instantaneous axes can be plotted for each portion within the arc of motion (see Figure 2-11, *B*). The path of the serial locations of the instantaneous axes of rotation is called the *evolute*. The path of the evolute is longer and more complex when the mating joint surfaces are less congruent or have greater differences in their radii of curvature, such as in the knee.

In many practical clinical situations it is necessary to make simple estimates of the location of the axis of rotation of a joint. These estimates are necessary when one performs *goniometry,* measures torque around a joint, or one constructs a prosthesis or an orthosis. A series of radiographs is required to precisely identify the instantaneous axis of rotation at a joint. This method is not practical in ordinary clinical situations. Instead, an *average axis of rotation* is assumed to occur throughout the entire arc of motion. This axis is located by an anatomic landmark that pierces the *convex* member of the joint.

HISTOLOGIC ORGANIZATION OF PERIARTICULAR CONNECTIVE TISSUES

There are only four primary types of tissue found in the body: connective tissue, muscle, nerve, and epithelium. Connective tissue, a derivative of the mesoderm, forms the basic structure of joints. The following section provides an overview of the histologic organization of the different kinds of connective tissues that form capsule, ligament, tendon, articular cartilage, and fibrocartilage. Throughout this textbook, these tissues are referred to as *periarticular connective tissues.* Bone is a very specialized form of connective tissue closely related to joints and is briefly reviewed later in this chapter.

Very generally, the fundamental materials that comprise all connective tissues in the body are *fibrous proteins, ground substance,* and *cells.* Even structures that are apparently as different as the capsule of the spleen, a fat pad, bone, and articular cartilage are made of these same fundamental materials. Each of these structures, however, consists of a unique composition, proportion, and arrangement of fibrous proteins, ground substance, and cells. The specific combination of these materials reflects the structures' unique mechanical or

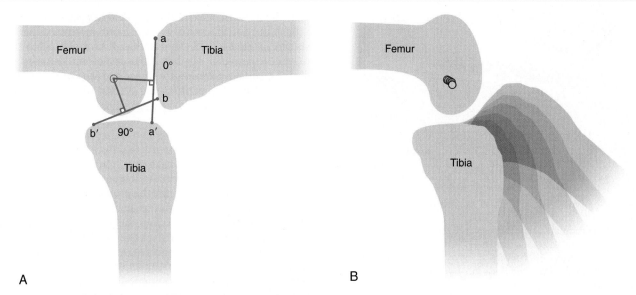

FIGURE 2-11. A method for determining the instantaneous axis of rotation for 90 degrees of knee flexion **(A).** With images retraced from a radiograph, two points (*a* and *b*) are identified on the proximal surface of the tibia. With the position of the femur held stationary, the same two points are again identified following 90 degrees of flexion (*a′* and *b′*). Lines are then drawn connecting a to a′, and b to b′. Next, two perpendicular lines are drawn from the midpoint of lines a to a′ and b to b′. The point of intersection of these two perpendicular lines identifies the instantaneous axis of rotation for the 90-degree arc of motion. This same method can be repeated for many smaller arcs of motion, resulting in several axes of rotation located in slightly different locations **(B).** At the knee, the average axis of rotation is oriented in the medial-lateral direction, generally through the lateral epicondyle of the femur.

physiologic functions. The following section describes the basic biologic materials that form periarticular connective tissues.

Fundamental Biologic Materials That Form Periarticular Connective Tissues

1. Fibrous Proteins
 Collagen (type I and II)
 Elastin

2. Ground Substance
 Glycosaminoglycans
 Water
 Solutes

3. Cells (Fibroblasts and Chondrocytes)

Fibrous Proteins

Collagen and elastin fibrous proteins are present in varying proportions in all periarticular connective tissues. Collagen is the most ubiquitous protein in the body, accounting for 30% of all proteins.[30] At the most basic level, collagen consists of amino acids wound in a triple helical fashion. These spiraled molecular threads, called *tropocollagen,* are placed together in a strand, several of which are cross-linked into ropelike *fibrils.* A collagen fibril may be 20 to 200 nm in diameter.[75] Many fibrils interconnect to form bundles or *fibers.* Although up to 28 specific types of collagen have been described based primarily on their amino acid sequences,[67] two types make up

the majority of collagen found in periarticular connective tissues: type I and type II.[75] *Type I collagen* consists of thick fibers that elongate little (i.e., stretch) when placed under tension. Being relatively stiff and strong, type I collagen is ideal for binding and supporting the articulations between bones. Type I collagen is therefore the primary protein found in ligaments and fibrous joint capsules. This type of collagen also makes up the parallel fibrous bundles that comprise tendons—the structures that transmit forces between muscle and bone. Figure 2-12 shows a high resolution and magnified image of type I collagen fibrils.

Type II collagen fibers are typically much thinner than type I fibers and possess slightly less tensile strength. These fibers provide a framework for maintaining the general shape and consistency of more complex structures, such as hyaline cartilage. Type II collagen still provides internal strength to the tissue in which it resides.

Two Predominant Types of Collagen Found in Periarticular Connective Tissues

Type I: thick, rugged fibers that elongate little when stretched; comprise ligaments, tendons, fascia, and fibrous joint capsules

Type II: thinner fibers than type I fibers; provide a framework for maintaining the general shape and consistency of structures, such as hyaline cartilage

---

In addition to collagen, periarticular connective tissues have varying amounts of *elastin fibers.* These protein fibers are composed of a net-like interweaving of small fibrils that resist

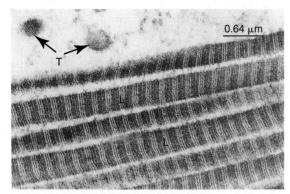

0.64 μm

FIGURE 2-12. Type I collagen fibers as viewed from a two-dimensional electron microscope (magnification ×32,000). Fibers are shown in longitudinal *(L)* and transverse *(T)* sections. The individual collagen fibrils display a characteristic cross-banding appearance. (From Young B, Lowe JS, Stevens A, et al: *Wheater's functional histology: a text and colour atlas*, ed 5, London, 2006, Churchill Livingstone.)

tensile (stretching) forces but have more "give" when elongated. Tissues with a high proportion of elastin readily return to their original shape after being greatly deformed. This property is useful in structures such as hyaline or elastic cartilage and certain spinal ligaments (such as the ligamentum flavum) that help realign the vertebrae to their original position after bending forward.

Ground Substance

Collagen and elastin fibers within periarticular connective tissues are embedded within a water-saturated matrix or gel known as *ground substance*. The ground substance of periarticular connective tissues consists primarily of *glycosaminoglycans* (GAGs), *water*, and *solutes*.[38,49,63] The GAGs are a family of large polymers of repeating polysaccharides that confer physical resilience to the ground substance. Figure 2-13 shows a stylized illustration of the ground substance within articular cartilage. Depicted at the bottom of Figure 2-13 are individual GAG chains attached to a core protein, forming a large complex *proteoglycan side unit*. Structurally, each proteoglycan side unit resembles a bottle brush—the wire stem of the brush being the core protein, and the bristles being the GAG chains. Many proteoglycan side units, in turn, are bonded to a central hyaluronan (hyaluronic acid), forming a *large proteoglycan complex*.[30,63,75]

Because the GAGs are highly negatively charged, the individual chains (or bristles on the brush) repel one another, greatly increasing three-dimensional volume of the proteoglycan complex. The negatively charged GAGs also make the proteoglycan complexes extremely hydrophilic, able to capture water equivalent to 50 times their weight.[38] The attracted water provides a fluid medium for diffusion of nutrients within the matrix. In addition, water and other positive ions confer a unique mechanical property to the tissue. The tendency of proteoglycans to imbibe and hold water causes the tissue to swell.[16] Swelling is limited by the embedded and entangled network of collagen (and elastin) fibers within the ground substance (see Figure 2-13, *top*). The interaction between the restraining fibers and the swelling proteoglycans

provides a turgid, semifluid structure that resists compression, much like a balloon or a water-filled mattress. The tissue shown in Figure 2-13 depicts the ground substance that is unique to articular cartilage. This important tissue provides an ideal surface covering for joints and is capable of dispersing millions of repetitive forces that likely affect joints throughout a lifetime.[7,8,38]

Cells

The primary cells within ligaments, tendons, and other supportive periarticular connective tissues are called *fibroblasts*. Chondrocytes, in contrast, are the primary cells within hyaline articular cartilage and fibrocartilage.[30,43,63] Both types of cells are responsible for synthesizing the specialized ground substance and fibrous proteins unique to the tissue, as well as conducting maintenance and repair. Damaged or aged components of periarticular connective tissues are constantly being removed, as new components are manufactured and remodeled. Cells of periarticular connective tissues are generally sparse and interspersed between the strands of fibers or embedded deeply in regions of high proteoglycan content. This sparseness of cells in conjunction with limited blood supply often results in poor or incomplete healing of damaged or injured joint tissues. In contrast to muscle cells, fibroblasts and chondrocytes do not confer significant mechanical properties on the tissue.

TYPES OF PERIARTICULAR CONNECTIVE TISSUES

Three types of periarticular connective tissues exist to varying degrees in all joints: *dense connective tissue, articular cartilage,* and *fibrocartilage* (Table 2-2).

Dense Connective Tissue

Dense connective tissue includes most of the nonmuscular "soft tissues" surrounding a joint: the fibrous (external) layer of the joint capsule, ligaments, and tendons. These tissues have few cells (fibroblasts), relatively low to moderate proportions of proteoglycan and elastin, and an abundance of tightly packed type I collagen fibers. As with most periarticular connective tissues, ligaments, tendons, and capsules possess a limited blood supply and therefore have a relatively low metabolism.[38] When physically loaded or stressed, however, the metabolism of these tissues can increase, often as a means of functionally adapting to a physical stimuli.[36,58,69,71] Such adaption has been well documented at the histologic level in tendons.[41,61] Strain placed on fibroblasts within the ground substance is believed to stimulate increased synthesis of collagen and GAGs, which can alter the tissue's structure and thereby modify its material properties, such as stiffness or ultimate failure point.[1,31,55,73]

Most anatomic or histologic texts[38,63,64] describe dense connective tissues as having two subsets, irregular and regular, based on the spatial orientation of the collagen fibers. The fibrous layer of the joint capsule is considered *irregular* dense connective tissue because of its irregular and often haphazard orientation of collagen fibers within its ground substance.[63] This type of tissue is well suited to resist tensile forces from multiple directions, such as what is often required by the

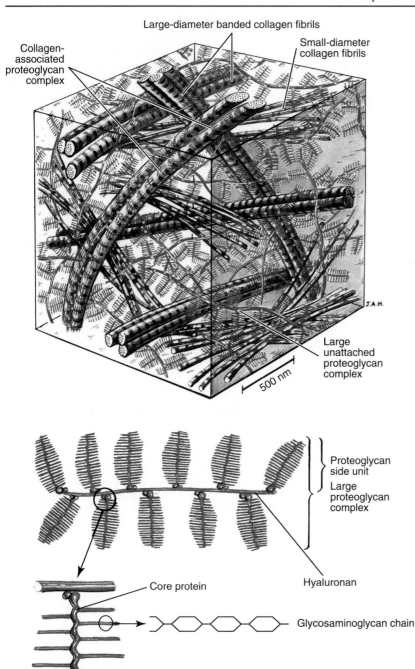

Collagen-associated proteoglycan complex

Large-diameter banded collagen fibrils

Small-diameter collagen fibrils

500 nm

Large unattached proteoglycan complex

Proteoglycan side unit

Large proteoglycan complex

Core protein

Hyaluronan

Glycosaminoglycan chain

FIGURE 2-13. Histologic organization of the ground substance of (hyaline) articular cartilage. The very bottom of the image shows the repeating disaccharide units that constitute a glycosaminoglycan chain *(GAG).* Many GAG chains attach to a core protein. The middle image shows the basic structure of a large proteoglycan complex, made up of many GAG chains. The three-dimensional image at the top of the figure shows the ground substance, which includes large quantities of proteoglycan complexes, interwoven within collagen fibers. Not depicted in the ground substance are interspersed cells (chondrocytes). In healthy tissue, water occupies much of the space between the proteoglycan complexes and fibers. (From Standring S: *Gray's anatomy: the anatomical basis of clinical practice,* ed 39, St Louis, 2005, Elsevier.)

spiraled nature of the joint capsules at the glenohumeral or hip joints. Ligaments and tendons are considered *regular* dense connective tissue because of the more orderly or near parallel orientation of their collagen fibers. The collagen fibers in most ligaments function most effectively when they are stretched nearly parallel to the long axis of the ligament. After the initial slack is pulled tight, the tissues provide immediate tension that restrains undesirable motion between bony partners.

When trauma or disease produces laxity in the joint capsules or ligaments, muscles take on a more dominant role in restraining joint movement. But even if muscles surrounding

a joint with loose supporting structures are strong, there is still potential for loss of joint stability. Compared with ligaments, muscles are slower to supply force because of reaction time and the electromechanical delay necessary to build active force. Also, muscle forces often have a less than ideal alignment for restraining undesirable joint movements and therefore cannot always provide the most optimal stabilizing force.

Tendons are designed to transfer large tensile loads between an activated muscle and the bone into which it inserts. The type I collagen fibers within tendons provide high tensile strength once they are fully elongated. Figure 2-14 illustrates

TABLE 2-2. Three Main Types of Periarticular Connective Tissues

Type	Histologic Consistency	Primary Function	Clinical Correlate
Dense connective tissue Ligaments Fibrous layer of the joint capsule Tendons	High proportion of parallel to slightly wavy type I collagen fibers; relative low elastin content Sparsely populated fibroblasts Relatively low to moderate proteoglycan content	Resists tension Ligaments and joint capsules protect and bind the joint Tendons transfer forces between muscle and bone	Repeated sprains of the lateral collateral ligament of the ankle may lead to chronic joint instability and potential posttraumatic osteoarthritis.
Articular cartilage (specialized hyaline cartilage)	High proportion of type II collagen fibers Sparsely to moderately populated chondrocytes Relatively high proteoglycan content	Distributes and absorbs joint forces (compression and shear) Reduces joint friction	During early stages of osteoarthritis, proteoglycans are lost from the ground substance, reducing the ability of the tissue to absorb water. The cartilage therefore loses its load attenuation property, leaving the subchondral bone vulnerable to damaging stresses.
Fibrocartilage Menisci (e.g., knee) Labra (e.g., hip) Discs (e.g., intervertebral, temporomandibular joint)	High proportion of multidirectional type I collagen fibers Sparsely to moderately populated fibroblasts and chondrocytes Relatively moderate proteoglycan content (depending on the structure)	Supports and mechanically stabilizes joints Dissipates loads across multiple planes Guides complex arthrokinematics	Torn or degenerated disc in temporomandibular joint may increase the stress on the adjacent bone, leading to degeneration, abnormal joint sounds, reduced jaw movements, and pain.

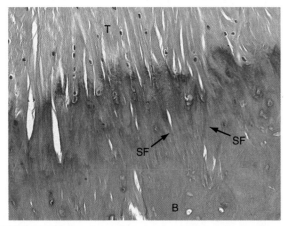

FIGURE 2-14. Light microscopic image of the collagen fibers of a tendon *(T)* blending with the collagen of the periosteum of a bone (pink-to-blue transition). Note the deeper collagen fibers known as *Sharpey's fibers (SF)* extending well into the bone tissue *(B).* (Hematoxylin-eosin stain; ×280.) (From Young B, Lowe JS, Stevens A, et al: *Wheater's functional histology: a text and colour atlas,* ed 5, London, 2006, Churchill Livingstone.)

a microscopic image of a tendon (T) as it inserts into bone (B). Note the near-parallel arranged collagen fibers, many of which are blending with the collagen of the periosteum. Some collagen fibers can be seen extending deeper into the bone material, often referred to as *Sharpey's fibers* (SF).[75]

Although structurally strong, tendons experience varying amounts of elongation when subjected to a high tensile force. The human Achilles tendon, for example, elongates up to 8%

of its resting length after a maximal contraction of the calf muscle.[40] This elastic property provides a mechanism to store and release energy during walking or jumping.[33,34,37] The property also allows the Achilles tendon to partially dissipate large or rapidly produced tensile force, which may offer some protection against injury.[41]

Articular Cartilage

Articular cartilage is a specialized type of hyaline cartilage that forms the load-bearing surface of joints. Articular cartilage covering the ends of the articulating bones has a thickness that ranges from 1 to 4 mm in areas of low compression and 5 to 7 mm in areas of high compression.[35] The tissue is avascular and aneural.[63,75] Unlike most hyaline cartilage throughout the body, articular cartilage lacks a perichondrium. This modification allows the opposing surfaces of the cartilage to form ideal load-bearing surfaces. Similar to periosteum on bone, perichondrium is a layer of connective tissue that covers most cartilage. It contains blood vessels and a ready supply of primitive cells that maintain and repair underlying tissue. This is an advantage not available to articular cartilage.

Chondrocytes of various shapes are located within the ground substance of different layers or zones of articular cartilage (Figure 2-15, *A*). These cells are bathed and nourished by nutrients contained within synovial fluid. Nourishment is facilitated by the "milking" action of articular surface deformation during intermittent joint loading. The chondrocytes are surrounded by predominantly type II collagen fibers. These fibers are arranged to form a restraining network or "scaffolding" that adds structural stability to the tissue (see

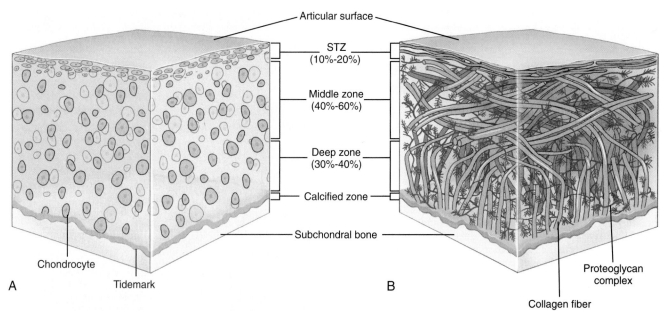

FIGURE 2-15. Two highly diagrammatic depictions of articular cartilage. **A,** The distribution of the cells (chondrocytes) is shown throughout the ground substance of the articular cartilage. The flattened chondrocytes near the articular surface are within the *superficial tangential zone (STZ)* and are oriented parallel to the joint surface. The STZ comprises about 10% to 20% of the articular cartilage thickness. The cells are more rounded in the *middle zone* and *deep zones*. A region of calcified cartilage *(calcified zone)* joins the deep zone with the underlying subchondral bone. The edge of the calcified zone that abuts the deep zone is known as the *tidemark* and forms a diffusion barrier between the articular cartilage and the underlying bone. Nutrients and gases must pass from the synovial fluid through all the layers of articular cartilage to nourish the chondrocytes, including those in the deep zone. **B,** The organization of the *collagen fibers* in articular cartilage is shown in this diagram. In the STZ, collagen is oriented nearly parallel to the articular surface, forming a fibrous grain that helps resist abrasion of the joint surface. The fibers become less tangential and more obliquely oriented in the *middle zone*, finally becoming almost perpendicular to the articular surface in the *deep zone*. The deepest fibers are anchored into the calcified zone to help tie the cartilage to the underlying subchondral bone. Proteoglycan complexes are also present throughout the ground substance.

Figure 2-15, *B*).[49] The deepest fibers in the calcified zone are firmly anchored to the subchondral bone. These fibers are linked to the vertically oriented fibers in the adjacent deep zone, which in turn are linked to the obliquely oriented fibers of the middle zone and finally to the transversely oriented fibers of the superficial tangential zone. The series of chemically interlinked fibers form a netlike fibrous structure that entraps the large proteoglycan complexes beneath the articular surface. The large amounts of proteoglycans, in turn, attract water, which provides a unique element of rigidity to articular cartilage. The rigidity increases the ability of cartilage to adequately withstand loads.[38]

Articular cartilage distributes and disperses compressive forces to the subchondral bone. It also reduces friction between joint surfaces. The coefficient of friction between two surfaces covered by articular cartilage and wet with synovial fluid is extremely low, ranging from 0.005 to 0.02 in the human knee, for example. This is 5 to 20 times lower and more slippery than ice on ice, which has a friction coefficient of 0.1.[45] The forces of normal weight-bearing activities therefore are reduced to a load level that typically can be absorbed without damaging the skeletal system.

The absence of a perichondrium on articular cartilage has the negative consequence of eliminating a ready source of primitive fibroblasts used for repair. Even though articular cartilage is capable of normal maintenance and replenishment of its matrix, significant damage to adult articular cartilage is often repaired poorly or not at all.

Fibrocartilage

As its name implies, fibrocartilage is a mixture of dense connective tissue and articular cartilage (Figure 2-16).[75] As such, fibrocartilage provides the resilience and shock absorption of articular cartilage and the tensile strength of ligaments and tendons. Dense bundles of type I collagen exist along with moderate amounts of proteoglycans. Depending on the tissue, fibrocartilage has varying numbers of chondrocytes and fibroblasts, located within a dense and often multidirectional collagen network.[30]

Fibrocartilage forms much of the substance of the intervertebral discs, the labra, and the discs located within the pubic symphysis, temporomandibular joint, and some joints of the extremities (e.g., the menisci of the knee). These structures help support and stabilize the joints, guide complex arthrokinematics, and help dissipate forces. Fibrocartilage is also found in some ligaments and tendons, especially at the point of insertion into bone.[63,75] The dense interwoven collagen fibers of fibrocartilage allow the tissue to resist multidirectional tensile, shear, and compressive forces. Fibrocartilage is therefore an ideal tissue to dissipate loads.

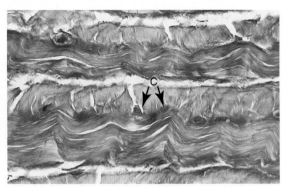

FIGURE 2-16. Photograph of a light microscopic image of fibrocartilage. (Hematoxylin-eosin and Alcian blue stain; ×320.) Note the alternating layers of hyaline cartilage matrix and thick collagen fibers. These layers are oriented in the direction of stress imposed on the tissues. Observe the pair of chondrocytes *(C)* located between a layer of collagen and hyaline cartilage. (From Young B, Lowe JS, Stevens A, et al: *Wheater's functional histology: a text and colour atlas,* ed 5, London, 2006, Churchill Livingstone.)

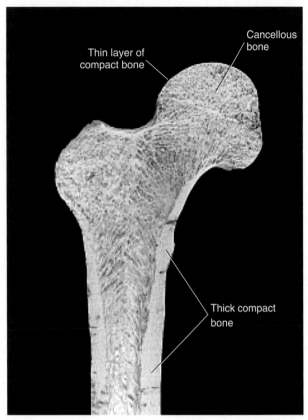

FIGURE 2-17. A cross-section showing the internal architecture of the proximal femur. Note the thicker areas of compact bone around the shaft and the lattice-like cancellous bone occupying most of the medullary region. (From Neumann DA: *An arthritis home study course: the synovial joint: anatomy, function, and dysfunction.* Orthopedic Section of the American Physical Therapy Association, LaCrosse, WI, 1998.)

Like articular cartilage, fibrocartilage typically lacks a perichondrium.[18,30] Fibrocartilage is also largely aneural and therefore does not produce pain or participate in proprioception, although a few neural receptors may be found at the periphery where fibrocartilage abuts a ligament or joint capsule. Most fibrocartilaginous tissues have a limited blood supply and are largely dependent on diffusion of nutrients from synovial fluid or from adjacent blood vessels. The diffusion of nutrients and removal of metabolic wastes in most fibrocartilaginous discs is assisted by the "milking" action of intermittent weight bearing.[26] This principle is readily apparent in adult intervertebral discs that are insufficiently nourished when the spine is held in fixed postures for extended periods. Without proper nutrition, the discs may partially degenerate and lose part of their protective function.[3]

A direct blood supply penetrates the outer rim of some fibrocartilaginous structures where they attach to joint capsules or ligaments, such as menisci in the knee or intervertebral discs. In adult joints, some repair of damaged fibrocartilage can occur near the vascularized periphery, such as the outer one third of menisci of the knee and the outermost lamellae of intervertebral discs. The innermost regions of fibrocartilage structures, much like articular cartilage, demonstrate poor or negligible healing as a result of the lack of a ready source of undifferentiated fibroblastic cells.[6,38,63]

BONE

Bone is a very specialized connective tissue, sharing several fundamental histologic characteristics with other periarticular connective tissues. Bone tissue consists of a highly cross-linked type 1 collagen, cells (such as osteoblasts), and a hard ground substance rich in mineral salts. The proteoglycans within the ground substance contain glycoproteins (such as osteocalcin) that strongly bind to calcium and phosphorous rich mineral salts–*calcium hydroxyapatite* $(Ca_{10}[PO_4]_6 [OH]_2)$.[49,63,75]

Bone gives rigid support to the body and provides the muscles with a system of levers. The outer cortex of the long bones of the adult skeleton has a shaft composed of thick, *compact bone* (Figure 2-17). The ends of long bones, however, are formed of a thinner layer of compact bone that surrounds a network of *cancellous bone*. Bones of the adult axial skeleton, such as the vertebral body, possess an outer shell of relatively thick compact bone that is filled with a supporting core of cancellous bone. As described earlier, articular cartilage covers the diarthrodial articular surfaces of all bones throughout the musculoskeletal system.

The structural subunit of compact bone is the *osteon (Haversian system)*, which organizes the collagen fibers and mineralized ground substance into a unique series of concentric spirals that form *lamellae* (Figure 2-18).[63,64,75] This infrastructure, made rigid by the calcium phosphate crystals, allows cortical bone to accept tremendous compressive loads. The osteoblasts eventually become surrounded by their secreted ground substance and become confined within narrow lacunae (i.e., spaces) positioned between the lamellae of the osteon.[49] (The confined osteoblasts are technically referred to as *osteocytes.*) Because bone deforms very little, blood vessels can pass into its substance from the outer periosteal and the inner endosteal surfaces. The blood vessels can then turn to travel along the long axis of the bone in a tunnel at the center of the *Haversian canals* (see Figure 2-18). This system allows a rich source of blood to reach the cells deep within the cortex. Furthermore, the connective tissue com-

Structure of Cortical (Compact) Bone

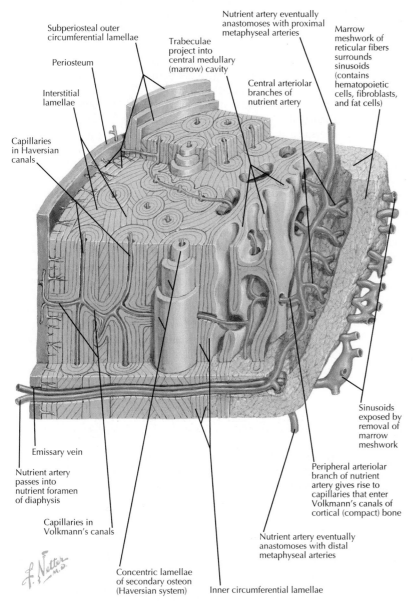

Subperiosteal outer circumferential lamellae

Periosteum

Interstitial lamellae

Capillaries in Haversian canals

Trabeculae project into central medullary (marrow) cavity

Nutrient artery eventually anastomoses with proximal metaphyseal arteries

Central arteriolar branches of nutrient artery

Marrow meshwork of reticular fibers surrounds sinusoids (contains hematopoietic cells, fibroblasts, and fat cells)

Emissary vein

Nutrient artery passes into nutrient foramen of diaphysis

Capillaries in Volkmann's canals

Concentric lamellae of secondary osteon (Haversian system)

Inner circumferential lamellae

Nutrient artery eventually anastomoses with distal metaphyseal arteries

Peripheral arteriolar branch of nutrient artery gives rise to capillaries that enter Volkmann's canals of cortical (compact) bone

Sinusoids exposed by removal of marrow meshwork

FIGURE 2-18. The ultrastructure of compact bone. Note the concentric lamellae that make up a single osteon (Haversian system). (From Ovalle WK, Nahirney PC: *Netter's essential histology,* Philadelphia, 2008, Saunders.)

prising the periosteum and endosteum of bone is also richly vascularized, as well as innervated with sensory receptors for pressure and pain.

Bone is a very dynamic tissue. Osteoblasts are constantly synthesizing ground substance and collagen as well as orchestrating the deposition of mineral salts. Remodeling occurs in response to forces applied through physical activity and in response to hormonal influences that regulate systemic calcium balance. The large-scale removal of bone is carried out by osteoclasts—specialized cells that originate from within the bone marrow. Primitive fibroblasts essential for the repair of fractured bone originate from the periosteum and endosteum and from the perivascular tissues that are woven throughout the bone's vascular canals. Of the tissues involved with joints, bone has by far the best capacity for remodeling, repair, and regeneration.

Bone demonstrates its greatest strength when compressed along the long axis of its shaft loading the Haversian systems longitudinally, which is comparable to compressing a straw along its long axis. The ends of long bones receive multidirectional compressive forces through the weight-bearing surfaces of articular cartilage. Stresses are spread to the subjacent subchondral bone and then into the network of cancellous bone, which in turn acts as a series of struts to redirect the forces into the long axis of the compact bone of the shaft. This structural arrangement redirects forces for absorption and transmission by taking advantage of bone's unique architectural design.

In contrast to periarticular connective tissues, bone has a rich blood supply coupled with a very dynamic metabolism. This allows bone to constantly remodel in response to physical stress. A rich blood supply also affords bone with a good potential for healing after fracture.

SPECIAL FOCUS 2-1

Wolff's Law

Bone is a very dynamic tissue, constantly altering its shape, strength, and density in response to external forces.[9,17,50] This general concept is often referred to as *Wolff's law,* named after the work and teachings of Julius Wolff (1839-1902), a German anatomist and orthopedic surgeon. Loosely translated, Wolff's law states that "bone is laid down in areas of high stress and reabsorbed in areas of low stress." This simple axiom has many clinical applications.[17] A deteriorated and dehydrated intervertebral disc, for example, may be unable to protect the underlying bone from stress. According to Wolff's law, bone responds to stress by synthesizing more bone. Bone "spurs" or osteophytes may form if the response is excessive. Occasionally osteophytes can block motion or compress an adjacent spinal nerve root, causing radiating pain in the lower extremity or weakness in associated muscles.

Wolff's law can also explain the *loss* of bone and its reduced strength after chronic unloading. For instance, bone mineral density in persons with spinal cord injury rapidly declines, likely caused by the unloading of bone stemming from the paralysis.[15] Reduced bone density can place the bones of the person with a spinal cord injury at a higher risk for fracture. Fractures are not uncommon, occurring from trauma such as falling out of a wheelchair, during daily activities such as performing "self" range-of-motion exercises to the lower extremities, or during a controlled transfer between a bathtub and chair. Researchers have shown that bone loss after spinal cord injury can be reduced by the appropriate use of electrical stimulation to the paralyzed limb muscles.[60] The forces produced by the stimulated muscle are transferred across the bone. Although not always practical, in theory the regular and appropriate application of electrical stimulation to paralyzed muscles may help prevent fractures in persons with chronic paralysis after a spinal cord injury. Additional research is needed to determine the feasibility and long-term benefits of using electrical stimulation as a regular part of rehabilitation for individuals with a spinal cord injury.[59]

SOME EFFECTS OF IMMOBILIZATION ON THE STRENGTH OF PERIARTICULAR CONNECTIVE TISSUE AND BONE

The amount and arrangement of the fibrous proteins, ground substance, and water that constitute periarticular connective tissues are influenced by physical activity.[9,41,72] At a normal level of physical activity, the composition of the tissues is typically strong enough to adequately resist the natural range of forces imposed on the musculoskeletal system. A joint immobilized for an extended period demonstrates marked changes in the structure and function of its associated connective tissues. The mechanical strength of the tissue is reduced in accordance with the decreased forces of the immobilized condition. This is a normal response to an abnormal condition. Placing a body part in a cast and confining a

person to a bed are examples in which immobilization dramatically reduces the level of force imposed on the musculoskeletal system. Although for different reasons, muscular paralysis or weakness also reduces the force on the musculoskeletal system.

The rate of decline in the strength of periarticular connective tissue is somewhat dependent on the normal metabolic activity of the specific tissue.[41,53] Chronic immobilization produces a marked decrease in tensile strength of the ligaments of the knee in a period of weeks.[47,72] The earliest biochemical markers of this remodeling can be detected within days after immobilization.[25,46] Even after the cessation of the immobilization and after the completion of an extended postimmobilization exercise program, the ligaments continue to have lower tensile strength than ligaments that were never subjected to immobilization.[25,72] Other tissues such as bone and articular cartilage also show a loss of mass, volume, and strength after immobilization.[9,10,21,28] The results from experimental studies imply that tissues rapidly lose strength in response to reduced loading. Full recovery of strength after restoration of loading is much slower and often incomplete.

Immobilizing a joint for an extended period is often necessary to promote healing after an injury such as a fractured bone. Clinical judgment is required to balance the potential negative effects of the immobilization with the need to promote healing. The maintenance of maximal tissue strength around joints requires judicious use of immobilization, a quick return to loading, and early rehabilitative intervention.

BRIEF OVERVIEW OF JOINT PATHOLOGY

Trauma to periarticular connective tissues can occur from a single overwhelming event (acute trauma) or in response to an accumulation of lesser injuries over an extended period (chronic trauma). *Acute trauma* often produces detectable pathology. A torn or severely stretched ligament or joint capsule causes an acute inflammatory reaction. The joint may also become structurally unstable when damaged periarticular connective tissues are not able to restrain the natural extremes of motion.

Joints most frequently affected by acute traumatic instability are typically associated with the longest external moment arms of the skeleton and therefore are exposed to high external torques. For this reason, the tibiofemoral, talocrural, and glenohumeral joints are frequently subjected to acute ligament damage with resultant instability.

Acute trauma can also result in intra-articular fractures involving articular cartilage and subchondral bone. Careful reduction or realignment of the fractured fragments helps to restore congruity to the joint and thereby facilitate smooth, low-friction sliding functions of articular surfaces. This is critical to maximal recovery of function. Although the bone adjacent to a joint has excellent ability to repair, the repair of fractured articular cartilage is often incomplete and produces mechanically inferior areas of the joint surface that are prone to degeneration. Focal increases in stress caused by poor surface alignment in conjunction with impaired articular cartilage strength can lead to posttraumatic osteoarthritis.

The repair of damaged fibrocartilaginous joint structures depends on the proximity and adequacy of blood supply. A tear of the outermost region of the meniscus of the knee adjacent to blood vessels embedded within the joint capsule may completely heal.[19,56] In contrast, tears of the innermost circumference of a meniscus do not typically heal. This is also the case in the inner lamellae of the adult intervertebral disc, which does not have the capacity to heal after significant damage.[3,20]

Chronic trauma is often classified as a type of "overuse syndrome" and reflects an accumulation of unrepaired, relatively minor damage. Chronically damaged joint capsules and ligaments gradually lose their restraining functions, although the instability of the joint may be masked by a muscular restraint substitute. In this case, joint forces may be increased because of an exaggerated muscular "guarding" of the joint. Only when the joint is challenged suddenly or forced by an extreme movement does the instability become apparent.

Recurring instability may cause abnormal loading conditions on the joint tissues, which can lead to their mechanical failure. The surfaces of articular cartilage and fibrocartilage may become fragmented, with a concurrent loss of proteoglycans and subsequent lowered resistance to compressive and shear forces.[13] Early stages of degeneration often demonstrate a roughened or "fibrillated" surface of the articular cartilage.[2] A fibrillated region of articular cartilage may later develop cracks, or clefts, that extend from the surface into the middle or deepest layers of the tissue. These changes reduce the shock absorption quality of the tissue.

Two disease states that commonly cause joint dysfunction are osteoarthritis (OA) and rheumatoid arthritis (RA). *Osteo-arthritis* is characterized by a gradual erosion of articular cartilage with a low inflammatory component.[5,24,32] Some clinicians and researchers refer to OA as "osteoarthrosis" to emphasize the lack of a distinctive inflammatory component.[11] As erosion of articular cartilage progresses, the underlying subchondral bone becomes more mineralized and in severe cases becomes the weight-bearing surface when the articular cartilage pad is completely worn. The fibrous joint capsule and synovium become distended and thickened. The severely involved joint may be completely unstable and dislocate or may fuse, allowing no motion.

The frequency of OA increases with age, and the disease has several manifestations.[12,16] *Idiopathic OA* occurs in the absence of a specific cause; it affects only one or a few joints, particularly those that are subjected to the highest weight-bearing loads: hip, knee, and lumbar spine. *Familial OA* or *generalized OA* affects joints of the hand and is more frequent in women. *Posttraumatic OA* may affect any synovial joint that has been exposed to a trauma of sufficient severity.

Rheumatoid arthritis differs markedly from OA, as it is a systemic, autoimmune connective tissue disorder with a strong inflammatory component. The destruction of multiple joints is a prominent manifestation of RA. The joint dysfunction is manifested by significant inflammation of the capsule, synovium, and synovial fluid. The articular cartilage is exposed to an enzymatic process that can rapidly erode the articular surface. The joint capsule is distended by the recurrent swelling and inflammation, often causing marked joint instability and pain.

SPECIAL FOCUS 2-2

A Brief Look at Some Effects of Advanced Aging on Periarticular Connective Tissue and Bone

Reaching an advanced age is associated with histologic changes in periarticular connective tissues and bone that, in turn, may produce mechanical changes in joint function. It is often not possible to separate the effects of aging in humans from the effects of reduced physical activity or immobilization. Furthermore, at a fundamental level, the physiologic effects of all three variables are remarkably similar.

The rate and process by which tissue ages is highly individualized and can be modified, positively or negatively, by the types and frequency of activities and by a host of medical, hormonal, and nutritional factors.[9,16,53] In the broadest sense, aging is accompanied by a slowing of the rate of fibrous proteins and proteoglycan replacement and repair in all periarticular connective tissues and bone.[16,42,61] Tissues therefore lose their ability to restrain and optimally disperse forces produced at the joint. The effects of microtrauma over the years can accumulate to produce subclinical damage that may progress to a structural failure or a measurable change in mechanical properties. A clinical example of this phenomenon is the age-related deterioration of the ligaments and articular capsule associated with the glenohumeral joint. Reduced structural support provided by these tissues may eventually culminate in tendonitis or tears in the rotator cuff muscles.[74]

The *glycosaminoglycan* (GAG) molecules produced by aging cells in connective tissues are fewer in number and smaller in size than those produced by young cells.[14,22,51,62] This reduced concentration of GAGs (and hence proteoglycans) reduces the water-binding capacity of the extracellular matrix. Aged articular cartilage, for instance, contains less water and is less able to attenuate and distribute imposed forces on subchondral bone. Dehydrated articular cartilage therefore may serve as a precursor to osteoarthritis.[12,16,27]

Less hydrated ligaments do not slide across one another as easily. As a result, the bundles of fibers within ligaments do not align themselves with the imposed forces as readily, hampering the ability of the tissue to maximally resist a rapidly applied force. The likelihood of adhesions forming between previously mobile tissue planes is increased, thus promoting range-of-motion restrictions in aging joints.[4,16,65]

Continued

A Brief Look at Some Effects of Advanced Aging on Periarticular Connective Tissue and Bone—cont'd

Interestingly, tendons have been shown to become *less* stiff with aging and with chronic unloading.[39,48,57] A significant increase in compliance therefore may reduce the mechanical efficiency and speed of transferring muscle force to bone. As a consequence, muscles may be less able to optimally stabilize a joint.

Bone becomes weaker with aging, in part because of decreased osteoblastic activity and a reduced differentiation potential of bone marrow stem cells.[9,29] The age-related alteration of connective tissue metabolism in bone contributes to the slower healing of fractures. The altered metabolism also contributes to osteoporo-

sis, particularly senile osteoporosis—a type that thins both trabecular and compact bone of individuals of both genders.

Fortunately, many of the potentially negative physiologic effects of aging periarticular connective tissues and bone can be mitigated, to an extent, through physical activity and resistance training.* These responses serve as the basis for many of the physical rehabilitation principles used in the treatment of persons of advanced age.

*References 23, 40, 41, 44, 52, 54, 66, 68.

SUMMARY

Joints provide the foundation of musculoskeletal motion and permit the stability and dispersion of forces between segments of the body. Several classification schemes exist to categorize joints and to allow discussion of their mechanical and kinematic characteristics. Motions of anatomic joints are often complex as a result of their asymmetrical shapes and incongruent surfaces. The axis of rotation is often estimated for purposes of clinical measurement.

The function and resilience of joints are determined by the architecture and the types of tissues that make up the joints. Interestingly, all periarticular connective tissues (and bone) share a fundamentally similar histologic organization. Each tissue contains cells, a ground substance or matrix, and fibrous proteins. The extent and proportion of these components vary considerably based on the primary functional demand imposed on the tissue. Joint capsules, ligaments, and tendons are designed to resist tension in multiple or single directions. Articular cartilage is extraordinarily suited to resist compression and shear within joints and, in the presence of synovial fluid, provides a remarkably smooth interface for joint movement. Fibrocartilage shares structural and functional characteristics of dense connective tissues and articular cartilage. The fibrocartilaginous menisci at the knee, for example, must resist large compression forces from the surrounding large muscles and tolerate the multidirectional shearing stress created by the sliding arthrokinematics within the joint. Bone is a highly specialized connective tissue, designed to support the body and its limbs and to provide a series of levers for the muscles to move the body.

The ability to repair damaged joint tissues is strongly related to the presence of a direct blood supply and the availability of progenitor cells. The functional health and longevity of joints are also affected by age, loading, immobilization, trauma, and certain disease states.

REFERENCES

1. Arnoczky SP, Lavagnino M, Whallon JH, Hoonjan A: In situ cell nucleus deformation in tendons under tensile load: A morphological analysis using confocal laser microscopy, *J Orthop Res* 20:29-35, 2002.

2. Bae WC, Wong VW, Hwang J, et al: Wear-lines and split-lines of human patellar cartilage: Relation to tensile biomechanical properties, *Osteoarthritis Cartilage* 16:841-845, 2008.

3. Beattie PF: Current understanding of lumbar intervertebral disc degeneration: A review with emphasis upon etiology, pathophysiology, and lumbar magnetic resonance imaging findings, *J Orthop Sports Phys Ther* 38:329-340, 2008.

4. Begg RK, Sparrow WA: Aging effects on knee and ankle joint angles at key events and phases of the gait cycle, *J Med Eng Technol* 30:382-389, 2006.

5. Brandt KD, Dieppe P, Radin EL: Etiopathogenesis of osteoarthritis, *Rheum Dis Clin North Am* 34:531-559, 2008.

6. Buckwalter JA, Brown TD: Joint injury, repair, and remodeling: Roles in post-traumatic osteoarthritis, *Clin Orthop Relat Res* 423:7-16, 2004.

7. Buckwalter JA, Kuettner KE, Thonar EJ: Age-related changes in articular cartilage proteoglycans: Electron microscopic studies, *J Orthop Res* 3:251-257, 1985.

8. Buckwalter JA, Mankin HJ, Grodzinsky AJ: Articular cartilage and osteoarthritis, *Instr Course Lect* 54:465-480, 2005.

9. Chen JS, Cameron ID, Cumming RG, et al: Effect of age-related chronic immobility on markers of bone turnover, *J Bone Miner Res* 21:324-331, 2006.

10. Demirbag D, Ozdemir F, Kokino S, Berkarda S: The relationship between bone mineral density and immobilization duration in hemiplegic limbs, *Ann Nucl Med* 19:695-700, 2005.

11. Dequeker J, Luyten FP: The history of osteoarthritis-osteoarthrosis, *Ann Rheum Dis* 67:5-10, 2008.

12. Ding C, Cicuttini F, Blizzard L, et al: A longitudinal study of the effect of sex and age on rate of change in knee cartilage volume in adults, *Rheumatology* 46:273-279, 2007.

13. Ding C, Cicuttini F, Scott F, et al: Association between age and knee structural change: A cross sectional MRI based study, *Ann Rheum Dis* 64:549-555, 2005.

14. Dudhia J: Aggrecan, aging and assembly in articular cartilage, *Cell Mol Life Sci* 62:2241-2256, 2005.

15. Dudley-Javoroski S, Shields RK: Dose estimation and surveillance of mechanical loading interventions for bone loss after spinal cord injury, *Phys Ther* 88:387-396, 2008.

16. Freemont AJ, Hoyland JA: Morphology, mechanisms and pathology of musculoskeletal aging, *J Pathol* 211:252-259, 2007.

17. Frost HM: A 2003 update of bone physiology and Wolff's Law for clinicians, *Angle Orthod* 74:3-15, 2004.

18. Gartner LP, Hiatt JL: *Color textbook of histology*, ed 3, Philadelphia, 2007, Saunders.

19. Greis PE, Bardana DD, Holmstrom MC, Burks RT: Meniscal injury: I. Basic science and evaluation, *J Am Acad Orthop Surg*, 10:168-176, 2002.

20. Grunhagen T, Wilde G, Soukane DM, et al: Nutrient supply and intervertebral disc metabolism, *J Bone Joint Surg Am* 88(Suppl 2):30-35, 2006.

21. Haapala J, Arokoski J, Pirttimaki J, et al: Incomplete restoration of immobilization induced softening of young beagle knee articular cartilage after 50-week remobilization, *Int J Sports Med* 21:76-81, 2000.

22. Hamerman D: Aging and the musculoskeletal system, *Ann Rheum Dis* 56:578-585, 1997.
23. Hanna F, Teichtahl AJ, Bell R, et al: The cross-sectional relationship between fortnightly exercise and knee cartilage properties in healthy adult women in midlife, *Menopause* 14:830-834, 2007.
24. Hardingham T: Extracellular matrix and pathogenic mechanisms in osteoarthritis, *Curr Rheumatol Rep* 10:30-36, 2008.
25. Hayashi K: Biomechanical studies of the remodeling of knee joint tendons and ligaments, *J Biomech* 29:707-716, 1996.
26. Humzah MD, Soames RW: Human intervertebral disc: Structure and function, *Anat Rec* 220:337-356, 1988.
27. Iannone F, Lapadula G: The pathophysiology of osteoarthritis, *Aging Clin Exp Res* 15:364-372, 2003.
28. Jortikka MO, Inkinen RI, Tammi MI, et al: Immobilisation causes longlasting matrix changes both in the immobilised and contralateral joint cartilage, *Ann Rheum Dis* 56:255-261, 1997.
29. Khosla S, Riggs BL: Pathophysiology of age-related bone loss and osteoporosis, *Endocrinol Metab Clin North Am* 34:1015-1030, 2005.
30. Kierszenbaum AL: *Histology and cell biology: An introduction to pathology*, ed 2, Philadelphia, 2007, Mosby.
31. Kjaer M, Magnusson P, Krogsgaard M, et al: Extracellular matrix adaptation of tendon and skeletal muscle to exercise, *J Anat* 208:445-450, 2006.
32. Krasnokutsky S, Samuels J, Abramson SB: Osteoarthritis in 2007, *Bull NYU Hosp Jt Dis* 65:222-228, 2007.
33. Kubo K, Kanehisa H, Takeshita D, et al: In vivo dynamics of human medial gastrocnemius muscle-tendon complex during stretch-shortening cycle exercise, *Acta Physiol Scand* 170:127-135, 2000.
34. Kurokawa S, Fukunaga T, Nagano A, Fukashiro S: Interaction between fascicles and tendinous structures during counter movement jumping investigated in vivo, *J Appl Physiol* 95:2306-2314, 2003.
35. Kurrat HJ, Oberlander W: The thickness of the cartilage in the hip joint, *J Anat* 126:145-155, 1978.
36. Langberg H, Skovgaard D, Petersen LJ, et al: Type I collagen synthesis and degradation in peritendinous tissue after exercise determined by microdialysis in humans, *J Physiol* 521(Pt 1):299-306, 1999.
37. Lieber RL, Leonard ME, Brown-Maupin CG: Effects of muscle contraction on the load-strain properties of frog aponeurosis and tendon, *Cells Tissues Organs* 166:48-54, 2000.
38. Lundon K: *Orthopaedic rehabilitation science: principles for clinical management of nonmineralized connective tissue*, St Louis, 2003, Butterworth-Heinemann.
39. Maganaris CN, Reeves ND, Rittweger J, et al: Adaptive response of human tendon to paralysis, *Muscle Nerve* 33:85-92, 2006.
40. Magnusson SP, Hansen P, Aagaard P, et al: Differential strain patterns of the human gastrocnemius aponeurosis and free tendon, in vivo, *Acta Physiol Scand* 177:185-195, 2003.
41. Magnusson SP, Narici MV, Maganaris CN, Kjaer M: Human tendon behaviour and adaptation, in vivo, *J Physiol* 586:71-81, 2008.
42. Martin JA, Brown TD, Heiner AD, Buckwalter JA: Chondrocyte senescence, joint loading and osteoarthritis, *Clin Orthop Relat Res* 427(Suppl):S96-S103, 2004.
43. Martin JA, Buckwalter JA: The role of chondrocyte senescence in the pathogenesis of osteoarthritis and in limiting cartilage repair, *J Bone Joint Surg Am* 85(Suppl 2):106-110, 2003.
44. Mikesky AE, Mazzuca SA, Brandt KD, et al: Effects of strength training on the incidence and progression of knee osteoarthritis, *Arthr Rheumat* 55:690-699, 2006.
45. Mow VC, Hayes WC: *Basic orthopaedic biomechanics*, New York, 1991, Raven Press.
46. Muller FJ, Setton LA, Manicourt DH, et al: Centrifugal and biochemical comparison of proteoglycan aggregates from articular cartilage in experimental joint disuse and joint instability, *J Orthop Res* 12:498-508, 1994.
47. Noyes FR: Functional properties of knee ligaments and alterations induced by immobilization: A correlative biomechanical and histological study in primates, *Clin Orthop Relat Res* 123:210-242, 1977.
48. Onambele GL, Narici MV, Maganaris CN: Calf muscle-tendon properties and postural balance in old age, *J Appl Physiol* 100:2048-2056, 2006.
49. Ovalle WK, Nahirney PC: *Netter's essential histology*, Philadelphia, 2008, Saunders.
50. Pearson OM, Lieberman DE: The aging of Wolff's "law": Ontogeny and responses to mechanical loading in cortical bone, *Am J Phys Anthropol* 39(Suppl):63-99, 2004.
51. Podichetty VK: The aging spine: The role of inflammatory mediators in intervertebral disc degeneration, *Cell Mol Biol* 53:4-18, 2007.
52. Racunica TL, Teichtahl AJ, Wang Y, et al: Effect of physical activity on articular knee joint structures in community-based adults, *Arthritis Rheum* 57:1261-1268, 2007.
53. Reeves ND: Adaptation of the tendon to mechanical usage, *J Musculoskelet Neuronal Interact* 6:174-180, 2006.
54. Reeves ND, Narici MV, Maganaris CN: Strength training alters the viscoelastic properties of tendons in elderly humans, *Muscle Nerve* 28:74-81, 2003.
55. Rosager S, Aagaard P, Dyhre-Poulsen P, et al: Load-displacement properties of the human triceps surae aponeurosis and tendon in runners and non-runners, *Scand J Med Sci Sports* 12:90-98, 2002.
56. Rubman MH, Noyes FR, Barber-Westin SD: Arthroscopic repair of meniscal tears that extend into the avascular zone. A review of 198 single and complex tears, *Am J Sports Med* 26:87-95, 1998.
57. Sargon MF, Doral MN, Atay OA: Age-related changes in human PCLs: A light and electron microscopic study, *Knee Surg Sports Traumatol Arthrosc* 12:280-284, 2004.
58. Setton LA, Chen J: Cell mechanics and mechanobiology in the intervertebral disc, *Spine* 29:2710-2723, 2004.
59. Shields RK, Dudley-Javoroski S: Musculoskeletal adaptations in chronic spinal cord injury: Effects of long-term soleus electrical stimulation training, *Neurorehabil Neural Repair* 21:169-179, 2007.
60. Shields RK, Dudley-Javoroski S, Law LA: Electrically induced muscle contractions influence bone density decline after spinal cord injury, *Spine* 31:548-553, 2006.
61. Smith K, Rennie MJ: New approaches and recent results concerning human-tissue collagen synthesis, *Curr Opin Clin Nutr Metab Care* 10:582-590, 2007.
62. Squires GR, Okouneff S, Ionescu M, Poole AR: The pathobiology of focal lesion development in aging human articular cartilage and molecular matrix changes characteristic of osteoarthritis, *Arthritis Rheum* 48:1261-1270, 2003.
63. Standring S: *Gray's anatomy: the anatomical basis of clinical practice*, ed 40, St Louis, 2009, Elsevier.
64. Stevens A, Lowe JS: *Human histology*, Philadelphia, 2005, Mosby.
65. Troke M, Moore AP, Maillardet FJ, Cheek E: A normative database of lumbar spine ranges of motion, *Man Ther* 10:198-206, 2005.
66. van Weeren PR, Firth EC, Brommer B, et al: Early exercise advances the maturation of glycosaminoglycans and collagen in the extracellular matrix of articular cartilage in the horse, *Equine Vet J* 40:128-135, 2008.
67. Veit G, Kobbe B, Keene DR, et al: Collagen XXVIII, a novel von Willebrand factor A domain-containing protein with many imperfections in the collagenous domain, *J Biol Chem* 281:3494-3504, 2006.
68. von SS, Kemmler W, Kalender WA, et al: Differential effects of strength versus power training on bone mineral density in postmenopausal women: A 2-year longitudinal study, *Br J Sports Med* 41:649-655, 2007.
69. Wackerhage H, Rennie MJ: How nutrition and exercise maintain the human musculoskeletal mass, *J Anat* 208:451-458, 2006.
70. Winter DA: *Biomechanics and motor control of human movement*, New Jersey, 2005, John Wiley & Sons.
71. Woo SL, Abramowitch SD, Kilger R, Liang R: Biomechanics of knee ligaments: Injury, healing, and repair, *J Biomech* 39:1-20, 2006.
72. Woo SL, Gomez MA, Sites TJ, et al: The biomechanical and morphological changes in the medial collateral ligament of the rabbit after immobilization and remobilization, *J Bone Joint Surg Am* 69:1200-1211, 1987.
73. Woo SL, Gomez MA, Woo YK, Akeson WH: Mechanical properties of tendons and ligaments. II. The relationships of immobilization and exercise on tissue remodeling, *Biorheology* 19:397-408, 1982.
74. Yamaguchi K, Sher JS, Andersen WK, et al: Glenohumeral motion in patients with rotator cuff tears: A comparison of asymptomatic and symptomatic shoulders, *J Shoulder Elbow Surg* 9:6-11, 2000.
75. Young B, Lowe JS, Stevens A: *Wheater's functional histology: a text and colour atlas*, ed 5, Philadelphia, 2006, Churchill Livingstone.

STUDY QUESTIONS

1 Describe the morphologic differences between ovoid and saddle joints. Provide an anatomic example of each type of joint.

2 Cite the major distinguishing structural and functional differences between a synarthrodial and a diarthrodial (synovial) joint.

3 Intra-articular discs (or menisci) are sometimes found in diarthrodial joints. Name three joints in the body that contain intra-articular discs. Describe the most likely function(s) of these structures at these joints.

4 List the four primary types of tissues that exist throughout the body.

5 Which of the joints illustrated in Figures 2-3 through 2-9 have (a) the greatest and (b) the least degrees of freedom?

6 Cite the major functional differences between type I collagen and elastin. Cite tissues that contain a high proportion of each protein.

7 What is the difference between an *evolute* and an *instantaneous axis of rotation?* Cite one biomechanical or practical conse-

quence of a joint that possesses a significantly large, although normal, evolute.

8 Define (a) perichondrium and (b) periosteum. What is the primary function of these tissues?

9 Describe the fundamental mechanism used by articular cartilage to repeatedly disperse compression forces across joints.

10 Describe the primary reasons why bone possesses a far superior healing potential than articular cartilage.

11 Describe the natural effects of advanced aging on periarticular connective tissues. In extreme cases, how could these changes manifest themselves clinically?

12 List three histologic features that are common to articular cartilage, tendon, and bone.

13 Briefly contrast osteoarthritis and rheumatoid arthritis.

14 List three structures *always* found in synovial joints. Cite common pathologies that may affect these structures, and comment on the nature of the resulting impairment.

15 What is the function of synovial fluid?

⊖ *Answers to the study questions can be found on the Evolve website.*

Muscle: the Primary Stabilizer and Mover of the Skeletal System

SANDRA K. HUNTER, PhD

DAVID A. BROWN, PT, PhD

CHAPTER AT A GLANCE

Stable posture results from a balance of competing forces. Movement, in contrast, occurs when competing forces are unbalanced. Force generated by muscles is the primary means for controlling the intricate balance between posture and movement. This chapter examines the role of muscle and tendon in generating, modulating, and transmitting force; these functions are necessary to stabilize and/or move skeletal structures. Specifically, this chapter investigates the following:

- How muscle stabilizes bones by generating an appropriate amount of force at a given length. Muscles generate force passively (i.e., by a muscle's resistance to stretch)

and, to a much greater extent, actively (i.e., by active contraction).
- The ways in which muscle modulates or controls force so that bones move smoothly and forcefully. Normal movement is highly regulated and refined, regardless of the infinite environmental constraints imposed on a given task.
- The use of electromyography (EMG) in the study of kinesiology.
- Basic mechanisms of muscle fatigue.
- Adaptations of muscle in strength training, immobilization, and advanced age.

The approach herein enables the student of kinesiology to understand the multiple roles of muscles in controlling the postures and movements that are used in daily tasks. In addition, the clinician also has the information needed to form clinical hypotheses about muscular impairments and adaptations that interfere or aid with functional activities. This understanding can lead to the judicious application of interventions to improve a person's functional abilities.

MUSCLE AS A SKELETAL STABILIZER: GENERATING AN APPROPRIATE AMOUNT OF FORCE AT A GIVEN LENGTH

Bones support the human body as it interacts with the environment. Although many tissues that attach to the skeleton support the body, only muscle can adapt to both immediate (acute) and repeated long-term (chronic) external forces that can destabilize the body. Muscle tissue is ideally suited for this function because it is coupled to both the external environment and the internal control mechanisms provided by the nervous system. Under the fine control of the nervous system, muscle generates the force required to stabilize skeletal structures under an amazingly wide array of conditions. For example, muscle exerts fine control to stabilize fingers wielding a tiny scalpel during eye surgery. Muscles also generate large forces during the final seconds of a "dead-lift" weightlifting task.

Understanding the special role of muscle in generating stabilizing forces begins with an introduction of the muscle fiber: the basic structural unit of muscle. This topic is followed by discussion of how muscle morphology and muscle-tendon architecture affect the range of force transferred to bone. The function of muscle is explored with regard to how it produces *passive tension* from being elongated (or stretched) or *active force* as it is stimulated, or "activated," by the nervous system. The relation between muscle force and length and how this influences the isometric torque generated about a joint are then examined. Box 3-1 is a summary of the major concepts addressed in this section.

BOX 3-1. Major Concepts: Muscle as a Skeletal Stabilizer

- Introduction to the structural organization of skeletal muscle
- Extracellular connective tissues within muscle
- Muscle morphology
- Muscle architecture: physiologic cross-sectional area and pennation angle
- Passive length-tension curve
- Parallel and series elastic components of muscle and tendon
- Elastic and viscoelastic properties of muscle
- Active length-tension curve
- Histologic structure of the muscle fiber
- Sliding filament theory
- Total length-tension curve: summation of the active and passive forces
- Isometric force and the internal torque–joint angle curve
- Mechanical and physiologic properties affecting the internal torque–joint angle curve

---

Introduction to the Structural Organization of Skeletal Muscle

Whole muscles throughout the body, such as the biceps or quadriceps, consist of many individual *muscle fibers,* ranging in thickness from about 10 to 100 μm and in length from about 1 to 50 cm.[109] The structural relationship between a muscle fiber and the muscle belly is shown in Figure 3-1. Each muscle fiber is actually an individual cell with multiple nuclei. Contraction or shortening of the individual muscle fiber is ultimately responsible for contraction of a whole muscle.

The fundamental unit within each muscle fiber is known as the *sarcomere.* Aligned in series throughout each fiber, the shortening of each sarcomere generates shortening of the fiber. For this reason the sarcomere is considered the ultimate force generator within muscle. The structure and function of the sarcomere is described in more detail later in the chapter. For now, it is important to understand that muscle contains proteins that may be considered as either contractile or noncontractile. *Contractile proteins* within the sarcomere, such as actin and myosin, interact to shorten the muscle fiber and generate an active force. (For this reason, the contractile proteins are also referred to as "active" proteins.) *Noncontractile proteins,* on the other hand, constitute much of the cytoskeleton within and between muscle fibers. These proteins are often referred to as "structural proteins" because of their role in supporting the structure of the muscle fibers. Although structural proteins do not directly cause contraction of the muscle fiber, they nevertheless play an important secondary role in the generation and transmission of force. For example, structural proteins such as *titin* provide some passive tension within the muscle fiber, whereas *desmin* stabilizes the alignment of adjacent sarcomeres. In general, structural proteins (1) generate passive tension when stretched, (2) provide internal and external support and alignment of the muscle fiber, and (3) help transfer active forces throughout the parent muscle. These concepts are further explained in upcoming sections of the chapter.

In addition to active and structural proteins introduced in the previous paragraph, a whole muscle consists of an extensive set of *extracellular connective tissues,* composed mostly of collagen and some elastin. Along with the structural proteins, these extracellular connective tissues are classified as noncontractile tissues, providing structural support and elasticity to the muscle.

Extracellular connective tissues within muscle are divided into three sets: epimysium, perimysium, and endomysium. Figure 3-1 shows these tissues as they surround the various components of muscle—from the muscle belly to the very small active proteins. The *epimysium* is a tough structure that surrounds the entire surface of the muscle belly and separates it from other muscles. In essence, the epimysium gives form to the muscle belly. The epimysium contains tightly woven bundles of collagen fibers that are resistive to stretch. The *perimysium* lies beneath the epimysium and divides muscle into fascicles (i.e., groups of fibers) that provide a conduit for blood vessels and nerves. This connective tissue, like epimysium, is tough and relatively thick and resistive to stretch. The *endomysium* surrounds individual muscle fibers, immediately external to the sarcolemma (cell membrane). The endomysium marks the location of the metabolic exchange between muscle fibers and capillaries.[95] This delicate tissue is com-

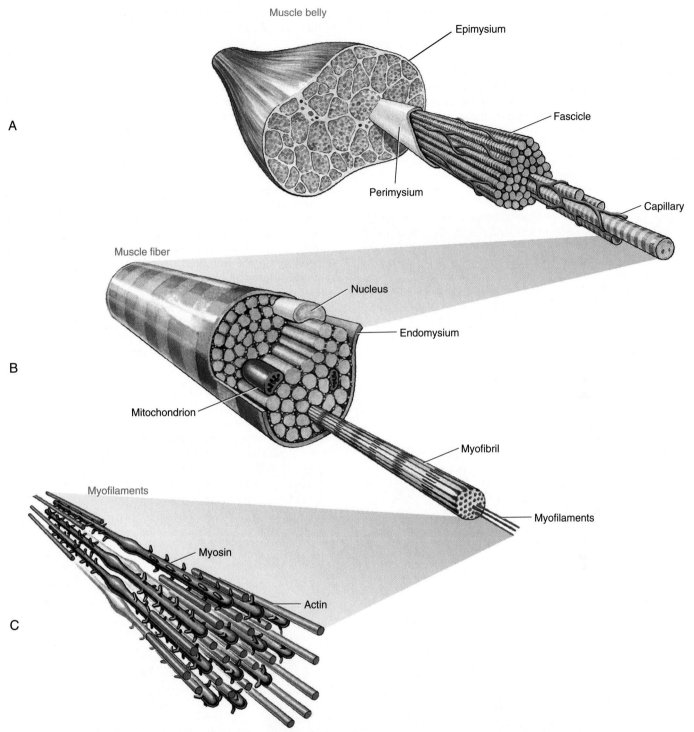

FIGURE 3-1. Basic components of muscle are shown, from the belly to the individual contractile, or active, proteins (myofilaments). Three sets of connective tissues are also depicted. **A,** The muscle belly is enclosed by the *epimysium;* individual fascicles (groups of fibers) are surrounded by the *perimysium.* **B,** Each muscle fiber is surrounded by the *endomysium.* Each *myofibril* within the muscle fibers contains many myofilaments. **C,** These filaments consist of the contractile proteins of actin and myosin. (Modified from Standring S: *Gray's anatomy: the anatomical basis of clinical practice,* ed 39, New York, 2005, Churchill Livingstone.)

posed of a relatively dense meshwork of collagen fibers that are partly connected to the perimysium. Through lateral connections from the muscle fiber, the endomysium conveys part of the muscle's contractile force to the tendon.

Muscle fibers within a muscle may be of varying length, with some extending from tendon to tendon and others only a fraction of this distance. Extracellular connective tissues help interconnect individual muscle fibers and therefore help transmit contractile forces throughout the entire length of the muscle.[65] Although the three sets of connective tissues are described as separate entities, they are interwoven as a continuous sheet of tissue. This arrangement confers strength, support, and elasticity to the whole muscle. Box 3-2 provides a summary of the functions of extracellular connective tissues within muscle.

Muscle Morphology

Muscle morphology describes the basic shape of a whole muscle. Muscles have many shapes, which influence their ultimate function (Figure 3-2). Two of the most common shapes are fusiform and pennate (from the Latin *penna,* meaning feather). *Fusiform muscles,* such as the biceps brachii, have fibers running parallel to one another and to the central tendon. *Pennate* muscles, in contrast, possess fibers that approach their central tendon obliquely. For reasons described in the next section, pennate muscles contain a larger number of fibers and therefore generate relatively large forces. Most muscles in the body are considered pennate and may be further classified as unipennate, bipennate, or multipennate, depending on the number of similarly angled sets of fibers that attach into the central tendon.

Muscle Architecture

This section describes two important architectural features of a muscle: *physiologic cross-sectional area* and *pennation angle.*

BOX 3-2. Summary of the Functions of Extracellular Connective Tissues within Muscle

- Provides gross structure to muscle
- Serves as a conduit for blood vessels and nerves
- Generates passive tension, most notably when the muscle is stretched to its near-maximal length
- Assists muscle to regain shape after it is stretched
- Conveys contractile force to the tendon and ultimately across the joint

---

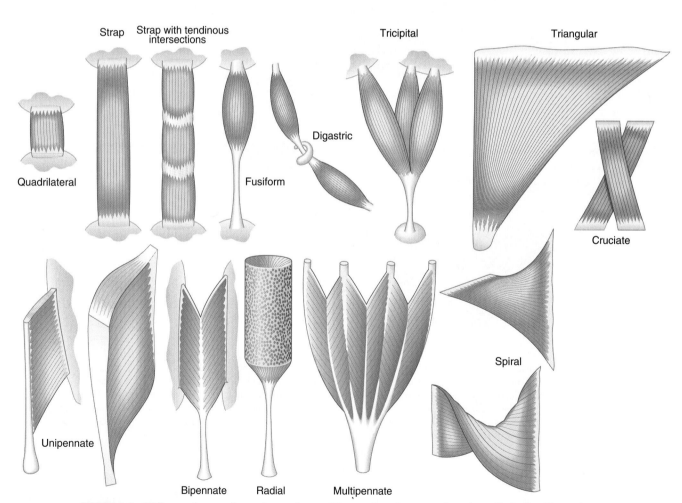

FIGURE 3-2. Different shapes of muscle are shown. The varying shapes are based on dissimilar fiber orientations relative to the tendon and the direction of pull. (Modified from Standring S: *Gray's anatomy: the anatomical basis of clinical practice,* ed 39, New York, 2005, Churchill Livingstone.)

These features significantly affect the amount of force that is transmitted through the muscle and its tendon, and ultimately to the skeleton.

The *physiologic cross-sectional area* of a whole muscle reflects the amount of active proteins available to generate a contraction force. The physiologic cross-sectional area of a fusiform muscle is determined by cutting through its muscle belly or by dividing the muscle's volume by its length. This value, expressed in square centimeters, represents the sum of the cross-sectional areas of all muscle fibers within the muscle. Assuming full activation, the *maximal force potential of a muscle is proportional to the sum of the cross-sectional area of all its fibers.* In normal conditions, therefore, a thicker muscle generates greater force than a thinner muscle of similar morphology. Measuring the physiologic cross-sectional area of a fusiform muscle is relatively simple because all fibers run essentially parallel. Caution needs to be used, however, when measuring the physiologic cross-section of pennate muscles, because fibers run at different angles to one another. For physiologic cross-sectional area to be measured accurately, the cross-section must be made perpendicular to each of the muscle fibers.

Pennation angle refers to the angle of orientation between the muscle fibers and tendon (Figure 3-3). If muscle fibers attach parallel to the tendon, the pennation angle is defined as 0 degrees. In this case essentially all of the force generated by the muscle fibers is transmitted to the tendon and across a joint. If, however, the pennation angle is greater than 0 degrees (i.e., oblique to the tendon), then less of the force produced by the muscle fiber is transmitted longitudinally through the tendon. Theoretically, a muscle with a pennation angle of 0 degrees transmits 100% of its contractile force through the tendon, whereas the same muscle with a pennation angle of 30 degrees transmits 86% of its force through the tendon. (The cosine of 30 degrees is 0.86.) Most human muscles have pennation angles that range from 0 to 30 degrees.[65]

In general, pennate muscles produce greater maximal force than fusiform muscles of similar volume. By orienting fibers obliquely to the central tendon, a pennate muscle can fit more fibers into a given length of muscle. This space-saving strategy provides pennate muscles with a relatively large physiologic cross-sectional area and hence a relatively large capability for generating high force. Consider, for example, the multipennate gastrocnemius muscle, which must generate very large forces during jumping. The reduced transfer of force from the pennate fiber to the tendon, because of the

---

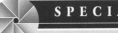

SPECIAL FOCUS 3-1

Method for Estimating the Maximal Force Potential of Muscle

*S*pecific force of skeletal muscle is defined as the maximum amount of active *force* produced *per unit physiologic cross-sectional area.* This value is typically expressed in units such as newtons per square meter (N/m^2) or pounds per square inch (lb/in^2). The specific force of human muscle is difficult to estimate, but studies indicate values between 15 and 60 N/cm^2 or, on average, 30 N/cm^2 (about 45 lb/in^2).[26] This large variability likely reflects the technical difficulty in measuring a person's true physiologic cross-sectional area, in addition to differences in fiber type composition across persons and muscles.[39] Generally, a muscle with a higher proportion of *fast twitch* fibers can have a slightly higher specific force than a muscle with a higher proportion of *slow twitch* fibers.

The fact that the maximal force generated by a healthy muscle is highly correlated with its cross-sectional area is a simple but very informative concept. Consider, for example, a quadriceps muscle in a healthy, average-sized man, with a physiologic cross-sectional area of 180 cm^2. Assuming a specific force of 30 N/cm^2, the muscle would be expected to exert a maximal force of about 5400 N (180 cm^2 × 30 N/cm^2), or about 1214 lb. Consider, in contrast, the much smaller adductor pollicis muscle in the hand—a muscle that has a similar specific force rating as the quadriceps. Because an average-sized adductor pollicis has a physiologic cross-sectional area of only about 2.5 cm^2, this muscle is capable of producing only about 75 N (17 lb) of contractile force.

The striking difference in maximal force potential in the two aforementioned muscles is not surprising considering their very different functional roles. Normally the demands on the quadriceps are large—this muscle is used routinely to lift much of the weight of the body against gravity. The architecture of the quadriceps significantly affects the amount of force that is transmitted through its tendon and ultimately to the skeleton across the knee. Assuming the quadriceps has an average angle of pennation of about 30 degrees, the maximal force expected to be transmitted through the tendon and across the knee would be about 4676 N (cosine 30 degrees × 5400 N), or 1051 lb. Although the magnitude of this force may seem implausible, it is actually within reason. Expressing this force in terms of *torque* may be more meaningful for the clinician who regularly works with strength-testing devices that measure knee extension strength. Assuming the quadriceps has a knee extensor moment arm of 4 cm,[61] the best estimate of the maximal knee extensor torque would be about 187 Nm (0.04 m × 4676 N)—a value that certainly falls within the range reported in the literature for an adult healthy male.[36,109]

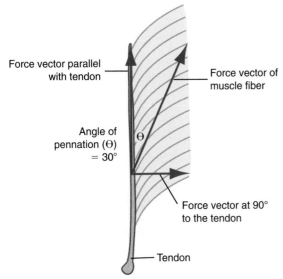

FIGURE 3-3. Unipennate muscle is shown with its muscle fibers oriented at a 30-degree pennation angle (θ).

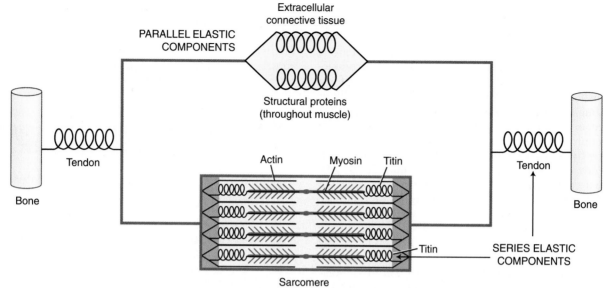

FIGURE 3-4. A highly diagrammatic model of a whole muscle attaching between two bones, depicting non-contractile elements (such as extracellular connective tissues and the protein titin) and contractile elements (such as actin and myosin). The model differentiates the noncontractile elements (as coiled springs) as either series or parallel elastic components. *Series elastic components* (aligned in series with the contractile components) are illustrated by the tendon and the structural protein titin, shown within the sarcomere. The *parallel elastic components* (aligned in parallel with the contractile components) are represented by extracellular connective tissues (such as perimysium) and other structural proteins located throughout the muscle.

greater pennation angle, is small compared with the large force potential gained in physiologic cross-sectional area. As shown in Figure 3-3, a pennation angle of 30 degrees still enables the fibers to transfer 86% of their force through to the long axis of the tendon.

Muscle and Tendon: Generation of Force

PASSIVE LENGTH-TENSION CURVE

On stimulation from the nervous system, the contractile (active) proteins within the sarcomeres cause a contraction or shortening of the entire muscle. These proteins—most notably actin and myosin—are physically supported by structural proteins, plus a network of other noncontractile extracellular connective tissues, namely, the epimysium, perimysium, endomysium. For functional rather than anatomic purposes, these noncontractile tissues have been described as parallel and series elastic components of muscle (Figure 3-4). *Series elastic components* are tissues that lie in series with the active proteins. Examples of these tissues are the tendon and large structural proteins, such as titin. The *parallel elastic components,* in contrast, are tissues that surround or lie in parallel with the active proteins. These noncontractile tissues include the extracellular connective tissues (such as the perimysium) and a family of other structural proteins that surround and support the muscle fiber.

Stretching a whole muscle by extending a joint elongates both the parallel and series elastic components, generating a springlike resistance, or stiffness, within the muscle. The resistance is referred to as *passive tension* because it is does not depend on active or volitional contraction. The concept of

parallel and serial elastic components is a simplified description of the anatomy; however, it is useful to explain the levels of resistance generated by a stretched muscle.

When the parallel and series elastic components are stretched within a muscle, a generalized *passive length-tension curve* is generated (Figure 3-5). The curve is similar to that

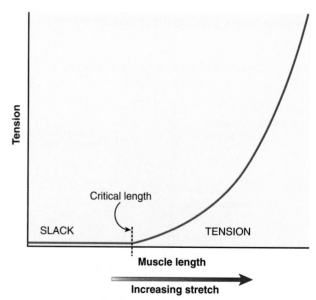

FIGURE 3-5. A generalized passive length-tension curve is shown. As a muscle is progressively stretched, the tissue is slack during the muscle's initial shortened length until it reaches a critical length at which it begins to generate passive tension. Beyond this critical length, the tension builds as an exponential function.

obtained by stretching a rubber band. Approximating the shape of an exponential mathematic function, the passive elements within the muscle begin generating passive tension after a *critical length* at which all of the relaxed (i.e., slack) tissue has been brought to an initial level of tension. After this critical length has been reached, tension progressively increases until the muscle reaches levels of very high stiffness. At even higher tension, the tissue eventually ruptures, or fails.

The passive tension in a stretched healthy muscle is attributed to the elastic forces produced by noncontractile elements, such as extracellular connective tissues, the tendon, and structural proteins. These tissues demonstrate different stiffness characteristics. When a muscle is only slightly or moderately stretched, structural proteins (in particular titin[62]) contribute most of the passive tension within the muscle. When a muscle is more extensively stretched, however, the extracellular connective tissues—especially those that compose the tendon—contribute much of the passive tension.[68]

The simple passive length-tension curve represents an important part of the overall force-generating capability of the musculotendinous unit. This capability is especially important at very long lengths where muscle fibers begin to lose their active force-generating capability because there is less overlap among the active proteins that generate force. The steepness of the passive length-tension curve varies among muscles depending on muscle architecture and fiber length.

Passive tension within stretched muscles serves many useful purposes, such as moving or stabilizing a joint against the forces of gravity, physical contact, or other activated muscles. Consider, for example, the passive elongation of the calf muscles and Achilles tendon at the end of the stance phase of fast-paced walking, just before push off. This passive tension assists with the transmission of muscular force through the foot and to the ground, thereby helping to initiate propulsion. Although passive tension within stretched muscles is typically useful, its functional effectiveness at times is limited because of (1) the slow adaptability of the tissue to rapidly changing external forces, and (2) the significant amount of initial lengthening that must occur before the tissue can generate sufficient passive tension.

Stretched muscle tissue exhibits the property of elasticity because it can temporarily store part of the energy that created the stretch. This stored energy, when released, can augment the overall force potential of a muscle. A stretched muscle also exhibits viscoelastic properties (see Chapter 1) because its passive resistance (stiffness) increases with increased velocity of stretch. Properties of both elasticity and viscoelasticity are important components of plyometric exercise.

Although the stored energy in a moderately stretched muscle may be relatively slight when compared with the full force potential of the muscle, it may help prevent a muscle from being damaged during maximal elongation.[69] Elasticity therefore can serve as a damping mechanism that protects the structural components of the muscle and tendon.

ACTIVE LENGTH-TENSION CURVE

Muscle tissue is uniquely designed to generate force actively (i.e., volitionally) in response to a stimulus from the nervous system. This section of the chapter describes the means by which a muscle generates active force. Active force is produced by an *activated* muscle fiber, that is, one that is being stimulated by the nervous system to contract. As diagramed in Figure 3-4, both active force and passive tension are ultimately transmitted to the bones that constitute the joint.

Muscle fibers are composed of many tiny strands called *myofibrils* (see Figure 3-1). *Myofibrils* contain the contractile (active) proteins of the muscle fiber and have a distinctive structure. Each myofibril is 1 to 2 μm in diameter and consists of many *myofilaments*. The two most important myofilaments within the myofibril are the proteins *actin* and *myosin*. As will be described, muscle contraction involves a complex physiologic and mechanical interaction between these two proteins. The regular organization of these filaments produces the characteristic banded appearance of the myofibril as seen under the microscope (Figure 3-6). The repeating functional subunits of the myofibril are the sarcomeres (Figure 3-7). The dark band within a single sarcomere, also called the *A band*, correspond to the presence of *myosin*—thick filaments. Myosin also contains projections, called *myosin heads*, which are arranged in pairs (Figure 3-8). The light bands, also called *I bands*, contain *actin*—thin filaments (see Figure 3-7). In a resting muscle fiber, actin filaments partially overlap the myosin filaments. Under an electron microscope, the bands reveal a more complex pattern that consists of an H band, M

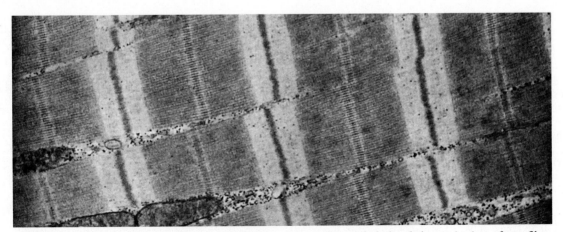

FIGURE 3-6. Electron micrograph of myofibrils demonstrates the regularly banded organization of myofilaments—actin and myosin. (From Fawcett DW: *The cell,* Philadelphia, 1981, Saunders.)

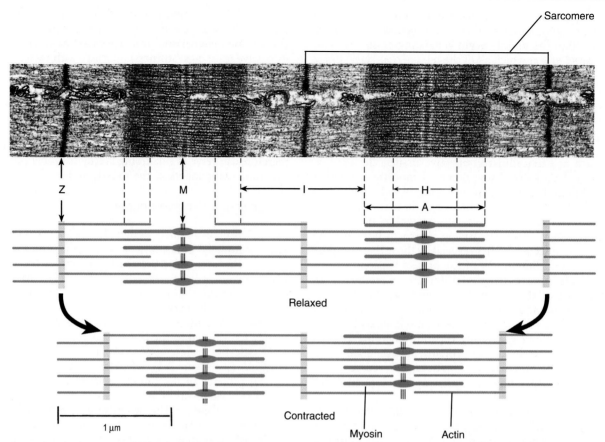

FIGURE 3-7. On top are electron micrographs of two full sarcomeres within a myofibril. The drawings below show relaxed and contracted (stimulated) myofibrils, indicating the position of the thick (myosin) and thin (actin) filaments. Detail of the regular, banded organization of the myofibril shows the position of the A band, I band, H band, M line, and Z discs. Relaxed and contracted states are shown to illustrate the changes that occur during shortening. (Modified from Standring S: *Gray's anatomy: the anatomical basis of clinical practice,* ed 39, New York, 2005, Churchill Livingstone. Photographs by Brenda Russell, Department of Physiology and Biophysics, University of Illinois at Chicago. Original art by Lesley Skeates.)

FIGURE 3-8. Further detail of a sarcomere showing the cross-bridge structure formed by the myosin heads and their attachment to the actin filaments. Note that the actin filament also contains the proteins troponin and tropomyosin. Troponin is responsible for exposing the actin filament to the myosin head, thereby allowing cross-bridge formation. (From Levy MN, Koeppen BM, Stanton BA: *Berne and Levy principles of physiology,* ed 4, St Louis, 2006, Mosby.)

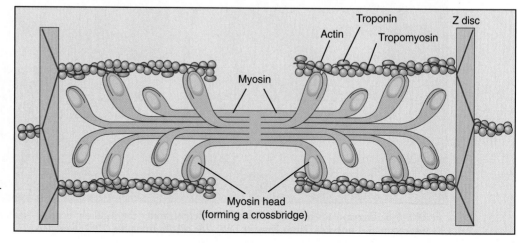

TABLE 3-1. **Defined Regions within a Sarcomere**	
Region	**Description**
A band	Dark bands caused by the presence of thick myosin myofilaments.
I bands	Light bands caused by the presence of thin actin myofilaments.
H band	Region within A band where actin and myosin do not overlap.
M line	Midregion thickening of thick myosin myofilaments in the center of H band.
Z discs	Connecting points between successive sarcomeres. Z discs help anchor the thin actin myofilaments.

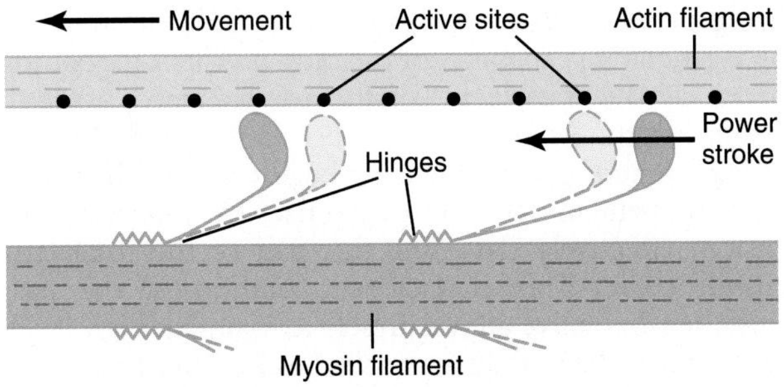

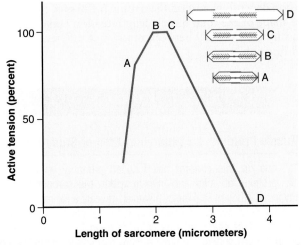

FIGURE 3-9. The sliding filament action showing myosin heads attaching and then releasing from the actin filament. This process is known as *crossbridge cycling*. Contractile force is generated during the power stroke of each crossbridge cycle. (From Guyton AC, Hall JE: *Textbook of medical physiology*, ed 10, Philadelphia, 2000, Saunders.)

line, and Z discs (defined in Table 3-1). Actin and myosin are aligned within the sarcomere with the help of structural proteins, providing mechanical stability to the fiber during contraction and stretch.[62,105] By way of the structural proteins and the endomysium, myofibrils ultimately connect with the tendon. This elegant connective web, formed between the proteins and connective tissues, allows force to be distributed longitudinally and laterally within a muscle.[74,75]

As described earlier, the sarcomere is the fundamental active force generator within the muscle fiber. Understanding the contractile events that take place in an individual sarcomere provides the basis for understanding the contraction process across the entire muscle. The contraction process is simply repeated from one sarcomere to the next. The model for describing active force generation within the sarcomere is called the *sliding filament hypothesis* and was developed independently by Hugh Huxley[54] and Andrew Huxley (no relation).[53] In this model, active force is generated as actin filaments slide past myosin filaments, causing approximation of the Z discs and narrowing of the H band. This action results in a progressive overlap of the actin and myosin filaments, which, in effect, produces a shortening of each sarcomere, although the active proteins themselves do not actually shorten (Figure 3-9). Each myosin head attaches to an adjacent actin filament, forming a *crossbridge*. The amount of force generated within each sarcomere therefore depends on the number of simultaneously formed crossbridges. The greater the number of crossbridges, the greater the force generated within the sarcomere.

As a consequence of the arrangement between the actin and myosin within a sarcomere, the amount of active force depends, in part, on the instantaneous *length* of the muscle fiber. A change in fiber length—from either active contraction or passive elongation—alters the amount of overlap between actin and myosin. The active length-tension curve for a sarcomere is presented in Figure 3-10. The ideal *resting length* of a muscle fiber (or individual sarcomere) is the length that allows the greatest number of crossbridges and therefore the greatest potential force. As the sarcomere is lengthened or shortened from its resting length, the number of potential crossbridges decreases so that lesser amounts of active force are generated, even under conditions of full activation or effort. The resulting active length-tension curve is described

FIGURE 3-10. Active length-tension curve of a sarcomere for four specified sarcomere lengths (upper right, *A* through *D*). Actin filaments *(A)* overlap so that the number of crossbridges is reduced. In *B* and *C*, actin and myosin filaments are positioned to allow an optimal number of crossbridges. In *D*, actin filaments are positioned out of the range of the myosin heads so that no crossbridges are formed. (From Guyton AC, Hall JE: *Textbook of medical physiology*, ed 10, Philadelphia, 2000, Saunders.)

by an inverted U-shape with its peak at the ideal resting length.

The term *length-force* relationship is more appropriate for considering the terminology established in this text (see definitions of force and tension in the glossary of Chapter 1). The phrase *length-tension* is used, however, because of its wide acceptance in the physiology literature.

SUMMATION OF ACTIVE FORCE AND PASSIVE TENSION: THE TOTAL LENGTH-TENSION CURVE

The active length-tension curve, when combined with the passive length-tension curve, yields the *total* length-tension curve of muscle. The combination of active force and passive tension allows for a large range of muscle forces over a wide range of muscle length. Consider the total length-tension curve for the muscle shown in Figure 3-11. At shortened lengths *(a)*, below active resting length and below the length that generates passive tension, active force dominates the force-generating capability of the muscle. The force continues to rise as the muscle is lengthened (stretched) toward its resting length. As the muscle fiber is stretched beyond its resting length *(b)*, passive tension begins to contribute so that the decrement in active force is offset by increased passive tension, effectively flattening this part of the total length-tension curve. This characteristic portion of the passive length-tension curve allows muscle to maintain high levels of force even as the muscle is stretched to a point at which active force generation is compromised. As the muscle fiber is further stretched *(c)*, passive tension dominates the curve so that connective tissues are under near-maximal stress. High levels of passive tension are most apparent in muscles that are stretched across multiple joints. For example, as the wrist is actively and fully extended, the fingers passively flex slightly because of the stretch placed on the finger flexor muscles as they cross the front of the wrist. The amount of passive tension depends in part on the natural stiffness of the muscle. The shape of the total muscle length-tension curve therefore can vary considerably between muscles of different structure and function.[8]

Isometric Muscle Force: Development of the Internal Torque–Joint Angle Curve

As defined in Chapter 1, isometric activation of a muscle produces force without a significant change in its length. This occurs naturally when the joint over which an activated muscle crosses is constrained from movement. Constraint often occurs from a force produced by an antagonistic muscle or an external source. Isometrically produced forces provide the necessary stability to the joints and body as a whole. The amplitude of an isometrically produced force from a given muscle reflects a summation of length-dependent active force and passive tension.

Maximal isometric force of a muscle is often used as a general indicator of a muscle's peak strength and can indicate neuromuscular recovery after injury.[57,84,110] In clinical settings it is not possible to directly measure length or force of maximally activated muscle. However, a muscle's internal *torque* generation can be measured isometrically at several joint angles. Figure 3-12 shows the internal torque versus the joint angle curve (so-called "torque-angle curve") of two muscle groups under isometric, maximal-effort conditions. (The

SPECIAL FOCUS 3-2

Muscle Proteins: an Expanding Area of Study for Muscle Physiologists

Thus far this chapter has focused primarily on the active proteins of actin and myosin within the sarcomere. More advanced study of this topic, however, reveals a far more complicated picture. Myosin, for example, is further classified into *heavy chain* or *light chain* proteins, with differing functions. The light chain myosin appears to have a more regulatory role in the contraction process, as do the proteins *tropomyosin* and *troponin*.

Furthermore, other proteins serve an important structural or supportive role within or between the sarcomeres. The importance of these noncontractile proteins has been realized in recent decades. The information contained in Table 3-2 is intended primarily as background material and summarizes the most likely function of the more commonly studied muscle proteins. The interested reader may consult other sources for more detail on this topic.[18]

TABLE 3-2. Summary of Functions of Selected Muscle Proteins

Proteins	Function
Active: Contractile	
Myosin heavy chain (several isoforms)	Molecular motor for muscle contraction–binds with actin to generate contraction force.
Actin	Binds with myosin to translate force and shorten the sarcomere
Active: Regulatory	
Tropomyosin	Regulates the interaction between actin and myosin; stabilizes actin filament
Troponin (several isoforms)	Influences the position of tropomyosin; binds with calcium ions
Myosin light chain (several isoforms for slow and fast light chains)	Influences the contraction velocity of the sarcomere; modulates the kinetics of crossbridge cycling
Structural	
Nebulin	Anchors actin to Z discs
Titin	Creates passive tension within the stretched sarcomere; acts as molecular "springs"
Desmin	Helps to stabilize the longitudinal and lateral alignment of adjacent sarcomeres
Vimentin	Helps maintain periodicity of Z discs
Skelemin	Helps stabilize the position of M lines
Dystrophin	Provides structural stability to the cytoskeleton and sarcolemma of the muscle fiber
Integrins	Stabilizes the cytoskeleton of the muscle fiber

Adapted from Caiozzo VJ, Rourke B: The muscular system: structural and functional plasticity. In Tipton CM, ed: *ACSM's advanced exercise physiology*, Philadelphia, 2006, Lippincott Williams & Wilkins.

torque-angle curve is the rotational equivalent of the total length-tension curve of a muscle group.) The internal torque produced isometrically by a muscle group can be determined by asking an individual to produce a maximal-effort contraction against a known external torque. As described in Chapter 4, an external torque can be determined by using an external force-sensing device (dynamometer) at a known distance from the joint's axis of rotation. Because the measurement is performed during an isometric activation, the internal torque is assumed equal to the external torque. When a maximal-strength test is performed in conjunction with considerable encouragement provided by the tester, most healthy adults can achieve near-maximal activation of their muscle.

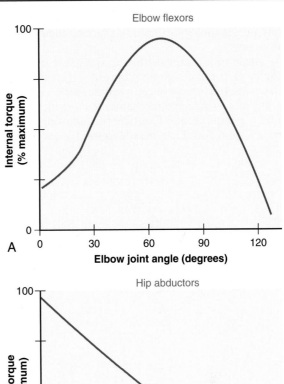

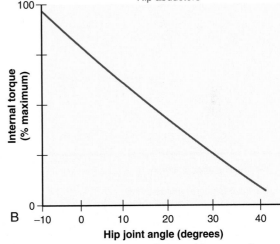

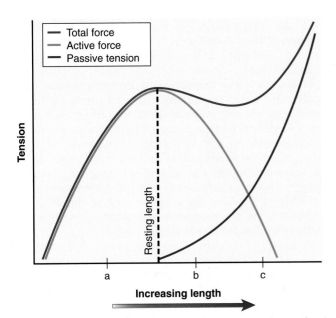

FIGURE 3-11. Total length-tension curve for a typical muscle. At shortened lengths *(a)*, all force is generated actively. As the muscle fiber is stretched beyond its resting length *(b)*, passive tension begins to contribute to the total force. In *(c)* the muscle is further stretched, and passive tension accounts for most of the total force.

FIGURE 3-12. Internal torque versus joint angle curve of two muscle groups under isometric, maximal-effort conditions. The shapes of the curves are very different for each muscle group. **A,** Internal torque of the elbow flexors is greatest at an angle of about 75 degrees of flexion. **B,** Internal torque of the hip abductors is greatest at a frontal plane angle of −10 degrees (i.e., 10 degrees of adduction).

SPECIAL FOCUS 3-3

Method of Measuring a Person's Maximal Voluntary Muscle Activation

In normal clinical strength-testing situations, it is difficult to know for certain if a person is actually maximally activating a given muscle, even when maximal effort and good health are assumed. A measure of *maximal voluntary activation* can be assessed by applying a brief electrical stimulus to the motor nerve or directly over the skin of a muscle while the person is attempting a maximal voluntary contraction. Any increase in measured force that immediately follows the electrical stimulus indicates that not all the muscle fibers were volitionally activated. This technique is known as the *interpolated stimulus technique*.[35] The magnitude of voluntary activation is typically expressed as a percent of a muscle's maximal activation potential (i.e., neural drive).

Most young healthy adults are able to achieve 95% to 100% of maximal isometric activation of the elbow flexor and dorsiflexors, although these values vary considerably among individuals and trials.[5,35] The average level of maximal voluntary isometric activation can also vary among muscles.[35] Significantly lower levels of maximal voluntary activation have also been reported in muscles after trauma or disease, such as in the quadriceps muscle after anterior cruciate ligament injury[107] or in the diaphragm muscle in persons with asthma.[6] Persons with multiple sclerosis have been shown to generate only 86% of maximum voluntary activation of their dorsiflexor muscles, compared with 96% activation in a healthy control group.[80]

Near-maximal activation is not always possible, however, in persons with pathology or trauma affecting their neuromuscular system.

The shape of a maximal-effort torque-angle curve is very specific to each muscle group (compare Figure 3-12, *A* and *B*). The shape of each curve can yield important information about the physiologic and mechanical factors that determine the muscle groups' torque. Consider the following two factors shown in Figure 3-13. First, muscle *length* changes as the joint

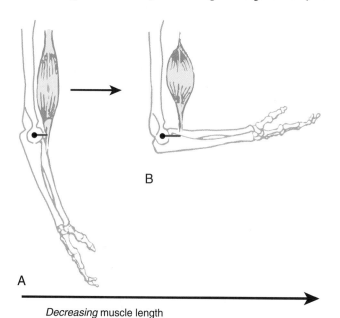

B

A

Decreasing muscle length

Increasing muscle moment arm

FIGURE 3-13. Muscle length and moment arm have an impact on the maximal-effort torque for a given muscle. **A,** Muscle is at its near-greatest length, and muscle moment arm *(brown line)* is at its near-shortest length. **B,** Muscle length is shortened, and muscle moment arm length is greatest. (Modified from LeVeau BF: *Williams and Lissner's biomechanics of human motion,* ed 3, Philadelphia, 1992, Saunders.)

angle changes. As previously described, a muscle's force output—in both active and passive terms—is highly dependent on muscle length. Second, the changing joint angle alters the length of the muscle's moment arm, or *leverage*.[104] For a given muscle force, a progressively larger moment arm creates a greater torque. Because both muscle length and leverage are altered simultaneously by rotation of the joint, it is not always possible to know which is more influential in determining the final shape of the torque-angle curve. A change in either variable—physiologic or mechanical—alters the clinical expression of a muscular-produced internal torque. Several clinically related examples are listed in Table 3-3.

The torque-angle curve of the hip abductors demonstrated in Figure 3-12, *B* depends primarily on muscle length, as shown by the linear reduction of maximal torque produced at progressively greater abduction angles of the hip. Regardless of the muscle group, however, the combination of high total muscle force (based on muscle length) and great leverage (based on moment arm length) results in the greatest relative internal torque.

In summary, the magnitude of isometric torque differs considerably based on the angle of the joint at the time of activation, even with maximal effort. Accordingly it is important that clinical measurements of isometric torque include the joint angle so that future comparisons are valid. The testing of isometric strength at different joint angles enables the characterizing of the functional range of a muscle's strength. This information may be required to determine the suitability of a person for a certain task at the workplace, especially if the task requires a critical internal torque to be produced at certain joint angles.

MUSCLE AS A SKELETAL MOVER: FORCE MODULATION

The previous sections considered how an isometrically activated muscle can stabilize the skeletal system; the next section considers how muscles actively grade forces while changing

TABLE 3-3. Clinical Examples and Consequences of Changes in Mechanical or Physiologic Variables That Influence the Production of Internal Torque

Changed Variable	Clinical Example	Effect of Internal Torque	Possible Clinical Consequence
Mechanical: Increased internal moment arm	Surgical displacement of greater trochanter to increase the internal moment arm of hip abductor muscles	Decrease in the amount of muscle force required to produce a given level of hip abduction torque	Decreased hip abductor force can reduce the force generated across an unstable or a painful hip joint; considered a means of "protecting" a joint from damaging forces
Mechanical: Decreased internal moment arm	Patellectomy after severe fracture of the patella	Increase in the amount of knee extensor muscle force required to produce a given level of knee extension torque	Increased force needed to extend the knee may increase the wear on the articular surfaces of the knee joint
Physiologic: Decreased muscle activation	Damage to the deep portion of the fibular nerve	Decreased strength in the dorsiflexor muscles	Reduced ability to walk safely
Physiologic: Significantly decreased muscle length at the time of neural activation	Damage to the radial nerve with paralysis of wrist extensor muscles	Decreased strength in wrist extensor muscles causing the finger flexor muscles to flex the wrist during grasping	Ineffective grasp because of overcontracted (shortened) finger flexor muscles

Exploring the Reasons for the Unique "Signature" of a Muscle Group's Isometric Torque-Angle Curve

Undoubtedly, the shape of a muscle group's torque-angle curve is related to the functional demands placed on the muscles and the joint. For the elbow flexors, for example, the maximal internal torque potential is *greatest* in the midranges of elbow motion and *least* near full extension and flexion (see Figure 3-12, *A*). Not coincidentally, in the upright position the external torque caused by gravity acting on the forearm and hand-held objects is also greatest in the midranges of elbow motion and least at the extremes of elbow motion.

For the hip abductor muscles, the internal torque potential is greatest near neutral (0 degrees of abduction) (see Figure 3-12, *B*). This hip joint angle coincides with the approximate angle at which the hip abductor muscles are most needed for frontal plane stability in the single-limb support phase of walking. Large amounts of hip abduction torque are rarely functionally required in a position of maximal hip abduction.

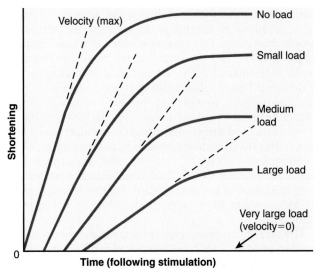

FIGURE 3-14. Relationship between muscle load (external resistance) and maximal shortening (contraction) velocity. (The velocity is equal to the slope of the dashed lines.) Without an external load, a muscle is capable of shortening at a high velocity. As the load on the muscle progressively increases, its maximal shortening velocity decreases. Eventually, at some very large load, the muscle is incapable of shortening and the velocity is zero. (Redrawn from McComas AJ: *Skeletal muscle: form and function,* Champaign, Ill, 1996, Human Kinetics.)

lengths, which is necessary to move the skeletal system in a highly controlled fashion.

Modulating Force through Concentric or Eccentric Activation: Introduction to the Force-Velocity Relationship of Muscle

As introduced in Chapter 1, the nervous system stimulates a muscle to generate or resist a force by *concentric, eccentric,* or *isometric* activation. During concentric activation, the muscle shortens (contracts). This occurs when the internal (muscle) torque exceeds the external (load) torque. During eccentric activation, the external torque exceeds the internal torque; the muscle is driven by the nervous system to contract but is elongated in response to a more dominating force, usually from an external source or from an antagonist muscle. During an isometric activation, the length of the muscle remains nearly constant, as the internal and external torques are equally matched.

During concentric and eccentric activations, a very specific relationship exists between a muscle's maximum force output and its velocity of contraction (or elongation). During concentric activation, for example, the muscle contracts at a maximum velocity when the load is negligible (Figure 3-14). As the load increases, the maximal contraction velocity of the muscle decreases. At some point, a very large load results in a contraction velocity of zero (i.e., the isometric state). Eccentric activation needs to be considered separately from concentric activation. With eccentric activation, a load that barely exceeds the isometric force level causes the muscle to lengthen slowly. Speed of lengthening increases as a greater load is applied. There is a maximal load that the muscle cannot resist, and beyond this load level the muscle uncontrollably lengthens.

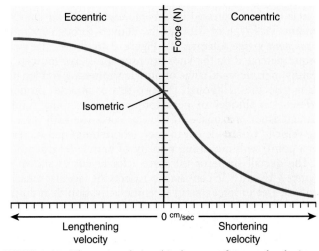

FIGURE 3-15. Theoretic relationship between force and velocity of muscle shortening or lengthening during maximal-effort muscle activation. Concentric (muscle-shortening) activation is shown on the right, and eccentric (muscle-lengthening) activation on the left. Isometric activation occurs at a velocity of zero.

FORCE-VELOCITY CURVE

The relationships between the velocity of a muscle's change in length and its maximum force output are most often expressed by the *force-velocity curve* plotted in Figure 3-15. This curve is shown during concentric, isometric, and eccentric activations, expressed with the force on the vertical axis and shortening and lengthening velocity of the muscle on the horizontal axis. This force-velocity curve demonstrates several important points about the physiology of muscle. During a maximal-effort *concentric* activation, the amount of muscle force produced is *inversely proportional* to the velocity of muscle shortening. This relation was first described by physiologist A.V. Hill in 1938 in skeletal muscle of the frog and is similar for humans.[41,42] The reduced force-generating capacity of muscle at higher velocities of contraction results primarily from the inherent limitation in the speed of attachment and reattachment of the crossbridges. At higher velocities of contraction, the number of attached crossbridges at any given time is less than when the muscle is contracting slowly. At a contraction velocity of zero (i.e., the isometric state), a maximum number of attached crossbridges exist within a given sarcomere at any given instant. For this reason, a muscle produces greater force isometrically than at any speed of shortening.

The underlying physiology behind the force-velocity relationship of *eccentrically active muscle* is very different from that of concentric muscle activation. During a maximal-effort eccentric activation, the muscle force is, to a point, *directly proportional* to the velocity of the muscle lengthening. For most individuals, however, the curve reaches a zero slope at lower lengthening velocities than that depicted in the theoretic curve of Figure 3-15. Although the reason is not completely understood, most humans (especially untrained) are unable to maximally activate their muscles eccentrically, especially at high velocities.[12,106] This may be a protective mechanism to guard against muscle damage produced by excessively large forces.

The clinical expression of a force-velocity relationship of muscle is often expressed by a *torque-joint angular velocity relationship*. This type of data can be derived through *isokinetic dynamometry* (see Chapter 4). Figure 3-16 shows the peak torque generated by the knee extensor and flexor muscles of healthy men, across a range of muscle shortening and lengthening velocities. Although the two sets of muscles produce different amplitudes of peak torque, each exhibits similar characteristics: maximal-effort torques decrease with increasing velocity of muscle contraction (shortening) and increase (to a point) with increasing velocity of muscle lengthening.

The overall shape of the force-velocity curves shown in Figures 3-15 and 3-16 consistently reflects the fact that muscles produce greater force during eccentric activation than during isometric or any velocity of concentric activation. Although the reason is not well understood, the relatively higher forces produced eccentrically result, in part, from (1) a greater average force produced per crossbridge, as each crossbridge is pulled apart and detached,[66] (2) a more rapid reattachment phase of crossbridge formation, and (3) passive tension produced by the viscoelastic properties of the stretched parallel and serial elastic components of the muscle.[25] Indirect evidence for the last factor is the well-known phenomenon of *delayed onset muscle soreness*, which is common after heavy bouts of eccentric muscle-based exercise, especially in untrained persons. One partial explanation for this characteristic soreness is based on strain-related injury to the forcefully (and rapidly) stretched muscle, which includes the myofibrils, cytoskeleton of the sarcomere, and extracellular connective tissues.[86]

The functional role of eccentrically active muscles is important to the metabolic and neurologic "efficiency" of movement. Eccentrically activated muscle stores energy when stretched; the energy is released only when the elongated

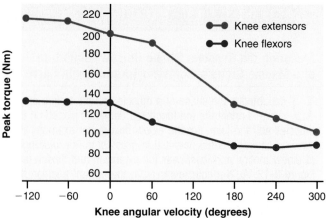

FIGURE 3-16. Peak torque generated by the knee extensor and flexor muscles. Positive velocities denote concentric activation, and negative velocities denote eccentric activation. Data are from 64 untrained, healthy men. (Data from Horstmann T, Maschmann J, Mayer F, et al: The influence of age on isokinetic torque of the upper and lower leg musculature in sedentary men, *Int J Sports Med* 20:362, 1999.)

muscle contracts. In addition, the ratio of electromyographic amplitude and oxygen consumption per force level is less for eccentrically activated muscle than for similar absolute workloads performed under concentric activation.[25] The mechanisms responsible for this efficiency are closely related to the three factors cited in the previous paragraph for why greater forces are produced through eccentric activation compared with noneccentric activation. The metabolic cost and electromyographic activity are less because, in part, a comparable task performed with eccentric activation requires slightly fewer active muscle fibers.

POWER AND WORK: ADDITIONAL CONCEPTS RELATED TO THE FORCE-VELOCITY RELATIONSHIP OF MUSCLE

The inverse relation between a muscle's maximal force potential and its shortening velocity is related to the concept of power. *Power,* or the rate of work, can be expressed as a product of force and contraction velocity. (Power of a muscle contraction is therefore related to area under the right side of the curve shown previously in Figure 3-15.) A constant power output of a muscle can be sustained by increasing the load (resistance) while proportionately decreasing the contraction velocity, or vice versa. This is very similar in concept to switching gears while riding a bicycle.

A muscle undergoing a concentric contraction against a load is doing *positive work* on the load. In contrast, a muscle undergoing eccentric activation against an overbearing load is doing *negative work*. In the latter case, the muscle is storing energy that is supplied by the load. A muscle therefore can act as either an active accelerator of movement against a load while the muscle is contracting (i.e., through concentric activation) or as a "brake" or decelerator when a load is applied and the activated muscle is lengthening (i.e., through eccentric activation). For example, the quadriceps muscles act concentrically when one ascends stairs and lifts the weight of the body, which is considered positive work. Negative work, however, is performed by these muscles as they lower the

SPECIAL FOCUS 3-5

Combining the Length-Tension and Force-Velocity Relationships

Although a muscle's length-tension and force-velocity relationships are described separately, in reality both are often in effect simultaneously. At any given time, an active muscle is functioning at a specific length and at a specific contraction velocity, including isometric. It is useful, therefore, to generate a plot that represents the three-dimensional relationship among muscle force, length, and contraction velocity (Figure 3-17). The plot does not, however, include the *passive length-tension* component of muscle. The plot shows, for example, that a muscle contracting at a high velocity at its shortened length produces relatively low force levels, even with maximal effort. In contrast, a muscle contracting at a low (near-isometric) velocity at a longer length (e.g., near its optimal muscle length) theoretically produces a substantially greater active force.

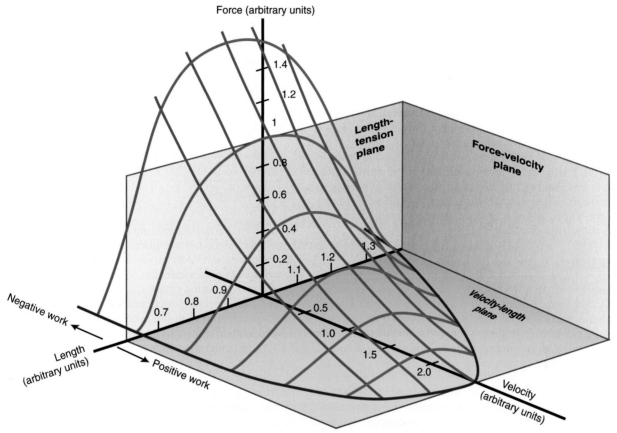

FIGURE 3-17. A theoretic plot representing the three-dimensional relationship among muscle force, muscle length, and muscle contraction velocity during a maximal effort. Positive work indicates concentric muscle activation, and negative work indicates eccentric muscle activation. (From Winter DA: *Biomechanics and motor control of human movement*, ed 2, New York, 1990, John Wiley & Sons.)

body down the stairs in a controlled fashion, under eccentric activation.

Activating Muscle via the Nervous System

Several important mechanisms underlying the generation of muscle force have been examined thus far in this chapter. Of utmost importance, however, is that muscle is excited by impulses generated from within the nervous system, specifically by *alpha motor neurons,* with their cell bodies located in the ventral (anterior) horn of the spinal cord. Each alpha motor neuron has an axon that extends from the spinal cord and connects with multiple muscle fibers located throughout a whole muscle. The single alpha motor neuron together with its entire family of innervated muscle fibers is called a *motor unit* (Figure 3-18). Excitation of alpha motor neurons arises from many sources, including cortical descending neurons, spinal interneurons, and other afferent (sensory) neurons. Each source can activate an alpha motor neuron by first *recruiting* a particular motor neuron and then driving it to higher rates of sequential activation—a process called *rate coding.* The process of rate coding provides a finely controlled mechanism of smoothly increasing muscle force. Recruitment and rate coding are the two primary strategies employed

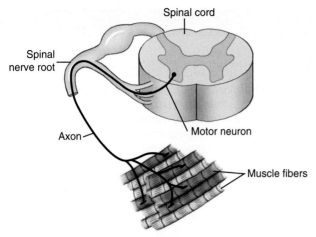

FIGURE 3-18. A motor unit consists of the (alpha) motor neuron and the muscle fibers it innervates.

by the nervous system to activate motor neurons. The spatial arrangement of motor units throughout a muscle and the strategies available to activate motor neurons allow for the production of very small forces involving only a few motor units, or very large forces involving most of the motor units within the muscle. Because motor units are distributed across an entire muscle, the forces from the activated fibers summate across the entire muscle and are then transmitted to the tendon and across the joint.

RECRUITMENT

Recruitment refers to the initial activation of specific motor neurons that cause excitation and activation of their associated muscle fibers. The nervous system recruits a motor unit by altering the voltage potential across the membrane of the cell body of the alpha motor neuron. This process involves a net summation of competing inhibitory and excitatory inputs. At a critical voltage, ions flow across the cell membrane and produce an electrical signal known as an *action potential*. The action potential is propagated down the axon of the alpha motor neuron to the motor endplate at the neuromuscular junction. Once the muscle fiber is activated, a muscle contraction (also called a *twitch*) occurs, and a small amount of force is generated. Box 3-3 lists the major sequence of events underlying muscle fiber activation. Through recruitment of more motor neurons, more muscle fibers are activated, and therefore more force is generated within the whole muscle.

The muscle fibers associated with each motor unit normally share similar contractile characteristics and are distributed randomly within a region of a muscle. Although each whole muscle may contain a few hundred motor units, each axon within a given motor unit may innervate 5 to 2000 muscle fibers. Muscles that require fine motor control and generate relatively low forces, such as those that control movement of the eye or digits of the hand, are usually associated with smaller-sized motor units. Typically these motor units have a small number of muscle fibers innervated per axon (i.e., possess a *low innervation ratio*). In contrast, muscles used to control less-refined movements involving the production of larger forces are generally associated with larger-sized

motor units. These motor units tend to innervate a relatively large number of muscle fibers per axon (i.e., possess a *high innervation ratio*).[28] Any given whole muscle, regardless of its functional role, possesses motor units with a wide variation of innervation ratios.

The size of the motor neuron influences the order in which it is recruited by the nervous system. Smaller neurons are generally recruited *before* the larger motor neurons (Figure 3-19). This principle is called the *Henneman Size Principle*, first experimentally demonstrated and developed by Elwood Henneman in the late 1950s.[40] The Size Principle accounts for much of the orderly recruitment of motor units, specified by size, which allows for smooth and controlled increments in force development.

Muscle fibers innervated by small motor neurons have *twitch responses* that are relatively long in duration ("slow twitch") and small in amplitude. Motor units associated with these fibers have been classified as *S* (for slow) because of the slower contractile characteristics of the muscle fibers. The associated fibers are referred to as *SO* fibers, indicating their slow and oxidative histochemical profile. Fibers associated with slow (S) motor units are relatively *fatigue resistant* (i.e., experience little loss of force during a sustained activation). Consequently, a muscle such as the soleus (which makes continuous and often small adjustments in the postural sway of the body over the foot) has a relatively large proportion of SO fibers.[55] This slow fiber type allows "postural muscles" such as the soleus to sustain low levels of force over a long duration.

In contrast, muscle fibers associated with larger motor neurons have twitch responses that are relatively brief in duration ("fast twitch") and higher in amplitude. Motor units associated with these fibers are classified as *FF* (fast and easily fatigable). The associated fibers are classified as *FG*, indicating

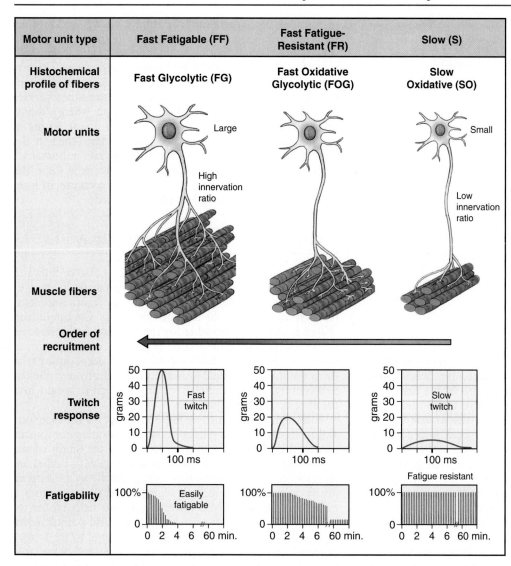

Motor unit type	Fast Fatigable (FF)	Fast Fatigue-Resistant (FR)	Slow (S)
Histochemical profile of fibers	Fast Glycolytic (FG)	Fast Oxidative Glycolytic (FOG)	Slow Oxidative (SO)
Motor units	Large / High innervation ratio		Small / Low innervation ratio
Muscle fibers			
Order of recruitment	←		
Twitch response	Fast twitch / 100 ms	100 ms	Slow twitch / 100 ms
Fatigability	Easily fatigable / 0 2 4 6 60 min.	0 2 4 6 60 min.	Fatigue resistant / 0 2 4 6 60 min.

FIGURE 3-19. Classification of motor unit types from muscle fibers based on histochemical profile, size, and twitch (contractile) characteristics. A theoretic continuum of differing contractile and morphologic characteristics is shown for each of the three motor unit types. It is important to note that the range of any single characteristic may vary considerably within any given motor unit (either within or between whole muscles).

their fast twitch, glycolytic histochemical profile. These fibers are easily fatigable. The larger FF motor units are generally recruited *after* the smaller SO motor units, when very large forces are required.

Figure 3-19 shows in a diagrammatic fashion the existence of a spectrum of intermediate motor units that have physiologic and histochemical profiles somewhere between "slow" and "fast fatigable." The more "intermediate" motor units are classified as *FR* (fast fatigue-resistant). The fibers are referred to as *FOG* fibers, indicating the utilization of oxidative and glycolytic energy sources.

The arrangement of the motor unit types depicted in Figure 3-19 allows for a broad continuum of physiologic responses from skeletal muscle. The smaller (slower) recruited motor units are typically recruited early during a movement and generate relatively low muscle forces that can be sustained over a relatively long time. The contractile characteristics associated with the muscle fibers are ideal for the control of fine or smoothly graded low-intensity contractions. Larger (faster) motor units are recruited after the smaller motor units, and add successively greater forces of shorter duration. Through this spectrum, the nervous system is able to activate muscle fibers that sustain stable postures over a long period of time and, when needed, produce large, short-duration bursts of force for more impulsive movements.

RATE CODING

After a specific motor neuron has been recruited, the force produced by the associated muscle fibers is strongly modulated by the rate of production of sequential action potentials. This process is referred to as *rate coding*. Although a single action potential in a skeletal muscle fiber lasts several milliseconds (ms), the resulting muscle fiber *twitch* (isolated contraction) may last for as long as 130 ms to 300 ms in a slow twitch fiber. When a motor unit is first recruited, it will discharge (or spike) at about 10 action potentials per second, or 10 Hz. (The average discharge rate of an action potential is indicated as a frequency [Hz], or by its reciprocal, the *interspike interval;* 10 Hz is equivalent to an interspike interval of 100 ms.) With increased excitation, the rate may increase to 50 Hz (20-ms interspike interval) during a high-force contraction, although this is usually sustained for only a brief period.[28] Because the twitch duration is often longer than the interval between discharges of action potentials, it is possible for a number of subsequent action potentials to begin during

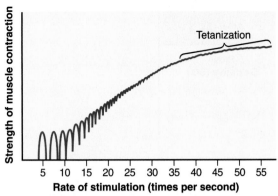

FIGURE 3-20. Summation of individual muscle twitches (contractions) is recorded over a wide range of stimulation frequencies. Note that at low frequencies of stimulation (5 to 10 per second), the initial twitch is relaxed before the next twitch can summate. At progressively higher frequencies, the twitches summate to generate higher force levels until a fused twitch (tetanization) occurs. (From Guyton AC, Hall JE: *Textbook of medical physiology*, ed 10, Philadelphia, 2000, Saunders.)

the initial twitch. If a fiber is allowed to relax completely before the subsequent action potential, the second fiber twitch generates a force equivalent to that of the first twitch (Figure 3-20). If the next action potential arrives before the preceding twitch has relaxed, however, the muscle twitches summate and generate an even greater peak force. Furthermore, if the next action potential arrives closer to the peak force level of the initial twitch, the force is even greater.

A set of repeating action potentials that each activates the muscle fiber before the relaxation of the previous twitch generates a series of summated mechanical twitches, referred to as an *unfused tetanus.* As the time interval between activation of successive twitches shortens, the unfused tetanus generates greater force until the successive peaks and valleys of mechanical twitches fuse into a single, stable level of muscle force, termed *fused tetanus (or tetanization)* (see Figure 3-20). Fused tetanus represents the greatest force level that is possible for a single muscle fiber. Motor units activated at high rates therefore are capable of generating greater overall force than the same number of motor units activated at lower rates.

The relation between the force and the frequency at which a motor unit is activated is curvilinear in shape, with a steep rise in force at low to moderate frequencies of activation, followed by a force plateau at high frequencies (usually by about 50 Hz for whole human muscle). The precise shape of the curve, however, depends on the duration of each twitch. A slow motor unit, for example, that generates a muscle twitch of a long duration will reach a fused tetany at a lower frequency than a fast motor unit.

The physiologic mechanisms of recruitment and rate coding of the motor unit operate simultaneously during the rise of a muscle force. The prevailing strategy (recruitment or rate coding) is highly specific to the particular demands and nature of a task. For example, motor unit recruitment during eccentric activation is different from that during concentric activation. During an eccentric activation, a relatively large force is generated per crossbridge. Consequently the number of motor units recruited is less for the same force produced during a concentric activation. Thus, a concentric activation requires the

recruitment of a larger number of motor units to produce the same force as an eccentric activation. Furthermore, rate coding is particularly important in production of a rapid force, especially in the early stages of an isometric activation. The rate coding may drive some motor units to discharge action potentials in quick succession (double discharges) to further increase force development. Double discharges occur when a motor unit discharges an action potential within about 20 ms of the previous—that is, at or more than 50 Hz, which is the upper limit of regular motor unit discharge rate in humans.[28] Regardless of the specific strategy used to increase force, the Henneman Size Principle (i.e., the order of recruitment from small to larger motor units) is still maintained.

INTRODUCTION TO ELECTROMYOGRAPHY

Electromyography (EMG) is the science of recording and interpreting the electrical activity that emanates from activated skeletal muscle. EMG is one of the most important research tools used in the field of kinesiology. On careful and skilled analysis, it is possible for the clinician and researcher to determine the timing and magnitude of activation of several whole muscles, both superficial and deep, during relatively complex functional movements. Especially over the last half-century, EMG studies have provided great insight into the specific actions of muscles.

Although EMG is also an important tool for the diagnosis and treatment of certain neuromuscular pathology or impairments, this chapter focuses on its use in the study of the kinesiology of the musculoskeletal system. EMG studies are regularly cited throughout this text, primarily as a means to justify a muscle's action or synergistic function during a movement or task. EMG research can also help explain or justify a wide range of other kinesiologic and pathokinesiologic phenomena, encompassing topics related to the fatigue of muscle, motor learning, protection of damaged or unstable joints, locomotion, ergonomics, and sport and recreation.[9,72] For this reason the reader needs to understand the basic technique, use, and limitations of kinesiologic EMG.

Recording of Electromyography

When a motor neuron is activated, the electrical impulse travels along the axon until it arrives at the motor endplates, and then it propagates in both directions away from the motor endplate along the length of the muscle fibers. The electrical signal that propagates along each muscle fiber is called the *motor unit action potential.* Sensitive electrodes are able to measure the sum of the change in voltage associated with all action potentials involved with the activated muscle fibers.[29] This voltage is often referred to as a *raw* or *interference EMG* signal. Raw EMG signals can be sensed by indwelling electrodes (fine wires inserted into the muscle) or by surface electrodes (placed on the skin overlying the muscle).

EMG recording electrodes are most often connected to a cable that attaches directly to the signal-processing hardware. More recent technical developments allow EMG signals to be recorded using telemetry systems. These systems are usually desired for monitoring and recording of muscle activity from long distances from the subject or patient, or during activities in which the cabling may disrupt freedom of move-

SPECIAL FOCUS 3-6

"Fiber Typing"—a Long History of Classification Nomenclature

As described in Figure 3-19, three types of motor units are recognized: slow (S), fast fatigue-resistant (FR), and fast fatigable (FF) motor units. Most muscle fibers associated with a given motor unit are physiologically similar and therefore have similar functional characteristics.

Over the years, researchers have attempted to identify via biopsy and histochemical or biochemical analysis muscle fibers that are physiologically associated with each of the main types of motor units. This process is referred to as "fiber typing." Several techniques of fiber typing have evolved over the last 50 years, three of which are highlighted in Table 3-4. The first method analyzed the histochemical profile of the fibers based on their relative *oxidative or glycolytic metabolism.* This system, as previously described in this chapter, conveniently links the contractile characteristics of the fibers with the classification nomenclature of the motor units (compare columns 1 and 2 in Table 3-4). This original method was developed from studies of animal motor units by Edgerton and colleagues in the 1960s, and later refined in the early 1970s.[82]

In 1970, Brooke and Kaiser[16] designed a technique of fiber typing human muscles. This technique studied the histochemical profile of fibers based on the activity of the enzyme *myosin ATPase* (column 3 in Table 3-4). The relative activity of this enzyme allowed the fast twitch (type II) fibers to be differentiated from the slow twitch (type I) fibers. In human muscle, the faster type II fibers can be furthered classified as type IIA and type IIX. (Note that type IIX in humans was originally identified as type IIB until in recent years, when the molecular composition of the myosin was truly identified as described subsequently.)

Until the early 1990s, histochemical techniques performed on cross-sections of muscle fibers were the dominant method for fiber typing human muscles. Biochemical analysis of protein molecules soon developed that allowed portions of muscle or single fibers to be analyzed based on the proportion of structurally similar isoforms of *myosin (heavy chain)*—a primary active (contractile) protein within the sarcomere. At least three isoforms of this myosin heavy chain (MHC) protein have been identified in humans: MHC I, MHC IIA, and MHC IIX (column 4 in Table 3-4). The dominant isoform found within a fiber is correlated with several of its mechanical properties, including maximal rate of shortening and force development, and force-velocity characteristics. This technique, currently considered the "gold standard" for fiber typing, is well correlated with the myosin ATPase histochemistry.[4,39,97]

TABLE 3-4. A Comparison of Three Methods of Fiber Typing Skeletal Muscle

Motor Unit Types	Histochemical Profile of Fibers Based on Relative Oxidative or Glycolytic Metabolism	Histochemical Profile of Fibers Based on Relative Activity of Myosin ATPase	Molecular Profile of Fibers Based on the Dominance of an Isoform of Myosin Heavy Chain (MHC)
Slow (S)	Slow oxidative (SO)	Type I (low activity)	MHC I
Fast fatigue-resistant (FR)	Fast oxidative glycolytic (FOG)	Type IIA (high activity)	MHC IIA
Fast fatigable (FF)	Fast glycolytic (FG)	Type IIX (high activity)	MHC IIX

ment. Surface EMG signals are transmitted to a recording computer by radio frequency waves and therefore are more susceptible to artifact than when cable electrodes are used.

The choice of electrodes depends on the particular situation and purpose of the EMG analysis. *Surface electrodes* are used most often because they are easy to apply, are noninvasive, and can detect signals from a relatively large area overlying the muscle. A common arrangement involves the placement of two surface electrodes over the muscle (each approximately 4 to 8 mm in diameter), side by side, on the skin overlying the muscle belly of interest. An additional reference (ground) electrode is placed over a bony area that has no muscle directly underneath. To ensure maximal amplitude of the EMG signal, the electrodes are placed in parallel with the long axis of the muscle fibers. This typical arrangement can usually detect action potentials within 2 cm of the electrodes.[73]

Fine wire electrodes inserted directly into the muscle belly permit a more specific region of a muscle to be monitored, as well as those deeper muscles not easily accessible through the use of surface electrodes, such as the brachialis, tibialis posterior, and transversus abdominis. Although the recording area is much smaller, fine wire electrodes can also discriminate single action potentials produced by one or a few motor units. Inserting fine wire electrodes into human muscle requires a relatively high level of technical skill and appropriate training before its safe implementation.

The voltage of the raw EMG signal is generally only a few millivolts, and therefore the signal can easily be distorted by other electrical sources caused by movement of electrodes and cables, adjacent or distant active muscles, and electromagnetic radiation from the surrounding environment. Several strategies can be used to minimize unwanted electrical artifact (often referred to as "noise"), including using the bipolar and ground electrode configuration described above. This arrangement minimizes common electrical artifact detected by both electrodes, a method electromyographers often refer to as "common mode rejection."[26,72]

Other strategies for reducing unwanted electrical artifact include adequate skin preparation and proper electrical shielding of the recording environment. Electrical signals can also be preamplified at the electrode site. This boost of the signal at the electrode site reduces artifact produced by movement of the electrode cables, which is a special concern when EMG is monitored during dynamic activities such as walking or running.[94] *Filtering* of the EMG signal can reduce certain interfering electrical signals by restricting the frequency range of the recorded EMG. A *band-pass filter* involves the combination of a high-pass filter (frequencies below a specified frequency are blocked, and higher frequencies are allowed to pass) and a low-pass filter (frequencies above a specified frequency are blocked, and lower frequencies are allowed to pass). A typical band-pass filter for surface EMG retains signals of 10 to 500 Hz and ignores the others.[71] Broader band-pass filtering of about 200 to 2000 Hz or even greater is often required for intramuscular recording of EMG. If needed, a filter can also be designed to eliminate common 60-Hz current that may exist in the recording environment.

To avoid losing parts of the EMG signal, it is important that the sampling rate be at least twice the rate of the highest frequency contained within the EMG signal. For example, using a band-pass filter set at 10 to 500 Hz ideally requires a sampling rate of at least 1000 samples per second.[71]

Analysis and Normalization of Electromyography

When combined with data such as time, joint kinematics, or external forces, the EMG signal can provide valuable insight into the actions of muscle.[98] In many kinesiologic analyses, the timing and amplitude of the EMG signal are of paramount interest. Consider, for example, the potential rele-

vance of studying the normal *timing* or sequencing of activation of the muscles associated with stabilization of the vertebral column. A delay or inhibition of the activation of a muscle such as the transversus abdominis or lumbar multifidi, for example, may suggest a cause for instability in the lower spine. Treatments can therefore be directed to concentrate on activities that specifically recruit and challenge these muscles.[43,44] Measuring the relative timing or order of muscle activation can be performed visually by using an oscilloscope or computer screen, or by more quantitative descriptive or mathematical or statistical methods.[94]

Assessing the demands placed on a muscle is usually determined by the relative *amplitude* of the EMG signal. Greater amplitude of EMG is generally assumed to indicate greater intensity of muscle activation and, in certain cases, greater relative muscle force. Figure 3-21, *A* and *B* depict a force generated by the isometric activation of an elbow flexor muscle producing a bipolar raw (interference) EMG signal. The raw EMG signal is a voltage that fluctuates on either side of zero and therefore often needs to be mathematically manipulated to serve as a useful quantitative measurement of muscle activation. One such method is called *full-wave rectification*, which converts the raw signal to positive voltages, resulting in the absolute value of the EMG (see Figure 3-21, *C*). The amplitude of the rectified EMG signal can be determined by averaging a sample of data collected over a specified time of activation. Furthermore, the rectified signal may be electronically filtered or *smoothed*, a process that flattens its "peaks and valleys" (see Figure 3-21, *D*). This smoothed signal is often referred to as a "linear envelope," which can be quantified as a "moving average," specified over a certain time frame or other event. Although not depicted in Figure 3-21,

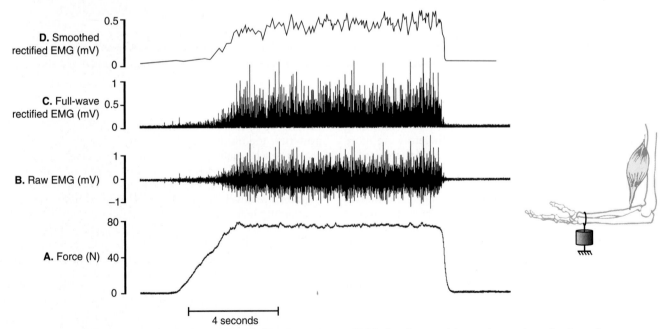

FIGURE 3-21. Diagram depicting several ways to process EMG signals caused by an isometric activation of the elbow flexor muscles at a submaximal effort performed by a young healthy woman. An external force produced by activation of the elbow flexor muscles is held at 80 N for about 10 seconds *(A)*. The EMG signal is recorded as a raw signal *(B)*, then is processed by full-wave rectification *(C)*, and finally is filtered and smoothed to delete the higher frequencies *(D)*.

the smoothed signal may also be *integrated,* a mathematic process that calculates the area under the (voltage-time) curve. This process allows for cumulative EMG quantification over a fixed period of time.

An alternative analysis for representing the raw EMG amplitude is to calculate the root mean squared *(RMS)* value over a period of time, which correlates with the standard deviation of the voltage relative to zero.[73] This mathematic analysis involves squaring the signal (to ensure a completely positive signal), averaging, and then calculating the square root. EMG voltages mathematically treated by any of the techniques described can also be used in biofeedback devices, such as visual meters or audio signals, or to trigger other devices, such as electrical stimulators, to activate a muscle at a preset threshold of voluntary contraction.

When the magnitude of a processed EMG signal is compared between different muscles, days, or conditions, it is usually necessary that the signal be *normalized* to some common reference signal. Expressing EMG amplitude in absolute voltage may produce meaningless data in many kinesiologic studies, especially when one is attempting to average data across different subjects and muscles. This is especially true when EMG data are collected across several sessions, requiring that the electrodes be reapplied. Even with the same muscular effort, absolute voltage will vary according to choice of electrode (including size), skin condition, and exact site of electrode placement. One common method of normalizing EMG involves referencing the signal produced by an activated muscle to that produced by the same muscle during a *maximal voluntary isometric contraction* (MVIC). Meaningful comparisons can then be made on the *relative* amplitude or intensity of muscle activation across different subjects or days, expressed as a percent of MVIC.[49] Alternatively, instead of using an MVIC as a reference signal, some electromyographers use the electrical response evoked from electrical stimulation of the muscle (i.e., M wave) under analysis. Also, a muscle's activation level can be referenced to some other meaningful reference task that does not involve maximal effort.[49,79]

Electromyographic Amplitude during Muscular Activation

To avoid the misinterpretation of EMG as it relates to a muscle's action or overall function, it is essential to understand the physiologic and technical factors that influence the amplitude of the EMG signal.

The amplitude of the EMG signal is generally proportional to the number and discharge rate of active motor units within the recording area of the EMG electrodes. These same factors also contribute to the force generated by a muscle. It is often tempting, therefore, to use a muscle's relative EMG magnitude as a measure of its relative *force* production. Although a generalized positive relationship may be assumed between these two variables during an isometric activation,[49,52] it cannot be assumed during all forms of nonisometric activations.[37,81] This caveat is based on several and often simultaneous factors, both physiologic and technical.

Physiologically, the EMG amplitude during a nonisometric activation can be influenced by the muscle's *length-tension* and *force-velocity* relationships. Consider the following two extreme hypothetic examples. Muscle A produces a 30% of maximal force via a high-velocity *eccentric* activation, across a muscle length that favors the production of relatively large active and passive forces. Muscle B, in contrast, produces an equivalent submaximal force via a high-velocity *concentric* activation, across a muscle length that favors the production of relatively small active and passive forces. Based on the combined influences of the muscle's length-tension and force-velocity relationships (depicted in Figures 3-11 and 3-15), Muscle A is assumed to operate at a relative *physiologic advantage* for producing force. Muscle A therefore requires fewer motor units to be recruited than Muscle B. EMG levels would therefore be less for the movement performed by Muscle A, although both muscles may be producing equivalent submaximal forces. In this extreme and hypothetic example, the EMG magnitude could not be used to reliably compare the relative forces produced by these two muscles.

Consider also that when an activated muscle is lengthening or shortening, the muscle fibers (the source for the electrical signal of EMG) change their spatial orientation to the recording electrodes. The EMG signal therefore may represent a compilation of several action potentials from different regions of a muscle or even from different muscles during the range of motion. This can alter the voltage signal recorded by the electrodes with a nonproportional change in the muscle force.

Other technical factors potentially affecting the magnitude of an EMG signal during movement are listed in the box. A detailed discussion of this topic can be found elsewhere.[29,72,73]

Technical Factors That May Affect the Magnitude of the EMG Signal
- Electrode configuration and size
- Range and type of filtering of the frequency content of the signal
- Magnitude of "cross-talk" from nearby muscles
- Location of the electrodes relative to the motor unit endplates
- Orientation of the electrodes relative to the muscle fiber

Throughout this textbook, EMG studies are cited that have compared average EMG amplitudes across different muscles from different subjects. Depending on the experimental design and technique (including appropriate normalization), specifics of the movement, and type and speed of the muscles' activation, it may be appropriate to assume that a greater relative amplitude of an EMG signal from a muscle is associated with a greater relative contractile force. In general, the confidence of this assumption is greatest when two muscles are compared while performing isometric activations. Confidence is less, however, when muscles are compared while performing movement that requires eccentric and concentric activations and when muscles are fatigued (see later).

In closing, although it may not be possible to predict the relative force in all muscles based on EMG amplitude, the amplitude (or timing) of the activation still provides very useful clues into the muscle's kinesiologic role in a given action. These clues are often reinforced through the analysis of other kinetic and kinematic variables, such as those provided by goniometers, accelerometers, video or other optical sensors, strain gauges, and force plates (see Chapter 4).

CAUSES OF MUSCLE FATIGUE IN HEALTHY PERSONS

Muscle fatigue is classically defined as an exercise-induced decline in maximal voluntary muscle force or power, despite maximal effort.[27] Even in healthy persons, muscle fatigue occurs during and after a sustained physical effort. Normally muscle fatigue is reversible with rest and should not be confused with being chronically "tired" or with muscle weakness that persists even with ample rest. Although muscle fatigue is a normal response to sustained physical effort, excessive or chronic muscle fatigue is not normal and is often a symptom of an underlying neuromuscular disorder.

In the healthy person, muscle fatigue can be subtle and is not always noticeable to the observer, especially during the performance of tasks involving prolonged, submaximal levels of effort.[48,93] This is apparent in Figure 3-22 (top panel), as a healthy subject is instructed to perform a series of elbow flexion contractions at a 50% submaximal effort, with every sixth effort (indicated by the arrows) being a maximum (100%) effort.[47] As observed in the figure, the magnitude of force produced by the maximal efforts gradually declines, although the person is still able to successfully generate the 50% level of maximal force. Continued performance of this repetitive submaximal effort, however, would eventually result in a decline in muscle force well below the 50% target level. Of interest, as evident in Figure 3-22 (bottom panel), the amplitude of the EMG signal gradually *increases* throughout the repeated submaximal efforts. This increased EMG signal reflects the recruitment of additional larger motor units as the other fatigued motor units cease or reduce their discharge rates.[88] This recruitment strategy is an attempt at maintaining a relatively stable force output.

In contrast to submaximal efforts depicted in Figure 3-22, a sustained muscle contraction at maximal effort results in a much more rapid rate of decline in maximal force. In this case, EMG amplitude *declines* as muscle force declines. This reduced EMG activity reflects a cessation or slowing of the discharge rate of the fatiguing motor units.[14] Because all motor units are presumably active during the initial stages of the maximal effort, there are no other motor units in reserve to compensate for the decline in muscle force, as is the case with prolonged submaximal efforts.

SPECIAL FOCUS 3-7

Frequency Shifts in the EMG Signal as an Indicator of Fatigue

As described, during prolonged or repeated *submaximal-effort* muscle contractions, EMG amplitude usually *increases* as the dormant motor units are recruited to assist or compensate for the fatigued motor units. Furthermore, during prolonged or repeated *maximal-effort* muscle contractions, EMG amplitude *decreases* as the population of activated motor units fails to adequately drive the muscle. These EMG responses may help to identify the onset of muscle fatigue during prolonged efforts.

Another method of indirectly assessing muscle fatigue during a maximal-effort task is based on the analysis of the frequency content of the raw EMG signal. When a muscle becomes progressively fatigued, such as during a prolonged effort, the EMG signal typically shows a shift to a *lower* median (or mean) frequency. Such analysis can be performed by applying a mathematic technique known as a *Fourier transformation* to obtain a power density spectrum of the EMG signal. A drop in the median frequency usually indicates that the action potentials contributing to the EMG signal are increasing in duration (conduction velocity is slowing) and reducing in amplitude.[73] The net effect is a shift in the median frequency of the EMG signal to lower frequencies.

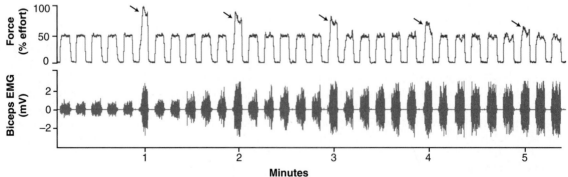

FIGURE 3-22 Isometric force of the elbow flexor muscles sustained intermittently (6 seconds on and 4 seconds off) at a magnitude 50% of initial maximal force. A maximal (100%) effort is performed every sixth effort (at 1-minute intervals) and is shown by the small arrows in the top panel. The bottom panel shows the surface raw EMG signal recorded from the biceps brachii during the fatiguing task. (Data from Hunter SK, Critchlow A, Shin IS, Enoka RM: Men are more fatigable than strength-matched women when performing intermittent submaximal contractions, *J Appl Physiol* 96:2125, 2004.)

The magnitude or rate of muscle fatigue is specific to the performance of the task, including the duration of the rest-work cycle.[27] A muscle that is rapidly fatigued by high-intensity and short-duration exercise can recover after a rest of only several minutes. In contrast, a muscle that is fatigued by low-intensity, long-duration exercise usually requires a much longer time to recover its force-generating capacity. Furthermore, the *type of activation* influences muscle fatigue. A muscle that is repeatedly activated eccentrically will exhibit less fatigue than when activated concentrically at the same velocity and under the same external load.[11] The relative fatigue-resistant nature of eccentric activation reflects the greater force generated per crossbridge and therefore the lower recruitment of motor units for a given submaximal load. Caution is required, however, when eccentric activation is employed as the primary rehabilitative training tool in a muscle that is unaccustomed to this type of activation. Delayed onset of muscle soreness (DOMS) experienced after repeated eccentric activations is usually more severe than after bouts of concentric or isometric activations.[85] DOMS tends to peak 24 to 72 hours after the bout of exercise and is ultimately caused by disruption of the sarcomeres and damage to the cytoskeleton within and around the fiber.[86]

There are several proposed mechanisms to explain the exact causes of fatigue. These mechanisms may be located at all points within and between the activation of the motor cortex and the sarcomere.[27,35] Mechanisms may occur in the muscle or the neuromuscular junction (often referred to as *muscular or peripheral mechanisms*). Alternatively, mechanisms may occur in the nervous system (often referred to as *neural or central mechanisms*). The distinction between muscular and neural mechanisms is not always clear. As an example, certain sensory neurons (group III and IV afferents) within muscle respond to the local metabolic byproducts associated with fatigue. Activation of these neurons in a fatiguing muscle can inhibit the discharge rate of the associated motor neurons,[70] paradoxically further reducing the force output of the fatigued muscle. In this example, the reason for the loss in force in the fatiguing muscle can be partially explained by both muscular and neural mechanisms.

Many mechanisms of fatigue in healthy persons are associated with the muscle itself. These mechanisms can be investigated by measuring the reduction in muscle force produced by electrical stimulation, which is independent of the central nervous system and voluntary effort.[13,31,32,35] These tests and others suggest that several muscular mechanisms may be responsible for fatigue (see list in box).[32]

Possible Muscular Mechanisms Contributing to Fatigue

- Reduced excitability at the neuromuscular junction
- Reduced excitability at the sarcolemma
- Changes in excitation-contraction coupling because of reduced sensitivity and availability of intracellular calcium
- Changes in contractile mechanics, including a slowing of crossbridge cycling
- Reduced energy source (metabolic origin)
- Reduced blood flow and oxygen supply

Several mechanisms of fatigue have been proposed that involve the nervous system—that is, regions proximal to the neuromuscular junction.[35,100] These neural mechanisms typically involve reduced excitatory input to supraspinal centers or a net decline in excitatory input to alpha motor neurons.[35] As a consequence, in healthy persons activation of the pool of motor neurons is reduced and muscle force declines. Persons with diseases of the nervous system such as multiple sclerosis may experience even greater muscle fatigue than healthy adults because of delays or blocks in the conduction of central neural impulses.[91]

In closing, considerable research is required to better understand the topic of muscle fatigue. Clarity in this area will benefit virtually any rehabilitation procedure that involves physical effort from the patient or client, regardless of whether there is an underlying pathologic process.

CHANGES IN MUSCLE WITH STRENGTH TRAINING, REDUCED USE, AND ADVANCED AGE

Changes in Muscle with Strength Training

The healthy neuromuscular system shows a remarkable ability to accommodate to different external demands or environmental stimuli. Such plasticity is evident in the robust and almost immediate alteration in the structure and function of the neuromuscular system after strength training. *Strength,* in the context of this chapter, refers to the maximal force or power produced by a muscle or muscle group during a maximal voluntary effort.

Repeated sessions of activating a muscle with progressively greater resistance will result in increased strength and hypertrophy.[58,60] Strength gains are commonly quantified by a *one-repetition maximum,* or 1 RM. By definition, 1 RM is the maximum load that can be lifted *once* as a muscle contracts through the joint's full or near-full range of motion. (For safety and practical reasons, formulas have been developed that allow a person's 1 RM strength to be determined by lifting a reduced load with a larger number of repetitions.[45]) The amount of resistance employed during strength training is often specified as a multiple of 1 RM; for example, the term *3 RMs* is the maximal load that can be lifted through a joint's full range of motion three times, and so on.

- *High-resistance training* for a specific muscle group usually involves a progressive increase in the magnitude of the load to 3 RMs to 12 RMs, performed over three bouts per exercise session.
- *Low-resistance training* involves lifting a lighter load greater than 15 RMs, usually performed over three bouts per exercise session.

  Note that these guidelines are general. The program details vary among patients and clients and will depend on specific goals of the training or rehabilitation. More detailed guidelines can be obtained from other sources.[58,60]

Increases in muscle strength from training are specific to the type and intensity of the exercise program. For example, high-resistance training involving concentric and eccentric activations performed three times a week for a 12-week period has been shown to increase 1 RM strength by 30% to 40%.[51] On average, this represents an increase of about 1% of strength per day of training. The same dynamic training regimen (concentric and eccentric activations), however, resulted in only a 10% increase in isometric strength.[51] Most strength-training programs should involve a component of eccentric activation. Because eccentric activations produce greater force per unit of muscle, this form of training can be more effective in promoting muscle hypertrophy than the same training using isometric and concentric activations.[89]

As expected, gains in 1 RM strength from low-resistance strength training are less than for high-resistance training,[59] but gains in muscle endurance can be greater.

One of the most dramatic responses to strength training is hypertrophy of muscle.[2,60,87,89,96] Hypertrophy results from increased protein synthesis within muscle fibers and therefore an increase in the physiologic cross-sectional area of the whole muscle. Increased pennation angles in hypertrophied muscles have been demonstrated, perhaps as a way to accommodate the larger amounts of contractile proteins.[2,56] Increased cross-sectional area in human muscle is primarily a result of fiber hypertrophy, with limited evidence of an increase in the actual number of fibers (hyperplasia). Staron and colleagues showed that the cross-sectional area of muscle increases as much as 30% in young adults after 20 weeks of high-resistance strength training, with increases in fiber size detected after only 6 weeks.[97] Although training causes hypertrophy in all exercised muscle fibers, it is usually greatest in the fast twitch (type II) fibers.[51,96,97,108] It has been proposed that increased strength in muscle may also be the result of an increase in the protein filament *desmin* (review Table 3-2 in Special Focus 3-2), which is believed to help transfer forces within and between muscle fibers.[108]

Strength gains from resistance training are also caused by adaptations within the nervous system.[24,34] Neural influences are especially evident during the first few training sessions. Some of the adaptations include an increased area of activity within the cortex of the brain during a motor task (as shown by functional magnetic resonance imaging), increased supraspinal motor drive, increased motor neuron excitability, and greater discharge frequency of motor units coupled with a decrease in neural inhibition at both spinal and supraspinal levels.[1,24,90] Perhaps the most convincing evidence of a neurogenic basis for strength training is documented increases in muscle strength through imagery training[111,112] or increases in the strength of control (nonexercised) muscles located contralateral to the exercised muscles.[20,76] Strength gains are often greater than what can be attributed to hypertrophy alone.[24] Although most of the neural adaptations cause greater activation of the agonist muscles, evidence suggests that training can result in *less* activation of the antagonist muscles.[34] The reduced force from opposing muscles would result in a greater net force produced by the agonist muscles.

Some of these concepts can be used by the clinician when more traditional methods of strength training are unsuccessful. This is especially relevant in persons with neurologic or neuromuscular pathologies who cannot tolerate the physical rigor of a strength-training regimen. Imagery training, for example, may be effective in very early stages of recovery of an injured limb after a stroke, when use of the affected limb is otherwise limited. Ultimately, the most effective method of strengthening a weakened muscle involves specific and adequate progressive overload to evoke changes not only in the nervous system but also in the structure of the muscle.

Changes in Muscle with Reduced Use

Trauma that requires a person's limb or joint to be rigidly immobilized for many weeks significantly reduces the use of the associated muscles. Periods of reduced muscle use (or disuse) also occur as a person confined to bed recovers from an illness or disease. These periods of reduced muscle activity lead to atrophy and usually marked reductions in strength, even in the first few weeks of inactivity.[3,7,21] The loss in strength can occur early, up to 3% to 6% per day in the first week alone.[7] After only 10 days of immobilization, healthy individuals can experience up to a 40% decrease of initial 1 RM strength.[101] Reduced strength after immobilization is usually twice that of the muscle atrophy—a 20% reduction in fiber cross-sectional area is associated with a 40% decline in strength. These relatively early changes suggest some neurologic basis for the reduced strength, in addition to the loss in the muscle's contractile proteins.

Protein synthesis is reduced in all muscle fiber types within a chronically immobilized limb,[3] but most notably in the slow twitch fibers.[7] Because slow twitch fibers are used so frequently throughout most routine daily activities, they are subjected to greater *relative* disuse when the limb is immobilized compared with fast twitch fibers. As a consequence, whole muscles of immobilized limbs tend to experience a relative transformation toward faster twitch characteristics,[38] and this shift can occur as early as 3 weeks after the onset of immobilization.[46]

The amount of neuromuscular adaptation after immobilization of a limb depends on several factors. The loss of strength is greatest when the muscle is maintained in its shortened position.[33,99] The greater slack placed on muscle fibers immobilized in a shortened length may specifically promote degradation of contractile proteins.[15] Furthermore, antigravity and single-joint muscles show a more rapid atrophy than other muscles within a chronically immobilized limb. These muscles include the soleus, vastus medialis, vastus intermedius, and multifidus.[64] In the lower extremity, the knee extensors generally demonstrate greater disuse atrophy and relative loss in strength than the knee flexor (hamstring) muscles.[78] The propensity for disuse atrophy in the quadriceps may be a concern when stability of the partially flexed knee is required, such as when a person is transferring to and from a chair, bed, or commode.

Resistive exercise is able to reverse or mitigate many of the changes that occur with chronic immobilization of a limb. A strengthening program incorporating eccentric activation demonstrates the greatest gains in strength and increases in fiber size.[46] Because the fibers associated with the smaller motor units are more prone to atrophy, a rehabilitation program should incorporate low-intensity, long-duration muscle activations early in the exercise program as a means to target these muscle fibers.

Changes in Muscle with Advanced Age

Even in healthy persons, reaching an advanced age is associated with reduced strength, power, and speed of muscle contraction. Although these changes can be subtle, they can be marked in very old age and they are measurable. Because of the relative rapid loss in the speed of muscle contraction, aged persons typically show greater loss in power (product of force and velocity) than in peak force alone.[10,92]

Although changes are highly variable, in general, healthy aged persons experience an approximate 10% per decade decline in peak strength after 60 years of age, with a more rapid decline after 75 years of age.[50,77] Loss in strength is generally more pronounced in the muscles of the lower limb, such as the quadriceps,[50,67] as compared with the upper limb. If marked, lower-limb weakness can interfere with functions required for independent living, such as safely walking, or rising from a chair.[83] Such age-related decrements in muscle strength are often accelerated in sedentary older adults or those with underlying pathology.[50]

The primary cause of reduced strength in healthy aged persons is *senile sarcopenia,* which is defined as a loss in muscle tissue with advanced age.[22,102] Sarcopenia may be dramatic, with a marked loss of muscle tissue and an infiltration of excessive amounts of connective tissue and intramuscular fat (compare muscles in Figure 3-23). The causes of senile sarcopenia are not fully understood and may be associated with the normal biologic processes of aging (such as programmed cell death–"apoptosis") or changes in physical activity, nutrition, and hormone levels.[17,78,87,102]

Sarcopenia occurs through a reduction in the actual number of muscle fibers as well as a decrease in size (atrophy) of all existing fibers.[87] Loss in the number of fibers is caused by a gradual demise of the associated motor units.[19,63,103] Initial studies using muscle biopsy suggested that there was a selective loss of type II (fast twitch) fibers in older adults. More recent evidence, however, indicates that the proportion of type II and type I fibers is usually maintained into old age, at least in healthy adults.[51,87] Because of the greater *atrophy* of the type II (fast) fibers, however, aged skeletal muscle typically has a greater proportional volume of muscle that expresses type I (slow twitch) characteristics compared with young adults. This phenomenon is apparent when excised cross-sections of stained muscle fibers of a young and a relatively older person are compared (Figure 3-24). The muscle fibers from both the young and older adult were stained using a similar fiber typing technique: type I (slow twitch) fibers are stained light, and type II (fast twitch) fibers are stained dark (see figure legend). The cross-section of the older muscle in Figure 3-24, *B* shows all fibers are smaller compared with the young muscle, especially the type II (fast twitch) fibers. The muscle sample obtained from the older subject in Figure 3-24, *B* demonstrates a greater proportional number of type I (slow twitch) fibers than the younger subject, although this is not typical of most recent findings. The more common occurrence is a proportional loss of both type I and type II fibers, with greater atrophy (reduced size) of the remaining type II fibers. This results in a net increase in the proportional area of type I fibers in old muscle compared with young muscle, which explains in part why whole muscles in aged adults take longer to contract and to relax and ultimately are less forceful and powerful.[23,51] Although a more sedentary lifestyle will accelerate these changes in muscle morphology, even the active older adult will experience these alterations to varying degrees.

Sarcopenia in aged persons explains most but not all of the loss in strength and power production. Loss of force with maximal effort may also involve a reduced ability of the nervous system to maximally activate the available muscle fibers. When given sufficient practice, some aged adults can learn to activate their available muscle to a greater level, nearly equivalent to that in younger adults. Clinically this

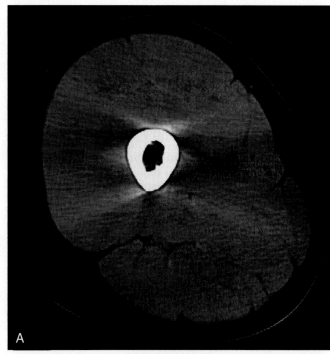

28-year-old female

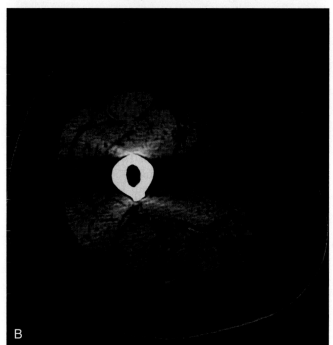

80-year-old female

FIGURE 3-23. Computed tomographic image showing a cross-section of the muscles of the mid-thigh in **A,** a healthy 28-year-old woman and **B,** a healthy but sedentary 80-year-old woman. The image of the older woman's thigh shows comparably less muscle mass and more intramuscular connective tissue.

may be an important consideration during initial assessment of the strength of an older individual.

The age-related alterations in muscle morphology can have marked effects on the ability of some older adults to effectively perform daily tasks. Fortunately, however, age in itself does not drastically alter the *plasticity* of the neuromuscular

27-year-old female

67-year-old female

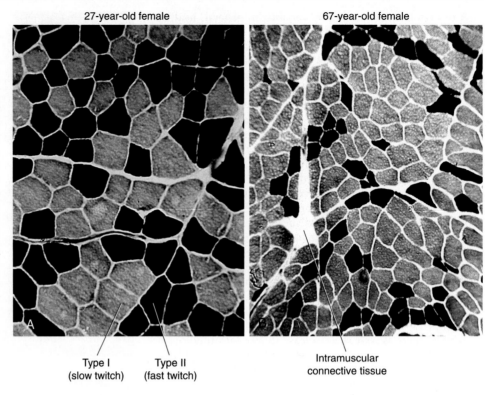

FIGURE 3-24. Cross-section of human muscle fibers from the vastus lateralis of **(A)** a healthy 27-year-old woman and **(B)** a healthy 67-year-old woman. The images are printed to similar scales. The fibers were histochemically stained for myosin ATPase activity to show the distribution of type I (slow twitch) fibers that stained light, and type II (fast twitch) fibers that stained dark. (The fibers were preincubated at pH 10.3.) Note the following in the older muscle: the reduced cross-sectional areas of the fibers, most notably the type II fibers, and greater intramuscular connective tissue.

Type I
(slow twitch)

Type II
(fast twitch)

Intramuscular
connective tissue

system. Strength training can theoretically compensate for some but certainly not all of the loss in strength and power in aged adults.[30] Resistive exercise, if performed safely, can be very helpful in maintaining the critical level of muscle force and power required for the performance of the basic activities of daily living.

SUMMARY

Skeletal muscle provides the primary forces that stabilize and move the bones and joints of the body. After activation by the nervous system via action potentials, muscles produce force by either contracting or resisting elongation. The contractile proteins of actin and myosin play a key role in driving this active process—referred to as the *sliding-filament hypothesis.* More recently appreciated is the important supportive and structural role of the noncontractile proteins. Proteins such as titin and desmin, for example, contribute to passive tension and provide elasticity, alignment, and stability to the sarcomeres and hence the whole of the muscle fiber. Furthermore, extracellular connective tissues surround individual and groups of muscle fibers, ultimately encasing the entire muscle belly before blending with the tendon and attaching to bone.

As described in Chapter 1, a muscle's action and ultimate function is based on its line of force relative to the axis of rotation at the joint. Chapter 3 focuses more on mechanisms responsible for the generation of the force. Ultimately, these mechanisms are governed by the nervous system, but also by the unique morphology (shape) and overall architecture of the individual muscles. Each individual muscle in the body has a unique form and therefore unique function. A small

fusiform muscle such as the lumbrical in the hand, for example, generates only a small force because of its small cross-sectional area. Because this muscle is well endowed with sensory receptors, it excels in providing the nervous system with proprioception. The larger gastrocnemius muscle, in contrast, produces large forces because of its larger cross-sectional area, resulting in part from the pennation arrangement of its fibers. A large force is required from this calf muscle to lift or propel the entire body during activities such as jumping and climbing.

Regardless of the shape or architecture of a muscle, the forces ultimately transferred through the tendon and to the bone are produced by a combination of active and passive mechanisms. Active mechanisms are typically under volitional control, based primarily on the interaction between actin and myosin. Passive mechanisms, in contrast, are based more on the inherent stiffness characteristics of the muscle, collectively due to the structural proteins and all connective tissues including those that constitute the tendon. Although relatively small within a muscle's midrange of movement, passive tension can be very large at the more extremes of the range, especially for muscles that cross multiple joints. Some passive tension produced in response to a muscle stretch is normal and performs useful physiologic functions, such as stabilizing the joint and protecting it from stretch-related injury. Excessive passive tension, however, is abnormal and can restrict the optimal postural alignment of the body as a whole, as well as reducing the ease and fluidity of movement. Increased stiffness in muscle can occur as a result of trauma or disease within the musculoskeletal system. In addition, excessive passive tension (or stiffness) within muscle may result from abnormal levels of involuntary activation by the nervous system. This impairment is often referred to as *spastic-*

ity or *rigidity* and is typically associated with injury or disease of the central nervous system.

Two of the most important clinically related principles of muscle physiology are the length-tension and force-velocity relationships. These basic principles, although originally formulated using isolated muscle fibers in the animal model, need to be applied clinically to whole muscles of patients or clients. The very relevant length-tension relationship of a single muscle fiber is expressed clinically as a torque–joint angle relationship of the whole muscle or muscle group, where torque is functionally analogous to force, and joint angle to length. The elbow flexor muscles, for example, produce their greatest elbow flexion torque near a 90-degree elbow joint angle. This joint angle corresponds approximately to where the biceps brachii has its greatest moment arm (leverage) as a flexor, but also approximately to the length at which this muscle produces its greatest force based on the action-myosin overlap of its individual fibers. Even with maximal effort, peak elbow flexion torque drops off considerably at full elbow extension or at full flexion because of these same leverage and physiologic factors.

In addition, a muscle's force-velocity relationship needs to be appreciated clinically within the scope of the muscle's torque–joint angular velocity relationship. For reasons described in this chapter, a muscle activated at a high joint angular velocity via eccentric activation produces greater force than any speed of concentric activation, including isometric. This principle can have important clinical implications, often physiologically linked to the muscle's length-tension relationship. Paralysis of proximal muscles, for example, often causes functional weakness in more distal but otherwise healthy muscles. Failure of proximal muscles to adequately stabilize the skeleton can cause a situation in which the more distal muscle is obligated to contract to an overly shortened length, at a quicker velocity than normal. This is evident, for example, by a weakened grasp after paralysis of the wrist extensor muscles. This and other kinesiologic examples are described in greater detail throughout this textbook.

The concept of the motor unit is an important premise behind much of the discussion of this chapter. A motor unit is a single cell body (located in the spinal cord), its axon, and all connected muscle fibers. Because all the fibers within a given motor unit maximally contract on stimulation of the cell body, a finite amount of force is generated from each motor unit. Forces are increased across the entire muscle through the recruitment of additional motor units. In addition, motor units can increase their force output by discharging at faster rates. The processes of recruitment and rate coding allow motor units to finely control the gradation of forces across the entire muscle.

Considerations for collecting, processing, and normalizing EMG data were introduced in this chapter. When interpreted correctly, the EMG signal can provide very useful information on the timing, level of activation, and ultimate function of muscles. Information obtained from EMG is often analyzed in conjunction with anatomic, biomechanical, kinetic, and kinematic data; this analysis serves as the foundation for much of the kinesiology described throughout this text.

This chapter concludes with a broad overview of selected topics that have important relevance to clinical practice. These topics include causes of muscle fatigue and the changes that occur in muscles with strength training, reduced use, and aging. Muscle fatigue for example, which is the exercise-induced reduction in muscle force of power, is necessary for effective neuromuscular adaptation during training and rehabilitation in healthy and clinical populations. Consequently, understanding the adaptation of muscle and its function to strength training, and in contrast to reduced use and aging, will aid the therapist in prescribing optimal therapies for rehabilitation to patient populations.

REFERENCES

1. Aagaard P: Training-induced changes in neural function, *Exerc Sport Sci Rev* 31:61-67, 2003.
2. Aagaard P, Andersen JL, Dyhre-Poulsen P, et al: A mechanism for increased contractile strength of human pennate muscle in response to strength training: changes in muscle architecture, *J Physiol* 534:613-623, 2001.
3. Adams GR, Caiozzo VJ, Baldwin KM: Skeletal muscle unweighting: spaceflight and ground-based models, *J Appl Physiol* 95:2185-2201, 2003.
4. Adams GR, Hather BM, Baldwin KM, Dudley GA: Skeletal muscle myosin heavy chain composition and resistance training, *J Appl Physiol* 74:911-915, 1993.
5. Allen GM, Gandevia SC, McKenzie DK: Reliability of measurements of muscle strength and voluntary activation using twitch interpolation, *Muscle Nerve* 18:593-600, 1995.
6. Allen GM, McKenzie DK, Gandevia SC, Bass S: Reduced voluntary drive to breathe in asthmatic subjects, *Respir Physiol* 93:29-40, 1993.
7. Appell HJ: Muscular atrophy following immobilisation. A review, *Sports Med* 10:42-58, 1990.
8. Baratta RV, Solomonow M, Best R, D'Ambrosia R: Isotonic length/force models of nine different skeletal muscles, *Med Biol Eng Comput* 31:449-458, 1993.
9. Basmajian J, Luca CD: *Muscles alive: their functions revealed by electromyography*, Baltimore, 1985, Williams & Wilkins.
10. Bassey EJ, Fiatarone MA, O'Neill EF, et al: Leg extensor power and functional performance in very old men and women, *Clin Sci* 82:321-327, 1992.
11. Baudry S, Klass M, Pasquet B, Duchateau J: Age-related fatigability of the ankle dorsiflexor muscles during concentric and eccentric contractions, *Eur J Appl Physiol* 100:515-525, 2006.
12. Beltman JG, Sargeant AJ, van Mechelen W, de Haan A: Voluntary activation level and muscle fiber recruitment of human quadriceps during lengthening contractions, *J Appl Physiol* 97:619-626, 2004.
13. Bigland-Ritchie B, Furbush F, Woods JJ: Fatigue of intermittent submaximal voluntary contractions: central and peripheral factors, *J Appl Physiol* 61:421-429, 1986.
14. Bigland-Ritchie B, Johansson R, Lippold OC, Woods JJ: Contractile speed and EMG changes during fatigue of sustained maximal voluntary contractions, *J Neurophysiol* 50:313-324, 1983.
15. Booth FW: Effect of limb immobilization on skeletal muscle, *J Appl Physiol* 52:1113-1118, 1982.
16. Brooke MH, Kaiser KK: Muscle fiber types: how many and what kind? *Arch Neurol* 23:369-379, 1970.
17. Brown M: Skeletal muscle and bone: effect of sex steroids and aging, *Adv Physiol Educ* 32:120-126, 2008.
18. Caiozzo VJ, Rourke B: The muscular system: structural and functional plasticity. In Tipton CM, editor: *ACSM'S advanced exercise physiology*, Philadelphia, 2006, Lippincott Williams & Wilkins.
19. Campbell MJ, McComas AJ, Petito F: Physiological changes in ageing muscles, *J Neurol Neurosurg Psychiatry* 36:174-182, 1973.
20. Carroll TJ, Herbert RD, Munn J, et al: Contralateral effects of unilateral strength training: evidence and possible mechanisms, *J Appl Physiol* 101:1514-1522, 2006.
21. Christensen B, Dyrberg E, Aagaard P, et al: Short-term immobilization and recovery affect skeletal muscle but not collagen tissue turnover in humans, *J Appl Physiol* 105:1845-1851, 2008.
22. Doherty TJ: Invited review: aging and sarcopenia, *J Appl Physiol* 95:1717-1727, 2003.
23. Doherty TJ, Brown WF: Age-related changes in the twitch contractile properties of human thenar motor units, *J Appl Physiol* 82:93-101, 1997.
24. Duchateau J, Enoka RM: Neural adaptations with chronic activity patterns in able-bodied humans, *Am J Phys Med Rehabil* 81:S17-S27, 2002.

25. Duchateau J, Enoka RM: Neural control of shortening and lengthening contractions: influence of task constraints, *J Physiol* 586:5853-5864, 2008.
26. Enoka RM: *Neuromechanics of human movement*, Champaign, Ill, 2008, Human Kinetics.
27. Enoka RM, Duchateau J: Muscle fatigue: what, why and how it influences muscle function, *J Physiol* 586:11-23, 2008.
28. Enoka RM, Fuglevand AJ: Motor unit physiology: some unresolved issues, *Muscle Nerve* 24:4-17, 2001.
29. Farina D, Merletti R, Enoka RM: The extraction of neural strategies from the surface EMG, *J Appl Physiol* 96:1486-1496, 2004.
30. Fiatarone MA, O'Neill EF, Ryan ND, et al: Exercise training and nutritional supplementation for physical frailty in very elderly people, *N Engl J Med* 330:1769-1775, 1994.
31. Fitts RH: The cross-bridge cycle and skeletal muscle fatigue, *J Appl Physiol* 104:551-558, 2008.
32. Fitts RH: The muscular system: fatigue processes. In Tipton CM, editor: *ACSM'S advanced exercise physiology*, Philadelphia, 2006, Lippincott Williams & Wilkins.
33. Fournier M, Roy RR, Perham H, et al: Is limb immobilization a model of muscle disuse? *Exp Neurol* 80:147-156, 1983.
34. Gabriel DA, Kamen G, Frost G: Neural adaptations to resistive exercise: mechanisms and recommendations for training practices, *Sports Med* 36:133-149, 2006.
35. Gandevia SC: Spinal and supraspinal factors in human muscle fatigue, *Physiol Rev* 81:1725-1789, 2001.
36. Ghena DR, Kurth AL, Thomas M, Mayhew J: Torque Characteristics of the Quadriceps and Hamstring Muscles during Concentric and Eccentric Loading, *J Orthop Sports Phys Ther* 14:149-154, 1991.
37. Graves AE, Kornatz KW, Enoka RM: Older adults use a unique strategy to lift inertial loads with the elbow flexor muscles, *J Neurophysiol* 83:2030-2039, 2000.
38. Haggmark T, Eriksson E: Cylinder or mobile cast brace after knee ligament surgery. A clinical analysis and morphologic and enzymatic studies of changes in the quadriceps muscle, *Am J Sports Med* 7:48-56, 1979.
39. Harridge SDR, Bottinelli R, Canepari M, et al: Whole-muscle and single-fibre contractile properties and myosin heavy chain isoforms in humans, *Pflugers Arch* 432:913-920, 1996.
40. Henneman E, Mendell L: Functional organization of motoneuron pool and its inputs. In Brookhart JM, Mountcastle VB, Brooks VB, editor: *Handbook of physiology*, vol 2, Bethesda, 1981, American Physiological Society.
41. Hill A: *The first and last experiments in muscle mechanics*, New York, 1970, Cambridge University Press.
42. Hill A: The heat of shortening and the dynamic constraints of muscle, *Proc R Soc Lond B Biol Sci* 126:136-195, 1938.
43. Hodges PW, Richardson CA: Contraction of the abdominal muscles associated with movement of the lower limb, *Phys Ther* 77:132, 1997.
44. Hodges PW, Richardson CA: Inefficient muscular stabilization of the lumbar spine associated with low back pain. A motor control evaluation of transversus abdominis, *Spine* 21:2640-2650, 1996.
45. Hoffman J: Resistance Training. In Hoffman J, editor: *Physiological aspects of sport training and performance*, Champaign, Ill, 2002, Human Kinetics.
46. Hortobagyi T, Dempsey L, Fraser D, et al: Changes in muscle strength, muscle fibre size and myofibrillar gene expression after immobilization and retraining in humans, *J Physiol* 524:293-304, 2000.
47. Hunter SK, Critchlow A, Shin IS, Enoka RM: Men are more fatigable than strength-matched women when performing intermittent submaximal contractions, *J Appl Physiol* 96:2125-2132, 2004.
48. Hunter SK, Duchateau J, Enoka RM: Muscle fatigue and the mechanisms of task failure, *Exerc Sport Sci Rev* 32:44-49, 2004.
49. Hunter SK, Ryan DL, Ortega JD, Enoka RM: Task differences with the same load torque alter the endurance time of submaximal fatiguing contractions in humans, *J Neurophysiol* 88:3087-3096, 2002.
50. Hunter SK, Thompson MW, Adams RD: Relationships among age-associated strength changes and physical activity level, limb dominance, and muscle group in women, *J Gerontol A Biol Sci Med Sci* 55:B264-B273, 2000.
51. Hunter SK, Thompson MW, Ruell PA, et al: Human skeletal sarcoplasmic reticulum Ca2+ uptake and muscle function with aging and strength training, *J Appl Physiol* 86:1858-1865, 1999.
52. Hunter SK, Yoon T, Farinella J, et al: Time to task failure and muscle activation vary with load type for a submaximal fatiguing contraction with the lower leg, *J Appl Physiol* 105:463-472, 2008.
53. Huxley AF, Niedergerke R: Structural changes in muscle during contraction; interference microscopy of living muscle fibres, *Nature* 173:971-973, 1954.
54. Huxley H, Hanson J: Changes in the cross-striations of muscle during contraction and stretch and their structural interpretation, *Nature* 173:973-976, 1954.
55. Johnson MA, Polgar J, Weightman D, Appleton D: Data on the distribution of fibre types in thirty-six human muscles. An autopsy study, *J Neurol Sci* 18:111-129, 1973.
56. Kawakami Y, Abe T, Fukunaga T: Muscle-fiber pennation angles are greater in hypertrophied than in normal muscles, *J Appl Physiol* 74:2740-2744, 1993.
57. Kesar TM, Ding J, Wexler AS, et al: Predicting muscle forces of individuals with hemiparesis following stroke, *J Neuroeng Rehabil* 5:7, 2008.
58. Kraemer WJ, Adams K, Cafarelli E, et al: American College of Sports Medicine position stand. Progression models in resistance training for healthy adults, *Med Sci Sports Exerc* 34:364-380, 2002.
59. Kraemer WJ, Deschenes MR, Fleck SJ: Physiological adaptations to resistance exercise. Implications for athletic conditioning, *Sports Med* 6:246-256, 1988.
60. Kraemer WJ, Ratamess NA: Fundamentals of resistance training: progression and exercise prescription, *Med Sci Sports Exerc* 36:674-688, 2004.
61. Krevolin JL, Pandy MG, Pearce JC: Moment arm of the patellar tendon in the human knee, *J Biomech* 37:785-788, 2004.
62. Labeit S, Kolmerer B: Titins: giant proteins in charge of muscle ultra-structure and elasticity, *Science* 270:293-296, 1995.
63. Lexell J, Taylor CC, Sjostrom M: What is the cause of the ageing atrophy? Total number, size and proportion of different fiber types studied in whole vastus lateralis muscle from 15- to 83-year-old men, *J Neurol Sci* 84:275-294, 1988.
64. Lieber RL: *Skeletal muscle structure, function and plasticity*, Baltimore, 2002, Lippincott Williams & Wilkins.
65. Lieber RL, Friden J: Clinical significance of skeletal muscle architecture, *Clin Orthop Relat Res* 383:140-151, 2001.
66. Lombardi V, Piazzesi G: The contractile response during steady lengthening of stimulated frog muscle fibres, *J Physiol* 431:141-171, 1990.
67. Lynch NA, Metter EJ, Lindle RS, et al: Muscle quality. I. Age-associated differences between arm and leg muscle groups, *J Appl Physiol* 86:188-194, 1999.
68. Magid A, Law DJ: Myofibrils bear most of the resting tension in frog skeletal muscle, *Science* 230:1280-1282, 1985.
69. Magnusson SP, Narici MV, Maganaris CN, Kjaer M: Human tendon behaviour and adaptation, in vivo, *J Physiol* 586:71-81, 2008.
70. Martin PG, Smith JL, Butler JE, et al: Fatigue-sensitive afferents inhibit extensor but not flexor motoneurons in humans, *J Neurosci* 26:4796-4802, 2006.
71. Merletti R, Hermens HJ: Detection and conditioning of the surface EMG signal. In Merletti R, Parker P, editors: *Electromyography: physiology, engineering and noninvasive applications*, Piscataway, NJ, 2004, IEEE Press, Wiley-Interscience.
72. Merletti R, Parker P: *Electromyography: physiology, engineering and noninvasive applications*, Piscataway, NJ, 2004, IEEE Press, Wiley-Interscience.
73. Merletti R, Rainoldi A, Farina D: Surface electromyography for noninvasive characterization of muscle, *Exerc Sport Sci Rev* 29:20-25, 2001.
74. Monti RJ, Roy RR, Edgerton VR: Role of motor unit structure in defining function, *Muscle Nerve* 24:848-866, 2001.
75. Monti RJ, Roy RR, Hodgson JA, Edgerton VR: Transmission of forces within mammalian skeletal muscles, *J Biomech* 32:371-380, 1999.
76. Munn J, Herbert RD, Hancock MJ, Gandevia SC: Training with unilateral resistance exercise increases contralateral strength, *J Appl Physiol* 99:1880-1884, 2005.
77. Narici MV, Bordini M, Cerretelli P: Effect of aging on human adductor pollicis muscle function, *J Appl Physiol* 71:1277-1281, 1991.
78. Narici MV, Maganaris CN: Plasticity of the muscle-tendon complex with disuse and aging, *Exerc Sport Sci Rev* 35:126-134, 2007.
79. Neumann DA: An electromyographic study of the hip abductor muscles as subjects with a hip prosthesis walked with different methods of using a cane and carrying a load, *Phys Ther* 79:1163, 1999.
80. Ng AV, Miller RG, Gelinas D, Kent-Braun JA: Functional relationships of central and peripheral muscle alterations in multiple sclerosis, *Muscle Nerve* 29:843-852, 2004.

81. Pasquet B, Carpentier A, Duchateau J, Hainaut K: Muscle fatigue during concentric and eccentric contractions, *Muscle Nerve* 23:1727-1735, 2000.

82. Peter JB, Barnard RJ, Edgerton VR, et al: Metabolic profiles of three fiber types of skeletal muscle in guinea pigs and rabbits, *Biochemistry* 11:2627-2633, 1972.

83. Petrella JK, Kim JS, Tuggle SC, et al: Age differences in knee extension power, contractile velocity, and fatigability, *J Appl Physiol* 98:211-220, 2005.

84. Petterson SC, Barrance P, Buchanan T, et al: Mechanisms underlying quadriceps weakness in knee osteoarthritis, *Med Sci Sports Exerc* 40:422-427, 2008.

85. Prasartwuth O, Taylor JL, Gandevia SC: Maximal force, voluntary activation and muscle soreness after eccentric damage to human elbow flexor muscles, *J Physiol* 567:337-348, 2005.

86. Proske U, Morgan DL: Muscle damage from eccentric exercise: mechanism, mechanical signs, adaptation and clinical applications, *J Physiol* 537:333-345, 2001.

87. Reeves ND, Narici MV, Maganaris CN: Myotendinous plasticity to ageing and resistance exercise in humans, *Exp Physiol* 91:483-498, 2006.

88. Riley ZA, Maerz AH, Litsey JC, Enoka RM: Motor unit recruitment in human biceps brachii during sustained voluntary contractions, *J Physiol* 586:2183-2193, 2008.

89. Roig M, O'Brien K, Kirk G, et al: The effects of eccentric versus concentric resistance training on muscle strength and mass in healthy adults: a systematic review with meta-analyses, *Br J Sports Med* 43:556-568, 2009.

90. Semmler JG, Enoka RM: Neural contributions to changes in muscle strength. In Zatsiorsky VM, editor: *Olympic encyclopaedia of sports medicine and science. Biomechanics in sport: the scientific basis of performance*, Oxford, UK, 2000, Blackwell Science.

91. Sheean GL, Murray NM, Rothwell JC, et al: An electrophysiological study of the mechanism of fatigue in multiple sclerosis, *Brain* 120:299-315, 1997.

92. Skelton DA, Kennedy J, Rutherford OM: Explosive power and asymmetry in leg muscle function in frequent fallers and non-fallers aged over 65, *Age Ageing* 31:119-125, 2002.

93. Smith JL, Martin PG, Gandevia SC, Taylor JL: Sustained contraction at very low forces produces prominent supraspinal fatigue in human elbow flexor muscles, *J Appl Physiol* 103:560-568, 2007.

94. Soderberg GL, Knutson LM: A guide for use and interpretation of kinesiologic electromyographic data, *Phys Ther* 80:485-498, 2000.

95. Standring S, Ellis H, Healy JC: *Gray's anatomy: the anatomical basis of clinical practice*, ed 40, New York, 2009, Churchill Livingstone.

96. Staron RS, Karapondo DL, Kraemer WJ, et al: Skeletal muscle adaptations during early phase of heavy-resistance training in men and women, *J Appl Physiol* 76:1247-1255, 1994.

97. Staron RS, Leonardi MJ, Karapondo DL, et al: Strength and skeletal muscle adaptations in heavy-resistance-trained women after detraining and retraining, *J Appl Physiol* 70:631-640, 1991.

98. Sutherland DH: The evolution of clinical gait analysis part l: Kinesiological EMG, *Gait Posture* 14:61-70, 2001.

99. Tabary JC, Tabary C, Tardieu C, et al: Physiological and structural changes in the cat's soleus muscle due to immobilization at different lengths by plaster casts, *J Physiol* 224:231-244, 1972.

100. Taylor JL, Todd G, Gandevia SC: Evidence for a supraspinal contribution to human muscle fatigue, *Clin Exp Pharmacol Physiol* 33:400-405, 2006.

101. Thom JM, Thompson MW, Ruell PA, et al: Effect of 10-day cast immobilization on sarcoplasmic reticulum calcium regulation in humans, *Acta Physiol Scand* 172:141-147, 2001.

102. Thompson LV: Age-related muscle dysfunction, *Exp Gerontol* 44:106-111, 2009.

103. Tomlinson BE, Irving D: The numbers of limb motor neurons in the human lumbosacral cord throughout life, *J Neurol Sci* 34:213-219, 1977.

104. van Mameren H, Drukker J: Attachment and composition of skeletal muscles in relation to their function, *J Biomech* 12:859-867, 1979.

105. Wang K, McCarter R, Wright J, et al: Viscoelasticity of the sarcomere matrix of skeletal muscles. The titin-myosin composite filament is a dual-stage molecular spring, *Biophys J* 64:1161-1177, 1993.

106. Westing SH, Seger JY, Thorstensson A: Effects of electrical stimulation on eccentric and concentric torque-velocity relationships during knee extension in man, *Acta Physiol Scand* 140:17-22, 1990.

107. Williams GN, Buchanan TS, Barrance PJ, et al: Quadriceps weakness, atrophy, and activation failure in predicted noncopers after anterior cruciate ligament injury, *Am J Sports Med* 33:402-407, 2005.

108. Woolstenhulme MT, Conlee RK, Drummond MJ, et al: Temporal response of desmin and dystrophin proteins to progressive resistance exercise in human skeletal muscle, *J Appl Physiol* 100:1876-1882, 2006.

109. Yamaguchi G, Sawa A, Moran D: A survey of human musculotendon actuator parameters. In Winters JW, Woo S-LY, editors: *Multiple muscle systems: biomechanics and movement organization*, New York, 1990, Springer-Verlag.

110. Yoshida Y, Mizner RL, Ramsey DK, Snyder-Mackler L: Examining outcomes from total knee arthroplasty and the relationship between quadriceps strength and knee function over time, *Clin Biomech* 23:320-328, 2008.

111. Yue G, Cole KJ: Strength increases from the motor program: comparison of training with maximal voluntary and imagined muscle contractions, *J Neurophysiol* 67:1114-1123, 1992.

112. Zijdewind I, Toering ST, Bessem B, et al: Effects of imagery motor training on torque production of ankle plantar flexor muscles, *Muscle Nerve* 28:168-173, 2003.

STUDY QUESTIONS

1 What functional purpose does pennation architecture serve within a muscle?

2 What tissues within a muscle are most responsible for the shape of the whole muscle's (a) passive, (b) active, and (c) total length-tension curve?

3 How does an activated muscle generate force without an actual shortening of its myofilaments?

4 The duration of a single action potential can be as little as 10 msec as it propagates along the muscle fiber. With such a short duration, how can a muscle develop and sustain a state of tetanization?

5 Define *muscle fatigue*. Explain how electromyographic amplitude can be used to detect the onset of muscle fatigue in a prolonged submaximal-effort muscle contraction.

6 What factors limit the ability of a muscle's electromyographic amplitude to be predictive of its relative force output in a freely activated muscle?

7 Define *physiologic cross-sectional area*.

8 Explain why internal torque produced by a muscle during isometric activation changes with a change in joint angle.

9 Consider the plot depicted in Figure 3-16.

a Explain possible reasons why the peak torque of the knee extensor muscles exceeds that of the knee flexor muscles, regardless of the velocity of muscle activation.

b Describe possible physiologic reasons for the nearly 40% reduction in peak torque of the knee extensor muscles at contraction velocities of 60 to 240 degrees/sec.

10 Describe the two fundamental strategies used by the nervous system to gradually increase muscle force.

11 Define *motor unit*. What is the Henneman Size Principle?

12 Describe how it is physiologically possible for a person to demonstrate clinically measurable increases in muscle strength *before* signs of muscle hypertrophy.

13 Explain how an otherwise healthy muscle within an immobilized limb can experience a relative transformation toward faster twitch characteristics.

14 What is the primary cause of reduced strength in healthy, aged persons?

15 What are some methods used to minimize unwanted "electrical noise" during collection of electromyographic signals?

⊖ *Answers to the study questions can be found on the Evolve website.*

4

Biomechanical Principles

PETER R. BLANPIED, PT, PhD
DEBORAH A. NAWOCZENSKI, PT, PhD

CHAPTER AT A GLANCE

Many treatment approaches used in physical rehabilitation depend on accurate analyses and descriptions of human movement. From the evaluation of these analyses and descriptions, impairments and functional limitations can be identified, diagnoses and prognoses of movement dysfunctions can be formulated, interventions can be planned, and progress can be evaluated. But human movement is often quite complex, frequently being influenced by a dizzying interplay of environmental, psychologic, physiologic, and mechanical factors. Most often, analyzing complex movements is simplified by starting with a basic evaluation of forces acting from within and outside of the body, and studying the effects of these forces on hypothetically rigid body segments. Newton's laws of motion help to explain the relationship between forces and their effect on individual joints, as well as on the entire body. Even at a basic level of analysis, this information can be used to guide treatment decisions and to understand mechanisms of injury. A simple planar force and torque analysis, for example, provides an estimate of hip joint forces during a straight-leg–raising exercise that may need to be modified in the presence of arthritis or injury. Practicing rehabilitation specialists rarely perform some of the more complex computations described in this chapter; however, understanding the conceptual framework of the computations, appreciating the magnitude of forces that exist within the body, and applying the concepts contained in this chapter are essential to understanding rehabilitation techniques. Such understanding makes clinical work interesting and provides the clinician with a flexible, varied, and rich source for treatment ideas.

NEWTON'S LAWS: UNDERLYING PRINCIPLES OF BIOMECHANICS

Biomechanics is the study of forces that are applied to the outside and inside of the body and the body's reaction to those forces. In the seventeenth century, Sir Isaac Newton observed that forces were related to mass and motion in a very predictable way. His *Philosophiae Naturalis Principia Mathematica* (1687) provided the basic laws and principles of mechanics that form the cornerstone for understanding human movement. These laws, referred to as the *law of inertia*, the *law of acceleration*, and the *law of action-reaction*, are collectively known as the *laws of motion* and form the framework from which advanced motion analysis techniques are derived.

Newton's Laws of Motion

This chapter uses Newton's laws of motion to introduce techniques for analysis of the relationship between the forces applied to the body and the consequences of those forces on human motion and posture. (Throughout the chapter, the term *body* is used when elaborating on the concepts related to the laws of motion and the methods of quantitative analysis. The reader should be aware that this term could also be used interchangeably with the entire human body; a segment or part of the body, such as the forearm segment; an object, such as a weight that is being lifted; or the system under consideration, such as the foot-floor interface. In most cases the simpler term, *body*, is used when describing the main concepts.) Newton's laws are described for both linear and rotational (angular) motion (Table 4-1).

NEWTON'S FIRST LAW: LAW OF INERTIA

Newton's first law states that a body remains at rest or at a constant linear velocity except when compelled by an external force to change its state. This means a force is required to start, stop, slow down, speed up, or alter the direction of *linear motion*. The application of Newton's first law to *rotational motion* states that a body remains at rest or at a constant angular velocity around an axis of rotation unless compelled by an external torque to change its state. This means a torque is required to start, stop, slow down, speed up, or alter the direction of *rotational motion*. Whether the motion is linear or rotational, Newton's first law describes the case in which a body is in equilibrium. A body is in *static equilibrium* when its linear and rotational velocities are zero—the body is not moving. Conversely, the body is in *dynamic equilibrium* when its linear and/or its rotational velocity is *not* zero, but is constant. In all cases of equilibrium, the linear and rotational *accelerations* of the body are zero.

Key Terms Associated with Newton's First Law
- Static equilibrium
- Dynamic equilibrium
- Inertia
- Mass
- Center of mass (gravity)
- Mass moment of inertia

Newton's first law is also called the law of inertia. *Inertia* is related to the amount of energy required to alter the velocity of a body. The inertia of a body is directly proportional to its *mass* (i.e., the amount of matter constituting the body). For example, more energy is required to speed up or slow down a moving 15-pound dumbbell than a 10-pound dumbbell.

Each body has a point, called the *center of mass*, about which its mass is evenly distributed in all directions. When subjected to gravity, the center of mass of a body closely coincides with its *center of gravity*. The center of gravity is the point about which the effects of gravity are completely balanced. The center of mass of the human body in the anatomic position lies just anterior to the second sacral vertebra, but the exact position of the center of mass will change as a person changes his or her body position.

In addition to the human body as a whole, each segment, such as the arm or trunk, also has a defined center of mass. In the lower extremity, for example, the major segments include the thigh, shank (lower leg), and foot. Figure 4-1 shows the center of mass of these segments for the lower extremities of a sprinter, indicated by black circles. The location of the center of mass within each segment remains fixed, approximately at its midpoint. In contrast, however, the location of the center of mass of the *entire* lower extremity changes with a change in spatial configuration of the segments

TABLE 4-1. Newton's Laws: Linear and Rotational Applications	
Linear Application	**Rotational Application**
First Law of Inertia	
A body remains at rest or at a constant linear velocity except when compelled by an external force to change its state.	A body remains at rest or at a constant angular velocity around an axis of rotation unless compelled by an external torque to change its state.
Second Law of Acceleration	
The linear acceleration of a body is directly proportional to the force causing it, takes place in the same direction in which the force acts, and is inversely proportional to the mass of the body.	The angular acceleration of a body is directly proportional to the torque causing it, takes place in the same rotary direction in which the torque acts, and is inversely proportional to the mass moment of inertia of the body.
Third Law of Action-Reaction	
For every force there is an equal and opposite directed force.	For every torque there is an equal and opposite directed torque.

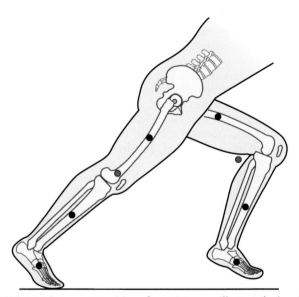

FIGURE 4-1. Lower extremities of a sprinter are illustrated, showing the centers of mass for the thigh, shank (lower leg), and foot segments as black circles. The center of mass for each lower extremity is shown as a red circle. The center of mass of the sprinter's left lower extremity exists outside of the body. The axis of rotation of the right hip is indicated by the smaller green circle.

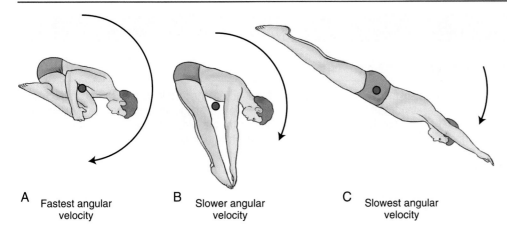

A   Fastest angular
    velocity

B   Slower angular
    velocity

C   Slowest angular
    velocity

FIGURE 4-2. A diver illustrates an example of how the mass moment of inertia around a medial-lateral axis *(red circle)* can be altered through changes in position of the extremities. In position **A,** the diver decreases the mass moment of inertia, which increases the angular velocity of the spin. In positions **B** and **C,** the extremities are positioned progressively farther from the axis, and the angular velocity is progressively slower.

(compare red circles in Figure 4-1). As shown for the left (flexed) lower extremity, the specific configuration of the segments can displace the center of mass of the lower limb *outside* the body. Additional information regarding the center of mass of body segments is discussed later in this chapter under the topic of anthropometry.

The *mass moment of inertia* of a body is a quantity that indicates its resistance to a change in *angular velocity.* Unlike inertia, its linear counterpart, the mass moment of inertia depends not only on the mass of the body, but, perhaps more important, on the distribution of its mass with respect to an axis of rotation.[7] (Mass moment of inertia is often indicated by I and is expressed in units of kilograms-meters squared [kg-m^2]). Because most human motion is angular rather than linear, the concept of mass moment of inertia is very relevant and important. Consider again the two positions of the lower extremities of the sprinter in Figure 4-1. Within each segment, the individual centers of mass of the thigh, shank, and foot are in the same location in both lower extremities; however, because of the different degrees of knee flexion, the *distances* of the centers of mass of the shank and foot segments have changed relative to the hip joint. As a consequence the mass moment of inertia of each entire limb changes; the right extended (and "longer") lower extremity has a greater mass moment of inertia than the left. (Another way of conceptualizing the increase is to note that as the knee extends, the center of mass of the entire right lower extremity, depicted by the red circle, moves farther from the hip, thereby increasing its mass moment of inertia.) The ability to actively change an entire limb's mass moment of inertia can profoundly affect the muscle forces and joint torques necessary for movement. For example, during the swing phase of running, the entire lower limb functionally shortens by the combined movements of knee flexion and ankle dorsiflexion (as in the left lower extremity in Figure 4-1). The lower limb's reduced mass moment of inertia reduces the torque required by the hip muscles to accelerate and decelerate the limb during swing phase. This concept can be readily appreciated during the swing phase while running with the knees held nearly extended (increased I), or almost fully flexed (decreased I).

The concept of mass moment of inertia applies to both rehabilitation and recreational settings. Consider, for example, the design of a prosthesis for the person with a lower limb amputation. The use of lighter components in the foot prosthesis, for example, not only reduces the overall mass (and weight) of the prosthesis, but also results in a change in the distribution of the mass to a more proximal location in the leg. As a result, less resistance is imposed on the remaining limb during the swing phase of gait. The benefit of these lighter components is realized in terms of lessened energy requirements for the person with an amputation. Changing footwear can also make a difference. Consider changes in the mass moment of inertia and resultant required torques for gait when the person changes from wearing a lightweight tennis shoe to a wearing a heavy winter boot.

Athletes often attempt to control the mass moment of inertia of their entire body by altering the position of their individual body segments relative to the axis of rotation. This concept is well illustrated by divers who reduce their moment of inertia in order to successfully complete multiple somersaults while in the air (Figure 4-2, *A*). The athlete can assume an extreme "tuck" position by placing the head near the knees, holding the arms and legs tightly together, thereby bringing their segments' centers of gravity closer to the axis of rotation. Based on the principle of "conservation of angular momentum," reducing the body's mass moment of inertia results in an increased angular velocity. Conversely, the athlete could slow the rotation by assuming a "pike" (see Figure 4-2, *B*) position and increasing the body's moment of inertia, or assuming a "layout" position (see Figure 4-2, *C*), which maximizes the body's mass moment of inertia and greatly slows the body's angular velocity.

NEWTON'S SECOND LAW: LAW OF ACCELERATION

Force (Torque)-Acceleration Relationship

Newton's second law states that the linear acceleration of a body is directly proportional to the force causing it, takes place in the same direction in which the force acts, and is inversely proportional to the mass of the body. Newton's second law generates an equation that relates force (F), mass (m), and acceleration (a) (Equation 4.1). Conceptually, Equation 4.1 defines a *force-acceleration relationship.* Considered a cause-and-effect relationship, the left side of the equation, force (F), can be regarded as a cause because it represents a pull or push exerted on a body; the right side, m × a, represents the effect of the pull or push. In this equation, ΣF designates the sum of, or net, forces acting on a body. If the

---

Newton's Second Law of Linear Motion Quantifying a Force
$$\Sigma F = m \times a \qquad \textbf{(Equation 4.1)}$$

A Closer Mathematic Look at the Concept of Mass Moment of Inertia

Thus far in this chapter, the concept of mass moment of inertia (I) has been described primarily from a functional standpoint. It may be instructive, however, to consider this physical property from a more mathematic perspective. I is formally defined in the following equation, in which n indicates the number of particles in a body, m_i is the mass of each particle in the body, and r_i is the distance of each particle to the axis of rotation.

Mass Moment of Inertia

$$I = \sum_{i=1}^{n} m_i r_i^2 \qquad \textbf{(Equation 4.2)}$$

As a way to further explore Equation 4.2, it will be used to determine how the grip applied to a baseball bat dramatically affects its mass moment of inertia and therefore the difficulty in swinging the bat. The bat illustrated in Figure 4-3 is considered to consist of six point masses (m_1 to m_6), ranging from 0.1 to 0.225 kg, each located 0.135 m from another. During the swing the batter rotates the bat; for illustration purposes the axis of this rotation is positioned as Y_1 (red line). If the bat is not sized correctly for the batter, the batter will often "choke up" by shifting his or her grip farther down the bat; again, for illustration purposes, the axis is now positioned as Y_2 (blue line). The calculations shown in the box demonstrate how the distribution of the mass particles, relative to a given axis of rotation, dramatically affects the mass moment of inertia of the rotating bat. First consider Y_1 as the axis of rotation. The mass moment of inertia of the bat is determined using Equation 4.2 and substituting known values. Next, consider Y_2 as the axis of rotation. The important point here is that the mass particles are distributed differently when each axis is considered separately. As seen in the calculations, the mass moment of inertia when considering Y_2 as the axis is 58% of that if Y_1 is the considered axis. This means that the batter could achieve the same angular acceleration with 58% less torque. Or, for the same torque, the bat would accelerate 1.72 times as fast. This is a significant functional advantage gained by choking up on the bat; the bat is easier to swing, although its mass and weight have not changed. The reason for the reduced moment of inertia is that mass points m_2 through m_6 are closer to the Y_2 axis. This is very significant mathematically when one considers that the mass moment of inertia of each point is related to the square of the distance to the axis.

Y_1 Axis of Rotation

$$
\begin{aligned}
I &= \sum_{i=1}^{n} m_i r_i^2 \\
&= m_1(r_1)^2 + m_2(r_2)^2 + m_3(r_3)^2 + m_4(r_4)^2 + m_5(r_5)^2 + m_6(r_6)^2 \\
&= 0.1\,kg\,(0.0\,m)^2 + 0.1\,kg\,(0.135\,m)^2 + 0.1\,kg\,(0.270\,m)^2 + \\
&\quad 0.15\,kg\,(0.405\,m)^2 + 0.175\,kg\,(0.54\,m)^2 + 0.225\,kg\,(0.675\,m)^2 \\
&= 0.187\,kg\text{-}m^2
\end{aligned}
$$

Y_2 Axis of Rotation

$$
\begin{aligned}
I &= \sum_{i=1}^{n} m_i r_i^2 \\
&= m_1(r_1)^2 + m_2(r_2)^2 + m_3(r_3)^2 + m_4(r_4)^2 + m_5(r_5)^2 + m_6(r_6)^2 \\
&= 0.1\,kg\,(0.135\,m)^2 + 0.1\,kg\,(0.0\,m)^2 + 0.1\,kg\,(0.135\,m)^2 + \\
&\quad 0.15\,kg\,(0.270\,m)^2 + 0.175\,kg\,(0.405\,m)^2 + 0.225\,kg\,(0.54\,m)^2 \\
&= 0.109\,kg\text{-}m^2
\end{aligned}
$$

The mass moment of inertia of human body segments is more difficult to determine than for the baseball bat, although they are based on the same mathematic principle. Much of the difficulty stems from the fact that segments in the human body are made up of different tissues, such as bone, muscle, fat, and skin and are not of uniform density. Values for the mass moment of inertia for each body segment have been generated from cadaver studies, mathematic modeling, and various imaging techniques.[3,8]

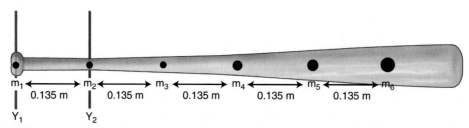

FIGURE 4-3. A baseball bat is shown with a potential to rotate around two separate axes of rotation (Y_1, Y_2). The set of calculations associated with each axis of rotation shows how the distribution of mass relative to the axis of rotation affects the mass moment of inertia. The bat is assumed to consist of six mass points (m_1 to m_6), ranging from 0.1 to 0.225 kg, located at equal distances from one another.

sum of the forces acting on a body is zero, acceleration is also zero and the body is in linear equilibrium. As previously discussed, this case is described by Newton's first law. If, however, the net force produces acceleration, the body will accelerate in the direction of the resultant force. In this case, the body is no longer in equilibrium.

Force is measured in newtons, where 1 newton (N) = 1 kg-m/sec².

The rotary or angular counterpart to Newton's second law states that a *torque* will cause an *angular acceleration* of a body around an axis of rotation. Furthermore, the *angular* acceleration of a body is directly proportional to the *torque* causing it, takes place in the same *rotary* direction in which the *torque* acts, and is inversely proportional to the *mass moment of inertia* of the body. (The italicized words denote the essential differences between the linear and angular counterparts of this law.) For the rotary condition, Newton's second law generates an equation that relates the torque (T), mass moment of inertia (I), and angular acceleration (α) (Equation 4.3). (This chapter uses the term *torque*. The reader should be aware that this term is interchangeable with terms *moment* and *moment of force*.) In this equation, ΣT designates the sum of, or net, torques acting to rotate a body. Conceptually, Equation 4.3 defines a *torque–angular acceleration relationship*. Within the musculoskeletal system, the primary torque producers are muscles. A contracting biceps muscle, for example, produces a net internal flexion torque at the elbow. Neglecting external influences such as gravity, the angular acceleration of the rotating forearm is proportional to the internal torque (i.e., the product of the muscle force and its internal moment arm) but is inversely proportional to the mass moment of inertia of the forearm-and-hand segment. Given a constant internal torque, the forearm-and-hand segment with the smaller mass moment of inertia will achieve a greater angular acceleration than one with a larger mass moment of inertia. (A smaller mass moment of inertia can be achieved by moving a cuff weight from the wrist to the mid-forearm, for example.) Understand that this inertial resistance to the angular acceleration of the limb applies even in the absence of gravity. For example, consider the positions of the lower limb in Figure 4-1 but with the person on his or her side in a "gravity eliminated" position. Because of changes in the mass moment of inertia, less muscular effort will be required to flex the hip with the knee also flexed than with the knee extended.

Newton's Second Law of Rotary Motion Quantifying a Torque
$$\Sigma T = I \times \alpha \qquad \textbf{(Equation 4.3)}$$

Torque is expressed in newton-meters, where 1 Nm = 1 kg-m^2 × radians/sec^2.

Impulse-Momentum Relationship

Additional relationships can be derived from Newton's second law through the broadening and rearranging of Equations 4.1 and 4.3. One such relationship is the *impulse-momentum relationship*.

Acceleration is the rate of change of velocity ($\Delta v/t$). Substituting this expression for linear acceleration in Equation 4.1 results in Equation 4.4. Equation 4.4 can be further rearranged to Equation 4.5.

$F = m \times \Delta v/t$	**(Equation 4.4)**
$F \times t = m \times \Delta v$	**(Equation 4.5)**

Application of a linear impulse (force multiplied by time) leads to a change in linear momentum (mass multiplied by a change in linear velocity).

The product of mass and velocity on the right side of Equation 4.5 defines the momentum of a moving body. *Momentum* describes the quantity of motion possessed by a

body. Momentum is generally represented by the letter *p* and has units of kilogram-meters per second (kg-m/sec). An *impulse* is a force applied over a period of time (the product of force and time on the left side of Equation 4.5). The linear momentum of an object such as a moving car is changed by the application of a force over a given time. When a quick change in momentum is required (during an emergency stop, for instance), a very large brake force is applied for a short time. Less brake force for the same time, or the same brake force for even less time, results in a smaller change in momentum. Impulse and momentum are vector quantities. Equation 4.5 defines the linear *impulse-momentum relationship*.

The impulse-momentum relationship provides another perspective from which to study human performance, as well as to gain insight into injury mechanisms. At certain locations the body develops mechanisms and structures to lessen peak external load forces. For example, when landing from a jump, peak forces can be reduced throughout the joints of the lower extremities if the impact of the landing is prolonged by more "give" in the muscles—through a lower level and prolonged eccentric activation. As another example, as the foot contacts the ground during normal gait, the fat pad over the plantar surface of the calcaneus cushions the interaction between the foot and the ground and works to decrease peak reaction forces. Running footwear often augments this function with shock-absorbing outsoles to further cushion the impact of the foot on the ground. Bicycle helmets, rubber or springed flooring, and protective padding are additional examples of equipment designs intended to reduce injuries by increasing the *duration* of impact in order to minimize the peak force of the impact.

Newton's second law involving torque can also apply to the rotary case of the impulse-momentum relationship. Similar to the substitutions and rearrangements for the linear relationship, the angular relationship can be expressed by substitution and rearrangement of Equation 4.3. Substituting $\Delta\omega/t$ (rate of change in angular velocity) for α (angular acceleration) results in Equation 4.6. Equation 4.6 can be rearranged to Equation 4.7–the angular equivalent of the impulse-momentum relationship. Torque and angular momentum are also vector quantities.

$T = I \times \Delta\omega/t$	**(Equation 4.6)**
$T \times t = I \times \Delta\omega$	**(Equation 4.7)**

Application of an angular impulse (torque multiplied by time) leads to a change in angular momentum (mass moment of inertia times a change in angular velocity).

Work-Energy Relationship

To this point, Newton's second law has been described using (1) the force (torque)-acceleration relationship (Equations 4.1 and 4.3) and (2) the impulse-momentum relationship (Equations 4.4 through 4.7). Newton's second law can also be restated to provide a *work-energy relationship*. This third approach can be used to study human movement by analyzing the extent to which work causes a change in an object's energy. Work occurs when a force or torque operates over some linear or angular displacement. *Work (W)* in a linear

SPECIAL FOCUS 4-2

A Closer Look at the Impulse-Momentum Relationship

Numerically, an impulse can be calculated as the product of the average force (N) and its time of application. Impulse can also be represented graphically as the area under a force-time curve. Figure 4-4 displays a force-time curve of the horizontal component of the anterior-posterior shear force applied by the ground against the foot *(ground reaction force)* as an individual runs across a force plate embedded in the floor. The curve is biphasic: the posterior-directed impulse during initial floor contact is negative, and the anterior-directed impulse during propulsion is positive. If the two impulses (i.e., areas under the curves) are equal, the net impulse is zero, and there is no change in the momentum of the system. In this example, however, the posterior-directed impulse is greater than the anterior, indicating that the runner's forward momentum is decreased.

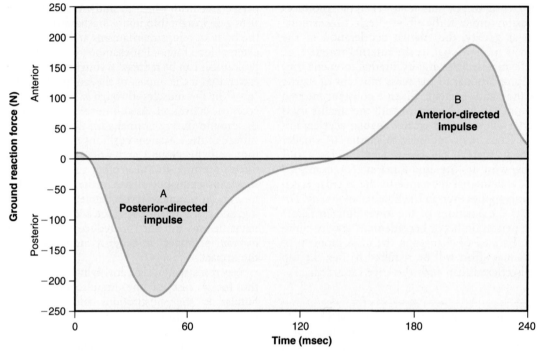

FIGURE 4-4. Graphic representation of the areas under a force-time curve showing the *(A)* posterior-directed and *(B)* anterior-directed impulses of the horizontal component of the ground reaction force while running.

sense is equal to the product of the magnitude of the *force (F)* applied against an object and the linear *displacement* of the object in the direction of the applied force (Equation 4.8). If no movement occurs in the direction of the applied force, no mechanical work is done. Similar to the linear case, angular work can be defined as the product of the magnitude of the torque (T) applied against the object, and the angular displacement of the object in the direction of the applied torque (Equation 4.9). Work is expressed in joules (J).

Related to the work-energy relationship, energy exists in two forms: potential energy and kinetic energy (see equations in box). *Potential energy* is a function of the height of the object's center of mass, within a gravitational field. Similar to momentum, *kinetic energy* is influenced by the object's mass and velocity, regardless of the influence of gravity. An object's angular kinetic energy is related to its mass moment of inertia (I) and its angular velocity. There is no angular correlate to potential energy.

Relationships between Work (W), Potential Energy (PE), and Kinetic Energy (KE)

$$W(\text{linear}) = F \times \text{linear displacement;} \qquad \textbf{(Equation 4.8)}$$
$$1 \text{ newton applied over } 1 \text{ m} = 1 \text{ J}$$

$$W(\text{angular}) = T \times \text{angular displacement;} \qquad \textbf{(Equation 4.9)}$$
$$1 \text{ Nm applied over } 1 \text{ radian} = 1 \text{ J}$$

$$PE = m \times g \times h, \text{ where } g = \text{gravity and } h = \text{height}$$

$$KE(\text{linear}) = \tfrac{1}{2} \, m \times v^2$$

$$KE(\text{angular}) = \tfrac{1}{2} \, I \times \omega^2$$

$$W(\text{angular or linear}) = KE_{\text{final}} - KE_{\text{initial}} + PE_{\text{final}} - PE_{\text{initial}}$$

Just as the impulse-momentum relationship describes the change in momentum caused by a force applied over a given *time,* the work-energy relationship describes the change in

Positive Work, Negative Work, and "Isometric Work"

As described, linear work is found by multiplying an applied force by the object's displacement in the direction of the applied force. Consider, for example, the linear force applied by the contracting elbow flexor muscles to flex the elbow and bring the hand to the mouth. In a linear sense, the work is the product of the muscles' contractile force and the distance the muscles shortened. In an angular sense, the rotary work is computed by the torque applied by the elbow flexors and the amount of flexion (in radians) occurring at the elbow. In this case the work is positive because the rotation of the forearm is in the same direction as the applied torque. In addition, the elbow flexors are shortening through concentric activation, and the work is being performed *by* the muscles. In contrast, when the elbow flexors are active, but the elbow is extending (e.g., when slowly lowering a weight), the elbow flexors are lengthening through an eccentric activation, and the work is being performed *on* the muscles. In this case, because the rotation is in a direction opposite to the applied torque, the work is negative. The final scenario is when the elbow flexors are active but no movement is taking place, as when a muscle is active isometrically. In this case, even though considerable metabolic energy may be expended, no mechanical work is being performed.

kinetic energy caused by a force applied over a given *displacement*. Using the example described earlier can illustrate the similarity in these concepts. The kinetic energy of an object such as a moving car is changed by the application of a force over a displacement. When a quick change in kinetic energy is required (e.g., for an emergency stop), a very large brake force is applied over a short displacement. Less brake force for the same displacement or the same brake force applied for even less displacement results in a smaller change in kinetic energy. Work and displacement are vector quantities.

The work-energy relationship does not take into account the *time* over which the forces or torques are applied. Yet in most daily activities it is often the rate of performing work that is important. The rate of performing work is defined as *power*. The ability for muscles to generate adequate power may be critical to the success of movement or to the understanding of the impact of a treatment intervention. On the basketball court, for example, it is often the player's vertical speed at takeoff that determines success in achieving a rebound. Another example of the importance of the rate of work can be appreciated in an elderly person with Parkinson's disease who must cross a busy street in the time determined by a pedestrian traffic signal.

Average power (P) is work (W) divided by time (Equation 4.10). Because work is the product of force (F) and displacement (d), the rate of work at any instant can be restated in Equation 4.11 as the product of force and velocity. Angular power may also be defined as in the linear case, using the angular analogs of force and linear velocity: torque (T) and angular velocity (ω), respectively (Equation 4.12). Angular power is often used as a clinical measure of muscle perfor-

mance. The mechanical power produced by the quadriceps, for example, is equal to the net internal torque produced by the muscle times the average angular velocity of knee extension. Power is often used to designate the net transfer of energy between active muscles and external loads. *Positive power* reflects the rate of work done by *concentrically active muscles* against an external load. *Negative power,* in contrast, reflects the rate of work done by the external load against *eccentrically active muscles.*

Power (P)	
Average power = W/t	(Equation 4.10)
Instantaneous power (linear) = $F \times v$	(Equation 4.11)
Instantaneous power (angular) = $T \times \omega$	(Equation 4.12)

Table 4-2 summarizes the definitions and units needed to describe many of the physical measurements related to Newton's second law.

NEWTON'S THIRD LAW: LAW OF ACTION-REACTION

Newton's third law of motion states that for every action there is an equal and opposite reaction. This law implies that every effect one body exerts on another is counteracted by an effect that the second body exerts on the first. The two bodies interact simultaneously, and the consequence is specified by Newton's law of acceleration ($\Sigma F = m \times a$); that is, each body experiences a different effect, and that effect depends on its mass. For example, a person who falls off the roof of a second-story building exerts a force on the ground, and the ground exerts an equal and opposite force on the person. Because of the huge discrepancies in mass between the earth and the person, the effect, or acceleration experienced by the person, is much greater than the effect "experienced" by the ground. As a result, the person may sustain significant injury.

Another example of Newton's law of action-reaction is the reaction force provided by the surface on which one is walking or standing. The foot produces a force against the ground, and in accordance with Newton's third law, the ground generates a *ground reaction force* in the opposite direction but of equal magnitude (Figure 4-5). The ground reaction force changes in magnitude, direction, and point of application on the foot throughout the stance period of gait. Newton's third law also has an angular equivalent. For example, during an isometric exercise, the internal and external torques are equal and in opposite rotary directions.

INTRODUCTION TO MOVEMENT ANALYSIS: SETTING THE STAGE FOR ANALYSIS

The previous section describes the nature of the cause-and-effect relationships between force and motion as outlined by Newton's laws. Now that this foundation has been established, this section introduces the steps and conventions used to formally analyze movement. Special attention is paid to the analysis of internal and external forces and torques and how these variables affect the body and its joints. This section should fully prepare the reader to follow the mathematic

TABLE 4-2. Physical Measurements Associated with Newton's Second Law

Physical Measurement	Linear Application Definition	Units	Conversion English → SI Units*	Rotational Application Definition	Units
Distance	Linear displacement	Meter (m)	ft × 0.305 = m	Angular displacement	Degrees (°)†
Velocity	Rate of linear displacement	Meters per second (m/sec)	ft/sec × 0.305 = m/sec	Rate of angular displacement	Degrees/sec
Acceleration	Rate of change in linear velocity	m/sec²	ft/sec² × 0.305 = m/sec²	Rate of change in angular velocity	Degrees/sec²
Mass	Quantity of matter in an object; influences the object's resistance to a change in linear velocity	Kilogram (kg)	lbm‡ × 0.454 = kg	Not applicable	
Mass moment of inertia	Not applicable		lbm-ft² × 0.042 = kg-m²	Quantity and distribution of matter around an object's axis of rotation; influences an object's resistance to a change in angular velocity	kg-m²
Force	A push or pull; mass times linear acceleration	Newton (N) = kg-m/sec²	lb × 4.448 = N	Not applicable	
Torque	Not applicable		ft-lb × 1.356 = Nm	A force times a moment arm; mass moment of inertia times angular acceleration	Newton-meter (Nm)
Impulse	Force times time	N-sec	lb-sec × 4.448 = N-sec ft-lb-sec × 1.356 = Nm-sec	Torque times time	Nm-sec
Momentum	Mass times linear velocity	kg-m/sec	lbm-ft/sec × 0.138 = kg-m/sec lbm-ft²/sec × 0.042 = kg-m²/sec	Mass moment of inertia times angular velocity	kg-m²/sec
Work	Force times linear displacement	Joule (J)	lb-ft × 1.356 = J	Torque times angular displacement	Joules (J)
Average power	Rate of linear work	Watt (W) = J/sec	lb-ft/sec × 1.356 = W	Rate of angular work	Watts (W) = J/sec

*To convert from English units to SI units, multiply the English value by the number in the table cell. To convert from SI units to English, divide by that number. If two equations are in the cell, the upper equation is used to convert the linear measure, and the lower equation is used to convert the angular measure.
†Radians, which are unitless, may be used instead of degrees (1 radian = about 57.3 degrees).
‡The English unit of a mass is a pound-mass (lbm) or slug.

solutions to three sample problems constructed in the next section.

Anthropometry

Anthropometry is derived from the Greek root *anthropos*, man, + *metron*, measure. In the context of human movement analysis, anthropometry may be broadly defined as the measurement of certain physical design features of the human body, such as length, mass, weight, volume, density, center of gravity, and mass moment of inertia. Knowledge of these parameters is often essential to conducting kinematic and kinetic analyses for both normal and pathologic motion. Variables such as mass and mass moment of inertia of individual limb segments, for example, are needed to determine the inertial properties that muscles must overcome to generate movement. Anthropometric information is also valuable

in the design of the work environment, furniture, tools, and sports equipment.

Much of the information pertaining to the body segments' center of gravity and mass moment of inertia has been derived from cadaver studies.[3,4] Other methods for deriving anthropometric data include mathematic modeling and imaging techniques, such as computed tomography and magnetic resonance imaging. Table 4-3 lists data on the weights of body segments and the location of the center of gravity. (The specific details contained in this table will be needed to solve selected parts of the biomechanical problems posed in Appendix I, Part B).

Free Body Diagram

The analysis of movement requires that all forces that act on the body be taken into account. Before any analysis, a *free*

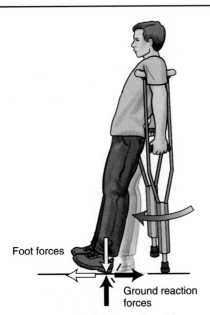

Foot forces

Ground reaction
forces

FIGURE 4-5. The action of the forces produced between the ground and foot are illustrated during the contact phase of the "swing-through" method of crutch-assisted walking. The action of the foot forces *(white arrows)* is counteracted by the ground reaction forces *(black arrows)*. If the horizontal component of the ground reaction force (caused by friction) is less than the horizontal component of the foot force, the foot will slide forward on the floor according to Newton's second law: $F = m \times a$.

body diagram is constructed to facilitate the process of solving biomechanical problems. The free body diagram is a "snapshot" or simplified sketch that represents the interaction between a body and its environment. The body under consideration may be a single rigid segment, such as the foot, or it may be several segments, such as the head, arms, and trunk. When the body consists of several segments, these are assumed to be rigidly connected together into a single rigid system.

A free body diagram requires that all relevant forces acting on the system are carefully drawn. These forces may be produced by muscle, gravity (as reflected in the weight of the segment), fluid, air resistance, friction, and ground reaction forces. Arrows are used to indicate force vectors.

How a free body diagram is configured depends on the intended purpose of the analysis. Consider the example presented in Figure 4-6. In this example, the free body diagram represents the shank-and-foot at the instant of initial heel contact during walking. The free body diagram involves figuratively "cutting through" the desired joint(s) to isolate or "free" the body of interest. In the example presented in Figure 4-6, the knee joint was cut through to isolate the shank-and-foot segment. The effects of active muscle force are usually distinguished from the effects of other soft tissues, such as passive tension created in stretched joint capsule and ligaments. Although the contribution of individual muscles acting across a joint may be determined, a single resultant muscle force (M) vector is often used to represent the sum total of all individual muscle forces. Other forces external to

TABLE 4-3. Anthropometric Data on Body Segments' Weight and Center of Gravity Location in the Anatomic Position (Extremity Data Are Unilateral Only)

Segment	Definition*	Segment Weight as a Percentage of Total Body Weight	Center of Gravity: Location from Proximal (or Cranial) End as a Percentage of Segment Length
Hand	Wrist axis to proximal interphalangeal (PIP) joint of third digit	0.6%	50.6%
Forearm	Elbow axis to ulnar styloid process	1.6%	43%
Upper arm	Glenohumeral axis to elbow axis	2.8%	43.6%
Forearm-and-hand	Elbow axis to ulnar styloid process	2.2%	68.2%
Total arm	Glenohumeral axis to ulnar styloid process	5%	53%
Foot	Lateral malleolus to head of second metatarsal	1.45%	50%
Shank (lower leg)	Femoral condyles to medial malleolus	4.65%	43.3%
Thigh	Greater trochanter to femoral condyles	10%	43.3%
Shank-and-foot	Femoral condyles to medial malleolus	6.1%	60.6%
Total leg	Greater trochanter to medial malleolus	16.1%	44.7%
Head-and-neck	Ear canal to C7-T1 (first rib)	8.1%	0% (at ear canal)
Trunk	Glenohumeral axis to greater trochanter	49.7%	50%
Trunk-head-and-neck	Glenohumeral axis to greater trochanter	57.8%	34%

Compiled results in Winter DA: *Biomechanics and motor control of human movement*, ed 3, New York, 2005, John Wiley & Sons. Mass moments of inertia are not included in this table because the focus of this chapter is limited to static analysis.

*Even though some definitions listed in this table do not represent the endpoints of the segment, they are easily identified locations on the human. The values for segment weight and center of gravity location in this table take into consideration the discrepancy between the definition of the segment and the true endpoints. For example, the segment definition for the forearm is the same for the forearm-and-hand, but the percentages listed for the segment weight and center of gravity location of the forearm-and-hand are higher, taking into consideration the mass of the hand.

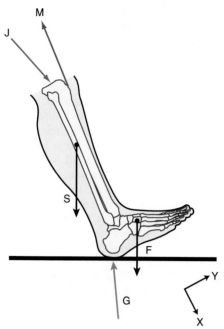

FIGURE 4-6. Free body diagram of the shank-and-foot at the instant of heel contact during walking. The segment is isolated by figuratively "cutting through" the knee joint. Relevant forces are drawn in as shown. The X-Y coordinate reference frame is placed so the X axis is parallel with the shank.

the system are added to the diagram, which may include the ground reaction force (G) and weight of the shank-and-foot segments (S and F). As specified by Newton's third law, the ground reaction force is the force developed in response to the foot striking the earth.

An additional force is identified in Figure 4-6: the *joint reaction force (J)*. This force includes joint contact forces as well as the net or cumulative effect of all other forces transmitted from one segment to another. Joint reaction forces are caused "in reaction" to other forces, such as those produced by activation of muscle, by passive tension in stretched periarticular connective tissues, and by gravity (body weight). As will be discussed, the free body diagram is completed by defining an X-Y coordinate reference frame and writing the governing equations of motion.

Clinically, reducing joint reaction force is often a major focus in treatment programs designed to lessen pain and prevent further joint degeneration in persons with arthritis. Frequently, treatments are directed toward reducing joint forces through changes in the magnitude of muscle activity and their activation patterns or through a reduction in the weight transmitted through a joint. Consider the patient with osteoarthritis of the hip joint as an example. The magnitude of the hip joint's reaction force may be decreased by having the person reduce walking velocity, thereby lessening the magnitude of muscle activation. Highly cushioned shoes may be recommended to reduce impact forces. In addition, a cane may be used to reduce forces through the hip joint.[1,10,13] If obesity is a factor, a weight-reduction program may be recommended.

STEPS FOR CONSTRUCTING THE FREE BODY DIAGRAM

The key elements needed to begin solving problems related to human movement are to determine the purpose of the analysis, identify the free body of interest, and indicate all the forces that act on that body. The following example presents steps to assist with construction of a free body diagram.

Consider the situation in which an individual is holding a weight out to the side, as shown in Figure 4-7. This free body is assumed to be in static equilibrium, and the sum of all forces and the sum of all torques acting on the body are equal to zero. One purpose of the analysis might be to determine how much muscle force is required by the glenohumeral joint abductor muscles (M) to keep the arm abducted to 90 degrees; another purpose might be to determine the magnitude of the glenohumeral joint reaction force (J) during this same activity.

Step I of constructing the free body diagram is to identify and isolate the free body under consideration. In this example, the glenohumeral joint was "cut through," and the free body is the combination of the entire arm and the resistance (exercise ball weight).

Step II involves defining a coordinate reference frame that allows the position and movement of a body to be defined with respect to a known point, location, or axis (see Figure 4-7, X-Y coordinate reference frame). More detail on establishing a reference frame is discussed ahead.

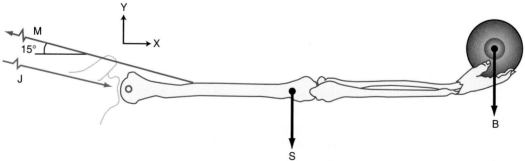

FIGURE 4-7. A frontal plane depiction of a free body diagram isolating the system as a right arm and ball combination: resultant shoulder abductor muscle force *(M)*; glenohumeral joint reaction force *(J)*; segment weight *(S)*; and ball weight *(B)*. The axis of rotation is shown as an open red circle at the glenohumeral joint. The X-Y coordinate reference frame is placed so the X axis is parallel with the upper extremity. (Modified from LeVeau BF: *Williams & Lissner's biomechanics of human motion*, ed 3, Philadelphia, 1992, Saunders.)

Step III involves identification and inclusion of all forces that act on the free body. Internal forces are those produced by muscle (M). External forces include the force of gravity on the mass of the exercise ball (B), as well as the force of gravity on the arm segment (S). Although not relevant to Figure 4-7, other examples of external forces could include forces applied by therapists, cables, resistance bands, the ground or other surface, air resistance, and orthotics. The forces are drawn on the figure while specifying their approximate point of application and spatial orientation. For example, vector S acts at the center of gravity of the upper extremity, a location determined by using anthropometric data, such as those presented in Table 4-3.

The direction of the muscle force (M) is drawn to correspond to the line of muscle pull and in a direction to generate torque that opposes the net torque produced by the external forces. In this example the torque produced by the external forces, S and B, tends to rotate the arm in a clockwise, adduction, or −Z direction. The line of force of M, therefore, in combination with its moment arm, creates a torque in a counterclockwise, abduction direction, or +Z direction. (The convention of using + or −Z to designate rotation direction is described ahead.)

Step IV of the procedure is to show the joint reaction force (J), in this case created across the glenohumeral articulation. Initially the direction of the joint reaction force may not be known, but, as explained later, it is typically drawn in a direction *opposite* to the pull of the dominant muscle force. The precise direction of J can be determined after static analysis is carried out and unknown variables are calculated.

Step V involves writing the three governing equations required to solve two-dimensional (2D) static equilibrium problems encountered in this chapter. The equations are: $\Sigma \text{Torque}_Z = 0$; $\Sigma \text{Force}_X = 0$; $\Sigma \text{Force}_Y = 0$. These equations are explained later in the chapter.

Steps in Constructing the Free Body Diagram

Step I: Identify and isolate the free body under consideration.
Step II: Establish a coordinate reference frame.
Step III: Draw the internal (muscular) and external forces that act on the system.
Step IV: Draw the joint reaction force.
Step V: Write the governing equations of motion.

SPATIAL REFERENCE FRAMES

In order to accurately describe motion or solve for unknown forces, a spatial reference frame needs to be established. This information allows the position and direction of movement of a body, a segment, or an object to be defined with respect to some known point, location, or segment's axis of rotation. If a reference frame is not identified, it becomes very difficult to interpret and compare measurements in clinical and research settings.

A spatial reference frame is arbitrarily established and may be placed inside or outside the body. Reference frames used to describe position or motion may be considered either relative or global. A *relative reference frame* describes the position of one limb segment with respect to an adjacent segment, such as the foot relative to the leg, the forearm relative to the upper arm, or the trunk relative to the thigh. A measurement is made by comparing motion of an anatomic landmark or coordinates between segments of interest. Goniometry provides one example of a relative reference frame used in clinical practice. Elbow joint range of motion, for example, describes a measurement using a relative reference frame defined by the long axes of the upper arm and forearm segments, with an axis of rotation through the elbow.

Relative reference frames, however, lack the information needed to define motion with respect to a fixed point or location in space. To analyze motion with respect to the ground, direction of gravity, or another type of externally defined reference frame in space, a *global (laboratory) reference frame* must be defined. Excessive anterior or lateral deviations of the trunk during gait are examples of a measurement made with respect to a global reference frame. In these examples, the position of the trunk is measured with respect to an external vertical reference.

Whether motion is measured via a relative or global reference frame, the location of a point or segment in space can be specified using a coordinate reference frame. In laboratory-based human movement analysis, the *Cartesian coordinate system* is most frequently employed. The Cartesian system uses coordinates for locating a point on a plane in 2D space by identifying the distance of the point from each of two intersecting lines, or in three-dimensional (3D) space by the distance from each of three planes intersecting at a point. A 2D coordinate reference frame is defined by two imaginary axes arranged perpendicular to each other *with the arrowheads pointed in positive directions*. The two axes (labeled, for example, X and Y) may be oriented in any manner that facilitates quantitative solutions (compare Figures 4-6 and 4-7, for example). A 2D reference frame is frequently used when the motion being described is predominantly planar (i.e., in one plane), such as knee flexion and extension during gait.

In most cases, human motion occurs in more than one plane. In order to fully describe this type of motion, a 3D coordinate reference frame is necessary. A 3D reference frame typically has three axes (X, Y, and Z), each perpendicular (or orthogonal) to another. As with the 2D system, *the arrowheads point in positive directions*. A universal convention for orienting this triplanar coordinate system in space is based on the *right-hand rule*. This rule is used throughout most quantitative biomechanical studies (see Special Focus 4-4).

Throughout most of this textbook, the terminology used to describe linear direction within planes (such as the direction of a muscle force or an axis of rotation around a joint) is less formal than that dictated by the right-hand rule. As described in Chapter 1, linear direction in space is loosely described relative to the human body standing in the anatomic position, using terms such as *anterior-posterior, medial-lateral,* and *vertical*. Although useful for most qualitative or anatomic-based descriptions, this convention is not well suited for quantitative analyses, such as those introduced later in this chapter. In these cases, the Cartesian coordinate system is used, and the orientation of its 3D axes is designated by the right-hand rule.

Rotary or angular movements or torques are often described as occurring in a plane, around a perpendicular axis of rota-

SPECIAL FOCUS 4-4

The "Right-Hand Rule": a Convention for Completely Describing the Spatial Orientation of a Three-Dimensional Coordinate Reference Frame

When a Cartesian coordinate system is set up, the direction or orientation of the orthogonal axes is not arbitrary. A convention must be used to facilitate the sharing of research from different laboratories throughout the worldwide scientific community. Using Figure 4-7 as an example, the X and Y axes are in the plane of the page or, relative to the subject, parallel with the frontal plane. (It is often most convenient, although not mandatory, to orient the X-Y axes so that the X axis is parallel with the body segment of interest.) A third axis, the Z axis, must be defined. Although not drawn in the figure, the Z axis is oriented perpendicular to the X-Y plane. By convention, the direction of the arrowheads shown on the X-Y coordinate reference frame indicates positive directions. As shown in Figure 4-7, positive X direction is to the right and positive Y direction is upward. The right-hand rule can be used to define the direction (+ or −) of the Z axis. Applying the *right-hand rule* is performed by laying the ulnar border of your *right* hand along the X axis, with the straight fingers pointing in a positive X direction (toward the ball on the model). Your hand should be positioned along the X axis so that when your fingers flex, they curl from the positive X direction toward the positive Y direction. Your extended thumb is pointing *out of the page,* thereby defining the direction of the positive Z axis. By necessity, the −Z axis is oriented perpendicularly *into the page.* Using the right-hand rule means that only two axes ever need to be defined and shown; use of the right-hand rule allows the third axis to be completely described.

SPECIAL FOCUS 4-5

Another Use of the "Right-Hand Rule": a Guide for Describing the Direction of Angular Motion and Torque

Another use of the right-hand rule is to define the *rotation direction* of angular motion and torque. Consider once again, the coordinate reference frame depicted in Figure 4-7. This reference frame indicates that the path of humeral motion (abduction) is in the X-Y (frontal) plane, around a perpendicular anterior-posterior axis (or, as described in Special Focus 4-4, the Z axis). The right-hand rule is again applied to Figure 4-7 as follows. Begin by aligning the ulnar side of your right hand parallel with the arm segment of the model, so that flexing your fingers curls them in the rotation path of shoulder abduction. The direction of your extended thumb points in the +Z direction, indicating abduction is a positive Z rotation. Shoulder adduction is in a negative Z direction.

This right-hand rule is also used to describe the rotary direction of torque. Again the right hand is used, curling your fingers in the path of motion produced by the torque. Returning to Figure 4-7, force M, produced by the shoulder abductor muscles, generates a +Z torque, whereas the shoulder adductor muscles (not shown) generate a −Z torque. With the coordinate reference frame oriented as shown, the shoulder abductors will always generate a +Z torque, regardless of concentric action (associated with a +Z motion), or eccentric action (associated with a −Z motion).

---

tion. In most kinesiologic literature, a segment's rotation direction is typically described by terms such as *flexion* and *extension* and, to a lesser extent, *clockwise* or *counterclockwise rotation.* Such a system is adequate for most clinical analysis and is used throughout this textbook. More formal, quantitative analysis, however, may be necessary to designate the direction of angular motion and torques. Such a system is based on the 3D Cartesian coordinate reference frame and uses another form of the *right-hand rule,*[4] as described in Special Focus 4-5.

In closing, analyzing movement within three dimensions is more complicated than in two dimensions, but it does provide a more comprehensive profile of human movement. There are excellent resources available that describe techniques for conducting 3D analysis, and some of these references are provided at the end of the chapter.[2,22,23] The quantitative analysis described in this chapter focuses on movements that are restricted to two dimensions.

Forces and Torques

As vector quantities, forces can be analyzed in different manners depending on the context of the analysis. Several forces can be combined into a single resultant force, repre-

sented by a single vector. Adding forces together uses processes called *vector composition.* Alternatively, a single force may be resolved or "decomposed" into two or more forces, the combination of which has the exact effect of the original force. This process of decomposing a single force into its components is termed *vector resolution.* The analysis of vectors using the processes of composition and resolution provides the means of understanding how forces rotate or translate body segments and subsequently cause rotation, compression, shear, or distraction at the joint surfaces.

GRAPHIC AND MATHEMATIC METHODS OF FORCE ANALYSIS

Composition and resolution of forces can be accomplished using graphic methods of analysis, or mathematic methods including the simple addition and subtraction of vectors or, in some cases, right-angle trigonometry. The graphic method of force analysis represents force or force component vectors as arrows and is performed by aligning them in a tip-to-tail fashion. A drawback to this method is that it requires a high degree of precision drawing. The length of the arrows must be precisely scaled to the magnitudes of the forces, and the orientations and directions of the arrows must match the forces exactly.

The trigonometric method does not require the same precision of drawing, and often provides a more accurate method of force analysis. This method uses rectangular components, and "right-angle trigonometry" to determine magnitudes and angles of forces. The trigonometric functions are based on the relationship that exists between the angles and sides of a right triangle. Refer to Appendix I, Part A, for a brief review of this material.

Proficiency in these techniques is needed to represent and subsequently calculate muscle and joint forces. Both graphic and trigonometric methods are illustrated next, but the remainder of the chapter will use only the trigonometric method.

Composition of Forces

Two or more forces are collinear if they share a common line of force. Vector composition allows several collinear forces to be simply combined graphically as a single *resultant force* (Figure 4-8). In Figure 4-8, *A,* the weight of the shank-and-foot segments (S) and the exercise weight (W) are added graphically by means of a ruler and a scale factor determined for the vectors. In this example, S and W act downward, so the resultant force (R) also acts downward and has the tendency to distract (pull apart) the knee joint. R is found graphically by aligning the tail of W to the tip of S. The resultant force R is depicted by the blue arrow that starts at the tail of S and ends at the tip of W. Figure 4-8, *B* illustrates a cervical traction device that employs a weighted pulley system, acting upward, opposite to the force created by gravity on the center of gravity of the head. Graphically, the tail of H is aligned to the tip of T, and the resultant arrow (R) starts at the tail of T and ends at the tip of H. The upward direction of R (in blue) indicates a net upward distraction force on the head and neck.

The collinear forces depicted in Figure 4-8 can also be combined by simply adding the force magnitudes of the vectors while paying attention to their directions. In Figure 4-8, *A,* the coordinate reference frame indicates both S and W are collinear and both acting entirely in a −Y direction. As indicated in the box, the result is found by adding the magnitudes of the collinear forces; in this case the result also acts

in a −Y direction. In Figure 4-8, *B,* the forces are collinear but acting in opposite directions (T acting in a +Y direction, H acting in a −Y direction). Adding the two magnitudes together while paying attention to the direction indicates the result is a 22 N force acting in a +Y direction. In this specific example, a traction force of at least 53 N is needed to offset the weight of the head. Using less force would result in no actual distraction (separation) or the cervical vertebrae. This technique may still, however, provide some therapeutic benefit.

Forces acting on a body may be coplanar (in the same plane), but they may not always be collinear. In this case the individual force vectors may be composed graphically using the *polygon method.* Figure 4-9 illustrates how the polygon method can be applied to a frontal plane model to estimate the joint reaction force on a prosthetic hip while the subject is standing on one limb. With the arrows drawn in proportion to their magnitude and in the correct orientation, the vectors of body weight (W) and hip abductor muscle force (M) are added in a tip-to-tail fashion (see Figure 4-9, *B*). The combined effect of the W and M vectors is determined by placing the tail of the M vector to the tip of the W vector. Completing the polygon yields the resultant force (R) starting at the tail of W and traveling to the tip of M. Figure 4-9, *B* illustrates this process, indicating the magnitude and direction of R. Note that R is equal in magnitude, but opposite in direction, to the prosthetic hip joint reaction force (J) depicted in Figure 4-9, *A.* An excessively large joint reaction force may, over time, contribute to premature loosening of the hip prosthesis.

A *parallelogram* can also be constructed to determine the resultant of two coplanar but noncollinear forces. Instead of placing the force vectors tip to tail, as discussed in the previous example, the resultant vector can be found by drawing a parallelogram based on the magnitude and direction of the two component force vectors. As with all graphic techniques of vector analysis, practice is required to be able to relatively accurately draw the size and orientation of the associated

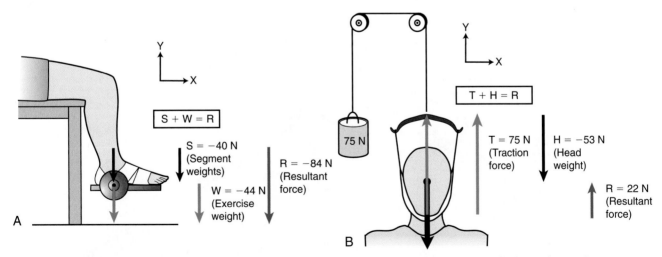

FIGURE 4-8. Vector composition of collinear forces. **A,** Two force vectors are acting on the knee: the weight of the shank-and-foot segment *(S)* and the exercise weight *(W)* applied at the ankle. These forces are added to determine the resultant force *(R).* The X-Y coordinate frame indicates +Y as upward; the negative sign assigned to the forces indicates a downward pull. **B,** The weight of the head *(H)* and traction force *(T)* act along the same line but in opposite directions. R is the algebraic sum of these vectors.

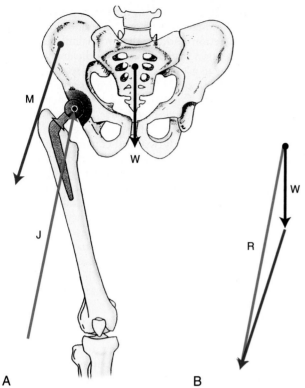

FIGURE 4-9. A, Three forces are shown acting on a pelvis that is involved in single-limb standing over a right prosthetic hip joint. The forces are hip abductor muscle force *(M)*, body weight *(W)*, and prosthetic hip joint reaction force *(J)*. **B,** The polygon (or tip-to-tail) method is used to determine the magnitude and direction of the resultant force *(R)*, based on the magnitude and direction of M and W. J in **A** is equal in magnitude and opposite in direction to R in **B.** (From Neumann DA: Hip abductor muscle activity in persons who walk with a hip prosthesis while using a cane and carrying a load, *Phys Ther* 79:1163, 1999.)

force vectors. Figure 4-10 provides an illustration of the parallelogram method used to combine several component vectors into one resultant vector. The component force vectors, F_1 and F_2 (black solid arrows), are generated by the pull of the flexor digitorum superficialis and profundus as they pass palmar (anterior) to the metacarpophalangeal joint. The diagonal, originating at the intersection of F_1 and F_2, represents the resultant force (R) (see Figure 4-10, thick red arrow). Because of the angle between F_1 and F_2, the resultant force tends to raise the tendons palmarly away from the joint. Clinically, this phenomenon is described as a *bowstringing force* because of the tendons' resemblance to a pulled cord connected to the two ends of a bow. Normally the bowstringing force is resisted by forces developed in the flexor pulley and collateral ligaments (see force P in blue in Figure 4-10). In severe cases of rheumatoid arthritis, for example, the bowstringing force may eventually rupture the ligaments and dislocate the metacarpophalangeal joints.

In summary, when two or more forces applied to a segment are combined into a single resultant force, the magnitude of the resultant force is considered equal to the sum of the component vectors. The resultant force can be determined graphically as summarized in the box.

Summary of How to Graphically Compose Force Vectors

- Collinear force vectors can be combined by simple addition or subtraction (see Figure 4-8).
- Nonparallel, coplanar force vectors can be composed by using the polygon (tip-to-tail) method (see Figure 4-9) or the parallelogram method (see Figure 4-10).

Resolution of Forces

The previous section illustrates the composition method of representing forces, whereby multiple coplanar forces acting

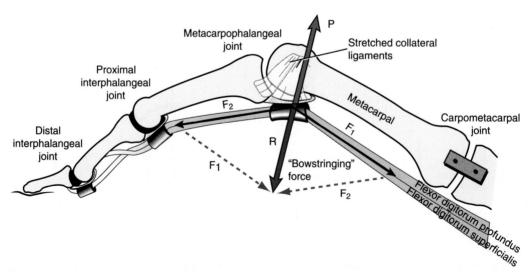

FIGURE 4-10. Parallelogram method is used to illustrate the effect of two force vectors (F_1 and F_2) produced by contraction of the flexor digitorum superficialis and profundus muscles across the metacarpophalangeal *(MCP)* joint. The resultant force *(R)* vector creates a bowstringing force resisted by the flexor pulley and collateral ligaments (force P in blue) at the MCP joint.

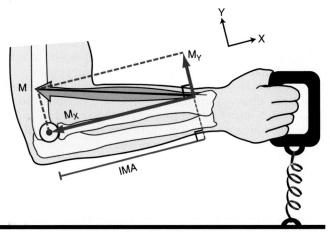

FIGURE 4-11. The muscle force *(M)* produced by the brachioradialis is represented as the hypotenuse (diagonal) of the rectangle. The X component *(M_X)* and the Y component *(M_Y)* are also indicated. The internal moment arm *(IMA)* is the perpendicular distance between the axis of rotation *(red circle)* and M_Y. The X-Y coordinate reference frame is placed so the X axis is parallel with the body segment of interest; the thin black arrowheads point toward positive directions.

Y Muscle Force Component	X Muscle Force Component
TABLE 4-4. Typical Characteristics of X and Y Components of a Muscle Force (as Illustrated in Figure 4-11)	
Acts perpendicular to a bony segment.	Acts parallel to a bony segment.
Often indicated as M_Y, depending on the choice of the reference system.	Often indicated as M_X, depending on the choice of the reference system.
Can cause translation of the bone and/or torque if moment arm >0.	Can cause translation of the bone. Often does not cause a torque because the chosen reference system reduces the moment arm to zero.
In a simple hinge joint model, M_Y creates a shear force between the articulating surfaces. (In reality, M_Y can create shear, compressive, and distractive forces depending on the anatomic complexity of the joint surfaces.)	In a simple hinge joint model, M_X creates a compression or distraction force between the articulating surfaces. (In reality, M_X can create shear, compressive, and distractive forces depending on the anatomic complexity of the joint surfaces.)

on a body are replaced by a single resultant force. In many clinical situations, however knowledge of the effect of the *individual components* that produce the resultant force may be more relevant to understanding the impact of these forces on motion and joint loading, as well as developing specific treatment strategies. *Vector resolution* is the process of replacing a single force with two or more forces that when combined are equivalent to the original force.

One of the most useful applications of the resolution of forces involves the description and calculation of the rectangular components of a muscle force. As depicted in Figure 4-11, the rectangular components of the muscle force are shown at right angles to each other and are referred to as the X and Y components (M_X and M_Y). (The X axis is set to be parallel to the long axis of the segment, with positive directed distally.) In the elbow model depicted in Figure 4-11, the *X component* represents the component of the muscle force that is directed *parallel* to the forearm. The effect of this force component is to compress and stabilize the joint or, in some cases, distract or separate the segments forming the joint. The X component of a muscle force does *not* produce a torque when it passes through the axis of rotation because it has no moment arm (see Figure 4-11, M_X). In the model depicted in Figure 4-11, the *Y component* represents the component of the muscle force that acts *perpendicularly* to the long axis of the segment. Because of the internal moment arm (see Chapter 1) associated with this force component, one effect of M_Y is to cause a rotation (i.e., produce a torque). In this example, the M_Y component may also create a shear force at the humeroradial joint that tends to cause a translation of the bony segment in the +Y direction.

For the purposes of this chapter, anatomic joints will be considered as frictionless hinge or pin joints with a stationary axis of rotation, allowing rotation in only one plane. Although it is fully recognized that even the simplest joint in the body is far more complex than this, consideration as pin joints

allows a much easier understanding of the concepts of this chapter. For example, if the X component of the muscle force (M_X) is directed *toward* the elbow joint as in Figure 4-11, it may be assumed that the muscle force causes compression of the radial head against the capitulum of the humerus. The Y component of the muscle force (M_Y in Figure 4-11) causes a shear, tending to move the forearm in the +Y direction (in this case upward and slightly posteriorly). As described later, these forces are opposed by the oppositely directed joint reaction forces. Table 4-4 summarizes the characteristics of the X and Y force components of a muscle, as illustrated in Figure 4-11.

CONTRASTING INTERNAL VERSUS EXTERNAL FORCES AND TORQUES

The previously described examples of resolving forces into X and Y components focused on the forces and torques produced by muscle. As described in Chapter 1, muscles, by definition, produce internal forces and torques. The resolution of forces into X and Y components can also be applied to *external forces* acting on the human body, such as those from gravity, physical contact, external loads and weights, and manual resistance as applied by a clinician. In the presence of an external moment arm, external forces produce an *external torque.* Generally, in a condition of equilibrium the external torque acts relative to the joint's axis of rotation in an opposite rotary direction as the net internal torque.

Figure 4-12 illustrates the resolution of both internal and external forces of an individual who is performing an isometric knee extension exercise. Three forces are depicted in Figure 4-12, *A:* the *internal* knee extensor muscle force (M), the *external* shank-and-foot segment weight (S), and the *external*

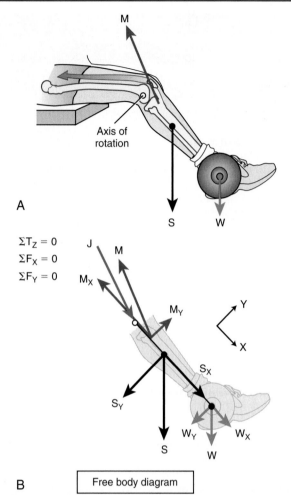

$\Sigma T_Z = 0$
$\Sigma F_X = 0$
$\Sigma F_Y = 0$

FIGURE 4-12. Resolution of internal forces *(red)* and external forces *(black and green)* for an individual performing an isometric knee extension exercise. **A,** The following resultant force vectors are depicted: muscle force *(M)* of the knee extensors; shank-and-foot segment weight *(S);* and exercise weight *(W)* applied at the ankle. **B,** The free body diagram shows the forces resolved into their X and Y components. The joint reaction force *(J)* is also shown *(blue).* In both **A** and **B,** the open circles mark the medial-lateral axis of rotation at the knee. (Vectors are not drawn to scale.) Observe that the X-Y coordinate reference frame is set so the X direction is parallel to the shank segment; thin black arrowheads point toward the positive direction.

exercise weight (W) applied at the ankle. Forces S and W act at the center of their respective masses.

Figure 4-12, *B* shows the free body diagram of the exercise performed in A, with M, S, and W resolved into their X and Y components. Assuming static rotary and linear equilibrium, the governing torque (T) and force (F) equations listed to the left of the figure may be used to solve unknown variables. This topic will be addressed in the final section of the chapter.

INFLUENCE OF CHANGING THE ANGLE OF THE JOINT

The relative magnitude of the X and Y components of internal and external forces applied to a bone depends on the position of the limb segment. Consider first how the change in angular position of a joint alters the *angle-of-insertion* of the muscle (see glossary, Chapter 1). Figure 4-13 shows the con-

stant magnitude biceps muscle force (M) at four different elbow joint positions, each with a different angle-of-insertion to the forearm (designated as α in each of the four parts of the figure). Note that each angle-of-insertion results in a different combination of M_X and M_Y force components. The M_X component creates compression force if it is directed *toward* the elbow, as in Figure 4-13, *A,* or distraction force if it is directed *away from* the elbow as in Figure 4-13, *C* and *D.* By acting with an internal moment arm (brown line labeled IMA), the M_Y *components* in Figure 4-13, *A* through *D* generate a +Z torque (flexion torque) at the elbow.

As shown in Figure 4-13, *A,* a relatively small angle-of-insertion of 20 degrees favors a relatively large X component force, which directs a larger percentage of the total muscle force to compress the joint surfaces of the elbow. Because the angle-of-insertion is less than 45 degrees in Figure 4-13, *A,* the magnitude of the M_X component exceeds the magnitude of the M_Y component. When the angle-of-insertion of the muscle is 90 degrees (as in Figure 4-13, *B*), 100% of M is in the Y direction and is available to produce an elbow flexion torque. At an angle-of-insertion of 45 degrees (Figure 4-13, *C*), the M_X and M_Y components have equal magnitude, with each about 71% of M. In Figure 4-13, *C* and *D,* the angle-of-insertion (shown to the right of M as α) produces a M_X component that is directed *away from* the joint, thereby producing a distracting or separating force on the joint.

In Figure 4-13, *A* through *D,* the internal torque is always in a +Z direction and is the product of M_Y and the internal moment arm (IMA). Even though the magnitude of M is assumed to remain constant throughout the range of motion, the change in M_Y (resulting from changes in angle-of-insertion) produces differing magnitudes of internal torque. Note that the +Z (flexion) torque ranges from 0.93 Nm at near full elbow flexion to 3.60 Nm at 90 degrees of elbow flexion—a near fourfold difference. This concept helps explain why people have greater strength (torque) in certain parts of the joint's range of motion. The torque-generating capabilities of the muscle depend not only on the angle-of-insertion, and subsequent magnitude of M_Y, but also on other physiologic factors, discussed in Chapter 3. These include muscle length, type of activation (i.e., isometric, concentric, or eccentric), and velocity of shortening or elongation of the activated muscle.

Changes in joint angle also can affect the amount of external or "resistance" torque encountered during an exercise. Returning to the example of the isometric knee extension exercise, Figure 4-14 shows how a change in knee joint angle affects the Y component of the external forces S and W. The external torque generated by gravity on the segment (S) and the exercise weight (W) is equal to the product of the external moment arm (brown line labeled EMA in *B* and *C*) and the Y component of the external forces (S_Y and W_Y). In Figure 4-14, *A,* no external torque exists in the sagittal plane because S and W force vectors are entirely in the +X direction (S_Y and $W_Y = 0$). The S and W vectors are directed through the knee's axis of rotation and therefore have no external moment arm. Because these external forces are pointed in the +X direction, they tend to distract the joint. Figure 4-14, *B* and *C* show how a greater external torque is generated with the knee fully extended (in *C*) compared with the knee flexed 45 degrees (in *B*). Although the magnitude of the external forces, S and W, are the same in all three cases, the −Z

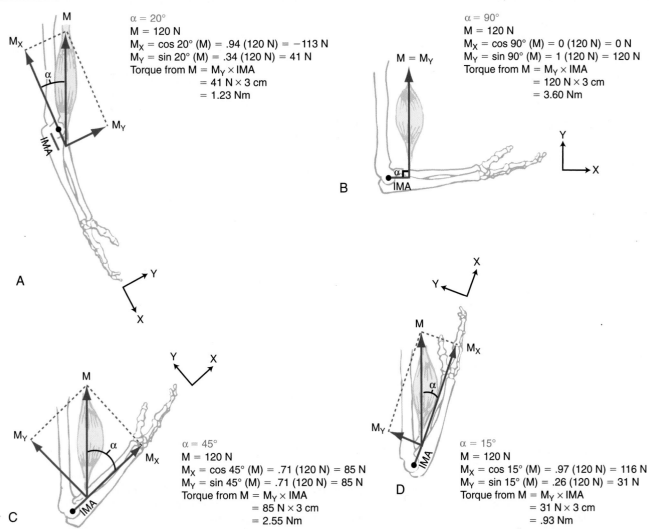

FIGURE 4-13. Changing the angle of the elbow joint alters the angle-of-insertion of the muscle to the forearm. These changes, in turn, alter the magnitude of the X (M_X) and Y (M_Y) components of the biceps muscle force *(M)*. Using trigonometric functions, the magnitudes of M_X and M_Y can be found for each position: **A,** angle-of-insertion of 20 degrees; **B,** angle-of-insertion of 90 degrees; **C,** angle-of-insertion of 45 degrees; and **D,** angle-of-insertion of 15 degrees. Although the magnitude of M is assumed to be constant (120 N), the changing magnitude of M_Y alters the internal torque significantly throughout the range of motion. The internal moment arm *(IMA)* is drawn as a brown line extending from the axis of rotation *(black dot)* to the point of application of M and remains constant throughout **A** to **D**. Note that the X-Y coordinate reference frame is set so the X direction is always parallel to the forearm segment; thin black arrowheads point toward the positive direction. (Modified from LeVeau BF: *Williams & Lissner's biomechanics of human motion,* ed 3, Philadelphia, 1992, Saunders.)

directed (flexion) external torque is greatest when the knee is in full extension. *As a general principle*, the external torque around a joint is greatest when the resultant external force vector intersects the bone or body segment at a *right angle* (as in Figure 4-14, *C*). When free weights are used, for example, external torque is generated by gravity acting vertically. Resistance torque from the weight is therefore greatest when the body segment is positioned horizontally. Alternatively, with use of a cable attached to a column of stacked weights, resistance torque from the cable is greatest in the position where the cable acts at a right angle to the segment. Note that this is often in a different position than where the torque caused by gravity acting on the segment is greatest. Resistive elastic bands and tubes present further complications, as resistance torque from these devices varies with the angle of the resis-

tance force vector and the amount of stretch in the device; both factors vary through a range of motion.[19,21]

COMPARING TWO METHODS FOR DETERMINING TORQUE AROUND A JOINT

In the context of kinesiology, a torque is the effect of a force tending to rotate a body segment around a joint's axis of rotation. *Torque is the rotary equivalent of a force.* Mathematically, torque is the product of a force and its moment arm and usually is expressed in units of newton-meters. Torque is a vector quantity, having both magnitude and direction.

Two methods for determining torque yield identical mathematic solutions. Understanding both methods provides valuable insight into the concept of torque, especially how it

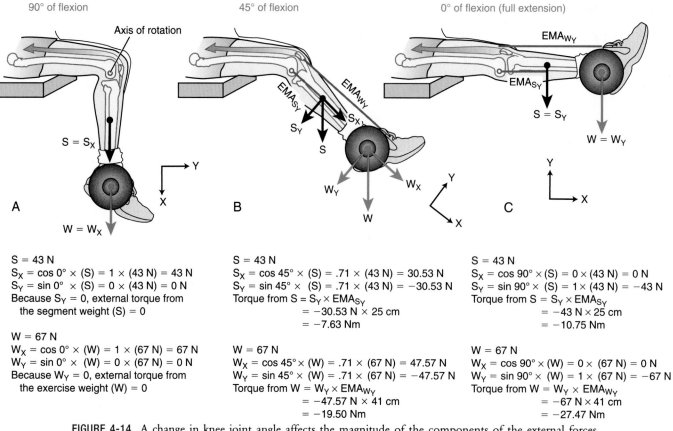

FIGURE 4-14. A change in knee joint angle affects the magnitude of the components of the external forces generated by the shank-and-foot segment weight *(S)* and exercise weight *(W)*. In **A,** all of W and S act in the +X direction and have no external moment arms to produce a sagittal plane external torque at the knee. In **B** and **C,** S_Y and W_Y act in a –Y direction, and each possesses an external moment arm (EMA_{S_Y} is equal to the external moment arm for S_Y; EMA_{W_Y} is equal to the external moment arm for W_Y). Different external torques are generated at each of the three knee angles. The X-Y coordinate reference frame is set so the X direction is parallel to the shank segment; thin black arrowheads point toward the positive direction.

relates to clinical kinesiology. The methods apply to both internal and external torque, assuming that the system in question is in rotational equilibrium (i.e., the angular acceleration around the joint is zero).

Internal Torque

The two methods for determining internal torque are illustrated in Figure 4-15. Method 1 calculates the internal torque as the product of M_Y and its internal moment arm (IMA_{M_Y}). Method 2 uses the entire muscle force (M) and therefore does not require this variable to be resolved into its rectangular components. In this method, internal torque is calculated as the product of the muscle force (the whole force, not a component) and IMA_M (i.e., the internal moment arm that extends perpendicularly between the axis of rotation and the line of action of M). Methods 1 and 2 yield the same internal torque because they both satisfy the definition of a torque (i.e., the product of a force and its associated moment arm). *The associated force and moment arm for any given torque must intersect each other at a 90-degree angle.*

External Torque

Figure 4-16 shows an external torque applied to the elbow through a resistance produced by an elastic band (depicted in green as R). The weight of the body segment is ignored in this example. Method 1 determines external torque as the product of R_Y times its external moment arm (EMA_{R_Y}). Method 2 uses the product of the band's entire resistive force (R) and its external moment arm (EMA_R). As with internal torque, both methods yield the same external torque because both satisfy the definition of a torque (i.e., the product of a resistance [external] force and its associated external moment arm). *The associated force and moment arm for any given torque must intersect each other at a 90-degree angle.*

MANUALLY APPLYING EXTERNAL TORQUES DURING EXERCISE AND STRENGTH TESTING

External or resistance torques are often applied manually during an exercise program. For example, if a patient is beginning a knee rehabilitation program to strengthen the quadriceps muscle, the clinician may initially apply manual resistance to the knee extensors at the midtibial region. As the patient's knee strength increases, the clinician can exert a greater force at the midtibial region, or the same force near the ankle.

Because external torque is the product of a force (resistance) and an associated external moment arm, an equivalent external torque can be applied by a relatively short external moment arm and a large external force, or a long external moment arm and a smaller external force. The knee extension resistance

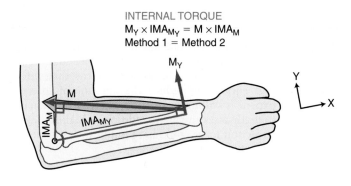

INTERNAL TORQUE
$M_Y \times IMA_{M_Y} = M \times IMA_M$
Method 1 = Method 2

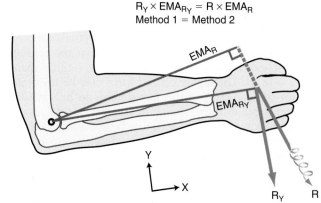

EXTERNAL TORQUE
$R_Y \times EMA_{R_Y} = R \times EMA_R$
Method 1 = Method 2

FIGURE 4-15. The internal (muscle-produced) flexion torque at the elbow can be determined using two different methods. Method 1 calculates torque as the product of the Y component of the muscle force (M_Y) times its internal moment arm (IMA_{M_Y}). Method 2 calculates torque as the product of the entire force of the muscle (M) times its internal moment arm (IMA_M). Both expressions yield equivalent internal torques. The axis of rotation is depicted as the open black circle at the elbow. The X-Y coordinate reference frame is set so the positive X direction is parallel to the forearm segment.

FIGURE 4-16. An external torque is applied to the elbow through a resistance generated by tension in a cable (R). The weight of the body segment is ignored. The external torque can be determined using two different methods. Method 1 uses the product of the Y component of the resistance (R_Y) times its external moment arm (EMA_{R_Y}). Method 2 calculates torque as product of the entire force of the resistance (R) times its external moment arm (EMA_R). Both expressions yield equivalent external torques. The axis of rotation is depicted as the open black circle at the elbow. The X-Y coordinate reference frame is set so the positive X direction is parallel to the forearm segment.

SPECIAL FOCUS 4-6

Designing Resistive Exercises So That the External and Internal Torque Potentials Are Optimally Matched

The concept of altering the angle of a joint is frequently used in exercise programs to adjust the magnitude of resistance experienced by the patient or client. It is often desirable to design an exercise program so that *the external torque matches the internal torque potential* of the muscle or muscle group. Consider a person performing a "biceps curl" exercise, shown in Figure 4-17, *A*. With the elbow flexed to 90 degrees, both the internal and external torque potentials are greatest, because the product of each resultant force (M and W) and their moment arms (IMA and EMA) are maximal. At this elbow position the internal and

external torque potentials are maximal as well as optimally matched. As the elbow position is altered in Figure 4-17, *B*, the external torque remains the same; however, the angle-of-insertion of the muscle is different, requiring a much larger muscle force, M, to produce the same internal +Z directed torque. Note the Y component of the muscle force (M_Y) in Figure 4-17, *B* has the same magnitude as the muscle force M in Figure 4-17, *A*. A person with significant weakness of the elbow flexor muscle may have difficulty holding an object in position *B* but may have no difficulty holding the same object in position *A*.

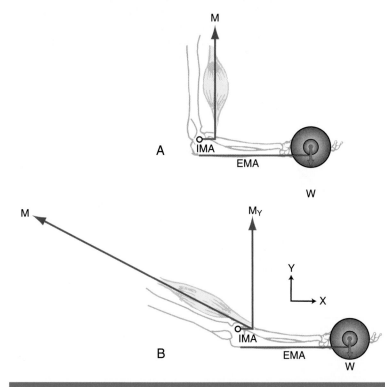

FIGURE 4-17. Changing the angle of elbow flexion can alter both internal and external torque potential. **A,** The 90-degree position of the elbow maximizes the potential for both the internal and the external torque. **B,** With the forearm horizontal and the elbow closer to extension, the external torque remains maximal but the overall biceps force (M) must increase substantially to yield sufficient M_Y force to support the weight. *EMA,* external moment arm; *IMA,* internal moment arm; *M,* muscle force; M_Y, Y component of the muscle force; *W,* exercise weight.

exercise depicted in Figure 4-18 shows that the same external torque (15 Nm) can be generated by two combinations of external forces and moment arms. Note that the resistance force applied to the leg is greater in Figure 4-18, *A* than in Figure 4-18, *B.* The higher contact force may be uncomfortable for the patient, and this factor needs to be considered during the application of resistance. A larger external moment arm, as shown in Figure 4-18, *B,* may be necessary if the clinician chooses to manually challenge a muscle group as potentially forceful as the quadriceps. Even using a long external moment arm, clinicians may be unable to provide enough torque to maximally resist large and strong muscle groups.[11]

A hand-held dynamometer is a device used to manually measure the maximal isometric strength of certain muscle groups. This device directly measures the force generated between the device and the limb during a maximal-effort muscle contraction. Figure 4-19 shows this device used to measure the maximal-effort, isometric elbow extension torque in an adult woman. The external force (R) measured by the dynamometer is in response to the internal force generated by the elbow extensor muscles (E). Because the test is performed isometrically, the measured external torque (R × EMA) will be equal in magnitude but opposite in direction to the actively generated internal torque (E × IMA). If the clinician is documenting external *force* (as indicated by the dial on the dynamometer), he or she needs to pay close attention to the position of the dynamometer relative to the person's limb. Changing the external moment arm of the device will alter the external force reading. This is shown by comparing the two placements of the dynamometer in Figure 4-19, *A* and *B.* The same elbow extension internal force (E) will result in two different external force readings (R). The longer external moment arm used in Figure 4-19, *A,* results in a lower external force than the shorter external moment arm used in Figure 4-19, *B.* On repeated testing, for example, before and after a strengthening program, the force dynamometer must be positioned with exactly the same external moment arm to allow a valid strength comparison to the prestrengthening values. Documenting external torques rather than forces does not require the external moment arm to be exactly the same for every testing session. The external moment arm does need to be measured each time, however, to allow conversion of the external force (as measured by the force dynamometer) to external torque (the product of the external force and the external moment arm).

Note also that although the elbow extension internal force and torque are the same in Figure 4-19, *A* and *B,* the joint reaction force (J) and external force (R) are higher in Figure

4-19, *B.* This means that the pressure between the force dynamometer pad and the patient's skin is higher and could potentially cause discomfort. In some cases the discomfort could be great enough to reduce the amount of internal torque the patient is willing to develop, thereby influencing a maximal strength assessment. In addition, a higher magnitude of joint reaction force could have implications in conditions of compromised articular cartilage.

INTRODUCTION TO BIOMECHANICS: FINDING THE SOLUTIONS

In the previous sections, concepts were introduced that provide the framework for quantitative methods of biomechanical analysis. Many approaches are applied when solving problems in biomechanics. These approaches can be employed to assess (1) the effect of a force at an instant in time *(force-acceleration relationship);* (2) the effect of a force applied over an interval of time *(impulse-momentum relationship);* and (3) the application of a force that causes an object to move through some distance *(work-energy relationship).* The particular approach selected depends on the objective of the analysis. The subsequent sections in this chapter are directed toward the analysis of forces or torques at one instant in time, or the *force (torque)-acceleration approach.*

When one considers the effects of a force, or forces, and the resultant acceleration at an instant in time, two situations can be defined. In the first case the effects of the forces cancel and there is no acceleration because the object is either stationary or moving at a constant velocity. This is the situation described previously as equilibrium and is analyzed using a branch of mechanics known as *statics.* In the second situation, linear and/or angular acceleration is occurring because the system is subjected to unbalanced forces or torques. In this situation the system is not in equilibrium, and analysis requires using a branch of mechanics known as *dynamics.* Static analysis is the simpler approach to problem solving in biomechanics and is the focus of this chapter. Although clinicians do not often mathematically complete the types of analyses contained in this chapter, a full appreciation of the biomechanics of normal and abnormal motion, including most treatment techniques, is facilitated through learning the components of the mathematic analysis. For example, recommendations for treatment of articular cartilage disorders are better made with consideration of the variables that influence compressive joint reaction force. Ligament reconstruction grafts often require a

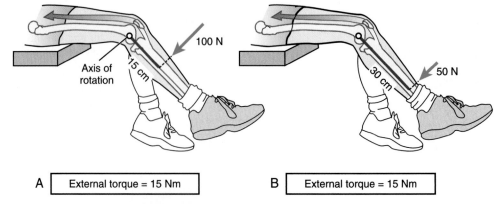

FIGURE 4-18. The same external torque (15 Nm) is applied against the quadriceps muscle by using a relatively large resistance (100 N) and small external moment arm **(A),** or a relatively small resistance (50 N) and large external moment arm **(B).** The external moment arms are indicated by the brown lines that extend from the medial-lateral axis of rotation at the knee.

Axis of rotation   15 cm   100 N

30 cm   50 N

A   External torque = 15 Nm

B   External torque = 15 Nm

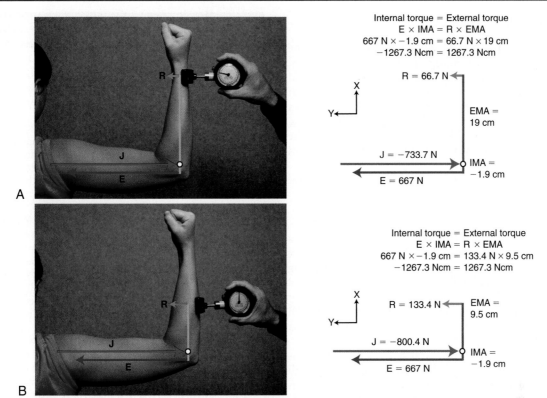

FIGURE 4-19. A dynamometer is used to measure the maximal, isometric strength of the elbow extensor muscles. The external moment arm *(EMA)* is the distance between the axis of rotation *(open circle)* and the point of external force *(R)* measured by the dynamometer. The different placement of the device on the limb creates different EMAs in **A** and **B.** Elbow extension force *(E)*, which is the same in **A** and **B,** generates equivalent internal torques through its internal moment arm *(IMA)*, which is equal in magnitude but opposite in direction to the external torques generated by the product of R and EMA. The joint reaction force *(J)*, shown in blue, is equal but opposite in direction to the sum of R + E. The distal application of the measuring device shown in **A** results in a longer EMA and a lower external force reading. Because R is less, J is also less. The more proximal application of the device in **B** results in a shorter EMA, a higher external force reading, and a greater J. Vectors are drawn to approximate scale. (The X-Y coordinate reference frame is set so the X direction is parallel to the forearm; thin black arrowheads point in positive directions. Based on conventions described in the next section [summarized in Box 4-1], the internal moment arm is assigned a negative number. This, in turn, appropriately assigns opposite rotational directions to the opposing torques.)

period of protective loading; this can be safely accomplished while strengthening muscles only if the magnitude and direction of muscle and joint forces are considered. The reader is encouraged to consider these types of clinical issues by answering the questions posed at the completion of each of the upcoming three sample problems.

Static Analysis

Biomechanical studies often induce conditions of static equilibrium in order to simplify the approach to the analysis of human movement. In static analysis the system is in equilibrium because it is not experiencing acceleration. As a consequence the sum of the forces and the sum of the torques acting on the system are zero. The forces and torques in any direction are completely balanced by the forces and torques acting in the opposite direction. Because in static equilibrium there is no linear or angular acceleration, the inertial effect of the mass and moment of inertia of the bodies can be ignored.

The force equilibrium equations, Equations 4.13 A and B, are used for static (uniplanar) translational equilibrium. In the case of static rotational equilibrium, the sum of the torques

around any axis of rotation is zero. The torque equilibrium equation, Equation 4.14, is also included. The equations previously depicted in Figure 4-19 provide a simplified example of static rotational equilibrium about the elbow. The muscle force of the elbow extensors (E) times the internal moment arm (IMA) creates a potential extension (clockwise, −Z) torque. This torque (product of E and IMA) is balanced by a flexion (counterclockwise, +Z) torque provided by the product of the transducer's force (R) and its external moment arm (EMA). Assuming no movement of the elbow, $\Sigma T_Z = 0$; in other words, the opposing torques at the elbow are assumed to be equal in magnitude and opposite in direction.

Governing Equations for Static Uniplanar Analysis: Forces and Torques Are Balanced

Force (F) Equilibrium Equations

$\Sigma F_X = 0$ **(Equation 4.13 A)**

$\Sigma F_Y = 0$ **(Equation 4.13 B)**

Torque (T) Equilibrium Equation

$\Sigma T_Z = 0$ **(Equation 4.14)**

GUIDELINES FOR PROBLEM SOLVING

The guidelines listed in Box 4-1 are necessary to follow the logic for solving the upcoming three sample problems. (Although most concepts listed in Box 4-1 have been described previously in this chapter, guideline 5 is new. This particular guideline describes the convention used to assign direction to moment arms.) In each of the three upcoming problems, an assumption of static equilibrium is required to solve the magnitude and direction of torque, muscle force, and joint reaction force.

Additional problem-solving examples and related clinical questions are available in Appendix I, Part B.

Problem 1

Consider the situation posed in Figure 4-20, *A*, in which a person generates an isometric elbow flexor muscle force at the elbow while holding a weight in the hand. Assuming equilibrium, the three unknown variables are the (1) internal (muscle-produced) elbow flexion torque, (2) elbow flexor muscle force, and (3) joint reaction force at the elbow. All abbreviations and pertinent data are included in the box associated with Figure 4-20.

To begin, a free body diagram and X-Y reference frame is constructed (see Figure 4-20, *B*). The axis of rotation and all moment arm distances are indicated. Although at this point the direction of the joint (reaction) force (J) is unknown, it is assumed to act in a direction *opposite* to the pull of muscle. This assumption generally holds true in an analysis in which the mechanical advantage of the system is less than one (i.e., when the muscle forces are greater than the external resistance forces) (see Chapter 1).

> ### BOX 4-1. Guidelines for Solving for Muscle Force, Torque, and Joint Reaction Force
>
> 1. Draw the free body diagram, isolating the body segment(s) under consideration. Draw in all forces acting on the free body, including, if appropriate, gravity, resistance, muscular, and joint reaction forces. Identify the axis of rotation at the center of the joint.
> 2. Establish an X-Y reference frame that will specify the desired orientation of the X and Y components of forces. Designate the X axis parallel with the isolated body segment (typically a long bone), positive pointing distally. The Y axis is oriented perpendicularly to the same body segment. (Use arrowheads on the X and Y axes to designate positive directions.)
> 3. Resolve all known forces into their X and Y components.
> 4. Identify the moment arms associated with each Y force component. The moment arm associated with a given Y force component is the perpendicular distance between the axis of rotation and the line of force. Note that joint reaction force and the X components of all forces will *not* have a moment arm, because the line of force of these forces typically passes through the axis of rotation (center of the joint).
> 5. Assign a direction to the moment arms. By convention, moment arms are measured *from* the axis of rotation *to* the Y component of the force. If this measurement travels in a positive X direction, it is assigned a positive value. If the measurement travels in a negative X direction, it is assigned a negative value.
> 6. Use $\Sigma T_Z = 0$ (Equation 4.14) to find the unknown muscle torque and force.
> 7. Use $\Sigma F_X = 0$ and $\Sigma F_Y = 0$ (Equations 4.13 A and B) to find the X and Y components of the unknown joint reaction force.
> 8. Compose X and Y components of the joint reaction force to find the magnitude of the total joint reaction force.
>
> *Note:* There are other, more elegant methods to determine torques and component forces in systems similar to those illustrated in this chapter. However, these methods require a working knowledge of cross products, dot products, and unit vectors, topics that are beyond the scope of this chapter.

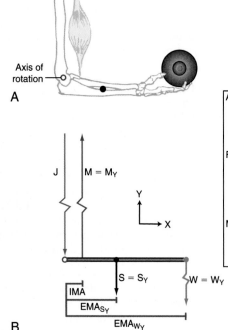

Angles:
Angle of forearm-hand segment relative to horizontal = 0°
Angle-of-insertion of M to forearm = 90°
Angle of J to X axis = unknown

Forces:
Forearm-hand segment weight (S) = 17 N
Exercise weight (W) = 60 N
Muscle force (M) = unknown
Joint reaction force (J) at the elbow = unknown

Moment arms:
External moment arm to S_Y (EMA_{S_Y}) = 0.15 m
External moment arm to W_Y (EMA_{W_Y}) = 0.35 m
Internal moment arm to M_Y (IMA) = 0.05 m

FIGURE 4-20. Problem 1. **A,** An isometric elbow flexion exercise is performed against an exercise weight held in the hand. The black dot marks the segment's center of gravity; the exercise weight's center of gravity is marked by the green dot. The forearm is held in the horizontal position. **B,** A free body diagram is shown of the exercise, including a box with the abbreviations and data required to solve the problem. The medial-lateral axis of rotation at the elbow is shown as an open red circle; the vectors are not drawn to scale. (The X-Y coordinate reference frame is set so the X direction is parallel to the forearm; black arrowheads point in positive directions.)

Resolving Known Forces into X and Y Components

In the elbow position depicted in Figure 4-20, all forces act parallel to the Y axis; there is no force acting in the X direction. This means the magnitude of the Y components of the forces is equal to the magnitude of the entire force, and the X components are all zero. This situation is unique to this position, in which muscle force and gravity are vertical and the segment is positioned horizontally.

The magnitude of the forces are determined through trigonometric functions, then the direction (+ or −) is applied.

$$S_Y = \sin 90° \times 17\,N = -17\,N$$
$$S_X = \cos 90° \times 17\,N = 0\,N$$
$$W_Y = \sin 90° \times 60\,N = -60\,N$$
$$W_X = \cos 90° \times 60\,N = 0\,N$$

Solving for Internal Torque and Muscle Force

The external torques originating from the weight of the forearm-hand segment (S_Y) and the exercise weight (W_Y) generate a −Z (clockwise, extension) torque about the elbow. In order for the system to remain in equilibrium, the elbow flexor muscles have to generate an opposing internal +Z (counterclockwise, flexion) torque. Summing the torques around the elbow axis allows the line-of-action of J to pass through the axis, thus making the moment arm of J equal to zero. This results in only one unknown in Equation 4.14: the magnitude of the muscle force:

$$\Sigma T_Z = 0 = T_S + T_W + T_M + T_J$$
$$0 = (S_Y \times EMA_{S_Y}) + (W_Y \times EMA_{W_Y}) + (M_Y \times IMA) + (J \times 0\,m)$$
$$0 = (-17\,N \times 0.15\,m) + (-60\,N \times 0.35\,m) + (M_Y \times 0.05\,m) + 0\,Nm$$
$$0 = -2.55\,Nm + -21\,Nm + (M_Y \times 0.05\,m) + 0\,Nm$$
$$23.55\,Nm = (M_Y \times 0.05\,m) = \text{internal torque}$$
$$471.00\,N = M_Y = M$$

The resultant muscle (internal) force is the result of all the active muscles that flex the elbow. This type of analysis does not, however, provide information about how the force is distributed among the various elbow flexor muscles. This requires more sophisticated procedures, such as muscle modeling and optimization techniques, which are beyond the scope of this text.

The magnitude of the muscle force is over six times greater than the magnitude of the external forces (i.e., forearm-hand weight and load weight). The larger force requirement can be explained by the disparity in moment arm length of the elbow flexors when compared with the moment arm lengths of the two external forces. The disparity in moment arm lengths is not unique to the elbow flexion model, but it is ubiquitous throughout the muscular-joint systems in the body. For this reason, most muscles of the body routinely generate force many times greater than the externally applied force. The combinations of external and muscular forces often require bone and articular cartilage to absorb and transmit very large joint forces, sometimes resulting from seemingly nonstressful activities. The next set of calculations determines the magnitude and direction of the joint reaction force.

Solving for Joint Reaction Force

Because the joint reaction force (J) is the only remaining unknown variable depicted in Figure 4-20, *B,* this variable is determined by Equations 4.13 A and B.

$$\Sigma F_X = 0 = M_X + S_X + W_X + J_X$$
$$0 = 0\,N + 0\,N + 0\,N + J_X$$
$$0\,N = J_X$$

Because there are no X components of M or either of the two external forces, the joint reaction force does not have an X component either.

$$\Sigma F_Y = 0 = M_Y + S_Y + W_Y + J_Y$$
$$0 = 471\,N + -17\,N + -60\,N + J_Y$$
$$-394\,N = J_Y$$

The negative Y component of the joint reaction force indicates that the joint force acts in a −Y direction (downward).

Total joint reaction force can be found by using the Pythagorean theorem with the X and Y components. (This step may not be necessary for problems such as this, where one of the component forces is zero, but it is included here for consistency of method.)

$$J^2 = (J_X)^2 + (J_Y)^2$$
$$J = \sqrt{[(J_X)^2 + (J_Y)^2]}$$
$$= \sqrt{[(0\,N)^2 + (-394.0\,N)^2]} = 394\,N$$

Because muscle force is usually the largest force acting about a joint, the direction of the net joint reaction force often opposes the pull of the muscle. Without such a force, for example, the muscle indicated in Figure 4-20 would accelerate the forearm upward, resulting in an unstable joint. In short, the joint reaction force in this case (largely supplied by the humerus pushing against the trochlear notch of the ulna) provides the required force to maintain linear static equilibrium at the elbow. As stated earlier, the joint reaction force does not produce a torque because it is assumed to act through the axis of rotation and therefore has a zero moment arm.

Clinical Questions Related to Problem 1

1. Assume a patient with osteoarthritis of the elbow is holding a load similar to that depicted in Figure 4-20. How would you respond to the question posed by a patient, "Why would my elbow be so painful from holding such a light weight?"
2. Describe a few clinical conditions in which the magnitude and direction of the joint reaction force could be biomechanically (physiologically) unhealthy for a patient.
3. Which variable is most responsible for the magnitude and direction of the joint reaction force at the elbow?
4. Assume a person with a recent elbow joint replacement needs to strengthen the elbow flexor muscles. Given the isometric situation depicted in Figure 4-20:
   a. How could the joint reaction force on the elbow be reduced while the same size exercise weight is used?
   b. How could the joint reaction force on the elbow be reduced while the same magnitude of external torque is created?

Answers to the clinical questions can be found on the Evolve website. ⊖

Problem 2

In Problem 1 the forearm is held horizontally, thereby orienting the internal and external forces perpendicular to the forearm. Although this presentation greatly simplifies the calculations, it does not represent a typical biomechanical situation. Problem 2 shows a more common situation, in which the forearm is held at a position other than the horizontal (Figure 4-21, *A*). As a result of the change in elbow angle, the angle-of-insertion of the elbow flexor muscles and the angle of application of the external forces are no longer right angles. In principle, all other aspects of this problem are identical to Problem 1. Assuming equilibrium, three unknown variables are once again to be determined: (1) the internal (muscular-produced) torque, (2) the muscle force, and (3) the joint reaction force at the elbow.

Figure 4-21, *B* illustrates the free body diagram of the forearm and hand segment held at 30 degrees below the horizontal (θ). The reference frame is established such that the X axis is parallel to the forearm-hand segment, positive pointed distally. All forces acting on the system are indicated, and each is resolved into their respective X and Y components. The angle-of-insertion of the elbow flexors to the forearm (α) is 60 degrees. All numeric data and abbreviations are listed in the box associated with Figure 4-21.

Resolving Known Forces into X and Y Components

Magnitudes of external forces are found through the use of trigonometric functions, then directions (+ or −) are applied based on the established X-Y axis reference frame:

$$S_Y = \cos 30° \times 17\,N = -14.72\,N$$
$$S_X = \sin 30° \times 17\,N = 8.5\,N$$
$$W_Y = \cos 30° \times 60\,N = -51.96\,N$$
$$W_X = \sin 30° \times 60\,N = 30\,N$$

Solving for Internal Torque and Muscle Force

$$\Sigma T_Z = 0 = T_S + T_W + T_M + T_J$$
$$0 = (S_Y \times EMA_{S_Y}) + (W_Y \times EMA_{W_Y}) + (M_Y \times IMA) + (J \times 0\,m)$$
$$0 = (-14.72\,N \times 0.15\,m) + (-51.96\,N \times 0.35\,m) + (M_Y \times 0.05\,m) + 0\,Nm$$
$$0 = -2.21\,Nm + -18.19\,Nm + (M_Y \times 0.05\,m)$$
$$20.40\,Nm = (M_Y \times 0.05\,m) = \text{internal torque}$$
$$408.00\,N = M_Y$$

Because an internal moment arm length of 0.05 m was used, the last calculation yielded the magnitude of its associated perpendicular vector, the Y component of M (M_Y), not the total muscle force M. The total muscle force M is determined as follows:

$$M = M_Y / \sin 60° = 408.00\,N / 0.866 = 471.13\,N$$

The X component of the muscle force, M_X, can be solved as follows:

$$M_X = M \times \cos 60°$$
$$= 471.13\,N \times 0.5$$
$$= -235.57\,N$$

The negative sign was added to indicate M_X is pointed in the −X direction.

Solving for Joint Reaction Force

The joint reaction force (J) and its X and Y components (J_Y and J_X) are shown separately in Figure 4-21, *C*. (This is done to increase the clarity of the illustration.) The directions of J_Y and J_X are assumed to act generally downward (negative Y) and to the right (positive X), respectively. These are directions that oppose the force of the muscle. The components (J_Y and J_X) of the joint force (J) can be readily determined by using Equations 4.13 A and B, as follows:

$$\Sigma F_X = 0 = M_X + S_X + W_X + J_X$$
$$0 = -235.57\,N + 8.50\,N + 30\,N + J_X$$
$$197.07\,N = J_X$$
$$\Sigma F_Y = 0 = M_Y + S_Y + W_Y + J_Y$$
$$0 = 408\,N + -14.72\,N + -51.96\,N + J_Y$$
$$-341.32\,N = J_Y$$

As depicted in Figure 4-21, *C*, J_Y and J_X act in directions that oppose the force of the muscle (M). This reflects the fact that muscle force, by far, is the largest of all the forces acting on the forearm-hand segment. J_X being positive indicates that the joint is under compression, whereas J_Y being negative indicates that the joint is under anterior and superior shear. In other words, if J_Y did not exist, the forearm would accelerate in an anterior and superior (+Y) direction.

The magnitude of the resultant joint force (J) can be determined using the Pythagorean theorem, as follows:

$$J = \sqrt{\left[(J_Y)^2 + (J_X)^2\right]}$$
$$J = \sqrt{\left[(-341.3\,N)^2 + (197.1\,N)^2\right]}$$
$$J = 394.1\,N$$

Another characteristic of the joint reaction force that is of interest is the direction of J with respect to the axis of the forearm (X axis). This can be calculated using the inverse cosine function as follows:

$$\text{Cos}\,\mu = J_X / J$$
$$\mu = \cos^{-1}(197.07\,N / 394.1\,N)$$
$$\mu = 60°$$

The resultant joint reaction force has a magnitude of 394.1 N and is directed toward the joint at an angle of 60 degrees to the forearm segment (i.e., the X axis). It is no coincidence that the angle of approach of J is the same as the angle-of-insertion of the elbow flexor muscles.

Clinical Questions Related to Problem 2

1. Assume the forearm (depicted in Figure 4-21) is held 30 degrees above rather than below the horizontal plane.
   a. Does the change in forearm angle alter magnitude of the external torque?
   b. Can you conclude that is it "easier" to hold the forearm 30 degrees above as compared with below the horizontal plane?
2. In what situation would a large force demand on the muscle be a clinical concern?

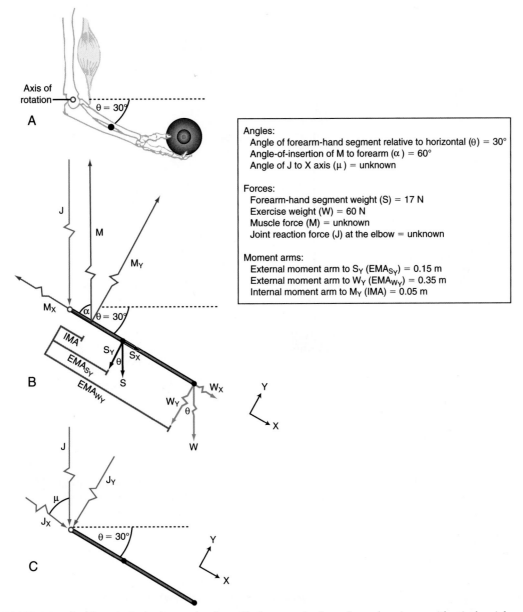

FIGURE 4-21. Problem 2. **A,** An isometric elbow flexion exercise is performed against an identical weight as that depicted in Figure 4-20. The forearm is held 30 degrees below the horizontal position. **B,** A free body diagram is shown, including a box with the abbreviations and data required to solve the problem. The vectors are not drawn to scale. **C,** The joint reaction force *(J)* vectors are shown in response to the biomechanics depicted in **B.** The X-Y coordinate reference frame is set so the X direction is parallel to the forearm; black arrowheads point in positive directions.

3. What would happen if, from the position depicted in Figure 4-21, *A,* the muscle force suddenly decreased or increased slightly?

Answers to the clinical questions can be found on the Evolve website. ⊝

Problem 3

Although the forearm was not positioned horizontally in Problem 2, all resultant forces were depicted as parallel. Problem 3 is complicated slightly by the forces not being parallel, and the bony lever system being a first-class (versus a third-class) lever (see Chapter 1). Problem 3 analyzes the isometric phase of a standing triceps-strengthening exercise using resistance applied by a cable (Figure 4-22, *A*). The patient can extend and hold her elbow partially flexed against the cable transmitting 15 pounds of force from the stack of weights. Assuming equilibrium, three unknown variables are once again to be determined using the same steps as before: (1) the internal (muscular-produced) torque, (2) the muscle force, and (3) the joint reaction force at the elbow.

Figure 4-22, *B* illustrates the free body diagram of the elbow held partially flexed, with the forearm oriented 25 degrees from the vertical (θ). The coordinate reference frame is again established such that the X axis is parallel to the forearm-hand segment, positive pointed distally. All forces acting on the system are indicated, and each is resolved into

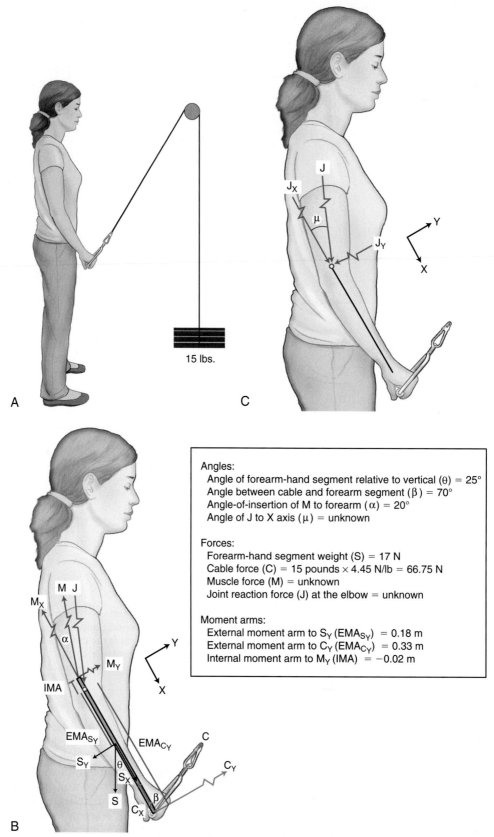

FIGURE 4-22. Problem 3. **A,** A standing isometric elbow extension exercise is performed against resistance provided by a cable. The forearm is held 25 degrees from the vertical position. **B,** A free body diagram is shown, including a box with the abbreviations and data required to solve the problem. The vectors are not drawn to scale. **C,** The joint reaction force *(J)* vectors are shown in response to the biomechanics depicted in **B.** (The X-Y coordinate reference frame is set so the X direction is parallel with the forearm; black arrowheads point in positive directions.)

The following appears in the box within the figure:

Angles:
  Angle of forearm-hand segment relative to vertical (θ) = 25°
  Angle between cable and forearm segment (β) = 70°
  Angle-of-insertion of M to forearm (α) = 20°
  Angle of J to X axis (μ) = unknown

Forces:
  Forearm-hand segment weight (S) = 17 N
  Cable force (C) = 15 pounds × 4.45 N/lb = 66.75 N
  Muscle force (M) = unknown
  Joint reaction force (J) at the elbow = unknown

Moment arms:
  External moment arm to S_Y (EMA_SY) = 0.18 m
  External moment arm to C_Y (EMA_CY) = 0.33 m
  Internal moment arm to M_Y (IMA) = −0.02 m

15 lbs.

their respective X and Y components. The angle-of-insertion of the elbow extensors to the forearm (α) is 20 degrees, and the angle between the cable and the long axis of the forearm (β) is 70 degrees. All numeric data and abbreviations are listed in the box associated with Figure 4-22.

Resolving Known Forces into X and Y Components

Magnitudes of forces are found through the use of trigonometric functions, then directions (+ or −) are applied as in previous problems, as follows:

$$S_Y = \sin 25° \times 17\,N = -7.18\,N$$
$$S_X = \cos 25° \times 17\,N = 15.41\,N$$
$$C_Y = \sin 70° \times 66.75\,N = 62.72\,N$$
$$C_X = \cos 70° \times 66.75\,N = -22.83\,N$$

Solving for Internal Torque and Muscle Force

This system is a first-class lever with the muscle force located on the opposite side of the elbow axis as the external forces. The internal moment arm IMA (as applied to M_Y) is assigned a negative value because the measurement of IMA from the axis of rotation to M_Y travels in a negative X direction (review no. 5 in Box 4-1).

$$\Sigma T_Z = 0 = T_S + T_C + T_M + T_J$$
$$0 = (S_Y \times EMA_{S_Y}) + (C_Y \times EMA_{C_Y}) + (M_Y \times IMA) + (J \times 0\,m)$$
$$0 = (-7.18\,N \times 0.18\,m) + (62.72\,N \times 0.33\,m) + (M_Y \times -0.02\,m) + 0\,Nm$$
$$0 = -1.29\,Nm + 20.70\,Nm + (M_Y \times -0.02\,m)$$
$$-19.41\,Nm = (M_Y \times -0.02\,m) = \text{internal torque}$$
$$970.5\,N = M_Y$$

This relatively large Y component of M is necessary because of the small IMA and the large external torque produced by C. The total muscle force, or M, is determined as follows:

$$M = M_Y / \sin 20° = 970.5\,N / 0.34 = 2854.41\,N$$

The X component of the muscle force, M_X, can be solved as follows:

$$M_X = M \times \cos 20°$$
$$= 2854.41\,N \times 0.94$$
$$= -2683.15\,N$$

The negative sign was added to indicate M_X is pointed in the −X direction.

Solving for Joint Reaction Force

The joint reaction force (J) and its X and Y components (J_Y and J_X) are shown separately in Figure 4-22, *C*. (This is done to increase the clarity of the illustration.) The directions of J_Y and J_X are assumed to act in −Y and +X directions, respectively. These directions oppose the Y and X components of the muscle force. This assumption can be verified by determining the J_Y and J_X components using Equations 4.13 A and B.

$$\Sigma F_X = 0 = M_X + S_X + C_X + J_X$$
$$0 = -2683.15\,N + 15.41\,N + -22.83\,N + J_X$$
$$2690.57\,N = J_X$$
$$\Sigma F_Y = 0 = M_Y + S_Y + C_Y + J_Y$$
$$0 = 970.5\,N + -7.18\,N + 62.72\,N + J_Y$$
$$-1026.04\,N = J_Y$$

As depicted in Figure 4-22, *C*, J_Y and J_X act in directions that oppose the force of the muscle. J_X being positive indicates that the joint is under compression, whereas J_Y being negative indicates that the joint is experiencing anterior shear. In other words, if J_Y did not exist, the forearm would accelerate in a general anterior (+Y) direction.

The magnitude of the resultant joint force (J) can be determined using the Pythagorean theorem:

$$J = \sqrt{[(J_Y)^2 + (J_X)^2]}$$
$$J = \sqrt{[(-1026.04\,N)^2 + (2690.57\,N)^2]}$$
$$J = 2879.57\,N$$

Another important characteristic of the joint reaction force is the direction of J with respect to the axis of the forearm (the X axis). This can be calculated using the inverse cosine function:

$$\cos \mu = J_X / J$$
$$\mu = \cos^{-1}(2690.57\,N / 2879.57\,N)$$
$$\mu = 21.57°$$

The resultant joint reaction force has a magnitude of 2879.57 N and is directed toward the elbow at an angle of over 21 degrees to the forearm segment (i.e., the X axis). The angle is almost the same as the angle-of-insertion of the muscle force (α), and the magnitude of J is similar to the magnitude of M. These similarities serve as a reminder of the dominant role of muscle in determining both the magnitude and direction of the joint reaction force. Note that if the M and J vector arrows were drawn to scale with the length of S, they would extend far beyond the limits of the page!

Clinical Questions Related to Problem 3

1. Figure 4-22 shows the pulley used by the resistance cable located at eye level. Assuming the subject maintains the same position of her upper extremity, what would happen to the required muscle force and components of the joint reaction force if the pulley was relocated at:
   a. Chest level?
   b. Floor level?
2. How would the exercise change if the pulley was located at floor level with the patient facing away from the pulley?
3. Note in Figure 4-22 that the angle (β) between the force in the cable (C) and the forearm is 70 degrees.
   a. At what angle of β would force C produce the greatest external torque?
   b. With the pulley at eye level, at what elbow angle would force C produce the greatest external torque?

Answers to the clinical questions can be found on the Evolve website. 🌐

Dynamic Analysis

Static analysis is the most basic approach to kinetic analysis of human movement. This form of analysis is used to evaluate forces and torques on a body when there are little or no significant linear or angular accelerations. External forces that act against a body at rest can be measured directly by various instruments, such as force transducers (shown in Figure 4-19), cable tensiometers, and force plates. Forces acting internal to the body are usually measured indirectly by knowledge of external torques and internal moment arms. This approach was highlighted in the previous three sample problems. In contrast, when linear or angular accelerations occur, a dynamic analysis must be undertaken. Walking is an example of a dynamic movement caused by unbalanced forces acting on the body; body segments are constantly speeding up or slowing down, and the body is in a continual state of losing and regaining balance with each step. A dynamic analysis therefore is required to calculate the forces and torques produced by or on the body during walking.

Solving for forces and torques under dynamic conditions requires knowledge of mass, mass moments of inertia, and linear and angular accelerations (for 2D dynamic analysis, see Equations 4.15 and 4.16). Anthropometric data provide the inertial characteristics of body segments (mass, mass moment of inertia), as well as the lengths of body segments and location of axis of rotation at joints. Kinematic data, such as displacement, velocity, and acceleration of segments, are measured through various laboratory techniques, which are described next.[2,18,20,22] This is followed by a description of the techniques commonly used to directly measure external forces, which may be used in static or dynamic analysis.

Two-Dimensional Dynamic Analyses of Force and Torque

Force Equations

$$\Sigma F_X = ma_X \qquad \textbf{(Equation 4.15 A)}$$
$$\Sigma F_Y = ma_Y \qquad \textbf{(Equation 4.15 B)}$$

Torque Equation

$$\Sigma T_Z = I \times \alpha_Z \qquad \textbf{(Equation 4.16)}$$

KINEMATIC MEASUREMENT SYSTEMS

Detailed analysis of movement requires a careful and objective evaluation of the motion of the joints and body as a whole. This analysis most frequently includes an assessment of position, displacement, velocity, and acceleration. Kinematic analysis may be used to assess the quality and quantity of motion of the body and its segments, the results of which describe the effects of internal and external forces and torques. Kinematic analysis can be performed in a variety of environments, including sport, ergonomics, and rehabilitation. There are several methods to objectively measure human motion, including electrogoniometry, accelerometry, imaging techniques, and electromagnetic tracking devices.

Electrogoniometer

An electrogoniometer measures joint angular rotation during movement. The device typically consists of an electrical potentiometer built into the pivot point (hinge) of two rigid arms. Rotation of a calibrated potentiometer measures the angular position of the joint. The related output voltage is

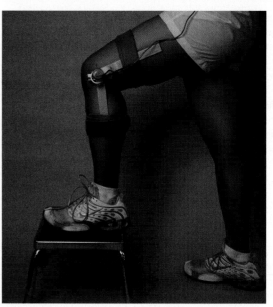

FIGURE 4-23. An electrogoniometer is shown strapped to the thigh and leg. The axis of the goniometer contains the potentiometer and is aligned over the medial-lateral axis of rotation at the knee joint. This particular instrument records a single plane of motion of the knee only.

typically measured by a computer data acquisition system. The arms of the electrogoniometer are strapped to the body segments, such that the axis of rotation of the goniometer is approximately aligned with the joint's axis of rotation (Figure 4-23). The position data obtained from the electrogoniometer combined with the time data can be mathematically converted to angular velocity and acceleration. Although the electrogoniometer provides a fairly inexpensive and direct means of capturing joint angular displacement, it encumbers the subject and is difficult to fit and secure over fatty and muscle tissues. In addition, a uniaxial electrogoniometer is limited to measuring range of motion in one plane. As shown in Figure 4-23, the uniaxial electrogoniometer can measure knee flexion and extension but is unable to detect the subtle but important rotation that also can occur in the horizontal plane. Other types of electrogoniometers exist. Figure 4-24 shows a different style that measures motion in two planes with sensors held onto the subject's skin by double-sided tape.

Accelerometer

An accelerometer is a device that measures acceleration of the object to which it is attached—either an individual segment or the whole body. Linear and angular accelerometers exist but measure accelerations only along a specific line or around a specific axis. Similar to electrogoniometers, multiple accelerometers are required for 3D or multi-segmental analyses. Data from accelerometers are used with body segment inertial information such as mass and mass moment of inertia to estimate net internal forces ($F = m \times a$) and torques ($T = I \times \alpha$). Whole-body accelerometers can be used to estimate an individual's relative physical activity during daily life.[5,6,9]

Imaging Techniques

Imaging techniques are the most widely used methods for collecting data on human motion. Many different types of imaging systems are available. This discussion is limited to the systems listed in the box.

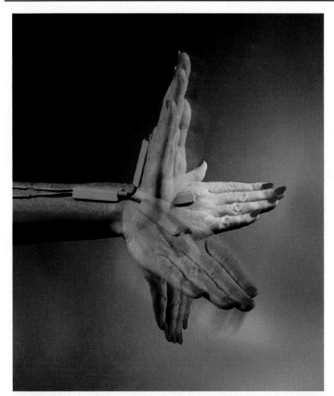

FIGURE 4-24. A biaxial electrogoniometer measuring wrist flexion and extension as well as radial and ulnar deviation. (Courtesy Biometrics, Ltd, Ladysmith, Virginia.)

Imaging Techniques
Photography
Cinematography
Videography
Optoelectronics

Unlike electrogoniometry and accelerometry, which measure movement directly from a body, imaging methods typically require additional signal conditioning, processing, and interpreting before meaningful output is obtained.

Photography is one of the oldest techniques for obtaining kinematic data. With the camera shutter held open, light from a flashing strobe can be used to track the location of reflective markers worn on the skin of a moving subject (see example in Chapter 15 and Figure 15-3). If the frequency of the strobe light is known, displacement data can be converted to velocity and acceleration data. In addition to using a strobe as an interrupted light source, a camera can use a constant light source and take multiple film or digital exposures of a moving event.

Cinematography, the art of movie photography, was once the most popular method of recording motion. High-speed cinematography, using 16-mm film, allowed for the measurement of fast movements. With the shutter speed known, a labor-intensive, frame-by-frame digital analysis on the movement in question was performed. Digital analysis was performed on movement of anatomic landmarks or of markers worn by subjects. Two-dimensional movement analysis was performed with the aid of one camera; 3D analysis, however, required two or more cameras.

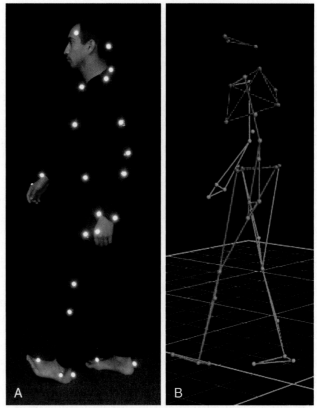

FIGURE 4-25. A, Reflective markers are used to indicate anatomic locations for determination of joint angular displacement of a walking individual. Marker location is acquired using video-based cameras that can operate at variable sampling rates. **B,** A computerized animated "stick figure" generated by data collected from the subject shown in **A.** (Courtesy Vicon Motion Systems, Inc., Centennial, Colorado.)

For the most part, still photography and cinematography analysis are rarely used today for the study of human motion. The methods are not practical because of the substantial time required for manually analyzing the data. Digital *videography* has replaced these systems and is one of the most popular methods for collecting kinematic information in both clinical and laboratory settings. The system typically consists of one or more digital video cameras, a signal processing device, a calibration device, and a computer. The procedures involved in video-based systems typically require markers to be attached to a subject at selected anatomic landmarks. Markers are considered passive if they are not connected to another electronic device or power source. Passive markers serve as a light source by reflecting the light back to the camera (Figure 4-25, *A*). Two-dimensional and 3D coordinates of markers are identified in space by a computer and are then used to reconstruct the image (or stick figure) for subsequent kinematic analysis (see Figure 4-25, *B*).

Video-based systems are quite versatile and are used to analyze human functional activities ranging from whole-body motion (e.g., swimming, running) to smaller motor tasks (e.g., typing, reaching). Some systems allow movement to be captured outdoors and processed at a later time, whereas others can process the signal almost in real time. Another desirable feature of most video-based systems is that the subject is not encumbered by wires or other electronic devices.

Optoelectronics is another popular type of kinematic acquisition system that uses active markers that are pulsed sequentially. The light is detected by special cameras that focus it on a semiconductor diode surface. The system enables collection of data at high sampling rates and can acquire real-time, 3D data. The system is limited in its ability to acquire data outside a controlled environment. Subjects may feel hampered by the wires that are connected to the active markers. Telemetry systems enable data to be gathered without the subjects being tethered to a power source, but these systems are vulnerable to ambient electrical interference.

Electromagnetic Tracking Devices

Electromagnetic tracking devices measure six degrees of freedom (three rotational and three translational), providing position and orientation data during both static and dynamic activities. Small sensors are secured to the skin overlying anatomic landmarks. Position and orientation data from the sensors located within a specified operating range of the transmitter are sent to the data capture system.

One disadvantage of this system is that the transmitters and receivers can be sensitive to metal in their vicinity that distorts the electromagnetic field generated by the transmitters. Although telemetry is available for these systems, most operate with wires that connect the sensors to the data capture system. The wires limit the volume of space from which motion can be recorded.

In any motion analysis system that uses skin sensors to record underlying bony movement, there is the potential for error associated with the extraneous movement of skin and soft tissue.

KINETIC MEASUREMENT SYSTEMS

Mechanical Devices

Mechanical devices measure an applied force by the amount of strain of a deformable material. Through purely mechanical means, the strain in the material causes the movement of a dial. The numeric values associated with the dial are calibrated to a known force. Some of the most common mechanical devices for measuring force include a bathroom scale, a grip strength dynamometer, and a hand-held dynamometer (as shown in Figure 4-19).

Transducers

Various types of transducers have been developed and widely used to measure force. Among these are strain gauges and piezoelectric, piezoresistive, and capacitance transducers. Essentially these transducers operate on the principle that an applied force deforms the transducer, resulting in a change in voltage in a known manner. Output from the transducer is converted to meaningful measures through a calibration process.

One of the most common transducers for collecting kinetic data while a subject is walking, stepping, or running is the *force plate*. Force plates use piezoelectric quartz or strain-gauge transducers that are sensitive to load in three orthogonal directions (an example of a force plate is shown in Figure 4-27, ahead, under the subject's forward right foot). The force plate measures the ground reaction forces in vertical, medial-lateral, and anterior-posterior components. The ground reaction force data are used in subsequent dynamic analysis.

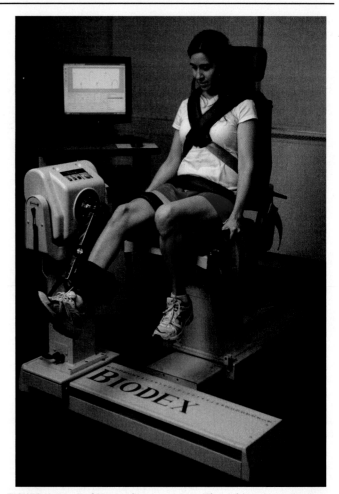

FIGURE 4-26. Isokinetic dynamometry. The subject is generating a maximal-effort knee extension torque at a joint angular velocity of 60 degrees/sec. The machine is functioning in its "concentric mode," providing resistance against the contracting right knee quadriceps muscle. Note that the medial-lateral axis of rotation of the tested knee is aligned with the axis of rotation of the dynamometer. (Courtesy of Biodex Medical Systems, Shirley, New York.)

Electromechanical Devices

A common electromechanical device used for dynamic strength assessment is the *isokinetic dynamometer*. During isokinetic testing, the device maintains a constant angular velocity of the tested limb while measuring the external torque applied to resist the subject's produced internal torque. The isokinetic system can often be adjusted to measure the torque produced by most major muscle groups of the body. Most isokinetic dynamometers can measure kinetic data produced by concentric, isometric, and eccentric activation of muscles. The angular velocity is determined by the user, varying between 0 degrees/sec (isometric) and 500 degrees/sec during concentric activations. Figure 4-26 shows a person who is exerting maximal-effort knee extension torque through a concentric contraction of the right knee extensor musculature. Isokinetic dynamometry provides an objective record of muscular kinetic data, produced during different types of muscle activation at multiple test velocities. The system also provides immediate feedback of kinetic data, which may serve as a source of biofeedback during training or rehabilitation.

SPECIAL FOCUS 4-7

Introduction to the Inverse Dynamic Approach for Solving for Internal Forces and Torques

Measuring joint reaction forces and muscle-produced net torques during *dynamic* conditions is often performed indirectly using a technique called the *inverse dynamic approach*.[22] A *direct* dynamic approach determines accelerations and external forces and torques through knowledge of internal forces and torques. Conversely, an *inverse* dynamic approach determines internal forces and torques through knowledge of accelerations and external forces and torques. The inverse dynamic approach relies on data from anthropometry, kinematics, and external forces, such as gravity and contact forces. Accelerations are determined employing the first and second derivatives of position-time data to yield velocity-time and acceleration-time data, respectively. The importance of acquiring accurate position data is a prerequisite to the soundness of this approach, because errors in measuring position data magnify errors in velocity and acceleration.

In the inverse dynamics approach, the system under consideration is often defined as a series of link segments. Figure 4-27, *A* illustrates the experimental setup for investigating the forces and torques in the right lower limb during different versions of a forward lunge exercise with three different trunk and upper extremity positions.[5] To simplify calculations, the subject's right lower limb is considered a linked segment model consisting of solid foot, leg, and thigh segments linked by frictionless hinges at the ankle and knee, and to the body at the hip (see Figure 4-27, *B*). The center of mass (CM) is located for each segment. In Figure 4-27, *C* the modeled segments of the right lower limb are disarticulated and the individual forces and torques (moments) are identified at each segment end point. The analysis on the series

of links usually begins with the analysis of the most distal segment, in this case the foot. Information gathered through motion analysis techniques, typically camera based, serves as input data for the dynamic equations of motion (Equations 4-15 and 4-16). This information includes the position and orientation of the segments in space and the acceleration of the segments and the segments' centers of mass. The ground reaction forces (components G_Y and G_X) acting on the distal end of the segment are measured in this example by a force plate built into the floor. From these data the ankle joint reaction force (components JA_Y and JA_X) and the net muscle torque (moments) at the ankle joint are determined. This information is then used as input for continued analysis of the next most proximal segment, the leg. Analysis takes place until all segments or links in the model are studied. Several assumptions made during the use of the inverse dynamic approach are included in the box.

Assumptions Made during the Inverse Dynamic Approach

1. Each segment or link has a fixed mass that is concentrated at its center of mass.
2. The location of each segment's center of mass remains fixed during the movement.
3. The joints in this model are considered frictionless hinge joints.
4. The mass moment of inertia of each segment is constant during the movement.
5. The length of each segment remains constant.

A   B   C

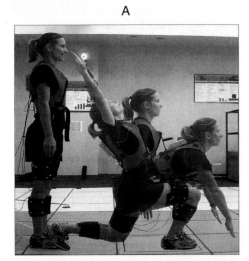
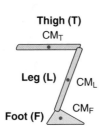
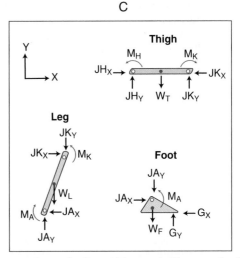

FIGURE 4-27. Example of an inverse dynamic approach to kinetic analysis of three versions of a forward lunge. **A,** Photograph of the experimental setup with the subject lunging onto the force plate with her right leg. Images were superimposed to show the three different trunk and upper extremity positions of interest. Videography-based passive reflective markers used to collect motion analysis data are visible on the lateral aspect of the subject's right shoe and on cuffs attached to her leg and thigh. Wires are also visible connecting electromyographic electrodes overlying the subject's muscles to a telemetry unit worn on the subject's back. **B,** The link model of the lower limb is shown as consisting of three articulated segments: thigh *(T),* leg *(L),* and foot *(F).* The center of mass *(CM)* of each segment is represented as a fixed point *(red circle):* CM_T, CM_L, and CM_F. **C,** The three link segments are disarticulated in order for the internal forces and torques to be determined, beginning with the most distal foot segment. The *red curved arrows* represent torque (moment) around each axis of rotation: M_A, M_K, and M_H are moments at the ankle, knee, and hip respectively; W_F, W_L, and W_T are segment weights of foot, leg, and thigh, respectively; JA_X and JA_Y, JK_X and JK_Y, and JH_X and JH_Y are joint reaction forces at the ankle, knee, and hip, respectively; G_X and G_Y are ground reaction forces acting on the foot. The coordinate system is set up with X horizontal and Y vertical; *arrowheads* point in positive directions. (**A** from Farrokhi S, Pollard C, Souza R, et al: Trunk position influences the kinematics, kinetics, and muscle activity of the lead lower extremity during the forward lunge exercise, *J Orthop Sports Phys Ther* 38:403, 2008.)

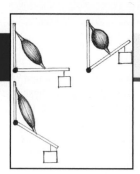

ADDITIONAL CLINICAL CONNECTIONS

CLINICAL CONNECTION 4-1
A Practical Method for Estimating Relative Torque Potential Based on Leverage

Earlier in this chapter, Figures 4-15 and 4-16 showed two methods for estimating internal and external torques. In both figures, Method 2 is considered a "shortcut" method because the resolution of the resultant forces into their component forces is unnecessary. Consider first *internal torque* (see Figure 4-15). The internal moment arm (depicted as IMA_M)—or leverage—of most muscles in the body can be qualitatively assessed by simply visualizing the shortest distance between a given whole muscle's line of force and the associated joint's axis of rotation. This experience can be practiced with the aid of a skeletal model and a piece of string that represents the resultant muscle's line of force (Figure 4-28). As apparent in the figure, the internal moment arm (shown in brown) is greater in position *A* than in position *B;* this means that for the same biceps force, more internal torque will be generated in position *A* than in position *B*. In general, the internal moment arm of any muscle is greatest when the angle-of-insertion of the muscle is 90 degrees to the bone.

Next, consider the shortcut method for determining *external torque.* Clinically, it is often necessary to quickly compare the relative external torque generated by gravity or other external forces applied to a joint. Consider, for example, the external torque at the knee during two squat postures (Figure 4-29). By visualizing the external moment arm between the knee joint axis of rotation and the line of gravity from body weight, it can be readily concluded that the external torque is greater in a deep squat *(A)* compared with a partial squat *(B)*. The ability to judge the relative demand placed on the muscles because of the external torque is useful in terms of protecting a joint that is painful or otherwise abnormal. For instance, a person with arthritic pain between the patella and femur is often advised to limit activities that involve lowering and rising from a deep squat position. This activity places large demands on the quadriceps muscle, which increases the compressive forces on the joint surfaces.

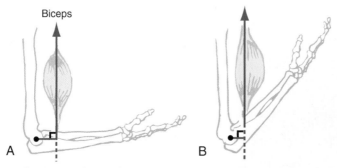

FIGURE 4-28. A piece of string can be used to mimic the line of force of the resultant force vector of an activated biceps muscle. The internal moment arm is shown as a brown line; the axis of rotation at the elbow is shown as a solid black circle. Note that the moment arm is greater when the elbow is in position **A** compared with position **B.** (Modified from LeVeau BF: *Williams & Lissner's biomechanics of human motion,* ed 3, Philadelphia, 1992, Saunders.)

ADDITIONAL CLINICAL CONNECTIONS

CLINICAL CONNECTION 4-1
A Practical Method for Estimating Relative Torque Potential Based on Leverage—cont'd

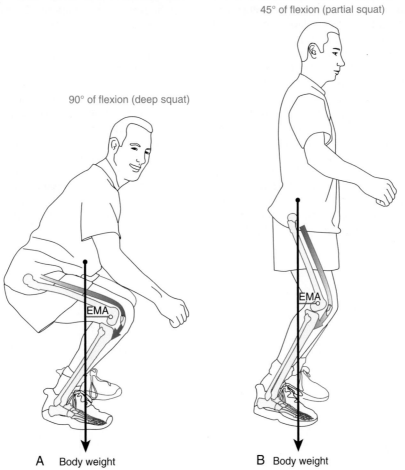

FIGURE 4-29. The depth of a squat significantly affects the magnitude of the external torque at the knee produced by superimposed body weight. The relative external torque, within the sagittal plane, can be estimated by comparing the distance that the body weight force vector falls posteriorly with the medial-lateral axis of rotation at the knee (shown as open circle). The external moment arm *(EMA)*–and thus the external torque created by body weight–is greater in **A** than in **B.** The external moment arms are shown as brown lines, originating at the axis of rotation and intersecting body weight force at right angles.

ADDITIONAL CLINICAL CONNECTIONS

CLINICAL CONNECTION 4-2
Modifying Internal Torque as a Means to Provide "Joint Protection"

Some treatments in rehabilitation medicine are directed at reducing the magnitude of force on joint surfaces during the performance of a physical activity. The purpose of such treatment is to protect a weakened or painful joint from large and potentially damaging forces. This result can be achieved by reducing the rate of movement (power), providing shock absorption (e.g., cushioned footwear), or limiting the mechanical force demands on the muscle.

Minimizing large muscular-based joint forces may be important for persons with a prosthesis (artificial joint replacement). A person with a hip replacement, for example, is often advised on ways to minimize unnecessarily large forces produced by the hip abductor muscles.[12,14,15] Figure 4-30 depicts a simple schematic representation of the pelvis and femur while a person with a prosthetic hip is in the single-limb support phase of gait. In order for equilibrium to be maintained within the frontal plane, the internal (counterclockwise, +Z) and the external (clockwise, −Z) torques around the stance hip must be balanced. As shown in both the anatomic *(A)* and see-saw *(B)* illustrations of Figure 4-30, the product of the body weight (W) times its moment arm D_1, must be equal in magnitude and opposite in direction to the hip abductor muscle force (M) times its moment arm (D): $W \times D_1 = M \times D$. Note that the external moment arm around the hip is almost twice the length of the internal moment arm.[16,17] This disparity in moment arm lengths requires that the muscle force be almost twice the force of superincumbent body weight in order to maintain equilibrium. In theory, reducing excessive body weight, carrying lighter loads, or carrying loads in certain fashions can decrease the external force and/or the external moment arm and therefore decrease the external torque about the hip. Reduction of large external torques substantially decreases large force demands from the hip abductors, thereby decreasing joint reaction forces on the prosthetic hip joint.

Certain orthopedic procedures illustrate how concepts of joint protection are used in rehabilitation practice. Consider the case of severe hip osteoarthritis, which results in destruction of the femoral head and a subsequent reduced size of the femoral neck and head. The bony loss shortens the internal moment arm length (D in Figure 4-30, *A*) available to the hip abductor muscles (M); thus, greater muscle forces are needed to maintain frontal plane equilibrium, and greater joint reaction forces result. A surgical procedure that attempts to reduce joint forces on the hip entails the relocation of the greater trochanter to a more lateral position. This procedure increases the length of the internal moment arm of the hip abductor muscles. An increase in the internal moment arm reduces the force required by the abductor muscles to generate a given torque during the single-limb support phase of gait.

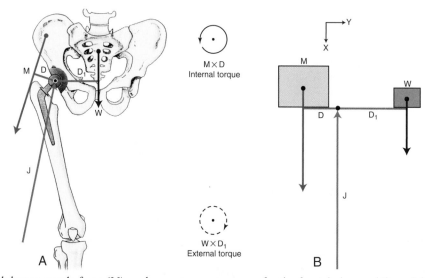

FIGURE 4-30. **A,** Hip abductor muscle force *(M)* produces a torque necessary for the frontal plane stability of the pelvis during the right single-limb support phase of gait. Rotary stability is established, assuming static equilibrium, when the external (clockwise, −Z) torque created by superincumbent body weight *(W)* is exactly balanced by the internal (counterclockwise, +Z) torque from the hip abductor muscles *(M)*. The counterclockwise torque equals M times its moment arm *(D)*, and the clockwise torque equals W times its moment arm *(D₁)*. **B,** This first-class lever seesaw model simplifies the model shown in **A.** The joint reaction force *(J)*, assuming that all force vectors act vertically, is shown as an upward-directed force with a magnitude equal to the sum of the hip abductor force and superimposed body weight. The X-Y coordinate reference frame is placed so the X axis is parallel with the body weight *(W)*; thin black arrowheads point toward the positive direction. (Modified from Neumann DA: Biomechanical analysis of selected principles of hip joint protection, *Arthritis Care Res* 2:146, 1989.)

ADDITIONAL CLINICAL CONNECTIONS

CLINICAL CONNECTION 4-3
The Influence of Antagonist Muscle Coactivation on the Clinical Measurement of Torque

When muscle strength is measured, care must be taken to encourage *activation* of the agonist muscles and relative *relaxation* of the antagonist muscles (review definitions of *agonist* and *antagonist* muscles in Chapter 1). Coactivation of antagonist muscles alters the net internal torque and decreases the ability to control or overcome external forces and torques. This concept is shown with the use of a hand-held dynamometer, similar to that previously described in Figure 4-19. Figure 4-31, *A* shows the measurement of elbow extension torque with activation *only* from the agonist (elbow extensor) muscles while the antagonist elbow flexors are relaxed. In contrast, Figure 4-31, *B* show a maximal-effort strength test of the elbow extensors with coactivation of both the agonist (E) and antagonist elbow flexor (F) muscles. (This situation may occur in a healthy person who is simply unable to relax the antagonist muscles or in a patient with neurologic pathology such as

Parkinson's disease or cerebral palsy.) The internal torque produced by the antagonist muscles actually *subtracts* from the internal torque produced by the agonist muscles. As a result, the *net* internal torque is reduced, as indicated by the reduced external force (R) applied against the dynamometer. Because the test condition is isometric, the measured external torque is equal in magnitude but opposite in direction to the reduced net internal torque. The important clinical point here is that even though the elbow extensor forces and torques may be equivalent in tests *A* and *B* of Figure 4-31, the external torque measures *less* in *B*. This scenario may give an erroneous impression of relative weakness of the agonist muscles when, in fact, they are not weak. As always, the joint reaction force (J) occurs in response to the sum of *all* forces across the joint and therefore will be *increased* in test *B* with antagonist activation.

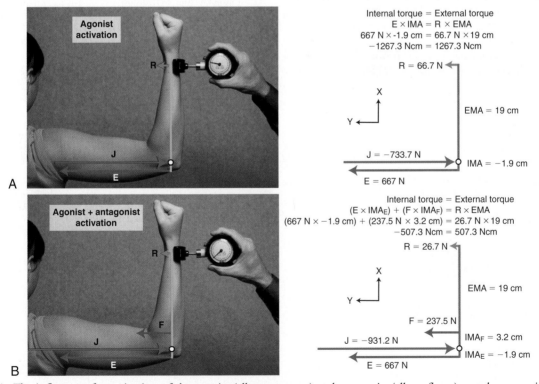

FIGURE 4-31. The influence of coactivation of the agonist (elbow extensor) and antagonist (elbow flexor) muscle groups is shown on the apparent strength (torque) of isometric elbow extension. **A,** Agonist (elbow extensor) activation only, with the same conditions and abbreviations used in Figure 4-19, *A.* **B,** Subject is simultaneously coactivating her elbow extensors and (antagonistic) elbow flexors muscles, producing a simultaneous elbow extension force *(E)* and an elbow flexion force *(F)*. Because F and E generate oppositely directed torques around the elbow, the *net* elbow extension torque is reduced. Note, however, that the magnitude of the joint reaction force *(J)* is increased in **B.** Vectors are drawn to approximate scale. Based on conventions summarized in Box 4-1, the internal moment arm used by the extensor muscles is assigned a negative number. This, in turn, assigns opposite rotational directions to the opposing internal torques. *EMA,* external moment arm; IMA_F and IMA_E, internal moment arms of the elbow flexors and extensor muscles, respectively; *R,* external force measured by the dynamometer.

SUMMARY

Many evaluation and treatment techniques used in rehabilitation involve the application or generation of forces and torques. A better understanding of the rationale and consequences of these techniques can be gained through the application of Newton's laws of motion and through static equilibrium or dynamic analyses. Although it is recognized that formal analyses are rarely completed in a clinic setting, principles learned from these analyses are clinically important and applied often. For example:

- Changing the moment of inertia of an arm by bending or straightening the elbow changes the required torque to move the shoulder.
- During an exercise the forces generated by muscles are often many times greater than the external forces used as resistance. This must be considered when a damaged muscle or tendon is being exercised.
- External torque is minimal when the line of force of the external force passes through or near the axis of motion.
- External torque is maximal when the line of force of the external force is at right angles to the limb. When gravity is used as a resistance force, this occurs when the limb is in a horizontal position.
- Internal torque produced by a muscle is maximal when its angle-of-insertion is 90 degrees.
- Exercises are often optimized when external and internal torques are matched through a range of motion.
- Forces at a joint occur as a necessary reaction to the combination of internal and external forces. Muscle force often plays the dominant role in the creation of these joint reaction forces.

Three quantitative-based sample problems were highlighted in this chapter. Two additional problems are available in Appendix I, Part B.

REFERENCES

1. Ajemian S, Thon D, Clare P, et al: Cane-assisted gait biomechanics and electromyography after total hip arthroplasty, *Arch Phys Med Rehabil* 85:1966-1971, 2004.
2. Allard P, Stokes IAF, Blanchi JP: *Three-dimensional analysis of human movement*, Champaign, 1995, Human Kinetics.
3. Dempster WT: *Space Requirements for the seated operator, WADC-TR-55-159*, Dayton, 1955, Wright Patterson Air Force Base.
4. Enoka RM: *Neuromechanical basis of kinesiology*, ed 2, Champaign, 1994, Human Kinetics.
5. Farrokhi S, Pollard CD, Souza RB, et al: Trunk position influences the kinematics, kinetics, and muscle activity of the lead lower extremity during the forward lunge exercise, *J Orthop Sports Phys Ther* 38:403-409, 2008.
6. Hale LA, Pal J, Becker I: Measuring free-living physical activity in adults with and without neurologic dysfunction with a triaxial accelerometer, *Arch Phys Med Rehabil* 89:1765-1771, 2008.
7. Hamill J, Knutzen KM: *Biomechanical basis of human movement*, ed 3, Philadelphia, 2008, Lippincott Williams & Wilkins.
8. Hatze H: A mathematical model for the computational determination of parameter values of anthropomorphic segments, *J Biomech* 13:833-843, 1980.
9. Lee Y, Lee M: Development of an integrated module using a wireless accelerometer and ECG sensor to monitor activities of daily living, *Telemed J E-Health* 14:580-586, 2008.
10. McGibbon CA, Krebs DE, Mann RW: In vivo hip pressures during cane and load-carrying gait, *Arthritis Care Res* 10:300-307, 1997.
11. Mulroy SJ, Lassen KD, Chambers SH, Perry J: The ability of male and female clinicians to effectively test knee extension strength using manual muscle testing, *J Orthop Sports Phys Ther* 26:192-199, 1997.
12. Münger P, Röder C, Ackermann-Liebrich U, Busato A: Patient-related risk factors leading to aseptic stem loosening in total hip arthroplasty: a case-control study of 5035 patients, *Acta Orthop* 77:567-574, 2006.
13. Neumann DA: Hip abductor muscle activity as subjects with hip prostheses walk with different methods of using a cane, *Phys Ther* 78:490-501, 1998.
14. Neumann DA: An electromyographic study of the hip abductor muscles as subjects with a hip prosthesis walked with different methods of using a cane and carrying a load, *Phys Ther* 79:1163-1173, 1999.
15. Neumann DA: Biomechanical analysis of selected principles of hip joint protection, *Arthritis Care Res* 2:146-155, 1989.
16. Neumann DA, Soderberg GL, Cook TM: Comparison of maximal isometric hip abductor muscle torques between hip sides, *Phys Ther* 68:496-502, 1988.
17. Olson VL, Smidt GL, Johnston RC: The maximum torque generated by the eccentric, isometric, and concentric contractions of the hip abductor muscles, *Phys Ther* 52:149-158, 1972.
18. Özkaya N, Nordin M: *Fundamentals of biomechanics: equilibrium, motion and deformation*, New York, 1999, Springer-Verlag.
19. Simoneau GG, Bereda SM, Sobush DC, Starsky AJ: Biomechanics of elastic resistance in therapeutic exercise programs, *J Orthop Sports Phys Ther* 31:16-24, 2001.
20. Soderberg GL: *Kinesiology: application to pathological motion*, ed 2, Baltimore, 1997, Williams & Wilkins.
21. Thomas M, Muller T, Busse MW: Quantification of tension in Thera-Band and Cando tubing at different strains and starting lengths, *J Sports Med Phys Fitness* 45:188-198, 2005.
22. Winter DA: *Biomechanics and motor control of human movement*, Hoboken, NJ, 2005, John Wiley & Sons.
23. Zatsiorsky VM, Seluyanov V: Estimation of the mass and inertia characteristics of the human body by means of the best predictive regression equations. In Winter DA, Norman RW, Wells RP, eds: *Biomechanics*, Champaign, 1985, Human Kinetics.

STUDY QUESTIONS

1 The first set of questions expands on the concepts introduced in Special Focus 4-6. In Figure 4-17, *A,* assume a constant 50% maximum effort:
   a Describe why internal torque would likely be reduced if the elbow were positioned in 110 degrees of flexion.
   b How does the external torque from gravity acting on the forearm-and-hand segment change if the elbow were to be positioned in 45 degrees of flexion?

2 The next set of questions expands on the concept of muscle coactivation introduced in Clinical Connection 4-3. Using Figure 4-31, *B,* what would happen to the magnitude of the external force (R) if:
   a F remained the same, but E increased?
   b F remained the same, but E decreased?
   c E remained the same, but F increased?
   d E remained the same, but F decreased?

3 How does an object's mass differ from its mass moment of inertia?
   a Provide an example of how the mass moment of inertia of a rotating limb could increase without an increase in its mass.
   b Describe a situation in which the mass moment of inertia of a rotating limb does not affect the force demands of the activated muscles.

4 Where is the approximate location of the center of mass of the human body in the anatomic position?
   a How would the location of the center of mass of the human body change if the arms were raised overhead?
   b How would the location of the center of mass of the human body change after a bilateral (transfemoral) amputation of the legs?

5 In which situation would a muscle produce a force across a joint that does not create a torque?

6 Figure 4-29 shows two levels of external (knee flexion) torque produced by body weight. At what knee angle would the external torque at the knee:
   a Be reduced to zero?
   b Cause a flexion torque?

7 Severe arthritis of the hip can cause a bony remodeling of the femoral head and neck. In some cases, this remodeling reduces the internal moment arm of the hip abductors (D in Figure 4-30).
   a In theory, while frontal plane rotary equilibrium around the right (stance) hip is maintained, how would a 50% reduction in internal moment arm affect the hip joint reaction force?
   b Assuming erosion of the articular surface of the femoral head, how would the reduction in internal moment arm affect the hip joint *pressure*?

8 Assume a person is preparing to quickly flex his hip while in a side-lying (essentially gravity-eliminated) position. What effect would keeping his knee extended have on the force requirements of the hip flexor muscles?

9 Assume the quadriceps muscle shown in Figure 4-18, *A* has an internal moment arm of 5 cm.
   a Based on the magnitude of the applied external torque, how much knee extensor muscle force is required to maintain static rotary equilibrium about the knee?
   b How much muscle force would be needed if the same external force (100 N) were applied 30 cm distal to the knee?

10 Assume a therapist is helping a patient with weak quadriceps stand up from a seated position from a standard chair. In preparation for this activity, the therapist often instructs the patient to bend as far forward from the hips as safely possible. How does this preparatory action likely increase the success of (or at least ease) the sit-to-stand activity?

⊖ *Answers to the study questions can be found on the Evolve website.*

Trigonometry Review and Additional Biomechanical Problems

Part A:
Basic Review of Right Angle Trigonometry

Part B:
Additional Biomechanical Problems

Part A: Basic Review of Right Angle Trigonometry

Trigonometric functions are based on the relationship that exists between the angles and sides of a right triangle. The sides of the triangle can represent distances, force magnitude, velocity, and other physical properties. Four of the common trigonometric functions used in quantitative analysis are found in Table I-1. Each trigonometric function has a specific value for a given angle. If the vectors representing two sides of a right triangle are known, the remaining side of the triangle can be determined by using the *Pythagorean theorem:* $a^2 = b^2 + c^2$, where a is the hypotenuse of the triangle. If one side and one angle other than the right angle are known, the remaining sides of the triangle can be determined by using one of the four trigonometric functions listed in the table paragraphs. Angles can be determined by knowing any two sides and using the inverse trigonometric functions (arcsine, arccosine, arctangent, and so on).

Figure I-1 illustrates the use of trigonometry to determine the force components of the posterior deltoid muscle during its isometric activation. The angle-of-insertion (α) of the muscle with the bone is 45 degrees. Based on the chosen X-Y coordinate reference frame, the rectangular components of the muscle force (M) are designated as M_X (parallel with the arm) and M_Y (perpendicular to the arm). Given a muscle force of 200 N, M_Y and M_X can be determined as follows:

$$M_X = M \cos 45° = 200 \text{ N} \times 0.707 = -141.4 \text{ N*}$$
$$M_Y = M \sin 45° = 200 \text{ N} \times 0.707 = 141.4 \text{ N}$$

If M_X and M_Y are known, M (hypotenuse) can be determined as follows, using the Pythagorean theorem:

$$M^2 = (M_X)^2 + (M_Y)^2$$
$$M = \sqrt{-141.4^2 + 141.4^2}$$
$$M = 200 \text{ N}$$

*The negative M_X value indicates that the force is directed *away from* the arrowhead of the X axis.

The rectangular components of *external forces,* such as those exerted by a wall pulley, by body weight, or by the clinician manually, are determined in a manner similar to that described for the muscle (internal) force.

Trigonometry can also be used to determine the magnitude of the resultant muscle force when one or more components and the angle-of-insertion (α in Figure I-1) are known. Consider the same example as given in Figure I-1, but now consider that the goal of the analysis is to determine the resultant muscle force of the posterior deltoid muscle if M_Y is known. As indicated in Figure I-1, the direction (angle-of-

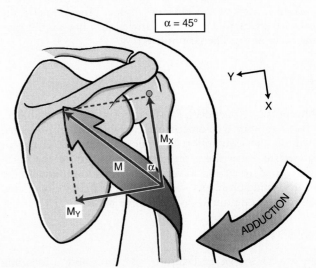

FIGURE I-1. Given the angle-of-insertion of the posterior deltoid (α = 45 degrees) and the resultant posterior deltoid muscle force (M), the two rectangular force components of the muscle force (M_X and M_Y) are determined using trigonometric relationships. The axis of rotation at the glenohumeral joint is indicated by the small circle at the head of the humerus.

TABLE I-1. Right-Angle Trigonometric Functions Commonly Used in Biomechanical Analysis	
Trigonometric Function	**Definition**
Sine (sin) α	Side opposite/hypotenuse
Cosine (cos) α	Side adjacent/hypotenuse
Tangent (tan) α	Side opposite/side adjacent
Cotangent (cot) α	Side adjacent/side opposite

α, Angle within a right triangle.

insertion) of muscle (M) is 45 degrees relative to the X axis. The magnitude of the resultant muscle force (hypotenuse of the triangle) can be derived using the relationship of the rectangular components, as follows:

$$\sin 45° = M_Y/M$$
$$M = 141.4 \, N/\sin 45°$$
$$M = 200 \, N$$

The direction (angle-of-insertion) of M relative to the X axis can be mathematically verified by any one of several trigonometric functions, such as the inverse sine function. If only M_Y and M_X are known, the direction of M can be determined using the inverse tangent function. Note that the components of the force always have a magnitude less than the magnitude of the resultant force.

Note: Resultant forces can arise from any combination of positive- or negative-directed X and Y component forces. Describing the *direction* of a resultant force (i.e., assigning it a positive or negative value) is therefore problematic. For the purposes of this this text, and particularly chapter 4, the direction of the resultant force will *not* be expressed with a positive or negative sign but as the absolute *angle* relative to the X or Y axis of the reference frame. (Trigonometrically solved resultant forces or their angles that have a negative value may be considered positive.)

Part B: Additional Biomechanical Problems

Conceptually, Appendix I, Part B is a continuation of Chapter 4. Two additional biomechanical problems are presented based on the assumption of static equilibrium. The steps required to solve these problems are similar to the three problems analyzed and solved in Chapter 4. Solutions to the two upcoming problems and the associated clinically related questions can be found on the Evolve website. ⊖

Problem 1

The subject shown in Figure I-2 is performing a standing *internal rotation* exercise of the shoulder muscles against a resistance supplied by a cable attached to a wrist cuff. The exercise is based on isometric activation of the internal rotator muscles with the shoulder in 35 degrees of external rotation. The shoulder remains in neutral flexion-extension and abduction-adduction throughout the effort. Using the data pro-

vided in the box and the conversion factors in Table 4-2, determine the muscle force (M) and the joint reaction force (J) in newtons.

CLINICAL QUESTIONS

1. At what rotary (horizontal plane) position of the shoulder is the resistance (external) torque the greatest?
2. How can the subject's body be repositioned so that maximal resistance (external) torque occurs at (a) 70 degrees of external rotation and (b) 30 degrees of internal rotation?
3. In previous problems encountered in Chapter 4, segment weight was included in the analyses of forces and torques. In this problem, does forearm-and-hand segment weight contribute to the horizontal plane torque (i.e., +Z- and −Z-directed torque)? Why or why not?
4. Consider the same exercise, but instead of standing as in Figure I-2, assume the subject is positioned supine. How does the forearm-and-hand segment weight now contribute to +Z- or −Z-directed torque as the shoulder moves through complete internal and external range of motion?

Problem 2

Figure I-3 is a sagittal plane view of a 180-pound subject performing shoulder flexion against the resistance supplied by an elastic band. Use the figure and data in the box to determine the muscle force (M) and the joint reaction force (J) in newtons.

This problem requires conversion and anthropometric information from Tables 4-2 and 4-3, respectively. For Table 4-3, use the anthropometric data for "total arm" segment, even though this does *not* include the length of the hand. This "total arm" segment is referred to as the 60-cm segment length in the data box.

CLINICAL QUESTIONS

1. What part of the capsule of the glenohumeral joint is likely being most stressed by this exercise?
2. At what sagittal plane position of the shoulder is the external torque due to the total arm weight maximal?
3. At what sagittal plane position of the shoulder would the external force of the elastic be at 90 degrees to the segment? Would this also be the position of maximal torque produced by the elastic? Why or why not?
4. While ignoring the weight of the upper limb, estimate the external torque produced in the −Z (extension) direction through 0 to 180 degrees of flexion while using (a) a hand-held weight of 27 N (about 6 lb) and (b) elastic force.

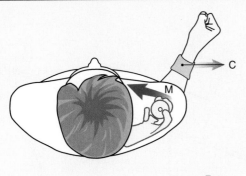

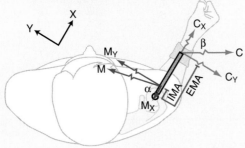

Angles:
  Angle-of-insertion of M to humerus (α) = 70°
  Angle between cable and X axis (β) = 55°
  Angle of J to X axis (μ) = unknown

Forces:
  Cable force (C) = 15 lbs
  Muscle force (M) = unknown
  Joint reaction force (J) at the shoulder = unknown

Moment arms:
  External moment arm to C_Y (EMA) = 8 inches
  Internal moment arm to M_Y (IMA) = 2.6 inches

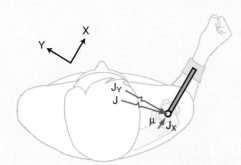

FIGURE I-2.

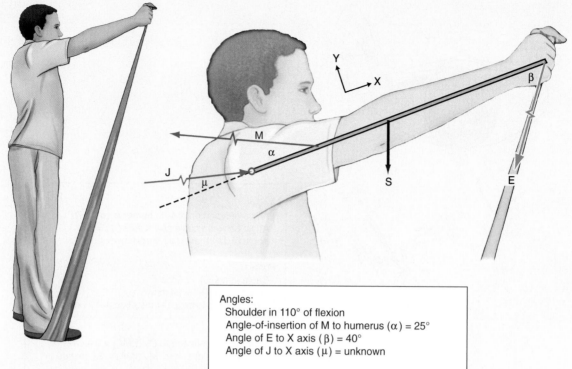

Angles:
  Shoulder in 110° of flexion
  Angle-of-insertion of M to humerus (α) = 25°
  Angle of E to X axis (β) = 40°
  Angle of J to X axis (μ) = unknown

Forces:
  Subject body weight = 180 lbs
  Elastic force (E) = 55 N
  Muscle force (M) = unknown
  Joint reaction force (J) at the shoulder = unknown

Moment arms:
  External moment arm to E_Y (EMA_{E_Y}) = 66 cm
  Internal moment arm to M_Y (IMA) = 10 cm
  Segment length (to ulnar styloid process) = 60 cm

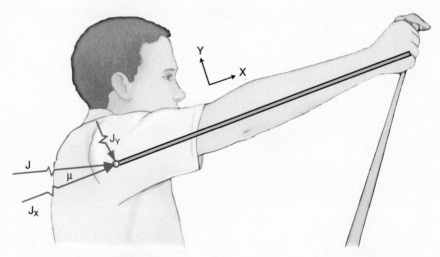

FIGURE I-3.

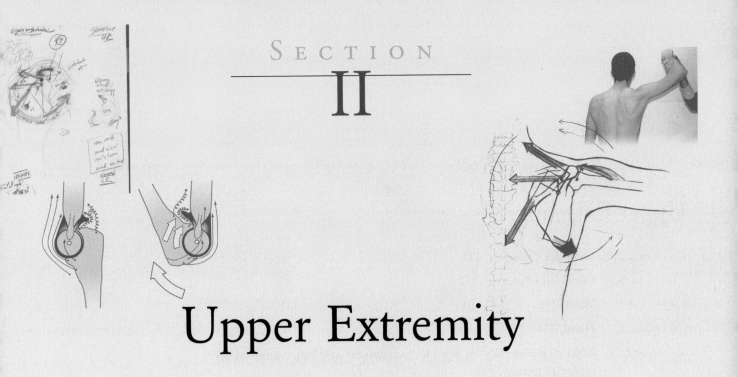

Upper Extremity

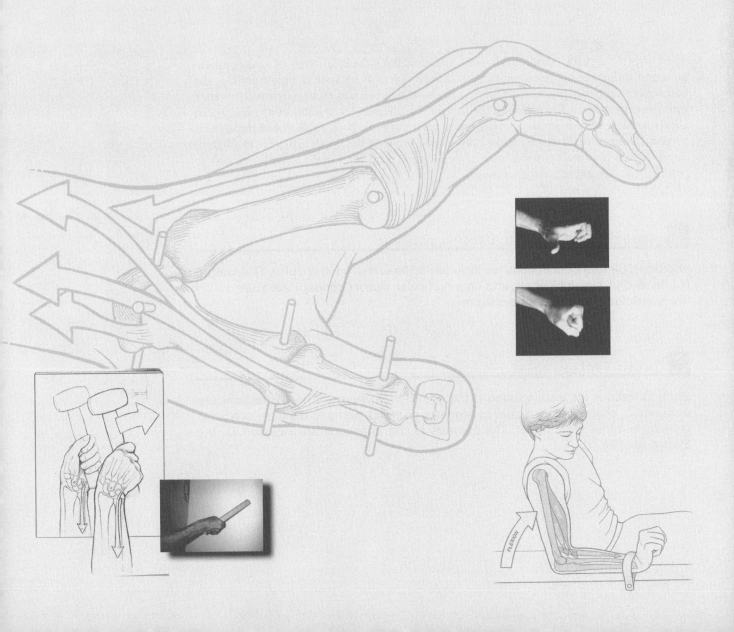

Section II

Upper Extremity

SECTION II is made up of four chapters, each describing the kinesiology of a major articular region within the upper extremity. Although presented as separate anatomic entities, the four regions cooperate functionally to place the hand in a position to most optimally interact with the environment. Disruption in the function of the muscles or joints of any region can greatly interfere with the capacity of the upper extremity as a whole. As described throughout Section II, impairments involving the muscles and joints of the upper extremity can significantly reduce the quality or the ease of performing many important activities related to personal care, livelihood, and recreation.

ADDITIONAL CLINICAL CONNECTIONS

Additional Clinical Connections are included at the end of each chapter. This feature is intended to highlight or expand on a particular clinical concept associated with the kinesiology covered in the chapter.

STUDY QUESTIONS

Study Questions are also included at the end of each chapter. These questions are designed to challenge the reader to review or reinforce some of the main concepts contained within the chapter. The answers to the questions are included on the Evolve website ⊖.

Shoulder Complex

DONALD A. NEUMANN, PT, PhD, FAPTA

The study of the upper extremity begins with the *shoulder complex*, a set of four articulations involving the sternum, clavicle, ribs, scapula, and humerus (Figure 5-1). This series of joints provides extensive range of motion to the upper extremity, thereby increasing the ability to reach and manipulate objects. Trauma or disease often limits shoulder motion, causing a significant reduction in the effectiveness of the entire upper limb.

Rarely does a single muscle act in isolation at the shoulder complex. Muscles work in "teams" to produce highly coordinated actions that are expressed over multiple joints. The very cooperative nature of shoulder muscles increases the versatility, control, and range of active movements. Paralysis, or weakness of *any single muscle*, therefore, often disrupts the natural kinematic sequencing of the entire shoulder. This chapter describes several of the important muscular synergies

that exist at the shoulder complex and how weakness in one muscle can affect the force generation potential in others. Muscles may weaken as a result of disease or injury affecting the neuromuscular or musculoskeletal systems.

OSTEOLOGY

Sternum

The sternum consists of the manubrium, body, and xiphoid process (Figure 5-2). The *manubrium* possesses a pair of oval-shaped *clavicular facets,* which articulate with the clavicles. The *costal facets,* located on the lateral edge of the manubrium, provide bilateral attachment sites for the first two ribs. The *jugular notch* is located at the superior aspect of the manubrium, between the clavicular facets.

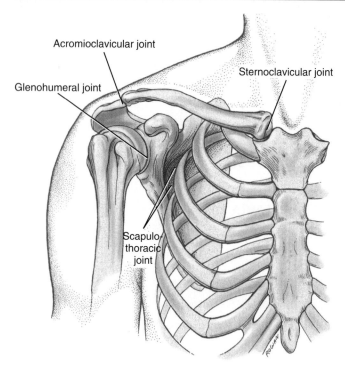

FIGURE 5-1. The joints of the right shoulder complex.

Osteologic Features of the Sternum
- Manubrium
- Clavicular facets
- Costal facets
- Jugular notch

Clavicle

When one looks from above, it is evident that the *shaft* of the clavicle is curved, with its anterior surface being generally convex medially and concave laterally (Figure 5-3). With the arm in the anatomic position, the long axis of the clavicle is oriented slightly above the horizontal plane and about 20 degrees posterior to the frontal plane (Figure 5-4; angle A). The rounded and prominent medial or *sternal end* of the clavicle articulates with the sternum (see Figure 5-3). The *costal facet* of the clavicle (see Figure 5-3; inferior surface) rests against the first rib. Lateral and slightly posterior to the costal facet is the distinct *costal tuberosity,* an attachment for the costoclavicular ligament.

Osteologic Features of the Clavicle
- Shaft
- Sternal end
- Costal facet
- Costal tuberosity
- Acromial end
- Acromial facet
- Conoid tubercle
- Trapezoid line

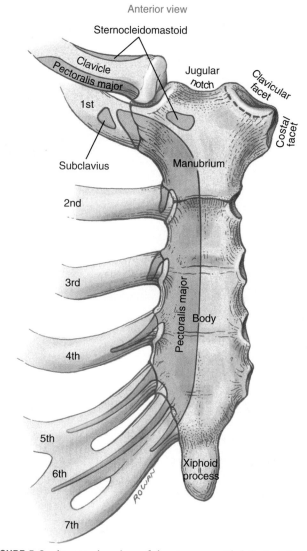

FIGURE 5-2. An anterior view of the sternum with left clavicle and ribs removed. The right side shows the first seven ribs and clavicle. The dashed line around the clavicular facet shows the attachments of the capsule at the sternoclavicular joint. Proximal attachments of muscle are shown in red.

The lateral or *acromial end* of the clavicle articulates with the scapula at the oval-shaped *acromial facet* (see Figure 5-3; inferior surface). The inferior surface of the lateral end of the clavicle is well marked by the *conoid tubercle* and the *trapezoid line.*

Scapula

The triangular-shaped scapula has three angles: *inferior, superior, and lateral* (Figure 5-5). Palpation of the inferior angle provides a convenient method for following the movement of the scapula during arm motion. The scapula also has three borders. With the arm resting by the side, the *medial or vertebral border* runs almost parallel to the spinal column. The *lateral or axillary border* runs from the inferior angle to the lateral angle of the scapula. The *superior border* extends from the superior angle laterally toward the coracoid process.

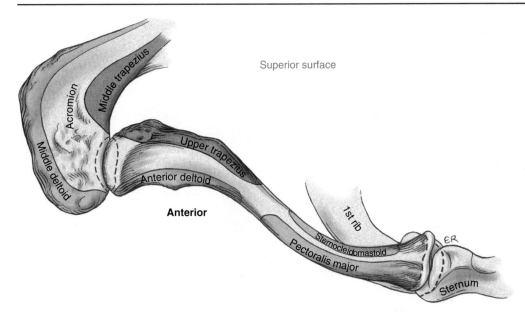

Superior surface

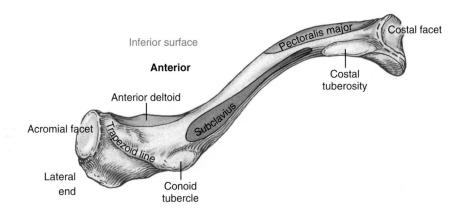

FIGURE 5-3. The superior and inferior surfaces of the right clavicle. The dashed line around the ends of the clavicle show attachments of the joint capsule. Proximal attachments of muscles are shown in red, distal attachments in gray.

Inferior surface

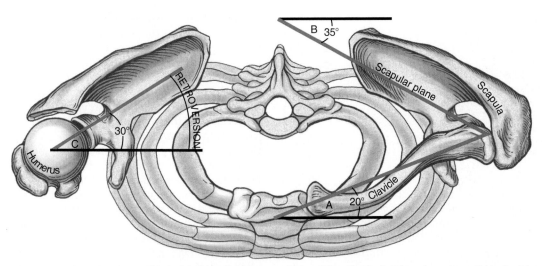

FIGURE 5-4. Superior view of both shoulders in the anatomic position. Angle A: The orientation of the clavicle deviated about 20 degrees posterior to the frontal plane. Angle B: The orientation of the scapula (scapular plane) deviated about 35 degrees anterior to the frontal plane. Angle C: Retroversion of the humeral head about 30 degrees posterior to the medial-lateral axis at the elbow. The right clavicle and acromion have been removed to expose the top of the right glenohumeral joint.

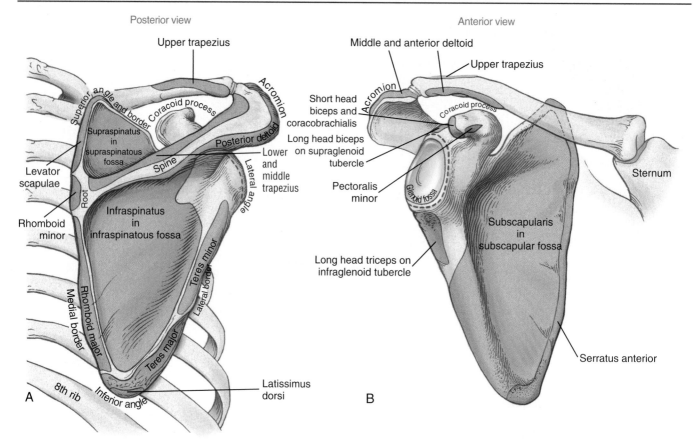

FIGURE 5-5. Posterior **(A)** and anterior **(B)** surfaces of the right scapula. Proximal attachments of muscles are shown in red, distal attachments in gray. The dashed lines show the capsular attachments around the gleno-humeral joint.

Osteologic Features of the Scapula
- Angles: inferior, superior, and lateral
- Medial or vertebral border
- Lateral or axillary border
- Superior border
- Supraspinatous fossa
- Infraspinatous fossa
- Spine
- Root of the spine
- Acromion
- Clavicular facet
- Glenoid fossa
- Supraglenoid and infraglenoid tubercles
- Coracoid process
- Subscapular fossa

The posterior surface of the scapula is separated into a *supraspinatous fossa* and an *infraspinatous fossa* by the prominent *spine*. The depth of the supraspinatous fossa is filled by the supraspinatus muscle. The medial end of the spine diminishes in height at the *root of the spine*. In contrast, the lateral end of the spine gains considerable height and flattens into the broad and prominent *acromion* (from the Greek *akros*, meaning topmost, highest). The acromion extends in a lateral and anterior direction, forming a horizontal shelf over the glenoid fossa. The *clavicular facet* on the acromion forms part of the acromioclavicular joint (see Figure 5-16, *B*).

The scapula articulates with the head of the humerus at the slightly concave *glenoid fossa* (from the Greek root *glene*, socket of joint, + *eidos*, resembling) (see Figure 5-5, *B*). The slope of the glenoid fossa is inclined upward about 4 degrees relative to a horizontal axis through the body of the scapula.[26] This inclination is highly variable, ranging from a downward inclination of 7 degrees to an upward inclination of nearly 16 degrees. At rest the scapula is normally positioned against the posterior-lateral surface of the thorax, with the glenoid fossa facing about 35 degrees anterior to the frontal plane (see Figure 5-4; angle B). This orientation of the scapula is referred to as the *scapular plane*. The scapula and humerus tend to follow this plane when the arm is naturally raised overhead.

Located at the superior and inferior rim of the glenoid fossa are the *supraglenoid* and *infraglenoid tubercles*. These tubercles serve as the proximal attachment for the long head of the biceps and triceps brachii, respectively (see Figure 5-5, *B*). Near the superior rim of the glenoid fossa is the prominent *coracoid process*, meaning "the shape of a crow's beak." The coracoid process projects sharply from the scapula, providing multiple attachments for ligaments and muscles (Figure 5-6). The *subscapular fossa* is located on the anterior surface of the scapula (see Figure 5-5, *B*). The concavity within the fossa is filled with the thick subscapularis muscle.

Proximal-to-Mid Humerus

The *head of the humerus,* nearly one half of a full sphere, forms the convex component of the glenohumeral joint (Figure 5-7).

The head faces medially and superiorly, forming an approximate 135-degree angle of inclination with the long axis of the humeral shaft (Figure 5-8, *A*). Relative to a medial-lateral axis through the elbow, the humeral head is rotated posteriorly about 30 degrees within the horizontal plane (see Figure 5-8,

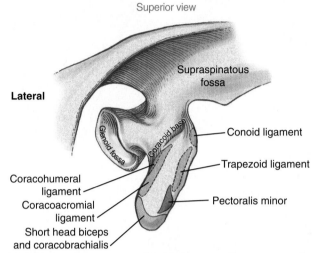

FIGURE 5-6. A close-up view of the right coracoid process seen from above. Proximal attachments of muscle are in red, distal attachments in gray. Ligamentous attachment is indicated by light blue outlined by dashed line.

B). This rotation, known as *retroversion* (from the Latin *retro,* backward, + *verto,* to turn) aligns the humeral head within the scapular plane for articulation with the glenoid fossa (see Figure 5-4; angle C). Interestingly, researchers have shown that the dominant shoulder in elite baseball pitchers possesses greater humeral retroversion than the nondominant limb.[24] This difference (which was not present in a control group of nonpitchers) was theorized to occur as an osseous adaptation to the large torsional stress generated during pitching.

The *anatomic neck* of the humerus separates the smooth articular surface of the head from the proximal shaft (see Figure 5-7, *A*). The prominent lesser and greater tubercles surround the anterior and lateral circumference of the extreme proximal end of the humerus (see Figure 5-7, *B*). The *lesser tubercle* projects rather sharply and anteriorly for attachment of the subscapularis. The large and rounded *greater tubercle* has an *upper, middle, and lower facet,* marking the distal attachment of the supraspinatus, infraspinatus, and teres minor, respectively (see Figure 5-7, *B* and Figure 5-9).

Sharp *crests* extend distally from the anterior side of the greater and lesser tubercles. These crests receive the distal attachments of the pectoralis major and teres major (see Figure 5-7, *A*). Between these crests is the *intertubercular (bicipital) groove,* which houses the tendon of the long head of the biceps brachii. The latissimus dorsi muscle attaches to the floor of the intertubercular groove, medial to the biceps tendon. Distal and lateral to the termination of the intertubercular groove is the *deltoid tuberosity.*

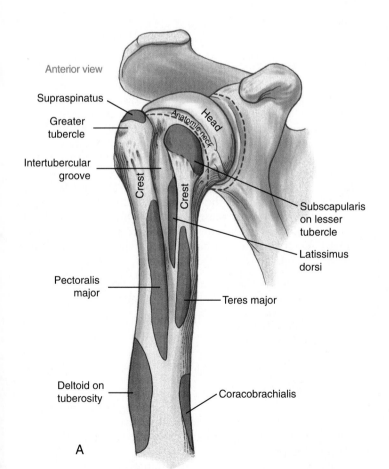

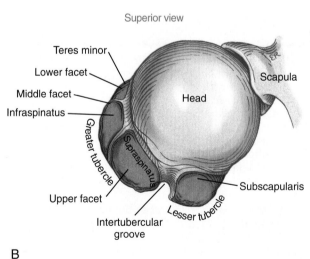

FIGURE 5-7. Anterior **(A)** and superior **(B)** aspects of the right humerus. The dashed line in **A** shows the capsular attachments around the glenohumeral joint. Distal attachment of muscles is shown in gray.

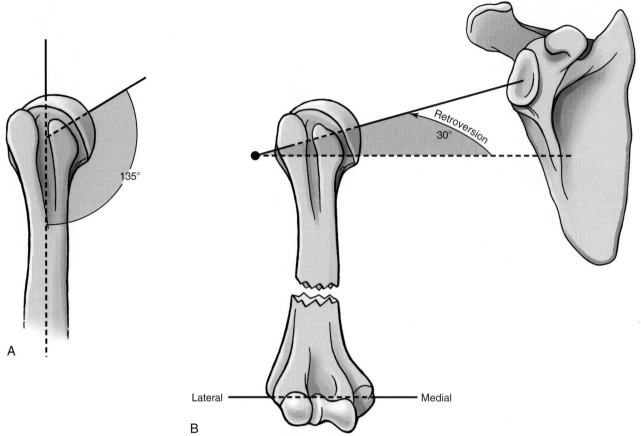

FIGURE 5-8. The right humerus showing a 135-degree "angle of inclination" between the shaft and head of the humerus in the frontal plane **(A)** and the retroversion of the humeral head relative to the distal humerus **(B).**

> **Osteologic Features of the Proximal-to-Mid Humerus**
> * Head of the humerus
> * Anatomic neck
> * Lesser tubercle and crest
> * Greater tubercle and crest
> * Upper, middle, and lower facets on the greater tubercle
> * Intertubercular (bicipital) groove
> * Deltoid tuberosity
> * Radial (spiral) groove

The *radial (spiral) groove* runs obliquely across the posterior surface of the humerus. The groove separates the proximal attachments of the lateral and medial head of the triceps (see Figure 5-9). Traveling distally, the radial nerve spirals around the posterior side of the humerus in the radial groove, heading toward the distal-lateral side of the humerus.

ARTHROLOGY

The most proximal articulation within the shoulder complex is the *sternoclavicular joint* (see Figure 5-1). The clavicle, through its attachment to the sternum, functions as a mechanical strut, or prop, holding the scapula at a relatively constant distance from the trunk. Located at the lateral end of the clavicle is the *acromioclavicular joint*. This joint, and

associated ligaments, firmly attaches the scapula to the clavicle. The anterior surface of the scapula rests against the posterior-lateral surface of the thorax, forming the *scapulothoracic joint*. This articulation is not a true anatomic joint; rather, it is an interface between bones. Movements at the scapulothoracic joint are mechanically linked to the movements at both the sternoclavicular and acromioclavicular joints. The position of the scapula on the thorax provides a base of operation for the *glenohumeral joint*, the most distal and mobile link of the complex. The term "shoulder movement" describes the combined motions at both the glenohumeral and the scapulothoracic joints.

> **Four Joints within the Shoulder Complex**
> * Sternoclavicular
> * Acromioclavicular
> * Scapulothoracic
> * Glenohumeral

The joints of the shoulder complex function as a series of links, all cooperating to maximize the range of motion available to the upper limb. A weakened, painful, or unstable link anywhere along the chain significantly decreases the effectiveness of the entire complex.

Before the kinematics of the sternoclavicular and acromioclavicular joints are described, the movements at the scapulothoracic joint must be defined (Figure 5-10). Primary movements at the scapulothoracic joint are traditionally described as elevation and depression, protraction and retraction, and upward and downward rotation. Additional movements of the scapula will be defined as the chapter unfolds.

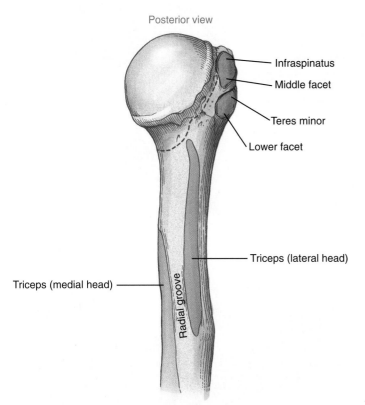

FIGURE 5-9. Posterior aspect of the right proximal humerus. Proximal attachments of muscles are in red, distal attachments in gray. The dashed line shows the capsular attachments of the glenohumeral joint.

> **Traditional Terminology for Describing the Primary Movements at the Scapulothoracic Joint**
>
> *Elevation*–The scapula slides superiorly on the thorax, as in the shrugging of the shoulders.
> *Depression*–From an elevated position, the scapula slides inferiorly on the thorax.
> *Protraction*–The medial border of the scapula slides anterior-laterally on the thorax away from the midline.
> *Retraction*–The medial border of the scapula slides posterior-medially on the thorax toward the midline, such as during "pinching" of the shoulder blades together.
> *Upward rotation*–The inferior angle of the scapula rotates in a superior-lateral direction, facing the glenoid fossa upward. This rotation occurs as a natural component of raising the arm upward.
> *Downward rotation*–From an upward rotated position, the inferior angle of the scapula rotates in an inferior-medial direction. This motion occurs as a natural component of lowering the arm down to the side.

Sternoclavicular Joint

GENERAL FEATURES

The sternoclavicular (SC) joint is a complex articulation, involving the medial end of the clavicle, the clavicular facet on the sternum, and the superior border of the cartilage of the first rib (Figure 5-11). The SC joint functions as the *basilar joint* of the entire upper extremity, linking the appendicular skeleton with the axial skeleton. The joint therefore must be firmly attached while simultaneously allowing considerable range of movement. These seemingly paradoxic functions are accomplished through extensive periarticular connective

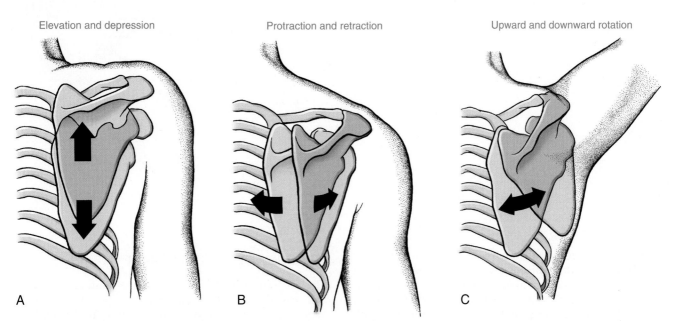

FIGURE 5-10. Motions of the right scapulothoracic joint. **A,** Elevation and depression. **B,** Protraction and retraction. **C,** Upward and downward rotation.

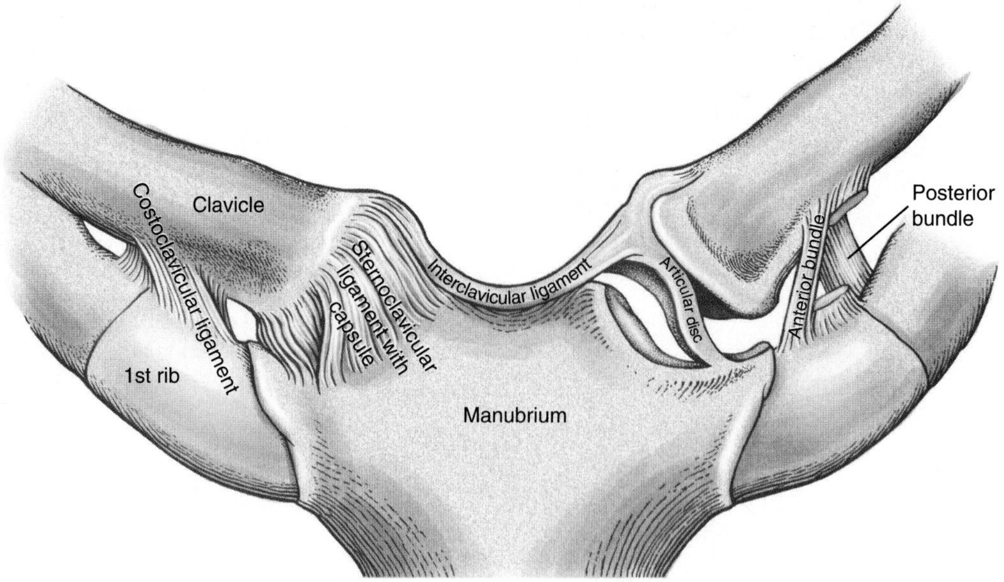

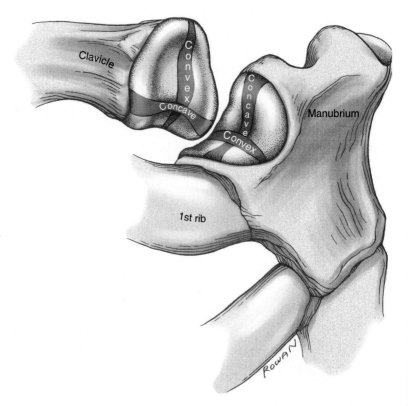

FIGURE 5-11. The sternoclavicular joints. The capsule and lateral section of the anterior bundle of the costoclavicular ligament have been removed on the left side.

FIGURE 5-12. An anterior-lateral view of the articular surfaces of the right sternoclavicular joint. The joint has been opened up to expose its articular surfaces. The longitudinal diameters *(purple)* extend roughly in the frontal plane between superior and inferior points of the articular surfaces. The transverse diameters *(blue)* extend roughly in the horizontal plane between anterior and posterior points of the articular surfaces.

tissues, and an irregular saddle-shaped articular surface (Figure 5-12). Although highly variable, the medial end of the clavicle is usually convex along its longitudinal diameter and concave along its transverse diameter.[178] The clavicular facet on the sternum typically is reciprocally shaped, with a slightly concave longitudinal diameter and a slightly convex transverse diameter.

PERIARTICULAR CONNECTIVE TISSUE

The SC joint is enclosed by a capsule reinforced by *anterior* and *posterior sternoclavicular ligaments* (see Figure 5-11).[177] When active, muscles add further stability to the joint: anteriorly by the sternocleidomastoid, posteriorly by the sternothyroid and sternohyoid, and inferiorly by the subclavius.

The *interclavicular ligament* spans the jugular notch, connecting the medial end of the right and left clavicles.

Tissues That Stabilize the Sternoclavicular Joint

- Anterior and posterior sternoclavicular joint ligaments
- Interclavicular ligament
- Costoclavicular ligament
- Articular disc
- Sternocleidomastoid, sternothyroid, sternohyoid, and subclavius muscles

---

The *costoclavicular ligament* is a strong structure extending from the cartilage of the first rib to the costal tuberosity on the inferior surface of the clavicle. The ligament has two distinct fiber bundles running perpendicular to each other.[178] The anterior bundle runs obliquely in a superior and lateral direction, and the posterior bundle runs obliquely in a superior and medial direction (see Figure 5-11). The crisscrossing of fibers assists with stabilizing the joint through all motions, except for a downward movement of the clavicle (i.e., depression).

The *articular disc* at the SC joint separates the joint into distinct medial and lateral joint cavities (see Figure 5-11).[178] The disc is a flattened piece of fibrocartilage that attaches inferiorly near the lateral edge of the clavicular facet and superiorly at the sternal end of the clavicle and interclavicular ligament. The remaining outer edge of the disc attaches to the internal surface of the capsule. The disc not only strengthens the articulation but functions as a shock absorber by increasing the surface area of joint contact. This absorption mechanism apparently works well because significant age-related degenerative arthritis is relatively rare at this joint.[35]

The tremendous stability at the SC joint is due to the arrangement of the periarticular connective tissues and, to a lesser extent, the interlocking of the articular surfaces. Large forces through the clavicle often cause fracture of the bone before the SC joint dislocates. Clavicular fractures are most common in males under 30 years old—most often as the result of contact-sport or road-traffic accidents.[164]

KINEMATICS

The osteokinematics of the clavicle involve a rotation in all three degrees of freedom. Each degree of freedom is associated with one of the three cardinal planes of motion: *sagittal, frontal,* and *horizontal.* The clavicle elevates and depresses, protracts and retracts, and rotates around the bone's longitudinal axis (Figure 5-13). The primary purpose of these movements is to place the scapula in an optimal position to accept the head of the humerus. Essentially all functional movements of the glenohumeral joint involve some movement of the clavicle around the SC joint. As described later in this chapter, the clavicle rotates in all three degrees of freedom as the arm is raised overhead.[110,115,125,169]

Elevation and Depression

Elevation and depression of the clavicle occur approximately parallel to the frontal plane, around a near anterior-posterior axis of rotation (see Figure 5-13). Maximums of approximately 45 degrees of elevation and 10 degrees of depression have been reported.[27,140] Elevation and depression of the clavicle produce a similar path of movement of the scapula.[73]

The arthrokinematics for elevation and depression of the clavicle occur along the SC joint's longitudinal diameter (see Figure 5-12). *Elevation* of the clavicle occurs as its convex articular surface rolls superiorly and simultaneously slides inferiorly on the concavity of the sternum (Figure 5-14, *A*). The stretched costoclavicular ligament helps limit as well as stabilize the elevated position of the clavicle. *Depression* of the clavicle occurs by action of its convex surface rolling inferiorly and sliding superiorly (see Figure 5-14, *B*).

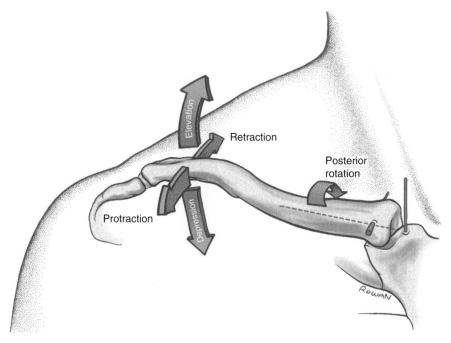

FIGURE 5-13. The osteokinematics of the right sternoclavicular joint. The motions are elevation and depression in a near frontal plane *(purple),* protraction and retraction in a near horizontal plane *(blue),* and posterior clavicular rotation in a near sagittal plane *(green).* The vertical and anterior-posterior axes of rotation are color-coded with the corresponding planes of movement. The longitudinal axis is indicated by the dashed green line.

FIGURE 5-14. Anterior view of a mechanical diagram of the arthrokinematics of roll and slide during elevation **(A)** and depression **(B)** of the clavicle around the right sternoclavicular joint. The axes of rotation are shown in the anterior-posterior direction near the head of the clavicle. Stretched structures are shown as thin elongated arrows; slackened structures are shown as wavy arrows. Note in **A** that the stretched costoclavicular ligament produces a downward force in the direction of the slide. *CCL,* costoclavicular ligament; *ICL,* interclavicular ligament; *SC,* superior capsule.

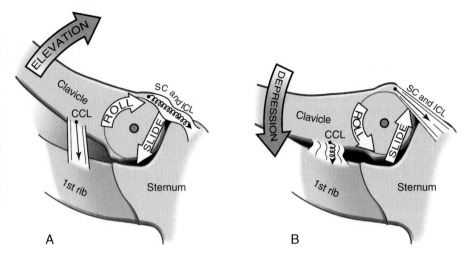

A fully depressed clavicle elongates and stretches the interclavicular ligament and the superior portion of the capsular ligaments.

Protraction and Retraction

Protraction and retraction of the clavicle occur nearly parallel to the horizontal plane, around a vertical axis of rotation (see Figure 5-13). (The axis of rotation is shown in Figure 5-13 as intersecting the sternum because, by convention, the axis of rotation for a given motion intersects the *convex* member of the joint.) A maximum of 15 to 30 degrees of motion have been reported in each direction.[27,140,179] The horizontal plane motions of the clavicle are strongly associated with protraction and retraction motions of the scapula.

The arthrokinematics for protraction and retraction of the clavicle occur along the SC joint's transverse diameter (see Figure 5-12). Retraction occurs as the concave articular surface of the clavicle rolls and slides posteriorly on the convex surface of the sternum (Figure 5-15). The end ranges of retraction elongate the anterior bundles of the costoclavicular ligament and the anterior capsular ligaments.

The arthrokinematics of protraction around the SC joint are similar to those of retraction, except that they occur in an anterior direction. The extremes of protraction occur during a motion involving maximal forward reach. Excessive tightness in the posterior bundle of the costoclavicular ligament, the posterior capsular ligament, and the scapular retractor muscles limit the extremes of clavicular protraction.

Axial (Longitudinal) Rotation of the Clavicle

The third degree of freedom at the SC joint is a rotation of the clavicle around the bone's longitudinal axis (see Figure 5-13). During shoulder abduction or flexion, a point on the superior aspect of the clavicle rotates *posteriorly* 20 to 35 degrees.[62,84,115,194] As the arm is returned to the side, the clavicle rotates back to its original position. The arthrokinematics of clavicular rotation involve a *spin* of its sternal end relative to the lateral surface of the articular disc.

Axial rotation of the clavicle is mechanically linked with the overall kinematics of abduction or flexion of the shoulder and cannot be independently performed with the arm resting at the side. The mechanics of this interesting

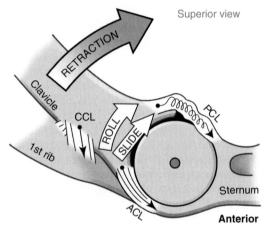

FIGURE 5-15. Superior view of a mechanical diagram of the arthrokinematics of roll and slide during retraction of the clavicle around the right sternoclavicular joint. The vertical axis of rotation is shown through the sternum. Stretched structures are shown as thin elongated arrows; slackened structures are shown as a wavy arrow. *ACL,* anterior capsular ligament; *CCL,* costoclavicular ligament; *PCL,* posterior capsular ligaments.

motion are further described later in this section on shoulder kinematics.

Acromioclavicular Joint

GENERAL FEATURES

The acromioclavicular (AC) joint is the articulation between the lateral end of the clavicle and the acromion of the scapula (Figure 5-16, *A*). The clavicular facet on the acromion faces medially and slightly superiorly, providing a point of attachment with the corresponding acromial facet on the clavicle. An articular disc of varying form is present in most AC joints.

The AC joint is a gliding or plane joint, reflecting the predominantly flat contour of the joint surfaces. Joint surfaces vary, however, from flat to slightly convex or concave (see Figure 5-16, *B*). Because of the predominantly flat joint surfaces, roll-and-slide arthrokinematics are not described.

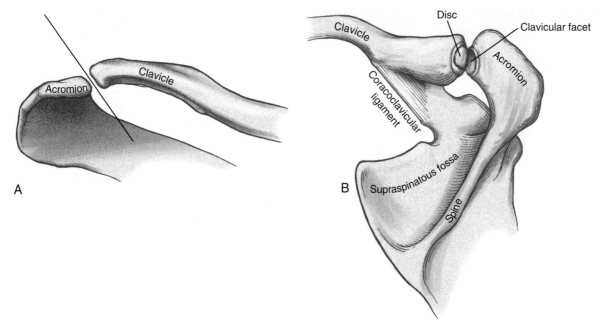

FIGURE 5-16. The right acromioclavicular joint. **A,** An anterior view showing the sloping nature of the articulation. **B,** A posterior view of the joint opened up from behind, showing the clavicular facet on the acromion and the disc.

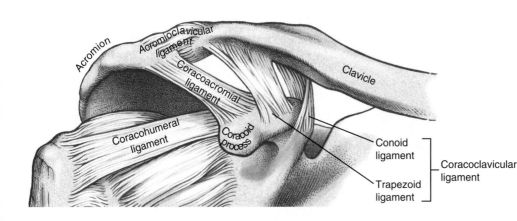

FIGURE 5-17. An anterior view of the right acromioclavicular joint including many surrounding ligaments.

PERIARTICULAR CONNECTIVE TISSUE

The AC joint is surrounded by a capsule that is directly reinforced by *superior* and *inferior ligaments* (Figure 5-17).[36,105] The superior capsular ligament is reinforced through attachments from the deltoid and trapezius.

Tissues That Stabilize the Acromioclavicular Joint
- Superior and inferior acromioclavicular joint ligaments
- Coracoclavicular ligament
- Articular disc (when present)
- Deltoid and upper trapezius

The *coracoclavicular ligament* provides an important extrinsic source of stability to the AC joint (see Figure 5-17). This extensive ligament consists of two parts: the trapezoid and

conoid ligaments. The *trapezoid ligament* extends in a superior-lateral direction from the superior surface of the coracoid process to the trapezoid line on the clavicle. The *conoid ligament* extends almost vertically from the proximal base of the coracoid process to the conoid tubercle on the clavicle.

Both parts of the coracoclavicular ligament are of similar length, cross-sectional area, stiffness, and tensile strength.[31] As a whole, the entire ligament is stronger and absorbs more energy at the point of rupture than most other ligaments of the shoulder. These structural features, in conjunction with the coracoclavicular ligament's near-vertical orientation, suggest an important role in suspending the scapula (and upper extremity) from the clavicle.

The articular surfaces at the AC joint are lined with a layer of fibrocartilage and often separated by a complete or incomplete *articular disc*. An extensive dissection of 223 sets of AC joints revealed complete discs in only about 10% of the joints.[35] The majority of joints possessed incomplete discs, which appeared fragmented and worn. According to

---

Acromioclavicular Joint Dislocation

The acromioclavicular (AC) joint is inherently susceptible to dislocation (separation) because of the sloped nature of the articulation and the high probability of receiving large shearing forces. Consider a person falling and striking the tip of the shoulder abruptly against the ground (Figure 5-18). The resulting medially and inferiorly directed ground reaction force may displace the acromion medially and under the sloped articular facet of the well-stabilized clavicle. Such horizontal shear is resisted primarily by the joint's superior and inferior capsular ligaments.[36] The coracoclavicular ligament, however, offers a secondary resistance to horizontal shear, especially if severe.[61] On occasion, the force applied to the scapula exceeds the tensile strength of all the ligaments, resulting in their rupture and complete dislocation of the AC joint. Trauma to the AC joint and associated ligaments can lead to instability and pain and possibly posttraumatic osteoarthritis. Extensive literature exists on the evaluation and the surgical and nonsurgical treatment of an injured AC joint, especially in athletes.[22,30,59,121]

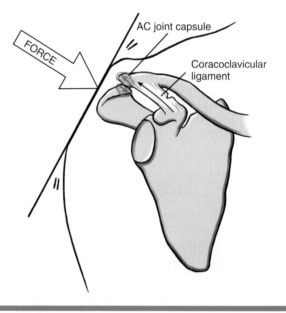

FIGURE 5-18. An anterior view of the shoulder striking the ground with the force of the impact directed at the acromion. The resulting shear force at the acromioclavicular (AC) joint is depicted by red arrows. Note the increased tension and partial tearing of the AC joint capsule and coracoclavicular ligament.

DePalma,[35] the incomplete discs are not structural anomalies but rather indications of the degeneration that often affects this joint.

KINEMATICS

Distinct differences exist in the function of the SC and AC joints. The SC joint permits extensive motion of the clavicle, which guides the general path of the scapula. The AC joint, in contrast, permits more subtle movements between the scapula and lateral end of the clavicle. The motions at the AC joint are kinesiologically important, however, and optimize the mobility and fit between the scapula and thorax.

The motions of the AC joint are described by the movement of the scapula relative to the lateral end of the clavicle. Motion has been defined for 3 degrees of freedom (Figure 5-19, *A*). The primary, or most obvious, motions are called *upward* and *downward rotation*. Secondary motions—referred to as *rotational adjustments*—fine-tune the position of the scapula, in both the horizontal and sagittal planes. Measuring isolated motions at the AC joint is difficult and is not done in typical clinical situations.

Upward and Downward Rotation

Upward rotation of the scapula at the AC joint occurs as the scapula "swings upwardly and outwardly" relative to the lateral end of the clavicle (see Figure 5-19, *A*). This motion occurs as a natural component of abduction or flexion of the shoulder. Reports vary widely, but up to 30 degrees of upward rotation at the AC joint occurs as the arm is raised fully over the head.[84,115,185,194] The motion contributes a significant component of the overall upward rotation at the scapulothoracic joint. Downward rotation at the AC joint returns the scapula back toward the anatomic position, a motion mechanically associated with shoulder adduction or extension. Figure 5-19, *A* depicts the upward and downward rotation of the scapula as a frontal plane motion, although most natural motions occur within the scapular plane.

Horizontal and Sagittal Plane "Rotational Adjustments" at the Acromioclavicular Joint

Kinematic observations of the AC joint during shoulder movement reveal pivoting or twisting type motions of the scapula around the lateral end of the clavicle. These so-called "rotational adjustment motions" optimally align the scapula

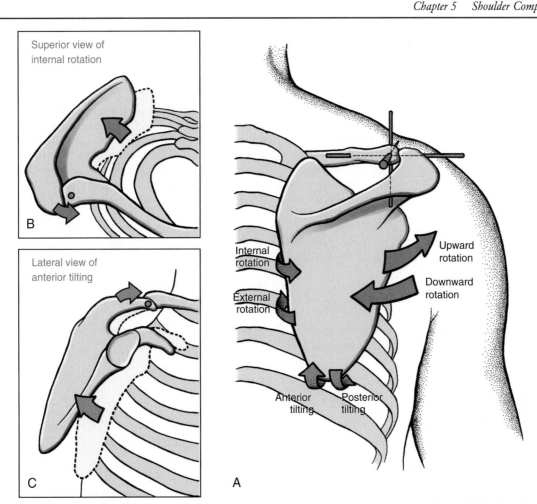

FIGURE 5-19. A, Posterior view showing the osteokinematics of the right acromioclavicular (AC) joint. The primary motions of upward and downward rotation are shown in purple. Horizontal and sagittal plane adjustments, considered as secondary motions, are shown in blue and green, respectively. Note that each plane of movement is color-coded with a corresponding axis of rotation. Images **B** and **C** show examples of rotational adjustments at the AC joint: internal rotation during scapulothoracic protraction **(B),** and anterior tilting during scapulothoracic elevation **(C).**

against the thorax, as well as adding to the total amount of its motion. Rotation adjustment motions at the AC joint are described within horizontal and sagittal planes (blue and green arrows in Figure 5-19, *A*, respectively).

Horizontal plane adjustments at the AC joint occur around a vertical axis, evident as the medial border of the scapula pivots away and toward the posterior surface of the thorax. These horizontal plane motions are described as *internal* and *external rotation*, defined by the direction of rotation of the glenoid fossa (see Figure 5-19, *A*). *Sagittal plane adjustments* at the AC joint occur around a near medial-lateral axis, evident as the inferior angle pivots away or toward the posterior surface of the thorax. The terms *anterior tilting* and *posterior tilting* describe the direction of this rotation, based on (as with horizontal plane motions) the direction of rotation of the glenoid fossa (see Figure 5-19).

The kinematics of the rotational adjustments at the AC joint are poorly understood, primarily because of the technical difficulties in isolating and measuring the relative small movements between the scapula and the clavicle. Moreover, the nomenclature used to describe these motions is not universally accepted. Differing magnitudes of motions have been reported

during shoulder abduction or flexion, generally ranging from 5 to 30 degrees per plane.* Although the kinematics at the AC joint are not well defined, certainly it enhances both the quality and quantity of movement at the scapulothoracic joint. Qualitatively, for instance, during protraction of the scapulothoracic joint, the AC joint internally rotates slightly within the horizontal plane (see Figure 5-19, *B*). This rotation helps align the anterior surface of the scapula to the curved contour of the thorax. For similar reasons of alignment, the scapula is allowed to tilt anteriorly slightly during elevation of the scapulothoracic joint, as during "shrugging" of the shoulders (see Figure 5-19, *C*). Without these rotational adjustments, the scapula would be obligated to follow the exact path of the moving clavicle, without any freedom to fine-tune its position on the thorax.

Scapulothoracic Joint

The scapulothoracic joint is not a true joint per se but rather a point of contact between the anterior surface of the scapula and the posterior-lateral wall of the thorax.[209] The two surfaces do

---

*References 47, 84, 113, 115, 123, 130, 135, 185, 194.

not make direct contact; rather, they are separated by muscles, such as the subscapularis, serratus anterior, and erector spinae. The relatively thick and moist surfaces of these muscles likely reduce shear within the articulation during movement. An audible clicking sound during scapular movements may indicate abnormal contact within the articulation.

In the anatomic position, the scapula is usually positioned between the second and the seventh ribs, with the medial border located about 6 cm lateral to the spine. Although highly variable, the average "resting" posture of the scapula is about 10 degrees of anterior tilt, 5 to 10 degrees of upward rotation, and about 35 degrees of internal rotation—a position consistent with the previously described *plane of the scapula*.[113,115]

Movements at the scapulothoracic joint are a very important element of shoulder kinesiology. The wide range of motion available to the shoulder is due, in part, to the large movement available to the scapulothoracic joint.

KINEMATICS

The movements that occur between the scapula and the thorax are a result of cooperation between the SC and the

AC joints. Restriction of motion at either joint can significantly limit motion of the scapula, and ultimately of the entire shoulder.

Elevation and Depression

Scapular elevation occurs as a composite of SC and AC joint rotations (Figure 5-20, *A*). For the most part, the motion of shrugging the shoulders is a direct result of the scapula following the path of the elevating clavicle around the SC joint (see Figure 5-20, *B*). Slight downward rotation of the scapula at the AC joint allows the scapula to remain nearly vertical throughout the elevation (see Figure 5-20, *C*). Additional adjustments at the AC joint help to keep the scapula flush with the slightly changing curvature of the thorax. Depression of the scapula occurs as the reverse action described for elevation.

Protraction and Retraction

Protraction of the scapula occurs through a summation of horizontal plane rotations at both the SC and AC joints (Figure 5-21, *A*). The scapula follows the general path of the protracting clavicle around the SC joint (see Figure 5-21, *B*).

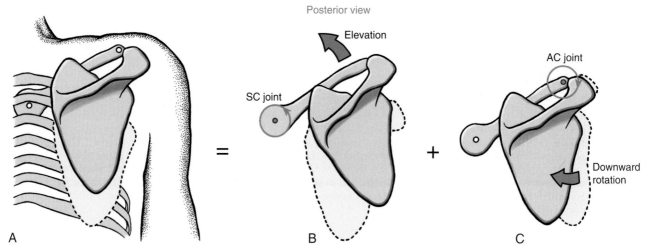

FIGURE 5-20. A, Scapulothoracic elevation shown as a summation of **B** (elevation at the sternoclavicular joint) and **C** (downward rotation at the acromioclavicular joint).

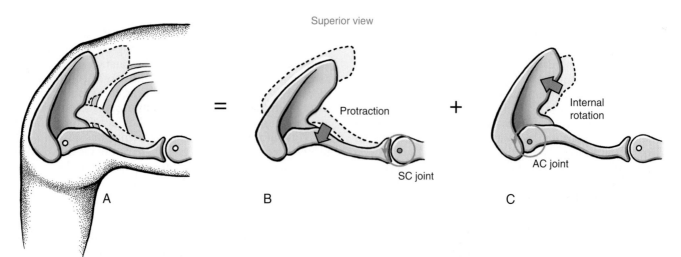

FIGURE 5-21. A, Scapulothoracic protraction shown as a summation of **B** (protraction at the sternoclavicular joint) and **C** (slight internal rotation at the acromioclavicular joint).

The AC joint can amplify, offset, or otherwise adjust the total amount of scapulothoracic protraction by contributing varying amounts of internal rotation (see Figure 5-21, *C*). Because scapulothoracic protraction occurs as a composite of motions at the SC and AC joints, a decrease in motion at one joint can be partially compensated for by an increase at the other. Consider, for example, an individual with severe degenerative arthritis and decreased motion at the AC joint. The SC joint may compensate by contributing a greater degree of protraction, thereby limiting the functional loss associated with forward reach of the upper limb.

Retraction of the scapula occurs in a similar but reverse fashion as protraction. Retraction of the scapula is often performed in the context of pulling an object toward the body, such as pulling on a wall pulley, climbing a rope, or putting the arm in a coat sleeve.

Upward and Downward Rotation

Upward rotation of the scapulothoracic joint is an integral part of raising the arm overhead (Figure 5-22, *A*). This motion places the glenoid fossa in a position to support and stabilize the head of the abducted (i.e., raised) humerus. Complete upward rotation of the scapula occurs by a summation of clavicular elevation at the SC joint (see Figure 5-22, *B*) *and* scapular upward rotation at the AC joint (see Figure 5-22, *C*).[62,84,110,115,169] These coupled rotations are essential to the full 60 degrees of upward rotation at the scapulothoracic joint.[49] The scapula may rotate upwardly and strictly in the frontal plane as in true abduction but more often follows a path closer to its own "scapular" plane. Normally the AC and SC joints have the mobility to adjust to the virtually infinite number of paths that the scapula may take during elevation of the arm.

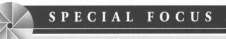

SPECIAL FOCUS 5-2

The Functional Importance of Full Upward Rotation of the Scapulothoracic Joint

The ability to raise the arm fully overhead is a prerequisite for many functional activities. A fully upward rotated scapula is an important component of this movement, accounting for approximately one third of the near 180 degrees of shoulder abduction or flexion.[5,84,123,134,194] As with all scapulothoracic motions, upward rotation is mechanically linked to the motions of the sternoclavicular and acromioclavicular joints.

The upward rotation of the scapula that occurs during full shoulder abduction in the plane of the scapula (about 35 degrees anterior to the frontal plane) serves at least three important functions. First, the upwardly rotated scapula projects the glenoid fossa upward and anterior-laterally, providing a structural base to maximize the upward and lateral reach of the upper limb. Second, the upwardly rotated scapula preserves the optimal length-tension relationship of the abductor muscles of the glenohumeral joint, such as the middle deltoid and supraspinatus. Third, the upwardly rotated scapula helps maintain the volume within the subacromial space: the area between the undersurface of the acromion and the humeral head (see Figures 5-24 and 5-25).[135] A reduced subacromial space during abduction may lead to a painful and damaging impingement of the residing tissues, such as the supraspinatus tendon.[116] Although more research is needed in this area, it is clear that the kinematics associated with upward rotation of the scapula are essential to optimal function of the shoulder, especially for full and pain-free range of abduction.

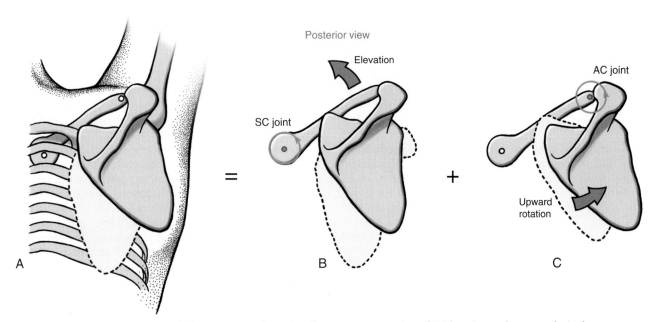

FIGURE 5-22. **A,** Scapulothoracic upward rotation shown as a summation of **B** (elevation at the sternoclavicular joint) and **C** (upward rotation at the acromioclavicular joint).

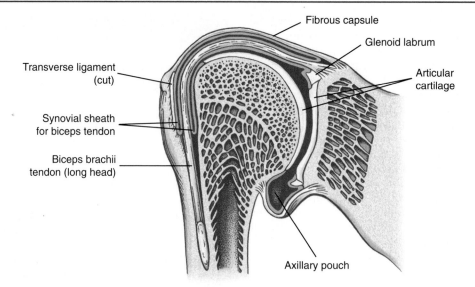

FIGURE 5-23. Anterior view of a frontal section through the right glenohumeral joint. Note the fibrous capsule, synovial membrane *(blue),* and the long head of the biceps tendon. The axillary pouch is shown as a recess in the inferior capsule.

Downward rotation of the scapula occurs as the arm is returned to the side from a raised position. The motion is described similarly to upward rotation, except that the clavicle depresses at the SC joint and the scapula downwardly rotates at the AC joint. The motion of downward rotation usually ends when the scapula has returned to the anatomic position.

Glenohumeral Joint

GENERAL FEATURES

The glenohumeral (GH) joint is the articulation formed between the large convex head of the humerus and the shallow concavity of the glenoid fossa (Figure 5-23). This joint operates in conjunction with the moving scapula to produce an extensive range of motion of the shoulder. In the anatomic position, the articular surface of the glenoid fossa is directed anterior-laterally in the scapular plane. In most people the glenoid fossa is upwardly rotated slightly: a position dependent on the amount of fixed upward inclination of the fossa and on the degree of upward rotation of the scapulothoracic joint.

In the anatomic position, the humeral head is directed medially and superiorly, as well as posteriorly because of its natural retroversion. This orientation places the head of the humerus directly into the scapular plane and therefore directly against the face of the glenoid fossa (see Figure 5-4, *B* and *C).*

PERIARTICULAR CONNECTIVE TISSUE AND OTHER SUPPORTING STRUCTURES

The GH joint is surrounded by a *fibrous capsule* that isolates the joint cavity from most surrounding tissues (see Figure 5-23). The capsule attaches along the rim of the glenoid fossa and extends to the anatomic neck of the humerus. A *synovial*

membrane lines the inner wall of the joint capsule. An extension of this synovial membrane lines the intracapsular portion of the tendon of the long head of the biceps brachii. This synovial membrane continues to surround the biceps tendon as it exits the joint capsule and descends into the intertubercular (i.e., bicipital) groove. The head of the humerus and the glenoid fossa are both lined with *articular cartilage.*

The potential volume of space within the GH joint capsule is about twice the size of the humeral head. The loose-fitting and expandable capsule provides extensive mobility to the GH joint. This mobility is evidenced by the amount of passive translation available at the GH joint. The humeral head can be pulled away from the fossa a significant distance without causing pain or trauma to the joint. In the anatomic or adducted position, the inferior portion of the capsule appears as a slackened or redundant recess called the *axillary pouch.*

The fibrous capsule of the GH joint is relatively thin and is reinforced by thicker external ligaments (described later). By crossing superiorly over the humeral head, the long head of the biceps also contributes to GH stability. The primary functional stability of the GH joint is based not only on passive tension within embedded ligaments, but on the active forces produced by local muscles, such as those of the rotator cuff (subscapularis, supraspinatus, infraspinatus, and teres minor). Unlike the capsular ligaments, which produce their greatest stabilizing tension only when stretched at relatively extreme motions, muscles generate large, active stabilizing tensions at virtually any joint position. The rotator cuff muscles are considered the "dynamic" stabilizers of the GH joint because of their predominant role in maintaining articular stability during active motions.

Capsular Ligaments

The external layers of the anterior and inferior walls of the joint capsule are thickened by fibrous connective tissue known

SPECIAL FOCUS 5-3

The "Loose Fit" of the Glenohumeral Joint: an Inherent Problem of Instability

Several anatomic features of the glenohumeral (GH) joint contribute to a design that favors mobility at the expense of stability. The articular surface of the glenoid fossa covers only about one third of the articular surface of the humeral head. This size difference allows only a small part of the humeral head to make contact with the glenoid fossa in any given shoulder position. In a typical adult, the longitudinal diameter of the humeral head is about 1.9 times larger than the longitudinal diameter of the glenoid fossa (Figure 5-24). The transverse diameter of the humeral head is about 2.3 times larger than the opposing transverse diameter of the glenoid fossa. The GH joint is often described as a ball-and-socket joint, although this description gives the erroneous impression that the head of the humerus fits *into* the glenoid fossa. The actual structure of the GH joint resembles more that of a golf ball pressed against a coin the size of a quarter. This bony fit offers little to no stability to the GH joint; instead, the mechanical integrity of the articulation is maintained primarily through mechanisms involving the surrounding muscles and capsular ligaments.

For a host of reasons, capsular ligaments may fail to adequately support and stabilize the GH joint. Such lack of support is manifested by excessive translation of the humeral head. Although some degree of laxity is normal at the GH joint, excessive laxity is not.[201] A condition of excessive laxity, or "joint play," associated with large translations of the proximal humerus relative to the glenoid is often referred to as *shoulder instability*. A diagnosis of shoulder instability typically means that the excessive laxity is associated with pain, apprehension, or a lack of function.[76]

Although GH joint instability can occur in multiple directions, most cases exhibit excessive motion anteriorly or inferiorly. In some cases, an unstable GH joint may contribute to subluxation or dislocation. *Subluxation* at the GH joint is defined as an incomplete separation of articular surfaces, often followed by spontaneous realignment. *Dislocation* at the GH joint, in contrast, is defined as a complete separation of articular surfaces *without* spontaneous realignment. Typically, a dislocated joint must be rearticulated by a special maneuver performed by another person or by the subject.

Instability of the GH joint is often associated with less than optimal alignment and disrupted arthrokinematics, which over time can place damaging stress on the joint's soft tissues. It is not always clear if shoulder instability is more the result or the cause of the abnormal arthrokinematics. The pathomechanics of shoulder instability are poorly understood and occupy the forefront of interest among clinicians, researchers, and surgeons.[16,25,201]

Ultimately, stability at the GH joint is achieved by a combination of passive and active mechanisms. *Active mechanisms* rely on the forces produced by muscle. These forces are provided primarily by the embracing nature of the rotator cuff group. *Passive mechanisms,* on the other hand, rely primarily on forces *other than* activated muscle. At the GH joint the passive mechanisms include (1) restraint provided by capsule, ligaments, glenoid labrum, and tendons; (2) mechanical support predicated on scapulothoracic posture; and (3) negative intracapsular pressure. Because of the variability and complexity of most movements of the shoulder, a combination of both passive and active mechanisms is typically required to ensure joint stability. This important and multifaceted topic of stability at the GH joint will be a recurring theme throughout the chapter.

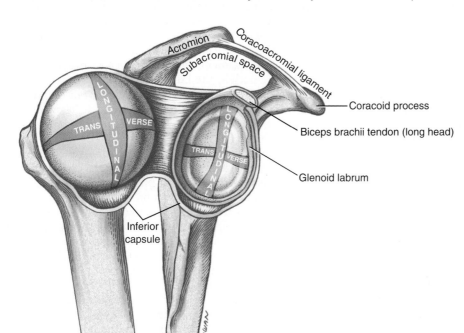

FIGURE 5-24. Side view of right glenohumeral joint with the joint opened up to expose the articular surfaces. Note the extent of the subacromial space under the coracoacromial arch. Normally this space is filled with the supraspinatus muscle and its tendon, and the subacromial bursa. The longitudinal and horizontal diameters are illustrated on both articular surfaces.

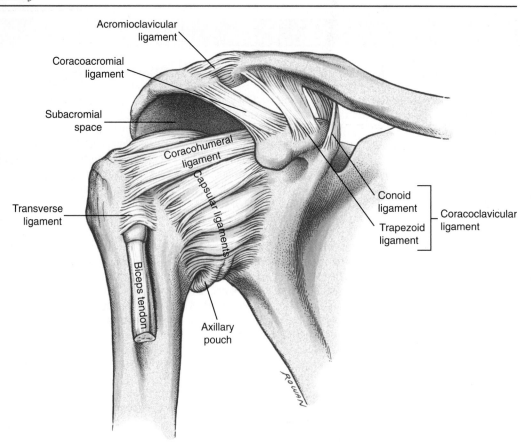

Acromioclavicular
ligament

Coracoacromial
ligament

Subacromial
space

Coracohumeral
ligament

Capsular ligaments

Conoid
ligament

Trapezoid
ligament

Coracoclavicular
ligament

Transverse
ligament

Biceps tendon

Axillary
pouch

FIGURE 5-25. Anterior view of the right glenohumeral joint showing the primary ligaments. Note the subacromial space located between the top of the humeral head and the underside of the acromion.

simply as the *glenohumeral capsular ligaments* (Figure 5-25). Most of the fibers within the ligaments attach to the humerus, although a few more circular fibers spiral around the joint and reattach within the capsule.[65] To generate stabilizing tensions across the joint, the inherently loose capsular ligaments must be elongated or twisted to varying degrees; the resulting passive tension generates mechanical support for the GH joint and limits the extremes of rotation and translation.

By reinforcing the walls of the capsule, the capsular ligaments also assist with maintaining a negative intra-articular pressure within the GH joint. This slight suction offers an additional source of stability.[85] Puncturing (or venting) of the capsule equalizes the pressure on both sides, removing the slight suction force between the head and the fossa. Experimental release of the pressure by piercing the capsule with a needle has been shown to cause inferior subluxation of the humeral head.[101]

The following discussion describes the essential anatomy and functions of the GH joint capsular ligaments. Although a separate entity, the coracohumeral ligament will be considered with this group. The following material is essential for determining which ligament, or part of the capsule, is most responsible for restricting a particular movement. Such information assists the clinician and surgeon understand the mechanisms responsible for capsular injury and joint instability, and also provides guidance for manual therapy and surgical intervention[38,88,139,202] Table 5-1 lists the distal attachments of the ligaments and specific motions that render each ligament taut. Considerably more detail exists on this subject and can be found in other sources.[11,19,33,39,100,201]

The GH joint's capsular ligaments consist of complex bands of interlacing collagen fibers, divided into superior, middle, and inferior bands.[65] The ligaments are best visualized from an internal view of the GH joint (Figure 5-26). The *superior glenohumeral ligament* has its proximal attachment near the supraglenoid tubercle, just anterior to the long head of the biceps. The ligament, with adjacent capsule, attaches near the anatomic neck of the humerus above the lesser tubercle. The ligament becomes particularly taut in full adduction. Once taut in adduction, the superior capsular ligament provides a restraint to inferior and anterior-posterior translations of the humeral head.[37]

The *middle glenohumeral ligament* has a wide proximal attachment to the superior and middle aspects of the anterior rim of the glenoid fossa. The ligament blends with the anterior capsule and broad tendon of the thick subscapularis muscle, then attaches along the anterior aspect of the anatomic neck. This ligament provides a substantial anterior restraint to the GH joint, especially in a position of 45 to 60 degrees of abduction.[37,54] Based on its location, the middle glenohumeral ligament is very effective at limiting the extremes of external rotation.[54,151]

The extensive *inferior glenohumeral ligament* attaches proximally along the anterior-inferior rim of the glenoid fossa, including the glenoid labrum. Distally the inferior glenohumeral ligament attaches as a broad sheet to the anterior-inferior and posterior-inferior margins of the anatomic neck.[128,129,182] The hammock-like inferior capsular ligament has three separate components: an *anterior band*, a *posterior band*, and a sheet of tissue connecting these bands known as

TABLE 5-1. Distal Attachments and Primary Functions of the Glenohumeral Joint Capsular Ligaments

Ligament	Distal (Humeral) Attachments	Primary Motions Drawing Structure Taut
Superior glenohumeral ligament	Anatomic neck, above the lesser tubercle	Adduction; inferior and anterior-posterior translations of the humeral head
Middle glenohumeral ligament	Along the anterior aspect of the anatomic neck; also blends with the subscapularis tendon	Anterior translation of the humeral head, especially in about 45-60 degrees of abduction; external rotation
Inferior glenohumeral ligament (three parts: anterior band, posterior band, and connecting axillary pouch)	As a broad sheet to the anterior-inferior and posterior-inferior margins of the anatomic neck	Axillary pouch: 90 degrees of abduction, combined with anterior-posterior and inferior translations Anterior band: 90 degrees of abduction and full external rotation; anterior translation of humeral head Posterior band: 90 degrees of abduction and full internal rotation
Coracohumeral ligament	Anterior side of the greater tubercle; also blends with the superior capsule and supraspinatus tendon	Adduction; inferior translation of the humeral head; external rotation

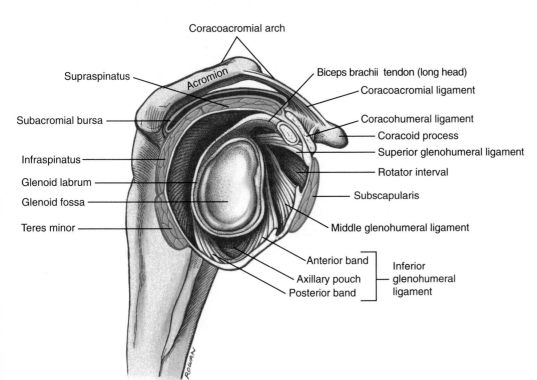

FIGURE 5-26. Lateral aspect of the internal surface of the right glenohumeral joint. The humerus has been removed to expose the capsular ligaments and the glenoid fossa. Note the prominent coracoacromial arch and underlying subacromial bursa *(blue)*. The four rotator cuff muscles are shown in red.

an *axillary pouch* (see Figure 5-26).[151] The axillary pouch and the surrounding inferior capsular ligaments become most taut in about 90 degrees of abduction. Acting as a sling, the taut axillary pouch supports the suspended humeral head and provides a cradling effect that resists inferior and anterior-posterior translations.[176,188,204] From this abducted position, the anterior and posterior bands become further taut at the extremes of external and internal rotation, respectively.[100,204] The anterior band—the strongest and thickest part of the entire capsule—is particularly important, as it furnishes the primary ligamentous restraint to anterior translation of the humeral head, both in an abducted and a neutral position.[65,152] Forceful and dynamic activities involving *abduction* and *external rotation* specifically stress the anterior band of

the inferior capsule. Such stress, for example, may occur during the "cocking phase" of throwing a baseball (Figure 5-27). Over many repetitions, this action can overstretch or tear the anterior band, thereby compromising one of the prime restraints to anterior translation of the humeral head.[10,100] Injury and increased laxity of this portion of the anterior and inferior capsule are indeed associated with recurrent anterior dislocations of the GH joint.[74,193] Whether the recurring anterior dislocation is caused by or results from tears or laxity in the anterior bands of the inferior capsule is not certain.[138,201]

The GH joint capsule is also strengthened by the *coracohumeral ligament* (see Figures 5-25 and 5-26). This ligament extends from the lateral border of the coracoid process to the

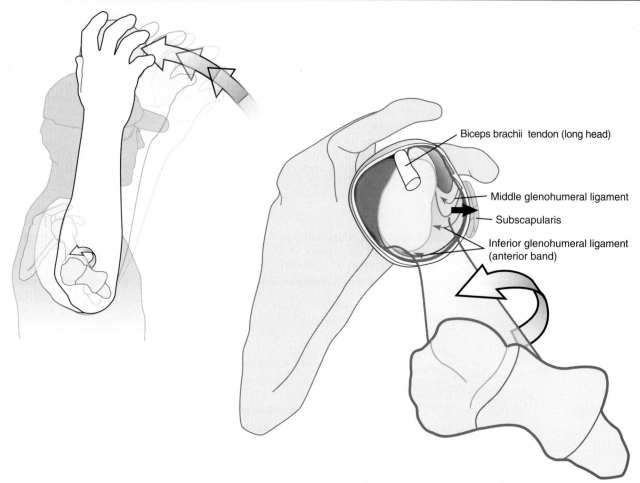

FIGURE 5-27. Illustration showing a high velocity abduction and external rotation motion of the glenohumeral joint during the cocking phase of pitching a baseball. This motion twists and elongates the middle GH ligament and anterior band of the inferior GH ligament (depicted as red thin arrows pointed toward the rim of the glenoid fossa). The humeral head has been removed to show the aforementioned stretched structures and glenoid fossa. This active motion tends to translate the humeral head anteriorly *(thick black arrow),* toward the anterior glenoid labrum and subscapularis muscle. Tension in the stretched ligaments and subscapularis muscles naturally resists this anterior translation.

anterior side of the greater tubercle of the humerus. The coracohumeral ligament also blends with the superior capsule and supraspinatus tendon. Similar to the superior capsular ligament, the position of adduction pulls the coracohumeral ligament taut. From this position, the coracohumeral ligament provides significant restraint to inferior translation and external rotation of the humeral head.[13,86,100]

Rotator Cuff Muscles and Long Head of the Biceps Brachii

As previously mentioned, the GH joint capsule receives significant structural reinforcement from the four *rotator cuff muscles* (see Figure 5-26). The subscapularis, the thickest of the four muscles,[90] lies just anterior to the capsule. The supraspinatus, infraspinatus, and teres minor lie superior and posterior to the capsule. These four muscles form a cuff that protects and actively stabilizes the GH joint, especially during dynamic activities. In addition to the belly of the rotator cuff muscles being located very close to the joint, the tendons of these muscles actually blend into the capsule.[178] This unique anatomic arrangement helps explain why the mechanical stability of the GH joint is so dependent on the innervation,

strength, and control of the rotator cuff muscles. It is clinically important to note that, as evidenced by Figure 5-26, the rotator cuff fails to cover two regions of the capsule: inferiorly, and a region between the supraspinatus and subscapularis known as the *rotator interval.*[83] The inherently weakened region of the rotator interval is, however, reinforced by the tendon of the long head of the biceps and the coracohumeral ligament.[86] The rotator interval is one common site for anterior dislocation of the GH joint.

The *long head of the biceps brachii* originates off the supraglenoid tubercle of the scapula and adjacent rim of connective tissue known as the glenoid labrum (see Figure 5-26). From this proximal attachment, this intracapsular tendon crosses over the humeral head as it courses toward the intertubercular groove on the anterior humerus. Cadaver studies strongly suggest that in an active state, the long head of the biceps restricts anterior translation of the humeral head.[100,154] In addition, the position of the tendon across the dome of the humeral head also suggests a role in resisting superior migration of the humeral head—an important force needed to control the natural arthrokinematics of abduction.[154]

Glenoid Labrum

The rim of the glenoid fossa is encircled by a fibrocartilage ring, or lip, known as the *glenoid labrum* (see Figure 5-26). About 50% of the overall depth of the glenoid fossa has been attributed to the glenoid labrum.[79] By deepening the concavity of the fossa, the labrum increases contact area with the humeral head and therefore helps stabilize the joint.[29]

Tissues That Reinforce or Deepen the Glenohumeral Joint

- Joint capsule and associated capsular ligaments
- Coracohumeral ligament
- Rotator cuff muscles (subscapularis, supraspinatus, infraspinatus, and teres minor)
- Long head of the biceps brachii
- Glenoid labrum

SCAPULOTHORACIC POSTURE AND ITS EFFECT ON STATIC STABILITY

Normally when one stands at complete rest with arms at the sides, the head of the humerus remains stable against the glenoid fossa. This stability is referred to as *static* because it exists at rest. One passive mechanism for controlling static stability at the GH joint is based on the analogy of a ball compressed against an inclined surface (Figure 5-28, *A*).[9] At rest, the superior capsular structures (SCS) provide the primary ligamentous support for the humeral head. These structures include the superior capsular ligament, the coracohumeral ligament, and the tendon of the supraspinatus. Combining the resultant capsular force vector with the force vector due to gravity yields a compressive locking force, oriented at right angles to the surface of the glenoid fossa. The compression force *(CF)* stabilizes the GH joint by compressing the humeral head firmly against the glenoid fossa, thereby resisting descent of the humerus.[86,87] The inclined plane of the glenoid also acts as a partial shelf that supports part of the weight of the arm.

Electromyographic (EMG) data suggest that the supraspinatus, and to a lesser extent the posterior deltoid, provides a secondary source of static stability by generating active forces that are directed nearly parallel to the superior capsular force vector. This secondary support may be required, for example, while supporting a hand-held load by the side at the waist. Of interest, a classic and early study by Basmajian and Bazant[9] showed that vertically running muscles, such as the biceps, triceps, and middle deltoid, are generally *not* actively involved in providing static stability, even when significant downward traction is applied to the arm.

An important component of the static locking mechanism is a scapulothoracic posture that maintains the glenoid fossa slightly upwardly rotated. A chronically downwardly rotated posture may be associated with "poor posture" or may be secondary to paralysis or weakness of certain muscles, such as the upper trapezius. Regardless of cause, loss of the upwardly rotated position increases the angle between the force vectors created by the superior capsular structures and gravity (see Figure 5-28, *B*). Adding the force vectors produced by the superior capsular structures and gravity now yields a *reduced* compressive force. Gravity can pull the humerus down the face of the glenoid fossa. Over time, and if not supported by external means, the downward pull can

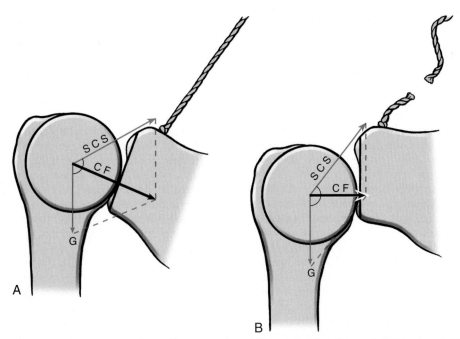

FIGURE 5-28. Scapular posture and its effect on static stability at the glenohumeral (GH) joint. **A,** The rope indicates a muscular force that holds the glenoid fossa in a slightly upward-rotated position. In this position the passive tension in the taut superior capsular structure *(SCS)* is added to the force produced by gravity *(G)*, yielding the compression force *(CF)*. The compression force applied against the slight incline of the glenoid "locks" the joint. **B,** With a loss of upward rotation posture of the scapula (indicated by the cut rope), the change in angle between the SCS and G vectors reduces the magnitude of the compression force across the GH joint. As a consequence, the head of the humerus may slide down the now vertically oriented glenoid fossa. The dashed lines indicate the parallelogram method of adding force vectors.

Why the Glenoid Labrum Is So Vulnerable to Injury

Several structural and functional factors explain why the glenoid labrum is so frequently involved in shoulder pathology. First, the superior part of the glenoid labrum is only loosely attached to the adjacent glenoid rim. Furthermore, approximately 50% of the fibers of the tendon of the long head of the biceps are direct extensions of the superior glenoid labrum; the remaining 50% arise from the supraglenoid tubercle.[197] Exceedingly large or repetitive forces within the biceps tendon can partially detach the loosely secured superior labrum from its near–12 o'clock position on the glenoid rim. The relatively high incidence of superior labral tears in throwing athletes, such as baseball pitchers, is likely related to the forces produced within the biceps during this activity.[100] The long head of the biceps is stressed (along with the anterior and inferior capsule) during the "cocking" phase of pitching, and again as the muscle rapidly decelerates the arm and forearm during the follow-through phase of the pitch.[4,100] This stress is transferred directly to the superior labrum. A weakening of the proximal attachment of the long head of the biceps likely limits the muscle's ability to restrain anterior translation of the humeral head.[42] These pathomechanics

may predispose the throwing athlete (or overhead laborer) to anterior instability and further associated stress.[156] Several other mechanisms of injury and biomechanical consequences of lesions of the superior labrum have been postulated.[144,145,208]

Lesions or detachments of the glenoid labrum are also common along the anterior-inferior rim of the glenoid fossa.[74,193] Normally this region of the labrum is firmly attached to the anterior band of the inferior capsular ligament.[29] As previously described, excessive laxity or tears in this portion of the capsule can lead to recurrent anterior dislocations of the humeral head.[170] A rapidly anteriorly translating humeral head can create damaging forces on the adjacent anterior-inferior capsule and glenoid labrum. The resulting frayed or partially torn labrum or adjacent capsule may create a vicious cycle of greater anterior GH joint instability and more frequent episodes of stress in this region. Conservative management of a detached or torn glenoid labrum is often unsuccessful, especially if the shoulder is also mechanically unstable. Surgical repair is often required, followed by a specific postoperative rehabilitation program.[156,208]

---

result in plastic deformation of the superior capsular structures. As a consequence, the inadequately supported head of the humerus may eventually sublux or dislocate inferiorly from the glenoid fossa.

CORACOACROMIAL ARCH AND ASSOCIATED BURSA

The *coracoacromial arch* is formed by the coracoacromial ligament and the acromion process of the scapula (see Figure 5-26). The *coracoacromial ligament* attaches between the anterior margin of the acromion and the lateral border of the coracoid process.

The coracoacromial arch forms the functional "roof" of the GH joint. The space between the coracoacromial arch and the underlying humeral head was referred to earlier in the chapter as the *subacromial space*. In the healthy adult, the subacromial space measures only about 1 cm in height.[157,189] The very clinically relevant subacromial space contains the supraspinatus muscle and tendon, the subacromial bursa, the long head of the biceps, and part of the superior capsule.

Multiple separate *bursa sacs* exist around the shoulder. Some of the sacs are direct extensions of the synovial membrane of the GH joint, such as the subscapular bursa, whereas others are separate structures. All are situated in regions where significant frictional forces develop, such as between tendons, capsule and bone, muscle and ligament, or two adjacent muscles. Two important bursa sacs are located superior to the humeral head (Figure 5-29). The *subacromial bursa* lies within the subacromial space above the supraspinatus muscle and below the acromion process. This bursa protects the relatively soft and vulnerable supraspinatus muscle and tendon from the rigid undersurface of the acromion. The *subdeltoid bursa* is a lateral extension of the subacromial bursa, limiting frictional forces between the deltoid and the underlying supraspinatus tendon and humeral head.

KINEMATICS

The GH joint is considered a universal joint because movement occurs in all three degrees of freedom. The primary motions at the GH joint are *flexion and extension, abduction and adduction, and internal and external rotation* (Figure 5-30). Often, a fourth motion is defined at the GH joint: *horizontal flexion and extension* (also called *horizontal adduction and abduction*). The motion occurs from a starting position of 90 degrees of abduction. The humerus moves anteriorly during horizontal flexion and posteriorly during horizontal extension.

Reporting the range of motion at the GH joint uses the anatomic position as the 0-degree or neutral reference point. In the sagittal plane, for example, flexion is described as the rotation of the humerus anterior to the 0-degree position. Extension, in contrast, is described as the rotation of the humerus posterior to the 0-degree position.

Virtually any purposeful motion of the GH joint involves motion at the scapulothoracic joint, including the associated movements at the SC and AC joints. The following discussion, however, focuses on the kinematics of the GH joint.

Abduction and Adduction

Abduction and adduction are traditionally defined as rotation of the humerus in the near frontal plane around an axis oriented in the near anterior-posterior direction (Figure 5-30). Normally, the healthy person has about 120 degrees of abduction at the GH joint, although a range of values has been reported.[5,84,115] External rotation of the GH joint naturally accompanies abduction—a point easily verifiable by palpation. This accompanying external rotation allows the greater tubercle of the humerus to pass posterior to the acromion process and therefore avoid jamming against the contents within the subacromial space, most notably the supraspinatus tendon. Full abduction of the shoulder complex

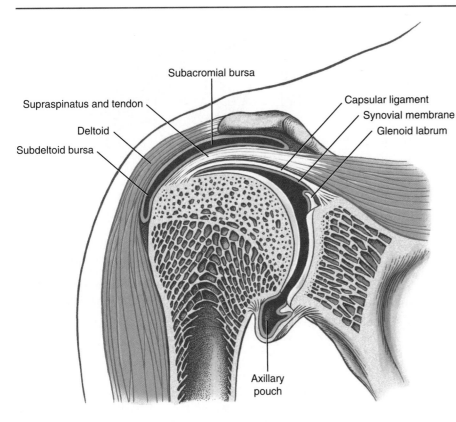

Subacromial bursa

Supraspinatus and tendon

Deltoid

Subdeltoid bursa

Capsular ligament

Synovial membrane

Glenoid labrum

Axillary pouch

FIGURE 5-29. An anterior view of a frontal plane cross-section of the right glenohumeral joint. Note the subacromial and subdeltoid bursa within the subacromial space. Bursa and synovial lining are depicted in blue. The deltoid and supraspinatus muscles are also shown.

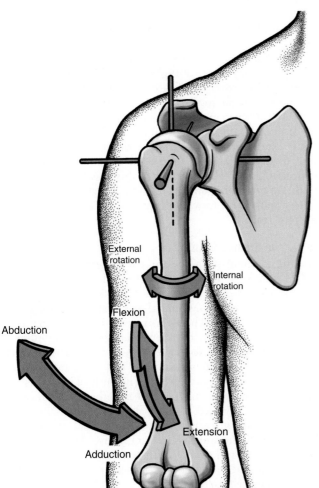

External rotation

Internal rotation

Flexion

Abduction

Adduction

Extension

FIGURE 5-30. The osteokinematics of the glenohumeral joint includes abduction and adduction *(purple)*, flexion and extension *(green)*, and internal and external rotation *(blue)*. Note that each axis of rotation is color-coded with its corresponding plane of movement.

requires a simultaneous approximate 60 degrees of upward rotation of the scapula; these kinematics were introduced previously in this chapter.

The arthrokinematics of abduction involve the convex head of the humerus rolling superiorly while simultaneously sliding inferiorly (see Figure 5-31). Roll-and-slide arthrokinematics occur along, or close to, the longitudinal diameter of the glenoid fossa (see Figure 5-24). With regard to arthrokinematics, adduction is similar to abduction but occurs in a reverse direction.

Figure 5-31 shows part of the supraspinatus muscle blending with the superior capsule of the GH joint. In addition to producing abduction, the active muscular contraction pulls the superior capsule taut, thereby protecting it from being pinched between the humeral head and undersurface of the acromion process. The muscular force also adds to the dynamic stability of the joint. (*Dynamic stability* refers to the stability achieved while the joint is moving.) As abduction proceeds, the prominent humeral head unfolds and stretches the axillary pouch of the inferior capsular ligament. The resulting tension within the inferior capsule acts as a hammock or sling, which supports the head of the humerus.

Importance of Roll-and-Slide Arthrokinematics at the Glenohumeral Joint

The roll-and-slide arthrokinematics depicted in Figure 5-31 are essential to the completion of full range abduction. Recall that the longitudinal diameter of the articular surface of the humeral head is almost twice the size of the longitudinal diameter on the glenoid fossa. The arthrokinematics of abduction demonstrate how a simultaneous roll and slide allow a larger convex surface to roll over a much smaller concave surface without running out of articular surface.

Without a sufficient concurrent inferior slide during abduction, the superior roll of the humeral head would ultimately lead to a jamming of the head against the unyielding coracoacromial arch. An adult-sized humeral head that is rolling up a glenoid fossa *without* a concurrent inferior slide would translate through the 10-mm subacromial space after only 22 degrees of GH joint abduction (Figure 5-32, *A*). This situation would create an impingement of the supraspinatus tendon and subacromial bursa between the head of the humerus and the coracoacromial arch.[67] Such an impingement can physically block further abduction (see Figure 5-32, *B*). In vivo measurements of the healthy shoulder show that throughout abduction in the scapular plane, the center of the humeral head remains essentially stationary, or it may translate superiorly only a few millimeters.[43,112,135,155,160] The concurrent inferior slide of the contact point of the humeral head offsets most of its inherent tendency to translate superiorly during abduction.

In healthy persons the offsetting effect of the roll-and-slide arthrokinematics in conjunction with a pliable inferior capsule contribute to the maintenance of a normal subacromial space during abduction. In cases of excessive stiffness and reduced volume of the axillary pouch, however, the humeral head is typically forced upward a considerable distance during abduction, and against the delicate tissues within the subacromial space. Such unnatural and repeated compression may damage and inflame the supraspinatus tendon, subacromial bursa, long head of the biceps tendon, and superior parts of the capsule. Over time, this repeated compression may lead to a painful condition known as *subacromial impingement syndrome*.[135,147]

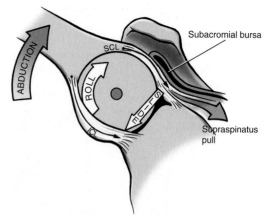

FIGURE 5-31. The arthrokinematics of the right glenohumeral joint during active abduction. The supraspinatus is shown contracting to direct the superior roll of the humeral head. The taut inferior capsular ligament (*ICL*) is shown supporting the head of the humerus like a hammock (see text). Note that the superior capsular ligament (*SCL*) remains relatively taut because of the pull from the attached contracting supraspinatus. Stretched tissues are depicted as long black arrows.

Flexion and Extension

Flexion and extension at the GH joint are defined as a rotation of the humerus within the near sagittal plane around a near medial-lateral axis of rotation (Figure 5-33). The arthrokinematics involve primarily a *spinning* motion of the humeral head around the glenoid fossa. As shown in Figure 5-33, the spinning of the humeral head draws most of the surrounding capsular structures taut. Tension within the stretched posterior capsule may cause a slight anterior translation of the humerus at the extremes of flexion.[75] At least 120 degrees of flexion are available to the GH joint. Flexing the shoulder to nearly 180 degrees includes an accompanying upward rotation of the scapulothoracic joint.[115]

Full extension of the shoulder occurs to a position of about 65 degrees actively (and 80 degrees passively) behind the frontal plane.[8] The extremes of this passive motion likely stretch the capsular ligaments, causing a slight anterior tilting of the scapula. This forward tilt may enhance the extent of a backward reach.

Internal and External Rotation

From the anatomic position, internal and external rotation at the GH joint is defined as an axial rotation of the humerus in the horizontal plane (see Figure 5-30). This rotation occurs around a vertical or longitudinal axis that runs through the shaft of the humerus. The arthrokinematics of external rotation take place over the transverse diameters of the humeral head and the glenoid fossa (see Figure 5-24). The humeral head simultaneously rolls posteriorly and slides anteriorly on the glenoid fossa (Figure 5-34). The arthrokinematics for internal rotation are similar, except that the direction of the roll and slide is reversed.

The simultaneous roll and slide of internal and external rotation allows the much larger transverse diameter of the humeral head to roll over a much smaller surface area of the glenoid fossa. The importance of these anterior and posterior slides is evidenced by returning to the model of the humeral head shown in Figure 5-32, *A*, but envisioning the humeral head rolling over the glenoid fossa's transverse diameter. If,

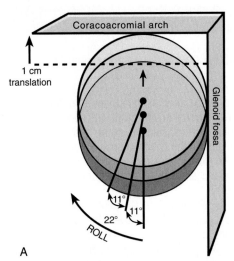
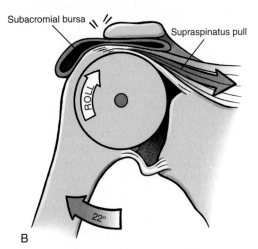

FIGURE 5-32. A, A model of the glenohumeral joint depicting a ball the size of a typical adult humeral head rolling across a flattened (glenoid) surface. Based on the assumption that the humeral head is a sphere with a circumference of 16.3 cm, the head of the humerus would translate upward 1 cm after a superior roll (abduction) of only 22 degrees. This magnitude of translation would cause the humeral head to press against the contents of the subacromial space. **B,** Anatomic representation of the model used in **A.** Note that abduction *without* a concurrent inferior slide causes the humeral head to impinge against the arch and block further abduction.

for example, 75 degrees of external rotation occur by a posterior roll *without* a concurrent anterior slide, the head displaces posteriorly, roughly 38 mm. This amount of translation completely disarticulates the joint because the *entire* transverse diameter of the glenoid fossa is only about 25 mm (about 1 inch). Normally, however, full external rotation results in only 1 to 2 mm of posterior translation of the center of the humeral head, demonstrating that an "offsetting" anterior slide accompanies the posterior roll.[75]

From an adducted position, about 75 to 85 degrees of internal rotation and 60 to 70 degrees of external rotation are usually possible, but much variation can be expected. In a position of 90 degrees of abduction, the external rotation range of motion usually increases to near 90 degrees. Regard-

less of the position at which these rotations occur, there is usually some associated movement at the scapulothoracic joint. From the anatomic position, full internal and external rotation of the shoulder includes varying amounts of scapular protraction and retraction, respectively.

As with all motions of the GH joint, the specific arthrokinematics depend on the exact plane of the osteokinematics. As previously described, from the anatomic position, internal and external rotation is associated with roll-and-slide arthrokinematics. Rotation of the GH joint from a position of about 90 degrees of abduction, however, requires primarily a spinning motion between a point on the humeral head and the glenoid fossa. Being able to visualize the relationship between the osteokinematics and arthrokinematics at a joint provides

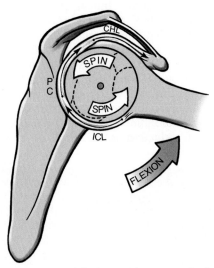

FIGURE 5-33. Side view of flexion in the near sagittal plane of the right glenohumeral joint. A point on the head of the humerus is shown spinning around a point on the glenoid fossa. Stretched structures are shown as *long thin arrows. PC,* posterior capsule; *ICL,* inferior capsular ligament; *CHL,* coracohumeral ligament.

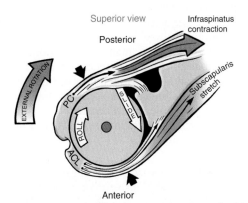

FIGURE 5-34. Superior view of roll-and-slide arthrokinematics during active external rotation of the right glenohumeral joint. The infraspinatus is shown contracting *(dark red),* causing the posterior roll of the humerus. The subscapularis muscle and anterior capsular ligament *(ACL)* generate passive tension from being stretched. The posterior capsule *(PC)* is pulled relatively taut because of the pull of the contracting infraspinatus muscle. The two large bold black arrows represent forces that centralize and thereby stabilize the humeral head during external rotation. Stretched tissues are depicted as *thin, elongated arrows.*

"Dynamic Centralization" of the Humeral Head: an Important Interaction between the Capsule and the Rotator Cuff Muscles

During all volitional motions at the glenohumeral (GH) joint, forces from activated rotator cuff muscles play a very important role in providing dynamic stability of the GH joint. Activated muscle forces combine with the passive forces from stretched capsular ligaments to maintain the humeral head in proper position on the glenoid fossa. Dynamic stability at the GH joint relies heavily on the interaction of these active and passive forces, particularly because of the natural incongruity and lack of bony containment of the joint. Figure 5-34 highlights an example of a dynamic stabilizing mechanism during active external rotation. The infraspinatus (one of the four rotator cuff muscles) is shown contracting to produce active external rotation torque at the GH joint. Because the infraspinatus attaches partially to the posterior capsule, its active contraction limits the amount of slack produced in this structure.[88] Maintenance of even relatively low-level tension in the posterior capsule, combined with the natural rigidity from the activated muscle, helps stabilize the posterior side of the joint during active external rotation. In the healthy shoulder, the anterior side of the joint is also stabilized during active external rotation. Passive tension in the stretched subscapularis muscle, middle glenohumeral capsular ligament, and coracohumeral ligament all add rigidity to the anterior capsule. Forces therefore are generated on both sides of the joint during active external rotation, serving to stabilize and centralize the humeral head against the glenoid fossa.[41]

An excessively tight GH joint capsule may interfere with the effectiveness of the centralization process just described. For instance, during active external rotation (as shown in Figure 5-34), an overly tight anterior capsule could create a large, passive force that positions the humeral head too far posteriorly. This mechanism could decentralize the humeral head relative to the glenoid, creating abnormal contact areas within the joint. Alternatively (and likely more commonly), during active internal rotation an overly tight posterior capsule can displace the humeral head too far anteriorly. This situation is a possible factor associated with GH joint instability and subacromial impingement syndrome.[111,122,192]

---

a useful mental construct for the treatment and evaluation of patients. These relationships are summarized in Table 5-2.

Overall Kinematics of Shoulder Abduction: Establishing the Six Kinematic Principles of the Shoulder Complex

To this point, the study of shoulder arthrology has focused primarily on the isolated kinematics of the various joints, or links, within the shoulder complex. The next and final discussion summarizes the kinematics across the entire region, with a focus on how the bones or joints contribute to full active abduction. This discussion will highlight six kinematic principles related to full active shoulder abduction, shown in a highly mechanical fashion in Figure 5-35. When performed in a pain-free and natural manner, full abduction usually indicates optimal kinematic sequencing across the shoulder complex. Understanding how the joints of the complex work together allows the clinician to appreciate how impairments in one part of the complex affect another. This understanding serves as an important foundation for effective evaluation and treatment of the shoulder.

SCAPULOHUMERAL RHYTHM

The most widely cited study on the kinematics of shoulder abduction was published by Inman and colleagues in 1944.[84] This classic work focused on shoulder abduction in the frontal plane. Data from this study were collected using two-dimensional radiographs and, most interesting, recording the movement of pins inserted directly into the bones of the shoulder in a live subject. This early study set the background for most subsequent studies on the kinematics of the shoulder.

In the healthy shoulder a natural kinematic rhythm or timing exists between glenohumeral abduction and scapulo-thoracic upward rotation. Inman popularized the term "scapulohumeral rhythm" to explain this kinematic relationship. He reported that after about 30 degrees of abduction this rhythm remained remarkably constant, occurring at a ratio of 2:1: for every 3 degrees of shoulder abduction, 2 degrees occurs by GH joint abduction and 1 degree occurs by scapulothoracic joint upward rotation. The first kinematic principle of shoulder abduction states that based on a generalized 2:1 scapulohumeral rhythm, a full arc of nearly 180 degrees of abduction is the result of a simultaneous

---

TABLE 5-2. Summary of the Kinematic Relationships at the Glenohumeral Joint

Osteokinematics	Plane of Motion/Axis of Rotation	Arthrokinematics
Abduction and adduction	Near frontal plane/near anterior-posterior axis of rotation	Roll and slide along joint's longitudinal diameter
Internal and external rotation	Horizontal plane/vertical axis of rotation	Roll and slide along joint's transverse diameter
Flexion and extension, internal and external rotation (in 90 degrees of abduction)	Near sagittal plane/near medial-lateral axis of rotation	Primarily a spin between humeral head and glenoid fossa

120 degrees of GH joint abduction and 60 degrees of scapulothoracic upward rotation (see two purple arcs in main illustration of Figure 5-35).

A significant amount of research on scapulohumeral rhythm has been published since Inman's classic in vivo work. Most of these studies used less invasive methods, including radiography, goniometry, photography, cinematography, and, more recently, fluoroscopy, magnetic resonance imaging, and electromechanical or electromagnetic tracking devices.* Published scapulohumeral rhythms vary across studies, ranging from 1.25:1 to 2.9:1, which are relatively close to Inman's reported 2:1 ratio.† Variations in scapulohumeral rhythms reflect differences in measurement technique, population sampled, speed and arc of measured motion, number of dimensions recorded, and amount of external load. Regardless of the differing ratios reported in the literature, Inman's classic 2:1 ratio remains a valuable axiom for evaluating shoulder abduction. It is simple to remember and helps to conceptualize the overall relationship between humeral and scapular movement considering the full 180 degrees of shoulder abduction.

---

*References 15, 32, 49, 68, 119, 132, 183, 191.
†References 5, 60, 70, 115, 125, 160, 183.

STERNOCLAVICULAR AND ACROMIOCLAVICULAR JOINTS DURING FULL ABDUCTION

Upward rotation of the scapula during full abduction is one of the essential components of shoulder kinematics. What dictates the overall path of the scapula, however, are the combined kinematics at the SC and AC joints.[84,115] These kinematics are plotted in Figure 5-36, based on data collected as a subject actively performed 180 degrees of frontal plane shoulder abduction. Although the preceding graph represents only one of many possible kinematic expressions at the SC and AC joints during abduction, it nicely introduces the next kinematic principle. The second kinematic principle of abduction states that the approximate 60 degrees of upward rotation of the scapula during full shoulder abduction are a result of a simultaneous elevation of the clavicle at the SC joint combined with upward rotation of the scapula at the AC joint. The precise angular motions that each joint contributes to scapular upward rotation are difficult to document with certainty. For mostly technical reasons, the kinematics at the SC joint have been more extensively studied in this regard. Inman reported that the SC joint elevates 30 degrees during 180 degrees of frontal plane abduction.[84] In contrast, Ludewig and co-workers reported an average of only 6 to 10 degrees of clavicular elevation; however, their data were collected throughout a more limited arc of abduction.[110,115] More definitive data are needed on the relative contributions of the SC and AC joints to upward rotation of the scapula, throughout a full range of shoulder abduction. It is clear, however, that each joint contributes significantly to the scapular motion, as depicted in the main illustration in Figure 5-35.

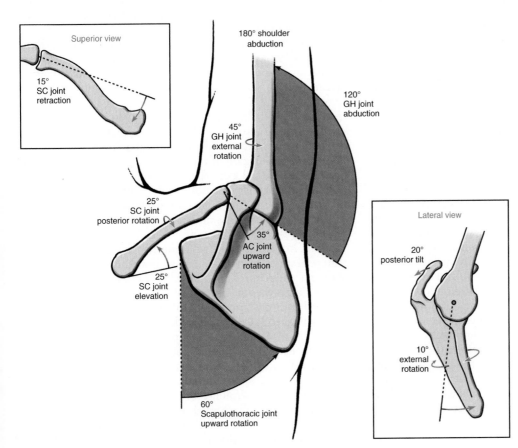

FIGURE 5-35. Posterior view of the right shoulder complex after the arm has abducted 180 degrees. The 60 degrees of scapulothoracic joint upward rotation and the 120 degrees of glenohumeral *(GH)* joint abduction are shaded in purple. Additional inserts contained in the boxes depict superior and lateral views of selected kinematics of the clavicle and scapula, respectively. All numeric values are chosen from a wide range of estimates cited across multiple literature sources (see text). Actual kinematic values vary considerably among persons and studies.

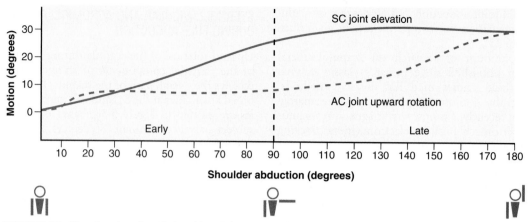

FIGURE 5-36. Plot showing the relationship of elevation at the sternoclavicular *(SC)* joint and upward rotation at the acromioclavicular *(AC)* joint during full shoulder abduction. The 180 degrees of abduction are divided into early and late phases. (Redrawn from data from Inman VT, Saunders M, Abbott LC: Observations on the function of the shoulder joint, *J Bone Joint Surg Am* 26:1, 1944.)

The third kinematic principle of abduction states that the clavicle retracts at the SC joint during full shoulder abduction. Recall that in the anatomic position the clavicle lies approximately horizontal, about 20 degrees posterior to the frontal plane (see Figure 5-4, *A*). During shoulder abduction the clavicle retracts about another 15 degrees (see Figure 5-35, top left inset). Of interest, these kinematics have been reported during active and passive abduction.[62,123,125,194] The retracting clavicle assists the AC joint with optimal positioning of the scapula within the horizontal plane.[110,115,174]

The fourth kinematic principle of abduction states that during full abduction, the scapula posteriorly tilts and externally rotates (Figure 5-35, lower right inset). (Although these kinematic terms were described previously in Figure 5-19, *A* for the AC joint, they are frequently used in the literature to describe the overall motion of the scapula relative to the thorax.) The magnitude of the posterior tilting and external rotation of the scapula vary widely and are determined by the combined kinematics at the SC and AC joints.[115,169,199] At rest in the anatomic position, the scapula is anteriorly tilted about 10 degrees and internally rotated approximately 35 degrees (i.e., in the scapular plane; see Figure 5-4, *B*). As shoulder abduction proceeds, the scapula posteriorly tilts primarily by motion at the AC joint. The external rotation of the scapula during full abduction, although relatively slight and variable, occurs as a *net* rotation based on movements at the SC and AC joints. According to Ludewig and colleagues, the AC joint actually internally rotates during shoulder abduction.[115] Any potential internal rotation of the scapula is normally offset, however, by a greater magnitude of retraction at the SC joint. As a result, the scapula usually undergoes a slight net external rotation, although the bone is still biased anteriorly in the scapular plane. It is important to realize that the magnitude and pattern of these scapular motions vary considerably among studies.* Nevertheless, these motions are important and function to move the coracoacromial arch *away* from the advancing humeral head. Most studies suggest that the posterior tilting and net external rotation of the scapula help preserve the volume of the subacromial space during abduction.† These motions may limit the likelihood of impingement of structures

in the subacromial space and thereby reduce mechanical stress on the shoulder capsule and rotator cuff muscles.[116]

The fifth kinematic principle of abduction states the clavicle rotates posteriorly around it own long axis. This motion was described earlier in this chapter as one of the primary SC joint motions (see Figure 5-13). Although actual measurements are scarce, the literature reports 20 to 35 degrees of clavicular rotation, depending on the plane and amount of shoulder abduction (see Figure 5-35, main illustration).[84,110,115,194] Data consistently show that most of the rotation occurs relatively late in the range of abduction.

The mechanism that drives the posterior rotation of the clavicle is based on a combination of interesting multi-joint kinematics and forces transferred from muscle to ligaments. Figure 5-37, *A* shows in a very highly diagrammatic fashion the relatively slackened coracoclavicular ligament while at rest in the anatomic position. At the early phases of shoulder abduction, the scapula begins to upwardly rotate at the AC joint, stretching the relatively stiff coracoclavicular ligament (see Figure 5-37, *B*). The inability of this ligament to significantly elongate restricts further upward rotation at this joint. Tension within the stretched ligament is transferred to the conoid tubercle region of the clavicle, a point posterior to the bone's longitudinal axis. The application of this force rotates the crank-shaped clavicle posteriorly. This rotation places the clavicular attachment of the coracoclavicular ligament closer to the coracoid process, unloading the ligament slightly and permitting the scapula to continue its final degrees of upward rotation. Inman[84] describes this mechanism as "a fundamental feature of shoulder motion," and without this motion complete shoulder abduction is not possible. Ludewig and colleagues report that posterior rotation of the clavicle is mechanically coupled with posterior tilting of the AC joint—motions that are essential to full-range shoulder abduction.[110]

The sixth kinematic principle of abduction states the humerus naturally externally rotates during shoulder abduction (see Figure 5-35, main illustration).[115] As stated earlier, external rotation allows the greater tubercle to pass posterior to the acromion, avoiding a potential impingement of the contents in the subacromial space. Stokdijk and colleagues have shown differing ratios of external rotation to humeral elevation based on the specific plane of elevation.[181] Pure frontal plane abduction had a higher ratio (i.e., greater exter-

---

*References 47, 113, 115, 123, 124, 125, 134, 169.
†References 92, 115, 123, 125, 135, 174.

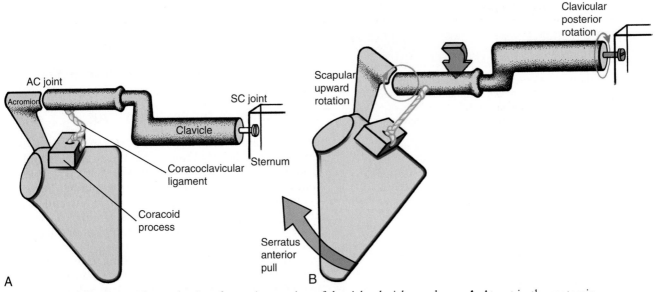

FIGURE 5-37. The mechanics of posterior rotation of the right clavicle are shown. **A,** At rest in the anatomic position, the acromioclavicular *(AC)* and sternoclavicular *(SC)* joints are shown with the coracoclavicular ligament represented by a slackened rope. **B,** As the serratus anterior muscle rotates the scapula upward, the coracoclavicular ligament is drawn taut. The tension created within the stretched ligament rotates the crank-shaped clavicle in a posterior direction, allowing the AC joint to allow full upward rotation.

Shoulder Abduction in the Frontal Plane versus the Scapular Plane

Shoulder abduction in the frontal plane is often used as a representative motion to evaluate overall shoulder function. Despite its common usage, however, this motion is not very natural. Abducting the shoulder in the scapular plane (about 35 degrees anterior to the frontal plane) is a more natural movement and generally allows greater elevation of the humerus than abducting in the pure frontal plane.[3] Furthermore, abducting in the scapular plane appears less mechanically coupled to an obligatory external rotation.[181] This can be demonstrated by the following example. Attempt to maximally abduct your shoulder in the pure frontal plane while consciously avoiding any accompanying external rotation. The difficulty or inability to complete the extremes of this motion results in part from the greater tubercle of the humerus compressing the contents of the subacromial space against a low point on the coracoacromial arch (Figure 5-38, *A*).[212] For natural completion of full frontal plane abduction, external rotation of the humerus must be combined with the abduction effort. This ensures that the prominent greater tubercle clears the posterior edge of the undersurface of the acromion.

Next, fully abduct your arm in the scapular plane. This abduction movement can usually be performed with greater ease and with less external rotation, at least in the early to mid ranges of shoulder motion. Impingement is avoided because scapular plane abduction places the apex of the greater tubercle under the relatively high point of the coracoacromial arch (see Figure 5-38, *B*). Abduction in the scapular plane also allows the naturally retroverted humeral head to fit more directly into the glenoid fossa. The proximal and distal attachments of the supraspinatus muscle are placed along a straight line. These mechanical differences between frontal plane and scapular plane abduction should be considered during evaluation and treatment of patients with shoulder dysfunction, particularly if subacromial impingement is suspected.

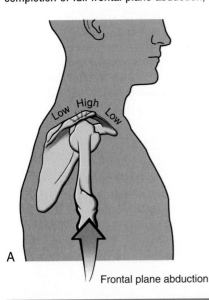

Frontal plane abduction

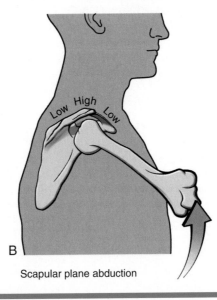

Scapular plane abduction

FIGURE 5-38. Side view of the right glenohumeral joint comparing abduction of the humerus in **A,** the true frontal plane and **B,** the scapular plane. In both **A** and **B,** the glenoid fossa is oriented in the scapular plane. The relative low and high points of the coracoacromial arch are also depicted. The line of force of the supraspinatus is shown in **B,** coursing under the coracoacromial arch.

BOX 5-1. Six Kinematic Principles Associated with Full Abduction of the Shoulder

Principle 1: Based on a generalized 2:1 scapulohumeral rhythm, active shoulder abduction of about 180 degrees occurs as a result of simultaneous 120 degrees of glenohumeral (GH) joint abduction and 60 degrees of scapulothoracic upward rotation.

Principle 2: The 60 degrees of upward rotation of the scapula during full shoulder abduction is the result of a simultaneous elevation at the sternoclavicular (SC) joint combined with upward rotation at the acromioclavicular (AC) joint.

Principle 3: The clavicle retracts at the SC joint during shoulder abduction.

Principle 4: The scapula posteriorly tilts and externally rotates during full shoulder abduction.

Principle 5: The clavicle posteriorly rotates around its own axis during shoulder abduction.

Principle 6: The GH joint externally rotates during shoulder abduction.

nal rotation per degree of abduction) than abduction in the scapular plane. The amount of external rotation that accompanies full active shoulder abduction is not known for certain but likely falls within the 25- to 55-degree range.

The six kinematic principles associated with the fully abducting shoulder are summarized in Box 5-1. These principles should provide a generalized guideline for organizing and highlighting the kinematics across the multiple joints of the shoulder. The actual magnitudes and pattern of motion associated with each principle will certainly vary for any individual person or study. This variability reflects the natural variability associated with human motion, and that caused by different methods of studying the topic.[187]

MUSCLE AND JOINT INTERACTION

Innervation of the Muscles and Joints of the Shoulder Complex

INTRODUCTION TO THE BRACHIAL PLEXUS

The entire upper extremity receives its innervation primarily through the *brachial plexus*–a consolidation of ventral rami from the C^5 to T^1 nerve roots (Figure 5-39). The basic anatomic plan of the brachial plexus as is follows. Nerve roots C^5 and C^6 form the upper trunk, C^7 forms the middle trunk, and C^8 and T^1 form the lower trunk. Trunks course a short distance before forming anterior or posterior subdivisions. The subdivisions then reorganize into three cords (lateral, posterior, and medial), named according to their relationship to the axillary artery. The cords finally branch into named major nerves, such as the ulnar, median, radial, axillary, and so on.

INNERVATION OF MUSCLE

The majority of the muscles that drive the shoulder complex receive their motor innervation from two regions of the brachial plexus: (1) nerves that branch from the posterior cord, such as the axillary, subscapular, and thoracodorsal nerves, and (2) nerves that branch from more proximal segments of the brachial plexus, such as the dorsal scapular, long thoracic, pectoral, and suprascapular nerves. This information is summarized in Table 5-3. An exception to this innervation scheme is the trapezius muscle, which is innervated primarily by cranial nerve XI, with lesser motor and sensory innervation from nerve roots of the upper cervical nerves.[178]

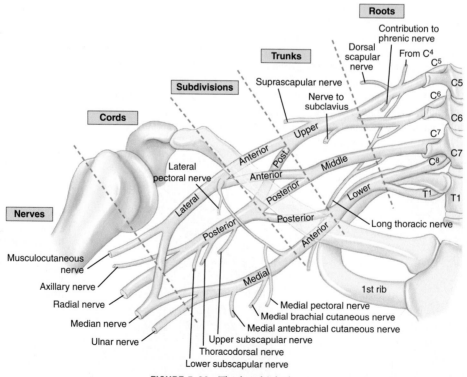

FIGURE 5-39. The brachial plexus.

TABLE 5-3. Nerves That Flow from the Brachial Plexus and Innervate the Primary Muscles of the Shoulder

Nerve	Relation to Brachial Plexus	Primary Nerve Root(s)	Muscles Supplied
Axillary	Posterior cord	C^5, C^6	Deltoid and teres minor
Thoracodorsal (middle subscapular)	Posterior cord	C^6, C^7, C^8	Latissimus dorsi
Upper subscapular	Posterior cord	C^5, C^6	Upper fibers of subscapularis
Lower subscapular	Posterior cord	C^5, C^6	Lower fibers of subscapularis and teres major
Lateral pectoral	At or proximal to lateral cord	C^5, C^6, C^7	Pectoralis major and occasionally the pectoralis minor
Medial pectoral	At or proximal to medial cord	C^8, T^1	Pectoralis major (sternocostal head) and pectoralis minor
Suprascapular	Upper trunk	C^5, C^6	Supraspinatus and infraspinatus
Subclavian	Upper trunk	C^5, C^6	Subclavius
Dorsal scapular	C^5 nerve root	C^5	Rhomboid major and minor; levator scapula*
Long thoracic	Proximal to trunks	C^5, C^6, C^7	Serratus anterior

Note: The primary spinal nerve roots that contribute to each nerve are listed.
*Also innervated by C^3 and C^4 nerve roots from the cervical plexus.

As a reference, the primary nerve roots that supply the muscles of the upper extremity are listed in Appendix II, Part A. In addition, Appendix II, Parts B to D include reference materials that may help with the clinical assessment of the functional status of the C^5 to T^1 nerve roots and several major peripheral nerves of the upper limb.

SENSORY INNERVATION TO THE JOINTS

The sternoclavicular joint receives sensory (afferent) innervation from the C^3 and C^4 nerve roots from the cervical plexus.[178] The acromioclavicular and glenohumeral joints receive sensory innervation via the C^5 and C^6 nerve roots via the suprascapular and axillary nerves.[63]

Action of the Shoulder Muscles

Most of the muscles of the shoulder complex fall into one of two functional categories: proximal stabilizers or distal mobilizers. The proximal stabilizers are muscles that originate on the spine, ribs, and cranium and insert on the scapula and clavicle. Examples of these muscles are the serratus anterior and the trapezius. The distal mobilizers consist of muscles that originate on the scapula and clavicle and insert on the humerus or the forearm. Examples of two distal mobilizers are the deltoid and biceps brachii muscles. As described subsequently, optimal function of the shoulder complex requires an interaction between the proximal stabilizers and the distal mobilizers. For example, for the deltoid to generate an effective abduction torque at the glenohumeral joint, the scapula must be firmly stabilized against the thorax by the serratus anterior and trapezius muscles. In cases of a paralyzed serratus anterior muscle, for example, the deltoid muscle is unable to express its full abduction function. Additional clinical examples of this important concept are presented in this chapter.

The proximal and distal attachments and nerve supply of the muscles of the shoulder complex are listed in Appendix II, Part E.

Primary Muscles Acting at the Scapulothoracic Joint

Elevators
- Upper trapezius
- Levator scapulae
- Rhomboids

Depressors
- Lower trapezius
- Latissimus dorsi
- Pectoralis minor
- Subclavius

Protractors
- Serratus anterior

Retractors
- Middle trapezius
- Rhomboids
- Lower trapezius

Upward Rotators
- Serratus anterior
- Upper and lower trapezius

Downward Rotators
- Rhomboids
- Pectoralis minor

Muscles of the Scapulothoracic Joint

The muscles of the scapulothoracic joint are categorized according to their actions as elevators or depressors, protractors or retractors, or upward and downward rotators. Some muscles act on the scapulothoracic joint indirectly by attaching to the clavicle or the humerus.

ELEVATORS

The muscles responsible for elevation of the scapulothoracic joint are the *upper trapezius, levator scapulae,* and, to a lesser extent, the *rhomboids* (Figure 5-40).[34] Functionally, these muscles support the posture of the shoulder girdle (scapula and clavicle) and upper extremity. Although variable, ideal posture of the shoulder girdle incorporates a slightly elevated and relatively retracted scapula, with the glenoid fossa facing slightly upward. The upper trapezius, by attaching to the lateral end of the clavicle, provides excellent leverage around the SC joint for maintenance of this ideal posture.

Several pathologies may cause a reduced muscular support of the shoulder girdle. For instance, isolated paralysis of the upper trapezius may occur from damage to the spinal accessory nerve (cranial nerve XI) or following polio (a virus

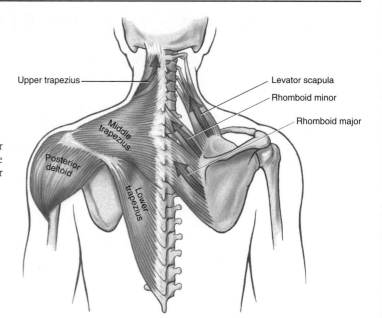

FIGURE 5-40. Posterior view showing the upper trapezius, levator scapula, rhomboid major, and rhomboid minor as elevators of the scapulothoracic joint. Parts of the middle deltoid, the posterior deltoid, and the middle and lower trapezius are also illustrated.

affecting the cells of motor nerves).[148] More generally, however, all the elevators of the scapulothoracic joint may be weakened or paralyzed after a stroke or from a disease such as muscular dystrophy. Regardless of the pathology, loss of muscular support of the shoulder girdle allows gravity to be the dominant force in determining the resting posture of the scapulothoracic joint. Such a posture typically includes a depressed, protracted, and excessively downwardly rotated scapula. Over time this posture can produce damaging stress on other structures located within the shoulder region. Figure 5-41, *A* shows the posture of a girl with paralysis of her left upper trapezius caused by the polio virus.[17] Over time, a depressed clavicle has resulted in superior dislocation of the SC joint (see arrow at medial end of clavicle in Figure 5-41, *A*). As the lateral end of the clavicle is lowered, the medial end is forced upward because of the fulcrum action of the underlying first rib. The depressed shaft of the clavicle may compress the subclavian vessels and part of the brachial plexus.

Another consequence of long-term paralysis of the upper trapezius is an inferior dislocation (or subluxation) of the GH joint (see arrow under lateral end of clavicle in Figure 5-41, *A*). Recall from earlier discussion that static stability of the GH joint is maintained in part by the humeral head being held firmly against the inclined plane of the glenoid fossa (see Figure 5-28, *A*). With long-term paralysis of the trapezius, the glenoid fossa loses its upwardly rotated position, allowing the humerus to slide inferiorly. The downward pull imposed by gravity on an unsupported arm may strain the capsular ligaments at the GH joint and eventually lead to an irreversible dislocation. This complication is often observed in persons with flaccid hemiplegia, which may necessitate a sling for external support of the arm.

The previous paragraphs highlight examples of abnormal scapular posturing occurring from a relatively extreme pathology involving denervation and subsequent muscular paralysis. Less extreme examples, however, are common in many clinical settings, often involving persons who have no history of neurologic or muscular pathology. For example, Figure 5-41, *B* features an otherwise healthy young woman with the classic "rounded shoulders" posture. Both scapulas are slightly depressed, downwardly rotated, and protracted. In principle, this posture can lead to similar (but usually far less damaging) biomechanical stress on the SC and GH joints as described for the girl with actual muscle paralysis. As evidenced by the position of the medial border and inferior angle in the subject in Figure 5-41, *B*, both scapulas are also slightly internally rotated and anteriorly tilted—postures believed to predispose to impingement of the tissues within the subacromial space.[14] Abnormal scapular posture in otherwise neurologically intact persons may be caused by or associated with a host of factors, including generalized laxity of connective tissues, muscle tightness, fatigue or weakness, GH joint capsule tightness, abnormal cervicothoracic posture, or simply habit or mood. It is often difficult to attribute abnormal posture of the scapula to any specific mechanical cause.

Regardless of the underlying cause or severity of abnormal posturing of the scapulothoracic joint, it is clear that this phenomenon affects the biomechanics of the entire shoulder complex.[94] Clinical inspection of the shoulder should always include an analysis of the support provided by the muscles that elevate the scapulothoracic joint. Treatment to improve abnormal scapulothoracic posture can vary depending on the underlying cause. In mild cases the condition may be improved by strengthening or stretching of selected muscles, combined with improving the patient's awareness of his or her postural fault.

DEPRESSORS

Depression of the scapulothoracic joint is performed by the *lower trapezius, latissimus dorsi, pectoralis minor,* and the *subclavius* (Figure 5-42).[163] The small subclavius muscle acts indirectly on the scapula through its inferior pull on the clavicle. The subclavius's near parallel line of force with the shaft of the clavicle suggests that this muscle has an important function in compressing and thereby stabilizing the SC joint. The lower trapezius and pectoralis minor act directly on the scapula. The latissimus dorsi, however, depresses the shoulder girdle indirectly, primarily by pulling the humerus inferiorly. The

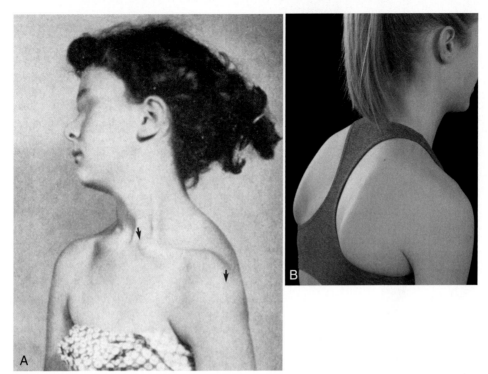

FIGURE 5-41. Examples of abnormal posture of the scapulothoracic joint. **A,** Photograph of a girl with paralysis of her left upper trapezius caused by polio virus. Such an example of isolated muscular paralysis was relatively common during the polio epidemic in the United States in the middle of the twentieth century. The *small arrows* indicate the secondary stress placed on the sternoclavicular (SC) and glenohumeral (GH) joints. **B,** Photograph of a healthy young woman with a posture of "rounded shoulders" without neurologic deficit. The prominence of the medial borders and inferior angles of the scapulas yields clues to the overall scapular posture. (**A** modified from Brunnstrom S: Muscle testing around the shoulder girdle, *J Bone Joint Surg Am* 23:263, 1941.)

FIGURE 5-42. A, A posterior view of the lower trapezius and the latissimus dorsi depressing the scapulothoracic joint. These muscles are pulling down against the resistance provided by the spring mechanism. **B,** An anterior view of the pectoralis minor and subclavius during the same activity described in **A.**

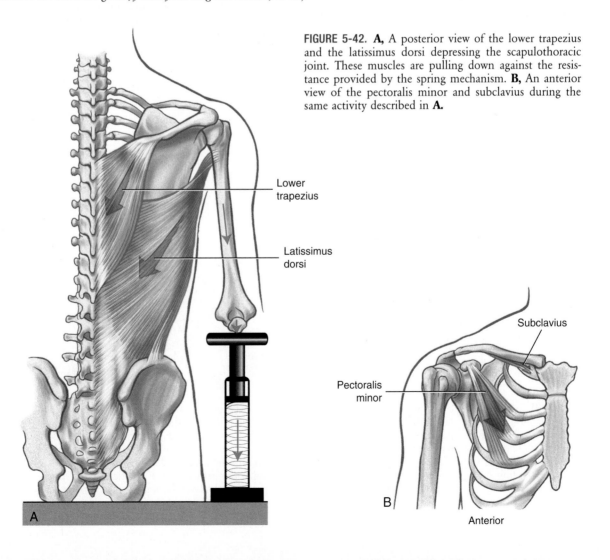

Lower trapezius

Latissimus dorsi

Subclavius

Pectoralis minor

Anterior

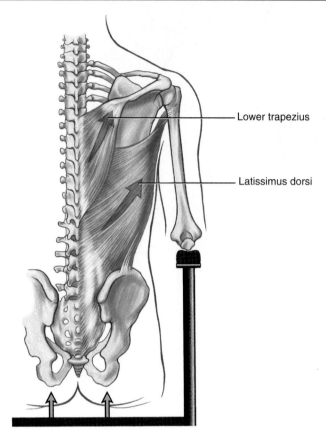

- Lower trapezius
- Latissimus dorsi

FIGURE 5-43. The lower trapezius and latissimus dorsi are shown indirectly elevating the ischial tuberosities away from the seat of the wheelchair. The contraction of these muscles lifts the pelvic-and-trunk segment up toward the fixed scapula-and-arm segment.

force generated by the depressor muscles can be directed through the scapula and upper extremity and applied against some object, such as the spring shown in Figure 5-42, *A.* Such an action can increase the overall functional length of the upper extremity.

If the arm is physically blocked from being depressed, force from the depressor muscles can raise the thorax relative to the fixed scapula and arm. This action can occur only if the scapula is stabilized to a greater extent than the thorax. For example, Figure 5-43 shows a person sitting in a wheelchair using the scapulothoracic depressors to relieve the contact pressure in the tissues superficial to the ischial tuberosities. With the arm firmly held against the armrest of the wheelchair, contraction of the lower trapezius and latissimus dorsi pulls the thorax and pelvis *up* toward the fixed scapula. This is a very useful movement especially for persons with quadriplegia who lack sufficient triceps strength to lift the body weight through elbow extension. This ability to partially unload the weight of the trunk and lower body is also a very important component of transferring between a wheelchair and bed.

PROTRACTORS

The serratus anterior is the prime protractor at the scapulothoracic joint (Figure 5-44, *A*). This extensive muscle has excellent leverage for protraction around the SC joint's vertical axis of rotation (Figure 5-44, *B*). The force of scapular protraction is usually transferred across the GH joint and employed for forward pushing and reaching activities. Persons with serratus anterior weakness have difficulty in performance of forward pushing motions. No other muscle can adequately provide this protraction effect on the scapula.

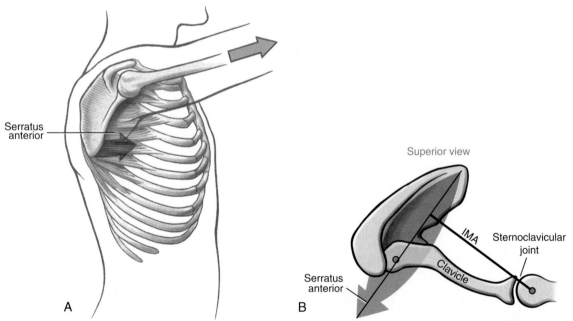

FIGURE 5-44. The right serratus anterior muscle. **A,** This expansive muscle passes anterior to the scapula to attach along the entire length of its medial border. The muscle's line of force is shown protracting the scapula and arm in a forward pushing or reaching motion. The fibers that attach near the inferior angle may assist with scapulothoracic depression. **B,** A superior view of the right shoulder girdle showing the protraction torque produced by the serratus anterior. The strength of the protraction torque is primarily the result of the muscle force multiplied by the internal moment arm *(IMA)* originating at the vertical axis of rotation at the sternoclavicular joint. The vertical axis of rotation is also shown at the acromioclavicular joint.

Another important action of the serratus anterior is to exaggerate the final phase of the standard prone push-up. The early phase of a push-up is performed primarily by the triceps and pectoral musculature. After the elbows are completely extended, however, the chest can be raised farther from the floor by a deliberate protraction of both scapulas. This final component of the push-up is performed primarily by contraction of the serratus anterior. Bilaterally, the muscles raise the thorax toward the fixed and stabilized scapulas. This so-called "push-up plus" action of the serratus anterior may be visualized by rotating Figure 5-44, *A* 90 degrees clockwise and reversing the direction of the arrow overlying the serratus anterior. Such a movement places specific demands on the serratus anterior and therefore is often incorporated into exercises for strengthening this important muscle.[40,50,95,114,141]

RETRACTORS

The *middle trapezius* has an optimal line of force to retract the scapula (Figure 5-45). The *rhomboids* and the *lower trapezius* muscles function as secondary retractors. All the retractors are particularly active during pulling activities, such as climbing and rowing. These muscles secure the scapula to the axial skeleton.

The secondary retractors are an excellent example of how muscles can share similar actions, but also function as direct antagonists to one another. During a vigorous retraction effort, the elevation tendency of the rhomboids is neutralized by the depression tendency of the lower trapezius. The line of forces of both muscles combine, however, to produce pure retraction (see Figure 5-45).

Complete paralysis of the trapezius, and to a lesser extent the rhomboids, significantly reduces the retraction potential of the scapula. The scapula tends to "drift" slightly into protraction as a result of the partially unopposed protraction action of the serratus anterior muscle.[17]

UPWARD AND DOWNWARD ROTATORS

Muscles that perform upward and downward rotation of the scapulothoracic joint are discussed next in the context of movement of the entire shoulder.

Muscles That Elevate the Arm

The term "elevation" of the arm describes the active movement of bringing the arm overhead without specifying the exact plane of the motion. Elevation of the arm is performed by muscles that typically fall into three groups: (1) muscles that elevate (i.e., abduct or flex) the humerus at the GH joint; (2) scapular muscles that control the upward rotation of the scapulothoracic joint; and (3) rotator cuff muscles that control the dynamic stability and arthrokinematics at the GH joint.

Muscles Primarily Responsible for Elevation of the Arm

Glenohumeral Joint Muscles
- Anterior and middle deltoid
- Supraspinatus
- Coracobrachialis
- Biceps (long head)

Scapulothoracic Joint Muscles
- Serratus anterior
- Trapezius

Rotator Cuff Muscles
- Supraspinatus
- Infraspinatus
- Teres minor
- Subscapularis

MUSCLES THAT ELEVATE THE ARM AT THE GLENOHUMERAL JOINT

The prime muscles that abduct the GH joint are the *anterior deltoid, middle deltoid,* and *supraspinatus* (Figure 5-46). Elevation of the arm through flexion is performed primarily by the

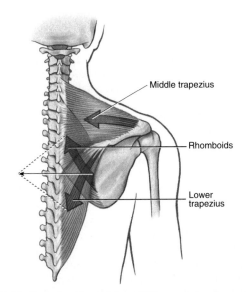

FIGURE 5-45. Posterior view of the middle trapezius, lower trapezius, and rhomboids cooperating to retract the scapulothoracic joint. The dashed line of force of both the rhomboid and lower trapezius combines to yield a single retraction force, shown by the thin straight arrow.

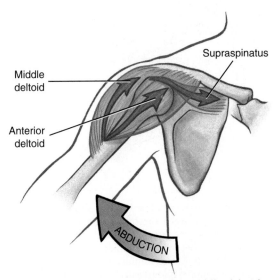

FIGURE 5-46. Anterior view showing the middle deltoid, anterior deltoid, and supraspinatus as abductors of the glenohumeral joint.

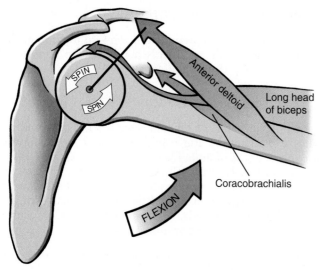

FIGURE 5-47. Lateral view of the anterior deltoid, coracobrachialis, and long head of the biceps flexing the glenohumeral joint in the pure sagittal plane. The medial-lateral axis of rotation is shown at the center of the humeral head. An internal moment arm is shown intersecting the line of force of the anterior deltoid only.

anterior deltoid, coracobrachialis, and *long head of the biceps brachii* (Figure 5-47).

The line of force of the middle deltoid and the supraspinatus are similar during shoulder abduction. Both muscles are activated at the onset of elevation, reaching a maximum level near 90 degrees of abduction.[98] During abduction, both muscles help stabilize the humeral head within the functional concavity formed by the inferior capsule of the joint.[1,96,106]

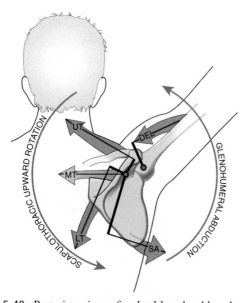

FIGURE 5-48. Posterior view of a healthy shoulder showing the muscular interaction between the scapulothoracic upward rotators and the glenohumeral abductors. Shoulder abduction requires a muscular "kinetic arc" between the humerus and the axial skeleton. Note two axes of rotation: the scapular axis, located near the acromion, and the glenohumeral joint axis, located at the humeral head. Internal moment arms for all muscles are shown as dark black lines. *DEL,* deltoid and supraspinatus; *LT,* lower trapezius; *MT,* middle trapezius; *SA,* serratus anterior; *UT,* upper trapezius.

The middle deltoid and supraspinatus possess a relatively significant moment arm for abduction, varying from 1 to 3 cm throughout most of the range of motion.[99,109,200]

The deltoid and the supraspinatus muscles contribute about equal shares of the total abduction torque at the GH joint.[80] With the deltoid paralyzed, the supraspinatus muscle is generally capable of fully abducting the GH joint, although the abduction torque is reduced. With the supraspinatus paralyzed or the tendon ruptured, full abduction is often difficult or not possible because of the altered arthrokinematics at the GH joint. Full active abduction is not possible with paralysis of both the deltoid and supraspinatus.

Research has shown that the extreme upper fibers of the infraspinatus and subscapularis muscles have a limited moment arm to abduct the GH joint.[64,109] This occurs because the upper fibers of these muscles pass slightly superior to the joint's anterior-posterior axis of rotation (see Figures 5-51 and 5-52). Although these muscles are considered only secondary abductors, they play a primary role in establishing dynamic stabilization and directing the joint's arthrokinematics, functions described later in this section.

UPWARD ROTATORS AT THE SCAPULOTHORACIC JOINT

Upward rotation of the scapula is an essential component of elevation of the arm. The primary upward rotator muscles are the *serratus anterior* and the *upper* and *lower fibers of the trapezius* (Figure 5-48). These muscles drive the upward rotation of the scapula and, equally important, provide stable attachments for the more distal mobilizers, such as the deltoid and rotator cuff muscles. In addition, the serratus anterior can posteriorly tilt and to a lesser degree externally rotate the scapula.[46,113,114] (These motions were described earlier in this chapter as the fourth kinematic principle of shoulder abduction; review Figure 5-35.) These secondary muscle actions are explained with the help of Figure 5-44. As noted in Figure 5-44, *A,* the line of force of the lower fibers of the serratus anterior pulls the inferior angle of the (upwardly rotated) scapula forward. Although speculative, this forward pull on inferior angle, in conjunction with other forces, may tilt the glenoid region of the scapula posteriorly. Also, the serratus anterior produces an external rotation torque on the scapula by generating a force that passes *medial* to the vertical axis of the AC joint (see Figure 5-44, *B*). This external rotation torque also helps secure the medial border of the scapula firmly against the thorax. Although not completely understood, both of the aforementioned secondary actions of the serratus anterior are likely important components in the overall kinematics of upward rotation of the scapula.[116]

Trapezius and Serratus Anterior Interaction during Upward Rotation of the Scapula

The axis of rotation for scapular upward rotation is depicted in Figure 5-48 as passing in an anterior-posterior direction through the scapula. This axis allows a convenient way to analyze the potential for the serratus anterior and trapezius to upwardly rotate the scapula. The axis of rotation of the upwardly rotating scapula is near the root of the spine during the early phase of shoulder abduction and near the acromion during the late phase of abduction.[5]

The upper and lower fibers of the trapezius and the lower fibers of the serratus anterior form a force-couple to effectively upwardly rotate the scapula (see Figure 5-48).[49,51] The

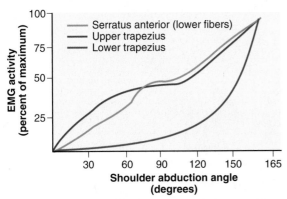

FIGURE 5-49. The electromyographic activation pattern of the upper trapezius and lower trapezius and the lower fibers of the serratus anterior during shoulder abduction in the scapular plane. (Data from Bagg SD, Forrest WJ: Electromyographic study of the scapular rotators during arm abduction in the scapula plane, *Am J Phys Med* 65:111, 1986.)

force-couple rotates the scapula in the same rotary direction as the abducting humerus. The mechanics of this force-couple assume that the force of each of the three muscles acts simultaneously. The pull of the lower fibers of the serratus anterior on the inferior angle of the scapula rotates the glenoid fossa upward and laterally. These fibers are the most effective upward rotators of the force-couple, primarily because of their larger moment arm for this action.

The upper trapezius upwardly rotates the scapula indirectly by its superior-and-medial pull on the clavicle.[49] The lower trapezius upwardly rotates the scapula by its inferior-and-medial pull on the root of the spine of the scapula. The lower trapezius has been shown to be particularly active during the later phase of shoulder abduction (Figure 5-49).[6,89] The upper trapezius, by comparison, shows a significant rise in EMG activation at the initiation of shoulder abduction, then continues a gradual rise in amplitude throughout the remainder of the range of motion. The upper trapezius elevates the clavicle throughout the early phase of abduction while simultaneously balancing the inferior pull of the lower trapezius during the late phase of abduction. The serratus anterior muscle shows a gradual increase in EMG amplitude throughout the entire range of shoulder abduction.

The middle trapezius is very active during shoulder abduction.[51] As depicted in Figure 5-48, the line of force of the middle trapezius runs *through* the rotating scapula's axis of rotation. In this case, the middle trapezius is robbed of its leverage to contribute upward rotation torque. This muscle, however, still contributes a needed retraction force on the scapula, which along with the rhomboid muscles, helps to neutralize the strong protraction effect of the serratus anterior. The net force dominance between the middle trapezius and the serratus anterior during elevation of the arm helps determine the final retraction-protraction position of the upward rotated scapula. During shoulder abduction (especially in the frontal plane), the scapular retractors typically dominate, as evidenced by the fact that the clavicle (and linked scapula) *retract* during shoulder abduction (review kinematic principle 3 in Box 5-1).

In summary, during elevation of the arm, the serratus anterior and trapezius control the mechanics of scapular upward rotation. The serratus anterior has the greater leverage for this motion. Both muscles are synergists in upward rotation but are

agonists and antagonists as they oppose, and thus partially limit, each other's strong protraction and retraction effect.

Paralysis of the Upward Rotators of the Scapulothoracic Joint
Trapezius Paralysis
Complete paralysis of the trapezius usually causes moderate to marked difficulty in elevating the arm overhead. The task typically can still be accomplished through full range of motion as long as the serratus anterior is fully innervated. Elevation of the arm in the pure frontal plane is particularly difficult with trapezius paralysis because this action requires that the middle trapezius generate a strong retraction force on the scapula.[17]

Serratus Anterior Paralysis
Paralysis of the serratus anterior muscle causes significant disruption in normal shoulder kinesiology. Disability may be slight with partial paralysis, or profound with complete paralysis. Paralysis of the serratus anterior can occur from injury to the long thoracic nerve, spinal cord, or cervical nerve roots.[180]

As a rule, persons with complete paralysis of the serratus anterior have great difficulty actively elevating the arm above the head. This difficulty exists even though the trapezius and glenohumeral abductor muscles are fully innervated. Attempts at shoulder abduction, especially against resistance, typically result in limited elevation of the arm, coupled with an excessively downwardly rotated scapula (Figure 5-50). Normally, contraction of a normal serratus anterior strongly upwardly rotates the scapula, thus allowing the contracting middle deltoid and supraspinatus to rotate the humerus in the same rotary direction as the scapula (see Figure 5-48). In cases of paralysis of the serratus anterior, however, the contracting middle deltoid and supraspinatus dominate the scapular kinetics, producing a paradoxic (and ineffective) *downward* rotation of the scapula. The combined active motions of downward rotation of the scapula and partial elevation of the arm cause the deltoid and supraspinatus to overshorten rapidly. As predicted by the force-velocity and length-tension relationships of muscle (see Chapter 3), the rapid overshortening of these muscles reduces their maximal force potential. This reduced force potential, in conjunction with the downward rotation position of the scapula, reduces both the range of motion and torque production of the elevating arm.

An analysis of the pathomechanics associated with paralysis of the serratus anterior provides a valuable lesson in the extreme kinesiologic importance of this muscle. Normally, during elevation of the arm, the serratus anterior produces a surprisingly large upward rotation torque on the scapula, one that must *exceed* the downward rotation torque produced by the active middle deltoid and supraspinatus. In addition, the serratus anterior must produce a subtle but important posterior tilting and external rotation torque to the upwardly rotating scapula. These secondary actions become clear when observing a person with serratus anterior paralysis, as depicted in Figure 5-50. In addition to the more obvious downwardly rotated position, the scapula is also slightly anteriorly tilted and internally rotated (evidenced by the "flaring" of the scapula's inferior angle and medial border, respectively). Such a distorted posture is often referred to clinically as a "winging" scapula. Such a position can eventually cause adaptive shortening of the pectoralis minor muscle—a direct antagonist to the serratus anterior. Increased passive tension in the pectoralis minor would further promote an anteriorly tilted and internally rotated position of the scapula.[15]

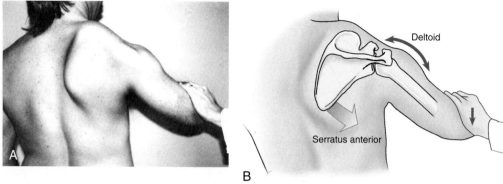

FIGURE 5-50. The pathomechanics of the right scapula after paralysis of the right serratus anterior caused by an injury of the long thoracic nerve. **A,** The dominant feature of the scapula is its paradoxic downwardly rotated position, which can be exaggerated by applying resistance against the shoulder abduction effort. Note also that the scapula is abnormally anteriorly tilted and internally rotated. **B,** Kinesiologic analysis of the extreme downward rotated position. Without an adequate upward rotation force from the serratus anterior *(fading arrow)*, the scapula is not properly stabilized against the thorax and cannot resist the pull of the deltoid. Subsequently the force of the deltoid *(bidirectional arrow)* causes the combined actions of downward rotation of the scapula and partial elevation (abduction) of the humerus.

It is surprising to note that even slight weakness of the serratus anterior can disrupt the normal arthrokinematics at the shoulder. Ludewig and Cook studied a group of overhead laborers diagnosed with subacromial impingement syndrome.[111] Of interest, during attempts at active abduction of the shoulder the researchers found a relationship between reduced serratus anterior activation and the combined kinematics of reduced upward rotation, reduced posterior tilting, and reduced external rotation of the scapula. As described throughout this chapter, these abnormal scapular kinematics are believed to be associated with reduced volume within the subacromial space. The reason why this muscle would show weakness in this otherwise healthy group of manual laborers is not certain. Whether the impingement is a cause or an effect of the weakness is also unclear.

FUNCTION OF THE ROTATOR CUFF MUSCLES DURING ELEVATION OF THE ARM

The rotator cuff group muscles include the subscapularis, supraspinatus, infraspinatus, and teres minor (Figures 5-51 and 5-52). These muscles show significant EMG activity when the arm is raised overhead.[41,98] The EMG activity primarily reflects the function of these muscles as regulators of dynamic joint stability and controllers of the arthrokinematics.

Regulators of Dynamic Stability at the Glenohumeral Joint

The loose fit between the head of the humerus and glenoid fossa permits extensive range of motion at the GH joint. The surrounding joint capsule therefore must be free of thick restraining ligaments that otherwise would restrict motion. As stated earlier in this chapter, the anatomic design of the GH joint favors mobility at the expense of stability. Although most muscles that cross the shoulder provide some dynamic stability to the GH joint, the rotator cuff group excels in this capacity.[198,203] An important design of the rotator cuff group is to compensate for the GH joint's natural laxity and propensity for instability. The distal attachment of the rotator cuff muscles blends into the GH joint capsule before attaching to the proximal humerus (see Figures 5-51 and 5-52). This anatomic arrangement forms a protective cuff around the joint,

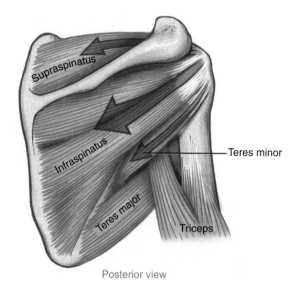

Posterior view

FIGURE 5-51. Posterior view of the right shoulder showing the activated supraspinatus, infraspinatus, and teres minor muscles. Note that the distal attachments of these muscles blend into and reinforce the superior and posterior aspects of the glenohumeral joint. The teres major and parts of the long and lateral heads of the triceps brachii are also illustrated.

becoming very rigid when activated by the nervous system. Nowhere else in the body do so many muscles form such an intimate structural part of a joint's periarticular structure.

Earlier in this chapter, the dynamic stabilizing function of the infraspinatus muscle during external rotation was discussed (see Figure 5-34). This dynamic stabilization is an essential function of all members of the rotator cuff. Forces produced primarily by the rotator cuff (and their attachments into the capsule) not only actively rotate the humeral head but also stabilize and centralize it against the glenoid fossa.[1,103] Dynamic stability at the GH joint therefore requires healthy neuromuscular and musculoskeletal systems. It is likely that these two systems are functionally integrated through proprioceptive sensory receptors located within the GH joint's periarticular connective tissues.[44,196] As part of a reflex loop,

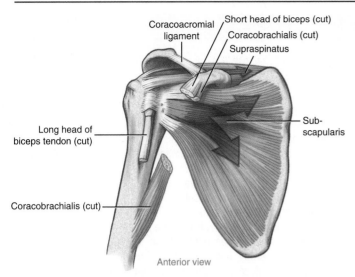

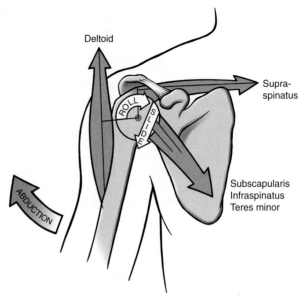

FIGURE 5-52. Anterior view of the right shoulder showing the subscapularis muscle blending into the anterior capsule of the glenohumeral joint before attaching to the lesser tubercle of the humerus. The subscapularis is shown with diverging arrows, reflecting two main fiber directions. The supraspinatus, coracobrachialis, tendon of the long head of the biceps, and coracohumeral and coracoacromial ligaments are also depicted.

FIGURE 5-53. Anterior view of the right shoulder emphasizing the actions of the rotator cuff muscles during abduction of the GH joint. The supraspinatus rolls the humeral head superiorly toward abduction while also compressing the joint for added stability. The remaining rotator cuff muscles (subscapularis, infraspinatus, and teres minor) exert a downward translational force on the humeral head to counteract excessive superior translation, especially that caused by deltoid contraction. Note the internal moment arm used by both the deltoid and supraspinatus.

these innervated connective tissues may provide rapid and important information to the participating muscles. This feedback could enhance the muscles' ability to control the arthrokinematics even at a subconscious level, as well as provide the needed dynamic stability. Challenging such a proprioceptive mechanism through functional exercise is a respected component of rehabilitation programs for persons with shoulder instability.[150]

Active Controllers of the Arthrokinematics at the Glenohumeral Joint

In the healthy shoulder the rotator cuff controls many of the active arthrokinematics of the GH joint (Figure 5-53). Contraction of the horizontally oriented supraspinatus produces a compression force directly into the glenoid fossa; this force stabilizes the humeral head firmly against the fossa during its superior roll into abduction.[211] Compression forces acting on the joint's surface increase linearly from 0 to 90 degrees of shoulder abduction, reaching a magnitude of 80% to 90% of body weight.[159,186] The surface area for dissipating joint forces increases to a maximum at a position of 60 to 120 degrees of shoulder elevation.[175] This increase in surface area assists with maintaining pressure at tolerable physiologic levels.

The horizontally aligned supraspinatus muscle is ideal for directing the arthrokinematics of abduction. During abduction the muscle's contractile force rolls the humeral head superiorly while simultaneously serving as a musculotendinous "spacer" that restricts any counterproductive superior translation of the humeral head.[186,207] In addition, the remaining rotator cuff muscles (subscapularis, infraspinatus, and teres minor) have a line of force that can exert an inferiorly directed force on the humeral head during abduction (see Figure 5-53).[72,127] The long head of the biceps also contributes in this fashion.[154]

Of interest, even passive forces from muscles being stretched during abduction, such as the latissimus dorsi and teres major, can exert a useful inferior-directed force on the humeral head.[72] These passive forces can help neutralize part of the contracting deltoid's near superior line of force.[43,155,171] Without the aforementioned sources of active and passive inferior-directed forces, the humeral head would otherwise jam or impinge against the coracoacromial arch, thereby blocking abduction.[155,161] This consequence is often observed after a complete rupture of the rotator cuff, especially of the supraspinatus and infraspinatus.[142]

Finally, during abduction the infraspinatus and teres minor muscles can also externally rotate the humerus to varying degrees to increase the clearance between the greater tubercle and the acromion.

Summary of the Functions of the Rotator Cuff Muscles in Controlling the Arthrokinematics of Abduction at the Glenohumeral Joint

Supraspinatus
- Drives the superior roll of the humeral head
- Compresses the humeral head firmly against the glenoid fossa
- Creates a semirigid spacer above the humeral head, restricting excessive superior translation of the humerus

Infraspinatus, Teres Minor, and Subscapularis
- Exert a depression force on the humeral head

Infraspinatus and Teres Minor
- Externally rotate the humerus

SPECIAL FOCUS 5-7

Shoulder Instability: a Final Look at This Important Clinical Issue

As described throughout this chapter, maintaining stability at the very mobile glenohumeral (GH) joint requires a unique interaction among active and passive mechanisms. For several reasons, these mechanisms sometimes fail, resulting in an unstable shoulder. The literature regarding the classification, cause, and treatment of shoulder instability is inconsistent. Such inconsistency reflects the multiple causes of the instability, as well as highly varied clinical expression. Although overlap is common, many authorities describe three types of shoulder instability: posttraumatic, atraumatic, and acquired.

Posttraumatic Instability

Many cases of shoulder instability are attributed to a specific event involving a traumatic dislocation of the GH joint.[76] The vast majority of traumatic dislocations occur in the anterior direction, typically related to a fall or forceful collision. The pathomechanics of anterior dislocation often involve the motion or position of extreme external rotation in an abducted position. With the shoulder in this vulnerable position, the force of impact can drive the humeral head off the anterior side of the glenoid fossa. This dislocation often injures or overstretches the rotator cuff muscles, middle and inferior GH ligaments, and anterior-inferior rim of the glenoid labrum.[138] Combined tears or lesions of this part of the capsule or labrum that are detached from the rim of the glenoid fossa are referred to as *Bankart lesions,* named after the physician who first described the injury.

Unfortunately, because of the associated injury to the labrum and capsular ligaments, posttraumatic dislocations frequently lead to future recurrences, often causing additional damage to the joint. This likelihood is far greater in adolescent persons as compared with persons in their middle and later years.[78] This difference is partially attributable to changes in activity level and the natural increase in stiffness of periarticular connective tissues that is associated with aging.

Young persons with recurrent dislocation often do not respond well to conservative therapy, such as immobilization, restricted activity, and exercise.[76] Surgery is commonly considered necessary, although opinions vary based on patient's age, activity level, degree of instability, and history of dislocation.[7] Surgery typically involves a repair of the damaged tissues, often including techniques to tighten the anterior and inferior regions of the capsule.[2] These techniques may include a surgical folding (plication) of the capsule. Loss of external rotation is always a possible consequence of tightening of structures on the anterior side of the joint.

Atraumatic Instability

Persons diagnosed with atraumatic instability typically display generalized and excessive ligamentous laxity throughout the body, often described as being congenital.[76,206] This relatively infrequent type of instability is usually not associated with a traumatic event. The instability may be unidirectional or multidirectional, and bilat-

eral. The cause of atraumatic instability is poorly understood and may involve several factors, as follows*:
- Bony dysplasia
- Abnormal scapular kinematics
- Weakness, poor control, or increased fatigability of GH joint or scapular muscles
- Unusually large rotator interval
- Redundant folds in the capsule
- Neuromuscular disturbances
- Increased laxity in connective tissue

Atraumatic instability has been shown to respond favorably to conservative therapy involving strengthening and coordination exercises.[21,206] Those who do not respond well to conservative therapy, however, may be candidates for an open or arthroscopic "capsular shift."[137] This surgery involves a tightening of the GH joint by selectively cutting, folding, and suturing redundant regions of the anterior and inferior capsule. At the time of surgery, persons with atraumatic instability have been shown to have a significant number of intra-articular lesions.[206] Although the actual percentage of lesions is lower than that observed with traumatic instability, this finding suggests that excessive laxity—even with minimal or no history of actual dislocation—can cause significant articular damage.

Acquired Shoulder Instability

The pathomechanics of acquired shoulder instability are related to overstretching and subsequent microtrauma of the capsular ligaments within the GH joint. This condition is often associated with repetitive, high-velocity shoulder motions that involve extreme external rotation and abduction.[76,102,202] These motions are common in throwing sports, swimming, tennis, and volleyball. Because of the biomechanics of the abducted and extremely externally rotated shoulder (see Figure 5-27), the anterior bands of the inferior GH ligament and to a lesser extent the middle GH ligament are most vulnerable to plastic deformation. Once weakened by this process, the soft tissues are less able to hold the humeral head against the glenoid fossa.[158] The tissue deformation leads to increased joint laxity, possibly predisposing other stress-related pathologies such as rotator cuff (syndrome) tendonitis and damage to the labrum and long head of the biceps.[162] Acquired shoulder instability has also been associated with *internal impingement syndrome.* This form of impingement typically occurs in a position of 90 degrees of abduction and full external rotation, as the undersurface of the posterior-superior rotator cuff is pinched between the greater tubercle and the adjacent edge of the glenoid fossa.[20]

Open surgical repair for acquired instability in overhead athletes is often associated with losses in shoulder external rotation and relatively low return to competition.[12,162,190] Arthroscopic repair is generally preferred. Although variable, this repair includes debridement of the rotator cuff, debridement or repair of the glenoid labrum, and anterior capsular plication.[165]

---

*References 48, 76, 112, 120, 153, 199, 205, 206.

SPECIAL FOCUS 5-8

Vulnerability of the Supraspinatus to Excessive Wear

The supraspinatus muscle is one of the most used muscles of the entire shoulder complex. This muscle assists the deltoid during abduction and also provides dynamic and, at times, static stability to the glenohumeral (GH) joint. Biomechanically the supraspinatus is subjected to large internal forces, even during routine activities. The muscle has an internal moment arm for shoulder abduction of about 2.5 cm (about 1 inch).[90] Supporting a load in the hand 50 cm (about 20 inches) distal to the GH joint creates a mechanical advantage of 1 : 20 (i.e., the ratio of internal moment arm of the muscle to the external moment arm of the load). A 1 : 20 mechanical advantage implies that the supraspinatus must generate a force 20 times greater than the weight of the load (see Chapter 1). These high forces, generated over many years, may partially tear the muscle's tendon as it inserts into the capsule and the greater tubercle of the humerus. Fortunately, the overlying deltoid muscle shares much of the demand placed on the vulnerable supraspinatus tendon. Nevertheless, the stress imposed on the supraspinatus is large, especially considering the muscle's small cross-sectional area compared with the deltoid.[90] Persons with a partially torn or inflamed supraspinatus tendon are advised to hold objects close to the body in order to reduce the external moment arm of the load and thereby minimize the force demands on the muscle. A partially torn tendon may eventually completely rupture, as shown by the magnetic resonance image in Figure 5-54.

Excessive deterioration of the tendon of the supraspinatus may be associated with similar pathology of the other tendons of the rotator cuff group. This more general condition is often referred to as "rotator cuff syndrome." Many factors can contribute to rotator cuff syndrome, such as trauma, overuse, or repeated impingement against the coracoacromial ligament, acromion, or the rim of the glenoid fossa.[66,82,97] The condition can include partial or full-thickness tears and inflammation of the rotator cuff tendons, inflammation and adhesions of the capsule (adhesive capsulitis), bursitis, degenerative osteoarthritis of the overlying acromioclavicular joint (as indicated in Figure 5-54), pain, and generalized shoulder weakness.[210] The supraspinatus tendon is particularly vulnerable to degeneration if associated with an age-related compromise in its blood supply.[23] Depending on the severity of the rotator cuff syndrome, the arthrokinematics at the GH joint may be completely disrupted, and the shoulder becomes so inflamed and painful that active or passive movement becomes very limited.

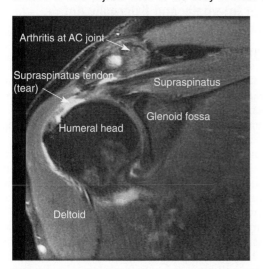

FIGURE 5-54. Frontal plane (T2 fat saturated) magnetic resonance image of the shoulder showing a full-thickness supraspinatus tendon tear. Also note the degenerative osteoarthritis of the acromioclavicular joint. (Courtesy Michael O'Brien, MD, Radiology Resident, University of Wisconsin.)

Muscles That Adduct and Extend the Shoulder

The primary adductor and extensor muscles of the shoulder are the *posterior deltoid, latissimus dorsi, teres major, long head of the triceps brachii,* and *sternocostal head of the pectoralis major* (review Figures 5-40, 5-42, 5-51, and 5-55, respectively). Pulling the arm against resistance offered by climbing a rope or propelling through water requires a forceful contraction of these powerful muscles. Of these muscles, the latissimus dorsi, teres major, and pectoralis major have the largest moment arms for the combined motions of adduction and extension.[99] The *infraspinatus* (lower fibers) and *teres minor* muscles likely assist with these movements. As depicted in Figure 5-56, the exten-

sor and adductor muscles are capable of generating the largest torques of any muscle group of the shoulder.[77,173]

With the humerus held stable, contraction of the latissimus dorsi can raise the pelvis upward. Persons with paraplegia often use this action during crutch- and brace-assisted ambulation as a substitute for weakened or paralyzed hip flexors.

Five of the seven adductor-extensor muscles have their primary proximal attachments on the inherently unstable scapula. It is the primary responsibility of the rhomboid muscles to stabilize the scapula during active adduction and extension of the GH joint. This stabilization function is evidenced by the downward rotation and retraction of the scapula that naturally occurs with combined adduction and extension

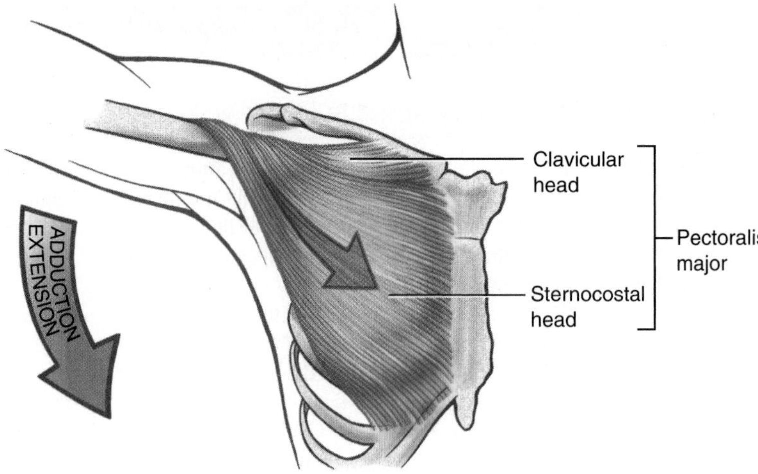

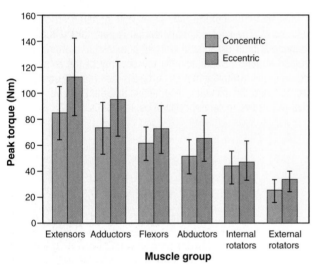

FIGURE 5-55. Anterior view of the right pectoralis major showing the adduction and extension function of the sternocostal head. The clavicular head of the pectoralis major is also shown.

FIGURE 5-56. Graph shows a sample of peak torque data produced by the six shoulder muscle groups from a set of nonathletic, healthy men (N = 15, aged 22 to 35 years). The peak torques are shown in descending order. Data were collected using an isokinetic device set at an angular velocity of 60 degree/sec. Data are reported as averages of three maximal-effort repetitions for both eccentric and concentric activations. Means are expressed in newton-meters; brackets indicate standard deviation of the mean. Consult reference source for more information on data from female subjects and other angular velocities. (Data from Shklar A, Dvir Z: Isokinetic strength measurements in shoulder muscles, *J Biomech* 10:369, 1995.)

of the shoulder. Figure 5-57 highlights the synergistic relationship between the rhomboids and the teres major during a strongly resisted adduction effort. Based on bony attachments, the pectoralis minor (see Figure 5-42, *B*) and the latissimus dorsi likely have a line of force to assist the rhomboids with downward rotation of the scapula. This speculation is most apparent when observed with the scapula already upwardly rotated and the shoulder abducted or flexed—positions that typically precede a vigorous shoulder adduction and extension effort, such as a propulsive swimming stroke.

As evident through palpation, full active extension of the shoulder beyond the neutral position is associated with anterior tilting of the scapula. This scapular motion, which is likely driven primarily by the pectoralis minor, functionally increases the extent of a backward reach.

The entire rotator cuff group is active during shoulder adduction and extension.[98] Forces produced by these muscles assist with the action directly or stabilize the head of the humerus against the glenoid fossa.[172]

Muscles That Internally and Externally Rotate the Shoulder

INTERNAL ROTATOR MUSCLES

The primary muscles that internally rotate the GH joint are the *subscapularis, anterior deltoid, pectoralis major, latissimus dorsi,* and *teres major.* Many of these internal rotators are also powerful extensors and adductors, such as those used during the propulsive phase of swimming.

The total muscle mass of the shoulder's internal rotators greatly exceeds that of the external rotators. This fact is reflected by the larger maximal-effort torque produced by the internal rotators, during both eccentric and concentric activations (see Figure 5-56).[52,136,173]

One activity requiring large torques by the internal rotator muscles is high-speed throwing. Of particular interest in sports medicine is the large torque generated by these muscles in professional baseball pitchers just before the maximal external rotation (end of cocking) phase of overhead pitching. At this phase of a pitch, the internal rotator muscles must strongly decelerate a large external rotation torque that peaks at approximately 70 to 90 Nm.[58,168] The opposing rotary torques create significant torsional shear on the shaft of the humerus. This magnitude of shear is likely involved in the pathomechanics of "ball-thrower's fracture"—an injury involving a spontaneous spiral fracture of the middle and distal thirds of the humerus.[168] Similar biomechanical studies have focused on the late cocking phase of pitching in 12-year-old elite baseball pitchers. Although the torsional shear is much less because of the greatly reduced pitching velocity, the forces are likely related to the pathomechanics of proximal humeral epiphysiolysis ("Little League shoulder") and the development of excessive retroversion of the child's humerus.[167]

The muscles that internally rotate the GH joint are often described as rotators of the humerus relative to the scapula

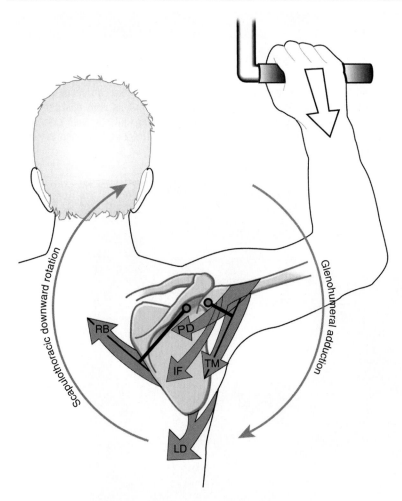

FIGURE 5-57. Posterior view of a shoulder showing the muscular interaction between the scapulothoracic downward rotators and the glenohumeral adductors (and extensors) of the right shoulder. For clarity, the long head of the triceps is not shown. The teres major is shown with its internal moment arm *(dark line)* extending from the glenohumeral joint. The rhomboids are shown with the internal moment arm extending from the scapula's axis (see text for further details.) *IF,* infraspinatus and teres minor; *LD,* latissimus dorsi; *PD,* posterior deltoid; *RB,* rhomboids; *TM,* teres major.

(Figure 5-58). The arthrokinematics of this motion are based on the convex humeral head rotating on the fixed glenoid fossa. Consider, however, the muscle function and kinematics that occur when the humerus is held in a fixed position and the scapula is free to rotate. As depicted in Figure 5-60, with sufficient muscle force the scapula and trunk can rotate around a fixed humerus. Note that the arthrokinematics of the scapula-on-humerus rotation involve a concave glenoid fossa rolling and sliding in similar directions on the convex humeral head (see Figure 5-60; box).

EXTERNAL ROTATOR MUSCLES

The primary muscles that externally rotate the GH joint are the *infraspinatus, teres minor,* and *posterior deltoid* (see Figures 5-40 and 5-51). The supraspinatus can assist with external rotation provided the GH joint is between neutral and full external rotation.[104]

The external rotator muscles constitute a relatively small percentage of the total muscle mass at the shoulder. The external rotators therefore produce the lowest maximal-effort torque of any muscle group at the shoulder (see Figure 5-56). Regardless of the muscles' relatively low maximal torque potential, the muscles frequently are used to generate high-velocity concentric contractions, such as during the cocking phase of pitching a baseball. Through eccentric activation, these same muscles must decelerate shoulder internal rotation

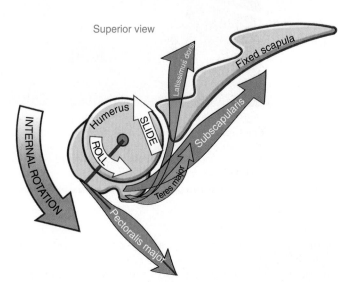

FIGURE 5-58. Superior view of the right shoulder showing the group action of the internal rotators around the glenohumeral joint's vertical axis of rotation. In this case the scapula is fixed and the humerus is free to rotate. The line of force of the pectoralis major is shown with its internal moment arm. Note the roll-and-slide arthrokinematics of the convex-on-concave motion. For clarity, the anterior deltoid is not shown.

SPECIAL FOCUS 5-9

A Closer Look at the Posterior Deltoid

The posterior deltoid is a shoulder extensor, adductor, and external rotator. In addition, this muscle is also the primary horizontal extensor at the shoulder. Vigorous contraction of the posterior deltoid during full horizontal extension requires that the scapula be firmly stabilized by the lower trapezius (Figure 5-59).

Complete paralysis of the posterior deltoid can occur from an overstretching of the axillary nerve. Persons with this paralysis frequently report difficulty in combining full shoulder extension and horizontal extension, such as that required to place the arm in the sleeve of a coat.

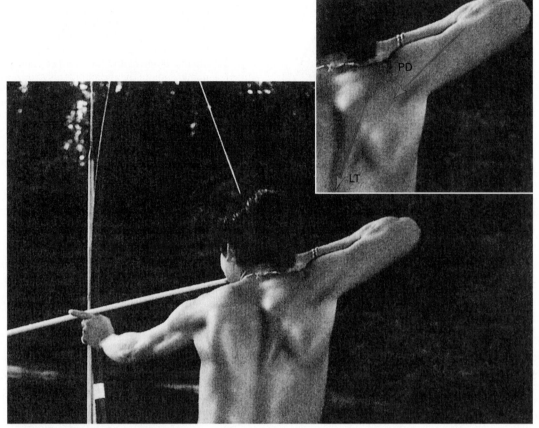

FIGURE 5-59. The hypertrophied right posterior deltoid of a Tirio Indian man engaged in bow fishing. Note the strong synergistic action between the right lower trapezius *(LT)* and right posterior deltoid *(PD)*. The lower trapezius must anchor the scapula to the spine and provide a fixed proximal attachment for the strongly activated posterior deltoid. (Courtesy of Plotkin MJ: *Tales of a shaman's apprentice,* New York, 1993, Viking-Penguin.)

at the release phase of pitching, which can reach a velocity of near 7000 degrees/sec.[45] These large force demands placed on the rapidly elongating infraspinatus and teres minor may cause tears and chronic inflammation at the point of their distal attachment, possibly leading to rotator cuff syndrome.[81]

SYNOPSIS

The four joints of the shoulder complex normally interact harmoniously to maximize the volume, stability, and ease of reach in the upper extremity. Each articulation contributes a

unique element to these functions. Most proximally, the SC joint firmly attaches the shoulder to the axial skeleton. This joint is well stabilized by its interlocking saddle-shaped surfaces, combined with a strong capsule and articular disc. The SC joint serves as the basilar pivot point for virtually all movements of the shoulder.

The overall kinematics of the scapula are guided primarily by movement of the clavicle. The more specific path of the scapula, however, is governed by additional and equally important movements at the AC joint. This relatively flat and shallow AC joint is dependent on local capsular ligaments as well as the extrinsically located coracoclavicular ligament for

Superior view

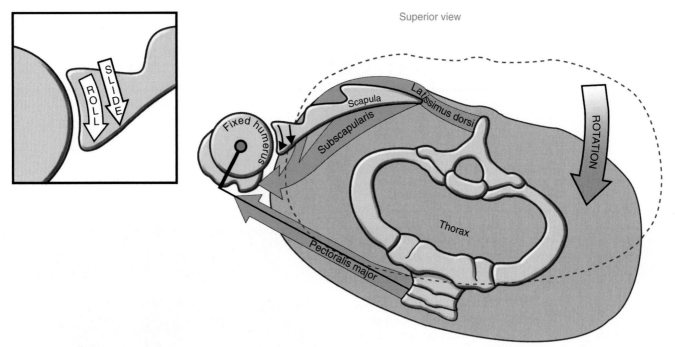

FIGURE 5-60. Superior view of the right shoulder showing actions of three internal rotators when the distal (humeral) segment is fixed and the trunk is free to rotate. The line of force of the pectoralis major is shown with its internal moment arm originating around the glenohumeral joint's vertical axis. Inset shows the roll-and-slide arthrokinematics during the concave-on-convex motion.

its stability. Unlike the more stable SC joint, the AC joint frequently dislocates after a strong medially and inferiorly directed force delivered to the shoulder. Both dislocation and degenerative osteoarthritis are more common at the AC joint than the SC joint.

The scapulothoracic joint serves as an important mechanical platform for all active movements of the humerus. Consider full shoulder abduction, for example, which consists of about 60 degrees of scapular upward rotation. Combined with the mechanically linked motions at the SC and AC joints, the upwardly rotated scapula provides a stable yet mobile base for the abducting the humeral head and maximizes the volume within the subacromial space.

The GH joint is the most distal and mobile link within the shoulder complex. Mobility is enhanced by the naturally loose articular capsule, in conjunction with a relatively flat and small glenoid fossa. Paradoxically, these same features that promote mobility at the GH joint often predispose it to instability, especially when associated with repetitive and vigorous, near–end range motions. Consequently, the GH joint is frequently involved with clinical conditions that involve excessive laxity, dislocation, or subluxation–generally referred to as *shoulder instability.*

In addition to being predisposed to instability, the GH joint is frequently affected by degenerative-related pathologies. A common causative factor underlying many of these pathologies is excessive stress placed on periarticular connective tissues and the adjacent rotator cuff muscles. Stressed and damaged tissues often become inflamed and painful, as demonstrated in subacromial bursitis, rotator cuff tendonitis, and adhesive capsulitis.

The goals of conservative treatment of many of the aforementioned degenerative or inflammatory conditions center around reducing the primary and secondary stresses on the joint, normalizing the arthrokinematics; restoring active and passive range of motion, improving strength, and reducing pain and inflammation. Accomplishing these goals typically leads to increased function of the shoulder.

Sixteen muscles power and control the wide range of movements available to the shoulder complex. Rather than working in isolation, these muscles most often interact synergistically to enhance their control over the multiple joints of the region. Consider, for example, the muscular interactions required to abduct the shoulder in the plane of the scapula. Muscles such as the deltoid and rotator cuff require coactivation of the serratus anterior and trapezius to effectively stabilize the scapula and clavicle. Furthermore, these scapulothoracic muscles can stabilize the scapula and clavicle only if their proximal skeletal attachments (cranium, ribs, and spine) are themselves well stabilized. Weakness anywhere along these links reduces the strength, ease, and control of active shoulder abduction. Factors that directly or indirectly disrupt these muscular-driven links include trauma, excessive stiffness of connective tissues, abnormal posture, joint instability, pain, peripheral nerve or spinal cord injuries, and diseases affecting the muscular or nervous system.

Appreciating how muscles naturally interact across the shoulder prepares the clinician to render an accurate diagnosis of the underlying pathomechanics of abnormal shoulder posture and movement. This knowledge is essential to the design of effective rehabilitation and treatment programs for the loss of normal muscle function.

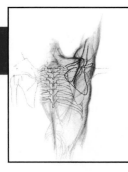

ADDITIONAL CLINICAL CONNECTIONS

CLINICAL CONNECTION 5-1
Subacromial Impingement Syndrome: a Closer Look at the Underlying Pathomechanics

Subacromial impingement syndrome is among the most common painful disorders of the shoulder.[195] The pathomechanics of this syndrome are primarily associated with repeated and unnatural compression of the tissues within the subacromial space. Specifically, the supraspinatus tendon, the tendon of the long head of the biceps, the superior capsule, and the subacromial bursa are compressed between the humeral head and the coracoacromial arch. Neer, who first introduced this topic in 1972, reported that possibly 95% of all tears within the rotator cuff can be attributed to the repetitive trauma caused by subacromial impingement.[146] Although this may be overstated, most researchers in this area believe that impingement is at least a very important factor in the cause of rotator cuff disease.[135] Because the site of the impingement is on the external surface of the rotator cuff, it is often referred to as an "external" impingement syndrome. In contrast, an "internal" impingement syndrome is characterized by compression of the *internal* surfaces of the rotator cuff between the greater tubercle and adjacent rim of the glenoid fossa.

Pain caused by subacromial impingement is typically concentrated in the anterior shoulder region, usually aggravated by active abduction of 60 to 120 degrees.[69] Tissues are more likely compressed within this arc of abduction because the greater tubercle of the humerus comes closest to the anterior acromion.[57] Indeed, subacromial pressures in symptomatic patients have been shown to rise sharply throughout this painful arc.[149] Because of the importance of raising the arm overhead, shoulder impingement syndrome can cause significant functional limitations.[112] This condition is most common in athletes and laborers who repeatedly abduct their shoulders over 90 degrees,[184] but it can also occur in relatively sedentary persons. Subacromial impingement can be detected on standard radiographic examination (Figure 5-61).

Michener and colleagues present a thorough review of the factors that may predispose a person to subacromial impingement syndrome.[135] One relevant kinesiologic factor involves abnormal arthrokinematics at the GH joint. As highlighted earlier, excessive superior migration of the humeral head during abduction can compress the contents within the subacromial space.[43] Why the humeral head migrates excessively superiorly is not known for certain but may be associated with the inability of muscles, such as the rotator cuff group, to coordinate the natural arthrokinematics.[72,111,127]

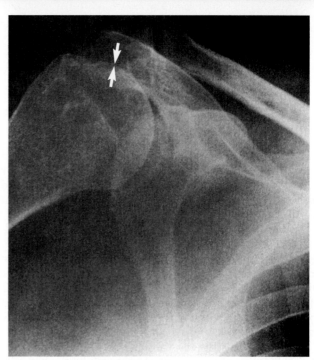

FIGURE 5-61. A radiograph of a person with subacromial impingement syndrome attempting abduction of the shoulder. The small arrows mark the impingement of the humeral head against the undersurface of the acromion. (Courtesy Gary L. Soderberg.)

Research on the causes of subacromial impingement syndrome has included the study of abnormal arthrokinematics at the GH joint from both humeral-on-scapular and scapular-on-humeral perspectives.* Theoretically, either kinematic perspective could compress the contents within the subacromial space. A considerable body of literature has implicated abnormal scapulothoracic kinematics as a possible contributing factor to impingement.[14,116,135] As described earlier in this chapter, in the healthy shoulder, abduction of the GH joint occurs in conjunction with scapulothoracic upward rotation, usually combined with more subtle scapular adjustment motions of posterior tilting and external rotation. Most

---

*References 15, 71, 94, 112, 126, 135, 143.

ADDITIONAL CLINICAL CONNECTIONS

CLINICAL CONNECTION 5-1
Subacromial Impingement Syndrome: a Closer Look at the Underlying Pathomechanics—cont'd

studies have shown that persons with subacromial impingement syndrome demonstrate less than normal upward rotation, less posterior tilting, and less external rotation of the scapula during shoulder abduction.[111,117,123] These abnormal kinematics are believed to contribute to subacromial impingement given that they reduce the clearance between the humeral head and coracoacromial arch.[57,91,117,135,174] Some groups of persons with a history of subacromial impingement syndrome, however, have shown slightly *greater* upward rotation and posterior tilting of the scapula during abduction. These seemingly paradoxic kinematics may likely be a compensatory mechanism employed to *increase* subacromial space and thereby reduce the severity of the impingement. Regardless of the specific pattern of scapular kinematics, an important point is that only a small deviation in scapular kinematics likely has a disproportionately large effect on a volume that is as small as the subacromial space, especially in light of other concomitant factors such as swelling of the bursa.[49]

"Faulty" posture of the scapula at rest has also been implicated as a contributing factor to reducing the volume of the subacromial space.[14,94,108,116] "Poor" or slouched posture in otherwise neurologically intact persons often is associated with a scapulothoracic joint that is abnormally downwardly rotated and excessively protracted—positions typically associated with excessive anterior tilting and internal rotation of the scapula. Such a posture has indeed been correlated with a tight or overshortened pectoralis minor muscle.[15] As described in the preceding paragraph, this abnormal scapular posture may contribute to the development of subacromial impingement syndrome. For years, anecdotal evidence has suggested such a causal relationship. Only more recently has objective evidence emerged that lends some support to this strongly held clinical notion.

The pathomechanics underlying poor or abnormal posture of the scapulothoracic joint are complex and not completely understood. In addition to a tight pectoralis minor, other causes may include altered posture of the cervical and thoracic spine; abnormal sitting posture; pain avoidance; fatigue, tightness, or weakness of shoulder muscles such as the serratus anterior and rotator cuff group; and reduced coordination of the muscles that naturally sequence the kinematics between the scapula and humerus.[†]

Subacromial impingement syndrome may also be caused by pathologies that are more directly associated with the GH joint. These pathologies may include ligamentous instability, adhesive capsulitis,[133,166] excessive tightness in the posterior capsule (and associated excessive anterior migration of the humeral head

toward the lower part of the coracoacromial arch), selected muscular tightness around the GH joint, and structurally induced changes in the volume of the subacromial space.[135] The last factor may result from osteophytes forming around the overlying AC joint,[118] an abnormal hook-shaped acromion, or swelling and fragmentation of structures in and around the subacromial space.

Regardless of cause, each time an impingement occurs, the delicate supraspinatus tendon and subacromial bursa become further traumatized, often leading to chronic inflammation or even rupture of the tendon.[18] The long head of the biceps and the superior capsule of the GH joint may also be traumatized. Therapeutic goals for the treatment of subacromial impingement syndrome include decreasing inflammation within the subacromial space, conditioning and increasing control of the rotator cuff and scapulothoracic muscles, improving kinesthetic awareness of movement and posture of the scapulothoracic joint, and attempting to restore the natural shoulder range of motion and arthrokinematics. Ergonomic education is also a factor in goal setting.

Ideally, the knowledge gained through continued research into the causes of subacromial impingement will help guide clinical decision making, ultimately increasing the quality of therapeutic intervention for persons with this pathology.[‡]

> **Ten Possible Direct or Indirect Causes of Shoulder Impingement Syndrome**
> - Abnormal kinematics at the glenohumeral (GH) and scapulothoracic joints
> - "Slouched" posture that affects the alignment of the scapulothoracic joint
> - Fatigue, weakness, poor control, or tightness of the muscles that govern motions at the GH or scapulothoracic joints
> - Inflammation and swelling of tissues within and around the subacromial space
> - Excessive wear and subsequent degeneration of the tendons of the rotator cuff muscles
> - Instability of the GH joint
> - Adhesions within the inferior GH joint capsule
> - Excessive tightness in the posterior capsule of the GH joint (and associated anterior migration of the humeral head toward the lower margin of the coracoacromial arch)
> - Osteophytes forming around the acromioclavicular joint
> - Abnormal shape of the acromion or coracoacromial arch

[†]References 15, 28, 47, 53, 55, 93, 107, 113, 131, 135.

[‡]References 15, 56, 108, 116, 123, 143.

REFERENCES

1. Abboud JA, Soslowsky LJ: Interplay of the static and dynamic restraints in glenohumeral instability. *Clin Orthop Relat Res* 48-57, 2002.
2. Alberta FG, Elattrache NS, Mihata T, et al: Arthroscopic anteroinferior suture plication resulting in decreased glenohumeral translation and external rotation. Study of a cadaver model. *J Bone Joint Surg Am* 88:179-187, 2006.
3. An KN, Browne AO, Korinek S, et al: Three-dimensional kinematics of glenohumeral elevation. *J Orthop Res* 9:143-149, 1991.
4. Andrews JR, Carson WG Jr, McLeod WD: Glenoid labrum tears related to the long head of the biceps. *Am J Sports Med* 13:337-341, 1985.
5. Bagg SD, Forrest WJ: A biomechanical analysis of scapular rotation during arm abduction in the scapular plane. *Am J Phys Med Rehabil* 67:238-245, 1988.
6. Bagg SD, Forrest WJ: Electromyographic study of the scapular rotators during arm abduction in the scapular plane. *Am J Phys Med* 65:111-124, 1986.
7. Barber FA, Ryu RK, Tauro JC: Should first time anterior shoulder dislocations be surgically stabilized? *Arthroscopy* 19:305-309, 2003.
8. Barnes CJ, Van Steyn SJ, Fischer RA: The effects of age, sex, and shoulder dominance on range of motion of the shoulder. *J Shoulder Elbow Surg* 10:242-246, 2001.
9. Basmajian JV, Bazant FJ: Factors preventing downward dislocation of the adducted shoulder joint. *J Bone Joint Surg Am* 41:1182-1186, 1959.
10. Bey MJ, Elders GJ, Huston LJ, et al: The mechanism of creation of superior labrum, anterior, and posterior lesions in a dynamic biomechanical model of the shoulder: The role of inferior subluxation. *J Shoulder Elbow Surg* 7:397-401, 1998.
11. Bigliani LU, Kelkar R, Flatow EL, et al: Glenohumeral stability. Biomechanical properties of passive and active stabilizers. *Clin Orthop Relat Res* 330:13-30, 1996.
12. Bigliani LU, Kurzweil PR, Schwartzbach CC, et al: Inferior capsular shift procedure for anterior-inferior shoulder instability in athletes. *Am J Sports Med* 22:578-584, 1994.
13. Boardman ND, Debski RE, Warner JJ, et al: Tensile properties of the superior glenohumeral and coracohumeral ligaments. *J Shoulder Elbow Surg* 5:249-254, 1996.
14. Borstad JD: Resting position variables at the shoulder: Evidence to support a posture-impairment association. *Phys Ther* 86:549-557, 2006.
15. Borstad JD, Ludewig PM: The effect of long versus short pectoralis minor resting length on scapular kinematics in healthy individuals. *J Orthop Sports Phys Ther* 35:227-238, 2005.
16. Brophy RH, Marx RG: Osteoarthritis following shoulder instability. *Clin Sports Med* 24:47-56, 2005.
17. Brunnstrom S: Muscle testing around the shoulder girdle. *J Bone Joint Surg Am* 23:263-272, 1941.
18. Budoff JE, Nirschl RP, Guidi EJ: Debridement of partial-thickness tears of the rotator cuff without acromioplasty. Long-term follow-up and review of the literature. *J Bone Joint Surg Am* 80:733-748, 1998.
19. Burkart AC, Debski RE: Anatomy and function of the glenohumeral ligaments in anterior shoulder instability. *Clin Orthop Relat Res* 32-39, 2002.
20. Burkhart SS, Morgan CD, Kibler WB: The disabled throwing shoulder: Spectrum of pathology. Part I: Pathoanatomy and biomechanics. *Arthroscopy* 19:404-420, 2003.
21. Burkhead WZ Jr, Rockwood CA Jr: Treatment of instability of the shoulder with an exercise program. *J Bone Joint Surg Am* 74:890-896, 1992.
22. Buttaci CJ, Stitik TP, Yonclas PP, Foye PM: Osteoarthritis of the acromioclavicular joint: A review of anatomy, biomechanics, diagnosis, and treatment. *Am J Phys Med Rehabil* 83:791-797, 2004.
23. Chansky HA, Iannotti JP: The vascularity of the rotator cuff. *Clin Sports Med* 10:807-822, 1991.
24. Chant CB, Litchfield R, Griffin S, Thain LM: Humeral head retroversion in competitive baseball players and its relationship to glenohumeral rotation range of motion. *J Orthop Sports Phys Ther* 37:514-520, 2007.
25. Chen S, Haen PS, Walton J, Murrell GA: The effects of thermal capsular shrinkage on the outcomes of arthroscopic stabilization for primary anterior shoulder instability. *Am J Sports Med* 33:705-711, 2005.
26. Churchill RS, Brems JJ, Kotschi H: Glenoid size, inclination, and version: An anatomic study. *J Shoulder Elbow Surg* 10:327-332, 2001.
27. Conway AM: Movements at the sternoclavicular and acromioclavicular joints. *Phys Ther* 41:421-432, 1961.
28. Cools AM, Witvrouw EE, Declercq GA, et al: Scapular muscle recruitment patterns: Trapezius muscle latency with and without impingement symptoms. *Am J Sports Med* 31:542-549, 2003.
29. Cooper DE, Arnoczky SP, O'Brien SJ, et al: Anatomy, histology, and vascularity of the glenoid labrum. An anatomical study. *J Bone Joint Surg Am* 74:46-52, 1992.
30. Corteen DP, Teitge RA: Stabilization of the clavicle after distal resection: A biomechanical study. *Am J Sports Med* 33:61-67, 2005.
31. Costic RS, Vangura A Jr, Fenwick JA, et al: Viscoelastic behavior and structural properties of the coracoclavicular ligaments. *Scand J Med Sci Sports* 13:305-310, 2003.
32. Crosbie J, Kilbreath SL, Hollmann L, York S: Scapulohumeral rhythm and associated spinal motion. *Clin Biomech (Bristol, Avon)* 23:184-192, 2008.
33. Curl LA, Warren RF: Glenohumeral joint stability. Selective cutting studies on the static capsular restraints. *Clin Orthop Relat Res* 330:54-65; 1996.
34. de Freitas V, Vitti M, Furlani J: Electromyographic analysis of the levator scapulae and rhomboideus major muscle in movements of the shoulder. *Electromyogr Clin Neurophysiol* 19:335-342, 1979.
35. DePalma AF: *Degenerative changes in sternoclavicular and acromioclavicular joints in various decades*. Springfield, Ill, 1957, Charles C Thomas.
36. Debski RE, Parsons IM, Woo SL, Fu FH: Effect of capsular injury on acromioclavicular joint mechanics. *J Bone Joint Surg* 83:1344-1351, 2001.
37. Debski RE, Sakone M, Woo SL, et al: Contribution of the passive properties of the rotator cuff to glenohumeral stability during anterior-posterior loading. *J Shoulder Elbow Surg* 8:324-329, 1999.
38. Debski RE, Weiss JA, Newman WJ, et al: Stress and strain in the anterior band of the inferior glenohumeral ligament during a simulated clinical examination. *J Shoulder Elbow Surg* 14:24S-31S, 2005.
39. Debski RE, Wong EK, Woo SL, et al: An analytical approach to determine the in situ forces in the glenohumeral ligaments. *J Biomech Eng* 121:311-315, 1999.
40. Decker MJ, Hintermeister RA, Faber KJ, Hawkins RJ: Serratus anterior muscle activity during selected rehabilitation exercises. *Am J Sports Med* 27:784-791, 1999.
41. Decker MJ, Tokish JM, Ellis HB, et al: Subscapularis muscle activity during selected rehabilitation exercises. *Am J Sports Med* 31:126-134, 2003.
42. Dessaur WA, Magarey ME: Diagnostic accuracy of clinical tests for superior labral anterior posterior lesions: A systematic review. *J Orthop Sports Phys Ther* 38:341-352, 2008.
43. Deutsch A, Altchek DW, Schwartz E, et al: Radiologic measurement of superior displacement of the humeral head in the impingement syndrome. *J Shoulder Elbow Surg* 5:186-193, 1996.
44. Diederichsen LP, Nørregaard J, Krogsgaard M, et al: Reflexes in the shoulder muscles elicited from the human coracoacromial ligament. *J Orthop Res* 22:976-983, 2004.
45. Dillman CJ, Fleisig GS, Andrews JR: Biomechanics of pitching with emphasis upon shoulder kinematics. *J Orthop Sports Phys Ther* 18:402-408, 1993.
46. Dvir Z, Berme N: The shoulder complex in elevation of the arm: a mechanism approach. *J Biomech* 11:219-225, 1978.
47. Ebaugh DD, McClure PW, Karduna AR: Effects of shoulder muscle fatigue caused by repetitive overhead activities on scapulothoracic and glenohumeral kinematics. *J Electromyogr Kinesiol* 16:224-235, 2006.
48. Ebaugh DD, McClure PW, Karduna AR: Scapulothoracic and glenohumeral kinematics following an external rotation fatigue protocol. *J Orthop Sports Phys Ther* 36:557-571, 2006.
49. Ebaugh DD, McClure PW, Karduna AR: Three-dimensional scapulothoracic motion during active and passive arm elevation. *Clin Biomech (Bristol, Avon)* 20:700-709, 2005.
50. Ekstrom RA, Bifulco KM, Lopau CJ, et al: Comparing the function of the upper and lower parts of the serratus anterior muscle using surface electromyography. *J Orthop Sports Phys Ther* 34:235-243, 2004.
51. Ekstrom RA, Donatelli RA, Soderberg GL: Surface electromyographic analysis of exercises for the trapezius and serratus anterior muscles. *J Orthop Sports Phys Ther* 33:247-258, 2003.
52. Ellenbecker TS, Mattalino AJ: Concentric isokinetic shoulder internal and external rotation strength in professional baseball pitchers. *J Orthop Sports Phys Ther* 25:323-328, 1997.
53. Endo K, Yukata K, Yasui N: Influence of age on scapulo-thoracic orientation. *Clin Biomech (Bristol, Avon)* 19:1009-1013, 2004.

54. Ferrari DA: Capsular ligaments of the shoulder. Anatomical and functional study of the anterior superior capsule. *Am J Sports Med* 18:20-24, 1990.

55. Finley MA, Lee RY: Effect of sitting posture on 3-dimensional scapular kinematics measured by skin-mounted electromagnetic tracking sensors. *Arch Phys Med Rehabil* 84:563-568, 2003.

56. Finley MA, McQuade KJ, Rodgers MM: Scapular kinematics during transfers in manual wheelchair users with and without shoulder impingement. *Clin Biomech (Bristol, Avon)* 20:32-40, 2005.

57. Flatow EL, Soslowsky LJ, Ticker JB, et al: Excursion of the rotator cuff under the acromion. Patterns of subacromial contact. *Am J Sports Med* 22:779-788, 1994.

58. Fleisig GS, Barrentine SW, Zheng N, et al: Kinematic and kinetic comparison of baseball pitching among various levels of development. *J Biomech* 32:1371-1375, 1999.

59. Fraser-Moodie JA, Shortt NL, Robinson CM: Injuries to the acromioclavicular joint. *J Bone Joint Surg Br* 90:697-707, 2008.

60. Freedman L, Munro RR: Abduction of the arm in the scapular plane: Scapular and glenohumeral movements. A roentgenographic study. *J Bone Joint Surg Am* 48:1503-1510, 1966.

61. Fukuda K, Craig EV, An KN, et al: Biomechanical study of the ligamentous system of the acromioclavicular joint. *J Bone Joint Surg Am* 68:434-440, 1986.

62. Fung M, Kato S, Barrance PJ, et al: Scapular and clavicular kinematics during humeral elevation: A study with cadavers. *J Shoulder Elbow Surg* 10:278-285, 2001.

63. Gelber PE, Reina F, Monllau JC, et al: Innervation patterns of the inferior glenohumeral ligament: Anatomical and biomechanical relevance. *Clin Anat* 19:304-311, 2006.

64. Gerber C, Blumenthal S, Curt A, Werner CM: Effect of selective experimental suprascapular nerve block on abduction and external rotation strength of the shoulder. *J Shoulder Elbow Surg* 16:815-820, 2007.

65. Gohlke F: The pattern of the collagen fiber bundles of the capsule of the glenohumeral joint. *J Shoulder Elbow Surg* 3:111-128, 1994.

66. Gomoll AH, Katz JN, Warner JJ, Millett PJ: Rotator cuff disorders: Recognition and management among patients with shoulder pain. *Arthritis Rheum* 50:3751-3761, 2004.

67. Graichen H, Bonel H, Stammberger T, et al: Three-dimensional analysis of the width of the subacromial space in healthy subjects and patients with impingement syndrome. *AJR Am J Roentgenol* 172:1081-1086, 1999.

68. Graichen H, Englmeier KH, Reiser M, Eckstein F: An in vivo technique for determining 3D muscular moment arms in different joint positions and during muscular activation–application to the supraspinatus. *Clin Biomech (Bristol, Avon)* 16:389-394, 2001.

69. Graichen H, Hinterwimmer S, von Eisenhart-Rothe R, et al: Effect of abducting and adducting muscle activity on glenohumeral translation, scapular kinematics and subacromial space width in vivo. *J Biomech* 38:755-760, 2005.

70. Graichen H, Stammberger T, Bonél H, et al: Magnetic resonance–based motion analysis of the shoulder during elevation. *Clin Orthop Relat Res* 370:154-163, 2000.

71. Graichen H, Stammberger T, Bonél H, et al: Three-dimensional analysis of shoulder girdle and supraspinatus motion patterns in patients with impingement syndrome. *J Orthop Res* 19:1192-1198, 2001.

72. Halder AM, Zhao KD, Odriscoll SW, et al: Dynamic contributions to superior shoulder stability. *J Orthop Res* 19:206-212, 2001.

73. Hallaceli H, Gunal I: Normal range of scapular elevation and depression in healthy subjects. *Arch Orthop Trauma Surg* 122:99-101, 2002.

74. Hara H, Ito N, Iwasaki K: Strength of the glenoid labrum and adjacent shoulder capsule. *J Shoulder Elbow Surg* 5:263-268, 1996.

75. Harryman DT, Sidles JA, Clark JM, et al: Translation of the humeral head on the glenoid with passive glenohumeral motion. *J Bone Joint Surg Am* 72:1334-1343, 1990.

76. Hayes K, Callanan M, Walton J, et al: Shoulder instability: Management and rehabilitation. *J Orthop Sports Phys Ther* 32:497-509, 2002.

77. Holzbaur KR, Delp SL, Gold GE, Murray WM: Moment-generating capacity of upper limb muscles in healthy adults. *J Biomech* 40:2442-2449, 2007.

78. Hovelius L, Eriksson K, Fredin H, et al: Recurrences after initial dislocation of the shoulder. Results of a prospective study of treatment. *J Bone Joint Surg Am* 65:343-349, 1983.

79. Howell SM, Galinat BJ: The glenoid-labral socket. A constrained articular surface. *Clin Orthop Relat Res* 122-125, 1989.

80. Howell SM, Imobersteg AM, Seger DH, Marone PJ: Clarification of the role of the supraspinatus muscle in shoulder function. *J Bone Joint Surg Am* 68:398-404, 1986.

81. Hughes RE, An KN: Force analysis of rotator cuff muscles. *Clin Orthop Relat Res* 330:75-83, 1996.

82. Hughes RE, Bryant CR, Hall JM, et al: Glenoid inclination is associated with full-thickness rotator cuff tears. *Clin Orthop Relat Res* 407:86-91, 2003.

83. Hunt SA, Kwon YW, Zuckerman JD: The rotator interval: Anatomy, pathology, and strategies for treatment. *J Am Acad Orthop Surg* 15:218-227, 2007.

84. Inman VT, Saunders M, Abbott LC: Observations on the function of the shoulder joint. *J Bone Joint Surg Am* 26:1-32, 1944.

85. Inokuchi W, Sanderhoff OB, Søjbjerg JO, Sneppen O: The relation between the position of the glenohumeral joint and the intraarticular pressure: An experimental study. *J Shoulder Elbow Surg* 6:144-149, 1997.

86. Itoi E, Berglund LJ, Grabowski JJ, et al: Superior-inferior stability of the shoulder: Role of the coracohumeral ligament and the rotator interval capsule. *Mayo Clin Proc* 73:508-515, 1998.

87. Itoi E, Motzkin NE, Morrey BF, An KN: Bulk effect of rotator cuff on inferior glenohumeral stability as function of scapular inclination angle: A cadaver study. *Tohoku J Exp Med* 171:267-276, 1993.

88. Johnson AJ, Godges JJ, Zimmerman GJ, Ounanian LL: The effect of anterior versus posterior glide joint mobilization on external rotation range of motion in patients with shoulder adhesive capsulitis. *J Orthop Sports Phys Ther* 37:88-99, 2007.

89. Johnson GR, Pandyan AD: The activity in the three regions of the trapezius under controlled loading conditions–an experimental and modelling study. *Clin Biomech (Bristol, Avon)* 20:155-161, 2005.

90. Johnson GR, Spalding D, Nowitzke A, Bogduk N: Modelling the muscles of the scapula morphometric and coordinate data and functional implications. *J Biomech* 29:1039-1051, 1996.

91. Karduna AR, Kerner PJ, Lazarus MD: Contact forces in the subacromial space: Effects of scapular orientation. *J Shoulder Elbow Surg* 14:393-399, 2005.

92. Karduna AR, McClure PW, Michener LA, Sennett B: Dynamic measurements of three-dimensional scapular kinematics: A validation study. *J Biomech Eng* 123:184-190, 2001.

93. Kebaetse M, McClure P, Pratt NA: Thoracic position effect on shoulder range of motion, strength, and three-dimensional scapular kinematics. *Arch Phys Med Rehabil* 80:945-950, 1999.

94. Kibler WB, McMullen J: Scapular dyskinesis and its relation to shoulder pain. *J Am Acad Orthop Surg* 11:142-151, 2003.

95. Kibler WB, Sciascia AD, Uhl TL, et al: Electromyographic analysis of specific exercises for scapular control in early phases of shoulder rehabilitation. *Am J Sports Med* 36:1789-1798, 2008.

96. Kido T, Itoi E, Lee SB, et al: Dynamic stabilizing function of the deltoid muscle in shoulders with anterior instability. *Am J Sports Med* 31:399-403, 2003.

97. Kim TK, McFarland EG: Internal impingement of the shoulder in flexion. *Clin Orthop Relat Res* 421:112-119, 2004.

98. Kronberg M, Nemeth G, Brostrom LA: Muscle activity and coordination in the normal shoulder. An electromyographic study. *Clin Orthop Relat Res* 257:76-85, 1990.

99. Kuechle DK, Newman SR, Itoi E, et al: Shoulder muscle moment arms during horizontal flexion and elevation. *J Shoulder Elbow Surg* 6:429-439, 1997.

100. Kuhn JE, Huston LJ, Soslowsky LJ, et al: External rotation of the glenohumeral joint: Ligament restraints and muscle effects in the neutral and abducted positions. *J Shoulder Elbow Surg* 14:39S-48S, 2005.

101. Kumar VP, Balasubramaniam P: The role of atmospheric pressure in stabilising the shoulder. An experimental study. *J Bone Joint Surg Br* 67:719-721, 1985.

102. Kvitne RS, Jobe FW: The diagnosis and treatment of anterior instability in the throwing athlete. *Clin Orthop Relat Res* 291:107-123, 1993.

103. Labriola JE, Lee TQ, Debski RE, McMahon PJ: Stability and instability of the glenohumeral joint: The role of shoulder muscles. *J Shoulder Elbow Surg* 14:32S-38S, 2005.

104. Langenderfer JE, Patthanacharoenphon C, Carpenter JE, Hughes RE: Variation in external rotation moment arms among subregions of supraspinatus, infraspinatus, and teres minor muscles. *J Orthop Res* 24:1737-1744, 2006.

105. Lee KW, Debski RE, Chen CH, et al: Functional evaluation of the ligaments at the acromioclavicular joint during anteroposterior and superoinferior translation. *Am J Sports Med* 25:858-862, 1997.

106. Lee SB, An KN: Dynamic glenohumeral stability provided by three heads of the deltoid muscle. *Clin Orthop Relat Res* 400:40-47, 2002.

107. Lewis JS, Green A, Wright C: Subacromial impingement syndrome: The role of posture and muscle imbalance. *J Shoulder Elbow Surg* 14:385-392, 2005.

108. Lewis JS, Wright C, Green A: Subacromial impingement syndrome: The effect of changing posture on shoulder range of movement. *J Orthop Sports Phys Ther* 35:72-87, 2005.

109. Liu J, Hughes RE, Smutz WP, et al: Roles of deltoid and rotator cuff muscles in shoulder elevation. *Clin Biomech (Bristol, Avon)* 12:32-38, 1997.

110. Ludewig PM, Behrens SA, Meyer SM, et al: Three-dimensional clavicular motion during arm elevation: Reliability and descriptive data. *J Orthop Sports Phys Ther* 34:140-149, 2004.

111. Ludewig PM, Cook TM: Alterations in shoulder kinematics and associated muscle activity in people with symptoms of shoulder impingement. *Phys Ther* 80:276-291, 2000.

112. Ludewig PM, Cook TM: Translations of the humerus in persons with shoulder impingement symptoms. *J Orthop Sports Phys Ther* 32:248-259, 2002.

113. Ludewig PM, Cook TM, Nawoczenski DA: Three-dimensional scapular orientation and muscle activity at selected positions of humeral elevation. *J Orthop Sports Phys Ther* 24:57-65, 1996.

114. Ludewig PM, Hoff MS, Osowski EE, et al: Relative balance of serratus anterior and upper trapezius muscle activity during push-up exercises. *Am J Sports Med* 32:484-493, 2004.

115. Ludewig PM, Phadke V, Braman JP, et al: Motion of the shoulder complex during multiplanar humeral elevation. *J Bone Joint Surg Am* 91:378-389, 2009.

116. Ludewig PM, Reynolds JF: The association of scapular kinematics and glenohumeral joint pathologies. J Orthop *Phys Ther* 39:90-104, 2009.

117. Lukasiewicz AC, McClure P, Michener L, et al: Comparison of 3-dimensional scapular position and orientation between subjects with and without shoulder impingement. *J Orthop Sports Phys Ther* 29:574-583, 1999.

118. Mahakkanukrauh P, Surin P: Prevalence of osteophytes associated with the acromion and acromioclavicular joint. *Clin Anat* 16:506-510, 2003.

119. Mandalidis DG, Mc Glone BS, Quigley RF, et al: Digital fluoroscopic assessment of the scapulohumeral rhythm. *Surg Radiol Anat* 21:241-246, 1999.

120. Matias R, Pascoal AG: The unstable shoulder in arm elevation: A three-dimensional and electromyographic study in subjects with glenohumeral instability. *Clin Biomech (Bristol, Avon)* 21(Suppl 1):S52-S58, 2006.

121. Mazzocca AD, Arciero RA, Bicos J: Evaluation and treatment of acromioclavicular joint injuries. *Am J Sports Med* 35:316-329, 2007.

122. McClure P, Balaicuis J, Heiland D, et al: A randomized controlled comparison of stretching procedures for posterior shoulder tightness. *J Orthop Sports Phys Ther* 37:108-114, 2007.

123. McClure PW, Bialker J, Neff N, et al: Shoulder function and 3-dimensional kinematics in people with shoulder impingement syndrome before and after a 6-week exercise program. *Phys Ther* 84:832-848, 2004.

124. McClure PW, Michener LA, Karduna AR: Shoulder function and 3-dimensional scapular kinematics in people with and without shoulder impingement syndrome. *Phys Ther* 86:1075-1090, 2006.

125. McClure PW, Michener LA, Sennett B, Karduna AR: Direct 3-dimensional measurement of scapular kinematics during dynamic movements in vivo. *J Shoulder Elbow Surg* 10:269-277, 2001.

126. McCully SP, Suprak DN, Kosek P, Karduna AR: Suprascapular nerve block disrupts the normal pattern of scapular kinematics. *Clin Biomech (Bristol, Avon)* 21:545-553, 2006.

127. McCully SP, Suprak DN, Kosek P, Karduna AR: Suprascapular nerve block results in a compensatory increase in deltoid muscle activity. *J Biomech* 40:1839-1846, 2007.

128. McMahon PJ, Dettling J, Sandusky MD, et al: The anterior band of the inferior glenohumeral ligament. Assessment of its permanent deformation and the anatomy of its glenoid attachment. *J Bone Joint Surg Br* 81:406-413, 1999.

129. McMahon PJ, Tibone JE, Cawley PW, et al: The anterior band of the inferior glenohumeral ligament: Biomechanical properties from tensile testing in the position of apprehension. *J Shoulder Elbow Surg* 7:467-471, 1998.

130. McQuade KJ: Effects of local muscle fatigue on the 3-dimensional scapulohumeral rhythm. *Clin Biomech (Bristol, Avon)* 10:144-148, 1995.

131. McQuade KJ, Dawson J, Smidt GL: Scapulothoracic muscle fatigue associated with alterations in scapulohumeral rhythm kinematics during maximum resistive shoulder elevation. *J Orthop Sports Phys Ther* 28:74-80, 1998.

132. McQuade KJ, Smidt GL: Dynamic scapulohumeral rhythm: The effects of external resistance during elevation of the arm in the scapular plane. *J Orthop Sports Phys Ther* 27:125-133, 1998.

133. Mengiardi B, Pfirrmann CW, Gerber C, et al: Frozen shoulder: MR arthrographic findings. *Radiology* 233:486-492, 2004.

134. Meskers CG, van der Helm FC, Rozing PM: The size of the supraspinatus outlet during elevation of the arm in the frontal and sagittal plane: A 3-D model study. *Clin Biomech (Bristol, Avon)* 17:257-266, 2002.

135. Michener LA, McClure PW, Karduna AR: Anatomical and biomechanical mechanisms of subacromial impingement syndrome (review). *Clin Biomech (Bristol, Avon)* 18:369-379, 2003.

136. Mikesky AE, Edwards JE, Wigglesworth JK, Kunkel S: Eccentric and concentric strength of the shoulder and arm musculature in collegiate baseball pitchers. *Am J Sports Med* 23:638-642, 1995.

137. Miller MD, Larsen KM, Luke T, et al: Anterior capsular shift volume reduction: An in vitro comparison of 3 techniques. *J Shoulder Elbow Surg* 12:350-354, 2003.

138. Mizuno N, Yoneda M, Hayashida K, et al: Recurrent anterior shoulder dislocation caused by a midsubstance complete capsular tear. *J Bone Joint Surg Am* 87:2717-2723, 2005.

139. Moore SM, Musahl V, McMahon PJ, Debski RE: Multidirectional kinematics of the glenohumeral joint during simulated simple translation tests: Impact on clinical diagnoses. *J Orthop Res* 22:889-894, 2004.

140. Moseley HF: The clavicle: Its anatomy and function. *Clin Orthop Relat Res* 58:17-27, 1968.

141. Moseley JB Jr, Jobe FW, Pink M, et al: EMG analysis of the scapular muscles during a shoulder rehabilitation program. *Am J Sports Med* 20:128-134, 1992.

142. Mura N, O'Driscoll SW, Zobitz ME, et al: The effect of infraspinatus disruption on glenohumeral torque and superior migration of the humeral head: A biomechanical study. *J Shoulder Elbow Surg* 12:179-184, 2003.

143. Myers JB, Laudner KG, Pasquale MR, et al: Scapular position and orientation in throwing athletes. *Am J Sports Med* 33:263-271, 2005.

144. Myers TH, Zemanovic JR, Andrews JR: The resisted supination external rotation test: A new test for the diagnosis of superior labral anterior posterior lesions. *Am J Sports Med* 33:1315-1320, 2005.

145. Nam EK, Snyder SJ: The diagnosis and treatment of superior labrum, anterior and posterior (SLAP) lesions. *Am J Sports Med* 31:798-810, 2003.

146. Neer CS: Anterior acromioplasty for the chronic impingement syndrome in the shoulder. *J Bone Joint Surg Am* 87:1399, 1972.

147. Neer CS: Impingement lesions. *Clin Orthop Relat Res* 173:70-77, 1983.

148. Neumann DA: Polio: Its impact on the people of the United States and the emerging profession of physical therapy. *J Orthop Sports Phys Ther* 34:479-492, 2004.

149. Nordt WE III, Garretson RB III, Plotkin E: The measurement of subacromial contact pressure in patients with impingement syndrome. *Arthroscopy* 15:121-125, 1999.

150. Nyland JA, Caborn DN, Johnson DL: The human glenohumeral joint. A proprioceptive and stability alliance. *Knee Surg Sports Traumatol Arthrosc* 6:50-61, 1998.

151. O'Brien SJ, Neves MC, Arnoczky SP, et al: The anatomy and histology of the inferior glenohumeral ligament complex of the shoulder. *Am J Sports Med* 18:449-456, 1990.

152. O'Brien SJ, Schwartz RS, Warren RF, Torzilli PA: Capsular restraints to anterior-posterior motion of the abducted shoulder: A biomechanical study. *J Shoulder Elbow Surg* 4:298-308, 1995.

153. Ozaki J: Glenohumeral movements of the involuntary inferior and multidirectional instability. *Clin Orthop Relat Res* 107-111, 1989.

154. Pagnani MJ, Deng XH, Warren RF, et al: Role of the long head of the biceps brachii in glenohumeral stability: A biomechanical study in cadavera. *J Shoulder Elbow Surg* 5:255-262, 1996.

155. Paletta GA Jr, Warner JJ, Warren RF, et al: Shoulder kinematics with two-plane x-ray evaluation in patients with anterior instability or rotator cuff tearing. *J Shoulder Elbow Surg* 6:516-527, 1997.

156. Panossian VR, Mihata T, Tibone JE, et al: Biomechanical analysis of isolated type II SLAP lesions and repair. *J Shoulder Elbow Surg* 14:529-534, 2005.

157. Petersson C: Degeneration of the acromioclavicular joint. *Acta Orthop Scand* 54:434, 1983.

158. Pollock RG, Wang VM, Bucchieri JS, et al: Effects of repetitive subfailure strains on the mechanical behavior of the inferior glenohumeral ligament. *J Shoulder Elbow Surg* 9:427-435, 2000.

159. Poppen NK, Walker PS: Forces at the glenohumeral joint in abduction. *Clin Orthop Relat Res* 165-170, 1978.

160. Poppen NK, Walker PS: Normal and abnormal motion of the shoulder. *J Bone Joint Surg Am* 58:195-201, 1976.

161. Reddy AS, Mohr KJ, Pink MM, Jobe FW: Electromyographic analysis of the deltoid and rotator cuff muscles in persons with subacromial impingement. *J Shoulder Elbow Surg* 9:519-523, 2000.

162. Reinold MM, Wilk KE, Hooks TR, et al: Thermal-assisted capsular shrinkage of the glenohumeral joint in overhead athletes: a 15- to 47-month follow-up. *J Orthop Sports Phys Ther* 33:455-467, 2003.

163. Reis FP, de Camargo AM, Vitti M, de Carvalho CA: Electromyographic study of the subclavius muscle. *Acta Anat (Basel)* 105:284-290, 1979.

164. Robinson CM: Fractures of the clavicle in the adult. Epidemiology and classification. *J Bone Joint Surg Br* 80:476-484, 1998.

165. Robinson CM, Jenkins PJ, White TO, et al: Primary arthroscopic stabilization for a first-time anterior dislocation of the shoulder. A randomized, double-blind trial. *J Bone Joint Surg Am* 90:708-721, 2008.

166. Rundquist PJ, Anderson DD, Guanche CA, Ludewig PM: Shoulder kinematics in subjects with frozen shoulder. *Arch Phys Med Rehabil* 84:1473-1479, 2003.

167. Sabick MB, Kim YK, Torry MR, et al: Biomechanics of the shoulder in youth baseball pitchers: Implications for the development of proximal humeral epiphysiolysis and humeral retrotorsion. *Am J Sports Med* 33:1716-1722, 2005.

168. Sabick MB, Torry MR, Kim YK, Hawkins RJ: Humeral torque in professional baseball pitchers. *Am J Sports Med* 32:892-898, 2004.

169. Sahara W, Sugamoto K, Murai M, Yoshikawa H: Three-dimensional clavicular and acromioclavicular rotations during arm abduction using vertically open MRI. *J Orthop Res* 25:1243-1249, 2007.

170. Saito H, Itoi E, Sugaya H, et al: Location of the glenoid defect in shoulders with recurrent anterior dislocation. *Am J Sports Med* 33:889-893, 2005.

171. Sharkey NA, Marder RA: The rotator cuff opposes superior translation of the humeral head. *Am J Sports Med* 23:270-275, 1995.

172. Sharkey NA, Marder RA, Hanson PB: The entire rotator cuff contributes to elevation of the arm. *J Orthop Res* 12:699-708, 1994.

173. Shklar A, Dvir Z: Isokinetic strength measurements in shoulder muscles. *J Biomech* 10:369-373, 1995.

174. Solem-Bertoft E, Thuomas KA, Westerberg CE: The influence of scapular retraction and protraction on the width of the subacromial space. An MRI study. *Clin Orthop Relat Res* 296:99-103, 1993.

175. Soslowsky LJ, Flatow EL, Bigliani LU, et al: Quantification of in situ contact areas at the glenohumeral joint: A biomechanical study. *J Orthop Res* 10:524-534, 1992.

176. Soslowsky LJ, Malicky DM, Blasier RB: Active and passive factors in inferior glenohumeral stabilization: A biomechanical model. *J Shoulder Elbow Surg* 6:371-379, 1997.

177. Spencer EE, Kuhn JE, Huston LJ, et al: Ligamentous restraints to anterior and posterior translation of the sternoclavicular joint. *J Shoulder Elbow Surg* 11:43-47, 2002.

178. Standring S: *Gray's anatomy: the anatomical basis of clinical practice*, ed 40, St Louis, 2009, Elsevier.

179. Steindler A: *Kinesiology of the human body: under normal and pathological conditions*. Springfield: Charles C Thomas, 1955.

180. Steinmann SP, Wood MB: Pectoralis major transfer for serratus anterior paralysis. *J Shoulder Elbow Surg* 12:555-560, 2003.

181. Stokdijk M, Eilers PH, Nagels J, Rozing PM: External rotation in the glenohumeral joint during elevation of the arm. *Clin Biomech (Bristol, Avon)* 18:296-302, 2003.

182. Sugalski MT, Wiater JM, Levine WN, Bigliani LU: An anatomic study of the humeral insertion of the inferior glenohumeral capsule. *J Shoulder Elbow Surg* 14:91-95, 2005.

183. Sugamoto K, Harada T, Machida A, et al: Scapulohumeral rhythm: Relationship between motion velocity and rhythm. *Clin Orthop Relat Res* 401:119-124, 2002.

184. Svendsen SW, Gelineck J, Mathiassen SE, et al. Work above shoulder level and degenerative alterations of the rotator cuff tendons: A magnetic resonance imaging study. *Arthritis Rheum* 50:3314-3322, 2004.

185. Teece RM, Lunden JB, Lloyd AS, et al: Three-dimensional acromioclavicular joint motions during elevation of the arm. *J Orthop Sports Phys Ther* 38:181-190, 2008.

186. Terrier A, Reist A, Vogel A, Farron A: Effect of supraspinatus deficiency on humerus translation and glenohumeral contact force during abduction. *Clin Biomech (Bristol, Avon)* 22:645-651, 2007.

187. Thigpen CA, Gross MT, Karas SG, et al: The repeatability of scapular rotations across three planes of humeral elevation. *Res Sports Med* 13:181-198,2005.

188. Ticker JB, Bigliani LU, Soslowsky LJ, et al: Inferior glenohumeral ligament: geometric and strain-rate dependent properties. *J Shoulder Elbow Surg* 5:269-279, 1996.

189. Tillander B, Norlin R: Intraoperative measurements of the subacromial distance. *Arthroscopy* 18:347-352, 2002.

190. Torg JS, Balduini FC, Bonci C, et al: A modified Bristow-Helfet-May procedure for recurrent dislocation and subluxation of the shoulder. Report of two hundred and twelve cases. *J Bone Joint Surg Am* 69:904-913, 1987.

191. Tsai NT, McClure PW, Karduna AR: Effects of muscle fatigue on 3-dimensional scapular kinematics. *Arch Phys Med Rehabil* 84:1000-1005, 2003.

192. Tyler TF, Nicholas SJ, Roy T, Gleim GW: Quantification of posterior capsule tightness and motion loss in patients with shoulder impingement. *Am J Sports Med* 28:668-673, 2000.

193. Urayama M, Itoi E, Sashi R, et al: Capsular elongation in shoulders with recurrent anterior dislocation. Quantitative assessment with magnetic resonance arthrography. *Am J Sports Med* 31:64-67, 2003.

194. van der Helm FC, Pronk GM: Three-dimensional recording and description of motions of the shoulder mechanism. *J Biomech Eng* 117:27-40, 1995.

195. van der Windt DA, Koes BW, de Jong BA, Bouter LM: Shoulder disorders in general practice: Incidence, patient characteristics, and management. *Ann Rheum Dis* 54:959-964, 1995.

196. Vangsness CT Jr, Ennis M, Taylor JG, Atkinson R: Neural anatomy of the glenohumeral ligaments, labrum, and subacromial bursa. *Arthroscopy* 11:180-184, 1995.

197. Vangsness CT Jr, Jorgenson SS, Watson T, Johnson DL: The origin of the long head of the biceps from the scapula and glenoid labrum. An anatomical study of 100 shoulders. *J Bone Joint Surg Br* 76:951-954, 1994.

198. Veeger HE, van der Helm FC: Shoulder function: The perfect compromise between mobility and stability. *J Biomech* 40:2119-2129, 2007.

199. von Eisenhart-Rothe R, Matsen FA, III, Eckstein F, et al: Pathomechanics in atraumatic shoulder instability: Scapular positioning correlates with humeral head centering. *Clin Orthop Relat Res* 433:82-89, 2005.

200. Walker PS, Poppen NK: Biomechanics of the shoulder joint during abduction in the plane of the scapula (proceedings). *Bull Hosp Joint Dis* 38:107-111, 1977.

201. Wang VM, Flatow EL: Pathomechanics of acquired shoulder instability: A basic science perspective. *J Shoulder Elbow Surg* 14:2S-11S, 2005.

202. Wang VM, Sugalski MT, Levine WN, et al: Comparison of glenohumeral mechanics following a capsular shift and anterior tightening. *J Bone Joint Surg Am* 87:1312-1322, 2005.

203. Ward SR, Hentzen ER, Smallwood LH, et al: Rotator cuff muscle architecture: implications for glenohumeral stability. *Clin Orthop Relat Res* 448:157-163, 2006.

204. Warner JJ, Deng XH, Warren RF, Torzilli PA: Static capsuloligamentous restraints to superior-inferior translation of the glenohumeral joint. *Am J Sports Med* 20:675-685, 1992.

205. Warner JJ, Micheli LJ, Arslanian LE, et al: Scapulothoracic motion in normal shoulders and shoulders with glenohumeral instability and impingement syndrome. A study using Moire topographic analysis. *Clin Orthop Relat Res* 285:191-199, 1992.

206. Werner AW, Lichtenberg S, Schmitz H, et al: Arthroscopic findings in atraumatic shoulder instability. *Arthroscopy* 20:268-272, 2004.

207. Werner CM, Weishaupt D, Blumenthal S, et al: Effect of experimental suprascapular nerve block on active glenohumeral translations in vivo. *J Orthop Res* 24:491-500, 2006.

208. Wilk KE, Reinold MM, Dugas JR, et al: Current concepts in the recognition and treatment of superior labral (SLAP) lesions. *J Orthop Sports Phys Ther* 35:273-291, 2005.

209. Williams GR Jr, Shakil M, Klimkiewicz J, Iannotti JP: Anatomy of the scapulothoracic articulation. *Clin Orthop Relat Res* 359:237-246, 1999.

210. Yamaguchi K, Ditsios K, Middleton WD, et al: The demographic and morphological features of rotator cuff disease. A comparison of asymptomatic and symptomatic shoulders. *J Bone Joint Surg Am* 88:1699-1704, 2006.

211. Yanagawa T, Goodwin CJ, Shelburne KB, et al: Contributions of the individual muscles of the shoulder to glenohumeral joint stability during abduction. *J Biomech Eng* 130:021024, 2008.

212. Yanai T, Fuss FK, Fukunaga T: In vivo measurements of subacromial impingement: substantial compression develops in abduction with large internal rotation. *Clin Biomech (Bristol, Avon)* 21:692-700, 2006.

STUDY QUESTIONS

1 How does the morphology (shape) of the sternoclavicular joint influence its arthrokinematics during elevation and depression and during protraction and retraction?

2 Which periarticular connective tissues and muscles associated with the sternoclavicular joint become taut after full depression of the clavicle?

3 Describe how the osteokinematics at the sternoclavicular and acromioclavicular joints can combine to augment protraction of the scapulothoracic joint. Include axes of rotation and planes of motion in your answer.

4 Contrast the arthrokinematics at the glenohumeral joint during internal rotation from (a) the anatomic position and (b) a position of 90 degrees of abduction.

5 Injury to which spinal nerve roots would most likely severely weaken the movement of protraction of the scapulothoracic joint? Hint: Refer to Appendix II, Part A.

6 With the arm well stabilized, describe the likely posture of the scapula following full activation of the teres major *without* activation of the rhomboids or pectoralis minor muscles.

7 Figure 5-58 shows several internal rotator muscles of the glenohumeral joint. What role, if any, do the muscles have in directing the posterior slide of the humerus?

8 List all the muscles of the shoulder complex that are likely contracting during active shoulder abduction from the anatomic position. Consulting Appendix II, Part A, which pair of spinal nerve roots is most likely associated with the innervation of most of these active muscles?

9 List the muscles of the shoulder that, if either tight or weak, could theoretically favor an *internally rotated* posture of the scapula.

10 List the muscles of the shoulder that, if either tight or weak, could theoretically favor an *anteriorly tilted* posture of the scapula.

11 In theory, how much active shoulder abduction is possible with a completely fused glenohumeral joint?

12 What motion increases tension in all parts of the inferior glenohumeral ligament?

13 Describe the exact path of the long head of the biceps, from its distal to its proximal attachment. Where is the tendon vulnerable to entrapment and associated inflammation?

14 What active motion or motions are essentially impossible after an avulsion injury of the upper trunk of the brachial plexus?

15 How does the posture of the scapula on the thorax affect the static stability at the glenohumeral joint?

Answers to the study questions can be found on the Evolve website.

Elbow and Forearm

DONALD A. NEUMANN, PT, PhD, FAPTA

CHAPTER AT A GLANCE

The elbow and forearm complex consists of three bones and four joints (Figure 6-1). The *humero-ulnar* and *humeroradial joints* form the elbow. The motions of flexion and extension of the elbow provide a means to adjust the overall functional length of the upper limb. This mechanism is used for many important activities, such as feeding, reaching, throwing, and personal hygiene.

The radius and ulna articulate with each other within the forearm at the *proximal* and *distal radio-ulnar joints*. This pair of articulations allows the palm of the hand to be turned up (supinated) or down (pronated), without requiring motion of the shoulder. Supination and pronation can be performed in conjunction with, or independent from, elbow flexion and

extension. The interaction between the elbow and forearm joints greatly increases the range of effective hand placement.

OSTEOLOGY

Mid-to-Distal Humerus

The anterior and posterior surfaces of the mid-to-distal humerus provide proximal attachments for the brachialis and the medial head of the triceps brachii (Figures 6-2 and 6-3). The distal end of the shaft of the humerus terminates medially as the trochlea and the medial epicondyle, and laterally as the capitulum and lateral epicondyle. The *trochlea* resembles a rounded, empty spool of thread. The medial and lateral borders of the trochlea flare slightly to form *medial and lateral lips*. The medial lip is prominent and extends farther distally than the adjacent lateral lip. Midway between the medial and lateral lips is the *trochlear groove*, which, when one looks from posterior to anterior, spirals slightly toward the medial direction (Figure 6-4). The *coronoid fossa* is located just proximal to the anterior aspect of the trochlea (see Figure 6-2).

**Four Articulations within the Elbow
and Forearm Complex**
1. Humero-ulnar joint
2. Humeroradial joint
3. Proximal radio-ulnar joint
4. Distal radio-ulnar joint

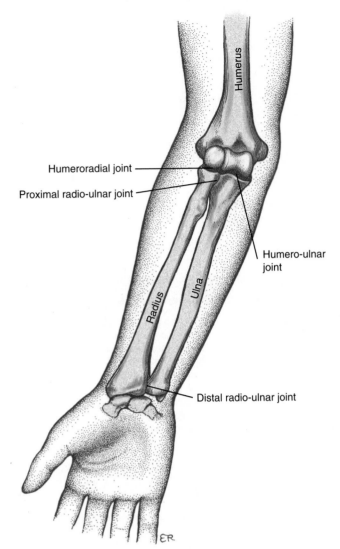

FIGURE 6-1. The articulations of the elbow and forearm complex.

Humeroradial joint

Proximal radio-ulnar joint

Humerus

Humero-ulnar joint

Radius

Ulna

Distal radio-ulnar joint

Osteologic Features of the Mid-to-Distal Humerus
- Trochlea including groove and medial and lateral lips
- Coronoid fossa
- Capitulum
- Radial fossa
- Medial and lateral epicondyles
- Medial and lateral supracondylar ridges
- Olecranon fossa

Directly lateral to the trochlea is the rounded *capitulum*. The capitulum forms nearly one half of a sphere. A small *radial fossa* is located proximal to the anterior surface of the capitulum.

The *medial epicondyle* of the humerus projects medially from the trochlea (see Figures 6-2 and 6-4). This prominent and easily palpable structure serves as the proximal attachment of the medial collateral ligament of the elbow as well as most forearm pronator and wrist flexor muscles.

The *lateral epicondyle* of the humerus, less prominent than the medial epicondyle, serves as the proximal attachment for

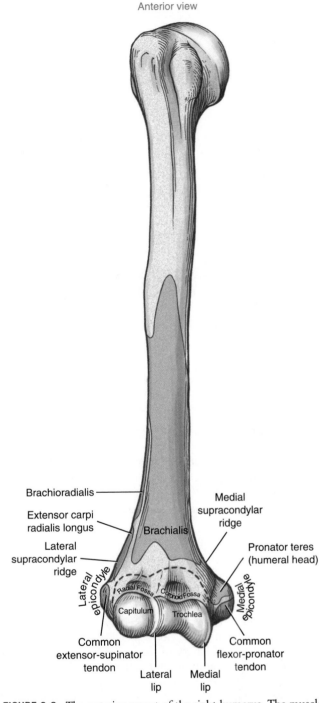

Anterior view

Brachioradialis

Extensor carpi radialis longus

Lateral supracondylar ridge

Lateral epicondyle

Radial Fossa

Capitulum

Common extensor-supinator tendon

Lateral lip

Brachialis

Coronoid Fossa

Trochlea

Medial lip

Medial supracondylar ridge

Pronator teres (humeral head)

Medial epicondyle

Common flexor-pronator tendon

FIGURE 6-2. The anterior aspect of the right humerus. The muscles' proximal attachments are shown in red. The dashed lines show the capsular attachments of the elbow joint.

the lateral collateral ligament complex of the elbow as well as most forearm supinator and wrist extensor muscles. Immediately proximal to both epicondyles are the *medial* and *lateral supracondylar ridges,* which are relatively superficial and easily palpated.

On the posterior aspect of the humerus, just proximal to the trochlea, is the very deep and broad *olecranon fossa.* Only

Posterior view

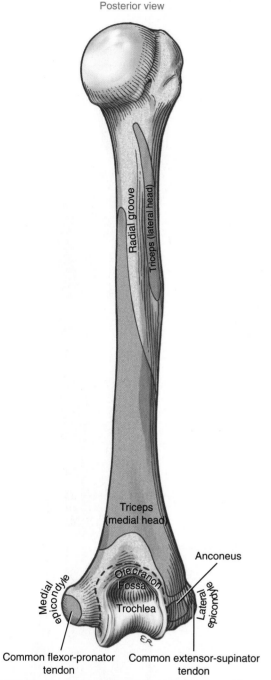

FIGURE 6-3. The posterior aspect of the right humerus. The muscles' proximal attachments are shown in red. The dashed lines show the capsular attachments around the elbow joint.

Right humerus: Inferior view

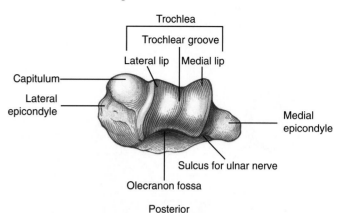

Posterior

FIGURE 6-4. The distal end of the right humerus, inferior view.

The *coronoid process* projects sharply from the anterior body of the proximal ulna.

Osteologic Features of the Ulna
- Olecranon process
- Coronoid process
- Trochlear notch and longitudinal crest
- Radial notch
- Supinator crest
- Tuberosity of the ulna
- Ulnar head
- Styloid process

The *trochlear notch* of the ulna is the large jawlike process located between the anterior tips of the olecranon and coronoid processes. This concave notch articulates firmly with the reciprocally shaped trochlea of the humerus, forming the humero-ulnar joint. A thin raised *longitudinal crest* divides the trochlear notch down its midline.

The *radial notch* of the ulna is an articular depression just lateral to the inferior aspect of the trochlear notch (see Figures 6-5 and 6-7). Extending distally and slightly dorsally from the radial notch is the *supinator crest,* marking the attachments for part of the lateral collateral ligament complex and the supinator muscle. The *tuberosity of the ulna* is a roughened impression just distal to the coronoid process, formed by the attachment of the brachialis muscle (see Figure 6-5).

The *ulnar head* is located at the distal end of the ulna (Figure 6-8). Most of the rounded ulnar head is covered with articular cartilage. The pointed *styloid process* (from the Greek root *stylos,* pillar) projects distally from the posterior-medial region of the extreme distal ulna.

Radius

In the fully supinated position, the radius lies parallel and lateral to the ulna (see Figures 6-5 and 6-6). The proximal end of the radius is small and therefore constitutes a relatively small structural component of the elbow. Its distal end, however, is enlarged, forming a major part of the wrist joint.

a thin sheet of bone or membrane separates the olecranon fossa from the coronoid fossa.

Ulna

The ulna has a very thick proximal end with distinct processes (Figures 6-5 and 6-6). The *olecranon process* forms the large, blunt, proximal tip of the ulna, making up the "point" of the elbow (Figure 6-7). The roughened posterior surface of the olecranon process accepts the insertion of the triceps brachii.

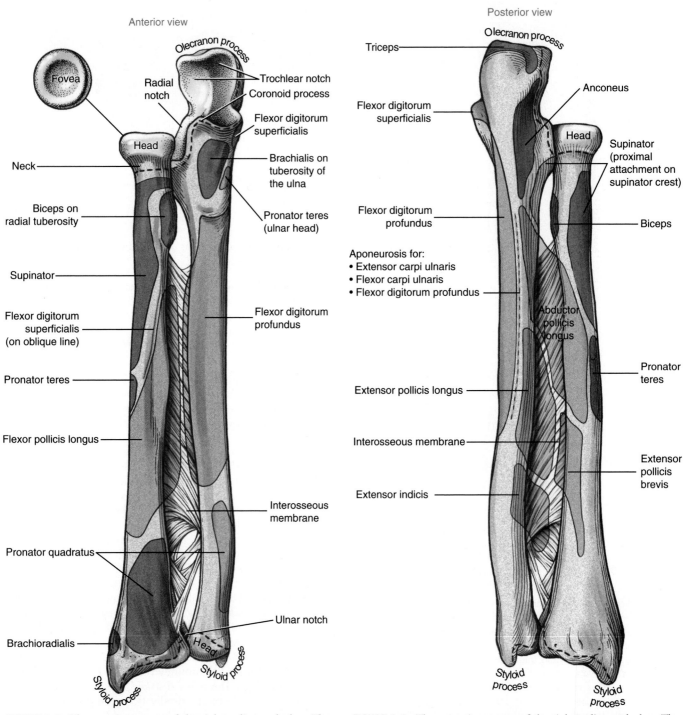

FIGURE 6-5. The anterior aspect of the right radius and ulna. The muscles' proximal attachments are shown in red and distal attachments in gray. The dashed lines show the capsular attachments around the elbow and wrist and the proximal and distal radio-ulnar joints. The radial head is depicted from above to show the concavity of the fovea.

FIGURE 6-6. The posterior aspect of the right radius and ulna. The muscles' proximal attachments are shown in red and distal attachments in gray. The dashed lines show the capsular attachments around the elbow and wrist and the proximal and distal radio-ulnar joints.

Lateral view

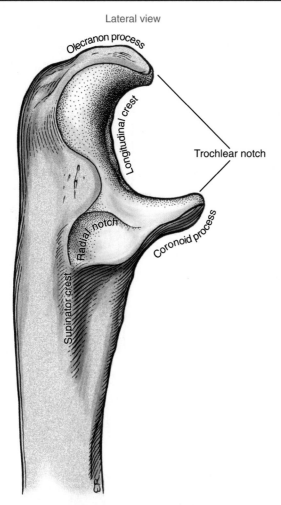

FIGURE 6-7. A lateral (radial) view of the right proximal ulna, with the radius removed. Note the jawlike shape of the trochlear notch.

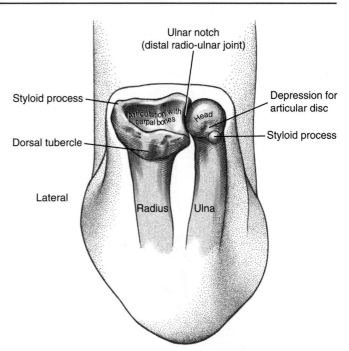

FIGURE 6-8. The distal end of the right radius and ulna with carpal bones removed. The forearm is in full supination. Note the prominent ulnar head and nearby styloid process of the ulna.

The distal end of the radius articulates with carpal bones to form the radiocarpal joint at the wrist (see Figure 6-8). The *ulnar notch* of the distal radius accepts the ulnar head at the distal radio-ulnar joint. The prominent *styloid process* projects from the lateral surface of the distal radius, extending approximately 1 cm farther distal than the ulnar styloid process.

ARTHROLOGY

Joints of the Elbow

GENERAL FEATURES OF THE HUMERO-ULNAR AND HUMERORADIAL JOINTS

The elbow consists of the humero-ulnar and humeroradial articulations. The tight fit between the trochlea and trochlear notch at the humero-ulnar joint provides most of the elbow's structural stability.

Early anatomists classified the elbow as a *ginglymus* or *hinged joint* owing to its predominant uniplanar motion of flexion and extension. The term *modified hinge joint* is actually more appropriate because the ulna experiences a slight amount of axial rotation (i.e., rotation around its own longitudinal axis) and side-to-side motion as it flexes and extends.[48] Bioengineers must account for these relatively small "extra-sagittal" accessory motions in the design of elbow joint prostheses. Without attention to this detail, the prosthetic implants are more likely to loosen prematurely.[13,29]

Normal "Valgus Angle" of the Elbow
Elbow flexion and extension occur around a relatively stationary medial-lateral axis of rotation, passing through the vicinity

---

Osteologic Features of the Radius

- Head
- Neck
- Fovea
- Radial (bicipital) tuberosity
- Ulnar notch
- Styloid process

The *radial head* is a disclike structure located at the extreme proximal end of the radius. Articular cartilage covers about 280 degrees of the rim of the radial head.[44] The rim of the radial head contacts the radial notch of the ulna, forming the proximal radio-ulnar joint. Immediately inferior to the radial head is the constricted *radial neck* (see Figure 6-5).

The superior surface of the radial head consists of a shallow, cup-shaped depression known as the *fovea*. This cartilage-lined concavity articulates with the capitulum of the humerus, forming the humeroradial joint. The biceps brachii muscle attaches to the radius at the *radial (bicipital) tuberosity,* a roughened region located at the anterior-medial edge of the proximal radius.

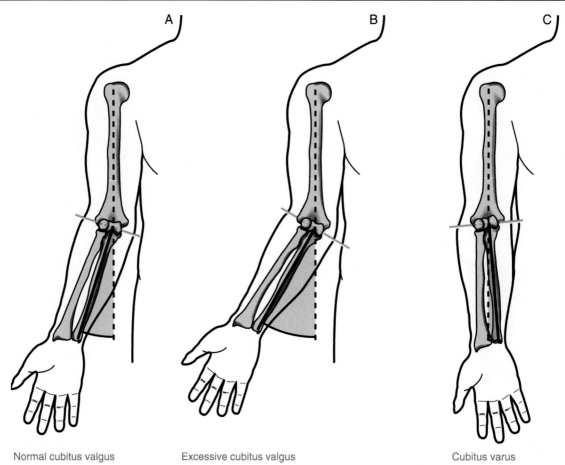

Normal cubitus valgus   Excessive cubitus valgus   Cubitus varus

FIGURE 6-9. A, The elbow's axis of rotation *(green line)* extends slightly obliquely in a medial-lateral direction through the capitulum and the trochlea. *Normal cubitus valgus* of the elbow is shown with an angle of about 15 degrees from the longitudinal axis of the humerus. **B,** *Excessive cubitus valgus* deformity is shown with the forearm deviated laterally 30 degrees. **C,** *Cubitus varus* deformity is depicted with the forearm deviated medially 5 degrees.

of the lateral epicondyle (Figure 6-9, *A*).[71] From medial to lateral, the axis courses slightly superiorly owing in part to the distal prolongation of the medial lip of the trochlea. This asymmetry in the trochlea causes the ulna to deviate laterally relative to the humerus. The natural frontal plane angle made by the extended elbow is referred to as *normal cubitus valgus.* (The term "carrying angle" is often used, reflecting the fact that the valgus angle tends to keep carried objects away from the side of the thigh during walking.) Paraskevas and co-workers reported an average cubitus valgus angle in healthy persons of about 13 degrees, with a standard deviation close to 6 degrees.[58] On average, women had a greater valgus angulation than men by about 2 degrees. Two studies using a large sample of normal subjects have shown that, regardless of gender, valgus angle is greater on the dominant arm.[58,85]

Occasionally the extended elbow may show an *excessive cubitus valgus* that exceeds about 20 or 25 degrees (see Figure 6-9, *B*). In contrast, the forearm may less commonly show a *cubitus varus* (or "gunstock") deformity, where the forearm is deviated toward the midline (see Figure 6-9, *C*). The terms *valgus* and *varus* are derived from the Latin *turned outward* (abducted) and *turned inward* (adducted), respectively.

A marked varus or valgus deformity may result from trauma, such as a severe fracture through the "growth plate" of the distal humerus in children. Excessive cubitus valgus may overstretch and damage the ulnar nerve as it crosses medial to the elbow.[11]

PERIARTICULAR CONNECTIVE TISSUE

The *articular capsule* of the elbow encloses the humero-ulnar joint, the humeroradial joint, and the proximal radio-ulnar joint (Figure 6-10). The articular capsule surrounding these joints is thin and reinforced anteriorly by oblique bands of fibrous tissue. A *synovial membrane* lines the internal surface of the capsule (Figure 6-11).

The articular capsule of the elbow is strengthened by collateral ligaments. These ligaments provide an important source of stability to the elbow joint. Motions that increase the tension in the ligaments are listed in Table 6-1. The *medial collateral ligament* consists of anterior, posterior, and transverse fiber bundles (Figure 6-12). The *anterior fibers* are the strongest and stiffest fibers of the medial collateral ligament.[63] As such,

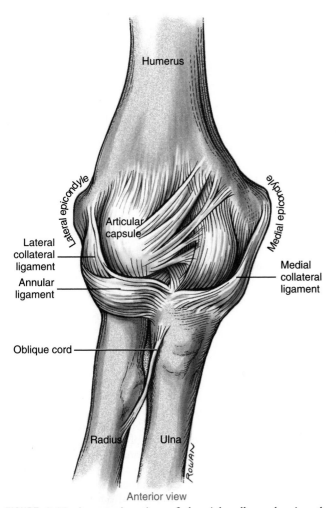

FIGURE 6-10. An anterior view of the right elbow showing the capsule and collateral ligaments.

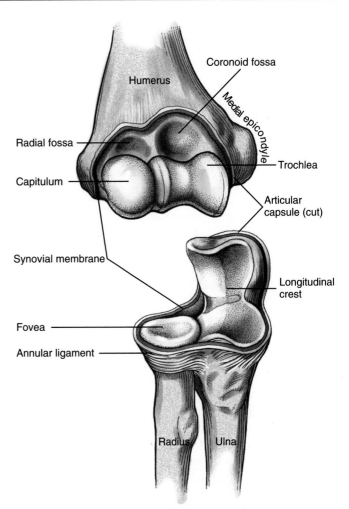

FIGURE 6-11. Anterior view of the right elbow disarticulated to expose the humero-ulnar and humeroradial joints. The margin of the proximal radio-ulnar joint is shown within the elbow's capsule. Note the small area on the trochlear notch lacking articular cartilage. The synovial membrane lining the internal side of the capsule is shown in blue.

TABLE 6-1. Motions That Increase Tension in the Collateral Ligaments of the Elbow	
Ligament	**Motions That Increase Tension**
Medial collateral ligament (anterior fibers*)	Valgus Extension and flexion
Medial collateral ligament (posterior fibers)	Valgus Flexion
Radial collateral ligament	Varus External rotation
Lateral (ulnar) collateral ligament*	Varus External rotation and flexion
Annular ligament	Distraction of the radius, external rotation

*Primary valgus or varus stabilizers.

these fibers provide the most significant resistance against a valgus (abduction) force to the elbow. The anterior fibers arise from the anterior part of the medial epicondyle and insert on the medial part of the coronoid process of the ulna.[18] Because the anterior fibers span both sides of the axis of rotation, at least some fibers are taut throughout sagittal plane movement. The anterior fibers therefore provide articular stability throughout the entire range of motion.[10]

The *posterior fibers* of the medial collateral ligament are less defined than the anterior fibers and are essentially thickenings of the posterior-medial capsule. As depicted in Figure 6-12, the posterior fibers attach on the posterior part of the medial epicondyle and insert on the medial margin of the olecranon process. The posterior fibers resist a valgus force, as well as become taut in the extremes of elbow flexion.[63] A third and poorly developed set of *transverse fibers* cross from the olecranon to the coronoid process of the ulna. Because these fibers originate and insert on the same bone, they do not provide significant articular stability.

In addition to the medial collateral ligaments, the proximal fibers of the wrist flexor and pronator group of muscles also resist excessive valgus-producing strain at the elbow, most notably by the flexor carpi ulnaris. For this reason, these

Medial aspect

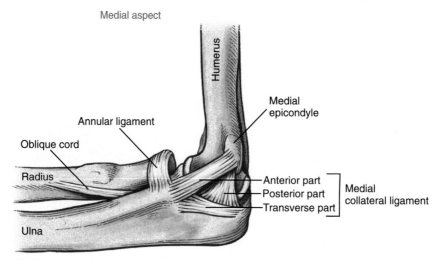

FIGURE 6-12. The components of the medial collateral ligament of the right elbow.

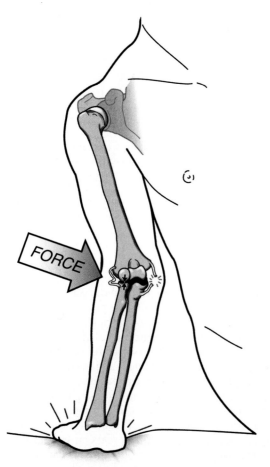

Anterior view

FIGURE 6-13. Attempts at catching oneself from a fall may create a severe valgus-producing force to the elbow, causing rupture of the medial collateral ligament and a potentially damaging compression force within the humeroradial joint.

muscles are referred to as *dynamic medial stabilizers* of the elbow.[38]

The medial collateral ligament is susceptible to injury when the fully extended elbow is violently forced into excessive valgus, often from a fall onto an outstretched arm and hand (Figure 6-13).[12] The ligamentous injury may be associated with a fracture within the humeroradial joint or anywhere along the length of the radius—the forearm bone that accepts 80% of the compression force applied through the wrist. A severe valgus-producing force may also injure the ulnar nerve or proximal attachments of the pronator–wrist flexor muscles. The anterior capsule may also be injured if the joint is excessively hyperextended. The medial collateral ligament is also susceptible to injury from repetitive, valgus-producing forces to the elbow in non–weight-bearing activities, such as pitching a baseball and spiking a volleyball.[65,83]

The *lateral collateral ligament complex* of the elbow is more variable in form than the medial collateral ligament (Figure 6-14). The ligamentous complex originates on the lateral epicondyle and immediately splits into two fiber bundles. One fiber bundle, traditionally known as the *radial collateral ligament,* fans out to blend with the annular ligament. A second fiber bundle, called the *lateral (ulnar) collateral ligament,* attaches distally to the supinator crest of the ulna. These fibers become taut during full flexion.[63] By attaching to the ulna, the lateral (ulnar) collateral ligament and the anterior fibers of the medial collateral ligament function as collateral "guy wires" to the elbow, providing medial-lateral stability to the ulna during sagittal plane motion.

The lateral collateral ligament complex and the posterior-lateral aspect of the capsule are primary stabilizers against a varus-producing force.[56] Often after a single traumatic sporting event, rupture of this ligament system can cause not only increased varus ("adduction") of the elbow, but also posterior-lateral rotary instability. This instability is expressed as exces-

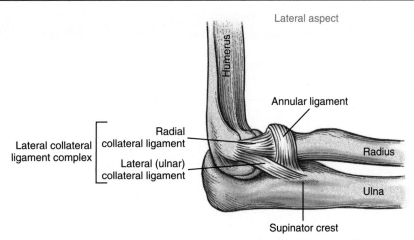

FIGURE 6-14. The components of the lateral collateral ligament complex of the right elbow.

sive external rotation of the forearm with subsequent subluxation of both the humero-ulnar and humeroradial joints.[19,54]

The ligaments around the elbow are endowed with mechanoreceptors consisting of Golgi organs, Ruffini terminals, Pacinian corpuscles, and free nerve endings.[59] These receptors may supply important information to the nervous system for augmenting proprioception and detecting safe limits of passive tension in the structures around the elbow.

As all joints do, the elbow joint has an intracapsular air pressure. This pressure, which is determined by the ratio of the volume of air to the volume of space, is lowest at about 80 degrees of flexion.[24] This joint position is often considered the "position of comfort" for persons with joint inflammation and swelling. Maintaining a swollen elbow in a flexed position may improve comfort but may predispose the person to an elbow flexion *contracture* (from the Latin root *contractura*, to draw together).

KINEMATICS

Functional Considerations of Flexion and Extension

Elbow flexion performs several important physiologic functions, such as pulling, lifting, feeding, and grooming.[77] The inability to actively bring the hand to the mouth for feeding, for example, significantly limits the level of functional independence. Persons with a spinal cord injury above the C^5 nerve root may experience this profound functional impairment because of paralysis of elbow flexor muscles.

Elbow extension occurs with activities such as throwing, pushing, and reaching. Loss of complete extension because of an elbow flexion contracture is often caused by marked stiffness in the elbow flexor muscles. The muscles become abnormally stiff after long periods of immobilization in a flexed and shortened position. Long-term flexion may be the result of casting for a fractured bone or of posttraumatic heterotopic ossification, osteophyte formation, elbow joint inflammation and effusion, muscle spasticity, paralysis of the

---

SPECIAL FOCUS 6-1

Elbow Flexion Contracture and Loss of Forward Reach

A *flexion contracture* is a tightening of muscular or nonmuscular tissues that restricts normal passive extension. One of the most disabling consequences of an elbow flexion contracture is reduced reaching capacity. The loss of forward reach varies with the degree of elbow flexion contracture. As shown in Figure 6-15, a fully extendable elbow (i.e., with a 0-degree contracture) demonstrates a 0-degree loss in area of forward reach. The area of forward reach diminishes only slightly (less than 6%) with a flexion contracture of less than 30 degrees. A flexion contracture that exceeds 30 degrees, however, results in a much greater loss of forward reach. As noted in the graph, a flexion contracture of 90 degrees reduces total reach by almost 50%. Minimizing a flexion

contracture to less than 30 degrees is therefore an important functional goal for patients. Therapeutics typically used to reduce an elbow flexion contracture include reducing inflammation and swelling, positioning the joint in more extension (through splinting, continuous passive-motion machines, or frequent encouragement), stretching structures located anterior to the joint's medial-lateral axis of rotation, manually mobilizing the joint, and strengthening muscles that produce elbow extension. If these relative conservative treatments are ineffective, then a surgical release may be indicated.[79] The most effective intervention for elbow flexion contracture, however, is prevention.

Continued

Elbow Flexion Contracture and Loss of Forward Reach—*cont'd*

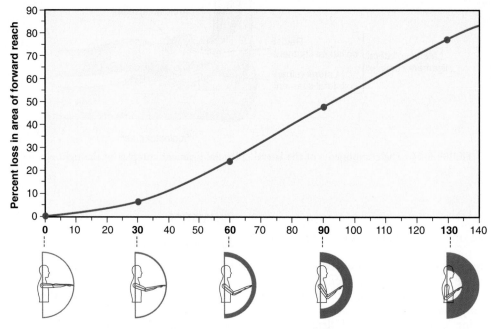

FIGURE 6-15. A graph showing the percent loss in area of forward reach of the arm, from the shoulder to finger, as a function of the severity of an elbow flexion contracture. Note the sharp increase in the reduction in reach as the flexion contracture exceeds 30 degrees. The figures across the bottom of the graph depict the progressive loss of reach, indicated by the increased semicircular area, as the flexion contracture becomes more severe.

triceps muscle, or scarring of the skin over the anterior elbow. In addition to the tightness in the flexor muscles, increased stiffness may occur in the anterior capsule and some anterior fibers of the medial collateral ligament.

The maximal range of passive motion generally available to the elbow is from 5 degrees beyond neutral (0 degree) extension through 145 degrees of flexion (Figure 6-16). Research indicates, however, that several common activities of daily living use a more limited "functional arc" of motion, usually between 30 and 130 degrees of flexion.[47] Unlike in lower extremity joints, such as the knee, the loss of the extremes of motion at the elbow usually results in only minimal functional impairment.

Arthrokinematics at the Humero-Ulnar Joint

The humero-ulnar joint is the articulation between the concave trochlear notch of the ulna and the convex trochlea of the humerus (Figure 6-17). Hyaline cartilage covers about 300 degrees of articular surface on the trochlea, compared with only 180 degrees on the trochlear notch. The natural congruency and shape of this joint limits motion primarily within the sagittal plane.

In order for the humero-ulnar joint to be fully extended, sufficient extensibility is required in the dermis anterior to

the elbow, flexor muscles, anterior capsule, and anterior fibers of the medial collateral ligament (Figure 6-18, *A*). Full extension also requires that the prominent tip of the olecranon process become wedged into the olecranon fossa. Excessive ectopic (from the Greek root *ecto,* outside, + *topos,* place) bone formation around the olecranon fossa can therefore limit full extension. Normally, once in extension, the healthy humero-ulnar joint is stabilized primarily by articular congruency and also by the increased tension in the stretched connective tissues.

During flexion at the humero-ulnar joint, the concave surface of the trochlear notch rolls and slides on the convex trochlea (see Figure 6-18, *B*). Full elbow flexion requires elongation of the posterior capsule, extensor muscles, ulnar nerve,[68,73] and certain portions of the collateral ligaments, especially the posterior fibers of the medial collateral ligament. Stretching of the ulnar nerve from prolonged or repetitive elbow flexion activities can lead to neuropathy. A common surgical treatment for this condition is to transfer the ulnar nerve anterior to the medial epicondyle, thereby reducing the tension in the nerve during flexion.[43]

In severe elbow injuries the trochlear notch of the ulna may dislocate posterior to the trochlea of the humerus. This dislocation is frequently caused from a fall onto an out-

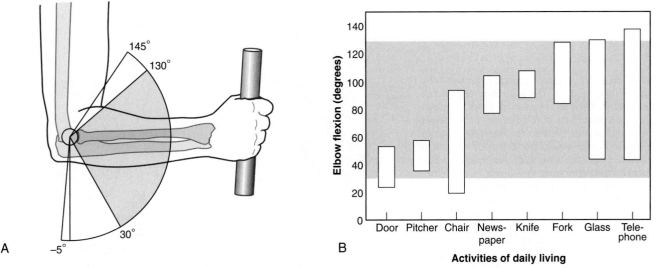

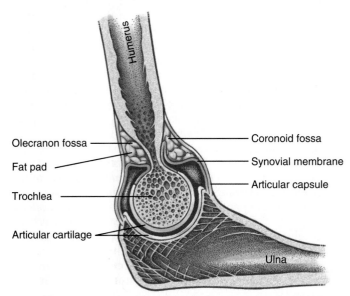

FIGURE 6-16. Range of motion at the elbow. **A,** A healthy person showing an average range of elbow motion from 5 degrees beyond neutral extension through 145 degrees of flexion. The 100-degree "functional arc" from 30 to 130 degrees of flexion (in red) is based on the data in the histogram. **B,** The histogram shows the range of motion at the elbow typically needed to perform the following activities of daily living: opening a *door,* pouring from a *pitcher,* rising from a *chair,* holding a *newspaper,* cutting with a *knife,* bringing a *fork* to the mouth, bringing a *glass* to the mouth, and holding a *telephone.* (Modified from Morrey BF, Askew LJ, Chao EY: A biomechanical study of normal functional elbow motion, *J Bone Joint Surg Am* 63:872, 1981.)

FIGURE 6-17. A sagittal section through the humero-ulnar joint showing the well-fitting joint surfaces between the trochlear notch and trochlea. The synovial membrane lining the internal side of the capsule is shown in blue.

stretched arm and hand and therefore may also be associated with a fracture of the radius.

Arthrokinematics at the Humeroradial Joint

The humeroradial joint is an articulation between the cuplike fovea of the radial head and the reciprocally shaped rounded capitulum. The arthrokinematics of flexion and extension consist of the fovea of the radius rolling and sliding across the convexity of the capitulum (Figure 6-19). During active flexion, the radial fovea is pulled firmly against the capitulum by contracting muscles.[46]

Compared with the humero-ulnar joint, the humeroradial joint provides minimal sagittal plane stability to the elbow. The humeroradial joint does, however, provide about 50% of the resistance against a valgus-producing force to the elbow.[49]

Structure and Function of the Interosseous Membrane

The radius and ulna are bound together by the *interosseous membrane* of the forearm (Figure 6-20). Although several accessory fibers have been described, the more prominent *central bands* are directed distal-medially from the radius, intersecting the shaft of the ulna at about 20 degrees.[69] The central bands are nearly twice the thickness of other fibers and have an ultimate tensile strength similar to that of the patellar tendon of the knee.[61] A few separate sparse and poorly defined bands flow perpendicular to the central bands of the interosseous membrane. One of these bands, the *oblique cord,* runs from the lateral side of the tuberosity of the ulna to just distal to the radial tuberosity. Another unnamed band is located at the extreme distal end of the interosseous membrane.

The primary functions of the interosseous membrane are to bind the radius to the ulna, serve as a stable attachment site for several extrinsic muscles of the hand, and provide a mechanism for transmitting force proximally through the upper limb. As illustrated in Figure 6-21, about 80% of the compression force that crosses the wrist is directed through the radiocarpal joint. (This fact accounts, in part, for the relatively high likelihood of fracturing the radius from a fall on an outstretched hand.) The remaining 20% of the force crosses the medial side of the wrist, through the soft tissues

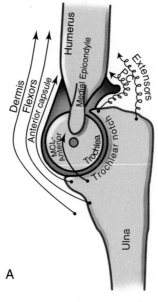

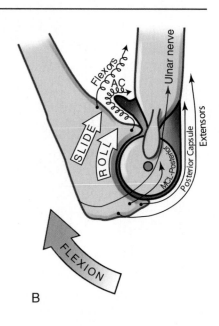

FIGURE 6-18. A sagittal section through the humero-ulnar joint. **A,** The joint is resting in full extension. **B,** The joint is passively flexed through full flexion. Note that in full flexion the coronoid process of the ulna fits into the coronoid fossa of the humerus. The medial-lateral axis of rotation is shown through the center of the trochlea. The stretched (taut) structures are shown as thin elongated arrows, and slackened structures are shown as wavy arrows. *AC,* anterior capsule; *MCL-Anterior,* some anterior fibers of the medial collateral ligament; *MCL-Posterior,* posterior fibers of the medial collateral ligament; *PC,* posterior capsule.

Resting in extension

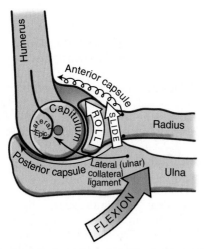

FIGURE 6-19. A sagittal section through the humeroradial joint during passive flexion. Note the medial-lateral axis of rotation in the center of the capitulum. The stretched (taut) structures are shown as thin elongated arrows, and slackened structures are shown as wavy arrows. Note the elongation of the lateral (ulnar) collateral ligament during flexion.

located within the "ulnocarpal space."[57] Because of the fiber direction of the central bands of the interosseous membrane, part of the proximal directed force through the radius is transferred across the membrane *to the ulna.*[60] This mechanism allows a significant portion of the compression force that naturally acts on the radius to cross the elbow via the humero-ulnar joint.[46] In this way, both the humero-ulnar and humeroradial joints more equally "share" the compression forces that cross the elbow, thereby reducing each individual joint's long-term wear and tear.

Most elbow flexors, and essentially all primary supinator and pronator muscles, have their distal attachment on the radius. As a consequence, contraction of these muscles pulls the radius proximally against the capitulum of the humerus, especially when the elbow is near full extension. Biomechanical analysis indicates that the resulting compression force at the humeroradial joint reaches three to four times body weight during maximal-effort activities.[2] Based on the mechanism described in Figure 6-21, the interosseous membrane helps shunt some of the muscular-produced compression forces *from the radius to the ulna.* In this way the interosseous membrane helps protect the humeroradial joint from large myogenic compression forces. Tears within the interosseous membrane can cause a measurable proximal migration of the radius due to activation of the regional muscles, leading to increased loading and possible degeneration at the humeroradial joint.[32,55] In cases where the head of the radius has been surgically removed because of trauma, the proximal migration is typically pronounced.[26] Over time, this proximal "drift" of the radius can cause bony asymmetry in the wrist or distal radio-ulnar joint, causing significant pain and loss of function.[16]

The predominant fiber direction of the interosseous membrane is *not* aligned to resist *distally applied* forces on the radius. For example, holding a heavy suitcase with the elbow extended causes a distracting force almost entirely through the radius (Figure 6-22). The distal pull on the radius slackens, rather than tenses, most of the interosseous membrane, thereby placing larger demands on other tissues, such as the oblique cord and annular ligament, to accept the weight of the load. Contraction of the brachioradialis or other muscles normally involved with grasp can assist with holding the radius and load firmly against the capitulum of the humerus. A deep aching in the forearm in persons who carry heavy loads for extended periods may be from fatigue in these muscles. Supporting loads through the forearm at shoulder

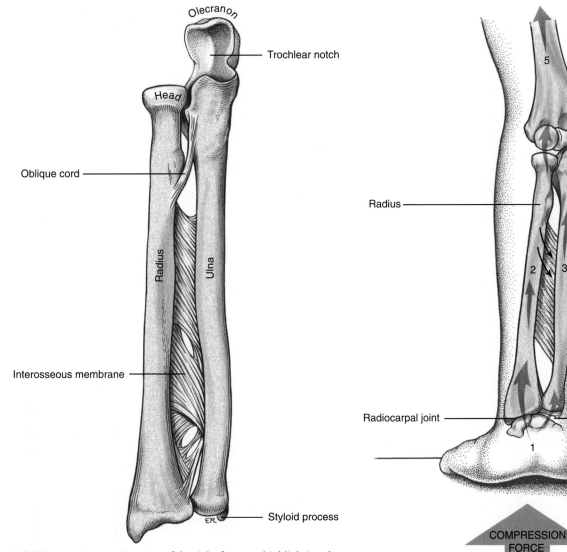

FIGURE 6-20. An anterior view of the right forearm, highlighting the components of the interosseous membrane.

FIGURE 6-21. A *compression force* through the hand is transmitted primarily through the wrist *(1)* at the radiocarpal joint and to the radius *(2)*. This force pulls the interosseous membrane taut (shown by *two black arrows*), thereby transferring a significant part of the compression force to the ulna *(3)* and across the elbow at the humero-ulnar joint *(4)*. The compression forces that cross the elbow are finally directed toward the shoulder *(5)*. The stretched (taut) structures are shown as *thin elongated arrows*.

level, for example, like a waiter carrying a tray of food, directs the weight proximally through the radius, so that the interosseous membrane can assist with dispersing the load more evenly through the forearm.

Joints of the Forearm

GENERAL FEATURES OF THE PROXIMAL AND DISTAL RADIO-ULNAR JOINTS

The radius and ulna are bound together by the interosseous membrane and the proximal and distal radio-ulnar joints. This set of joints, situated at either end of the forearm, allows the forearm to rotate into pronation and supination. Forearm supination places the palm up, or supine, and pronation places the palm down, or prone. This forearm rotation occurs around an *axis of rotation* that extends from the radial head through the ulnar head—an axis that intersects and connects both radio-ulnar joints (Figure 6-23).[31] Pronation and supina-

tion provide a mechanism that allows independent "rotation" of the hand without an obligatory rotation of the ulna or humerus.

The kinematics of forearm rotation are more complicated than those implied by the simple "palm-up and palm-down" terminology. The palm does indeed rotate, but only because the hand and wrist connect firmly *to the radius* and not to the ulna. The space between the distal ulna and the medial side of the carpus allows the carpal bones to rotate freely, along with the radius, without interference from the distal ulna.

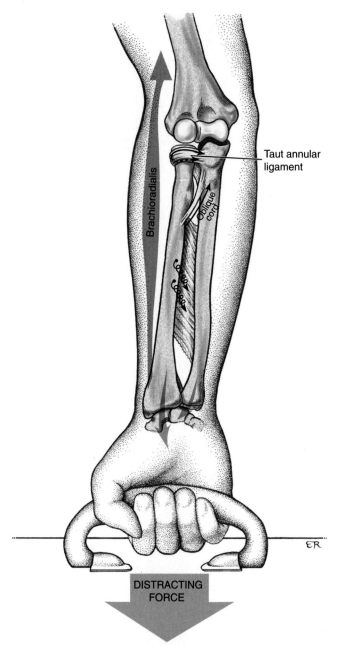

Taut annular ligament

FIGURE 6-22. Holding a load, such as a suitcase, places a distal-directed *distracting force* predominantly through the radius. This distraction slackens most of the interosseous membrane (shown by *wavy arrows* over the membrane). Other structures, such as the oblique cord, the annular ligament, and the brachioradialis, must assist with the support of the load. The stretched (taut) structures are shown as *thin elongated arrows*, and the slackened structures are shown as *wavy arrows*.

In the anatomic position the forearm is fully supinated when the ulna and radius lie parallel to each other (see Figure 6-23, *A*). During pronation the distal segment of the forearm complex (i.e., the radius and hand) rotates and crosses over an essentially fixed ulna (see Figure 6-23, *B*). The ulna, through its firm attachment to the humerus at the humero-ulnar joint, remains nearly stationary during an isolated pro-

nation and supination movement. A stable humero-ulnar joint provides an essential rigid link that the radius, wrist, and hand can pivot on. Movement of the humero-ulnar joint during pronation and supination has been described, but only as a very slight counter-rotation of the ulna relative to the radius.[35] It certainly is possible for the ulna to rotate freely during pronation and supination, but only if the humerus is also freely rotating at the glenohumeral joint.

JOINT STRUCTURE AND PERIARTICULAR CONNECTIVE TISSUE

Proximal Radio-Ulnar Joint

The proximal radio-ulnar joint, the humero-ulnar joint, and the humeroradial joint all share one articular capsule. Within this capsule the radial head is held against the proximal ulna by a fibro-osseous ring. This ring is formed by the radial notch of the ulna and the annular ligament (Figure 6-24, *A*). About 75% of the ring is formed by the annular ligament and 25% by the radial notch of the ulna.

The *annular* (from the Latin *annulus*, ring) *ligament* is a thick circular band of connective tissue attaching to the ulna on either side of the radial notch (see Figure 6-24, *B*). The ligament fits snugly around the radial head, holding the proximal radius against the ulna. The internal circumference of the annular ligament is lined with cartilage to reduce the friction against the radial head during pronation and supination. The external surface of the ligament receives attachments from the elbow capsule, the radial collateral ligament, and the supinator muscle.[8] The *quadrate ligament* is a thin, fibrous ligament that arises just below the radial notch of the ulna and attaches to the medial surface of the neck of the radius (see Figure 6-24, *B*). This function of the poorly defined ligament is not clear, although it may support the capsule of the proximal radio-ulnar joint throughout forearm rotation.[70]

Distal Radio-Ulnar Joint

The distal radio-ulnar joint consists of the convex head of the ulna resting on the shallow concavity formed by the ulnar notch on the radius and the proximal surface of an articular disc (Figure 6-26). This important joint firmly connects the distal ends of the radius and ulna. The shallow and often irregularly shaped ulnar notch of the radius affords only marginal osseous containment to the joint. The stability of the distal radio-ulnar joint is furnished through activation of muscles,[28] plus an elaborate set of local connective tissues.

The articular disc at the distal radio-ulnar joint is also known as the *triangular fibrocartilage*, indicating its shape and predominant tissue type. As depicted in Figure 6-26, *A*, the lateral side of the disc attaches along the entire rim of the ulnar notch of the radius. The main body of the disc fans out horizontally into a triangular shape, with its apex attaching medially into the depression on the ulnar head and adjacent styloid process. The anterior and posterior edges of the disc are continuous with the *palmar (anterior)* and *dorsal (posterior) radio-ulnar joint capsular ligaments* (see Figure 6-26). The proximal surface of the disc, along with the attached capsular ligaments, holds the head of the ulna snugly against the ulnar notch of the radius during pronation and supination.[51,81]

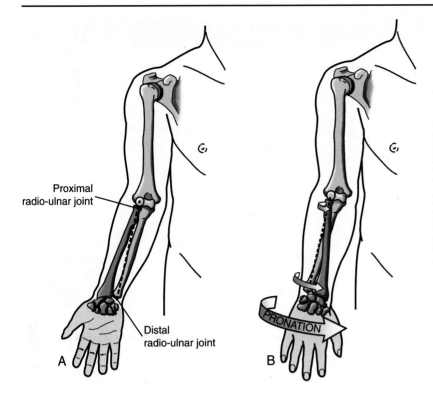

FIGURE 6-23. Anterior view of the right forearm. **A,** In full supination the radius and ulna are parallel. **B,** Moving into full pronation, the radius crosses over the ulna. The axis of rotation *(dashed line)* extends obliquely across the forearm from the radial head to the ulnar head. The radius and carpal bones (shown in brown) form the distal segment of the forearm complex. The humerus and ulna (shown in yellow) form the proximal segment of the forearm complex. Note that the thumb stays with the radius during pronation.

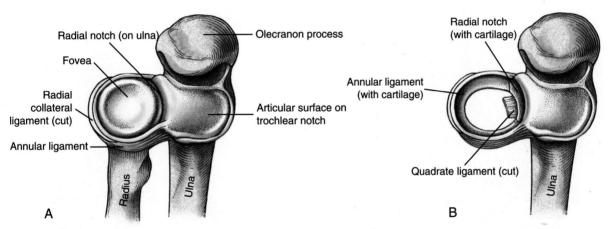

FIGURE 6-24. The right proximal radio-ulnar joint as viewed from above. **A,** The radius is held against the radial notch of the ulna by the annular ligament. **B,** The radius is removed, exposing the internal surface of the concave component of the proximal radio-ulnar joint. Note the cartilage lining the entire fibro-osseous ring. The quadrate ligament is cut near its attachment to the neck of the radius.

Experimentally cutting the capsular ligaments in fresh cadaver specimens causes marked increases in multidirectional translations of the distal radius in all positions of supination and pronation.[80]

Introduction to the Triangular Fibrocartilage Complex

The articular disc is part of a larger set of connective tissue known as the *triangular fibrocartilage complex*–typically abbreviated *TFCC*.[25,34,67] The TFCC occupies most of the "ulnocarpal space" between the head of the ulna and the ulnar side of the wrist. Several adjacent connective tissues are typically included with this complex, such as the capsular ligaments of the distal radio-ulnar joint and ulnar collateral ligament (see Figure 6-26, *B*). The TFCC is the primary stabilizer of the distal radio-ulnar joint.[80]

Other structures that provide stability to the distal radio-ulnar joint are the pronator quadratus, the tendon of the extensor carpi ulnaris, and the more distal fibers of the interosseous membrane.[22,82] Tears or disruptions of the TFCC, especially the disc,[39] may cause complete dislocation or gen-

SPECIAL FOCUS 6-2

Dislocations of the Proximal Radio-Ulnar Joint: the "Pulled-Elbow" Syndrome

A strenuous pull on the forearm through the hand can cause the radial head to slip through the distal end of the annular ligament. Young children are particularly susceptible to this "pulled-elbow" syndrome because of ligamentous laxity, a nonossified radial head, relative reduced strength and slowed reflexes, and the increased likelihood of others forcefully pulling on their arms—such as a parent, or even a pet dog (Figure 6-25). One of the best ways to prevent this dislocation is to explain to parents how a sharp pull on the child's hand can cause such a dislocation.

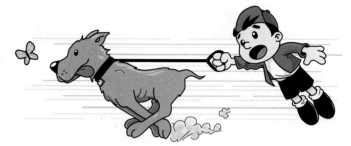

FIGURE 6-25. An example of a cause of "pulled-elbow syndrome" in a child. (Redrawn from Letts RM: Dislocations of the child's elbow. In Morrey BF, ed: *The elbow and its disorders*, ed 3, Philadelphia, 2000, Saunders. By permission of the Mayo Foundation for Medical Education and Research.)

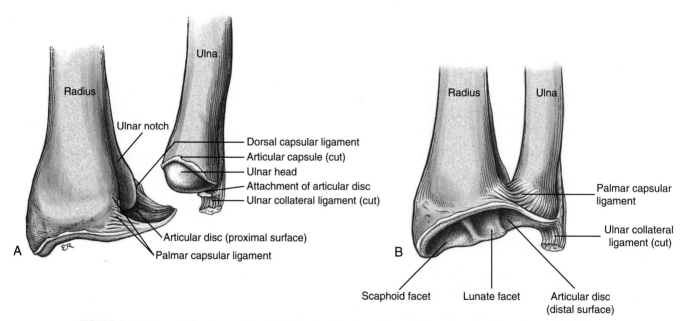

FIGURE 6-26. An anterior view of the right distal radio-ulnar joint. **A,** The ulnar head has been pulled away from the concavity formed by the proximal surface of the articular disc and the ulnar notch of the radius. **B,** The distal forearm has been tilted slightly to expose part of the distal surface of the articular disc and its connections with the palmar capsular ligament of the distal radio-ulnar joint. The scaphoid and lunate facets on the distal radius show impressions made by these carpal bones at the radiocarpal joint of the wrist.

eralized instability of the distal radio-ulnar joint, making pronation and supination motions, as well as motions of the wrist, painful and difficult to perform. (The triangular fibrocartilage complex is anatomically and functionally associated with other structures of the wrist, and hence is discussed further in Chapter 7.)

Stabilizers of the Distal Radio-Ulnar Joint
- Triangular fibrocartilage complex (TFCC)
- Pronator quadratus
- Tendon of the extensor carpi ulnaris
- Distal fibers of the interosseous membrane

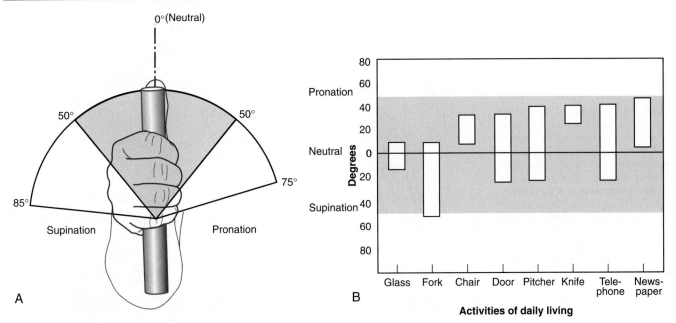

FIGURE 6-27. Range of motion at the forearm complex. **A,** A healthy person generally allows 0 to 85 degrees of supination and 0 to 75 degrees of pronation. The 0-degree neutral position is shown with the thumb pointing straight up. As in the elbow, a 100-degree "functional arc" exists (shown in red). This arc is derived from the data in the histogram in **B. B,** Histogram showing the amount of forearm rotation usually required for healthy persons to perform the following activities of daily living: bringing a *glass* to the mouth, bringing a *fork* to the mouth, rising from a *chair*, opening a *door*, pouring from a *pitcher*, cutting with a *knife*, holding a *telephone*, and reading a *newspaper*. (Modified from Morrey BF, Askew LJ, Chao EY: A biomechanical study of normal functional elbow motion, *J Bone Joint Surg Am* 63:872, 1981.)

KINEMATICS

Functional Considerations of Pronation and Supination

Forearm supination occurs during many activities that involve rotating the palmar surface of the hand toward the face, such as feeding, washing, and shaving. Forearm pronation, in contrast, is used to place the palmar surface of the hand down on an object, such as grasping a coin or pushing up from a chair.

The neutral or zero reference position of forearm rotation is the "thumb-up" position, midway between complete pronation and supination. On average the forearm rotates through about 75 degrees of pronation and 85 degrees of supination (Figure 6-27, *A*). As shown in Figure 6-27, *B*, several activities of daily living require only about 100 degrees of forearm rotation—from about 50 degrees of pronation through 50 degrees of supination.[47] As in the elbow joint, a 100-degree functional arc exists—an arc that does not include the terminal ranges of motion. Persons who lack the last 30 degrees of complete forearm rotation, for example, are still capable of performing many routine activities of daily living. To some extent, reduced pronation and supination can be compensated for by internally and externally rotating the shoulder, respectively.

Arthrokinematics at the Proximal and Distal Radio-Ulnar Joints

Pronation and supination require simultaneous movements at both the proximal and distal radio-ulnar joints. As will be explained, pronation and supination also require movement at the adjacent humeroradial joint. A restriction at any one

TABLE 6-2. Structures That Can Restrict Supination and Pronation

Restriction	Structures
Limit supination	Pronator teres, pronator quadratus TFCC, especially the palmar capsular ligament at the distal radio-ulnar joint Interosseous membrane
Limit pronation	Biceps or supinator muscles TFCC, especially the dorsal capsular ligament at the distal radio-ulnar joint

TFCC, triangular fibrocartilage complex.

of these joints would restrict the overall movement of forearm rotation. Restrictions in passive range of motion can occur from tightness in muscle and/or connective tissues. Table 6-2 lists a sample of these tissues.

Supination

Supination at the *proximal radio-ulnar joint* occurs as a rotation of the radial head within the fibro-osseous ring formed by the annular ligament and radial notch of the ulna (Figure 6-28, bottom box). The tight constraint of the radial head by the fibro-osseous ring prohibits standard roll-and-slide arthrokinematics.[5]

Supination at the *distal radio-ulnar joint* occurs as the concave ulnar notch of the radius rolls and slides in similar

FIGURE 6-28. Illustration on the left shows the anterior aspect of a right forearm after completing full *supination*. During supination, the radius and carpal bones rotate around the fixed humerus and ulna. The inactive but stretched pronator teres is also shown. *Viewed as though looking down at your own right forearm,* the two insets depict the arthrokinematics at the proximal and distal radio-ulnar joints. The stretched (taut) structures are shown as *thin elongated arrows,* and slackened structures are shown as *wavy arrows.* See text for further details.

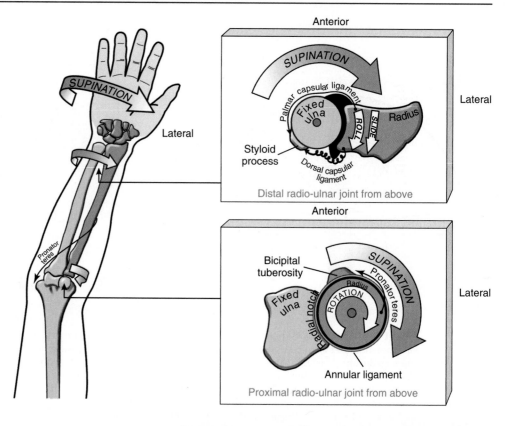

directions on the head of the ulna (see Figure 6-28, top box).[5] During supination the proximal surface of the articular disc remains in contact with the ulnar head. At the end range of supination, the palmar capsular ligament is stretched to its maximal length, creating a stiffness that naturally stabilizes the joint.[17,67,78] This stiffness provides increased stability at a position of reduced joint congruency. At the extremes of both supination and pronation, only about 10% of the surface of the ulnar notch of the radius is in direct contact with the ulnar head.[20] This is in sharp contrast to the 60% contact area in the neutral (midposition) of pronation and supination.

Pronation

The arthrokinematics of pronation at the proximal and distal radio-ulnar joints occur by mechanisms similar to those described for supination (Figure 6-29). As depicted in the top inset of Figure 6-29, full pronation elongates and thereby increases the tension in the dorsal capsular ligament at the distal radio-ulnar joint.[17] Full pronation slackens the palmar capsular ligament to about 70% of its original length.[67] In addition, full pronation exposes the articular surface of the ulnar head (see the asterisk in Figure 6-29, top inset), making it readily palpable.

Humeroradial Joint: a "Shared" Joint between the Elbow and the Forearm

During pronation and supination, the proximal end of the radius rotates at both the *proximal radio-ulnar* and *humeroradial joints.* Both joints have distinctive arthrokinematics during pronation and supination. The arthrokinematics at the proximal radio-ulnar joint were explained previously. The arthrokinematics at the humeroradial joint involve a *spin* of the fovea

---

SPECIAL FOCUS 6-3

Preventing Forearm Pronation Contractures

The axis of rotation for pronation and supination is oriented roughly parallel with the central bands of the interosseous membrane (compare Figures 6-20 and 6-23,*A*), deviating by only about 10 to 12 degrees. This relatively parallel arrangement limits the change in length (or tension) of the membrane throughout a pronation to supination movement. (Recall from Chapter 1 that any force that acts exactly *parallel to* an axis of rotation produces no resistive torque.) Because the axis and the membrane are not precisely parallel, however, some change in length occurs throughout a full arc of forearm rotation. Although some data conflict, most studies indicate that the interosseous membrane, as a whole, is most slack in *pronation.*[32,42] Long-term splinting or casting of the forearm often requires the forearm to be immobilized in partial pronation, typically as a means to optimize the use of the hand. A relatively slackened membrane in pronation is theoretically more likely to develop tightness over time and predispose the person to a pronation contracture. Pronation contractures may also occur because of tightness in the pronator teres, pronator quadratus, extrinsic finger flexor muscles, and the palmar radio-ulnar joint capsular ligaments. Although not always practical or even possible, clinicians should nevertheless be aware of the possible therapeutic benefit of immobilizing a forearm in a neutral or partially supinated position, in which the interosseous membrane is relatively stretched.[16,41,82] Increased resting tension in the interosseous membrane, albeit small, should theoretically limit adaptive shortening of the tissue over time.

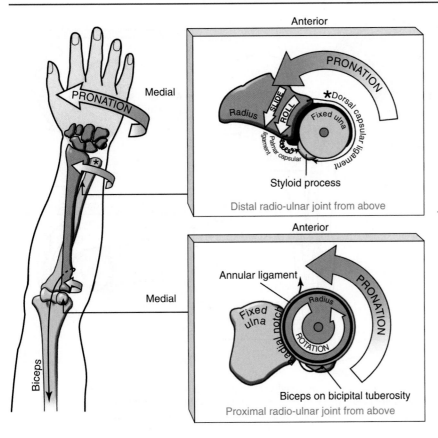

FIGURE 6-29. Illustration on the left shows the right forearm after completing full *pronation*. During pronation the radius and carpal bones rotate around the fixed humerus and ulna. The inactive but stretched biceps muscle is also shown. *Viewed as though looking down at your own right forearm,* the two insets show a superior view of the arthrokinematics at the proximal and distal radio-ulnar joints. The stretched (taut) structures are shown as thin elongated arrows, and slackened structures are shown as wavy arrows. The asterisks mark the exposed point on the anterior aspect of the ulnar head, which is apparent once the radius rotates fully around the ulna into complete pronation. See text for further details.

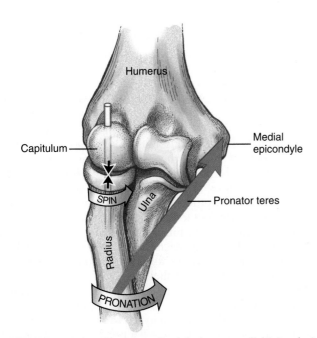

FIGURE 6-30. An anterior view of a right humeroradial joint during active pronation of the forearm. During pronation the fovea of the radial head spins against the capitulum. The spinning occurs around an axis that is nearly coincident with the axis of rotation through the proximal and distal radio-ulnar joints. The pronator teres muscle is shown active as it pronates the forearm and pulls the radius proximally against the capitulum. The opposing small arrows indicate an increased compression force at the humeroradial joint.

of the radial head against the rounded capitulum of the humerus. Figure 6-30 shows the arthrokinematics during active pronation under the power of the pronator teres muscle. Contraction of this muscle—as well as others inserting into the radius—can generate significant compression forces on the humeroradial joint, especially when the joint is near extension. This compression force is associated with a proximal migration of the radius, which is greater during active *pronation* than during supination.[46] Because the interosseous membrane as a whole is relatively slackened in pronation,[32,42] it is likely less able to resist the proximal pull on the radius imparted by pronator muscle contraction. The natural proximal migration of the radius and associated increased joint compression of the humeroradial joint during active pronation has been referred to as the "screw home" mechanism of the elbow.[45]

Based on location, the humeroradial joint is mechanically linked to the kinematics of both the elbow and forearm. *Any motion performed at the elbow or forearm requires movement at this joint.* A postmortem study of 32 cadavers (age at death ranging from 70 to 95 years) showed more frequent and severe degeneration across the humeroradial than the humero-ulnar joint.[1] The increased wear on the lateral compartment of the elbow can be explained in part by the frequent and complex arthrokinematics (spin and roll-and-slide), combined with varying amounts of muscular-produced compression force. Pain or limited motion at the humeroradial joint can significantly disrupt the functional mobility of the entire distal upper extremity.

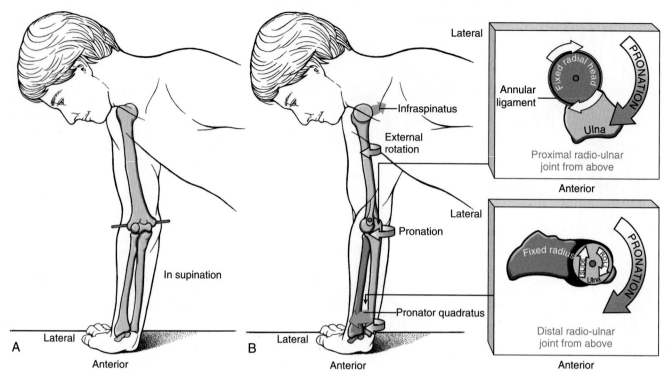

FIGURE 6-31. **A,** A person is shown supporting his upper body weight through his right forearm, which is in full supination (i.e., the bones of the forearm are parallel). The radius is held fixed to the ground through the wrist; however, the humerus and ulna are free to rotate. **B,** The humerus and ulna have rotated about 80 to 90 degrees externally from the initial position shown in **A.** This rotation produces pronation at the forearm as the ulna rotates around the fixed radius. Note the activity depicted in the infraspinatus and pronator quadratus muscles. The two insets show a superior view of the arthrokinematics at the proximal and distal radio-ulnar joints.

Pronation and Supination with the Radius and Hand Held Fixed

Up to this point in this chapter, the kinematics of pronation and supination have been described as a rotation of the *radius and hand* relative to a stationary, or fixed, humerus and ulna (see Figures 6-28 and 6-29). The forearm rotation occurs when the upper limb is in a *non–weight-bearing position.* Pronation and supination are next described when the upper limb is in a weight-bearing position. In this case the humerus and ulna rotate relative to a stationary, or fixed, radius and hand.

Consider a person bearing weight through an upper extremity with elbow and wrist extended (Figure 6-31, *A*). The person's right glenohumeral joint is held partially internally rotated. The ulna and radius are positioned parallel in full supination. (The "rod" placed through the epicondyles of the humerus helps with the orientation of this position.) With the radius and hand held firmly fixed with the ground, pronation of the forearm occurs by an *external rotation* of the humerus and ulna (see Figure 6-31, *B*). Because of the naturally tight structural fit of the humero-ulnar joint, rotation of the humerus is transferred, nearly degree for degree, to the rotating ulna. Moving back to the fully supinated position involves internal rotation of the humerus and ulna relative to the fixed radius and hand. It is important to note that these pronation and supination kinematics are essentially *an expres-sion of active external and internal rotation of the glenohumeral joint, respectively.*

Figure 6-31, *B* depicts an interesting muscle "force-couple" used to pronate the forearm from the weight-bearing position. The infraspinatus rotates the humerus relative to a fixed scapula, whereas the pronator quadratus rotates the ulna relative to a fixed radius. Both muscles, acting at either end of the upper extremity, produce forces that contribute to a pronation torque at the forearm. From a therapeutic perspective, an understanding of the muscular mechanics of pronation and supination from this weight-bearing perspective provides additional exercise strategies for strengthening or stretching muscles of the forearm and shoulder.

The far right side of Figure 6-31, *B* illustrates the arthrokinematics at the radio-ulnar joints during pronation while the radius and hand are stationary. At the *proximal radio-ulnar joint* the annular ligament *and* radial notch of the ulna rotate around the fixed radial head (see Figure 6-31, *B*, top inset). Although not depicted, the capitulum of the humerus is spinning relative to the fovea of the fixed radius. At the *distal radio-ulnar joint* the head of the ulna rotates around the fixed ulnar notch of the radius (see Figure 6-31, bottom inset). Table 6-3 summarizes and compares the arthrokinematics at the radio-ulnar joints for both weight-bearing and non–weight-bearing conditions of the upper limb.

TABLE 6-3. Arthrokinematics of Pronation and Supination		
	Weight-Bearing (Radius and Hand Fixed)	**Non–Weight-Bearing (Radius and Hand Free to Rotate)**
Proximal radio-ulnar joint	Annular ligament *and* radial notch of the ulna rotate around a fixed radial head.	Radial head rotates within a ring formed by the annular ligament *and* the radial notch of the ulna.
Distal radio-ulnar joint	Convex ulnar head rolls and slides in opposite directions on the concave ulnar notch of the radius.	Concavity of the ulnar notch of the radius rolls and slides in similar directions on the convex ulna head.

MUSCLE AND JOINT INTERACTION

Neuroanatomy Overview: Paths of the Musculocutaneous, Radial, Median, and Ulnar Nerves throughout the Elbow, Forearm, Wrist, and Hand

The musculocutaneous, radial, median, and ulnar nerves provide motor and sensory innervation to the muscles, ligaments, joint capsules, and skin of the elbow, forearm, wrist, and hand. The anatomic path of these nerves is described as a background for this chapter and the following two chapters on the wrist and the hand.

The *musculocutaneous nerve*, formed from the C^5-C^7 spinal nerve roots, innervates the biceps brachii, coracobrachialis, and brachialis muscles (Figure 6-32, *A*). As its name implies, the musculocutaneous nerve innervates muscle then continues distally as a sensory nerve to the skin, supplying the lateral forearm.

The *radial nerve*, formed from the C^5-T^1 spinal nerve roots, is a direct continuation of the posterior cord of the brachial plexus (see Figure 6-32, *B*). This large nerve courses within the radial groove of the humerus to innervate the triceps and the anconeus. The radial nerve then emerges laterally at the distal humerus to innervate muscles that attach on or near the lateral epicondyle. Proximal to the elbow, the radial nerve innervates the brachioradialis, a small lateral part of the brachialis, and the extensor carpi radialis longus. Distal to the elbow, the radial nerve consists of superficial and deep branches. The *superficial branch* is purely sensory, supplying the posterior-lateral aspects of the distal forearm, including the dorsal "web space" of the hand. The *deep branch* contains the remaining motor fibers of the radial nerve. This motor branch supplies the extensor carpi radialis brevis and the supinator muscle. After piercing through an intramuscular tunnel in the supinator muscle, the final section of the radial nerve courses toward the posterior side of the forearm. This terminal branch, often referred to as the *posterior interosseous nerve*, supplies the extensor carpi ulnaris and several muscles of the forearm, which function in extension of the digits.

The *median nerve*, formed from the C^6-T^1 spinal nerve roots, courses toward the elbow to innervate most muscles attaching on or near the medial epicondyle of the humerus. These muscles include the wrist flexors and forearm pronators (pronator teres, flexor carpi radialis, and palmaris longus) and the deeper flexor digitorum superficialis (see Figure 6-32, *C*). A deep branch of the median nerve, often referred to as *anterior interosseous nerve*, innervates the deep muscles of the forearm: the lateral half of the flexor digitorum profundus, the flexor pollicis longus, and the pronator quadratus. The terminal part of the median nerve continues distally to cross the wrist through the carpal tunnel, under the cover of the transverse carpal ligament. The nerve then innervates several of the intrinsic muscles of the thumb and the lateral fingers. The median nerve provides a rich source of sensation to the lateral palm, palmar surface of the thumb, and lateral two and one-half fingers (see Figure 6-32, *C,* inset on median nerve sensory distribution).

The *ulnar nerve,* formed from the spinal nerve roots C^8-T^1, is formed by a direct branch of the medial cord of the brachial plexus (see Figure 6-32, *D*). After passing posterior to the medial epicondyle, the ulnar nerve innervates the flexor carpi ulnaris and the medial half of the flexor digitorum profundus. The nerve then crosses the wrist external to the carpal tunnel and supplies motor innervation to many of the intrinsic muscles of the hand. The ulnar nerve supplies sensation to the skin on the ulnar side of the hand, including the medial side of the ring finger and entire small finger.

Innervation of Muscles and Joints of the Elbow and Forearm

Knowledge of the specific innervation to the muscle, skin, and joints is useful clinical information for treatment of persons who have sustained injury to the peripheral nerves or nerve roots. The informed clinician can anticipate not only the extent of the sensory and motor involvement after injury, but also the likely complications. Therapeutic activities, such as splinting, selective strengthening, range-of-motion exercise, and patient education, can often be initiated early after injury, provided there are no contraindications. This proactive approach minimizes the potential for permanent deformity and damage to insensitive skin and joints, thereby minimizing functional limitations.

INNERVATION OF MUSCLE

The *elbow flexors* have three different sources of peripheral nerve supply: the musculocutaneous nerve to the biceps brachii and brachialis, the radial nerve to the brachioradialis and lateral part of the brachialis, and the median nerve to the pronator teres. In contrast, the *elbow extensors*—the triceps brachii and anconeus—have a single source of nerve supply through the radial nerve. Injury to this nerve can result in complete paralysis of the elbow extensors. Because three different nerves must be affected for all four elbow flexors to be paralyzed, important functions such as feeding and grooming are often preserved.

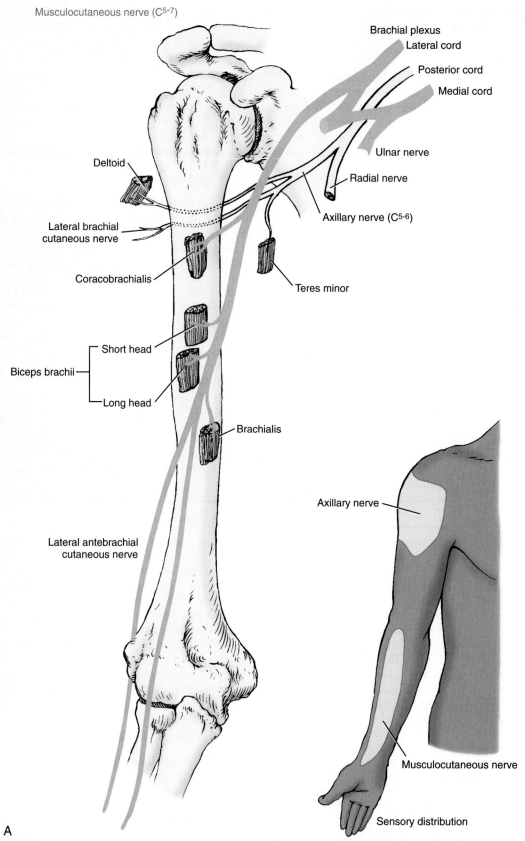

Musculocutaneous nerve (C^{5-7})

Brachial plexus
Lateral cord
Posterior cord
Medial cord

Deltoid

Ulnar nerve
Radial nerve

Lateral brachial cutaneous nerve

Axillary nerve (C^{5-6})

Coracobrachialis

Teres minor

Short head
Biceps brachii
Long head

Brachialis

Axillary nerve

Lateral antebrachial cutaneous nerve

Musculocutaneous nerve

A

Sensory distribution

FIGURE 6-32. Paths of the peripheral nerves throughout the elbow, wrist, and hand. The following illustrate the path and general proximal-to-distal order of muscle innervation. The location of some muscles is altered slightly for illustration purposes. The primary nerve roots that form each nerve are shown in parentheses. **A,** The path of the musculocutaneous nerve is shown as it innervates the coracobrachialis, biceps brachii, and brachialis muscles. The sensory distribution of this nerve is shown as the lighter region along the lateral forearm. The motor and sensory components of the axillary nerve are also shown.

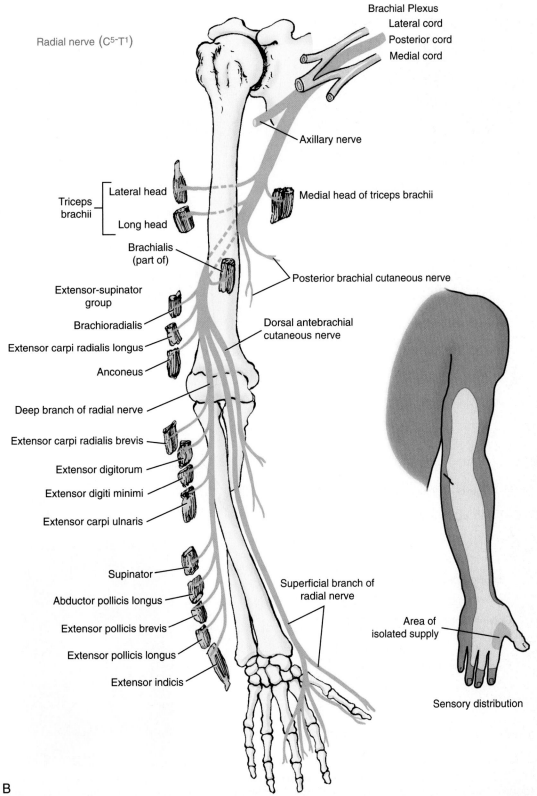

Radial nerve (C⁵-T¹)

Brachial Plexus
Lateral cord
Posterior cord
Medial cord

Axillary nerve

Triceps brachii
Lateral head
Long head

Medial head of triceps brachii

Brachialis (part of)

Extensor-supinator group

Brachioradialis

Extensor carpi radialis longus

Anconeus

Posterior brachial cutaneous nerve

Dorsal antebrachial cutaneous nerve

Deep branch of radial nerve

Extensor carpi radialis brevis

Extensor digitorum

Extensor digiti minimi

Extensor carpi ulnaris

Supinator

Abductor pollicis longus

Extensor pollicis brevis

Extensor pollicis longus

Extensor indicis

Superficial branch of radial nerve

Area of isolated supply

Sensory distribution

B

FIGURE 6-32, cont'd B, The path of the radial nerve is shown as it innervates most of the extensors of the arm, forearm, wrist, and digits. See text for more detail on the proximal-to-distal order of muscle innervation. The general sensory distribution of this nerve is shown as the lighter region along the dorsal aspect of the upper extremity. The dorsal "web space" of the hand is innervated solely by sensory branches of the radial nerve (depicted in green). This area of "isolated" nerve supply makes it a preferred location for testing the sensory function of this nerve.

Continued

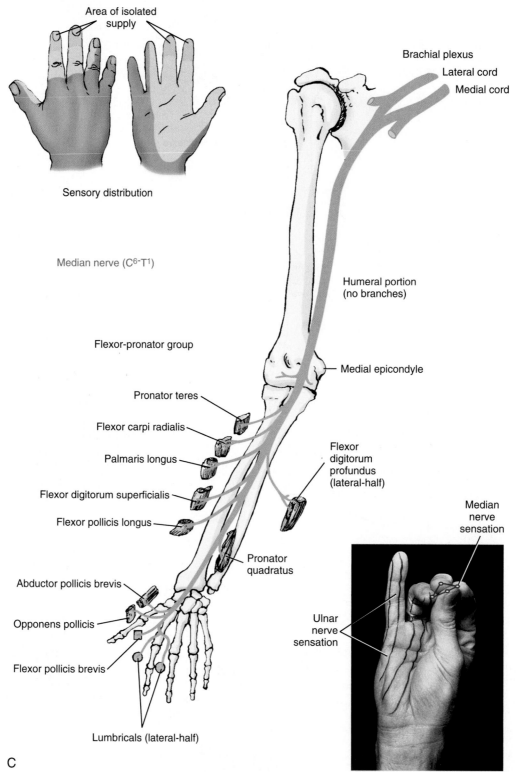

Area of isolated supply

Sensory distribution

Median nerve (C⁶-T¹)

Brachial plexus
Lateral cord
Medial cord

Humeral portion (no branches)

Medial epicondyle

Flexor-pronator group

Pronator teres

Flexor carpi radialis

Palmaris longus

Flexor digitorum superficialis

Flexor pollicis longus

Flexor digitorum profundus (lateral-half)

Pronator quadratus

Abductor pollicis brevis

Opponens pollicis

Flexor pollicis brevis

Median nerve sensation

Ulnar nerve sensation

Lumbricals (lateral-half)

C

FIGURE 6-32, cont'd C, The path of the median nerve is shown supplying the pronators, wrist flexors, long (extrinsic) flexors of the digits (except the flexor digitorum profundus to the ring and small finger), most intrinsic muscles to the thumb, and two lateral lumbricals. The general sensory distribution of this nerve is shown as the lighter region within the hand. The area of skin that receives isolated median nerve sensation is indicated (in green) along the distal end of the index and middle fingers. *Inset,* The median nerve supplies the sensation of the skin that naturally makes contact in a pinching motion between the thumb and fingers.

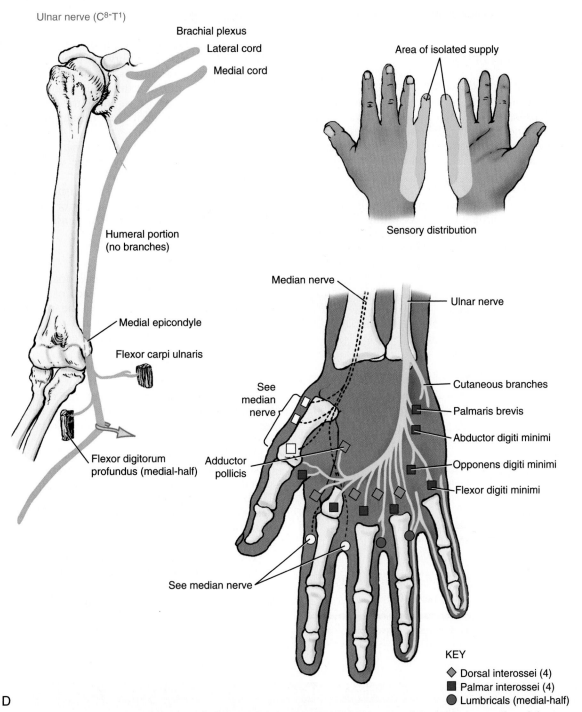

D

FIGURE 6-32, cont'd **D,** The path of the ulnar nerve is shown supplying most of the intrinsic muscles of the hand, including the two medial lumbricals. The general sensory distribution of this nerve covers the skin on the ulnar side of the hand, including the medial side of the ring finger and entire small finger. The area of skin that receives isolated ulnar nerve sensation is depicted in green, which includes the entire small finger and the extreme ulnar side of the hand. (**A** to **D** modified from de Groot JH: *Correlative neuroanatomy,* ed 21, Norwalk, 1991, Appleton & Lange. Photograph by Donald A. Neumann.)

The muscles that *pronate the forearm* (pronator teres, pronator quadratus, and other secondary muscles that originate from the medial epicondyle) are innervated through the median nerve. *Supination of the forearm* is driven by the biceps brachii via the musculocutaneous nerve and the supinator muscle, plus secondary muscles that arise from the lateral epicondyle and dorsal forearm, via the radial nerve.

Table 6-4 summarizes the peripheral nerve and primary spinal nerve root innervation to the muscles of the elbow and forearm. This table was derived primarily from Appendix II, Part A, which lists the primary nerve roots that innervate the muscles of the upper extremity. Appendix II, Parts B to D include additional reference items to help guide the clinical assessment of the functional status of the C^5-T^1 spinal nerve roots and several major peripheral nerves of the upper limb.

SENSORY INNERVATION OF JOINTS

Humero-Ulnar and Humeroradial Joints

The humero-ulnar and humeroradial joints and the surrounding connective tissues receive their sensory innervation from the C^6-C^8 spinal nerve roots.[33] Fibers from these afferent nerve roots are carried primarily by the musculocutaneous and radial nerves and by the ulnar and median nerves.[70]

Proximal and Distal Radio-Ulnar Joints

The proximal radio-ulnar joint and surrounding elbow capsule receive sensory innervation from fibers within the median nerve that enter the C^6-C^7 spinal nerve roots.[70] The distal radio-ulnar joint receives most of its sensory innervation from fibers of the ulnar nerve that enter the C^8 nerve root.[33]

TABLE 6-4. Motor Innervation to the Muscles of the Elbow and Forearm

Muscle	Innervation
Elbow Flexors	
Brachialis	Musculocutaneous nerve (C^5, C^6)
Biceps brachii	Musculocutaneous nerve (C^5, C^6)
Brachioradialis	Radial nerve (C^5, C^6)
Pronator teres	Median nerve (C^6, C^7)
Elbow Extensors	
Triceps brachii	Radial nerve (C^7, C^8)
Anconeus	Radial nerve (C^7, C^8)
Forearm Pronators	
Pronator quadratus	Median nerve (C^8, T^1)
Pronator teres	Median nerve (C^6, C^7)
Forearm Supinators	
Biceps brachii	Musculocutaneous nerve (C^5, C^6)
Supinator	Radial nerve (C^6)

The primary spinal nerve root innervation of the muscles is in parentheses.

Function of the Elbow Muscles

Muscles that attach distally on the ulna flex or extend the elbow but possess no ability to pronate or supinate the forearm. In contrast, muscles that attach distally on the radius may, in theory, flex or extend the elbow, but also have a potential to pronate or supinate the forearm. This basic concept serves as the underlying theme through much of the remainder of this chapter.

Muscles acting primarily on the wrist also cross the elbow joint. For this reason, many of the wrist muscles have a potential to flex or extend the elbow.[3] This potential is relatively minimal and is not discussed further. The proximal and distal attachments and nerve supply of the muscles of the elbow and forearm are listed in Appendix II, Part E.

ELBOW FLEXORS

The biceps brachii, brachialis, brachioradialis, and pronator teres are primary elbow flexors. Each of these muscles produces a force that passes anterior to the medial-lateral axis of rotation at the elbow. Structural and related biomechanical variables of these muscles are included in Table 6-5.

Individual Muscle Action of the Elbow Flexors

The *biceps brachii* attaches proximally on the scapula and distally on the radial tuberosity on the radius (Figure 6-33). Secondary distal attachments include the deep fascia of the forearm through an aponeurotic sheet known as the *fibrous lacertus*.

The biceps produces its maximal electromyographic (EMG) signal when performing both flexion and supination simultaneously,[6] such as when bringing a spoon to the mouth. The biceps exhibits relatively low levels of EMG activity when flexion is performed with the forearm deliberately held in pronation. This lack of muscle activation can be verified by self-palpation.

The *brachialis* lies deep to the biceps, originating on the anterior humerus and attaching distally on the extreme proximal ulna (Figure 6-34). This muscle's sole function is to flex the elbow. As shown in Table 6-5, the brachialis has an average physiologic cross-section of 7 cm², the largest of any muscle crossing the elbow. For comparison, the long head of the

TABLE 6-5. Structural and Related Biomechanical Variables of the Primary Elbow Flexor Muscles*

Muscle	Work Capacity	Contraction Excursion	Peak Force	Leverage
	Volume (cm³)	Length (cm)[†]	Physiologic Cross-sectional Area (cm²)	Internal Moment Arm (cm)[‡]
biceps brachii (long head)	33.4	13.6	2.5	3.20
biceps brachii (short head)	30.8	15.0	2.1	3.20
brachialis	59.3	9.0	7.0	1.98
brachioradialis	21.9	16.4	1.5	5.19
pronator teres	18.7	5.6	3.4	2.01

Data from An KN, Hui FC, Morrey BF, et al: Muscles across the elbow joint: a biomechanical analysis, *J Biomech* 14:659, 1981.
*Structural properties are indicated by italics. The related biomechanical variables are indicated in bold.
[†]Muscle belly length measured at 70 degrees of flexion.
[‡]Internal moment arm measured with elbow flexed to 100 degrees and forearm fully supinated.

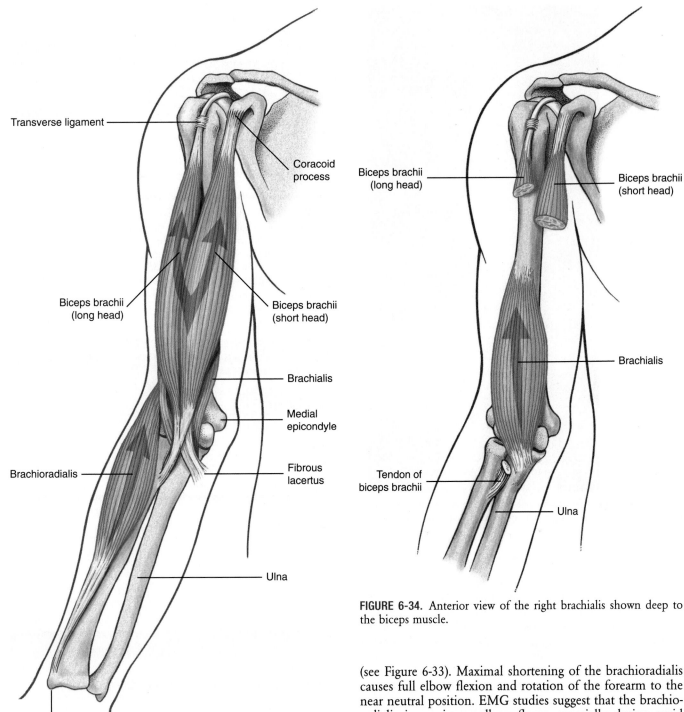

FIGURE 6-33. Anterior view of the right biceps brachii and brachio-radialis muscles. The brachialis is deep to the biceps.

FIGURE 6-34. Anterior view of the right brachialis shown deep to the biceps muscle.

biceps has a cross-sectional area of only 2.5 cm². Based on its large physiologic cross-section, the brachialis is expected to generate the greatest force of any muscle crossing the elbow.

The *brachioradialis* is the longest of all elbow muscles, attaching proximally on the lateral supracondylar ridge of the humerus and distally near the styloid process of the radius (see Figure 6-33). Maximal shortening of the brachioradialis causes full elbow flexion and rotation of the forearm to the near neutral position. EMG studies suggest that the brachio-radialis is a primary elbow flexor, especially during rapid movements against a high resistance.[6,15,21]

The brachioradialis muscle can be readily palpated on the anterior-lateral aspect of the forearm. Resisted elbow flexion, from a position of about 90 degrees of flexion and neutral forearm rotation, causes the muscle to stand out or "bow-string" sharply across the elbow (Figure 6-35). The bowstring-ing of this muscle increases its flexion moment arm to a length that exceeds that of the other flexors (see Table 6-5).

The anatomy of the *pronator teres* is described under the section on pronator muscles (see Figure 6-48). As a point of comparison, the pronator teres has a similar flexor moment arm as the brachialis, but only about 50% of its physiologic cross-sectional area (see Table 6-5).

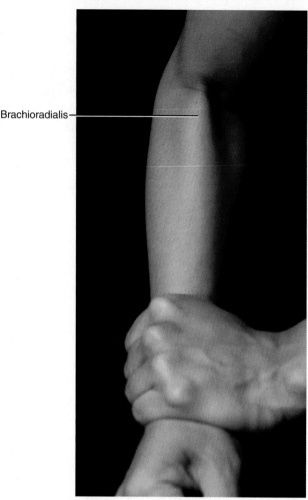

FIGURE 6-35. The right brachioradialis muscle is shown "bowstringing" over the elbow during a maximal-effort isometric activation.

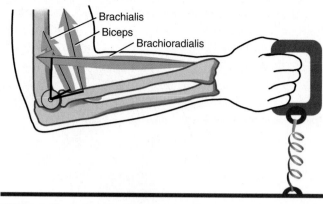

FIGURE 6-36. A lateral view showing the line of force of three primary elbow flexors. The internal moment arm *(thick dark lines)* for each muscle is drawn to approximate scale. Note that the elbow has been flexed about 100 degrees, placing the biceps tendon at 90 degrees of insertion with the radius. See text for further details. The elbow's medial-lateral axis of rotation is shown piercing the capitulum.

TABLE 6-6. Average Maximal Isometric Internal Torques across the Elbow and Forearm

Movement	Torque (kg-cm)	
	Males	Females
Flexion	725 (154)	336 (80)
Extension	421 (109)	210 (61)
Pronation	73 (18)	36 (8)
Supination	91 (23)	44 (12)

Data from Askew LJ, An KN, Morrey BF, Chao EY: Isometric elbow strength in normal individuals, *Clin Orthop Relat Res* 222:261, 1987.
Standard deviations are in parentheses. Data are from 104 healthy subjects; $\overline{X}$ age male = 41 yr, $\overline{X}$ age female = 45.1 yr. The elbow is maintained in 90 degrees of flexion with neutral forearm rotation. Data are shown for dominant limb only.
Conversions: 0.098 N-m/kg-cm.

Torque Generated by the Elbow Flexor Muscles

Figure 6-36 shows the line of force of three primary elbow flexors. The strength of the flexion torque varies considerably based on age,[23] gender, weightlifting experience,[76] speed of muscle contraction, and position of the joints across the upper extremity.[84] According to a study reported by Gallagher and colleagues,[23] the dominant side produced significantly higher levels of flexion torque, work, and power. No significant differences, however, were found for elbow extension and forearm pronation and supination.

Maximal-effort flexion torques of 725 kg-cm for men and 336 kg-cm for women have been reported for healthy middle-aged persons (Table 6-6).[4] These data show that flexion torques are about 70% greater than extensor torques. In the knee, however, which is functionally analogous to the elbow in the lower extremity, the strength differential favors the extensor muscles, by an approximately similar magnitude. This difference likely reflects the greater relative functional demands typically placed on the flexors of the elbow as compared with the flexors of the knee.

Elbow flexor torques produced with the forearm supinated are about 20% to 25% greater than those produced with the forearm fully pronated.[62] This difference is due primarily to the increased flexor moment arm of the biceps[50] and

---

SPECIAL FOCUS 6-4

Brachialis: the Workhorse of the Elbow Flexors

In addition to a large cross-sectional area, the brachialis muscle also has the largest volume of all elbow flexors (see Table 6-5). Muscle volume can be measured by recording the volume of water displaced by the muscle.[3] Large muscle volume suggests that the muscle has a large *work capacity*. For this reason, the brachialis has been called the "workhorse" of the elbow flexors.[6] This name is due in part to the muscle's large work capacity, but also to its active involvement in all types of elbow flexion activities, whether performed quickly or slowly or combined with pronation or supination. Because the brachialis attaches distally to the ulna, the motion of pronation or supination has no influence on its length, line of force, or internal moment arm.

the brachioradialis when the forearm is in or approaches supination.

Biomechanical and physiologic data can be used to predict the maximal flexion torque produced by the three primary elbow flexor muscles across a full range of motion (Figure 6-37, *A*). The predicted maximal torque for all muscles occurs at about 90 degrees of flexion, which agrees in general with actual torque measurements in healthy persons.[62,76] The two primary factors responsible for the overall shape of the maximal torque-angle curve of the elbow flexors are (1) the muscle's maximal flexion *force* potential and (2) the internal *moment arm* length. The data plotted in Figure 6-37, *B* predict that the maximal force of all muscles occurs at a muscle length that corresponds to about 80 degrees of flexion. The data plotted in Figure 6-37, *C* predict that the average maximal moment arm of all three muscles occurs at about 100 degrees

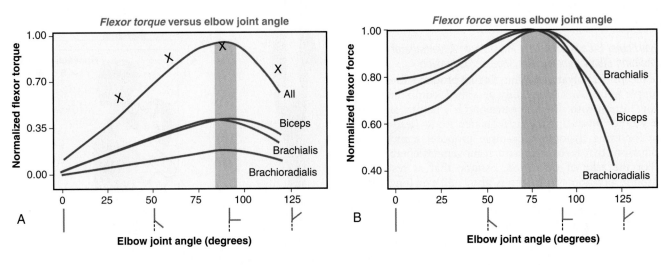

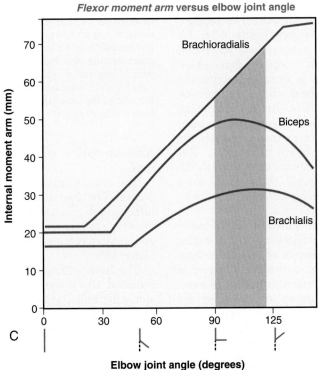

FIGURE 6-37. A, Predicted maximal isometric *torque* versus joint angle curves for three primary elbow flexors based on a theoretic model that incorporates each muscle's architecture, length-tension relationship, and internal moment arm. **B,** The length-tension relationships of the three muscles are shown as a normalized *flexor force* plotted against elbow joint angle. Note that muscle length decreases as joint angle increases. **C,** The length of each muscle's *internal moment arm* is plotted against the elbow joint angle. The joint angle where each predicted variable is greatest is shaded in red. (Data for **A** and **B** from An KN, Kaufman KR, Chao EY: Physiological considerations of muscle force through the elbow joint, *J Biomech* 22:1249, 1989. Data for **C** from Amis AA, Dowson D, Wright V: Muscle strengths and musculoskeletal geometry of the upper limb, *Eng Med* 8:41, 1979.)

of flexion. At about this joint angle, the insertion of the biceps tendon to the radius is near 90 degrees (see Figure 6-36). This mechanical condition maximizes the internal moment arm of a muscle and thereby maximizes the conversion of a muscle force to a joint torque. It is interesting that the data presented in Figure 6-37, *B* and *C* predict peak torques across generally similar joint angles. The natural ability to produce maximal elbow flexion torque at about 90 degrees of flexion functionally corresponds to the angle at which the greatest *external* torque (due to gravity) typically acts against the forearm, at least while standing or in an upright sitting position.

Polyarticular Biceps Brachii: a Physiologic Advantage of Combining Elbow Flexion with Shoulder Extension

The biceps is a polyarticular muscle that produces force across multiple joints. As subsequently described, combining active elbow flexion with shoulder extension is a natural and effective way for producing biceps-generated elbow flexor torque. The following hypothetic example proposes a physiologic mechanism that favors this natural movement combination.

For the sake of discussion, assume that at rest in the anatomic position the biceps is about 30 cm long (Figure 6-38, *A*). The biceps then shortens to about 23 cm after an active motion that combines 90 degrees of elbow flexion with 45 degrees of shoulder flexion (see Figure 6-38, *B*). If the motion took 1 second to perform, the muscle experiences an average contraction velocity of 7 cm/sec. In contrast, consider a more natural and effective activation pattern involving both the biceps and posterior deltoid to produce *elbow flexion* with *shoulder extension* (see Figure 6-38, *C*). During an activity such as pulling a heavy load up toward the side, for example, the activated biceps produces elbow flexion while at the same time it is elongated across the extending shoulder. By extending the shoulder, the contracting posterior deltoid, in effect, reduces the net shortening of the biceps. Based on the example in Figure 6-38, *C*, combining elbow flexion with shoulder extension reduces the average contraction velocity of the biceps to 5 cm/sec. This is 2 cm/sec slower than combining elbow flexion with shoulder flexion. As described in Chapter 3, the maximal force output of a muscle is greater when its contraction velocity is closer to zero, or isometric.

The simple model described here illustrates one of many examples in which a one-joint muscle, such as the posterior deltoid, can enhance the force potential of another polyarticular muscle. In the example, the posterior deltoid serves as a powerful shoulder extensor for a vigorous pulling motion. In addition, the posterior deltoid assists in controlling the optimal contraction velocity and operational length of the biceps throughout the elbow flexion motion. The posterior deltoid, especially during high-power activities, is a very important synergist to the elbow flexors. Consider the consequences of performing the lift described in Figure 6-38, *C* with total paralysis of the posterior deltoid.

ELBOW EXTENSORS

Muscular Components

The primary elbow extensors are the *triceps brachii* and the *anconeus* (Figures 6-39 and 6-40). The triceps converge to a

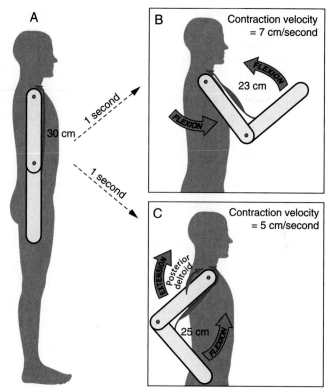

FIGURE 6-38.   A, This model is showing a person with a 30-cm long biceps muscle. **B,** After a 1-sec contraction, the biceps has contracted to a length of 23 cm, causing a simultaneous motion of 90 degrees of *elbow flexion* and 45 degrees of *shoulder flexion*. The biceps has shortened at a contraction velocity of 7 cm/sec. **C,** The biceps *and* posterior deltoid are shown active in a typical pulling motion, which combines the simultaneous motions of 90 degrees of *elbow flexion* with 45 degrees of *shoulder extension*. The biceps is depicted as experiencing a net contraction to a length of 25 cm, over a 1-sec interval. Because of the simultaneous contraction of the posterior deltoid, the biceps shortened only 5 cm, at a contraction velocity of 5 cm/sec.

common tendon attaching to the olecranon process of the ulna.

The triceps brachii has three heads: long, lateral, and medial. The *long head* has its proximal attachment on the infraglenoid tubercle of the scapula, thereby allowing the muscle to extend and adduct the shoulder. The long head has an extensive volume, exceeding all other muscles of the elbow (Table 6-7).

The *lateral* and *medial heads* of the triceps muscle have their proximal attachments on the humerus, on either side and along the radial groove. The medial head has an extensive proximal attachment on the posterior side of the humerus, occupying a location relatively similar to that of the brachialis on the bone's anterior side. Some of the more distal fibers of the medial head attach directly into the posterior capsule of the elbow. These fibers may be analogous to the articularis genu muscle at the knee, with a similar function in drawing the capsule taut during extension.[70] Indeed, these muscle fibers are often referred to as the *articularis cubiti*.

The *anconeus* is a small triangular muscle spanning the posterior side of the elbow. The muscle is located between the lateral epicondyle of the humerus and a strip along the posterior aspect of the proximal ulna (see Figure 6-39). Compared with the triceps muscle, the anconeus has a relatively

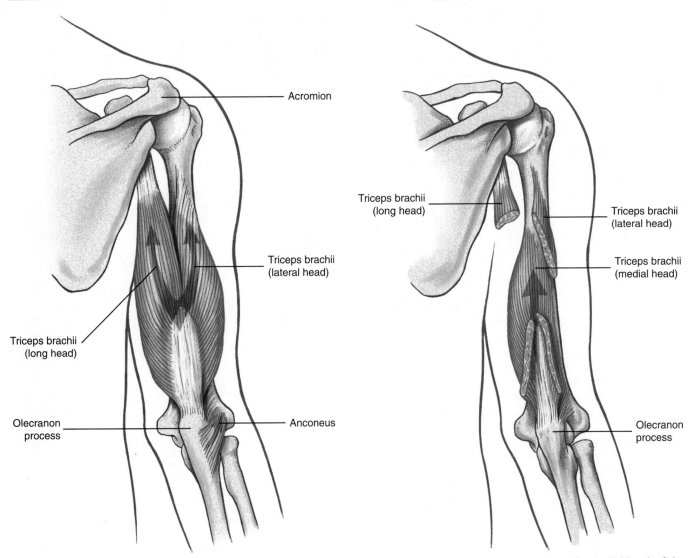

FIGURE 6-39. A posterior view shows the right triceps brachii and anconeus muscles. The medial head of the triceps is deep to the long and lateral heads and therefore not entirely visible.

FIGURE 6-40. A posterior view shows the right medial head of the triceps brachii. The long head and lateral head of the triceps are partially removed to expose the deeper medial head. The anconeus is not illustrated.

TABLE 6-7. Structural and Related Biomechanical Variables of the Primary Elbow Extensor Muscles*

Muscle	Work Capacity	Contraction Excursion	Peak Force	Leverage
	Volume (cm³)	Length (cm)†	Physiologic Cross-sectional Area (cm²)	Internal Moment Arm (cm)‡
Triceps brachii (long head)	66.6	10.2	6.7	1.87
Triceps brachii (medial head)	38.7	6.3	6.1	1.87
Triceps brachii (lateral head)	47.3	8.4	6.0	1.87
Anconeus	6.7	2.7	2.5	0.72

Data from An KN, Hui FC, Morrey BF, Chao EY: Muscles across the elbow joint: a biomechanical analysis, *J Biomech* 14:659, 1981.

*Structural properties are indicated by italics. The related biomechanical variables are indicated in bold.

†Muscle belly length measured at 70 degrees of flexion.

‡Internal moment arm measured with elbow flexed to 100 degrees.

small cross-sectional area and a small moment arm for extension (see Table 6-7). Although the anconeus is not capable of producing large elbow extension torque, it still provides important longitudinal and medial-lateral stability across the humero-ulnar joint. This stability is beneficial during extension activities, but also during active pronation and supination. The anconeus has a similar topographic orientation at the elbow as the oblique fibers of the vastus medialis have at the knee. This orientation is best appreciated by visually internally rotating the upper limb by 180 degrees, such that the olecranon faces anteriorly—a position more structurally and functionally analogous to the lower limb.

Electromyographic Analysis of Elbow Extension

Maximal-effort elbow extension generates near maximum levels of EMG activity from all components of the elbow extensor group. During submaximal efforts of elbow extension, however, different parts of muscles are recruited only at certain levels of effort.[74] The anconeus is usually the first muscle to initiate and maintain low levels of elbow extension force.[36] As extensor effort gradually increases, the medial head of the triceps is usually next in line to join the anconeus.[74] The medial head remains active for most elbow extension movements.[21] The medial head has therefore been termed the "workhorse" of the extensors, functioning as the extensor counterpart to the brachialis.[74]

Only after extensor demands at the elbow increase to moderate-to-high levels does the nervous system recruit the lateral head of the triceps, followed closely by the long head. The long head functions as a "reserve" elbow extensor, equipped with a large volume suited for tasks that require high work performance.

Torque Generation by the Elbow Extensors

The elbow extensor muscles provide static stability to the elbow, similar to the way the quadriceps muscles are often used to stabilize the knee. Consider the common posture of bearing weight through the upper limb with elbows held partially flexed. The extensors stabilize the flexed elbow through isometric contraction or very-low–velocity eccentric activation. In contrast, these same muscles are required to generate much larger and dynamic extensor torques through high-velocity concentric or eccentric activations. Consider activities such as throwing a ball, pushing up from a low chair, or rapidly pushing open a door. As with many explosive pushing activities, elbow extension is typically combined with some degree of shoulder flexion (Figure 6-41). The shoulder

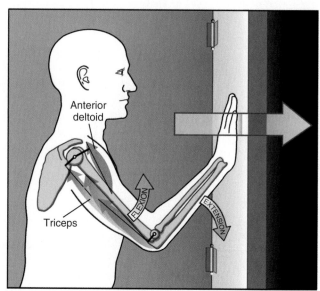

FIGURE 6-41. The triceps muscle is shown generating an extensor torque across the elbow to rapidly push open a door. Note that the elbow is extending as the anterior deltoid is flexing the shoulder. The anterior deltoid must oppose and exceed the shoulder extensor torque produced by the long head of the triceps. See text for further description. The internal moment arms are shown as bold lines originating at the joints' axes of rotation.

SPECIAL FOCUS 6-5

Law of Parsimony

The hierarchic recruitment pattern described by the actions of the various members of the elbow extensors is certainly not the only strategy used by the nervous system to modulate the levels of extensor torque. As with most active movements, the pattern of muscle activation varies greatly from muscle to muscle and from person to person. It appears, however, that a general hierarchic recruitment pattern exists for the elbow extensors. This method of muscle group activation illustrates the *law of parsimony,* a principle alluded to in other works.[40,53] In the present context, the law of parsimony states that the nervous system tends to activate the fewest muscles or muscle fibers possible for the control of a given joint action. Recall that it is the responsibility of the small anconeus and medial head of the triceps to control activities that require lower level extensor torque. Not until more dynamic or highly resisted extensor torque is needed does the

nervous system select the larger, polyarticular, long head of the triceps. This hierarchic pattern of muscle recruitment makes practical sense from an energy perspective. Consider, for example, the inefficiency of having only the long head of the triceps, instead of the anconeus or medial head of the triceps, performing very low level maintenance types of stabilization functions at the elbow. Additional muscular forces would be required from shoulder flexors, assuming gravitation forces are inadequate, to neutralize the undesired shoulder extension potential of the long head of the triceps. A simple task would require greater muscle activity than what is absolutely necessary. As electromyographic evidence and general intuition suggest, tasks with low-level force demands are often accomplished by one-joint muscles. As force demands increase, larger polyarticular muscles are recruited, along with the necessary neutralizer muscles.

flexion function of the anterior deltoid is an important synergistic component of the forward push. The anterior deltoid produces a shoulder flexion torque that drives the limb forward and neutralizes the shoulder extension tendency of the long head of the triceps. From a physiologic perspective, combining shoulder flexion with elbow extension minimizes the rate and amount of shortening required by the long head of the triceps to completely extend the elbow.

The elbow extensor muscles produce maximal-level torque when the elbow is flexed to about 90 degrees.[14,62] This is approximately the same angle at which the elbow flexor muscles, as a group, produce maximum-flexion torque. The 90-degree flexed elbow therefore is the most actively isometric stable position of the joint. Of interest, although both muscle groups produce peak, maximal-effort torques at roughly similar joint angles, the largest internal moment arms for the two groups occur at very different joint angles: about 90 degrees of flexion for the elbow flexors, and near full extension for the triceps and anconeus.[3] Full extension places the thick olecranon process between the joint's axis of rotation and the line of force of the tendon of the triceps (Figure 6-42). The fact that peak elbow extensor torque occurs near 90 degrees of flexion instead of near extension suggests that muscle length, not leverage, is very influential in determining where in the range of motion that peak elbow extension torque naturally occurs.

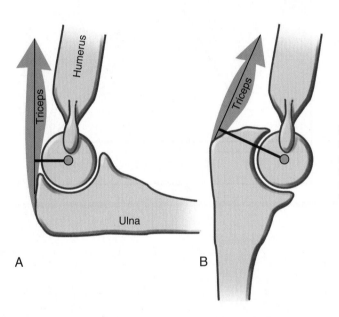

A   B

FIGURE 6-42. The moment arm of the triceps is shown with the elbow flexed to 90 degrees **(A)** and fully extended to near 0 degrees **(B).** The moment arms are shown as thick black lines. Note that the moment arm increases in extension **(B)** because the olecranon process extends the distance between the axis of rotation and the perpendicular intersection with the line of force of the triceps.

SPECIAL FOCUS 6-6

Using Shoulder Muscles to Substitute for Triceps Paralysis

Fractures of the cervical spine may result in C[6] quadriplegia, with loss of motor and sensory function below the C[6] nerve root level. Symptoms may include total paralysis of the trunk and lower extremity muscles with partial paralysis of the upper extremity muscles. Because of the sparing of certain muscles innervated by C[6] and above, persons with this level of quadriplegia may still be able to perform many independent functional activities. Examples are moving up to the sitting position, dressing, and transferring between a wheelchair and bed. Therapists who specialize in mobility training for persons with quadriplegia design movement strategies that allow an innervated muscle to substitute for part of the functional loss imposed by a paralyzed muscle.[52] This art of "muscle substitution" is an essential component to maximizing the movement efficiency in a person with paralysis.

Persons with C[6] quadriplegia have marked or total paralysis of elbow extensors, because these muscles receive most of their nerve root innervation below C[6]. Loss of elbow extension reduces the ability to reach away from the body. Activities such as sitting up in bed or transferring to and from a wheelchair become very difficult and labor intensive. A valuable method of muscle substitution uses innervated proximal shoulder muscles, such as the clavicular head of the pectoralis major and/or the anterior deltoid, to actively extend and lock the elbow (Figure 6-43).[27,30] This ability of a proximal muscle to extend the elbow requires that the hand be firmly fixed distally to some object. Under these circumstances, contraction of the shoulder musculature adducts and/or horizontally flexes the glenohumeral joint, pulling the humerus toward the midline. Controlling the stability of the elbow by using more proximal musculature is a very useful clinical concept. This concept also applies to the lower limb, because the hip extensors are able to extend the knee even in the absence of the quadriceps muscle, as long as the foot is firmly fixed to the ground.

Continued

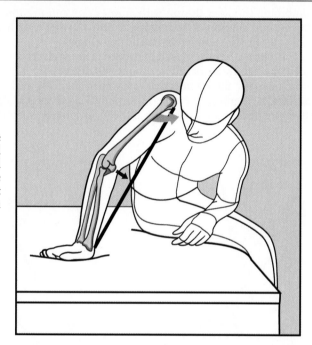

FIGURE 6-43. A depiction of a person with C⁶ quadriplegia using the innervated clavicular portion of the pectoralis major and anterior deltoid *(red arrow)* to pull the humerus toward the midline. With the wrist and hand fixed to the bed, the muscles rotate the elbow into extension. Once locked into extension, the stable elbow allows the entire limb to accept weight without buckling at its middle link. The model in the illustration is assumed to have total paralysis of the triceps.

Function of the Supinator and Pronator Muscles

The lines of force of most pronator and supinator muscles of the forearm are shown in Figure 6-44. In order to be even considered as a pronator or a supinator, a given muscle must possess two fundamental features. *First,* the muscle must attach on both sides of the axis of rotation—that is, a proximal attachment on the humerus or the ulna and a distal attachment on the radius or the hand. Muscles such as the brachialis or extensor pollicis brevis therefore cannot pronate or supinate the forearm, regardless of any other biomechanical variable. *Second,* the muscle must produce a force that acts with an *internal moment arm* around the axis of rotation for pronation and supination. The muscle's moment arm is greatest if its line of force is perpendicular to the axis of rotation. Although no pronator or supinator muscle (at least when considered in the anatomic position) has such an ideal line of force, the pronator quadratus comes very close (see Figure 6-44, *B*).

Pronation and supination of the forearm are functionally associated with internal and external rotation at the shoulder. Shoulder internal rotation often occurs with pronation, whereas shoulder external rotation often occurs with supination. Combining these shoulder and forearm rotations allows the hand to rotate nearly 360 degrees in space, rather than only 170 to 180 degrees by pronation and supination alone. A functional association in strength has also been demonstrated, at least between shoulder external rotation and forearm supination. Supination torques are 9% greater when performed with the shoulder externally rotated as compared with internally rotated.[66] The mechanism for this difference

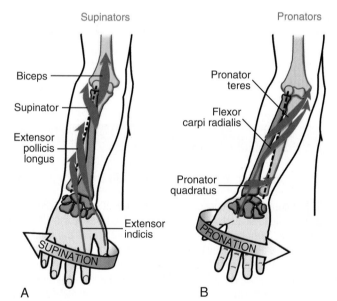

FIGURE 6-44. The line of force of supinators **(A)** and pronators **(B)** of the forearm. Note the degree to which all muscles intersect the forearm's axis of rotation *(dashed line)*.

is not clear but may involve the biceps muscle—the primary supinator of the forearm. External rotation may elongate the long head of the biceps slightly as its tendon crosses the humeral head, thereby augmenting the muscle's force-generating ability.

When forearm muscle strength and range of motion are tested clinically, care must be taken to eliminate contributing motion or torque that has originated from the shoulder. To accomplish this, forearm pronation and supination are tested with the elbow held flexed to 90 degrees, with the medial epicondyle of the humerus pressed against the side of the body. In this position any undesired rotation at the shoulder is easily detected.

SUPINATOR MUSCLES

The primary supinator muscles are the *supinator* and *biceps brachii*.[9] Secondary muscles with a limited potential to supinate are the radial wrist extensors, which attach near the lateral epicondyle of the humerus, the extensor pollicis longus, and the extensor indicis (see Figure 6-44, *A*). The brachioradialis is considered a secondary supinator *and* a secondary pronator, especially during short-arc, high-power motions.[6,15,21] Regardless of the position of the forearm, contraction of the brachioradialis rotates the forearm *to* the neutral, thumb-up position.[9] From a fully pronated position, therefore, the muscle supinates; from a fully supinated position, the muscle pronates. Of interest, contraction of the brachioradialis biases the forearm toward a position that maximizes its moment arm as an elbow flexor.

Primary Supinator Muscles
- Supinator
- Biceps brachii

Secondary Supinator Muscles
- Radial wrist extensors
- Extensor pollicis longus
- Extensor indicis
- Brachioradialis (from a pronated position)

Supinator versus Biceps Brachii

The *supinator muscle* has an extensive proximal muscle attachment (Figure 6-45). A superficial set of fibers arises from the lateral epicondyle of the humerus and the radial collateral and annular ligaments. A deeper set of fibers arises from the ulna near and along the supinator crest. Both sets of muscle fibers attach distally along the proximal one third of the radius. From a pronated position, the supinator is twisted and elongated around the radius and therefore is in excellent position to supinate the forearm. The supinator has only minimal attachments to the humerus and passes too close to the medial-lateral axis of rotation at the elbow to produce significant flexion or extension torque.

The supinator muscle is a relentless forearm supinator, similar to the brachialis during elbow flexion. The supinator muscle generates significant EMG activity during forearm supination, regardless of the elbow angle or the speed or power of the action.[75] The biceps muscle, also a primary supinator, is normally recruited during higher power supination activities, especially those associated with elbow flexion.

The nervous system usually recruits the supinator muscle for low-power tasks that require a supination motion only,

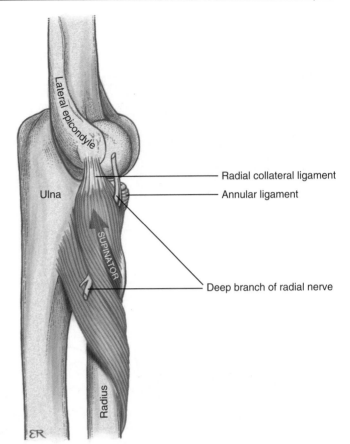

FIGURE 6-45. A lateral view of the right supinator muscle. The deep branch of the radial nerve is shown exiting between the superficial and deep fibers of the muscle. The radial nerve courses distally, as the posterior interosseous nerve, to innervate the finger and thumb extensors.

while the biceps remains relatively inactive. (This is in accord with the law of parsimony described earlier in this chapter.) Only during moderate- or high-power supination motions does the biceps show significant EMG activity. Using the large polyarticular biceps to perform a simple, low-power supination task is not an efficient motor response. Additional muscles, such as the triceps and posterior deltoid, would be required to neutralize any undesired biceps action at the shoulder and elbow. A simple movement then becomes increasingly more complicated and more energy-consuming than necessary.

The *biceps brachii* is a powerful supinator muscle of the forearm. The biceps has about three times the physiologic cross-sectional area as the supinator muscle.[37] The dominant role of the biceps as a supinator can be verified by palpating the biceps during a series of rapid and forceful pronation-to-supination motions, especially with the elbow flexed to 90 degrees. As the forearm is pronated, the biceps tendon wraps around the proximal radius. From a fully pronated position, active contraction of the biceps "spins" the radius sharply into supination.

The effectiveness of the biceps as a supinator is greatest when the elbow is flexed to about 90 degrees.[9] For this reason, the elbow is naturally held flexed to about 90 degrees during many high-powered supination tasks. At a 90-degree elbow

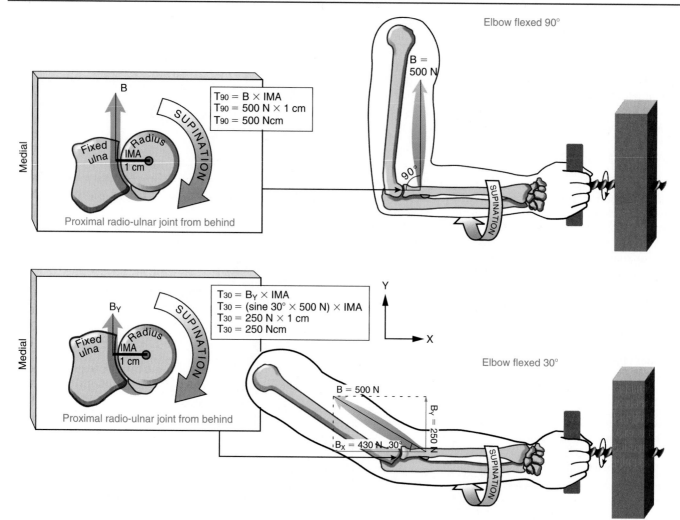

FIGURE 6-46. The difference in the mechanical ability of the biceps to produce a supination torque is illustrated when the elbow is flexed 90 degrees and when the elbow is flexed 30 degrees. *Top,* Lateral view shows the biceps attaching to the radius at a 90-degree angle. The muscle *(B)* is contracting to supinate the forearm with a maximal-effort force of 500 N. As shown from a superior view, 100% of the biceps force can be multiplied by the estimated 1-cm internal moment arm available for supination, producing 500 Ncm of torque (500 N × 1 cm). *Bottom,* Lateral view shows that when the elbow is flexed to 30 degrees, the angle-of-insertion of the biceps to the radius is reduced to about 30 degrees. This change in angle reduces the force that the biceps can use to supinate (i.e., that generated perpendicular to the radius) to 250 N *(B$_Y$)*. An even larger force component of the biceps, labeled B$_X$, is directed proximally through the radius in a direction nearly parallel with the forearm's axis of rotation. This force component has essentially no moment arm to supinate. The calculations show that the maximum supination torque with the elbow flexed 30 degrees is reduced to 250 Ncm (250 N × 1 cm) (sine 30 degrees = 0.5, and cosine 30 degrees = 0.86).

angle, the tendon of the biceps approaches a 90-degree angle-of-insertion into the radius. This biomechanical situation allows the *entire* magnitude of a maximal-effort biceps force to intersect nearly perpendicular to the axis of rotation of the forearm. When the elbow is flexed to only 30 degrees, for example, the tendon of the biceps loses its right-angle intersection with the axis of rotation. As depicted by the calculations shown in Figure 6-46, this change in angle reduces the mechanical supinator torque potential of the biceps by 50%. Clinically, this difference is important during evaluation of the torque output from a strength-testing apparatus or when providing advice about ergonomics.

When high-power supination torque is required to vigorously turn a screw, for example, the biceps is recruited by the nervous system to assist other muscles, such as the smaller supinator muscle and extensor pollicis longus. For reasons described previously, this task typically requires that the elbow be held flexed to about 90 degrees (Figure 6-47). Maintaining this elbow posture during the task requires that the triceps muscle co-contract synchronously with the biceps muscle. The triceps muscle supplies an essential force during this activity because it prevents the biceps from actually flexing the elbow and shoulder during every supination effort. Unopposed biceps action causes the screwdriver to be pulled away from the screw on every effort—hardly effective. By attaching to the ulna versus the radius, the triceps is able to neutralize the elbow flexion tendency of the biceps *without* interfering with the supination task. This muscular coopera-

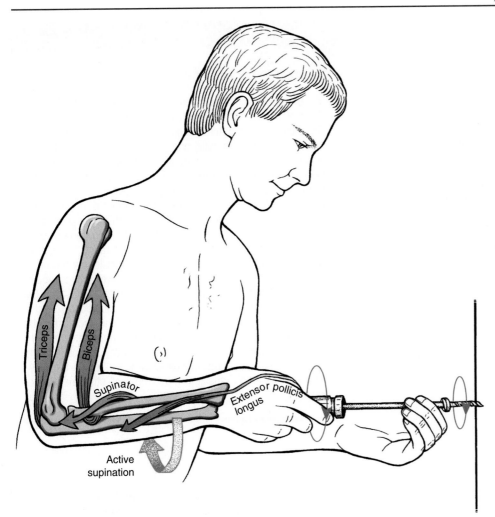

Triceps

Biceps

Supinator

Extensor pollicis longus

Active supination

FIGURE 6-47. Vigorous contraction is shown of the right biceps, supinator, and extensor pollicis longus muscles to tighten a screw using a clockwise rotation with a screwdriver. The triceps muscle is activated isometrically to neutralize the strong elbow flexion tendency of the biceps.

tion is an excellent example of how two muscles can function as synergists for one activity while at the same time remaining as direct antagonists.

PRONATOR MUSCLES

The primary muscles for pronation are the *pronator teres* and the *pronator quadratus* (Figure 6-48). The flexor carpi radialis and the palmaris longus are secondary pronators, both attaching to the medial epicondyle of the humerus (see Figure 6-44, *B*).

Primary Pronator Muscles
- Pronator teres
- Pronator quadratus

Secondary Pronator Muscles
- Flexor carpi radialis
- Palmaris longus
- Brachioradialis (from a supinated position)

SPECIAL FOCUS 6-7

Supination versus Pronation Torque Potential

As a group, the supinators produce about 25% greater isometric torque than the pronators (see Table 6-6). This difference is partially explained by the fact that the supinator muscles possess about twice the physiologic cross-sectional area as the pronator muscles.[37] Many functional activities rely on the relative strength of supination. Consider the activity of using a screwdriver to tighten a screw. When performed by the right hand, a clockwise tightening motion is driven by a concentric contraction of the supinator muscles. The direction of the threads on a standard screw reflects the dominance in strength of the supinator muscles. Unfortunately for the left-hand dominant person, a clockwise rotation of the left forearm must be performed by the *pronator muscles*. Left-handed persons often use the right hand for this activity, explaining why so many are somewhat ambidextrous.

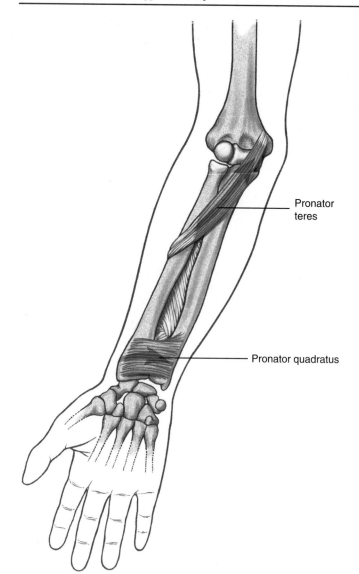

FIGURE 6-48. Anterior view of the right pronator teres and pronator quadratus.

Pronator Teres versus Pronator Quadratus

The *pronator teres* has two heads: humeral and ulnar. The median nerve passes between these two heads and therefore is a site for possible nerve compression.[64] The pronator teres functions as a primary forearm pronator, as well as an elbow flexor. The pronator teres produces its greatest EMG activity during higher-power pronation actions,[7] such as attempting to unscrew an overtightened screw with the right hand or pitching a baseball. The triceps is an important synergist to the pronator teres, often required to neutralize the ability of the pronator teres to flex the elbow.

In cases of median nerve injury proximal to the elbow, all pronator muscles are paralyzed, and active pronation is essentially lost. The forearm tends to remain chronically supinated owing to the unopposed action of the innervated supinator and biceps muscles.

The *pronator quadratus* is located at the extreme distal end of the anterior forearm, deep to all the wrist flexors and extrinsic finger flexors. This flat, quadrilateral muscle attaches

between the anterior surfaces of the distal one quarter of the ulna and the radius. Overall, from proximal to distal, the pronator quadratus has a slight obliquity in fiber direction, similar to, but not quite as angled as, the pronator teres. The pronator quadratus is the most active and consistently used pronator muscle, involved during all pronation movements, regardless of the power demands or the amount of associated elbow flexion.[7]

The pronator quadratus is well designed biomechanically as an effective torque producer and a stabilizer of the distal radio-ulnar joint.[25,72] The pronator quadratus has a line of force oriented almost perpendicular to the forearm's axis of rotation (Figure 6-49, *A*). This design maximizes the potential of the muscle to produce a torque. In addition to effectively producing a pronation torque, the muscle simultaneously compresses the ulnar notch of the radius directly against the ulnar head (see Figure 6-49, *B*). This compression force stabilizes the distal radio-ulnar joint throughout the range of pronation (see Figure 6-49, *C*). This active force augments the passive force produced by the triangular fibrocartilage complex. The force of the pronator quadratus also guides the joint through its natural arthrokinematics.

In the healthy joint, the compression force from the pronator quadratus and other muscles is absorbed by the joint without difficulty. In cases of severe rheumatoid arthritis, the articular cartilage, bone, and periarticular connective tissue lose their ability to adequately absorb joint forces. These myogenic compressive forces can become detrimental to joint stability. The same forces that help stabilize the joint in the healthy state may cause joint destruction in the diseased state.

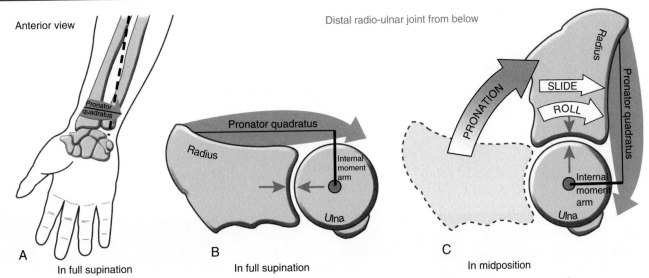

FIGURE 6-49. A, Anterior view of the distal radio-ulnar joint shows the line of force of the pronator quadratus intersecting the forearm's axis of rotation *(dashed line)* at a near right angle. **B,** The line of force of the pronator quadratus, with its internal moment arm, is shown with the carpal bones removed and forearm in full supination. The pronator quadratus produces a pronation torque, which is the product of the pronator muscle's force times the internal moment arm, *and* a compression force between the joint surfaces *(opposing arrows)*. **C,** This dual function of the pronator quadratus is shown as the muscle pronates the forearm to the midposition. The roll-and-slide arthrokinematics are also indicated.

SYNOPSIS

The shape of the proximal and distal ends of the radius and ulna provides insightful clues to the kinesiology of the regions. The large, C-shaped *proximal end of the ulna* provides a rigid, hingelike stability to the humero-ulnar joint. The kinematics therefore are limited primarily to the sagittal plane. The rounded head of the *distal end of the ulna* articulates with the concave ulnar notch of the radius to form the distal radio-ulnar joint. Unlike the distal end of the radius, the distal ulna is *not* firmly articulated with the carpal bones. Any firm connection in this region would physically restrict pronation and supination.

The *proximal end of the radius* possesses a disclike head designed primarily to rotate against the capitulum and within the fibro-osseous ring of the proximal radio-ulnar joint. This rotation of the radius is the main kinematic component of pronation and supination. The ulna, in contrast, serves as a stable base for the rotating radius by virtue of its firm linkage to the humerus via the humero-ulnar joint. The relatively large *distal end of the radius* expands in both medial-lateral and anterior-posterior dimensions to accept the proximal row of carpal bones. This expanded surface area provides an excellent path for transmission of forces through the hand to the radius. Based on the prevailing fiber direction of the interosseous membrane, proximally directed forces acting on the radius are ultimately transmitted nearly equally across both medial and lateral compartments of the elbow.

Four major peripheral nerves cross the elbow: musculocutaneous, median, radial, and ulnar. With the exception of the musculocutaneous nerve, these nerves are injured with relative frequency, causing marked loss of sensory and muscle function distal to the site of trauma. Reduced muscular forces resulting from injury to any one of these nerves create a kinetic imbalance across the joints, which, if untreated, typically lead to deformity.

Essentially all muscles acting on the elbow and forearm have their distal attachment on either the ulna or the radius. Those muscles that attach to the *ulna*—namely the brachialis and triceps—flex or extend the elbow but have no ability to pronate or supinate the forearm. The remaining muscles, in contrast, have their distal attachment on the *radius*. These muscles flex the elbow and, depending on their line of force, also pronate or supinate the forearm. This anatomic arrangement allows the elbow to actively flex and extend while allowing the forearm to simultaneously pronate or supinate without any mechanical interference among muscles. This design greatly enhances the ability of the upper extremity to interact with the surrounding environment, during activities that range from feeding, grooming, or preparing food to grosser actions such as thrusting the body upwards from a chair.

About half of the muscles studied in this chapter control multiple regions of the arm or forearm. For this reason, movements that appear quite simple and limited to just one region—such as the forearm, for example—are typically more complex and involve a larger than expected set of participating muscles. Reconsider the forceful biceps-driven supination action required to tighten a screw (previously highlighted in Figure 6-47). During this task, triceps activation is also required to neutralize the strong (and unwanted) elbow flexion component of the biceps. The co-contraction of the long head of the biceps and triceps muscles must also kinetically balance and stabilize the glenohumeral joint. In addition, axial-scapular muscles, such as the trapezius, rhomboids, and serratus anterior, are needed to stabilize the scapula against the strong pull of the biceps and triceps muscles. Without this stabilization—be it from selective nerve injury, loss of motor control, pain, or simple disuse—the muscles of the elbow and forearm are less effective at performing their tasks.

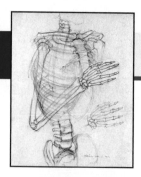

ADDITIONAL CLINICAL CONNECTIONS

CLINICAL CONNECTION 6-1
"Reverse Action" of the Elbow Flexor Muscles

During most typical activities of daily living, contraction of the elbow flexor muscles is performed to rotate the forearm toward the arm. Contraction of the same muscles, however, can rotate the arm *to* the forearm, provided that the distal aspect of the upper extremity is well fixed. A clinical example of the usefulness of such a "reverse contraction" of the elbow flexors is shown for a person with C^6 quadriplegia (Figure 6-50). The person has complete paralysis of the trunk and lower extremity muscles but near-normal strength of the shoulder, elbow flexor, and wrist extensor muscles. With the distal aspect of the upper limb well fixed with

the assistance of the wrist extensor muscles and a strap, the elbow flexor muscles can generate sufficient force to rotate the arm toward the forearm. This maneuver allows the elbow flexor muscles to assist the person in moving up to a sitting position. For this person, coming up to a sitting position is an essential step in preparing for other functional activities, such as dressing or transferring from the bed into a wheelchair.

Of interest, the arthrokinematics at the humero-ulnar joint during this action involve a roll and slide in *opposite* directions.

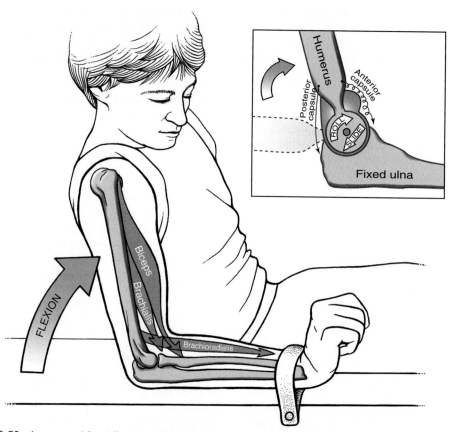

FIGURE 6-50. A person with midlevel quadriplegia (tetraplegia) using his elbow flexor muscles to flex the elbow and bring his trunk off the mat. Note that the distal forearm is securely stabilized. *Inset,* The arthrokinematics at the humero-ulnar joint are shown during this movement. The anterior capsule is in a slackened position, and the posterior capsule is taut.

ADDITIONAL CLINICAL CONNECTIONS

CLINICAL CONNECTION 6-2
The "Lap Test": a Specialized Clinical Test of the Innervation Status of the Supinator Muscle

The radial nerve spirals obliquely around the posterior side of the humerus within the shallow radial groove of the humerus (see Figure 6-32, *B*). Fractures or other trauma to the humerus in this region of the bone often injure the radial nerve. If the injury is severe enough, all radial nerve–innervated muscles distal to the site of injury may be paralyzed. The paralysis may be extensive, including the triceps, anconeus, brachioradialis, wrist extensor group, supinator, and all extrinsic extensor muscles to the digits. Loss of normal sensation typically includes the skin of the dorsal surface of the arm, most notably that covering the dorsal web space of the hand.

Because of the potential for regeneration of an injured peripheral nerve, the muscles may, in time, recover from the paralysis in an orderly proximal-to-distal fashion. Clues to whether the nerve has regenerated can be gained through electrophysiologic testing, in conjunction with palpation and manual testing of the strength of the affected musculature. One key muscle in this regard is the supinator muscle (see Figure 6-45); reinnervation of this muscle would strongly suggest that the radial nerve has regenerated distally to the proximal forearm. The deep lying supinator muscle, however, is difficult to palpate or isolate from other surrounding muscles.

Based on the law of parsimony, a clinical test exists that may help determine the function of the supinator muscle in cases in which reinnervation is suspected. The "lap test," as it is sometimes called, requires the patient to support the forearm on the lap and *very slowly* supinate the forearm, free of any external resistance. Normally, with adequate practice, this very-low–power supination can be performed without, or with very little, activation of the biceps. (You may want to practice this on yourself). If the supinator muscle is innervated and functioning, the patient will usually be able to supinate *without* an accompanying contraction of the biceps. If, however, the supinator muscle is still paralyzed, even slow, low-power supination effort causes the biceps tendon to stand out sharply as it contracts to compensate for supinator muscle paralysis. Exaggerated biceps response to a very-low–level supination task is a positive "lap test" result, suggesting marked weakness in the supinator muscle.

Although the predictive validity of this test is unknown, the test does nevertheless show an example of applying kinesiologic and anatomic knowledge to clinical practice.

REFERENCES

1. Ahrens PM, Redfern DR, Forester AJ: Patterns of articular wear in the cadaveric elbow joint, *J Shoulder Elbow Surg* 10:52-56, 2001.
2. Amis AA, Dowson D, Wright V: Elbow joint force predictions for some strenuous isometric actions, *J Biomech* 13:765-775, 1980.
3. An KN, Hui FC, Morrey BF, et al: Muscles across the elbow joint: a biomechanical analysis. *J Biomech* 14:659-669, 1981.
4. Askew LJ, An KN, Morrey BF, Chao EY: Isometric elbow strength in normal individuals, *Clin Orthop Relat Res* 222:261-266, 1987.
5. Baeyens JP, Van GF, Goossens M, et al: In vivo 3D arthrokinematics of the proximal and distal radioulnar joints during active pronation and supination, *Clin Biomech (Bristol, Avon)* 21(Suppl 1):S9-S12, 2006.
6. Basmajian JV, Latif A: Integrated actions and functions of the chief flexors of the elbow: A detailed electromyographic analysis, *J Bone Joint Surg Am* 39:1106-1118, 1957.
7. Basmajian JV, Travill A: Electromyography of the pronator muscles of the forearm, *Anat Rec* 139:45-49, 1961.
8. Bozkurt M, Acar HI, Apaydin N, et al: The annular ligament: an anatomical study, *Am J Sports Med* 33:114-118, 2005.
9. Bremer AK, Sennwald GR, Favre P, Jacob HA: Moment arms of forearm rotators, *Clin Biomech (Bristol, Avon)* 21:683-691, 2006.
10. Callaway GH, Field LD, Deng XH, et al: Biomechanical evaluation of the medial collateral ligament of the elbow, *J Bone Joint Surg Am* 79:1223-1231, 1997.
11. Chang CW, Wang YC, Chu CH: Increased carrying angle is a risk factor for nontraumatic ulnar neuropathy at the elbow, *Clin Orthop Relat Res* 466:2190-2195, 2008.
12. Cohen MS, Bruno RJ: The collateral ligaments of the elbow: Anatomy and clinical correlation, *Clin Orthop Relat Res* 383:123-130, 2001.
13. Cooney WP: Reconstructive procedures of the elbow: Joint replacement arthroplasty. In Morrey BF, editor: *The elbow and its disorders*, ed 3, Philadelphia, 2000, Saunders.
14. Currier DP: Maximal isometric tension of the elbow extensors at varied positions. I. Assessment by cable tensiometer, *Phys Ther* 52:1043-1049, 1972.
15. de Sousa OM, de Moraes JL, Vieira FL: Electromyographic study of the brachioradialis muscle, *Anat Rec* 139:125-131, 1961.
16. DeFrate LE, Li G, Zayontz SJ, Herndon JH: A minimally invasive method for the determination of force in the interosseous ligament, *Clin Biomech (Bristol, Avon)* 16:895-900, 2001.
17. DiTano O, Trumble TE, Tencer AF: Biomechanical function of the distal radioulnar and ulnocarpal wrist ligaments, *J Hand Surg [Am]* 28:622-627, 2003.
18. Dugas JR, Ostrander RV, Cain EL, et al: Anatomy of the anterior bundle of the ulnar collateral ligament, *J Shoulder Elbow Surg* 16:657-660, 2007.
19. Dunning CE, Zarzour ZD, Patterson SD, et al: Ligamentous stabilizers against posterolateral rotatory instability of the elbow, *J Bone Joint Surg Am* 83:1823-1828, 2001.
20. Ekenstam F, Hagert CG: Anatomical studies on the geometry and stability of the distal radio ulnar joint, *Scand J Plastic Reconstruct Surg* 19:17-25, 1985.
21. Funk DA, An KN, Morrey BF, Daube JR: Electromyographic analysis of muscles across the elbow joint, *J Orthop Res* 5:529-538, 1987.
22. Gabl M, Zimmermann R, Angermann P, et al: The interosseous membrane and its influence on the distal radioulnar joint. An anatomical investigation of the distal tract, *J Hand Surg [Br]* 23:179-182, 1998.
23. Gallagher MA, Cuomo F, Polonsky L, et al: Effects of age, testing speed, and arm dominance on isokinetic strength of the elbow, *J Shoulder Elbow Surg* 6:340-346, 1997.
24. Gallay SH, Richards RR, O'Driscoll SW: Intraarticular capacity and compliance of stiff and normal elbows, *Arthroscopy* 9:9-13, 1993.
25. Garcia-Elias M: Soft-tissue anatomy and relationships about the distal ulna, *Hand Clin* 14:165-176, 1998.
26. Geel CW, Palmer AK: Radial head fractures and their effect on the distal radioulnar joint. A rationale for treatment, *Clin Orthop Relat Res* 275:79-84, 1992.
27. Gefen JY, Gelmann AS, Herbison GJ, et al: Use of shoulder flexors to achieve isometric elbow extension in C6 tetraplegic patients during weight shift, *Spinal Cord* 35:308-313, 1997.
28. Gordon KD, Kedgley AE, Ferreira LM, et al: Effect of simulated muscle activity on distal radioulnar joint loading in vitro, *J Orthop Res* 24:1395-1404, 2006.
29. Hargreaves D, Emery R: Total elbow replacement in the treatment of rheumatoid disease, *Clin Orthop Relat Res* 366:61-71, 1999.
30. Hoffmann G, Laffont I, Hanneton S, Roby-Brami A: How to extend the elbow with a weak or paralyzed triceps: Control of arm kinematics for aiming in C6-C7 quadriplegic patients, *Neuroscience* 139:749-765, 2006.
31. Hollister AM, Gellman H, Waters RL: The relationship of the interosseous membrane to the axis of rotation of the forearm, *Clin Orthop Relat Res* 298: 272-276, 1994.
32. Hotchkiss RN, An KN, Sowa DT, et al: An anatomic and mechanical study of the interosseous membrane of the forearm: pathomechanics of proximal migration of the radius, *J Hand Surg [Am]* 14:256-261, 1989.
33. Inman VT, Saunders JB: Referred pain from skeletal structures, *J Nerv Ment Dis* 99:660-667, 1944.
34. Ishii S, Palmer AK, Werner FW, et al: An anatomic study of the ligamentous structure of the triangular fibrocartilage complex, *J Hand Surg [Am]* 23:977-985, 1998.
35. Kleinman WB, Graham TJ: The distal radioulnar joint capsule: Clinical anatomy and role in posttraumatic limitation of forearm rotation, *J Hand Surg [Am]* 23:588-599, 1998.
36. Le Bozec S, Maton B, Cnockaert JC: The synergy of elbow extensor muscles during static work in man, *Eur J Appli Physiol Occup Physiol* 43:57-68, 1980.
37. Lehmkuhl LD, Smith LK: *Brunnstrom's clinical kinesiology*, ed 4, Philadelphia, 1983, FA Davis.
38. Lin F, Kohli N, Perlmutter S, et al: Muscle contribution to elbow joint valgus stability, *J Shoulder Elbow Surg* 16:795-802, 2007.
39. Lindau T, Adlercreutz C, Aspenberg P: Peripheral tears of the triangular fibrocartilage complex cause distal radioulnar joint instability after distal radial fractures, *J Hand Surg [Am]* 25:464-468, 2000.
40. MacConaill MA, Basmajian JV: *Muscles and movements: a basis for human kinesiology*, New York, 1977, Robert E. Krieger.
41. Mandelbaum BR, Silvers HJ, Watanabe DS, et al: Effectiveness of a neuromuscular and proprioceptive training program in preventing anterior cruciate ligament injuries in female athletes: 2-year follow-up, *Am J Sports Med* 33:1003-1010, 2005.
42. Manson TT, Pfaeffle HJ, Herdon JH, et al: Forearm rotation alters interosseous ligament strain distribution, *J Hand Surg [Am]* 25:1058-1063, 2000.
43. Matei CI, Logigian EL, Shefner JM: Evaluation of patients with recurrent symptoms after ulnar nerve transposition, *Muscle Nerve* 30:493-496, 2004.
44. Miyasaka KC: Anatomy of the elbow, *Orthop Clin North Am* 30:1-13, 1999.
45. Morrey BF: Radial head fracture. In Morrey BF, editor: *The elbow and its disorders*, ed 3, Philadelphia, 2000, Saunders.
46. Morrey BF, An KN, Stormont TJ: Force transmission through the radial head, *J Bone Joint Surg [Am]* 70:250-256, 1988.
47. Morrey BF, Askew LJ, Chao EY: A biomechanical study of normal functional elbow motion, *J Bone Joint Surg [Am]* 63:872-877, 1981.
48. Morrey BF, Chao EY: Passive motion of the elbow joint, *J Bone Joint Surg [Am]* 58:501-508, 1976.
49. Morrey BF, Tanaka S, An KN: Valgus stability of the elbow. A definition of primary and secondary constraints, *Clin Orthop Relat Res* Apr:187-195, 1991.
50. Murray WM, Delp SL, Buchanan TS: Variation of muscle moment arms with elbow and forearm position, *J Biomech* 28:513-525, 1995.
51. Nakamura T, Yabe Y, Horiuchi Y: Dynamic changes in the shape of the triangular fibrocartilage complex during rotation demonstrated with high resolution magnetic resonance imaging, *J Hand Surg [Br]* 24:338-341, 1999.
52. Neumann DA: Use of diaphragm to assist rolling for the patient with quadriplegia, *Phys Ther* 59:39, 1979.
53. Neumann DA, Soderberg GL, Cook TM: Electromyographic analysis of hip abductor musculature in healthy right-handed persons, *Phys Ther* 69:431-440, 1989.
54. O'Driscoll SW, Jupiter JB, King GJ, et al: The unstable elbow, *Instr Course Lect* 50:89-102, 2001.
55. Ofuchi S, Takahashi K, Yamagata M, et al: Pressure distribution in the humeroradial joint and force transmission to the capitulum during rotation of the forearm: Effects of the Sauve-Kapandji procedure and incision of the interosseous membrane, *J Orthop Sci* 6:33-38, 2001.
56. Olsen BS, Søjbjerg JO, Dalstra M, Sneppen O: Kinematics of the lateral ligamentous constraints of the elbow joint, *J Shoulder Elbow Surg* 5:333-341, 1996.
57. Palmer AK, Werner FW: Biomechanics of the distal radioulnar joint, *Clin Orthop Relat Res* 187:26-35, 1984.

58. Paraskevas G, Papadopoulos A, Papaziogas B, et al: Study of the carrying angle of the human elbow joint in full extension: A morphometric analysis, *Surg Radiol Anat* 26:19-23, 2004.

59. Petrie S, Collins JG, Solomonow M, et al: Mechanoreceptors in the human elbow ligaments, *J Hand Surg [Am]* 23:512-518, 1998.

60. Pfaeffle HJ, Fischer KJ, Manson TT, et al: Role of the forearm interosseous ligament: Is it more than just longitudinal load transfer? *J Hand Surg [Am]* 25:683-688, 2000.

61. Pfaeffle HJ, Tomaino MM, Grewal R, et al: Tensile properties of the interosseous membrane of the human forearm, *J Orthop Res* 14:842-845, 1996.

62. Provins K.A., Salter N: Maximum torque exerted about the elbow joint, *J Appl Physiol* 7:393-398, 1955.

63. Regan WD, Korinek SL, Morrey BF, et al: Biomechanical study of ligaments around the elbow joint, *Clin Orthop Relat Res* 271:170-179, 1991.

64. Rehak DC: Pronator syndrome, *Clin Sports Med* 20:531-540, 2001.

65. Sabick MB, Torry MR, Lawton RL, Hawkins RJ: Valgus torque in youth baseball pitchers: A biomechanical study, *J Shoulder Elbow Surg* 13:349-355, 2004.

66. Savva N, McAllen CJ, Giddins GE: The relationship between the strength of supination of the forearm and rotation of the shoulder, *J Bone Joint Surg Br* 85:406-407, 2003.

67. Schuind F, An KN, Berglund L, et al: The distal radioulnar ligaments: a biomechanical study, *J Hand Surg [Am]* 16:1106-1114, 1991.

68. Schuind FA, Goldschmidt D, Bastin C, Burny F: A biomechanical study of the ulnar nerve at the elbow, *J Hand Surg [Br]* 20:623-627, 1995.

69. Skahen JR 3rd, Palmer AK, Werner FW, Fortino MD: The interosseous membrane of the forearm: anatomy and function, *J Hand Surg [Am]* 22:981-985, 1997.

70. Standring S: *Gray's anatomy: the anatomical basis of clinical practice*, ed 40, St Louis, 2009, Elsevier.

71. Stokdijk M, Meskers CG, Veeger HE, et al: Determination of the optimal elbow axis for evaluation of placement of prostheses, *Clin Biomech* 14:177-184, 1999.

72. Stuart PR. Pronator quadratus revisited, *J Hand Surg [Br]* 21:714-722, 1996.

73. Topp KS, Boyd BS: Structure and biomechanics of peripheral nerves: Nerve responses to physical stresses and implications for physical therapist practice, *Phys Ther* 86:92-109, 2006.

74. Travill A: Electromyographic study of the extensor apparatus, *Anat Rec* 144:373-376, 1962.

75. Travill A., Basmajian JV: Electromyography of the supinators of the forearm, *Anat Rec* 139:557-560, 1961.

76. Tsunoda N, O'Hagan F, Sale DG, MacDougall JD: Elbow flexion strength curves in untrained men and women and male bodybuilders, *Eur J Appl Physiol Occup Physiol* 66:235-239, 1993.

77. van Andel CJ, Wolterbeek N, Doorenbosch CA, et al: Complete 3D kinematics of upper extremity functional tasks, *Gait Posture* 27:120-127, 2008.

78. Van der Heijden EP, Hillen B: A two-dimensional kinematic analysis of the distal radioulnar joint, *J Hand Surg [Br]* 21:824-829, 1996.

79. Vardakas DG, Varitimidis SE, Goebel F, et al: Evaluating and treating the stiff elbow, *Hand Clin* 18:77-85, 2002.

80. Ward LD, Ambrose CG, Masson MV, Levaro F.: The role of the distal radioulnar ligaments, interosseous membrane, and joint capsule in distal radioulnar joint stability, *J Hand Surg [Am]* 25:341-351, 2000.

81. Watanabe H, Berger RA, An KN et al. Stability of the distal radioulnar joint contributed by the joint capsule, *J Hand Surg [Am]* 29:1114-1120, 2004.

82. Watanabe H, Berger RA, Berglund LJ, et al: Contribution of the interosseous membrane to distal radioulnar joint constraint, *J Hand Surg [Am]* 30:1164-1171, 2005.

83. Williams RJ III, Urquhart ER, Altchek DW: Medial collateral ligament tears in the throwing athlete, *Instr Course Lect* 53:579-586, 2004.

84. Winters JM, Kleweno DG: Effect of initial upper-limb alignment on muscle contributions to isometric strength curves, *J Biomech* 26:143-153, 1993.

85. Yilmaz E, Karakurt L, Belhan O, et al: Variation of carrying angle with age, sex, and special reference to side, *Orthopedics* 28:1360-1363, 2005.

STUDY QUESTIONS

1 List both muscular and nonmuscular tissues that are able to resist a distal pull (distraction) of the radius.

2 Describe how the different fibers of the medial collateral ligament of the elbow provide useful tension throughout the *entire* range of flexion and extension.

3 Describe the arthrokinematics at the humeroradial joint during a combined motion of elbow flexion and supination of the forearm.

4 Based on moment arm alone, which tissue shown in Figure 6-18, *A* could generate the greatest resistive torque opposing an elbow extension movement?

5 How many nerves innervate muscles that flex the elbow?

6 Based on data provided in Table 6-7, which head of the triceps produces the greatest elbow extension torque?

7 Why was the extensor pollicis brevis muscle *not* included in this chapter as a secondary supinator muscle of the forearm?

8 What is the kinesiologic role of the anterior deltoid during a "pushing" motion that combines elbow extension and shoulder flexion?

9 What muscle is the most direct antagonist to the brachialis muscle?

10 A patient has a 10-degree elbow flexion contracture that is assumed to originate because of muscular tightness. At the patient's end range of extension, you apply an extension torque and note that the forearm passively "drifts" into supination. What clue does this observation provide as to which muscle or muscles are most tight (stiff)?

11 How would a radial nerve lesion in the axilla affect the task depicted in Figure 6-47?

12 What position of the upper extremity maximally elongates the biceps brachii muscle?

13 Why would a surgeon be concerned about the integrity of the interosseous membrane prior to a radial head resection?

14 A patient has a median nerve injury at the level of the middle of the humerus. Would you expect any weakness in active flexion of the elbow? Over time, what deformity or "tightness pattern" is most likely to develop at the forearm?

15 Assume you want to maximally stretch (elongate) the brachialis muscle by passively extending the elbow. Would the effectiveness of the stretch be enhanced by combining full passive pronation or supination of the forearm to the elbow extension?

⊖ *Answers to the study questions can be found on the Evolve website.*

Wrist

DONALD A. NEUMANN, PT, PhD, FAPTA

CHAPTER AT A GLANCE

The wrist, or carpus, contains eight carpal bones that, as a group, act as a functional "spacer" between the forearm and hand. In addition to numerous small intercarpal joints, the wrist consists of two primary articulations: the radiocarpal and midcarpal joints (Figure 7-1). The *radiocarpal joint* is located between the distal end of the radius and the proximal row of carpal bones. Just distal to this joint is the *midcarpal joint,* joining the proximal and distal rows of carpal bones. The two joints allow the wrist to flex and extend and to move from side to side in motions called radial and ulnar deviation. The nearby distal radio-ulnar joint is considered part of the forearm complex rather than the wrist because of its role in pronation and supination (see Chapter 6).

The position of the wrist significantly affects the function of the hand. This is because many muscles that control the digits originate extrinsic to the hand, with their proximal attachments located in the forearm. A painful, unstable, or weak wrist often assumes a position that interferes with the optimal length and passive tension of the extrinsic musculature, thereby reducing the effectiveness of grasp.

Several new terms are introduced here to describe the relative position, or topography, within the wrist and the hand.

Palmar and *volar* are synonymous with *anterior; dorsal* is synonymous with *posterior.* These terms are used interchangeably throughout this chapter and the next chapter on the hand.

OSTEOLOGY

Distal Forearm

The dorsal surface of the distal radius has several grooves and raised areas that help guide or stabilize the tendons that course toward the wrist and hand (Figure 7-2). For example, the palpable *dorsal (Lister's) tubercle* separates the tendon of the extensor carpi radialis brevis from the tendon of the extensor pollicis longus.

The palmar or volar surface of the distal radius is the location of the proximal attachments of the wrist capsule and the thick palmar radiocarpal ligaments (Figure 7-3, *A*). The *styloid process of the radius* projects distally from the lateral side of the radius. The *styloid process of the ulna,* sharper than its radial counterpart, extends distally from the posterior-medial corner of the distal ulna.

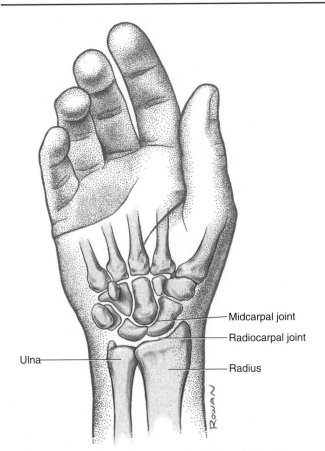

Dorsal view

Extensor carpi radialis longus

Extensor carpi radialis brevis

Trapezium

Trapezoid

Capitate

Hamate

Scaphoid

Lunate

Triquetrum

Extensor carpi ulnaris

Pisiform

Groove for extensor carpi ulnaris

Groove for extensor pollicis longus

Groove for extensor carpi radialis brevis

Tubercle

Brachioradialis

Radius

Ulna

FIGURE 7-2. The dorsal aspect of the bones of the right wrist. The muscles' distal attachments are shown in gray. The dashed lines show the proximal attachment of the dorsal capsule of the wrist.

Midcarpal joint

Radiocarpal joint

Ulna

Radius

FIGURE 7-1. The bones and major articulations of the wrist.

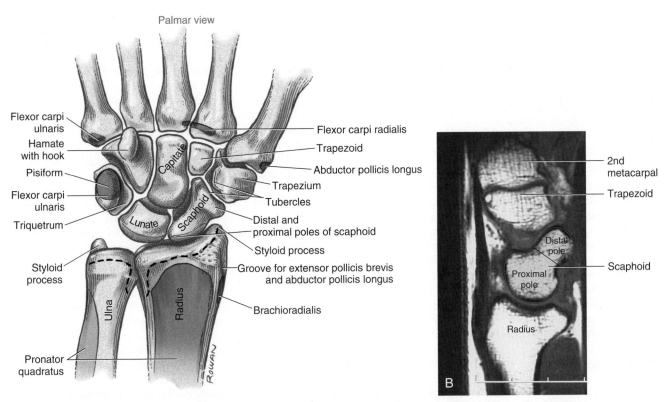

Palmar view

Flexor carpi ulnaris

Hamate with hook

Pisiform

Flexor carpi ulnaris

Triquetrum

Styloid process

Ulna

Pronator quadratus

Capitate

Lunate

Scaphoid

Radius

Flexor carpi radialis

Trapezoid

Abductor pollicis longus

Trapezium

Tubercles

Distal and proximal poles of scaphoid

Styloid process

Groove for extensor pollicis brevis and abductor pollicis longus

Brachioradialis

A

2nd metacarpal

Trapezoid

Distal pole

Proximal pole

Scaphoid

Radius

B

FIGURE 7-3. A, The palmar aspect of the bones of the right wrist. The muscles' proximal attachments are shown in red and distal attachments in gray. The dashed lines show the proximal attachment of the palmar capsule of the wrist. **B,** The full appreciation of the shape of the scaphoid is provided through a sagittal plane cross-section MRI (magnetic resonance image). The thin black line marks the "waist" region of the bone, midway between the proximal and distal poles.

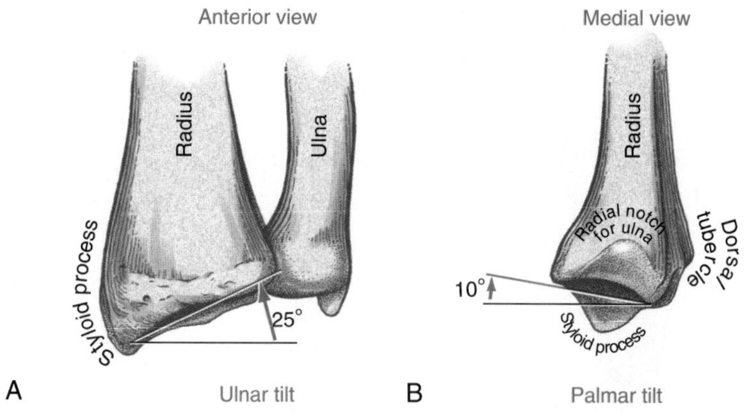

FIGURE 7-4. A, Anterior view of the distal radius showing an *ulnar tilt* of about 25 degrees. **B,** A medial view of the distal radius showing a *palmar tilt* of about 10 degrees.

The *distal articular surface of the radius* is concave in both medial-lateral and anterior-posterior directions (see Figure 6-26, *B*). Facets are formed in the articular cartilage from indentations made by the scaphoid and lunate bones of the wrist.

Fractures of the distal end of the radius with a dorsal displacement of the distal fragment are very common. A frequent mechanism for this injury is a fall over an outstretched hand. A fracture that heals in an abnormally aligned fashion can significantly alter the congruence, or fit, of both the distal radio-ulnar joint and the radiocarpal joint of the wrist.[36,59] Depending on the nature of the incongruence, the joints may become unstable (especially the distal radio-ulnar joint) or may develop degenerative arthritis from altered contact pressure at the articular surfaces.

Abnormal alignment of the distal radius also can change the relationship between the axis of rotation of the forearm and the interosseous membrane. If the misalignment is severe, the interosseous membrane may restrict the full extent of pronation or supination.[36]

Osteologic Features of the Distal Forearm
- Dorsal tubercle of the radius
- Styloid process of the radius
- Styloid process of the ulna
- Distal articular surface of the radius

The distal end of the radius has two configurations of biomechanical importance. First, the distal end of the radius angles about 25 degrees toward the ulnar (medial) direction (Figure 7-4, *A*). This *ulnar tilt* allows the wrist and hand to rotate farther into ulnar deviation than into radial deviation. As a result of this tilt, radial deviation of the wrist is limited by impingement of the lateral side of the carpus against the styloid process of the radius. Second, the distal articular surface of the radius is angled about 10 degrees in the palmar direction (see Figure 7-4, *B*). This *palmar tilt* accounts, in part, for the greater amounts of flexion than extension at the wrist.

Carpal Bones

From a radial (lateral) to ulnar direction, the proximal row of carpal bones includes the scaphoid, lunate, triquetrum, and pisiform. The distal row includes the trapezium, trapezoid, capitate, and hamate (Figures 7-2 and 7-3).

The proximal row of carpal bones is joined in a relatively loose fashion. In contrast, the distal row of carpal bones is bound tightly by strong ligaments, providing a rigid and stable base for articulation with the metacarpal bones.

The following section presents a general anatomic description of each carpal bone. The ability to visualize each bone's relative position and shape is helpful in an understanding of the ligamentous anatomy and wrist kinematics.

SCAPHOID

The naming of the scaphoid is based on its vague resemblance to a boat (*scaphoid* from the Greek *skaphoeides*, like a boat). Most of the "hull" or undersurface of the boat rides on the radius; the cargo area of the "boat" is filled with part of the head of the capitate (see Figure 7-3, *A*). The scaphoid contacts four carpal bones and the radius.

The scaphoid has two convex surfaces called *poles*. The *proximal pole* articulates with the *scaphoid facet* of the radius (see Figure 6-26, *B*). The *distal pole* has a slightly rounded surface, which articulates with the trapezium and trapezoid. The distal pole projects obliquely palmarly, which can be well appreciated from a sagittal plane slice provided by magnetic resonance imaging (MRI) (see Figure 7-3, *B*). The distal pole has a blunt *tubercle*, which is palpable at the palmar base of the thenar musculature. Because of its elongated shape, the scaphoid is functionally and anatomically associated with both rows of carpal bones.[7]

The distal-medial surface of the scaphoid is deeply concave to accept the lateral half of the prominent head of the capitate bone (see Figure 7-3, *A*). A small facet on the scaphoid's medial side articulates with the lunate. This articulation, reinforced primarily by the scapholunate ligament, provides an important mechanical link within the proximal row of carpal bones—a point to be revisited later in this chapter.

LUNATE

The lunate (from the Latin *luna*, moon) is the central bone of the proximal row, wedged between the scaphoid and triquetrum. The lunate is the most inherently unstable of the carpal bones, in part because of its shape, but primarily because of its lack of firm ligamentous attachments to the relatively rigid capitate bone.

Like the scaphoid, the lunate's proximal surface is convex, fitting into the concave facet on the radius (see Figure 6-26, *B*). The distal surface of the lunate is deeply concave, giving the bone its crescent moon–shaped appearance (see Figure

7-3, *A*). This articular surface accepts two convexities: the medial half of the head of the capitate and part of the apex of the hamate.

TRIQUETRUM

The triquetrum, or triangular bone, occupies the most ulnar position in the wrist, just medial to the lunate. It is easily palpable, just distal to the ulnar styloid process, especially with the wrist radially deviated. The lateral surface of the triquetrum is long and flat for articulation with a similarly shaped surface on the hamate.

The triquetrum is the third most frequently fractured bone of the wrist, after the scaphoid and lunate.

PISIFORM

The pisiform, meaning "shaped like a pea," articulates loosely with the palmar surface of the triquetrum. The bone is easily moveable and palpable. The pisiform is embedded within the tendon of the flexor carpi ulnaris and therefore has the characteristics of a sesamoid bone. In addition, this bone serves as an attachment for the abductor digiti minimi muscle, transverse carpal ligament, and several other ligaments.

CAPITATE

The capitate is the largest of all carpal bones. This bone occupies a central location within the wrist, making articular contact with seven surrounding bones when considering the metacarpals (see Figure 7-3, *A*). The word *capitate* is derived from the Latin root meaning *head*, which describes the shape of the bone's prominent proximal surface. The large head articulates with the deep concavity provided by the scaphoid and lunate. The capitate is well stabilized between the hamate and trapezoid by short but strong ligaments.

The capitate's distal surface is rigidly joined to the base of the third and, to a lesser extent, the second and fourth metacarpal bones. This rigid articulation allows the capitate and the third metacarpal to function as a single column, providing significant longitudinal stability to the entire wrist and hand. The axis of rotation for all wrist motions passes through the capitate.

TRAPEZIUM

The trapezium has an asymmetric shape. The proximal surface is slightly concave for articulation with the scaphoid. Of particular importance is the distal saddle-shaped surface, which articulates with the base of the first metacarpal. The first carpometacarpal joint is a highly specialized saddle-type articulation allowing a wide range of motion to the human thumb.

A slender and sharp *tubercle* projects from the palmar surface of the trapezium. This tubercle, along with the palmar tubercle of the scaphoid, provides attachment for the lateral side of the transverse carpal ligament (see Figure 7-5). Immediately medial to the palmar tubercle is a distinct groove for the tendon of the flexor carpi radialis.

TRAPEZOID

The trapezoid is a small bone wedged tightly between the capitate and the trapezium. The trapezoid, like the trapezium,

has a proximal surface that is slightly concave for articulation with the scaphoid. The bone makes a relatively firm articulation with the base of the second metacarpal bone.

HAMATE

The hamate is named after the large hooklike process that projects from its palmar surface. The hamate has the general shape of a pyramid. Its base, or distal surface, articulates with the bases of the fourth and fifth metacarpals. This articulation provides important functional mobility to the ulnar aspect of the hand, most noticeably when the hand is cupped.

The apex of the hamate—its proximal surface—projects toward the concave surface of the lunate. The hook of the hamate (along with the pisiform) provides bony attachments for the medial side of the transverse carpal ligament (see Figure 7-5).

Carpal Tunnel

As illustrated in Figure 7-5, the palmar side of the carpal bones forms a concavity. Arching over this concavity is a thick fibrous band of connective tissue known as the *transverse carpal ligament.* This ligament is connected to four raised points on the palmar carpus, namely, the pisiform and the hook of the hamate on the ulnar side, and the tubercles of the scaphoid and the trapezium on the radial side. The transverse carpal ligament serves as a primary attachment site for many muscles located within the hand and the palmaris longus, a wrist flexor muscle.

The transverse carpal ligament converts the palmar concavity made by the carpal bones into a *carpal tunnel.* The tunnel serves as a passageway for the median nerve and the tendons of extrinsic flexor muscles of the digits. Furthermore, the transverse carpal ligament restrains the enclosed tendons from "bowstringing" anteriorly and out of the carpal tunnel, most notably during grasping actions performed with a partially flexed wrist.

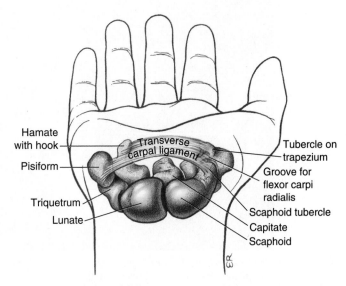

FIGURE 7-5. A view through the carpal tunnel of the right wrist with all contents removed. The transverse carpal ligament is shown as the roof of the tunnel.

SPECIAL FOCUS 7-1

Scaphoid and Lunate: Vulnerability to Injury and Clinical Complications

It is likely that more has been written in the medical literature on the scaphoid and lunate than on all other carpal bones combined. Both bones are lodged between two rigid structures: the distal forearm and the distal row of carpal bones. Like a nut within a nutcracker, the scaphoid and lunate are vulnerable to compression-related injuries. As will be explained, it is not uncommon for either bone to develop avascular necrosis, which interferes with the healing process after fracture.

The Scaphoid Bone and Its Vulnerability to Fracture

The scaphoid is located in the direct path of force transmission through the wrist. For this reason, the scaphoid accounts for 60% to 70% of all carpal fractures.[65] A common mechanism for fracturing this bone is to fall on a fully supinated forearm with wrist fully extended and radially deviated. Persons with a fractured scaphoid typically show tenderness within the anatomic "snuffbox" of the wrist. Most fractures occur near or along the scaphoid's "waist," midway between the bone's two poles (Figure 7-6, *A*). Because most blood vessels enter the scaphoid at and distal to its waist, fractures proximal to the waist may result in a delayed union or nonunion.[21,24] If the fracture is untreated, the proximal pole may develop avascular necrosis. Fractures of the proximal pole typically require surgery, followed by immobilization for at least 12 weeks or until there is evidence of radiographic union. Fractures of the distal pole typically do not require surgery, especially if nondisplaced, and generally require only 5 to 6 weeks of immobilization. Actual times of immobilization can vary greatly, based on the specific circumstances of the patient and the fracture.

Often a fractured scaphoid is associated with other injuries along the weight-bearing path of the wrist and hand.[44] Associated injuries often involve fracture and/or dislocation of the lunate and fracture of the trapezium and distal radius.

Kienböck's Disease: Avascular Necrosis of the Lunate

The condition of lunatomalacia (meaning literally "softening of the lunate") was first described by Kienböck in 1910.[61] *Kienböck's disease,* as it is called today, is described as a painful orthopedic disorder of unknown cause, characterized by avascular necrosis of the lunate.[71] A history of trauma is frequently, but not universally, associated with the onset of the condition. Trauma may be linked with an isolated dislocation or fracture or with repetitive or near-constant lower-magnitude compression forces. It is not understood how the trauma, compression, and avascular necrosis are interrelated in the pathogenesis of the disease.[65] What is clear, however, is that as avascular necrosis develops, the lunate often becomes fragmented and shortened, which may alter its relationship with the other adjoining carpal bones (see Figure 7-6, *B*).[2] In severe cases the lunate may totally collapse, disrupting the kinematics and kinetics of the entire wrist. This tends to occur more often in those involved in manual labor, such as pneumatic drill operators.

Treatment of Kienböck's disease may be conservative or radical, depending on the amount of functional limitation and pain, as well as the progression of the disease. In relatively mild forms of the disease—before the lunate fragments and becomes sclerotic—treatment may involve immobilization by casting or splinting.[71] If the disease progresses, the length of the ulna or radius may be surgically altered as a means to reduce the contact stress on the lunate.[71] In more advanced cases, treatments may include partial fusion of selected carpal bones, lunate excision, or proximal row carpectomy.[9,21]

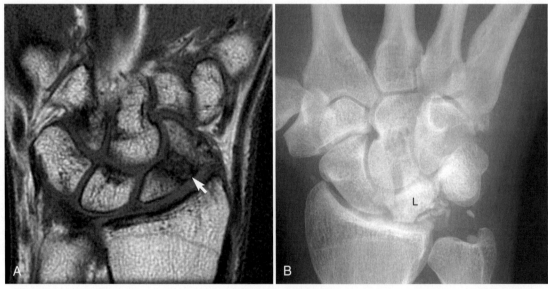

FIGURE 7-6. A, A frontal (coronal) plane T1-weighted magnetic resonance image of the wrist of a patient showing a fracture of the scaphoid at the region of its waist. **B,** An anterior-posterior view of a radiograph of the wrist of a patient with Kienböck's disease. Note that the lunate (*L*) is sclerotic, malformed, and fragmented. (From Helms CA: *Fundamentals of skeletal radiology,* ed 3, Philadelphia, 2005, Elsevier.)

ARTHROLOGY

Joint Structure and Ligaments of the Wrist

JOINT STRUCTURE

As illustrated in Figure 7-1, the two primary articulations within the wrist are the *radiocarpal* and *midcarpal joints*. Many other *intercarpal joints* also exist between adjacent carpal bones (see Figure 7-7). Intercarpal joints contribute to wrist motion through small gliding and rotary motions. Compared with the large range of motion permitted at the radiocarpal and midcarpal joints, motion at the intercarpal joints is relatively small but nevertheless essential for normal wrist motion.

Joints of the Wrist
- Radiocarpal joint
- Midcarpal joint
  - Medial compartment
  - Lateral compartment
- Intercarpal joints

Radiocarpal Joint

The *proximal components* of the radiocarpal joint are the concave surfaces of the radius and an adjacent articular disc (Figures 7-7 and 7-8). As described in Chapter 6, this articular disc (also called the *triangular fibrocartilage*) is an integral part of the distal radio-ulnar joint. The *distal components* of the radiocarpal joint are the convex proximal surfaces of the scaphoid and the lunate. The triquetrum is also considered part of the radiocarpal joint because at full ulnar deviation its medial surface contacts the articular disc.

The thick articular surface of the distal radius and the articular disc accept and disperse the forces that cross the wrist. Approximately 20% of the total compression force that crosses the radiocarpal joint passes through the articular disc.

The remaining 80% passes directly through the scaphoid and lunate to the radius.[58] The contact areas at the radiocarpal joint tend to be greatest when the wrist is partially extended and ulnarly deviated.[42] This is also the wrist position at which maximal grip strength is obtained.

Midcarpal Joint

The midcarpal joint is the articulation between the proximal and distal rows of carpal bones (see Figure 7-8). The capsule that surrounds the midcarpal joint is continuous with each of the many intercarpal joints.

The midcarpal joint can be divided descriptively into medial and lateral joint compartments.[78] The larger *medial compartment* is formed by the convex head of the capitate and apex of the hamate, fitting into the concave recess formed by the distal surfaces of the scaphoid, lunate, and triquetrum (see Figure 7-8). The head of the capitate fits into this concave recess much like a ball-and-socket joint.

The *lateral compartment* of the midcarpal joint is formed by the junction of the slightly convex distal pole of the scaphoid with the slightly concave proximal surfaces of the trapezium and the trapezoid (see Figure 7-8). The lateral compartment lacks the pronounced ovoid shape of the medial compartment. Cineradiography of wrist motion shows less movement at the lateral than the medial compartment.[52] For this reason, subsequent arthrokinematic analysis of the midcarpal joint focuses on the medial compartment.

WRIST LIGAMENTS

Many of the ligaments of the wrist are small and difficult to isolate. Their inconspicuous nature should not, however, minimize their extreme kinesiologic importance. Wrist ligaments are essential to maintaining the natural intercarpal alignment and for transferring forces within and across the carpus. Muscle-produced forces stored in stretched ligaments

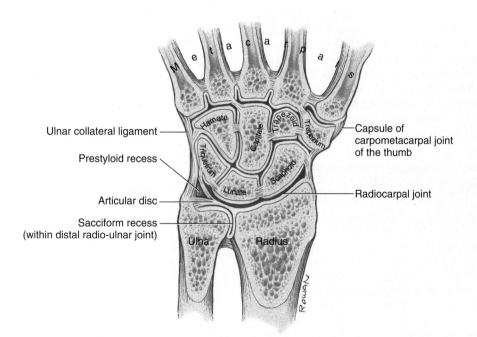

FIGURE 7-7. A frontal plane cross-section through the right wrist and distal forearm showing the shape of the bones and connective tissues. Observe the many individual intercarpal joints.

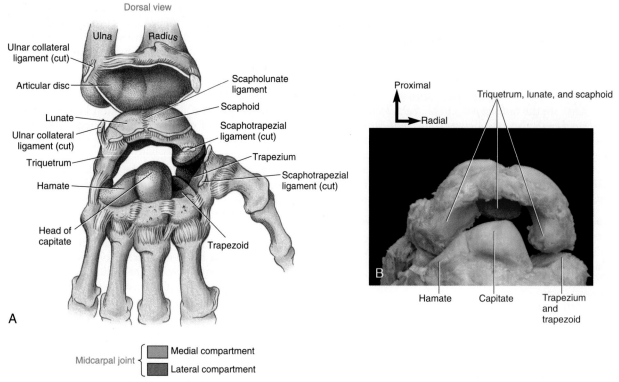

FIGURE 7-8. A, Illustration of a dorsal view of a dissected right wrist showing several key structures associated with the radiocarpal and midcarpal joints. Red and gray colors highlight the medial and lateral compartments of the midcarpal joint, respectively. **B,** Photograph of a dissected right wrist (as in **A**), emphasizing the articular surfaces of the midcarpal joint. (Dissection prepared by Anthony Hornung, PT, and Rolandas Kesminas, PT, Marquette University.)

provide important control to the complex arthrokinematics of the wrist. Ligaments also supply sensory feedback to activated muscles.[28] Ligaments damaged through injury and disease leave the wrist vulnerable to weakness, deformity, instability, and degenerative arthritis.

Wrist ligaments are classified as extrinsic or intrinsic (Box 7-1). Extrinsic ligaments have their proximal attachments on the forearm but attach distally within the wrist. As noted in Box 7-1, the triangular fibrocartilage complex (introduced previously in Chapter 6) includes structures associated with the wrist *and* the distal radio-ulnar joint. Intrinsic ligaments have both their proximal and distal attachments within the wrist. More detailed or alternative descriptions of these ligaments can be found in other sources.[6,78]

SPECIAL FOCUS 7-2

Total Wrist Arthroplasty

Total wrist arthroplasty (replacement) has not reached the level of success of arthroplasty of other joints in the body, such as the hip or knee.[12,74] One obstacle is the small size of the replacement components, which concentrates high stress on the implanted material. Over time, high stress contributes to premature loosening or dislocation. The success rate of total wrist replacement will likely improve with continued advances in surgical technique, preoperative and postoperative management, knowledge of the natural biomechanics, and design of implants.

BOX 7-1. Extrinsic and Intrinsic Ligaments

EXTRINSIC LIGAMENTS OF THE WRIST
Dorsal radiocarpal
Radial collateral
Palmar radiocarpal
- Radioscaphocapite
- Radiolunate
- Radioscapholunate
Triangular fibrocartilage complex (TFCC)
- Articular disc (triangular fibrocartilage)
- Radio-ulnar joint capsular ligament
- Palmar ulnocarpal ligament
  - Ulnotriquetral
  - Ulnolunate
- Ulnar collateral ligament
- Meniscus homologue

INTRINSIC LIGAMENTS OF THE WRIST
Short (distal row)
- Dorsal
- Palmar
- Interosseous
Intermediate
- Lunotriquetral
- Scapholunate
- Scaphotrapezial
Long
- Palmar intercarpal ("inverted V")
  - Lateral leg (capitate to scaphoid)
  - Medial leg (capitate to triquetrum)
- Dorsal intercarpal (trapezium-scaphoid-lunate-triquetrum)

Extrinsic Ligaments

A fibrous capsule surrounds the external surfaces of both the wrist and the distal radio-ulnar joint. Dorsally, the capsule thickens slightly to form the *dorsal radiocarpal ligament* (Figure 7-9). This ligament is thin and not easily distinguishable from the capsule itself. In general, the dorsal radiocarpal ligament courses distally in an ulnarly direction, attaching primarily between the distal radius and the dorsal surfaces of the lunate and triquetrum.[73,77] The dorsal radiocarpal ligament reinforces the posterior side of the radiocarpal joint and helps guide the natural arthrokinematics, especially of the bones in the proximal row.[77] The fibers that attach to the lunate provide an especially important restraint against anterior (volar) dislocation of this inherently unstable bone.[86]

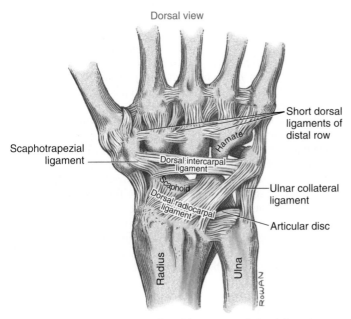

Dorsal view

Scaphotrapezial ligament

Short dorsal ligaments of distal row

Hamate

Dorsal intercarpal ligament

Scaphoid

Dorsal radiocarpal ligament

Ulnar collateral ligament

Articular disc

Radius

Ulna

FIGURE 7-9. The primary dorsal ligaments of the right wrist.

Taleisnik originally described the thickening of the external surface of the lateral-palmer part of the capsule of the wrist as the *radial collateral ligament* (Figure 7-10).[80] More recent anatomic descriptions, however, typically do not include the radial collateral ligament as a distinct anatomic entity.[6] This connective tissue, regardless of its name, likely provides little lateral stability to the wrist. Extrinsic muscles, such as the abductor pollicis longus and the extensor pollicis brevis, perform most of this function.

Deep and separate from the palmar capsule of the wrist are several stout and extensive ligaments known collectively as the *palmar radiocarpal ligaments.* Three ligaments are typically described within this set: the *radioscaphocapitate,* the *radiolunate,* and, in a deeper plane, the *radioscapholunate* (see Figure 7-10).[78] The palmar radiocarpal ligaments are much stronger and thicker than their dorsal counterparts.[80] In general, each ligament arises from a roughened area on the distal radius, travels distally in a generally ulnar direction, and attaches to the palmar surface of several carpal bones. The radioscaphocapitate—the most lateral ligament of this set—often partially blends with the radial collateral ligament.

The palmar radiocarpal ligaments become maximally taut at full wrist extension.[44] Passive tension exists in these ligaments even in the relaxed neutral wrist position.[88] An example of the role these ligaments play in guiding the arthrokinematics of the wrist will be provided later in this chapter.

Although the ulnocarpal space appears empty on a standard radiograph (Figure 7-11, *A*), it is actually filled with at least five interconnected tissues, known collectively as the *triangular fibrocartilage complex* (TFCC) (see Box 7-1). The primary component of the TFCC is the *triangular fibrocartilage*—the previously described *articular disc* located within both the distal radio-ulnar and the radiocarpal joints (see Figure 7-11, *B*).

The primary global function of the TFCC is to securely bind the distal ends of the radius and ulna while simultaneously permitting the radius, with attached carpus, to freely rotate (pronate and supinate) around a fixed ulna. A summary

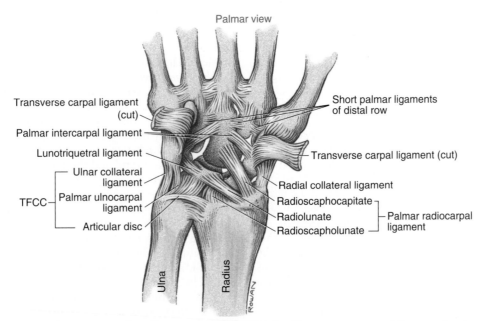

Palmar view

Transverse carpal ligament (cut)

Palmar intercarpal ligament

Lunotriquetral ligament

TFCC
- Ulnar collateral ligament
- Palmar ulnocarpal ligament
- Articular disc

Short palmar ligaments of distal row

Transverse carpal ligament (cut)

Radial collateral ligament

Radioscaphocapitate
Radiolunate
Radioscapholunate
— Palmar radiocarpal ligament

Ulna

Radius

FIGURE 7-10. The primary palmar ligaments of the right wrist. The transverse carpal ligament has been cut and reflected to show the underlying ligaments. *TFCC,* triangular fibrocartilage complex.

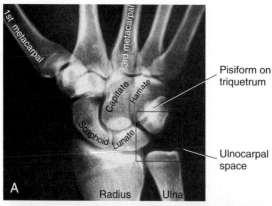

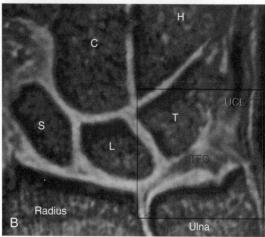

FIGURE 7-11. A, Radiograph of the wrist showing the carpal bones and the "ulnocarpal space." **B,** Magnetic resonance image of the wrist highlighting the ulnocarpal space (in red box) and two components of the triangular fibrocartilage complex: (1) TFC, triangular fibrocartilage, and (2) UCL, ulnar collateral ligament. *C,* capitate; *H,* hamate; *L,* lunate; *S,* scaphoid; *T,* triquetrum.

of the more specific functions of the TFCC is included in Box 7-2. Anatomic details of the components of the TFCC are described in the following paragraphs.

The triangular fibrocartilage (TFC) attaches directly or indirectly to all components of the TFCC and therefore forms the structural backbone of the entire complex. The TFC is a biconcave articular disc, composed chiefly of fibrocartilage.[78] The name "triangular" refers to the shape of the disc: its base attaches along the ulnar notch of the radius, and its apex attaches near the styloid process of the ulna (see Figure 6-26, *A*). The sides of the "triangle" are formed by the *palmar* and *dorsal capsular ligaments* of the distal radio-ulnar joint.[25] The disc's proximal surface accepts the head of the ulna at the distal radio-ulnar joint, and its distal surface accepts the convex surfaces of part of the lunate and the triquetrum at the radiocarpal joint (see Figures 6-26, 7-7, and 7-8, *A*). The central 80% of the disc is avascular with little or no healing potential.[13]

The *palmar ulnocarpal ligament* originates from the palmar edge of the articular disc and adjacent palmar aspect of the distal radio-ulnar joint capsule (see Figure 7-10).[31] From this common proximal attachment the tissue splits into two distinct ligaments: ulnolunate and ulnotriquetral.

The *ulnar collateral ligament* represents a thickening of the medial aspect of the capsule of the wrist[31,80] (see Figure 7-10).

(According to the British edition of *Gray's Anatomy,* the ulnar collateral ligament and the juxtaposed ulnotriquetral ligament are part of the same structure.[78]) Along with the flexor and extensor carpi ulnaris muscles, the palmar ulnocarpal and ulnar collateral ligaments reinforce the ulnar side of the wrist. These ligaments must be sufficiently flexible, however, to allow the radius and hand to rotate freely around the fixed ulna during pronation and supination.

The final component yet to be described within the TFCC is a poorly organized and defined connective tissue substance known as the *meniscus homologue.*[31] This tissue likely represents the vestige of a more primitive embryonic connective tissue within the ulnar side of the wrist.[78] Referred to as a "cartilaginous filler,"[80] the meniscus homologue fills gaps within and immediately medial to the prestyloid recess of the ulnocarpal space (see Figure 7-7). The synovial lining within this recess often becomes distended and painful with rheumatoid arthritis. Tears in the articular disc may permit synovial fluid to spread from the radiocarpal joint to the distal radio-ulnar joint.

Intrinsic Ligaments

The primary intrinsic ligaments of the wrist can be classified into three sets: short, intermediate, or long (see Box 7-1).[80] *Short ligaments* connect the bones of the distal row by their palmar, dorsal, or interosseous surfaces (see Figures 7-9 and 7-10). The short ligaments firmly stabilize and unite the distal row of bones, permitting them to function essentially as a single mechanical unit.

Three *intermediate ligaments* exist within the wrist. The *lunotriquetral ligament* is a fibrous continuation of the palmar radiolunate ligament (see Figure 7-10). The *scapholunate ligament* is a broad collection of fibers that forms the primary bond between the scaphoid and the lunate (see Figure 7-8, *A*).[76] Several *scaphotrapezial ligaments* reinforce the articulation between the scaphoid and the trapezium (see Figure 7-9).

Two relatively *long ligaments* are present within the wrist. The *palmar intercarpal ligament* firmly attaches to the palmar surface of the capitate bone (see Figure 7-10). From this common attachment the ligament bifurcates proximally, forming two discrete fiber groups that resemble the shape of an inverted V. The *lateral leg* of the inverted V attaches to the scaphoid, and the *medial leg* to the triquetrum. These ligaments help guide the arthrokinematics of the wrist.

Lastly, a thin *dorsal intercarpal ligament* provides transverse stability to the wrist by interconnecting the trapezium, scaphoid, lunate, and triquetrum (see Figure 7-9).[46,85]

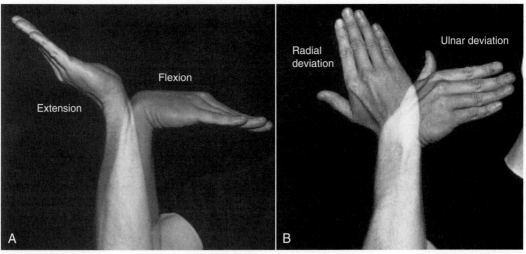

FIGURE 7-12. Osteokinematics of the wrist. **A,** Flexion and extension. **B,** Ulnar and radial deviation. Note that flexion exceeds extension and ulnar deviation exceeds radial deviation.

Kinematics of Wrist Motion

OSTEOKINEMATICS

The osteokinematics of the wrist are defined for 2 degrees of freedom: flexion-extension and ulnar-radial deviation (Figure 7-12). Wrist circumduction—a full circular motion made by the wrist—is a combination of the aforementioned movements, not a distinct third degree of freedom.

Most natural dynamic movements of the wrist combine elements of both frontal and sagittal planes: extension tends to occur with radial deviation, and flexion with ulnar deviation.[41] The resulting natural path of motion for the wrist follows a slightly oblique path, similar to a dart thrower's motion.[50] This natural combination of movements occurs with other functions, such as tying shoelaces or combing hair. These natural kinematics should be considered during rehabilitation of the wrist after injury.

The axis of rotation for wrist movements is reported to pass through the head of the capitate (Figure 7-13).[94] Generally, the axis runs in a near medial-lateral direction for flexion and extension and near anterior-posterior direction for radial and ulnar deviation. Although the axes are depicted as stationary, in reality they migrate slightly throughout the full range of motion.[60] The firm articulation between the capitate and the base of the third metacarpal bone causes the rotation of the capitate to direct the osteokinematic path of the entire hand.

The wrist rotates in the sagittal plane about 130 to 160 degrees (see Figure 7-12, *A*). On average, the wrist flexes from 0 degrees to about 70 to 85 degrees and extends from 0 degrees to about 60 to 75 degrees.[67,69] As with any diarthrodial joint, wrist range of motion varies with age and health and whether the motion is performed actively or passively. Total flexion normally exceeds extension by about 10 to 15 degrees. End-range extension is naturally limited by stiffness in the thick palmar radiocarpal ligaments. In some persons, a greater than average palmar tilt of the distal radius may also limit extension range (see Figure 7-4, *B*).

The wrist rotates in the frontal plane approximately 50 to 60 degrees (see Figure 7-12, *B*).[67,94] Radial and ulnar deviation of the wrist is measured as the angle between the radius and the shaft of the third metacarpal. Ulnar deviation occurs from 0 degrees to about 35 to 40 degrees. Radial deviation occurs from 0 degrees

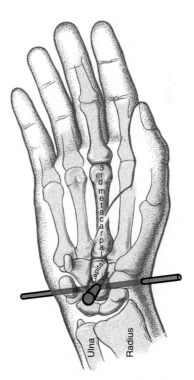

FIGURE 7-13. The medial-lateral *(green)* and anterior-posterior *(purple)* axes of rotation for wrist movement are shown piercing the head of the capitate bone.

to about 15 to 20 degrees. Primarily because of the ulnar tilt of the distal radius (see Figure 7-4, *A*), maximum ulnar deviation normally is double the maximum amount of radial deviation.

Ryu and colleagues tested 40 healthy subjects using a biaxial electrogoniometer to determine the range of wrist motion needed to perform 24 activities of daily living (ADLs).[67] The ADLs included personal care, hygiene, food preparation, writing, and using various tools or utensils. The researchers concluded that these ADLs could be comfortably performed using 40 degrees of flexion, 40 degrees of extension, 10 degrees of radial deviation, and 30 degrees of ulnar deviation. These functional ranges were 50% to 80% of the subjects' maximal range of wrist motion.

Medical management of a severely painful or unstable wrist may require surgical fusion.[14] To minimize the functional impairment associated with this procedure, the wrist is often fused in an "average" *position of function:* about 10 to 15 degrees of extension and 10 degrees of ulnar deviation.[68] Although permanently fusing a wrist (even partially) may seem like a radical option, the procedure may be the only treatment that can achieve stability and relieve pain.

ARTHROKINEMATICS

Many different methodologies have been used to study the kinematics of the wrist; these include in vitro and, more recently, in vivo techniques.[47,51] These techniques include the following:

- Radiography
- Cineradiography
- Anatomic dissection
- Placement of pins in bones
- Three-dimensional (3D) computer imaging
- Sonic digitizing
- Roentgen-stereophotography
- Optoelectric systems
- Electromagnetic tracking devices
- 3D Computed tomography (CT)
- Electromechanical linkage systems

Even with these sophisticated techniques, the resulting data describing the kinematics across the regions of the wrist are inconsistent. Precise and repeatable descriptions of the kinematics are hampered by the complexity of the anatomy and the movement (up to eight small bones experiencing multiplanar rotations and translations) and by natural human variation. Although much has been learned over the last two decades, the study of carpal kinematics continues to evolve.*

Perhaps the most fundamental and accepted premise of carpal kinematics is that the wrist is a double-joint system, with movement occurring simultaneously at both the radiocarpal and midcarpal joints. The following discussion on arthrokinematics focuses on the dynamic relationship between these two joints.

Wrist Extension and Flexion

The essential kinematics of sagittal plane motion at the wrist can be appreciated by visualizing the wrist as an articulated *central column,* formed by the linkages between the distal radius, lunate, capitate, and third metacarpal (Figure 7-14). Within this column, the *radiocarpal joint* is represented by the articulation between the radius and lunate, and the medial compartment of the *midcarpal joint* is represented by the articulation between the lunate and capitate. The carpometacarpal joint is a semirigid articulation formed between the capitate and the base of the third metacarpal.

Dynamic Interaction within the Joints of the Central Column of the Wrist

The arthrokinematics of extension and flexion are based on synchronous convex-on-concave rotations at both the radiocarpal and the midcarpal joints. At the radiocarpal joint depicted in red in Figure 7-15, *extension* occurs as the convex surface of the lunate rolls dorsally on the radius and simultaneously slides palmarly. The rolling motion directs the lunate's distal surface dorsally, toward the direction of extension. At the midcarpal joint, illustrated in white in Figure

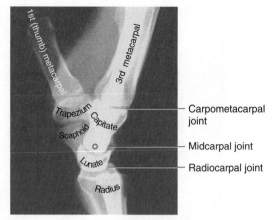

FIGURE 7-14. A lateral view of a radiograph of the central column of the wrist. The axis of rotation for flexion and extension is shown as a small circle at the base of the capitate. Observe the crescent shape of the lunate. For illustrative purposes, the lunate and capitate bones have been digitally enhanced.

7-15, the head of the capitate rolls dorsally on the lunate and simultaneously slides in a palmar direction. Combining the arthrokinematics over both joints produces full wrist extension. This two-joint system has the advantage of yielding a significant total range of motion by requiring only moderate amounts of rotation at the individual joints. Mechanically, therefore, each joint moves within a relatively limited—and therefore more stable—arc of motion.

Full wrist extension elongates the palmar radiocarpal ligaments and all muscles that cross on the palmar side of the wrist. Tension within these stretched structures helps stabilize the wrist in its close-packed position of full extension.[43,44] Stability in full wrist extension is useful when weight is borne through the upper extremity during activities such as crawling on the hands and knees and transferring one's own body from a wheelchair to a bed.

The arthrokinematics of wrist *flexion* are similar to those described for extension but occur in a reverse fashion (see Figure 7-15).

Studies quantifying the individual angular contributions of the radiocarpal and midcarpal joints to the total sagittal plane motion of the wrist cite inconsistent data.* With few exceptions, however, most studies report synchronous and roughly equal—or at least significant—contributions from both joints.

Using the simplified central column model to describe flexion and extension of the wrist offers an excellent conceptualization of a rather complex event. A limitation of the model, however, is that it does not account for *all* the carpal bones that participate in the motion. For instance, the model ignores the kinematics of the scaphoid bone at the radiocarpal joint. In brief, the arthrokinematics of the scaphoid on the radius are similar to those of the lunate during flexion and extension, except for one feature. Based on the different size and curvature of the two bones, the scaphoid rolls on the radius at a different speed than the lunate.[66] This difference causes a slight displacement between the scaphoid and lunate by the end of full motion. Normally, in the healthy wrist, the amount of displacement is minimized by the restraining action of ligaments, especially the scapholunate ligament (see Figure 7-8, *A*). Rupture of this important ligament occurs relatively frequently and can significantly alter the

---

*References 23, 48, 49, 60, 70, 90.

*References 15, 34, 47, 67, 79, 92.

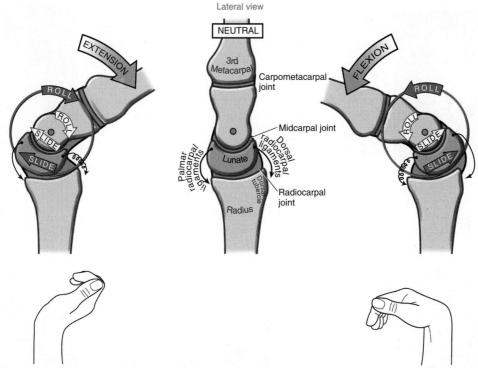

FIGURE 7-15. A model of the central column of the right wrist showing flexion and extension. The wrist in the center is shown at rest, in a neutral position. The roll-and-slide arthrokinematics are shown in red for the radiocarpal joint and in white for the midcarpal joint. During wrist extension *(left)*, the dorsal radiocarpal ligaments become slackened and the palmar radiocarpal ligaments taut. The reverse arthrokinematics occur during wrist flexion *(right)*.

arthrokinematics and transfer of force within the proximal row of carpal bones.[81,91] Damage to this ligament can occur through trauma, chronic synovitis from rheumatoid arthritis,[5] or even surgical removal of a ganglion cyst.

Ulnar and Radial Deviation of the Wrist
Dynamic Interaction between the Radiocarpal and Midcarpal Joints
Like flexion and extension, ulnar and radial deviation occurs through synchronous convex-on-concave rotations at both radiocarpal and midcarpal joints. During *ulnar deviation*, the midcarpal joint and, to a lesser extent, the radiocarpal joint contribute to overall wrist motion (Figure 7-16).[35] At the radiocarpal joint shown in red in Figure 7-16, the scaphoid, lunate, and triquetrum roll ulnarly and slide a significant distance radially. The extent of this radial slide is apparent by the final position of the lunate relative to the radius at full ulnar deviation. Ulnar deviation at the midcarpal joint occurs primarily from the capitate rolling ulnarly and sliding slightly radially.

Full range of ulnar deviation causes the triquetrum to contact the articular disc. Compression of the hamate against the triquetrum pushes the proximal row of carpal bones against the styloid process of the radius. This compression helps stabilize the wrist for activities that require large gripping forces.

Radial deviation at the wrist occurs through similar arthrokinematics as described for ulnar deviation (see Figure 7-16). The amount of radial deviation at the radiocarpal joint is limited as the radial side of the carpus impinges against the styloid process of the radius. Consequently, a greater amount of the radial deviation occurs at the midcarpal joint.[35]

Using magnetic resonance imaging, Moritomo and colleagues specifically measured the three-dimensional movement at the midcarpal joint during radial and ulnar deviation.[51] They reported a kinematic association between radial devia-

tion and slight extension, and ulnar deviation and slight flexion. This "dart-throwing" movement pattern observed at the midcarpal joint is similar to that observed during many natural wrist movements.

Additional Arthrokinematics Involving the Proximal Row of Carpal Bones
Careful observation of ulnar and radial deviation using cineradiography or serial static radiographs reveals more complicated arthrokinematics than previously described. During these frontal plane movements, the proximal row of carpal bones "rock" slightly into flexion and extension and, to a much lesser extent, "twist." The rocking motion is most noticeable in the scaphoid and, to a lesser extent, the lunate. During radial deviation the proximal row flexes slightly; during ulnar deviation the proximal row extends slightly.[35,37] Note in Figure 7-16, especially on the radiograph, the change in position of the scaphoid tubercle between the extremes of ulnar and radial deviation. According to Moojen and coworkers, at 20 degrees of ulnar deviation the scaphoid is rotated about 20 degrees into extension, relative to the radius.[47] The scaphoid appears to "stand up" or to lengthen, which projects its tubercle distally. At 20 degrees of radial deviation, the scaphoid flexes beyond neutral about 15 degrees, taking on a shortened stature with its tubercle having approached the radius. A functional shortening of the scaphoid allows a few more degrees of radial deviation before complete blockage against the styloid process of the radius. The exact mechanism responsible for the flexion and extension of the proximal carpal row during ulnar and radial deviation is not fully understood, but many explanations have been offered.[66] Most likely, the mechanism is driven by passive forces in ligaments and compressions between adjacent carpal bones.

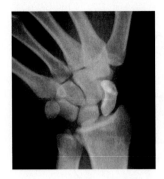
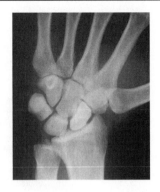

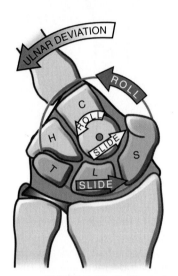
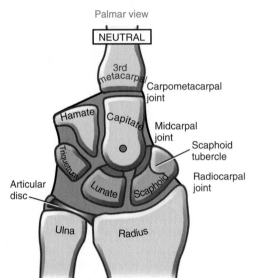
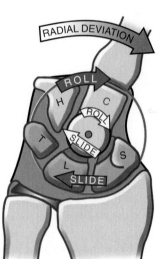

FIGURE 7-16. Radiographs and mechanical depiction of the arthrokinematics of ulnar and radial deviation for the right wrist. The roll-and-slide arthrokinematics are shown in red for the radiocarpal joint and in white for the midcarpal joint.

SPECIAL FOCUS 7-3

Passive Axial Rotation at the Wrist: How Much and Why?

I n addition to flexion-extension and radial-ulnar deviation, the wrist possesses some passive axial rotation between the carpal bones and forearm. This accessory motion (or joint "play") can be appreciated by firmly grasping your right fist with your left hand. While securely holding your right hand from moving, strongly attempt to actively pronate and supinate the right forearm. The passive axial rotation at the right wrist is demonstrated by the rotation of the distal radius relative to the base of the hand. Gupta and Moosawi have measured an average of 34 degrees of total passive axial rotation in 20 asymptomatic wrists; the midcarpal joint permitted on average three times more passive axial rotation than the radiocarpal joint.[27]

The axial rotation at the wrist is limited by the shapes of the joints, especially the elliptic fit of the radiocarpal joint, and the tension in the obliquely oriented radiocarpal ligaments.[64] The relatively limited axial rotation permitted at the radiocarpal joint has important kinesiologic implications. With the wrist's potential third degree of freedom mostly restricted, the hand ultimately must *follow* the pronating and supinating radius; and furthermore, the restriction allows the pronator and supinator muscles to transfer their torques across the wrist to the working hand.

Accessory motions within the wrist—as in all synovial joints—enhance the overall function of the joint. For instance, axial rotation at the wrist amplifies the total extent of functional pronation and supination of the hand relative to the forearm, as well as dampening the impact of reaching these end-range movements. These functions are useful for activities such as wringing out clothes or turning doorknobs.

Carpal Instability

An unstable wrist demonstrates malalignment of one or more carpal bones, typically associated with abnormal and painful kinematics. The primary cause of carpal instability is laxity or rupture of specific ligaments. Although the intrinsic ligaments can tolerate greater relative stretch before rupture than can the extrinsic ligaments, they are more frequently injured.[55] The clinical manifestation of carpal instability depends on the injured

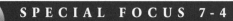

SPECIAL FOCUS 7-4

Guiding Tensions within the "Double-V" System of Ligaments

The arthrokinematics of wrist motion are ultimately driven by muscle but guided or controlled by passive tension within ligaments. Figure 7-17 illustrates one example of how a system of ligaments helps control the arthrokinematics of ulnar and radial deviation. In the neutral position, four ligaments appear as two inverted Vs, which have been referred to as the *double-V system of ligaments*.[80] The *distal inverted V* is formed by the medial and lateral legs of the palmar intercarpal ligament; the *proximal inverted V* is formed by the lunate attachments of the palmar ulnocarpal and palmar radiocarpal ligaments (see Figure 7-10). All four legs of the ligamentous mechanism are under slight tension

even in the neutral position. During ulnar deviation, passive tension rises diagonally across the wrist by the stretch placed in the lateral leg of the palmar intercarpal ligament and fibers of the palmar ulnocarpal ligament.[88] During *radial deviation,* tension is created in the opposite diagonal by a stretch in the medial leg of the palmar intercarpal ligament and fibers of the palmar radiocarpal ligament. A gradual increase in tension within these ligaments provides an important source of control to the movement, as well as dynamic stability to the carpal bones. Tensions in stretched collateral ligaments of the wrist may assist the double-V system in determining the end range of radial and ulnar deviation.

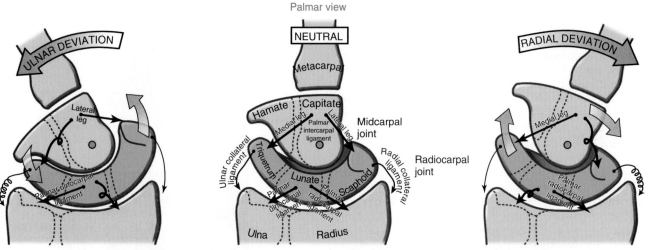

FIGURE 7-17. The tensing and slackening of the "double-V" system ligaments of the wrist are illustrated. The collateral ligaments are also shown. The bones have been blocked together for simplicity. Taut lines represent ligaments under increased tension.

ligament (or ligaments) and the severity of the damage. Carpal instability may be static (demonstrated at rest) or dynamic (demonstrated only during free or resisted movement).

The following examples describe two of many forms of carpal instability. More detail on this subject is contained in other sources.[18]

Two Common Forms of Carpal Instability
1. Rotational collapse of wrist: the "zigzag" deformity
   • Dorsal intercalated segment instability (DISI)
   • Volar intercalated segment instability (VISI)
2. Ulnar translocation of the carpus

ROTATIONAL COLLAPSE OF THE WRIST

Mechanically, the wrist consists of a mobile proximal row of carpal bones intercalated or interposed between two rigid structures: the forearm and the distal row of carpal bones. Like cars of a freight train that are subject to derailment, the proximal row of carpal bones is susceptible to a rotational collapse in a "zigzag" fashion when compressed from both ends (Figure 7-18). The compression forces that cross the wrist arise from

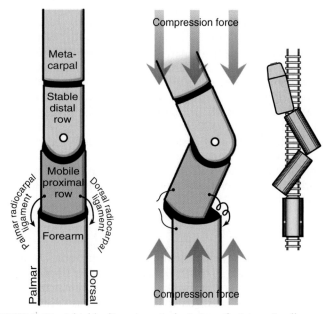

FIGURE 7-18. A highly diagrammatic depiction of a "zigzag" collapse of the central column of the wrist after a large compression force.

FIGURE 7-19. Highly mechanical model showing factors that maintain stability of the lunate. **A,** Acting through ligaments, the scaphoid provides a mechanical linkage between the relatively mobile lunate and the rigid distal row of carpal bones. **B,** Compression forces through the wrist from a fall may fracture the scaphoid and tear the scapholunate ligament. Loss of the mechanical link provided by the scaphoid often leads to lunate instability and/or dislocation.

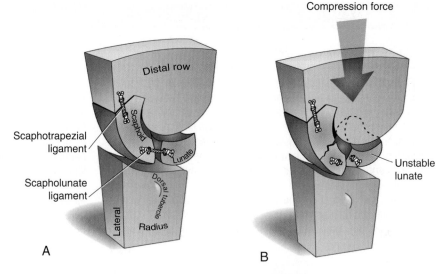

muscle activation and contact with the surrounding environment. In most healthy persons the wrist remains stable throughout life. Collapse and subsequent joint dislocation are prevented primarily by resistance from ligaments and from forces in tendons and the shapes of the adjoining carpal bones.

The lunate is the most frequently dislocated carpal bone.[65] Normally its stability is provided by ligaments and articular contact with adjacent bones of the proximal row, most notably the scaphoid (Figure 7-19, *A*). By virtue of its two poles, the scaphoid forms an important mechanical link between the lunate and the more stable, distal row of carpal bones. The continuity of this link requires that the scaphoid and adjoining ligaments be intact.[46,76,81] Consider, as an example, a fall over an outstretched hand with a resulting fracture in the waist region of the scaphoid, and tearing of the scapholunate ligament (see Figure 7-19, *B*). Disruption of the mechanical link between the two bones can result in *scapholunate dissociation* and subsequent malalignment of either or both bones.[39] As shown in Figure 7-19, *B*, the more unstable lunate most often dislocates, or subluxes, so its distal articular surface faces *dorsally*. This condition is referred to clinically as *dorsal intercalated segment instability* (DISI) (Figure 7-20). Injury to other ligaments, such as the lunotriquetral ligament, may cause the lunate to dislocate such that its distal articular surface faces *volarly* (palmarly). This condition is referred to as *volar (palmar) intercalated segment instability* (VISI).[75] Regardless of the type of rotational collapse, the consequences can be painful and disabling. Changes in the natural arthrokinematics may create regions of high stress, eventually leading to joint destruction, chronic inflammation, and changes in the shapes of the bones. A painful and unstable wrist may fail to provide a stable platform for the hand. A collapsed wrist may also alter the length-tension relationship and moment arms of the muscles that cross the region.[81]

ULNAR TRANSLOCATION OF THE CARPUS

As pointed out earlier, the distal end of the radius is angled from side to side so that its articular surface is sloped ulnarly about 25 degrees (see Figure 7-4, *A*). This ulnar tilt of the radius creates a natural tendency for the carpus to slide (translate) in an ulnar direction.[3] Figure 7-21 shows that a wrist with an ulnar tilt of 25 degrees has an ulnar translation force of 42% of the total compression force that crosses the wrist. This

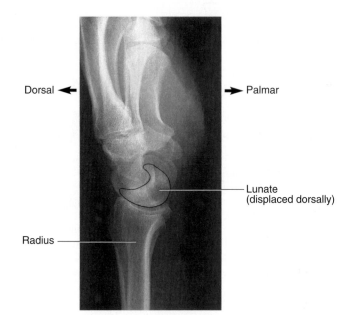

FIGURE 7-20. Lateral radiograph showing an abnormal *dorsal* position of the distal surface of the lunate, a condition referred to as *dorsal intercalated segment instability* (DISI). (Radiograph courtesy Jon Marion, CHT, OTR, and Thomas Hitchcock, MD. Marshfield Clinic, Marshfield, Wisconsin.)

translational force is naturally resisted by passive tension from various extrinsic ligaments, such as palmar radiocarpal ligament. A disease such as rheumatoid arthritis may weaken the ligaments of the wrist. Over time, the carpus may migrate ulnarly. An excessive ulnar translocation can significantly alter the biomechanics of the entire wrist and hand.

MUSCLE AND JOINT INTERACTION

Innervation of the Wrist Muscles and Joints

INNERVATION OF MUSCLE

The *radial nerve* innervates all the muscles that cross the dorsal side of the wrist (see Figure 6-32, *B*). The primary wrist extensors are the extensor carpi radialis longus, extensor carpi radialis

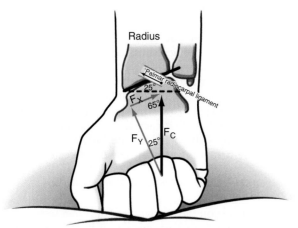

FIGURE 7-21. This shows how the ulnar tilt of the distal radius can predispose to ulnar translocation of the carpus. Compression forces *(F$_C$)* that cross the wrist are resolved into (1) a force vector acting perpendicularly to the radiocarpal joint *(F$_Y$)* and (2) a force vector *(F$_X$)* running parallel to the radiocarpal joint. The F$_Y$ force compresses and stabilizes the radiocarpal joint with a magnitude of about 90% of F$_C$ (cosine 25° × F$_C$). The F$_X$ force tends to translate the carpus in an ulnar direction, with a magnitude of 42% of F$_C$ (sine 25° × F$_C$). Note that the fiber direction of the palmar radiocarpal ligament resists this natural ulnar translation of the carpus. The greater the ulnar tilt and/or compression force across the wrist, the greater the potential for the ulnar translation.

brevis, and extensor carpi ulnaris. The *median and ulnar nerves* innervate all muscles that cross the palmar side of the wrist, including the primary wrist flexors (see Figure 6-32, *C* and *D*). The flexor carpi radialis and palmaris longus are innervated by the median nerve; the flexor carpi ulnaris is innervated by the ulnar nerve. As a reference, the primary spinal nerve roots that supply the muscles of the upper extremity are listed in Appendix II, Part A. In addition, Appendix II, Parts B to D include additional reference items to help guide the clinical assessment of the functional status of the C^5 to T^1 spinal nerve roots and several major peripheral nerves of the upper limb.

SENSORY INNERVATION OF THE JOINTS

The radiocarpal and midcarpal joints receive sensory fibers from the C^6 and C^7 spinal nerve roots carried in the median and radial nerves.[19,26,30] (This terminal sensory branch of the radial nerve often develops a painful neuroma within the wrists' dorsal capsule.) The midcarpal joint is also innervated by sensory nerves traveling to the C^8 spinal nerve root via the deep branch of the ulnar nerve.

Function of the Muscles at the Wrist

The wrist is controlled by a primary and a secondary set of muscles. The tendons of the muscles within the *primary set* attach distally within the carpus, or the adjacent proximal end of the metacarpals; these muscles act essentially on the wrist only. The tendons of the muscles within the *secondary set* cross the carpus as they continue distally to attach to the digits. The secondary muscles therefore act on the wrist *and* the hand. This chapter focuses more on the muscles of the primary set. The anatomy and kinesiology of the muscles of the secondary set—such as the extensor pollicis longus and the flexor digitorum superficialis—are considered in detail in Chapter 8. The

proximal and distal attachments and nerve supply of the muscles of the wrist are listed in Appendix II, Part E.

As depicted in Figure 7-13, the medial-lateral and anterior-posterior axes of rotation of the wrist intersect within the head of the capitate bone. With the possible exception of the palmaris longus, no muscle has a line of force that passes precisely *through* either axis of rotation. At least from the anatomic position, essentially all wrist muscles therefore are equipped with moment arms to produce torques in both sagittal and frontal planes. The extensor carpi radialis longus, for example, passes dorsally to the medial-lateral axis of rotation and laterally to the anterior-posterior axis of rotation. Contraction of only this muscle would produce a combination of wrist extension *and* radial deviation. Using the extensor carpi radialis longus to produce a pure radial deviation motion, for example, would necessitate the activation of other muscles to neutralize the undesired wrist extension potential of the aforementioned muscle. Muscles of the wrist and hand rarely act in isolation when producing a meaningful movement. This theme of intermuscular cooperation will be further developed in this chapter and Chapter 8.

FUNCTION OF THE WRIST EXTENSORS

Muscular Anatomy

The primary wrist extensors are the *extensor carpi radialis longus*, the *extensor carpi radialis brevis*, and the *extensor carpi ulnaris* (Figure 7-22). The extensor digitorum is also capable

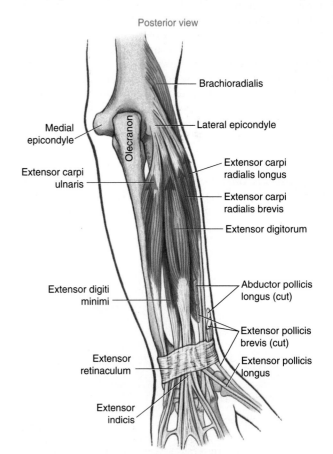

FIGURE 7-22. A posterior view of the right forearm showing the primary wrist extensors: extensor carpi radialis longus, extensor carpi radialis brevis, and extensor carpi ulnaris. The extensor digitorum and other secondary wrist extensors are also evident.

of generating significant wrist extension torque but is mainly involved with extension of the fingers. Other secondary wrist extensors are the extensor indicis, extensor digiti minimi, and extensor pollicis longus.

Wrist Extensor Muscles

Primary Set (Act on Wrist Only)
- Extensor carpi radialis longus
- Extensor carpi radialis brevis
- Extensor carpi ulnaris

Secondary Set (Act on Wrist and Hand)
- Extensor digitorum
- Extensor indicis
- Extensor digiti minimi
- Extensor pollicis longus

The proximal attachments of the primary wrist extensors are located on and near the lateral ("extensor-supinator") epicondyle of the humerus and dorsal border of the ulna (see Figures 6-2 and 6-6). Distally, the extensor carpi radialis longus and brevis attach side by side to the dorsal bases of the second and third metacarpals, respectively; the extensor carpi ulnaris attaches to the dorsal base of the fifth metacarpal.

The tendons of the muscles that cross the dorsal and dorsal-radial side of the wrist are secured in place by the *extensor retinaculum* (Figure 7-23). Ulnarly, the extensor retinaculum wraps around the styloid process of the ulna to attach palmarly to the tendon of the flexor carpi ulnaris, pisiform bone, and pisometacarpal ligament. Radially, the retinaculum attaches to the styloid process of the radius and the radial collateral ligament. The extensor retinaculum prevents the underlying tendons from "bowstringing" up and away from the radiocarpal joint during active movements of the wrist.

Between the extensor retinaculum and the underlying bones are six *fibro-osseus compartments* that house the tendons along with their synovial sheaths.[32] Clinicians frequently refer to these compartments by Roman numerals I to VI (see Figure 7-23). Each compartment houses a specific set of tendons. Tenosynovitis frequently occurs within one or more of these compartments, often from repetitive or forceful activities that increase tension on the associated tendons. The tendons and surrounding synovial membranes within compartment I are

particularly susceptible to inflammation, a condition called *de Quervain's tenosynovitis*. Activities that frequently cause this painful condition include repetitively pressing the trigger switch on a power tool, gripping tools while simultaneously supinating and pronating the forearm, or wringing out clothes. De Quervain's tenosynovitis is typically treated conservatively by phonophoresis or iontophoresis, cortisone injections, ice, wearing a hand-wrist–based thumb splint, and modifying the activity that caused the inflammation. If conservative therapy fails to reduce the inflammation, surgical release of the first compartment may be indicated.

Biomechanical Assessment of Wrist Muscles' Action and Torque Potential

Data are available on the relative position, cross-sectional area, and length of the internal moment arms of most muscles that cross the wrist.[40,83] By knowing the approximate location of the axes of rotation of the wrist, these data provide a useful method for estimating the action and relative torque potential of the wrist muscles (Figure 7-24). Consider, for instance, the extensor carpi ulnaris and the flexor carpi ulnaris. By noting the location of each tendon from the axis of rotation, it is evident that the extensor carpi ulnaris is an extensor and ulnar deviator and the flexor carpi ulnaris is a flexor and ulnar deviator. Because both muscles have similar cross-sectional areas, they likely produce comparable levels of maximal force. In order to estimate the relative *torque* production of the two muscles, however, each muscle's cross-sectional area must be multiplied by each muscle's specific moment arm length. The extensor carpi ulnaris therefore is considered a more potent ulnar deviator than an extensor; the flexor carpi ulnaris is considered both a potent flexor and a potent ulnar deviator.

Wrist Extensor Activity while Making a Fist

The main function of the wrist extensors is to position and stabilize the wrist during activities involving active flexion of the fingers. Of particular importance is the role of the wrist extensor muscles in making a fist or producing a strong grip. To demonstrate this, rapidly tighten and release the fist and note the strong synchronous activity from the wrist extensors. The extrinsic finger flexor muscles, namely the flexor digitorum profundus and flexor digitorum superficialis, possess a significant internal moment arm as *wrist* flexors. The leverage

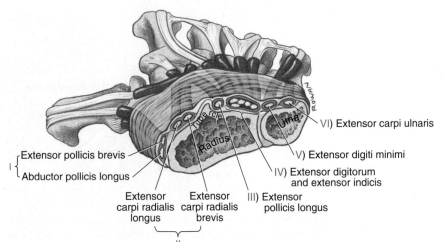

FIGURE 7-23. A dorsal oblique view shows a cross-section of the tendons of the extensor muscles of the wrist and digits passing through the extensor retinaculum of the wrist. All tendons that cross the dorsal aspect of the wrist travel within one of six fibro-osseus compartments embedded within the extensor retinaculum. Roman numerals indicate the specific fibro-osseus compartment, along with their associated set of tendons. See text for more discussion. Synovial linings are indicated in blue.

I) Extensor pollicis brevis / Abductor pollicis longus

II) Extensor carpi radialis longus / Extensor carpi radialis brevis

III) Extensor pollicis longus

IV) Extensor digitorum and extensor indicis

V) Extensor digiti minimi

VI) Extensor carpi ulnaris

Radius

Ulna

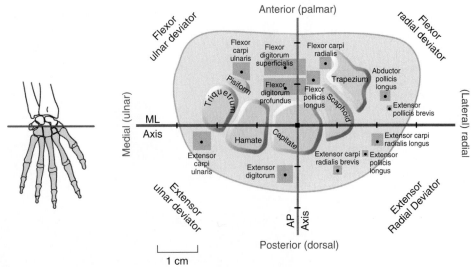

FIGURE 7-24. A cross-sectional view looking distally through the right carpal tunnel, similar to the perspective shown in Figure 7-5. The plot depicts the *cross-sectional area, position,* and length of the *internal moment arms* for most muscles that cross the wrist at the level of the head of the capitate. The area within the red boxes on the grid is proportional to the cross-sectional area of the muscle's belly and therefore indicative of the maximal force production. The small black dot within each red box indicates the position of the muscle's tendon. The wrist's medial-lateral *(ML)* axis of rotation *(dark gray)* and anterior-posterior *(AP)* axis of rotation *(red)* intersect within the head of the capitate bone. Each muscle's moment arm for a particular action is equal to the perpendicular distance between either axis and the position of the muscle's tendon. The length of each moment arm (expressed in centimeters) is indicated by the major tick marks. Assume that the wrist is held in a neutral position.

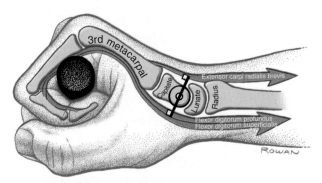

FIGURE 7-25. Muscle mechanics involved with the production of a strong grip. Contraction of the extrinsic finger flexors (flexor digitorum superficialis and profundus) flexes the fingers but also creates a simultaneous *wrist flexion* torque. Activation of the wrist extensors, such as the extensor carpi radialis brevis, is necessary to block the wrist flexion tendency caused by the activated finger flexor muscles. In this manner the wrist extensors maintain the optimal length of the finger flexors to effectively flex the fingers. The internal moment arms for the extensor carpi radialis brevis and extrinsic finger flexors are shown in dark bold lines. The small circle within the capitate marks the medial-lateral axis of rotation at the wrist.

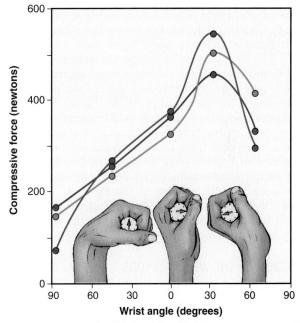

FIGURE 7-26. The compression forces produced by a maximal-effort grip are shown for three different wrist positions (for three subjects). Maximal grip force occurs at about 30 degrees of extension. (With permission from Inman VT, Ralston HJ, Todd F: *Human walking,* Baltimore, 1981, Williams & Wilkins.)

of these muscles for wrist flexion is evident in Figure 7-24. The wrist extensor muscles must counterbalance the significant wrist flexion torque produced by the finger flexor muscles (Figure 7-25). As a strong grip is applied to an object, the wrist extensors typically hold the wrist in about 30 to 35 degrees of extension and about 5 degrees of ulnar deviation.[56] This position optimizes the length-tension relationship of the extrinsic finger flexors, thereby facilitating maximal grip strength (Figure 7-26).

As evident in Figure 7-26, grip strength is significantly reduced when the wrist is fully flexed. The decreased grip strength is caused by a combination of two factors. First, and likely foremost, the finger flexors cannot generate adequate force because they are functioning at an extremely shortened length respective to their length-tension curve. Second, the overstretched finger extensors, particularly the extensor digitorum, create a passive extensor torque at the fingers, which

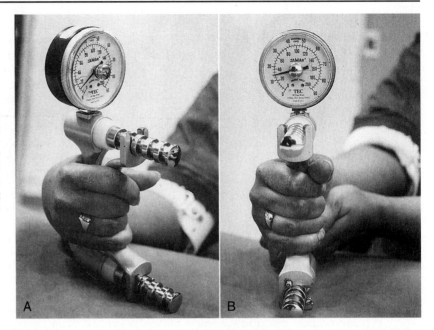

FIGURE 7-27. A person with paralysis of her right wrist extensor muscles (after a radial nerve injury) is performing a maximal-effort grip using a dynamometer. **A,** Despite normally innervated finger flexor muscles, maximal grip strength measures only 10 pounds (about 4.5 kg). **B,** The same person is shown stabilizing her wrist in order to prevent it from flexing during the grip effort. Note that the grip force has nearly tripled.

further reduces effective grip force. This combination of physiologic and biomechanic events explains why a person with paralyzed wrist extensor muscles has difficulty producing an effective grip, even though the finger flexor muscles remain fully innervated. Trying to produce a maximal-effort grip when the wrist extensors are paralyzed results in an abnormal posture of finger flexion *and* wrist flexion (Figure 7-27, *A*). Stabilizing the wrist in greater extension enables the finger flexor muscles to nearly triple their grip force (see Figure 7-27, *B*). Manually or orthotically preventing the wrist from flexing maintains the extrinsic finger flexors at an elongated length more conducive to a higher force production.

Ordinarily the person depicted in Figure 7-27 wears a splint that holds the wrist in 10 to 20 degrees of extension. If the radial nerve fails to reinnervate the wrist extensor muscles, a tendon from another muscle is often surgically transferred to provide wrist extension torque. For example, the pronator teres muscle, innervated by the median nerve, is connected to the tendon of the extensor carpi radialis brevis. Of the three primary wrist extensors, the extensor carpi radialis brevis is located most centrally at the wrist and has the greatest moment arm for wrist extension (see Figure 7-24).

FUNCTION OF THE WRIST FLEXORS

Muscular Anatomy

The three primary wrist flexors are the *flexor carpi radialis,* the *flexor carpi ulnaris,* and the *palmaris longus* (Figure 7-28). The palmaris longus is absent in about 10% to 15% of people.[82] Even when present, the muscle often exhibits variation in shape and number of tendons. The tendon of this muscle is often used as a donor in tendon grafting surgery.

The tendons of the three primary wrist flexor muscles are easily identified on the anterior distal forearm, especially during strong isometric activation. The *palmar carpal ligament,* not easily identified by palpation, is located proximal to the transverse carpal ligament. This structure, analogous to the extensor retinaculum, stabilizes the tendons of the wrist flexors and prevents excessive bowstringing during flexion.

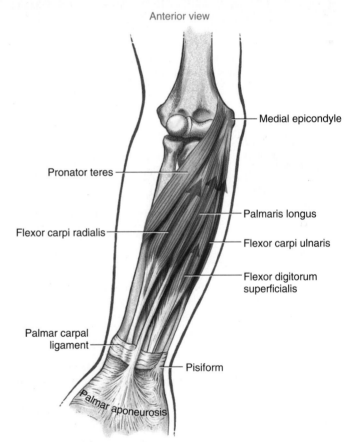

Anterior view

Pronator teres

Flexor carpi radialis

Palmar carpal ligament

Palmar aponeurosis

Medial epicondyle

Palmaris longus

Flexor carpi ulnaris

Flexor digitorum superficialis

Pisiform

FIGURE 7-28. Anterior view of the right forearm showing the primary wrist flexor muscles: flexor carpi radialis, palmaris longus, and flexor carpi ulnaris. The flexor digitorum superficialis (a secondary wrist flexor) and pronator teres muscles are also shown.

Other secondary muscles capable of flexing the wrist are the extrinsic flexors of the digits: the flexor digitorum profundus, flexor digitorum superficialis, and flexor pollicis longus. (The classification of these muscles as "secondary" wrist flexors should *not* imply they have a limited potential to perform this

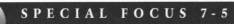

SPECIAL FOCUS 7-5

Overuse Syndrome of the Wrist Extensor Muscles: "Lateral Epicondylalgia"

The most active wrist extensor muscle during light closure of the fist is the extensor carpi radialis brevis. As grip force increases, the extensor carpi ulnaris, followed closely in time by the extensor carpi radialis longus, joins the activated extensor brevis.[63] Activities that require repetitive forceful grasp, such as hammering or playing tennis,[8] may stress the proximal attachment site of the wrist extensor muscles, often leading to a painful condition called *lateral epicondylalgia* or, more informally, "tennis elbow." The stress on this region may be great, considering the high forces in the muscles during a maximal grasp and, with regard to the extensor carpi radialis brevis, the relatively small muscular attachment site on the lateral epicondyle. Furthermore, the proximal tendon of the extensor carpi radialis brevis naturally contacts the lateral margin of the capitulum (of the distal humerus) during flexion and extension of the elbow. This contact may actually cause an abrasion of the undersurface of this muscle.[10]

The symptoms of this relatively frequently reported syndrome include pain during passive wrist flexion and forearm pronation, tenderness over the lateral epicondyle, and reduced grip strength.

Traditional treatment includes splinting, rest, stretching and mobilization of the muscles, laser therapy, and other physical modalities specifically aimed at reducing inflammation, such as ultrasound, ice, electrotherapy, iontophoresis, and so on.[84]

The pathophysiology of lateral epicondylalgia is not well understood. Until relatively recently, the condition was called *lateral epicondylitis,* reflecting the belief that the stressed proximal tendon of the wrist extensors, especially the extensor carpi radialis brevis, was actually inflamed (hence the suffix -*itis*).[87] Several different lines of research have recently reported, however, that the affected tendon does not show indicators of inflammation, but of degeneration.[1,38,53,62] What has traditionally been thought to be a primary inflammatory process may actually be a degenerative one, similar to that observed with aging, vascular compromise, and microtrauma.[4] Regardless of the actual pathologic process, the root cause of the problem is likely of biomechanical origin: a large stress is placed on the wrist extensor muscles to balance the strong wrist flexion potential of the extrinsic finger flexors.

---

task. Actually, based on the muscles' cross-sectional areas and wrist flexor moment arms [see Figure 7-24], the wrist flexion torque potential of extrinsic flexors of the digits may *exceed* that of the primary wrist flexors.) With the wrist in a neutral position, the abductor pollicis longus and extensor pollicis brevis have a small moment arm for wrist flexion (see Figure 7-24).

Wrist Flexor Muscles

Primary Set (Act on Wrist Only)
- Flexor carpi radialis
- Flexor carpi ulnaris
- Palmaris longus

Secondary Set (Act on Wrist and Hand)
- Flexor digitorum profundus
- Flexor digitorum superficialis
- Flexor pollicis longus
- Abductor pollicis longus
- Extensor pollicis brevis

The proximal attachments of the primary wrist flexors are located on and near the medial ("flexor-pronator") epicondyle of the humerus and dorsal border of the ulna (see Figures 6-2 and 6-6). Technically, the tendon of the flexor carpi radialis does not cross the wrist *through* the carpal tunnel; rather, the tendon passes in a separate tunnel formed by a groove in the trapezium and fascia from the adjacent transverse carpal ligament (Figure 7-29). The tendon of the flexor carpi radialis attaches distally to the palmar base of the second and sometimes the third metacarpal. The palmaris longus has a distal attachment primarily to the thick aponeurosis of the palm. The tendon of the flexor carpi ulnaris courses distally to attach to the pisiform bone and, in a plane superficial to the transverse carpal ligament, into the pisohamate and pisometacarpal ligaments and the base of the fifth metacarpal bone.

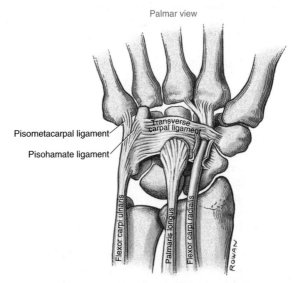

FIGURE 7-29. The palmar aspect of the right wrist showing the distal attachments of the primary wrist flexor muscles. Note that the tendon of the flexor carpi radialis courses through a sheath located within the superficial fibers of the transverse carpal ligament. Most of the distal attachment of the palmaris longus has been removed with the palmar aponeurosis.

Functional Considerations

Based on moment arm and cross-sectional area (see Figure 7-24), the flexor carpi ulnaris produces the greatest wrist flexion torque potential of the three primary wrist flexor muscles. During active wrist flexion, the flexor carpi radialis and flexor carpi ulnaris act together as synergists while simultaneously opposing each other's radial and ulnar deviation ability.

As indicated in Table 7-1, data indicate that the wrist flexor muscles produce about 70% greater isometric torque than the wrist extensor muscles—12.2 Nm versus 7.1 Nm, respectively.[17] The greater total cross-sectional area of the wrist flexor muscles as a group can account for much of this disparity.[29] It is noteworthy that the extrinsic finger flexors (flexors digitorum superficialis and profundus) account for about two thirds of the total cross-sectional area of the wrist flexors.[40] Activities such as lifting or pulling heavy objects normally demand strength in both the wrist flexor and finger flexor musculature. Strong coactivation of the wrist extensor muscles is required during these activities to prevent a relatively ineffective position of combined wrist *and* finger flexion.

TABLE 7-1. Magnitude and Wrist Joint Position of Peak Isometric Torque Produced by Healthy Males			
Wrist Muscle Group	Mean Peak Torque (Nm)	Joint Angle of Peak Torque
Flexors	12.2 (3.7)	40 degrees of flexion
Extensors	7.1 (2.1)	From 30 degrees of flexion to 70 degrees of extension
Radial deviators	11.0 (2.0)	0 degrees (neutral)
Ulnar deviators	9.5 (2.2)	0 degrees (neutral)

Data from Delp SL, Grierson AE, Buchanan TS: Maximum isometric moments generated by the wrist muscles in flexion-extension and radial-ulnar deviation, *J Biomech* 29:1371, 1996.
Standard deviations in parentheses.
Conversions: 1.36 Nm/ft-lb.

FUNCTION OF THE RADIAL AND ULNAR DEVIATORS

Muscles capable of producing *radial deviation* of the wrist are the extensor carpi radialis brevis and longus, extensor pollicis longus and brevis, flexor carpi radialis, abductor pollicis longus, and flexor pollicis longus (review Figure 7-24). In the neutral wrist position, the extensor carpi radialis longus and abductor pollicis longus possess the largest product of cross-sectional area and moment arm for radial deviation torque. The extensor pollicis brevis has the greatest moment arm of all radial deviators; however, because of a relatively small cross-sectional area, this muscle's torque production is relatively small. The abductor pollicis longus and extensor pollicis brevis provide important stability to the radial side of the wrist, augmenting that produced passively by the radial collateral ligament. As shown in Table 7-1, the radial deviator muscles generate about 15% greater isometric torque than the ulnar deviator muscles—11.0 Nm versus 9.5 Nm, respectively.[17]

Radial Deviators of the Wrist
• Extensor carpi radialis longus
• Extensor carpi radialis brevis
• Extensor pollicis longus
• Extensor pollicis brevis
• Flexor carpi radialis
• Abductor pollicis longus
• Flexor pollicis longus

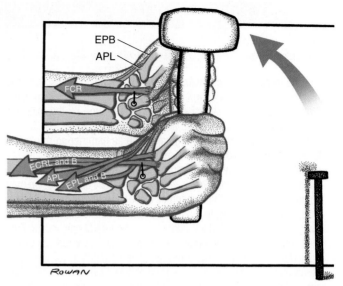

FIGURE 7-30. The muscles that perform radial deviation of the wrist are shown preparing to strike a nail with a hammer. The image in the background is a mirror reflection of the palmar surface of the wrist. The axis of rotation is through the capitate with the internal moment arms shown for the extensor carpi radialis brevis *(ECRB)* and the flexor carpi radialis *(FCR)* only. The flexor pollicis longus is not shown. *APL,* abductor pollicis longus; *ECRL and B,* extensor carpi radialis longus and brevis; *EPL and B,* extensor pollicis longus and brevis.

Figure 7-30 shows the radial deviator muscles contracting during use of a hammer. All these muscles pass laterally to the wrist's anterior-posterior axis of rotation. The action of the extensor carpi radialis longus and the flexor carpi radialis, shown with moment arms, illustrates a fine example of two muscles cooperating as synergists for one motion but as antagonists for another. The net effect of this muscular cooperation produces a radially deviated wrist, well stabilized in slight extension for optimal grasp of the hammer.

Muscles capable of *ulnar deviation* of the wrist are the extensor carpi ulnaris, flexor carpi ulnaris, flexor digitorum profundus and superficialis, and extensor digitorum (see Figure 7-24). Because of moment arm length, however, the muscles most capable of this action, by far, are the extensor carpi ulnaris and flexor carpi radialis. Figure 7-31 shows this strong pair of ulnar deviator muscles contracting as a nail is struck with a hammer. Both the flexor and extensor carpi ulnaris contract synergistically to perform the ulnar deviation but also stabilize the wrist in a slightly extended position. Because of the strong functional association between the flexor and extensor carpi ulnaris muscles, injury to either muscle can incapacitate the overall kinetics of ulnar deviation. For example, rheumatoid arthritis often causes inflammation and pain in the extensor carpi ulnaris tendon near its distal attachment. Attempts at active ulnar deviation with minimal to no activation in the painful extensor carpi ulnaris cause the action of the flexor carpi ulnaris to go unopposed. The resulting flexed posture of the wrist is thereby not suitable for an effective grasp.

Ulnar Deviators of the Wrist
• Extensor carpi ulnaris
• Flexor carpi ulnaris
• Flexor digitorum profundus and superficialis
• Extensor digitorum

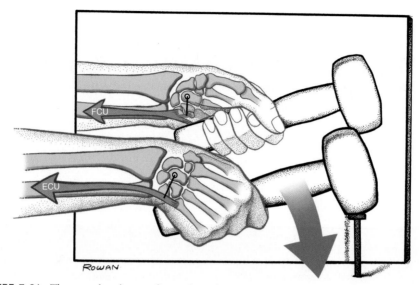

FIGURE 7-31. The muscles that perform ulnar deviation are shown as a nail is struck with a hammer. The image in the background is a mirror reflection of the palmar surface of the wrist. The axis of rotation is shown through the capitate with internal moment arms shown for the flexor carpi ulnaris *(FCU)* and the extensor carpi ulnaris *(ECU)*.

SYNOPSIS

The wrist consists of two primary articulations: the radiocarpal and the midcarpal joints. The radiocarpal joint joins the distal end of the radius with bones of the proximal carpus; the midcarpal joint unites the proximal and distal rows of carpal bones. Forces produced by active muscle and subsequently stretched ligaments guide the arthrokinematics across both joints. The resulting biplanar movements of the wrist optimize hand placement. Reduced or painful movement of the wrist can dramatically compromise the function of the hand and thus the entire upper limb.

In addition to effective placement of the hand, the wrist is associated with two other important functions of the upper extremity: load acceptance and the kinematics of pronation and supination of the forearm. First, the wrist must be able to accept large compression forces that impact the distal end of the upper limb, similar to the way the ankle accepts forces during standing or walking. Compression forces that impact the wrist, however, occur not only from contact with the environment, such as pushing up from an armrest of a chair, but also from muscle forces produced to make a grasp. The naturally broadened shape of the distal radius helps reduce the contact stress against the carpal bones. The interosseous membrane and the relative flexible articulations within the proximal row of carpal bones further dissipate the compression forces that cross the wrist. Often, external forces may exceed the ability of these load dispersal mechanisms to protect the region, resulting in trauma such as fracture of the distal radius, tears in part of the interosseous membrane, rupture of the scapholunate ligament, and fracture or dislocation of the scaphoid and lunate bones.

The design of the wrist is also strongly associated with the kinematics of pronation and supination of the forearm. Elements of this design are present on both sides of the wrist. Radially, the radiocarpal joint restricts axial rotation between the carpus and the radius. By restricting this motion, the hand is obligated to follow the path of the pronating and supinating radius. As the wrist limits axial rotation radially, it selectively permits this motion ulnarly. The large ulnocarpal space and associated soft tissues loosely bind the ulnar side of the carpus to the ulna. Acting as a semi-elastic tether, the triangular fibrocartilage complex allows the radius, with firmly attached carpus, to pronate and supinate freely about the distal end of the ulna. Without this freedom of motion on the ulnar side of the wrist, pronation and supination of the forearm would be significantly restricted.

Essentially all muscles that cross the wrist have multiple actions—either at the wrist itself or at the more distal digits. Consequently, relatively simple, uniplanar motions demand relatively complex muscular interactions. Consider, for example, that extending the wrist requires at least a pair of muscles to neutralize unwanted radial or ulnar deviations. Consider also the need for strong muscle activation from the wrist extensor muscles to stabilize the wrist during grasping. Without such proximal stability, the finger flexors are typically rendered ineffective. Loss of proximal stability of the wrist can occur from several sources: injury or disease of the peripheral or central nervous center, or pain in the region of the lateral epicondyle—the proximal attachment site of the wrist extensor muscles, or one of the six fibro-osseous compartments located on the dorsal side of the wrist. Understanding how these impairments affect the kinesiology of the wrist is a fundamental element of providing the most effective therapeutic intervention.

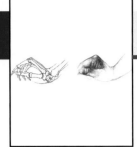

ADDITIONAL CLINICAL CONNECTIONS

CLINICAL CONNECTION 7-1
"Ulnar Variance" at the Wrist: Associated Kinesiology and Clinical Implications

DEFINING "ULNAR VARIANCE": The distal ends of the radius and the ulna approach the proximal side of the carpus at two locations: the radiocarpal joint and the ulnocarpal space. Excessive asymmetry in the length of either the radius or the ulna can place large and damaging stress on the soft tissues and bones of the wrist. Often, and especially when combined with excessive manual labor, increased carpal stress can cause chronic inflammation, pain, rupture or deformation of ligaments, change in shape of the bones and articular surfaces, reduced grip strength, and altered hemodynamics.

Variation in the length or position of the forearm bones can occur congenitally or can be acquired through trauma or disease. A method for quantifying the relative lengths of these bones at the wrist is referred to as *ulnar variance*.[57] This quantification is typically determined from a posterior-anterior (PA) radiograph, as shown in Figure 7-32. An ulnar variance of zero, as indicated in the asymptomatic specimen illustrated in the figure, implies that the forearm bones extend distally the same length. *Positive ulnar variance* is the distance the ulnar head extends *distal* to the reference line; *negative ulnar variance* is the distance the ulnar head lies *proximal* to this line. Normative mean values for ulnar variance are generally reported to be between 0 and −1 mm, with a standard deviation of about 1.5 mm.[72,89]

A near neutral ulnar variance is expected in a healthy person when the variance is measured on a static radiograph. During certain active movements, however, ulnar variance fluctuates to varying degrees. As described in Chapter 6, the radius naturally "pistons" proximally and distally during forearm pronation and supination, respectively.[22] Although relatively slight, this translation of the radius is evident at both the elbow and the wrist. As depicted in Figure 6-30, the proximal migration of the radius during pronation increases the compression force at the humeroradial joint. The natural, muscular-driven proximal migration of the radius creates a *positive* ulnar variance at the wrist (i.e., the ulnar head aligns more distally relative to the translated radius).[33] Muscle contraction involved with making a grip also pulls the radius proximally, increasing positive ulnar variance by 1 to 2 mm.[20] (Although the term *ulnar variance* implies displacement of the ulna, most often the variance is created by displacement of the *radius;* the stable humero-ulnar joint typically restricts migration of the ulna.)

Although pronation naturally creates a greater positive ulnar variance, supination creates a greater negative ulnar variance.[33] This is because of the natural *distal* migration of the radius with supination, an action that also reduces the compression force at the humeroradial joint.

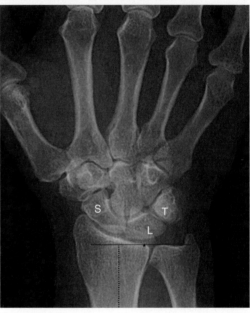

FIGURE 7-32. A posterior-anterior (PA) radiograph of an asymptomatic wrist, illustrating the measurement of ulnar variance. A dashed black line is drawn parallel with the long axis of the radius. Next, a red reference line is drawn perpendicular to the long axis of the radius at the level of the subchondral bone of the lunate facet of the radius (indicated by the asterisk). The distance between this reference line and the most distal portion of the ulnar head is the measure of ulnar variance. This image indicates an ulnar variance of zero—often referred to as "neutral" ulnar variance. *L,* lunate; *S,* scaphoid; *T,* triquetrum. (Radiograph courtesy of Jon Marion, OTR, CHT, and Thomas Hitchcock, MD, Marshfield Clinic, Marshfield, Wisconsin.)

Natural Consequences of Active Pronation
- Proximal migration of the radius
- Increased ulnar variance at the wrist
- Increased compression at the humeroradial joint

Natural Consequences of Active Supination
- Distal migration of the radius
- Decreased ulnar variance at the wrist
- Decreased compression at the humeroradial joint

ADDITIONAL CLINICAL CONNECTIONS

CLINICAL CONNECTION 7-1
"Ulnar Variance" at the Wrist: Associated Kinesiology and Clinical Implications—cont'd

The natural change in ulnar variance with forearm pronation and supination is indeed small—on the order of 1 to 2 mm. The pliability of the triangular fibrocartilage complex and articular cartilage covering the adjacent bones typically accommodates to this small movement without negative physiologic consequence. Ulnar variance that significantly exceeds the natural 1 to 2 mm, however, can cause functional impairments at the wrist and distal radio-ulnar joint, which can be severe and disabling. The following sections highlight examples of such cases, including the relevant kinesiology and implications for medical treatment.

EXAMPLES OF CAUSE OF AND PATHOMECHANICS ASSOCIATED WITH EXCESSIVE ULNAR VARIANCE

Positive Ulnar Variance
Several factors can cause the ulna to extend farther distally than the radius. Figure 7-33 shows an example of a patient who had dislocated her distal radio-ulnar joint and later developed 6 mm of positive ulnar variance. The patient experienced severe pain in the ulnocarpal space for 9 months, resulting in frequent loss of work. The patient ultimately required a surgical shortening of her ulna, thereby realigning the distal radio-ulnar joint.

Excessive positive ulnar variance is often associated with "ulnar impaction syndrome," characterized by distal encroachment of the ulna against the more central, avascular part of the triangular fibrocartilage (TFC), triquetrum, or lunate. When severe, ulnar impaction often progresses to inflammation and degeneration of the TFC.[93] Figure 7-34 illustrates a case of ulnar impaction syndrome in a physical 54-year-old mill worker. The patient's pain was exacerbated by activities performed in ulnar deviation and by those that naturally increased his positive ulnar variance, such as weight bearing through the upper extremity or making a strong

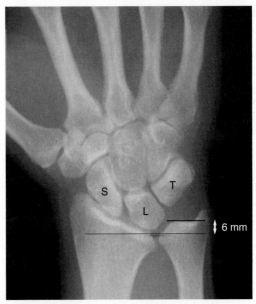

FIGURE 7-33. A posterior-anterior (PA) radiograph of a wrist with 6 mm of positive ulnar variance. Note the displaced distal radio-ulnar joint. *L,* lunate; *S,* scaphoid; *T,* triquetrum. (Radiograph courtesy of Jon Marion, OTR, CHT, and Thomas Hitchcock, MD, Marshfield Clinic, Marshfield, Wisconsin.)

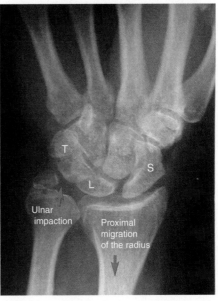

FIGURE 7-34. A posterior-anterior (PA) radiograph of the wrist of a patient diagnosed with "ulnar impaction syndrome." The patient has 5 mm of positive ulnar variance, secondary to a shortening (fracture) of the radius with subsequent proximal migration. Note the relative distal projection of the ulnar head into the ulnocarpal space. Also observe (1) the large osteophyte just distal to the ulnar head, (2) the loss of joint space between the lunate and the triquetrum, and (3) the scapholunate diastasis (separation of bones without fracture), likely involving rupture of the scapholunate ligament. *L,* lunate; *S,* scaphoid; *T,* triquetrum. (Radiograph courtesy of Ann Porretto-Loehrke, DPT, CHT, and John Bax, MD, PhD, Hand and Upper Extremity Center of Northeast Wisconsin, Appleton, Wisconsin.)

Continued

grip while pronating the forearm. This patient had fractured his radius while in his teens, resulting in a shortened radius with subsequent proximal migration. A shortened radius, from either a compression fracture or surgical removal of the radial head, is a common precursor to ulnar impaction syndrome. In general, the likelihood of proximal migration of the radius is increased if the interosseous membrane is also torn. As described in Chapter 6, an important but subtle function of the interosseous membrane is to resist proximal migration of the radius.[16]

Negative Ulnar Variance

Figure 7-35 shows a severe case of negative ulnar variance of the wrist secondary to a congenitally short ulna. The shortened ulna altered the natural congruence of the distal radio-ulnar joint, likely increasing intra-articular stress.[54] The increased stress placed on the joint, coupled with the patient's physically demanding occupation, eventually led to instability and degenerative arthritis, including rupture of most components of her triangular fibrocartilage cartilage complex (TFCC). The chief complaint of this 42-year-old woman was unmanageable pain in the ulnar region of the wrist, instability ("popping sounds"), and a significant loss of rotation of the forearm, especially supination.

Surgical intervention is often required in cases of severe pain and degeneration and loss of function in the distal radio-ulnar joint and ulnar side of the wrist. One such surgery to restore function primarily at the distal radio-ulnar joint is the *Sauve-Kapandji* procedure. The first step of the surgery is to fuse the unstable and painful distal radio-ulnar joint through the use of a screw (Figure

7-36). Next, a small 1-cm section of the ulna is removed at a point 1 to 2 cm proximal to the fused joint. This resulting space forms a "pseudo-arthrosis" (false joint), which serves as the "new" distal radio-ulnar joint. Pronation and supination now occur as the radius, carpal bones, and remaining distal ulna all rotate—as a fixed unit—about the more proximal ulna. Efforts are usually taken to stabilize the remaining proximal "stump" of ulna, typically by using attachments of the pronator quadratus and extensor carpi ulnaris muscles.[45] An intact interosseous membrane also provides stability to the proximal ulna.

A successful Sauve-Kapandji operation typically restores at least functional, pain-free motion at the ulnar side of the wrist and distal forearm. Together with an intact TFCC, the short, distal (fused) segment of ulna acts as a stable base for the ulnar side of the wrist, which is especially useful during weight-bearing activities.[11]

In addition to degeneration of the distal radio-ulnar joint and the TFCC, negative ulnar variance is often associated with *Kienböck's disease,* that is, fragmentation of the lunate (review Special Focus 7-1).[71] As was also the case in the patient discussed in Figure 7-35, the more distally projected radius jams against the lunate, perpetuating its fragmentation and avascular necrosis. Surgical treatment for Kienböck's disease may involve lengthening of the ulna, shortening of the radius, or, in very severe cases, partial or complete excision of the proximal row of carpal bones.[71] These procedures are all aimed at reducing the damaging stress on the lunate.

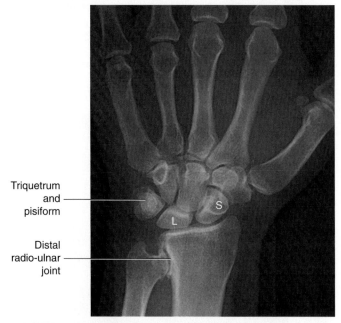

FIGURE 7-35. A posterior-anterior (PA) radiograph of a wrist with negative ulnar variance and associated degeneration of the distal radio-ulnar joint. *L,* lunate; *S,* scaphoid; *T,* triquetrum. (Radiograph courtesy of Jon Marion, OTR, CHT, and Thomas Hitchcock, MD, Marshfield Clinic, Marshfield, Wisconsin.)

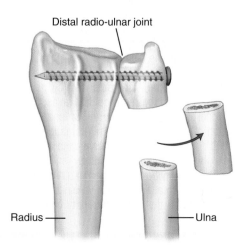

FIGURE 7-36. Sauve-Kapandji procedure performed on the wrist. The distal radio-ulnar joint is fused, and a pseudo-arthrosis is created in the ulna. (From Burke SL, Higgins J, McClinton MA, et al: *Hand and upper extremity rehabilitation: a practical guide,* ed 3, St Louis, 2006, Churchill Livingstone.)

REFERENCES

1. Alfredson H, Ljung BO, Thorsen K, Lorentzon R: In vivo investigation of ECRB tendons with microdialysis technique—no signs of inflammation but high amounts of glutamate in tennis elbow, *Acta Orthop Scand* 71:475-479, 2000.
2. Allan CH, Joshi A, Lichtman DM: Kienböck's disease: diagnosis and treatment, *J Am Acad Orthop Surg* 9:128-136, 2001.
3. Arimitsu S, Murase T, Hashimoto J, et al: A three-dimensional quantitative analysis of carpal deformity in rheumatoid wrists, *J Bone Joint Surg [Br]* 89:490-494, 2007.
4. Ashe MC, McCauley T, Khan KM: Tendinopathies in the upper extremity: A paradigm shift, *J Hand Ther* 17:329-334, 2004.
5. Bathala EA, Murray PM: Long-term follow-up of an undiagnosed transscaphoid perilunate dislocation demonstrating articular remodeling and functional adaptation, *J Hand Surg [Am]* 32:1020-1023, 2007.
6. Berger RA: The anatomy of the ligaments of the wrist and distal radioulnar joints, *Clin Orthop Relat Res* 383:32-40, 2001.
7. Berger RA: The anatomy of the scaphoid, *Hand Clin* 17:525-532, 2001.
8. Blackwell JR, Cole KJ: Wrist kinematics differ in expert and novice tennis players performing the backhand stroke: Implications for tennis elbow, *J Biomech* 27:509-516, 1994.
9. Blankenhorn BD, Pfaeffle HJ, Tang P, et al: Carpal kinematics after proximal row carpectomy, *J Hand Surg [Am]* 32:37-46, 2007.
10. Bunata RE, Brown DS, Capelo R: Anatomic factors related to the cause of tennis elbow, *J Hand Surg [Am]* 89:1955-1963, 2007.
11. Carter PB, Stuart PR: The Sauve-Kapandji procedure for post-traumatic disorders of the distal radio-ulnar joint, *J Bone Joint Surg [Br]* 82:1013-1018, 2000.
12. Cavaliere CM, Chung KC: A systematic review of total wrist arthroplasty compared with total wrist arthrodesis for rheumatoid arthritis, *Plast Reconstr Surg* 122:813-825, 2008.
13. Chidgey LK, Dell PC, Bittar ES, Spanier SS: Histologic anatomy of the triangular fibrocartilage, *J Hand Surg [Am]* 16:1084-1100, 1991.
14. Dacho AK, Baumeister S, Germann G, Sauerbier M: Comparison of proximal row carpectomy and midcarpal arthrodesis for the treatment of scaphoid nonunion advanced collapse (SNAC-wrist) and scapholunate advanced collapse (SLAC-wrist) in stage II, *J Plast Reconstr Aesthet Surg* 61:1210-1218, 2008.
15. de Lange A, Kauer JM, Huiskes R: Kinematic behavior of the human wrist joint: A roentgen-stereophotogrammetric analysis, *J Orthop Res* 3:56-64, 1985.
16. DeFrate LE, Li G, Zayontz SJ, Herndon JH: A minimally invasive method for the determination of force in the interosseous ligament, *Clin Biomech (Bristol, Avon)* 16:895-900, 2001.
17. Delp SL, Grierson AE, Buchanan TS: Maximum isometric moments generated by the wrist muscles in flexion-extension and radial-ulnar deviation, *J Biomech* 29:1371-1375, 1996.
18. Dobyns JH, Cooney WP: Classification of carpal instability. In Cooney WP, Linscheid R, Dobyns JH, editors: The Wrist, St Louis, 1998, Mosby.
19. Ferreres A, Suso S, Ordi J, et al: Wrist denervation. Anatomical considerations, *J Hand Surg [Br]* 20:761-768, 1995.
20. Friedman SL, Palmer AK, Short WH, et al: The change in ulnar variance with grip, *J Hand Surg [Am]* 18:713-716, 1993.
21. Frykman GK, Kroop WE: Fractures and traumatic conditions of the wrist. In Hunter JM, Mackin EJ, Callahan AD, editors: *Rehabilitation of the hand: surgery and therapy*, ed 4, St Louis, 1995, Mosby.
22. Garcia-Elias M: Soft-tissue anatomy and relationships about the distal ulna, *Hand Clin* 14:165-176, 1998.
23. Gardner MJ, Crisco JJ, Wolfe SW: Carpal kinematics, *Hand Clin* 22:413-420, 2006.
24. Gelberman RH, Gross MS: The vascularity of the wrist. Identification of arterial patterns at risk, *Clin Orthop Relat Res* 202:40-49, 1986.
25. Gofton WT, Gordon KD, Dunning CE, et al: Soft-tissue stabilizers of the distal radioulnar joint: an in vitro kinematic study, *J Hand Surg [Am]* 29:423-431, 2004
26. Gray DJ, Gardner E: The innervation of the joints of the wrist and hand, *Anat Rec* 151:261-266, 1965.
27. Gupta A, Moosawi NA: How much can carpus rotate axially? An in vivo study. *Clin Biomech (Bristol, Avon)* 20:172-176, 2005.
28. Hagert E, Ljung BO, Forsgren S: General innervation pattern and sensory corpuscles in the scapholunate interosseous ligament, *Cells Tissues Organs* 177:47-54, 2004.
29. Holzbaur KR, Delp SL, Gold GE, Murray WM: Moment-generating capacity of upper limb muscles in healthy adults, *J Biomech* 40:2442-2449, 2007.
30. Inman VT, Saunders JB: Referred pain from skeletal structures, *J Nerv Ment Dis* 99:660-667, 1944.
31. Ishii S, Palmer AK, Werner FW, et al: An anatomic study of the ligamentous structure of the triangular fibrocartilage complex, *J Hand Surg [Am]* 23:977-985, 1998.
32. Iwamoto A, Morris RP, Andersen C, et al: An anatomic and biomechanic study of the wrist extensor retinaculum septa and tendon compartments, *J Hand Surg [Am]* 31:896-903, 2006.
33. Jung JM, Baek GH, Kim JH, et al: Changes in ulnar variance in relation to forearm rotation and grip, *J Bone Joint Surg Br* 83:1029-1033, 2001.
34. Kauer JM: The mechanism of the carpal joint, *Clin Orthop Relat Res* 202:16-26, 1986.
35. Kaufmann R, Pfaeffle J, Blankenhorn B, et al: Kinematics of the midcarpal and radiocarpal joints in radioulnar deviation: an in vitro study, *J Hand Surg [Am]* 30:937-942, 2005.
36. Kihara H, Palmer AK, Werner FW, et al: The effect of dorsally angulated distal radius fractures on distal radioulnar joint congruency and forearm rotation, *J Hand Surg [Am]* 21:40-47, 1996.
37. Kobayashi M, Berger RA, Nagy L, et al: Normal kinematics of carpal bones: A three-dimensional analysis of carpal bone motion relative to the radius, *J Biomech* 30:787-793, 1997.
38. Kraushaar BS, Nirschl RP: Tendinosis of the elbow (tennis elbow). Clinical features and findings of histological, immunohistochemical, and electron microscopy studies, *J Bone Joint Surg [Am]* 81:259-278, 1999.
39. Kuo CE, Wolfe SW: Scapholunate instability: current concepts in diagnosis and management, *J Hand Surg [Am]* 33:998-1013, 2008.
40. Lehmkuhl LD, Smith LK: Brunnstrom's clinical kinesiology, ed 4, Philadelphia, 1983, FA Davis.
41. Li ZM, Kuxhaus L, Fisk JA, Christophel TH: Coupling between wrist flexion-extension and radial-ulnar deviation, *Clin Biomech (Bristol, Avon)* 20:177-183, 2005.
42. Linscheid RL: Kinematic considerations of the wrist, *Clin Orthop Relat Res* 202:27-39, 1986.
43. MacConaill MA, Basmajian JV: *Muscles and movements: a basis for human kinesiology*, New York, 1977, Robert E. Krieger.
44. Majima M, Horii E, Matsuki H, et al: Load transmission through the wrist in the extended position, *J Hand Surg [Am]* 33:182-188, 2008.
45. Minami A, Kato H, Iwasaki N: Modification of the Sauve-Kapandji procedure with extensor carpi ulnaris tenodesis, *J Hand Surg [Am]* 25:1080-1084, 2000.
46. Mitsuyasu H, Patterson RM, Shah MA, et al: The role of the dorsal intercarpal ligament in dynamic and static scapholunate instability, *J Hand Surg [Am]* 29:279-288, 2004.
47. Moojen TM, Snel JG, Ritt MJ, et al: In vivo analysis of carpal kinematics and comparative review of the literature, *J Hand Surg [Am]* 28:81-87, 2003.
48. Moojen TM, Snel JG, Ritt MJ, et al: Three-dimensional carpal kinematics in vivo, *Clin Biomech (Bristol, Avon)* 17:506-514, 2002.
49. Moore DC, Crisco JJ, Trafton TG, Leventhal EL: A digital database of wrist bone anatomy and carpal kinematics, *J Biomech* 40:2537-2542, 2007.
50. Moritomo H, Apergis EP, Herzberg G, et al: 2007 IFSSH committee report of wrist biomechanics committee: biomechanics of the so-called dart-throwing motion of the wrist, *J Hand Surg [Am]* 32:1447-1453, 2007.
51. Moritomo H, Murase T, Goto A, et al: Capitate-based kinematics of the midcarpal joint during wrist radioulnar deviation: an in vivo three-dimensional motion analysis, *J Hand Surg [Am]* 29:668-675, 2004.
52. Neumann DA: *Observations from cineradiography analysis*, 2000, unpublished work.
53. Nirschl RP, Pettrone FA: Tennis elbow. The surgical treatment of lateral epicondylitis, *J Bone Joint Surg [Am]* 61:832-839, 1979.
54. Nishiwaki M, Nakamura T, Nagura T, et al: Ulnar-shortening effect on distal radioulnar joint pressure: A biomechanical study, *J Hand Surg [Am]* 33:198-205, 2008.
55. Nowalk MD, Logan SE: Distinguishing biomechanical properties of intrinsic and extrinsic human wrist ligaments, *J Biomech Eng* 113:85-93, 1991.
56. O'Driscoll SW, Horii E, Ness R, et al: The relationship between wrist position, grasp size, and grip strength, *J Hand Surg [Am]* 17:169-177, 1992.
57. Palmer AK, Glisson RR, Werner FW: Ulnar variance determination, *J Hand Surg [Am]* 7:376-379, 1982.
58. Palmer AK, Werner FW: Biomechanics of the distal radioulnar joint, *Clin Orthop Relat Res* 187:26-35, 1984.

59. Park MJ, Cooney WP 3rd, Hahn ME, et al: The effects of dorsally angulated distal radius fractures on carpal kinematics, *J Hand Surg [Am]* 27:223-232, 2002.

60. Patterson RM, Nicodemus CL, Viegas SF, et al: High-speed, three-dimensional kinematic analysis of the normal wrist, *J Hand Surg [Am]* 23:446-453, 1998.

61. Peltier LF: The classic. Concerning traumatic malacia of the lunate and its consequences: degeneration and compression fractures. Translation of 1910 article. Privatdozent Dr. Robert Kienbock, *Clin Orthop Relat Res* 150:4-8, 1980.

62. Potter HG, Hannafin JA, Morwessel RM, et al: Lateral epicondylitis: Correlation of MR imaging, surgical, and histopathologic findings, *Radiology* 196:43-46, 1995.

63. Radonjic D, Long C: Kinesiology of the wrist, *Am J Phys Med* 50:57-71, 1971.

64. Ritt MJ, Stuart PR, Berglund LJ, et al: Rotational stability of the carpus relative to the forearm, *J Hand Surg [Am]* 20:305-311, 1995.

65. Ruby LK: Fractures and dislocations of the carpus. In Browner BD, Jupiter JB, Levine AM, editors: *Skeletal trauma: fractures, dislocations, ligamentous injuries*, vol 2, ed 2, Philadelphia, 1998, Saunders.

66. Ruby LK, Cooney WP 3rd, An KN, et al: Relative motion of selected carpal bones: a kinematic analysis of the normal wrist, *J Hand Surg [Am]* 13:1-10, 1988.

67. Ryu JY, Cooney WP 3rd, Askew LJ, et al: Functional ranges of motion of the wrist joint, *J Hand Surg [Am]* 16:409-419, 1991.

68. Safaee-Rad R, Shwedyk E, Quanbury AO, Cooper JE: Normal functional range of motion of upper limb joints during performance of three feeding activities, *Arch Phys Med Rehabil* 71:505-509, 1990.

69. Sarrafian SK, Melamed JL, Goshgarian GM: Study of wrist motion in flexion and extension, *Clin Orthop Relat Res* Jul-126:153-159, 1977.

70. Savelberg HH, Kooloos JG, de Lange A, et al: Human carpal ligament recruitment and three-dimensional carpal motion, *J Orthop Res* 9:693-704, 1991.

71. Schuind F, Eslami S, Ledoux P: Kienböck's disease, *J Bone Joint Surg Br* 90:133-139, 2008.

72. Schuind FA, Linscheid RL, An KN, Chao EY: A normal data base of posteroanterior roentgenographic measurements of the wrist, *J Bone Joint Surg Am* 74:1418-1429, 1992.

73. Shaaban H, Giakas G, Bolton M, et al: Contact area inside the distal radioulnar joint: effect of axial loading and position of the forearm, *Clin Biomech (Bristol, Avon)* 22:313-318, 2007.

74. Shepherd DE, Johnstone A: A new design concept for wrist arthroplasty. Proceedings of the Institution of Mechanical Engineers. 2005; Part H, *J Eng Med* 219:43-52, 2005.

75. Shin AY, Battaglia MJ, Bishop AT: Lunotriquetral instability: diagnosis and treatment, *J Am Acad Orthop Surg* 8:170-179, 2000.

76. Short WH, Werner FW, Green JK, Masaoka S: Biomechanical evaluation of ligamentous stabilizers of the scaphoid and lunate, *J Hand Surg [Am]* 27:991-1002, 2002.

77. Short WH, Werner FW, Green JK, et al: The effect of sectioning the dorsal radiocarpal ligament and insertion of a pressure sensor into the radiocarpal joint on scaphoid and lunate kinematics, *J Hand Surg [Am]* 27:68-76, 2002.

78. Standring S: *Gray's anatomy: The anatomical basis of clinical practice*, ed 40, St Louis, 2009, Elsevier.

79. Sun JS, Shih TT, Ko CM, et al: In vivo kinematic study of normal wrist motion: an ultrafast computed tomographic study, *Clin Biomech (Bristol, Avon)* 15:212-216, 2000.

80. Taleisnik J: The ligaments of the wrist. In Taleisnik J, editor: *The wrist*, New York, 1985, Churchill Livingstone.

81. Tang JB, Ryu J, Omokawa S, Wearden S: Wrist kinetics after scapholunate dissociation: the effect of scapholunate interosseous ligament injury and persistent scapholunate gaps, *J Orthop Res* 20:215-221, 2002.

82. Thompson NW, Mockford BJ, Rasheed T, Herbert KJ: Functional absence of flexor digitorum superficialis to the little finger and absence of palmaris longus—is there a link? *J Hand Surg [Br]* 27:433-434, 2002.

83. Tolbert JR, Blair WF, Andrews JG, Crowninshield RD: The kinetics of normal and prosthetic wrists, *J Biomech* 18:887-897, 1985.

84. Trudel D, Duley J, Zastrow I, et al: Rehabilitation for patients with lateral epicondylitis: A systematic review, *J Hand Ther* 17:243-266, 2004.

85. Viegas SF: The dorsal ligaments of the wrist, *Hand Clin* 17:65-75, 2001.

86. Viegas SF, Yamaguchi S, Boyd NL, Patterson RM: The dorsal ligaments of the wrist: anatomy, mechanical properties, and function, *J Hand Surg [Am]* 24:456-468, 1999.

87. Waugh EJ: Lateral epicondylalgia or epicondylitis: What's in a name? *J Orthop Sports Phys Ther* 35:200-202, 2005.

88. Weaver L, Tencer AF, Trumble TE: Tensions in the palmar ligaments of the wrist. I. The normal wrist, *J Hand Surg [Am]* 19:464-474, 1994.

89. Werner FW, Palmer AK, Fortino MD, Short WH: Force transmission through the distal ulna: effect of ulnar variance, lunate fossa angulation, and radial and palmar tilt of the distal radius, *J Hand Surg [Am]* 17:423-428, 1992.

90. Werner FW, Short WH, Fortino MD, Palmer AK: The relative contribution of selected carpal bones to global wrist motion during simulated planar and out-of-plane wrist motion, *J Hand Surg [Am]* 22:708-713, 1997.

91. Werner FW, Short WH, Green JK, et al: Severity of scapholunate instability is related to joint anatomy and congruency, *J Hand Surg [Am]* 32:55-60, 2007.

92. Wolfe SW, Crisco JJ, Katz LD: A non-invasive method for studying in vivo carpal kinematics, *J Hand Surg [Br]* 22:147-152, 1997.

93. Yoshioka H, Tanaka T, Ueno T, et al: Study of ulnar variance with high-resolution MRI: correlation with triangular fibrocartilage complex and cartilage of ulnar side of wrist, *J Magn Reson Imaging* 26:714-719, 2007.

94. Youm Y, McMurthy RY, Flatt AE, Gillespie TE: Kinematics of the wrist. I. An experimental study of radial-ulnar deviation and flexion-extension, *J Bone Joint Surg Am* 60:423-431, 1978.

STUDY QUESTIONS

1 How does the tendon of the flexor carpi radialis reach the base of the metacarpal bones without actually entering the carpal tunnel?

2 Cite factors that justify the greater range of ulnar deviation as compared with radial deviation of the wrist.

3 Assume that trauma associated with a fractured distal radius created a permanent 25 degree *dorsal tilt* of the distal radius (review Figure 7-4, *B*). What are some probable functional impairments that may result from this malalignment?

4 Describe the arthrokinematic pattern for flexion and extension at the radiocarpal joint.

5 Justify the importance of the capitate bone with regard to the osteokinematics of the entire wrist and hand.

6 The following questions are based on the data presented in Figure 7-24.

 a Which muscle would produce the greatest flexion torque at the wrist, the flexor carpi radialis, or the flexor digitorum superficialis?

 b Which muscle has the longest moment arm for ulnar deviation torque?

 c Which muscle is the *most* direct antagonist to the flexor carpi ulnaris?

7 Which two tendons of the thumb share the same fibrous tunnel within the extensor reticulum of the wrist?

8 What is the role of the scaphoid in providing mechanical stability to the lunate?

9 How would you *maximally* stretch the extensor carpi radialis longus muscle?

10 Which extrinsic ligaments naturally resist an ulnar translocation of the carpus?

11 A patient had severe trauma to the proximal radius and adjacent interosseous membrane that necessitated a partial resection of the radial head. Describe possible functional impairments or pathologies that might result from a subsequent 6- to 7-mm proximal migration of the radius.

12 Which carpal bones normally do *not* contact the capitate bone?

13 Compare the convex-concave joint relationships that exist within the medial and lateral compartments of the *midcarpal joint* of the wrist. Describe how these relationships affect the arthrokinematics of the joint during flexion and extension.

14 List all muscles that have a full or partial proximal attachment to the lateral epicondyle of the humerus. Which nerve innervates all these muscles?

15 Describe the muscular interaction between the flexor carpi ulnaris and flexor carpi radialis during active flexion of the wrist?

Answers to the study questions can be found on the Evolve website.

Similar to the eye, the hand serves as a very important sensory organ for the perception of one's surroundings (Figure 8-1). The hand is also a primary effector organ for our most complex motor behaviors, and the hand helps to express emotions through gesture, touch, music, and art.

Twenty-nine muscles drive the 19 bones and 19 articulations within the hand. Biomechanically, these structures interact with superb proficiency. The hand may be used in a very primitive fashion, as a hook or a club, or, more often, as a highly specialized instrument performing very complex manipulations requiring multiple levels of force and precision.

Because of the hand's enormous biomechanical complexity, its function involves a disproportionately large region of the cortex of the brain (Figure 8-2). Diseases or injuries affecting the hand often create a disproportionate disability. A

hand totally incapacitated by rheumatoid arthritis, stroke, or nerve or bone injury, for instance, can dramatically reduce the function of the entire upper limb. This chapter describes the kinesiologic principles behind many of the musculoskeletal impairments of the hand frequently encountered in medical and rehabilitation settings. These principles often serve as the basis for treatment.

TERMINOLOGY

The wrist, or carpus, has eight carpal bones. The hand has five metacarpals, often referred to collectively as the "metacarpus." Each of the five digits contains a set of phalanges. The digits are designated numerically from one to five, or as the thumb and the index, middle, ring, and small (little)

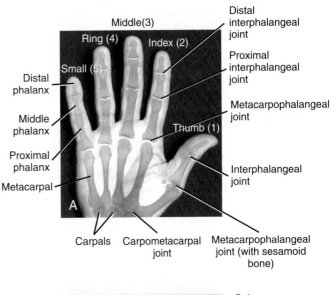

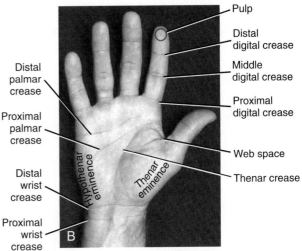

FIGURE 8-3. A palmar view of the basic anatomy of the hand. **A,** Major bones and joints. **B,** External landmarks.

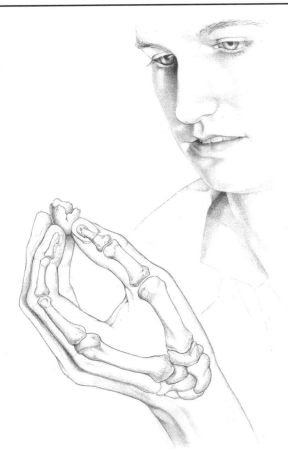

FIGURE 8-1. A very strong functional relationship exists between the hand and the eyes.

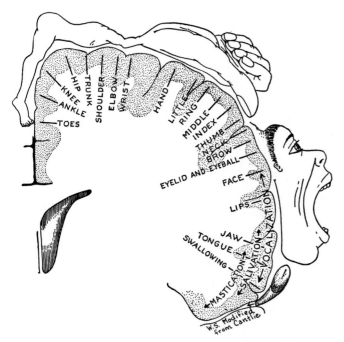

FIGURE 8-2. A motor homunculus of the brain showing the somatotopic representation of body parts. The sensory homunculus of the human brain has a similar representation. (From Penfield and Rosnussen: Cerebral cortex of man, New York, Macmillan, 1950.)

fingers (Figure 8-3, *A*). A *ray* describes one metacarpal bone and its associated phalanges.

The articulations between the proximal end of the metacarpals and the distal row of carpal bones form the *carpometacarpal (CMC) joints* (see Figure 8-3, *A*). The articulations between the metacarpals and the proximal phalanges form the *metacarpophalangeal (MCP) joints.* Each finger has two *interphalangeal joints:* a proximal interphalangeal (PIP) and a distal interphalangeal (DIP) joint. The thumb has only two phalanges and therefore only one interphalangeal (IP) joint.

Articulations Common to Each "Ray" of the Hand

- Carpometacarpal (CMC) joint
- Metacarpophalangeal (MCP) joint
- Interphalangeal (IP) joints
  - Thumb has one IP joint
  - Fingers have a proximal interphalangeal (PIP) joint and a distal interphalangeal (DIP) joint

Figure 8-3, *B* shows several features of the external anatomy of the hand. Note the *palmar creases,* or lines, that exist in the skin of the palm. They function as dermal "hinges," marking where the skin folds on itself during movement, and to increase palmar skin adherence for enhancing the security of grasp. The location of the creases also serves as a useful clinical reference for the underlying anatomy. On the palmar (anterior) side of the wrist are the proximal and distal *wrist creases.* Of clinical interest is the fact that the distal wrist crease marks the location of the proximal margin of the underlying transverse carpal ligament. The *thenar crease* is formed by the folding of the dermis as the thumb is moved across the palm. The proximal *digital creases* are located distal to the actual joint line of the MCP joints. The distal and middle digital creases are superficial to the DIP and PIP joints, respectively.

OSTEOLOGY

Metacarpals

The metacarpals, like the digits, are designated numerically as one through five, beginning on the radial (lateral) side.

Each metacarpal has similar anatomic characteristics (Figures 8-4 and 8-5). The first metacarpal (the thumb) is the shortest and stoutest; the second is usually the longest, and the length of the remaining three bones decreases from the radial to ulnar (medial) direction.

Osteologic Features of a Metacarpal
* Shaft
* Base
* Head
* Neck
* Posterior tubercles

Each metacarpal has an elongated *shaft* with articular surfaces at each end (Figure 8-6). The palmar surface of the shaft is slightly concave longitudinally to accommodate many muscles and tendons in this region. Its proximal end, or *base,* articulates with one or more of the carpal bones. The bases of the second through the fifth metacarpals possess small facets for articulation with adjacent metacarpal bases.

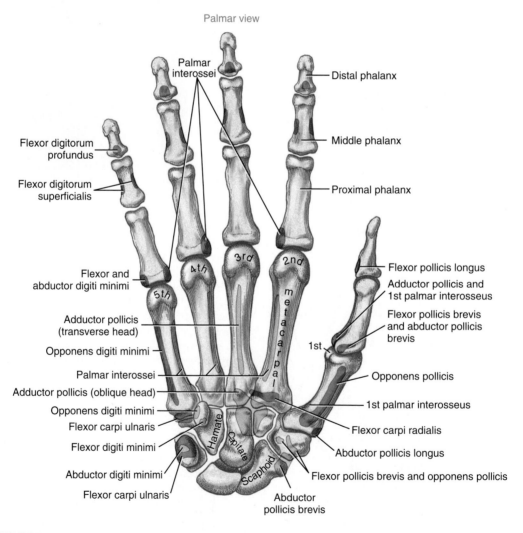

Palmar view

FIGURE 8-4. A palmar view of the bones of the right wrist and hand. Proximal attachments of muscles are indicated in red and distal attachments in gray.

Dorsal view

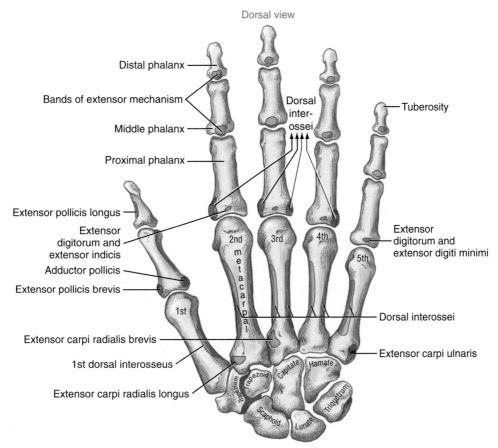

FIGURE 8-5. A dorsal view of the bones of the right wrist and hand. Proximal attachments of muscles are indicated in red and distal attachments in gray.

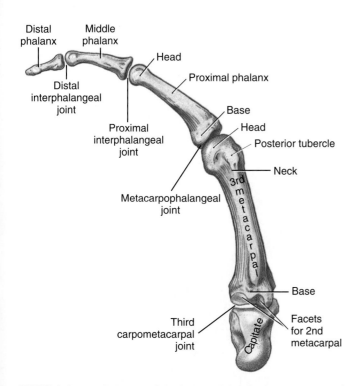

FIGURE 8-6. A radial view of the bones of the third ray (metacarpal and associated phalanges), including the capitate bone of the wrist.

The distal end of each metacarpal has a large convex *head.* The heads of the second through fifth metacarpals are evident as "knuckles" on the dorsal side of a clenched fist. Immediately proximal to the head is the metacarpal *neck*–a common site of fracture, especially of the fifth digit. A pair of *posterior tubercles* marks the attachment sites for the collateral ligaments of the MCP joints.

With the hand at rest in the anatomic position, the thumb's metacarpal is oriented in a different plane than the other digits. The second through the fifth metacarpals are aligned generally side by side, with their palmar surfaces facing anteriorly. The position of the thumb's metacarpal, however, is rotated almost 90 degrees medially (i.e., internally), relative to the other digits (see Figure 8-3). Rotation places the very sensitive palmar surface of the thumb *toward* the midline of the hand. Optimum prehension depends on the thumb flexing in a plane that intersects, versus parallels, the plane of the flexing fingers. In addition, the thumb's metacarpal is positioned well anterior, or palmar, to the other metacarpals (Figure 7-14). This position of the first metacarpal and trapezium is strongly influenced by the palmar projection of the distal pole of the scaphoid.

The location of the first metacarpal allows the entire thumb to sweep freely across the palm toward the fingers. Virtually all prehensile motions, from pinch to precision handling, require the thumb to interact with the fingers. In the absence of a healthy and mobile thumb, the overall function of the hand is substantially reduced.

The medially rotated thumb requires unique terminology to describe its movement as well as position. In the anatomic position the dorsal surface of the bones of the thumb (i.e., the surface where the thumbnail resides) faces laterally (Figure 8-7). The palmar surface therefore faces medially, the radial surface anteriorly, and the ulnar surface posteriorly. The terminology to describe the surfaces of the carpal bones and all other digital bones is standard: a palmar surface faces anteriorly, a radial surface faces laterally, and so forth.

Phalanges

The hand has 14 phalanges (from the Greek root *phalanx,* a line of soldiers). The phalanges within each finger are referred to as *proximal, middle,* and *distal* (see Figure 8-3, *A*). The thumb has only a proximal and a distal phalanx.

Osteologic Features of a Phalanx
* Base
* Shaft
* Head (proximal and middle phalanx only)
* Tuberosity (distal phalanx only)

Except for differences in sizes, all phalanges within a particular digit have similar morphology (see Figure 8-5). The proximal and middle phalanges of each finger have a concave *base, shaft,* and convex *head.* As in the metacarpals, their palmar surfaces are slightly concave longitudinally. The distal phalanx of each digit has a concave base. At its distal end is a rounded *tuberosity* that anchors the fleshy pulp of soft tissue to the bony tip of each digit.

Arches of the Hand

Observe the natural concavity of the palmar surface of your relaxed hand. Control of this concavity allows the human hand to securely hold and manipulate objects of many and varied shapes and sizes. This palmar concavity is supported by three integrated arch systems: two transverse and one longitudinal (Figure 8-8). The *proximal transverse arch* is formed by the distal row of carpal bones. This is a static, rigid arch that forms the *carpal tunnel* (see Chapter 7). Like most arches in buildings and bridges, the arches of the hand are supported by a central *keystone* structure. The capitate bone is the keystone of the proximal transverse arch, reinforced by multiple contacts with other bones, and strong intercarpal ligaments.

The *distal transverse arch* of the hand passes through the MCP joints. In contrast to the rigidity of the proximal arch, the sides of the distal arch are mobile. To appreciate this mobility, imagine transforming your hand from a completely flat surface to a cup-shaped surface that surrounds a baseball. Transverse flexibility within the hand occurs as the peripheral metacarpals (first, fourth, and fifth) "fold" around the more stable central (second and third) metacarpals. The keystone of the distal transverse arch is formed by the MCP joints of these central metacarpals.

The *longitudinal arch* of the hand follows the general shape of the second and third rays. The proximal end of this arch is firmly linked to the carpus by the carpometacarpal (CMC) joints. These relatively rigid articulations provide an important element of longitudinal stability to the hand. The distal end of the arch is very mobile, which can be demonstrated by actively flexing and extending the fingers. The keystone of the longitudinal arch consists of the second and third MCP joints; note that these joints serve as keystones to *both* the longitudinal and distal transverse arches.

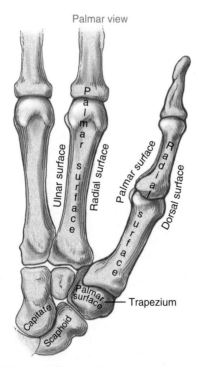 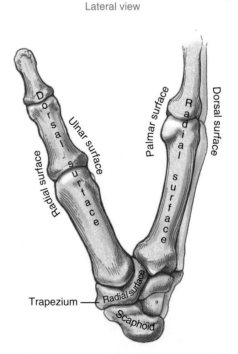

FIGURE 8-7. Palmar and lateral views of the hand showing the orientation of the bony surfaces of the right thumb. Note that the bones of the thumb are rotated approximately 90 degrees relative to the other bones of the wrist and the hand.

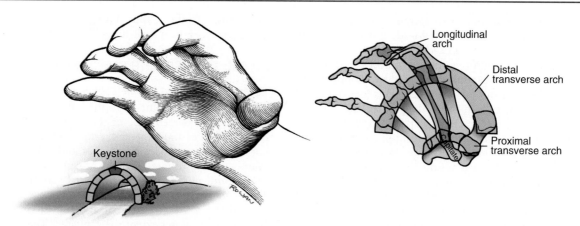

FIGURE 8-8. The natural concavity of the palm of the hand is supported by three integrated arch systems: one longitudinal and two transverse.

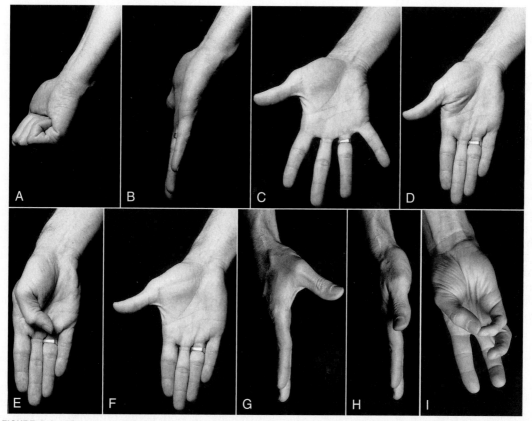

FIGURE 8-9. The system for naming the movements within the hand. **A** to **D,** Finger motion. **E** to **I,** Thumb motion. (**A,** Finger flexion; **B,** finger extension; **C,** finger abduction; **D,** finger adduction; **E,** thumb flexion; **F,** thumb extension; **G,** thumb abduction; **H,** thumb adduction; and **I,** thumb opposition.)

ARTHROLOGY

As depicted in Figure 8-8, all three arches of the hand are mechanically interlinked. Both transverse arches are joined together by a "rigid tie-beam" provided by the second and third metacarpals.[27] In the healthy hand, this mechanical linkage reinforces the entire arch system. In the hand with joint disease, however, a structural failure at any arch may weaken another. A classic example is the destruction of the MCP joints from severe rheumatoid arthritis. This topic will be revisited at the end of this chapter.

Before progressing to the study of the structure and function of the joints, the terminology that describes the movement of the digits must be defined. The following descriptions assume that a particular movement starts from the anatomic position, with the elbow extended, forearm fully supinated, and wrist in a neutral position. Movement of the fingers is described in the standard fashion using the cardinal planes of the body: *flexion* and *extension* occur in the sagittal plane, and *abduction* and *adduction* occur in the frontal plane (Figure 8-9,

A to D). The middle finger is the reference digit for naming abduction and adduction. The side-to-side movement of the middle finger is called *radial* and *ulnar deviation*.

Because the entire thumb is rotated almost 90 degrees in relation to the fingers, the terminology used to describe thumb movement is different from that for the fingers (see Figure 8-9, *E to I*). *Flexion* is the movement of the palmar surface of the thumb in the frontal plane across the palm. *Extension* returns the thumb back toward its anatomic position. *Abduction* is the forward movement of the thumb away from the palm in a near sagittal plane. *Adduction* returns the thumb to the plane of the hand. (Although not used in this text, other terms frequently used to describe the movements of the thumb include *ulnar adduction* for flexion, *radial abduction* for extension, and *palmar abduction* for abduction.) *Opposition* is a special term describing the movement of the thumb across the palm, making direct contact with the tip of any of the fingers. *Reposition* is a movement from full opposition back to the anatomic position. This special terminology used to define the movement of the thumb serves as the basis for the naming of the muscles that act on the thumb (e.g., the opponens pollicis, extensor pollicis longus, and adductor pollicis).

Carpometacarpal Joints

The carpometacarpal (CMC) joints of the hand form the articulation between the distal row of carpal bones and the bases of the five metacarpal bones. These joints are positioned at the very proximal region of the hand.

Figure 8-10 shows a mechanical illustration of the relative mobility at the CMC joints. The joints of the second and third digits are rigidly joined to the distal carpus, forming a stable *central pillar* throughout the hand. In contrast, the more peripheral CMC joints form mobile radial and ulnar borders, which are capable of folding around the hand's central pillar. The function of the CMC joints allows the concavity of the palm to fit around many objects. This feature is one of the most impressive functions of the human hand. Cylindric objects, for example, can fit snugly into the palm, with the index and middle digits positioned to rein-

force grasp. Without this ability, the dexterity of the hand is reduced to a primitive hingelike grasping motion.

SECOND THROUGH FIFTH CARPOMETACARPAL JOINTS

General Features and Ligamentous Support

The *second* CMC joint is formed through the articulation between the enlarged base of the second metacarpal and the distal surface of the trapezoid, and to a lesser extent the capitate and trapezium (see Figures 8-4 and 8-5). The *third* CMC joint is formed primarily by the articulation between the base of the third metacarpal and the distal surface of the capitate. The *fourth* CMC joint consists of the articulation between the base of the fourth metacarpal and the distal surface of the hamate and to lesser extent the capitate.[70] The *fifth* CMC joint consists of the articulation between the base of the fifth metacarpal and the distal surface of the hamate only. (The hamate accepts both the fourth and fifth metacarpals, similar to the manner in which the cuboid bone of the foot accepts both the fourth and fifth metatarsals.) The bases of the second through fifth metacarpals have small facets for attachments to one another through *intermetacarpal joints*. These joints help stabilize the bases of the second through fifth metacarpals, thereby reinforcing the carpometacarpal joints.

All CMC joints of the fingers are surrounded by articular capsules and strengthened by multiple dorsal, palmar, and interosseous ligaments.[70] The dorsal ligaments are particularly well developed (Figure 8-11).

Joint Structure and Kinematics

The CMC joints of the second and third digits are difficult to classify, ranging from planar to complex saddle joints (Figure 8-12).[101] Their jagged interlocking articular surfaces, coupled with strong ligaments, permit very little movement. As mentioned earlier, stability at these joints forms the central pillar of the hand. The inherent stability of these radial-central metacarpals also provides a very firm attachment for several key muscles, including the extensor carpi radialis longus and brevis, the flexor carpi radialis, and the adductor pollicis.

The slightly convex bases of the fourth and fifth metacarpals articulate with a slightly concave articular surface formed by the hamate. These two ulnar CMC joints contribute a subtle but important element of mobility to the hand. As depicted in Figure 8-10, the fourth and fifth CMC joints allow the ulnar border of the hand to fold toward the center of the hand, thereby deepening the palmar concavity. This mobility—often referred to as a "cupping" motion—occurs primarily by flexion and "internal" rotation of the ulnar metacarpals toward the middle digit. Measurements of maximal passive mobility on cadaver hands have shown that, on average, the fourth CMC joint flexes and extends about 20 degrees and rotates internally about 27 degrees.[21] The fifth CMC joint (when tested with the fourth CMC joint firmly constrained) flexes and extends about 28 degrees and rotates internally 22 degrees. The range of flexion and extension of the fifth CMC joint increases to an average of 44 degrees when the closely positioned fourth CMC joint is unconstrained and free to move. This research demonstrates the strong mechanical link between the kinematics of the fourth and fifth CMC joints. This point should be considered when evaluating and treating limitations of motion in this region of the hand.

The greater relative mobility allowed at the ulnar CMC joints is evidenced by the movement of the fourth and fifth

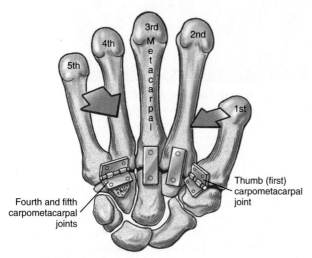

FIGURE 8-10. Palmar view of the right hand showing a highly mechanical depiction of the mobility across the five carpometacarpal joints. The peripheral joints—the first, fourth, and fifth—are much more mobile than the central two joints.

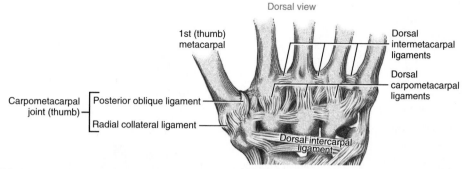

Dorsal view

1st (thumb)
metacarpal

Dorsal
intermetacarpal
ligaments

Dorsal
carpometacarpal
ligaments

Carpometacarpal
joint (thumb) ⎡ Posterior oblique ligament

⎣ Radial collateral ligament

Dorsal intercarpal
ligament

FIGURE 8-11. Dorsal side of the right hand showing the capsule and ligaments that stabilize the carpometa-carpal joints.

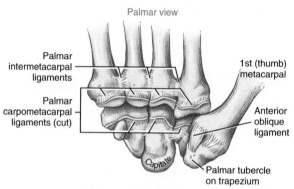

Palmar view

Palmar
intermetacarpal
ligaments

Palmar
carpometacarpal
ligaments (cut)

1st (thumb)
metacarpal

Anterior
oblique
ligament

Capitate

Palmar tubercle
on trapezium

FIGURE 8-12. The palmar side of the right hand showing the articular surfaces of the second through the fifth carpometacarpal joints. The capsule and palmar carpometacarpal ligaments of digits 2 to 5 have been cut.

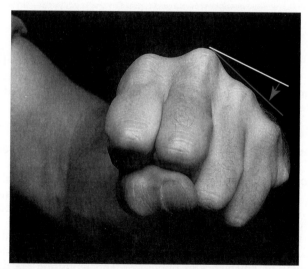

FIGURE 8-13. Mobility of the ulnar (fourth and fifth) carpometacarpal joints of the left hand. White line indicates the relaxed position of the distal metacarpals; red line indicates their position after the fist is clenched.

metacarpal heads while clenching a fist (Figure 8-13). The increased mobility of the fourth and fifth CMC joints improves the effectiveness of grasp, as well as enhancing the functional interaction with the opposable thumb. The irregular and varied shapes of these CMC joint surfaces prohibit standard roll-and-slide arthrokinematic descriptions.

CARPOMETACARPAL JOINT OF THE THUMB

The CMC joint of the thumb is located at the base of the first ray, between the metacarpal and the trapezium (see Figure 8-7). This joint is by far the most complex of the CMC joints, enabling extensive movements of the thumb. Its unique saddle shape allows the thumb to fully oppose, thereby easily contacting the tips of the other digits. Through this action, the thumb is able to encircle objects held within the palm. Opposition greatly enhances the dexterity of human prehension.

Capsule and Ligaments of the Thumb Carpometacarpal Joint

The capsule at the CMC joint of the thumb is naturally loose to accommodate a large range of motion. The capsule, however, is strengthened by the action of ligaments and by the forces produced by the overriding musculature.

Many names have been used to describe the ligaments at the CMC joint of the thumb.[6,20,37,80] The number of named, distinct ligaments reported to cross the base of the thumb ranges from three to perhaps as many as seven.[72] This text focuses on five capsular ligaments, each adding an important element of stability to the CMC joint (Figure 8-14). As a set, the ligaments help control the extent and direction of joint motion, maintain joint alignment, and dissipate forces produced by activated muscle.[76] Table 8-1 summarizes the major attachments of these ligaments and the motions that pull or wind them taut. In general, extension, abduction, and opposition of the thumb elongate most of the ligaments. Although all five ligaments listed in Table 8-1 are important stabilizers of the thumb's CMC joint, the anterior oblique ligament warrants distinction.[6,44,83] Rupture of this ligament secondary to severe arthritis or trauma often results in a radial dislocation of the joint, forming a characteristic "hump" at the base of the thumb.[76]

Saddle Joint Structure

The CMC joint of the thumb is the classic saddle joint of the body (Figure 8-15). The characteristic feature of a saddle joint is that each articular surface is convex in one dimension and concave in the other. The longitudinal diameter of the articular surface of the *trapezium* is generally concave from a palmar-to-dorsal direction. This surface is analogous to the front-to-rear contour of a horse's saddle. The transverse diameter on the articular surface of the trapezium is generally convex in a medial-to-lateral direction—a shape analogous to the side-to-side contour of a horse's saddle. The contour of the proximal articular surface of the *thumb metacarpal* has the reciprocal shape of that described for the trapezium (see

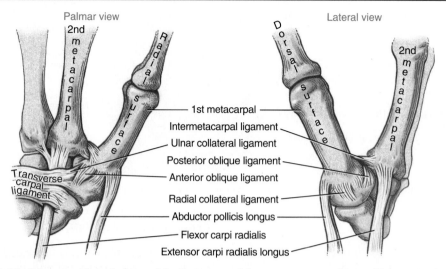

FIGURE 8-14. Palmar and lateral views of the ligaments of the carpometacarpal joint of the right thumb.

TABLE 8-1. Ligaments of the Carpometacarpal Joint of the Thumb*

Name	Proximal Attachment	Distal Attachment	Most Taut Positions
Anterior oblique†	Palmar tubercle on trapezium	Palmar base of thumb metacarpal	Abduction, extension, and opposition
Ulnar collateral	Transverse carpal ligament	Palmar-ulnar base of thumb metacarpal	Abduction, extension, and opposition
First intermetacarpal	Dorsal-radial side of base of second metacarpal	Palmar-ulnar base of thumb metacarpal with ulnar collateral	Abduction and opposition
Posterior oblique	Posterior surface of trapezium	Palmar-ulnar base of thumb metacarpal	Abduction and opposition
Radial collateral	Radial surface of trapezium	Dorsal surface of thumb metacarpal	All movements to varying degrees except extension

*Ligament names are based on attachment to trapezium surfaces, *not* the thumb metacarpal.
†Often described as having superficial and deep ("beak") fibers.

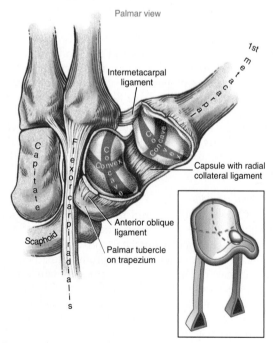

FIGURE 8-15. The carpometacarpal joint of the right thumb is exposed to show its saddle-shaped appearance. The longitudinal diameters are shown in purple, and the transverse diameters in green.

Figure 8-15). The longitudinal diameter along the articular surface of the metacarpal is convex in a palmar-to-dorsal direction; its transverse diameter is concave in a medial-to-lateral direction.

Kinematics

The motions at the CMC joint occur primarily in two degrees of freedom. Abduction and adduction occur generally in the sagittal plane, and flexion and extension occur generally in the frontal plane. The axis of rotation for each plane of movement passes through the convex member of the articulation.[38]

Opposition and reposition of the thumb are mechanically derived from the two primary planes of motion at the CMC joint. The kinematics of opposition and reposition are discussed after the description of the two primary motions.

Abduction and Adduction at the Thumb Carpometacarpal Joint

In the position of adduction of the CMC joint, the thumb lies within the plane of the hand. Maximum abduction, in contrast, positions the thumb metacarpal about 45 degrees anterior to the plane of the palm. Full abduction opens the web space of the thumb, forming a wide concave curvature useful for grasping large objects.

The arthrokinematics of abduction and adduction are based on the convex articular surface of the thumb metacar-

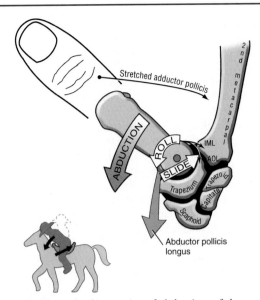

FIGURE 8-16. The arthrokinematics of abduction of the carpometacarpal joint of the thumb. Full abduction stretches the anterior oblique ligament *(AOL)*, the intermetacarpal ligament *(IML)*, and the adductor pollicis muscle. The axis of rotation is depicted as a small circle at the base of the metacarpal. The muscle primarily responsible for the active rolling of the articular surface of the thumb metacarpal is the abductor pollicis longus. Note the analogy between the arthrokinematics of abduction and a cowboy falling forward on the horse's saddle: as the cowboy falls forward (toward abduction), a point on his chest "rolls" anteriorly, but a point on his rear end "slides" posteriorly.

pal moving on the fixed concave (longitudinal) diameter of the trapezium (review Figure 8-15). During *abduction*, the convex articular surface of the metacarpal rolls palmarly and slides dorsally on the concave surface of the trapezium (Figure 8-16). Full abduction at the CMC joint elongates the adductor pollicis muscle and most ligaments at the CMC joint. The arthrokinematics of *adduction* occur in the reverse order from those described for abduction.

Flexion and Extension at the Thumb Carpometacarpal Joint
Actively performing flexion and extension of the CMC joint of the thumb is associated with varying amounts of axial rotation of the metacarpal. During flexion, the metacarpal rotates *medially* (i.e., toward the third digit); during extension, the metacarpal rotates *laterally* (i.e., away from the third digit). The "automatic" axial rotation is apparent by the change in orientation of the nail of the thumb between full extension and full flexion. This rotation is not considered a third degree of freedom because it cannot be executed independently of the other motions.

In the anatomic position the CMC joint can be extended an additional 10 to 15 degrees.[15] From full extension the thumb metacarpal flexes across the palm about 45 to 50 degrees.

The arthrokinematics of flexion and extension at the CMC joint are based on the concave articular surface of the metacarpal moving across the convex (transverse) diameter on the trapezium (review Figure 8-15). During *flexion*, the concave surface of the metacarpal rolls and slides in an ulnar (medial) direction (Figure 8-17, *A*).[38] A shallow groove in the transverse

---

SPECIAL FOCUS 8-1

Osteoarthritis of the Carpometacarpal Joint of the Thumb: a Common and Potentially Disabling Condition

The large functional demand placed on the carpometacarpal (CMC) joint of the thumb is often considering a predisposing factor in the development of local osteoarthritis.[76] This common condition receives more surgical attention than any other osteoarthritis-related condition of the upper limb.[84] Osteoarthritis may develop at the CMC joint secondary to acute injury or, perhaps more commonly, from the cumulative low-level trauma associated with an arduous occupation or hobby.[28,69] An interesting anthropologic study of skeletal remains from the United Arab Emirates (2300 BC) found that 20% of the sample had moderate to severe osteoarthritis of the CMC joint.[16] This high incidence of degeneration was attributed to excessive use of the thumbs related to occupation.

Other factors besides stress and overuse can cause osteoarthritis at the base of the thumb, including genetics or subtle natural asymmetry of the articular surfaces. Regardless of the specific cause, persons who require medical attention for arthritis of the first CMC joint typically report pain as the foremost presenting symptom, but also experience joint instability.[85] A painful and unstable base of the thumb markedly reduces the functional potential of the entire hand, and therefore the entire upper extremity. Persons with advanced osteoarthritis of the base of the thumb often develop a weakened pinch, osteophyte formation, swelling, subluxation or dislocation, and crepitation. The literature strongly suggests that idiopathic osteoarthritis of the CMC joint of the thumb is disproportionally more common in women, typically in their fifth and sixth decades.[82,98] This gender-related propensity

may be associated with postmenopausal-induced laxity in the joint's ligaments. Studies also suggest that the trapeziums of women are, in general, less congruent and have a smaller surface area than those of men.[48,114] These factors may also contribute to the higher incidence of arthritis in the CMC joints of women.

Common conservative therapeutic interventions for osteoarthritis of the thumb CMC joint include splinting; judicious use of exercise; physical modalities such as cold and heat; nonsteroidal anti-inflammatory drugs (NSAIDs); and corticosteroid injections.[76] In addition, patients are instructed in ways to modify their activities of daily living to "protect" the base of the thumb from unnecessarily large forces.[67]

Surgical intervention is typically used when conservative therapy is unable to retard the progression of pain or instability.[76,78,106] Surgery often involves arthroplasty with reconstruction of the damaged ligaments, such as the anterior oblique ligament. The joint is often stabilized by weaving the tendon of the flexor carpi radialis between and through adjacent bones.[68] The degenerated trapezium may be left intact or replaced with a "spacer" consisting of a coiled tendon or other material. Although patients typically report significant improvement of function after surgery, long-term success is often hindered by the complex arthrokinematics coupled with the large forces that naturally occur at the CMC joint.[78] In certain cases, partial or full fusion (arthrodesis) of the carpometacarpal joint is indicated, especially for young and physically active persons.

diameter of the trapezium helps guide the slight medial rotation of the metacarpal. Full flexion elongates tissues such as the radial collateral ligament.[115]

During *extension* of the CMC joint, the concave metacarpal rolls and slides in a lateral (radial) direction across the transverse diameter of the joint (see Figure 8-17, *B*). The groove on the articular surface of the trapezium guides the metacarpal into slight lateral rotation.[15,51] Full extension stretches ligaments situated on the ulnar side of the joint, such as the anterior oblique ligament. Table 8-2 shows a summary of the kinematics for flexion-extension and abduction-adduction at the CMC joint of the thumb.

Opposition of the Thumb Carpometacarpal Joint

The ability to deliberately and precisely oppose the thumb to the tips of the other fingers is perhaps the ultimate expression of functional health of this digit—and arguably of the entire hand. This complex motion is a composite of the other primary motions already described for the CMC joint.[57]

For ease of discussion, Figure 8-18, *A* shows the full arc of *opposition* divided into two phases. In *phase one*, the thumb metacarpal abducts. In *phase two*, the abducted metacarpal flexes and medially rotates across the palm toward the small finger. Figure 8-18, *B* shows the detail of the kinematics of this complex movement. During abduction, the base of the thumb metacarpal takes a path in a palmar direction across the surface of the trapezium. During flexion–medial rotation, the base of this metacarpal turns slightly medially, led by the groove on the surface of the trapezium.[115] Muscle force, especially from the opponens pollicis, helps guide and rotate the metacarpal to the medial side of the articular surface of the trapezium. The partially abducted CMC joint increases passive tension in most connective tissues associated with the CMC joint. Increased tension in the stretched posterior oblique ligament, for instance, promotes the medial rotation (spin) of the thumb metacarpal.[115]

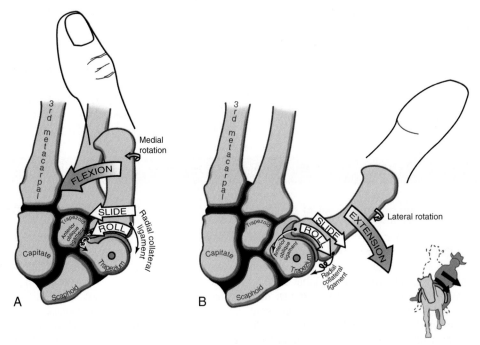

FIGURE 8-17. The arthrokinematics of flexion and extension at the carpometacarpal joint of the thumb. **A,** Flexion is associated with a slight medial rotation, causing elongation in the radial collateral ligament. The anterior oblique ligament is slack. **B,** Extension is associated with slight lateral rotation, causing elongation of the anterior oblique ligament. The axis of rotation is depicted as a small circle through the trapezium. Note the analogy between the arthrokinematics of extension and a cowboy falling sideways on the horse's saddle: As the cowboy falls sideways (toward extension), points on his chest and rear end both "roll and slide" in the same lateral direction.

TABLE 8-2. Factors Associated with Kinematics of the Primary Motions of the Carpometacarpal Joint of the Thumb*			
Motion	**Osteokinematics**	**Joint Geometry**	**Arthrokinematics**
Abduction and adduction	Sagittal plane movement around a medial-lateral axis of rotation through the metacarpal	Convex (longitudinal) diameter of metacarpal moving on a concave surface of the trapezium	Abduction: palmar roll and dorsal slide Adduction: dorsal roll and palmar slide
Flexion and extension	Frontal plane movement around an anterior-posterior axis of rotation through the trapezium	Concave (transverse) diameter of the metacarpal moving on a convex surface of the trapezium	Flexion: medial roll and slide Extension: lateral roll and slide

*Opposition and reposition are not shown because they are derived from the two primary planes of motions (see text for further explanation).

Reposition of the CMC joint returns the metacarpal from full opposition back to the anatomic position. This motion involves arthrokinematics of both adduction and extension–lateral rotation of the thumb metacarpal.

Metacarpophalangeal Joints

FINGERS

General Features and Ligaments

The metacarpophalangeal (MCP) joints of the fingers are relatively large, ovoid articulations formed between the convex heads of the metacarpals and the shallow concave proximal surfaces of the proximal phalanges (Figure 8-19). Motion at the MCP joint occurs predominantly in two planes: flexion and extension in the sagittal plane, and abduction and adduction in the frontal plane.

Mechanical stability at the MCP joint is critical to the overall biomechanics of the hand. As discussed earlier, the MCP joints serve as keystones that support the mobile arches of the hand. In the healthy hand, stability at the MCP joints is achieved by an elaborate set of interconnecting connective tissues. Embedded within the capsule of each MCP joint are a pair of radial and ulnar collateral ligaments and one palmar plate (Figure 8-20). Each *collateral ligament* has its proximal attachment on the posterior tubercle of the metacarpal head. Crossing the MCP joint in an oblique palmar direction, the ligament forms two distinct parts. The more dorsal *cord part* of the ligament is thick and strong, attaching distally to the palmar aspect of the proximal end of the phalanx. The *accessory part* consists of fan-shaped fibers, which attach distally along the edge of the palmar plate.

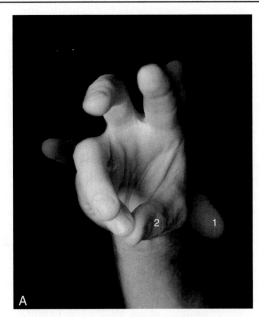
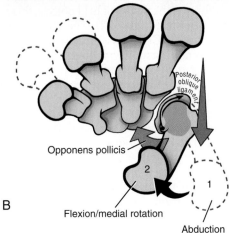

FIGURE 8-18. The arthrokinematics of opposition of the carpometacarpal joint of the thumb. **A,** Two phases of opposition are shown: (1) abduction and (2) flexion with medial rotation **B,** The detailed kinematics of the two phases of opposition: the posterior oblique ligament is shown taut; the opponens pollicis is shown contracting *(red).*

As evidenced by the change in orientation of the thumbnail, full opposition incorporates 45 to 60 degrees of medial rotation of the thumb.[13] The CMC joint of the thumb accounts for most but not all of this rotation. Lesser amounts of axial rotation occur in the form of accessory motions at the MCP and IP joints. The trapezium also medially rotates slightly against the scaphoid and the trapezoid, thereby amplifying the final magnitude of the metacarpal rotation.[75] The small finger contributes indirectly to opposition through a cupping motion at the fifth CMC joint. This motion allows the tip of the thumb to more easily contact the tip of the small finger.

Full opposition is often considered the CMC joint's close-packed position.[63,101] This position is stabilized not only by a twisting of several ligaments, but by activation of muscle. Although maximum in full opposition, only about half of the surface area within the joint makes articular contact. Considering the large and frequent forces that cross this joint, the relatively small contact area may naturally predispose the joint to large and potentially damaging pressures.

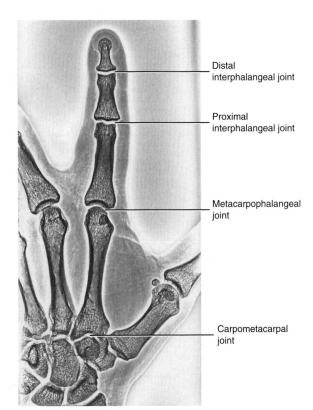

FIGURE 8-19. The joints of the index finger.

Located palmar to each MCP joint are ligamentous-like structures called *palmar* (or *volar*) *plates* (see Figure 8-20). The term *plate* describes a composition of dense, thick fibrocartilage. The distal end of each plate attaches to the base of each proximal phalanx. At this region the plates are relatively thick and stiff. The thinner and more elastic proximal end attaches to the metacarpal bone, just proximal to the head. *Fibrous digital sheaths*, which form tunnels or pulleys for the extrinsic finger flexors, are anchored on the palmar (anterior) surface of the palmar plates. The primary function of the palmar plates is to strengthen the structure of the MCP joints, and limit the extremes of extension.

Figure 8-21 illustrates several anatomic aspects of the MCP joints. The concave component of an MCP joint is formed

by the articular surface of the proximal phalanx, the collateral ligaments, and the dorsal surface of the palmar plate. These tissues form a three-sided receptacle aptly suited to accept the large metacarpal head. This structure adds to the stability of the joint while also increasing the area of articular contact. Attaching between the palmar plates of each MCP joint are three *deep transverse metacarpal ligaments*. The three ligaments merge into a wide, flat structure that interconnects and loosely binds the second through the fifth metacarpals.

Kinematics
Osteokinematics

In addition to the volitional motions of flexion-extension and abduction-adduction at the MCP joints, substantial accessory motions are possible. With the MCP joint relaxed and nearly extended, the ample passive mobility of the proximal phalanx relative to the head of the metacarpal can be appreciated. The joint can be distracted-compressed, translated in anterior-to-posterior and side-to-side directions, and axially rotated. The extent of passive axial rotation is particularly remarkable. These ample accessory motions at the MCP joints permit the fingers to better conform to the shapes of held objects, thereby increasing control of grasp (Figure 8-22). The range of this passive axial rotation at the MCP joints is greatest at the ring and small fingers, with average rotations of about 30 to 40 degrees.[50]

The overall range of flexion and extension at the MCP joints increases gradually from the second to the fifth digit: the second (index) flexes to about 90 degrees, and the fifth to about 110 to 115 degrees.[4] The greater mobility allowed at the more ulnar MCP joints is similar to that expressed at the CMC joints. The MCP joints can be passively extended beyond the neutral (0-degree) position for a considerable range of 30 to 45 degrees. Abduction and adduction at the MCP joints occur to about 20 degrees on both sides of the midline reference formed by the third metacarpal.

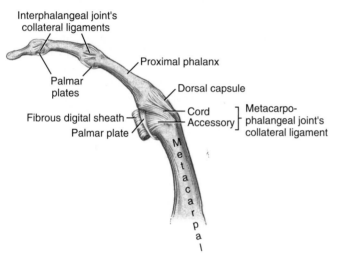

FIGURE 8-20. A lateral view of the collateral ligaments and associated connective tissues of the metacarpophalangeal, proximal interphalangeal, and distal interphalangeal joints of the finger.

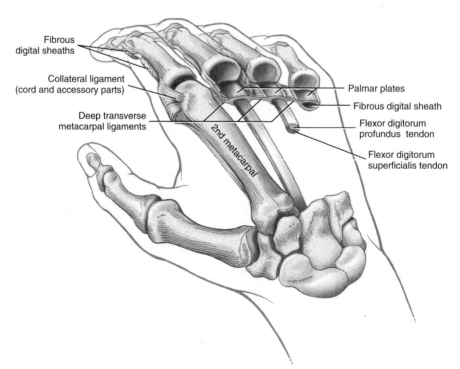

FIGURE 8-21. A dorsal view of the hand with an emphasis on the periarticular connective tissues at the metacarpophalangeal joints. Several metacarpal bones have been removed to expose various joint structures.

The Metacarpophalangeal Joints of the Fingers Permit Volitional Movements Primarily in Two Degrees of Freedom

- *Flexion* and *extension* occur in the sagittal plane around a medial-lateral axis of rotation.
- *Abduction* and *adduction* occur in the frontal plane around an anterior-posterior axis of rotation.

The axis of rotation for each movement passes through the head of the metacarpal.

Arthrokinematics

The head of each metacarpal has a slightly different shape but in general is rounded at the apex and nearly flat on the palmar surface (see Figure 8-6). Articular cartilage covers the entire head and most of the palmar surface. The convex-concave relationship of the joint surfaces is readily apparent (Figure 8-23). The longitudinal diameter of the joint follows the sagittal plane; the shorter transverse diameter follows the frontal plane.

The arthrokinematics at the MCP joint are based on the concave articular surface of the phalanx moving against the convex metacarpal head. Figure 8-24, *A* shows the arthrokinematics of active *flexion*, driven by one of the extrinsic flexor muscles: the flexor digitorum profundus. Flexion stretches and therefore increases the passive tension in both the dorsal capsule and the collateral ligaments. In the healthy state this passive tension helps guide the joint's natural arthrokinematics.[7] For example, as depicted in Figure 8-24, *A*, the increased tension in the stretched dorsal capsule (depicted by the thin elongated arrow) prevents the joint from unnaturally "hinging" outward on its dorsal side. The tension helps maintain firm contact between the articular surfaces as the proximal phalanx slides and rolls in a palmar direction. The increased tension in the dorsal capsule and collateral ligaments stabilizes the joint in flexion, which is useful during grasp.

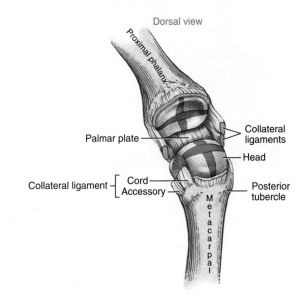

FIGURE 8-23. A dorsal view of the metacarpophalangeal joint opened to expose the shape of the articular surfaces. The longitudinal diameter of the joint is shown in green; the transverse diameter in purple.

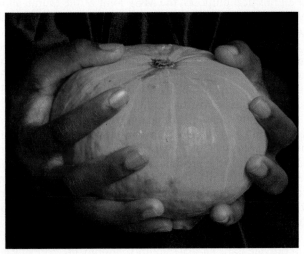

FIGURE 8-22. The accessory motions of axial rotation at the metacarpophalangeal joints are evident across several fingers during a grasp of a large, round object.

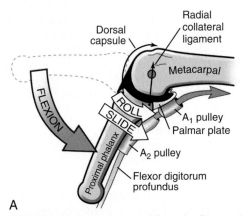

A

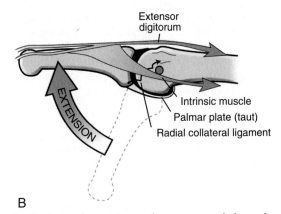

B

FIGURE 8-24. Lateral view of the arthrokinematics of active flexion and extension at the metacarpophalangeal (MCP) joint. **A,** Flexion is shown during activation of the flexor digitorum profundus muscle. The tendon of this muscle is shown coursing through the A$_1$ and A$_2$ pulleys (specifically named pulleys within the fibrous digital sheaths). Flexion draws both the dorsal capsule and radial collateral ligament relatively taut. The arthrokinematics are shown as a roll and slide in similar directions. **B,** Extension is shown controlled by coactivation of the extensor digitorum and one of the intrinsic muscles of the finger. The extended position draws the palmar plate taut while simultaneously creating relative slack in the radial collateral ligament. Taut or stretched tissues are shown as thin elongated arrows; slack structures are shown as wavy arrows. The axis of rotation for this motion is in the medial-lateral direction, shown piercing the head of the metacarpal.

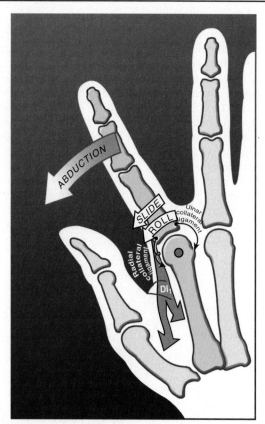

FIGURE 8-25. The arthrokinematics of active abduction at the metacarpophalangeal joint. Abduction is shown powered by the first dorsal interosseus muscle *(DI₁)*. At full abduction, the ulnar collateral ligament is taut and the radial collateral ligament is slack. Note that the axis of rotation for this motion is in an anterior-posterior direction, through the head of the metacarpal.

Figure 8-24, *B* illustrates active *extension* of the MCP joint, driven through a coordinated coactivation of the extensor digitorum and one of the intrinsic muscles (to be further described later in this chapter). The arthrokinematics of extension are similar to those illustrated for flexion except that the roll and slide of the proximal phalanx occur in a dorsal direction. By 0 degrees of extension, the collateral ligaments have slackened while the palmar plate has elongated and unfolded to support the head of the metacarpal. The relative slackness created in the collateral ligaments accounts, in part, for the increased passive mobility ("play") within the joint in the extended position. Extension beyond the 0-degree position is normally blocked by contraction of an intrinsic muscle, such as a lumbrical.

The arthrokinematics of *abduction* and *adduction* of the MCP joints are similar to those described for flexion and extension. During abduction of the index MCP joint, for instance, the proximal phalanx rolls and slides in a radial direction (Figure 8-25). The first dorsal interosseus muscle not only directs the arthrokinematics of abduction, but stabilizes the joint radially as the radial collateral ligament progressively slackens.[7]

The extent of active abduction and adduction at the MCP joints is significantly less when the motions are performed in full flexion compared with full extension. (This can be readily verified on your own hand.) Two factors can account for this difference. First, the collateral ligaments are taut near full flexion. Stored passive tension in these ligaments theoretically increases the compression force between the joint surfaces, thereby reducing available motion. Second, in the position of about 70 degrees of flexion, the articular surface of the proximal phalanges contacts the flattened palmar part of the metacarpal heads (see Figure 8-24, *A*). This relatively flat surface blocks the natural arthrokinematics required for maximal abduction and adduction range of motion.

THUMB

General Features and Ligaments

The MCP joint of the thumb consists of the articulation between the convex head of the first metacarpal and the concave proximal surface of the proximal phalanx of the thumb (Figure 8-27). The basic structure and arthrokinematics of the MCP joint of the thumb are similar to those of the fingers. Marked differences exist, however, in osteokinematics. Active and passive motions at the MCP joint of the thumb are significantly less than those at the MCP joints of the fingers. For all practical purposes, the MCP joint of the thumb allows only one degree of freedom: flexion and extension within the frontal plane.[94] Unlike the MCP joints of the fingers, extension of the thumb MCP joint is usually limited to just a few degrees. The arthrokinematics of active flexion at the metacarpophalangeal joint of the thumb is illustrated in Figure 8-28. From full extension, the proximal phalanx of the thumb can actively flex about 60 degrees across the palm toward the middle digit.[41]

Active abduction and adduction of the thumb MCP joint are very limited and therefore are considered accessory motions. This limitation can be observed by attempting to actively abduct or adduct the proximal phalanx while firmly stabilizing the thumb metacarpal. The structure of the collateral ligaments and bony configuration of this joint are most likely responsible for restricting this motion—a restriction that lends natural longitudinal stability throughout the entire ray of the thumb.

Although the limited abduction and adduction at the MCP joint provide some natural stability to thumb, the normally taut collateral ligaments at the joint are particularly vulnerable to injury from excessively large external torques. This is well exemplified by the relatively common "skier's injury" in which the handle and strap of the ski pole of a falling skier create a large abduction torque against the MCP joint, damaging the joint's ulnar collateral ligament. The rupture point of this ligament occurs at about 45 degrees of abduction.[25] Furthermore, the ligament is most vulnerable to rupture when the abduction torque is applied with the MCP joint flexed to about 30 degrees, a scenario likely present at the time of the skiing accident.

Interphalangeal Joints

FINGERS

Distal to the MCP joints are the proximal and distal interphalangeal joints of the fingers (see Figure 8-27). Each joint allows only one degree of freedom: flexion and extension. From both structural and functional perspectives, these joints are simpler than the MCP joints.

General Features and Ligaments

The *proximal interphalangeal (PIP) joints* are formed by the articulation between the heads of the proximal phalanges and the bases of the middle phalanges. The articular surface of

Clinical Relevance of the Flexed Position of the Metacarpophalangeal Joints of the Fingers

It has long been recognized that the flexed MCP joint is more stable and exhibits less passive, accessory movement than an extended joint.[26] Accordingly, flexion is considered the MCP joint's *close-packed position*.[101] As described in Chapter 1, the close-packed position of most joints is that unique position at which accessory movements (joint "play") are minimal and congruency within the joint is greatest. The close-packed position of the MCP joint is associated with increased tension in many of the surrounding ligaments. The increased tension in the collateral ligaments provides added stability to the base of the fingers during activities such as gripping or pinching, or the use of a key— activities that are typically performed in about 60 to 70 degrees of flexion.[36]

Although specific research is lacking on this topic, it is likely that the increased stability associated with flexion of the MCP joint is a result of, at least in large part, the elongation and subsequent stretch placed on the collateral ligaments. The stretch is caused by the eccentric or "out-of-round" cam shape of the metacarpal head. Because of this shape, flexion increases the distance between the proximal and distal attachments of the ligament (Figure 8-26).[18]

After trauma or surgery, the hand is often immobilized by a cast or splint to promote healing and relieve pain. If the period of immobilization is prolonged, periarticular connective tissues positioned at a shortened (slackened) length will often remodel in this position and subsequently generate greater resistance to elongation. In contrast, connective tissues immobilized in an elongated position are more likely to retain their normal stiffness. Consider, for example, a patient whose hand must be immobilized for 3 or 4 weeks after a fracture of the neck of the fourth or fifth metacarpal. A clinician will typically splint the hand with *the MCP joints flexed to about 70 degrees.* The flexed position of the MCP joints is designed to place a relative stretch on the collateral ligaments and thereby prevent their tightness. Preventing tightness within the collateral ligaments reduces the likelihood of developing an "extension contracture" of the MCP joints.

In some cases, however immobilizing the MCP joints in full flexion is contraindicated.[7] For example, after surgical reconstruction of the dorsal capsule or implantation of a total joint arthroplasty, the MCP joints must be immobilized in an extended (near 0-degree) position. This position reduces the strain on the healing tissues located on the dorsal aspect of the joint.

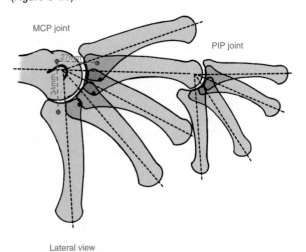

FIGURE 8-26. Because of the cam-shaped metacarpal head, flexion at the metacarpophalangeal (MCP) joint increases the distance between the attachment points of the collateral ligaments (27 mm in extension and 34 mm in 90 degrees of flexion). This is in contrast to the proximal interphalangeal (PIP) joint, where the distances between the proximal and distal attachments of the collateral ligaments remain essentially constant throughout flexion. (From Dubousset JF: The digital joints. In Tubiana R, ed: *The hand,* Philadelphia, Saunders, 1981.)

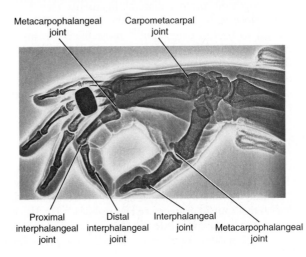

FIGURE 8-27. A side view of many of the joints of the wrist and hand. Note the sesamoid bone on the palmar side of the metacarpophalangeal joint of the thumb.

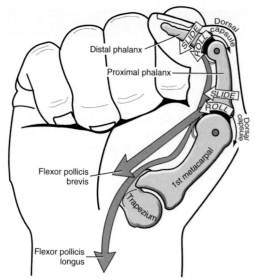

FIGURE 8-28. The arthrokinematics of active flexion are depicted for the metacarpophalangeal and interphalangeal joints of the thumb. Flexion is shown powered by the flexor pollicis longus and flexor pollicis brevis. The axis of rotation for flexion and extension at these joints is in the anterior-posterior direction, through the convex member of the joints. Taut or stretched tissues are shown as thin elongated arrows.

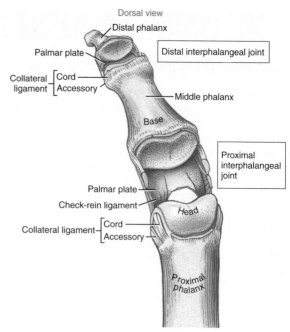

FIGURE 8-29. A dorsal view of the proximal interphalangeal and distal interphalangeal joints opened to expose the shape of the articular surfaces.

the joint appears as a tongue-in-groove articulation similar to that used in carpentry to join planks of wood (Figure 8-29). The head of the proximal phalanx has two rounded condyles separated by a shallow central groove. The opposing surface of the middle phalanx has two shallow concave facets separated by a central ridge. The tongue-in-groove articulation helps guide the motion of flexion and extension as it restricts axial rotation.

Each PIP joint is surrounded by a capsule that is reinforced by radial and ulnar *collateral ligaments*.[101] The cord portion of the collateral ligament at the PIP joint significantly limits abduction and adduction motion. As with the MCP joint, the accessory portion of the collateral ligament blends with and reinforces the *palmar plate* (see Figure 8-29). The anatomic connections between the palmar plate and collateral ligaments form a secure seat for the head of the proximal phalanx.[53] The palmar plate is the primary structure that limits hyperextension of the PIP joint.[113] In addition, the palmar surface of the plate serves as the attachment for the base of the *fibrous digital sheath*—the structure that houses the tendons of the extrinsic finger flexor muscles (see index and small fingers, Figure 8-21).

The proximal lateral regions of each palmar plate at the PIP joints thicken longitudinally, forming a fibrous tissue referred to as *check-rein ligaments* (see Figure 8-29).[101,113] These tissues reinforce the proximal attachments of the palmar plate, as well as assist in limiting hyperextension of the joint. When enlarged, check-rein ligaments are often considered a pathologic tissue and as such are often excised during surgical release of a flexion contracture at the PIP joint.

The *distal interphalangeal (DIP) joints* are formed through the articulation between the heads of the middle phalanges and the bases of the distal phalanges (see Figure 8-29). The structure of the DIP joint and the surrounding connective tissue are similar to those of the PIP joint, except for the absence of the check-rein ligaments.

Kinematics

The PIP joints flex to about 100 to 120 degrees. The DIP joints allow less flexion, to about 70 to 90 degrees. As with the MCP joints, flexion at the PIP and DIP joints is greater in the more ulnar digits. Minimal hyperextension is usually allowed at the PIP joints. The DIP joints, however, normally allow up to about 30 degrees of extension beyond the neutral (0 degree) position.

Similarities in joint structure cause similar arthrokinematics at the PIP and DIP joints. During active flexion at the PIP joint, for instance, the concave base of the middle phalanx rolls and slides in a palmar direction by the pull of the extrinsic finger flexors (Figure 8-30). During flexion, the passive tension created in the dorsal capsule helps guide and stabilize the roll-and-slide arthrokinematics.

In contrast to the MCP joints, passive tension in the collateral ligaments at the IP joints remains relatively constant throughout the range of motion.[62] Perhaps the more spheric shape of the heads of the phalanges prevents a significant change in length in these collateral ligaments (see Figure 8-26).[18] The close-packed position of the PIP and DIP joints is considered to be full extension,[101] most likely because of the stretch placed on the palmar plates. During periods of immobilization of the hand, the PIP and DIP joints are often splinted in near extension. This position places a stretch on the palmar plates, reducing the likelihood of a flexion contracture developing in these joints.

THUMB

The structure and function of the interphalangeal (IP) joint of the thumb are similar to those of the IP joints of the fingers. Motion is limited primarily to one degree of freedom, allowing active flexion to about 70 degrees (see Figure 8-28).[41] The IP joint of the thumb can be passively extended beyond neutral to about 20 degrees. This motion is often employed to apply a force

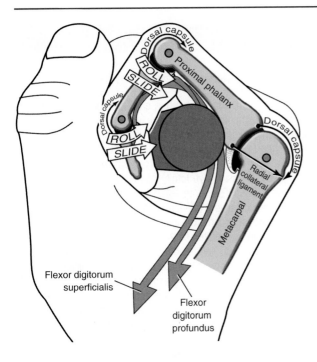

FIGURE 8-30. Illustration highlighting the arthrokinematics of active flexion at the proximal and distal interphalangeal joints of the index finger. Flexion elongates the dorsal capsules of the interphalangeal joints. The metacarpophalangeal and interphalangeal joints are shown flexing under the power of the flexor digitorum superficialis and the flexor digitorum profundus. The axis of rotation for flexion and extension at all three finger joints is in the medial-lateral direction, through the convex member of the joint. Taut or stretched tissues are shown as thin elongated arrows.

SPECIAL FOCUS 8-3

"Position of Function" of the Wrist and Hand

Some medical conditions, such as a traumatic head injury, stroke, or high-level quadriplegia, can result in a permanent deformity of the wrist and hand. The deformity is caused by a combination of long-term paralysis, disuse, or abnormal tone in the muscles. Clinicians therefore, often use splints that favor a position of the wrist and hand that maximally preserves functional potential. This splinted position, often called the *position of function,* is shown in Figure 8-31. This position provides a slightly opened and cupped hand, with the wrist in position to maintain optimal length of the finger flexor muscles.

FIGURE 8-31. A splint is used to support the wrist and hand in a "position of function." The person has flaccid paralysis from a stroke. The position of function incorporates the following: *wrist,* 20 to 30 degrees of extension with slight ulnar deviation; *fingers,* 35 to 45 degrees of metacarpophalangeal (MCP) joint flexion and 15 to 30 degrees of proximal interphalangeal (PIP) and distal interphalangeal (DIP) joint flexion; and *thumb,* 35 to 45 degrees of carpometacarpal (CMC) joint abduction. These positions may vary based on the patient's underlying physical or medical condition. (Courtesy of Teri Bielefeld, PT, CHT, Zablocki VA Hospital, Milwaukee, Wisconsin.)

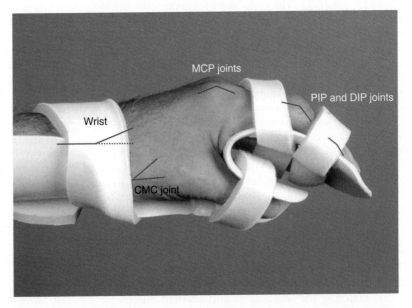

between the pad of the thumb and an object, such as pushing a thumbtack into a board. The amount of passive hyperextension often increases throughout life owing to years of stretch placed on palmar structures, including the palmar plate.

MUSCLE AND JOINT INTERACTION

Innervation of Muscles, Skin, and Joints of the Hand

The highly complex and coordinated functions of the hand require a rich source of motor and sensory innervation of the region's muscles, skin, and joints. Consider, for instance, the very precise and delicate movements of the digits performed by a concert violinist. One fact allowing such precision is that a single axon traveling to an intrinsic muscle of the hand, such as the thumb, may innervate as few as 100 muscle fibers.[74] In this case, one axon would simultaneously activate *all* 100 muscle fibers. By contrast, a single axon traveling to the medial head of the gastrocnemius muscle–a muscle not involved with fine movements–may innervate about 2000 muscle fibers.[24] The smaller fiber-per-axon ratio typical of most intrinsic muscles of the hand allows for a more precise gradation between levels of force, ultimately permitting finer control of movement.

Fine control over the muscles and movements of the digits also requires a constant stream of sensory information. Consider the importance of this sensory information for a person who quickly peels and eats a piece of fruit, with very little eye contact. This activity is controlled primarily through input from sensory nerves in the hands; much of the muscular activity is in *response* to this sensory information. Muscle activation devoid of sensory input typically results in a crude and uncoordinated movement. This is frequently observed in diseases that spare the motor system but affect primarily the sensory system, such as *tabes dorsalis,* a condition that affects the (sensory) afferent tracts within the spinal cord.

MUSCLE AND SKIN INNERVATION

Innervation to the muscles and the skin of the hand is illustrated in Figure 6-32. The *radial nerve* innervates the extrinsic extensor muscles of the digits. These muscles, located on the dorsal aspect of the forearm, are the extensor digitorum, extensor digiti minimi, extensor indicis, extensor pollicis longus, extensor pollicis brevis, and abductor pollicis longus. The radial nerve is responsible for the sensation on the dorsal aspect of the wrist and hand, especially around the dorsal region of the thenar web space.

The *median nerve* innervates most of the extrinsic flexors of the digits. In the forearm the median nerve innervates the flexor digitorum superficialis. A branch of the median nerve (anterior interosseous nerve) then innervates the lateral half of the flexor digitorum profundus and the flexor pollicis longus.

Continuing distally, the median nerve enters the hand through the carpal tunnel, deep to the transverse carpal ligament. Once in the hand, it innervates the muscles that form the thenar eminence (flexor pollicis brevis, abductor pollicis brevis, and opponens pollicis) and the lateral two lumbricals. The median nerve is responsible for the sensation on the palmar-lateral aspect of the hand, including the tips and the palmar region of the lateral three and one-half digits.

The *ulnar nerve* innervates the medial half of the flexor digitorum profundus. Distally the ulnar nerve crosses the

SPECIAL FOCUS 8-4

The "Protective" Role of Normal Sensation

Normal sensation to the hand is essential for its protection against mechanical and thermal injury. Persons with peripheral neuropathy, spinal cord injury, and uncontrolled diabetes, for example, often lack sensation in their extremities, making them very vulnerable to injury. Persons with Hansen's disease (formerly called "leprosy"[111]) may have totally insensitive digits, as well as dermatologic lesions. Over time—and especially without medical care—persons with severe or uncontrolled Hansen's disease may experience a partial or complete loss of their digits. This phenomenon is only indirectly related to the infecting bacteria; the more direct cause stems from the unnecessarily large, and often damaging, contact forces applied to the insensitive digits. With normal sensation, persons generally apply a relatively low amount of force to their hands while performing routine activities—usually just the minimum needed to adequately perform a given task. In Hansen's disease, however, a greater than normal force is often applied as a means to compensate for the diminished sensation. Although the increased force may be slight for any given application, multiple applications over an extended period of time can damage skin and other connective tissue. Regardless of the pathology that causes the loss of sensation, clinicians must educate their patients about their increased vulnerability to injury and suggest methods for protecting the region.[64]

wrist superficial to the carpal tunnel. In the hand the deep motor branch of the ulnar nerve innervates the hypothenar muscles (flexor digiti minimi, abductor digiti minimi, opponens digiti minimi, and palmaris brevis) and the medial two lumbricals. The deep motor branch continues laterally, deep in the hand, to innervate all palmar and dorsal interossei and finally the adductor pollicis. The ulnar nerve is responsible for the sensation on the ulnar border of the hand, including most of the skin of the ulnar one and one-half digits.

As a reference, the primary nerve roots that supply the muscles of the upper extremity are listed in Appendix II, Part A. In addition, Appendix II, Parts B to D include additional reference items to help guide the clinical assessment of the functional status of the C^5-T^1 nerve roots and several major peripheral nerves of the upper limb.

SENSORY INNERVATION TO THE JOINTS

For the most part, the *joints of the hand* receive sensation from sensory nerve fibers that supply the overlying dermatomes. (See dermatome chart in Appendix II, Part D.) These afferent nerve fibers merge with the following dorsal nerve roots at the spinal cord: C^6, carrying sensation from the thumb and index finger; C^7, carrying sensation from the middle finger; and C^8, carrying sensation from the ring and small fingers.[30,39,101]

Muscular Function of the Hand

Muscles that operate the digits are classified as either *extrinsic* or *intrinsic* to the hand (Table 8-3). Extrinsic muscles have their proximal attachments in the forearm or, in some cases, as far proximal as the epicondyles of the humerus. Intrinsic

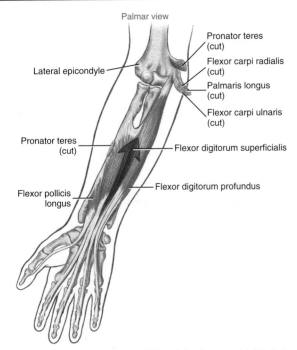

Palmar view

Lateral epicondyle

Pronator teres (cut)

Flexor carpi radialis (cut)

Palmaris longus (cut)

Flexor carpi ulnaris (cut)

Pronator teres (cut)

Flexor digitorum superficialis

Flexor digitorum profundus

Flexor pollicis longus

FIGURE 8-32. An anterior view of the right forearm highlighting the action of the flexor digitorum superficialis muscle. Note the cut proximal ends of the wrist flexors and pronator teres muscles.

TABLE 8-3. **Extrinsic and Intrinsic Muscles to the Hand**	
Muscles	
Extrinsic Muscles	
Flexors of the digits	Flexor digitorum superficialis Flexor digitorum profundus Flexor pollicis longus
Extensors of the fingers	Extensor digitorum Extensor indicis Extensor digiti minimi
Extensors of the thumb	Extensor pollicis longus Extensor pollicis brevis Abductor pollicis longus
Intrinsic Muscles	
Thenar eminence	Abductor pollicis brevis Flexor pollicis brevis Opponens pollicis
Hypothenar eminence	Abductor digiti minimi Flexor digiti minimi Opponens digiti minimi Palmaris brevis
Other	Adductor pollicis (two heads) Lumbricals (four) Interossei (four palmar and four dorsal)

muscles, in contrast, have both their proximal and distal attachments within the hand. As a summary and reference, the detailed anatomy and nerve supply of the muscles of the hand are included in Appendix II, Part E.

Most active movements of the hand, such as opening and closing the fingers, require precise cooperation between the extrinsic and the intrinsic muscles of the hand and the muscles of the wrist. This topic is addressed in detail later in this chapter.

EXTRINSIC FLEXORS OF THE DIGITS

Anatomy and Joint Action of the Extrinsic Flexors of the Digits

The extrinsic flexor muscles of the digits are the flexor digitorum superficialis, flexor digitorum profundus, and flexor pollicis longus (Figures 8-32 and 8-33). These muscles have extensive proximal attachments from the medial epicondyle of the humerus and regions of the forearm.

The muscle belly of the *flexor digitorum superficialis* is located in the anterior forearm, just deep to the three wrist flexors and the pronator teres muscle (see Figure 8-32). Its four tendons cross the wrist and enter the palmar aspect of the hand. At the level of the proximal phalanx, each tendon splits to allow passage of the tendon of the flexor digitorum profundus (Figure 8-34, middle and index finger). The two split parts of each tendon partially reunite, cross the PIP joint, and attach on the sides of the palmar aspect of the middle phalanx.

The primary action of the flexor digitorum superficialis is to flex the PIP joints. This muscle, however, flexes all the joints it crosses. In general, with the exception of the small finger, each tendon can be controlled relatively independently of the other. This independence of function is especially evident at the index finger.

The muscle belly of the *flexor digitorum profundus* is located in the deepest muscular plane of the forearm, deep to the flexor digitorum superficialis muscle (see Figure 8-33). Once in the digit, each tendon passes through the split tendon of the

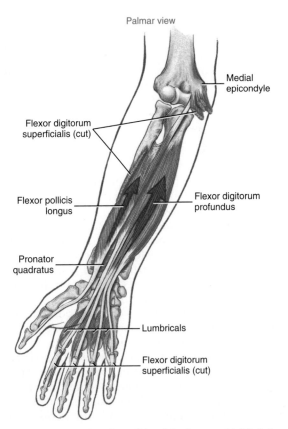

Palmar view

Medial epicondyle

Flexor digitorum superficialis (cut)

Flexor pollicis longus

Flexor digitorum profundus

Pronator quadratus

Lumbricals

Flexor digitorum superficialis (cut)

FIGURE 8-33. An anterior view of the right forearm highlighting the action of the flexor digitorum profundus and the flexor pollicis longus muscles. The lumbrical muscles are shown attaching to the tendons of the flexor digitorum profundus. Note the cut proximal and distal ends of the flexor digitorum superficialis.

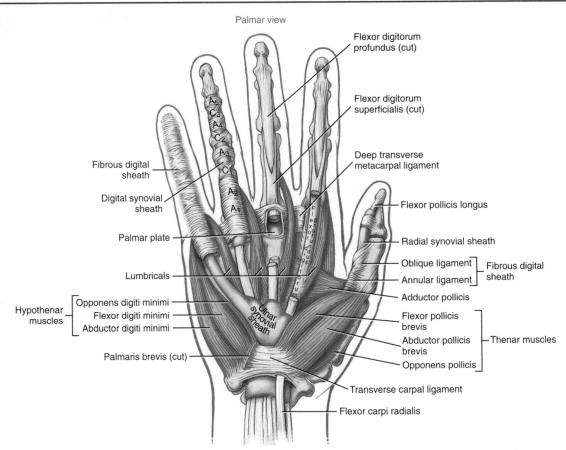

Palmar view

Flexor digitorum profundus (cut)

Flexor digitorum superficialis (cut)

Deep transverse metacarpal ligament

Fibrous digital sheath

Digital synovial sheath

Palmar plate

Lumbricals

Hypothenar muscles
- Opponens digiti minimi
- Flexor digiti minimi
- Abductor digiti minimi

Palmaris brevis (cut)

Flexor pollicis longus

Radial synovial sheath

Oblique ligament ⎫ Fibrous digital
Annular ligament ⎭ sheath

Adductor pollicis

Flexor pollicis brevis

Abductor pollicis brevis ⎤ Thenar muscles

Opponens pollicis

Transverse carpal ligament

Flexor carpi radialis

FIGURE 8-34. A palmar view illustrates several important structures of the hand. Note the *small finger* showing the fibrous digital sheath and ulnar synovial sheath encasing the extrinsic flexor tendons. The *ring finger* has the fibrous digital sheath removed, thereby highlighting the digital synovial sheath *(blue)* and the annular (A_1 to A_5) and cruciate (C_1 to C_3) pulleys. The *middle finger* shows the pulleys removed to expose the distal attachments of the flexor digitorum superficialis and profundus. The *index finger* has a portion of flexor digitorum superficialis tendon removed, thereby exposing the deeper tendon of the flexor digitorum profundus and attached lumbrical. The *thumb* highlights the oblique and annular pulleys, along with the radial synovial sheath surrounding the tendon of the flexor pollicis longus. (The thenar and hypothenar muscles are also drawn.)

flexor digitorum superficialis. Each profundus tendon then continues distally to attach to the palmar side of the base of the distal phalanx. The flexor digitorum profundus is the sole flexor of the DIP joint, but, like the superficialis, can assist in flexing every joint it crosses.

The flexor digitorum profundus to the index finger can be controlled relatively independently of the other profundus tendons. The remaining three tendons, however, are interconnected through various muscular fasciculi, which usually prohibit isolated DIP joint flexion of a single finger. To appreciate this interconnection, grasp the middle finger and maximally extend all of its joints. While holding this position, attempt to actively flex *only* the DIP joint of the ring finger. The inability or difficulty in performing this motion is caused by the excessive elongation placed on the entire muscle belly of the flexor digitorum profundus by the full extension of the middle finger. During manual muscle testing, this maneuver is often used to inhibit profundus action, thereby allowing the flexor digitorum superficialis to be the more dominant flexor of the PIP joint.

The *flexor pollicis longus* resides in the deepest muscular plane of the forearm, just lateral to the flexor digitorum profundus (see Figure 8-33). This muscle crosses the wrist and attaches distally to the palmar side of the base of the distal phalanx of the thumb. The flexor pollicis longus is the sole flexor at the IP joint of the thumb, and it also exerts a substantial flexion torque at the MCP and CMC joints of the thumb. If not opposed, the flexor pollicis longus also flexes the wrist.

All three of the aforementioned extrinsic flexors of the digits often contract in unison, especially when a firm grip of the entire hand is required. The actions of these muscles curl the digits into flexion while also assisting with opposition of the first, fourth, and fifth digits' CMC joints. This action is most evident when a fist is alternately tightly clenched and released. Although subtle, these opposition actions assist certain intrinsic muscles in raising the borders of the hand, thereby improving the effectiveness and security of grasp.

Distal to the carpal tunnel, the *ulnar synovial sheath* surrounds the flexor digitorum superficialis and profundus tendons. This sheath ends in the proximal palm, except for a distal continuation around the tendons of the small finger (see Figure 8-34). The *radial synovial sheath* remains in contact with the tendon of the flexor pollicis longus to its distal insertion on the thumb.

The extrinsic flexor tendons of the digits travel to their distal attachment in protective fibro-osseous tunnels known

SPECIAL FOCUS 8-5

Anatomic Basis for "Carpal Tunnel Syndrome"

All nine extrinsic flexor tendons of the digits and the median nerve pass through the carpal tunnel (Figure 8-35). These tendons are surrounded by synovial sheaths, designed to reduce friction between the structures. An *ulnar synovial sheath* surrounds the eight tendons of the flexors digitorum superficialis and profundus, and a separate *radial synovial sheath* surrounds the tendon of the flexor pollicis longus. Hand activities that require repetitive, prolonged, or extreme wrist positions can irritate the tendons and their sheaths. Because of the closed and relatively small compartment of the carpal tunnel, swelling of the synovial membranes may increase the pressure on the median nerve. *Carpal tunnel syndrome* may result, which is characterized by pain and paresthesia in the sensory distribution of the median nerve.

With progression of the syndrome, muscular weakness and atrophy can occur in the muscles of the thenar eminence. Persons with carpal tunnel syndrome often experience abnormally large increases in carpal tunnel pressure, especially during extreme wrist motions,[46] including making a fist. Activities that create repetitive movement of the tendons and median nerve within the carpal tunnel, such as prolonged use of a computer keyboard, have been implicated as a cause of carpal tunnel syndrome.[108] Pressures have been shown to increase significantly when typing is performed with greater wrist extension or radial deviation.[87] Alternative design of the standard computer keyboard may provide a less stressful position for the wrist and thereby reduce the severity of this painful condition.[65,95]

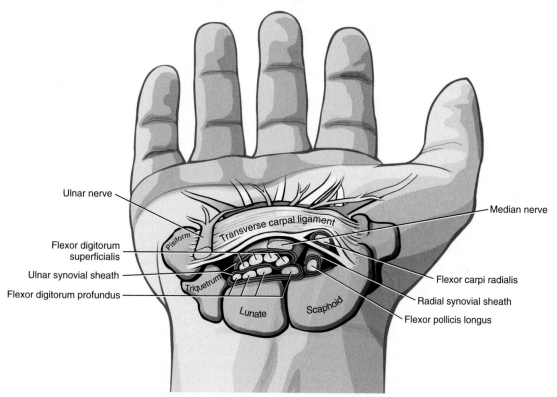

FIGURE 8-35. A transverse view through the entrance of the carpal tunnel of the right wrist. The ulnar synovial sheath *(blue)* surrounds the tendons of the flexors digitorum superficialis and profundus. The radial synovial sheath surrounds the tendon of the flexor pollicis longus. Note the position of the median and ulnar nerves relative to the transverse carpal ligament.

as *fibrous digital sheaths* (see Figure 8-34, small finger). Sheaths start proximally as a continuation of the thick aponeurosis just under the skin of the palm. Throughout the length of each digit, the sheaths are anchored to the phalanges and the palmar plates (see Figure 8-21, index finger). Embedded within each digital sheath are discrete bands of tissue called *flexor pulleys* (see Figure 8-34, A₁ to A₅, C₁ to C₃ in ring finger). Deep to these pulleys is a *digital synovial sheath*, surrounding the flexor tendons from the distal palmar crease to the DIP joint. This sheath serves as a nutritional and lubrication

source for the enclosed tendons. The synovial fluid secreted from the sheath reduces the friction between the flexor digitorum superficialis and profundus tendons. After injury or laceration, adhesions may develop between the tendon and adjacent digital sheath or between tendons. After surgical repair of a lacerated tendon, the therapist usually initiates a closely monitored exercise program to facilitate gliding of the tendon. This therapy is performed according to a strict time schedule as determined by the surgeon and the therapist, depending on the type of repair and other parameters.

The flexor tendons and surrounding synovial membranes may become inflamed—a condition known as *tenosynovitis.* Associated swelling limits the space within the sheath and thereby restricts the gliding action of the tendons. The inflamed region of the tendon may also develop a nodule that occasionally becomes wedged within the stenosed region of the sheath, thereby blocking movement of the digit. With additional force, the tendon may suddenly slip through the constriction with a snap, a condition often referred to as a "trigger finger." Conservative management that includes activity modification, splinting, and cortisone injection may be effective in early stages, but surgical release of the constricted region of the sheath is usually required in chronic cases.

Anatomy and Function of the Flexor Pulleys

Figure 8-34 shows the flexor pulleys that are embedded within the fibrous digital sheath. Five *annular pulleys* have been described for each finger, designated as A_1 to A_5.[17] The major pulleys (A_2 and A_4) attach to the shafts of the proximal and middle phalanges. The minor pulleys (A_1, A_3, and A_5) attach directly to the palmar plate at each of the three joints within a finger. Three less distinct *cruciate pulleys* (C_1 to C_3) have also been described.[17] The cruciate pulleys are made of thin, flexible fibers that crisscross over the tendons at regions where the digital sheaths bend during flexion.

The *annular and oblique ligaments* of the thumb function as pulleys for the passage of the tendon of the flexor pollicis longus (see Figure 8-34).

Flexor pulleys, palmar aponeurosis, and skin share a similar function of holding the underlying tendons at a relatively close distance to the joints.[29] Without the restraint provided by these tissues, the force of a strong contraction of the extrinsic finger flexors causes the tendon to pull away from the joint's axis of rotation, a phenomenon referred to as "bowstringing" of the tendon.

The flexor pulleys of the digits have a particularly important role in stabilizing the position of the tendons relative to the underlying joints.[90] The pulleys may be overstretched or torn secondary to trauma, overuse, or disease. (Of interest, overstretching and subsequent bowstringing of the flexor tendons have been observed in 26% of elite rock climbers, most often in the ring and middle fingers.[89,109]) A severing or overstretching of the major A_2 or A_4 pulley significantly alters the moment arms of the flexor tendons and subsequently alters the biomechanics at the MCP and PIP joints.[29] Preservation of these two major pulleys is therefore a major goal of hand surgeons.

Role of Proximal Stabilizer Muscles during Active Finger Flexion

The extrinsic digital flexors are mechanically capable of flexing multiple joints, from the DIP joint to, at least theoretically for the flexor digitorum superficialis, the elbow. In order for these muscles to isolate their flexion potential across a single joint, other muscles contract synergistically with the extrinsic digital flexors. Consider the flexor digitorum superficialis performing isolated PIP joint flexion (Figure 8-36). At the onset of contraction, the extensor digitorum must act as a proximal stabilizer to prevent the flexor digitorum superficialis from flexing the MCP joint and the wrist. Because the flexor moment arm length of the flexor digitorum superficialis progressively increases at the more proximal joints, a relatively small force applied to a distal joint is amplified to a greater torque at the more proximal joints. Figure 8-36 shows that a

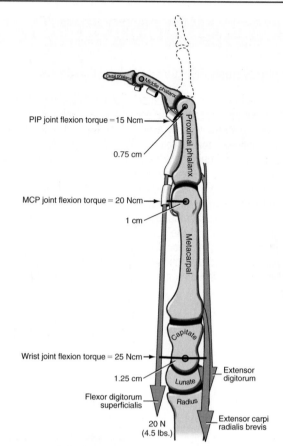

FIGURE 8-36. The muscle activation required to produce the simple motion of proximal interphalangeal joint flexion. A 20-N (4.5-lb) force produced by the flexor digitorum superficialis creates a flexion torque across every joint it crosses. Because of the progressively larger moment arms in the more proximal joints, the flexor torques progressively increase in a proximal direction from 15 to 25 Ncm. For only proximal interphalangeal joint flexion to be isolated, the extensor digitorum and the extensor carpi radialis brevis must resist the flexion effect of the flexor digitorum superficialis across the wrist and metacarpophalangeal joints.

20-N (4.5-lb) force within the superficialis tendon produces a 15-Ncm torque at the PIP joint, a 20-Ncm torque at the MCP joint, and a 25-Ncm torque at the midcarpal joint of the wrist. *The greater the force produced by the flexor digitorum superficialis, the greater the force demands placed on the proximal stabilizers.* The proximal stabilizers include the extensor digitorum and, if needed, the wrist extensors. The amount of muscle force and muscular coordination required for a simple action of PIP joint flexion is actually more than what it first appears. Paralysis or weakness of proximal stabilizers can significantly disrupt the effectiveness of more distal muscle function.

Passive Finger Flexion via "Tenodesis Action" of the Extrinsic Digital Flexors

The extrinsic flexors of the digits—namely, the flexor digitorum profundus and superficialis and the flexor pollicis longus—cross anterior to the wrist. The position of the wrist therefore significantly alters the length and subsequent passive tension in these muscles. One implication of this arrangement can be appreciated by actively extending the wrist and observing the *passive flexion* of the fingers and thumb (Figure 8-37). The digits automatically flex because of the increased

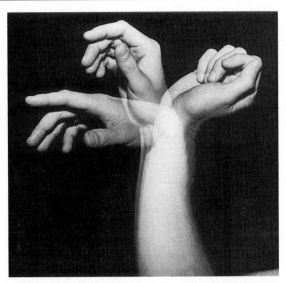

passive tension in the stretched flexor muscles. The stretching of a polyarticular muscle across one joint, which generates a passive movement at other joints, is referred to as a *tenodesis action* of a muscle.

The amount of passive flexion of the fingers caused by the aforementioned tenodesis action is surprisingly large; in healthy subjects, on average, completely extending the wrist from full flexion automatically flexes the DIP joint about 20 degrees, the PIP joint about 50 degrees, and the MCP joint about 35 degrees.[104] Figure 8-37 also demonstrates that in the position of full wrist flexion, the fingers, most notably the index, passively extend owing to a similar tenodesis action of the stretched extrinsic digital extensor muscles. Essentially all polyarticular muscles in the body demonstrate some degree of tenodesis action.

EXTRINSIC EXTENSORS OF THE FINGERS

Muscular Anatomy

The extrinsic extensors of the fingers are the extensor digitorum, the extensor indicis, and the extensor digiti minimi (see Figure 7-22). The extensor digitorum and the extensor digiti

FIGURE 8-37. "Tenodesis action" of the finger flexors in a healthy person. As the wrist is extended, the thumb and fingers automatically flex because of the stretch placed on the extrinsic digital flexors. The flexion occurs passively, without effort from the subject.

SPECIAL FOCUS 8-6

The Usefulness of Tenodesis Action in Some Persons with Quadriplegia

The natural tenodesis action of the extrinsic digital flexor muscles has important clinical implications. One example involves a person with C[6] quadriplegia who has near or complete paralysis of his digital flexors and extensors, but well-innervated wrist extensors. People with this level of spinal cord injury often employ a tenodesis action for many functions, such as holding a cup of water. In order to open the hand to grasp the cup, the person allows gravity to first flex the wrist. This, in turn, stretches the partially paralyzed extensors of the fingers and thumb (see

"taut" muscles in Figure 8-38, *A*). In Figure 8-38, *B, active contraction of a wrist extensor muscle* (shown in red) slackens the extensor digitorum but also, more important, stretches the paralyzed finger and thumb flexor muscles, such as the flexor digitorum profundus and flexor pollicis longus. The stretch in these flexor muscles creates enough passive tension to effectively flex the digits and grasp the cup. The amount of passive tension in the digital flexors is controlled indirectly by the degree of active wrist extension.

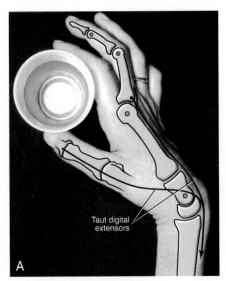

Taut flexor digitorum profundus and flexor pollicis longus

Taut digital extensors

Slack extensor digitorum

Active extensor carpi radialis brevis

FIGURE 8-38. A person with C[6] level quadriplegia using "tenodesis action" to grasp a cup of water. **A,** Gravity-induced wrist flexion causes the hand to open. **B,** Active wrist extension by contraction of the innervated extensor carpi radialis brevis (shown in red) creates enough passive tension in the paralyzed digital flexors to hold the cup of water. See full description above.

Dorsal view

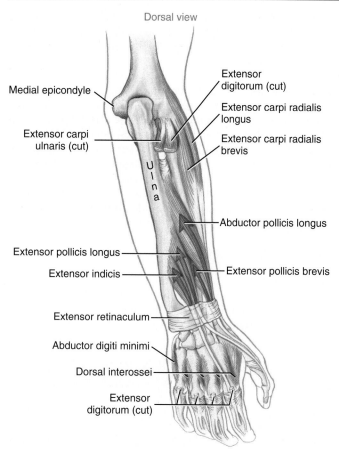

Medial epicondyle

Extensor carpi ulnaris (cut)

Ulna

Extensor digitorum (cut)

Extensor carpi radialis longus

Extensor carpi radialis brevis

Abductor pollicis longus

Extensor pollicis longus

Extensor indicis

Extensor pollicis brevis

Extensor retinaculum

Abductor digiti minimi

Dorsal interossei

Extensor digitorum (cut)

FIGURE 8-39. A dorsal view of the right upper extremity highlighting the digital extensors: the extensor indicis, extensor pollicis longus, extensor pollicis brevis, and abductor pollicis longus. Note the cut proximal ends of extensor carpi ulnaris and the extensor digitorum.

minimi originate from a common tendon off the lateral epicondyle of the humerus. The extensor indicis has its proximal attachment on the dorsal region of the forearm. The *extensor digitorum,* in terms of cross-sectional area, is by far the predominant finger extensor. In addition to functioning as a finger extensor, the extensor digitorum has an excellent moment arm as a wrist extensor (see Figure 7-24).

Dissecting away the extensor digitorum and extensor minimi exposes the deeper *extensor indicis* and the extrinsic extensor muscles of the thumb (Figure 8-39). The extensor indicis muscle has only one tendon, which serves the index finger. The *extensor digiti minimi* is a small fusiform muscle often interconnected with the extensor digitorum. As depicted in Figure 8-40, the extensor digiti minimi often has two tendons.

Tendons of the extensor digitorum, extensor indicis, and extensor digiti minimi cross the wrist in synovial-lined compartments located within the extensor retinaculum (see Figure 7-23). Distal to the extensor retinaculum, the tendons course toward the fingers, dorsal to the metacarpals (see Figure 8-40). The tendons of the extensor digitorum are interconnected by several *juncturae tendinae.* These thin strips of connective tissue stabilize the angle of approach of the tendons to the base of the MCP joints and may limit independent movement of the individual tendons.

The anatomic organization of the extensor tendons of the fingers is very different from that of the finger flexors. The flexor tendons travel in well-defined digital sheaths toward single bony attachments. In contrast, distal to the wrist, the extensor tendons lack a defined digital sheath or pulley system. The extensor tendons eventually become integrated into a fibrous expansion of connective tissues, located along the length of the dorsum of each finger (see Figure 8-40). The complex set of connective tissue is called the *extensor mechanism,* although other terms have been used over the years,

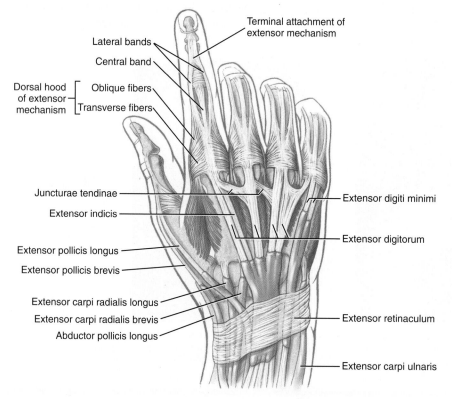

Terminal attachment of extensor mechanism

Lateral bands

Central band

Dorsal hood of extensor mechanism

Oblique fibers

Transverse fibers

Juncturae tendinae

Extensor indicis

Extensor pollicis longus

Extensor pollicis brevis

Extensor carpi radialis longus

Extensor carpi radialis brevis

Abductor pollicis longus

Extensor digiti minimi

Extensor digitorum

Extensor retinaculum

Extensor carpi ulnaris

FIGURE 8-40. A dorsal view of the muscles, tendons, and extensor mechanism of the right hand. The synovial sheaths (in blue) and the extensor retinaculum are also depicted. The dorsal interosseus muscles and abductor digiti minimi muscles are also evident on the dorsal aspect of the hand.

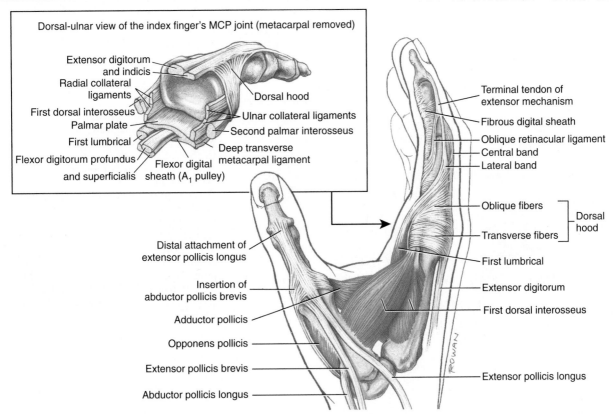

FIGURE 8-41. A lateral view of the muscles, tendons, and extensor mechanism of the right hand. The illustration in the box highlights the anatomy associated with the metacarpophalangeal joint of the index finger.

including the *extensor expansion, extensor apparatus,* and *extensor assembly.*[14,100] The extensor mechanism serves as a primary distal attachment for the extensor digitorum, indicis, and digiti minimi and for most of the intrinsic muscles acting on the fingers. The following section describes the anatomy of the extensor mechanism. A similar but less organized extensor mechanism exists for the thumb.

Extensor Mechanism of the Fingers

A small slip of the tendon of the extensor digitorum attaches to the base of the dorsal side of the proximal phalanx. The remaining tendon flattens into a *central band,* forming the "backbone" of the extensor mechanism to each finger (see Figures 8-40 and 8-41). The central band courses distally to attach to the dorsal base of the middle phalanx. Before crossing the PIP joint, two *lateral bands* diverge from the central band. More distally, the lateral bands fuse into a single terminal tendon that attaches to the dorsal base of the distal phalanx. The multiple attachments of the extensor mechanism into the phalanges allow the extensor digitorum to transfer extensor force distally throughout the entire finger.

The position of lateral bands relative to the PIP joint is stabilized bilaterally on each finger by a set of thin connective tissues, generally known as retinacular ligaments.[93,110] The more substantial of these connective tissues is a pair of oblique retinacular ligaments. Figure 8-41 shows the radial *oblique retinacular ligament* of the index finger. The slender fibers arise proximally from the fibrous digital sheath, just proximal to the PIP joint, and course obliquely and distally to insert into the lateral bands. The ligaments help coordinate

movement between the PIP and DIP joints of the fingers, a point to be discussed later in this chapter.

The most prominent feature of the proximal end of the extensor mechanism is the *dorsal hood* (see Figures 8-40 and 8-41). This specialized tissue consists of a nearly triangular sheet of thin aponeurosis that contains both transverse and oblique fibers. The *transverse fibers* (also called "sagittal" bands) run nearly perpendicular to the long axis of the tendon of the extensor digitorum. The transverse fibers from both sides of the extensor tendon attach into the palmar plate, forming a "sling" around the base of the proximal phalanx (Figure 8-42). This sling is used by the extensor digitorum muscle to extend the MCP joint. In addition, the transverse fibers stabilize the tendon of the extensor digitorum over the dorsum of the MCP joint. The *oblique fibers* of the dorsal hood course distally and dorsally to fuse primarily with the lateral bands (see Figure 8-41).

As a general rule, the intrinsic muscles of the hand (specifically the lumbricals and interossei) attach into the extensor mechanism via the oblique fibers and, to a lesser extent, the transverse fibers of the dorsal hood. Figure 8-41 shows this arrangement for the first dorsal interosseus and lumbrical of the index finger. Via these important connections, the intrinsic muscles assist the extensor digitorum with extension of the PIP and DIP joints.

The anatomic and functional components of the extensor mechanism are summarized in Table 8-4.

Action of the Extrinsic Finger Extensors

Isolated contraction of the extensor digitorum produces hyperextension of the MCP joints. Only in the presence of

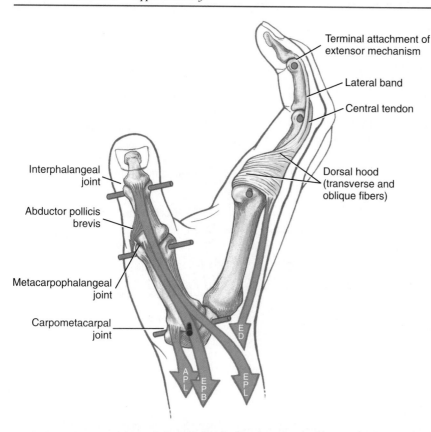

Terminal attachment of extensor mechanism

Lateral band

Central tendon

Interphalangeal joint

Abductor pollicis brevis

Dorsal hood (transverse and oblique fibers)

Metacarpophalangeal joint

Carpometacarpal joint

ED

APL

EPB

EPL

FIGURE 8-42. The function of the extrinsic extensor muscles of the hand is demonstrated. Each muscle's action is determined by the orientation of the line of force relative to the axes of rotation at each joint. (The axes of rotation for all flexion and extension movements are depicted in green. The axis of rotation for abduction and adduction movements at the base of the thumb is indicated in purple.) Isolated contraction of the extensor digitorum *(ED)* hyperextends the metacarpophalangeal joints. The extensor pollicis longus *(EPL)*, the extensor pollicis brevis *(EPB)*, and the abductor pollicis longus *(APL)* are all primary thumb extensors. Attachments of the abductor pollicis brevis are shown blending into the distal tendon of the extensor pollicis longus.

TABLE 8-4. Anatomy and Primary Function of the Components of the Extensor Mechanism

Component	Pertinent Anatomy	Primary Function
Central band	Direct continuation of the tendon of the extensor digitorum; attaches to the dorsal side of the base of the middle phalanx	Serves as the "backbone" of the extensor mechanism Transmits extensor force from the extensor digitorum across the PIP joint
Lateral bands	Formed from divisions off the central band; pair of bands fuse as a single attachment to the dorsal side of the distal phalanx	Transmit extensor force from the extensor digitorum, lumbricals, and interossei across the PIP and DIP joints
Dorsal hood (transverse and oblique fibers)	*Transverse fibers:* Connect the extensor tendon with the palmar plate at the MCP joint	Stabilize the extensor digitorum tendon over the dorsal aspect of the MCP joint Form a sling around the proximal end of the proximal phalanx, thereby assisting the extensor digitorum in extending the MCP joint
	Oblique fibers: Course distally and dorsally to fuse with the lateral bands	Transfer force from lumbricals and interossei to the lateral bands of the extensor mechanism, thereby assisting with extension of the PIP and DIP joints
Oblique retinacular ligament	Slender, oblique-running fibers connecting the fibrous digital sheaths to the lateral bands of the extensor mechanism	Helps coordinate movement between the PIP and DIP joints of the fingers

DIP, Distal interphalangeal; *MCP,* metacarpophalangeal; *PIP,* proximal interphalangeal.

activated intrinsic muscles of the fingers can the extensor digitorum fully extend the PIP and DIP joints. This important point will be reinforced later in this chapter.

EXTRINSIC EXTENSORS OF THE THUMB

Anatomic Considerations

The extrinsic extensors of the thumb are the *extensor pollicis longus, extensor pollicis brevis,* and *abductor pollicis longus* (see Figures 8-39 and 8-41). These radial innervated muscles have

their proximal attachments on the dorsal region of the forearm. The tendons of these muscles compose the "anatomic snuffbox" located on the radial side of the wrist. The tendons of the abductor pollicis longus and the extensor pollicis brevis together pass through first dorsal compartment within the extensor retinaculum of the wrist (see Figure 7-23). Distal to the extensor retinaculum, the tendon of the abductor pollicis longus inserts primarily into the radial-dorsal surface of the base of the thumb metacarpal. Additional distal attachments of this muscle have been observed attaching into the trapezium and blending with fibers of the intrinsic thenar muscles.[91] The extensor pollicis brevis attaches distally to the dorsal base of the proximal phalanx of the thumb. The tendon of the extensor pollicis longus crosses the wrist in the third compartment in a groove just medial to the dorsal tubercle of the radius (see Figure 7-23). The extensor pollicis longus attaches distally to the dorsal base of the distal phalanx of the thumb. Fibers from both extrinsic extensor tendons contribute to the central tendon of the extensor mechanism of the thumb.

Functional Considerations

The multiple actions of the extensor pollicis longus, extensor pollicis brevis, and abductor pollicis longus can be understood by noting their line of force relative to the axes of rotation at the joints they cross (see Figure 8-42). The *extensor pollicis longus* extends the IP, MCP, and CMC joints of the thumb. The muscle passes to the dorsal side of the medial-lateral axis of the CMC joint and is therefore also capable of adducting this joint. The extensor pollicis longus is unique in its ability to perform all three actions that compose the repositioning of the thumb to the anatomic position: extension (with slight lateral rotation) and adduction of the first metacarpal.

Figure 8-42 also illustrates that the *extensor pollicis brevis* is an extensor of the MCP and CMC joints of the thumb; the *abductor pollicis longus* extends only at the CMC joint. The long abductor muscle is also a prime abductor of the CMC joint, based on its line of force passing anterior (palmar) to the joint's medial-lateral axis of rotation. The combined extension-abduction action of the abductor pollicis longus reflects its attachment on the radial-dorsal corner of the base of the thumb metacarpal. The actions of all the muscles that cross the joints of the thumb are summarized in Box 8-1.

The extensor pollicis longus and the abductor pollicis longus are potent radial deviators at the wrist (see Figure 7-24). During extension of the thumb, therefore, an ulnar deviator muscle must be activated to stabilize the wrist against unwanted

---

BOX 8-1. Actions of Muscles That Cross the Joints of the Thumb

CARPOMETACARPAL JOINT

Flexion	Extension
Adductor pollicis	Extensor pollicis brevis
Flexor pollicis brevis	Extensor pollicis longus
Flexor pollicis longus	Abductor pollicis longus
Opponens pollicis	
Abductor pollicis brevis*	

Abduction	Adduction
Abductor pollicis brevis	Adductor pollicis
Abductor pollicis longus	Extensor pollicis longus
Flexor pollicis brevis*	First dorsal interosseus*
Opponens pollicis*	

Opposition	Reposition
Opponens pollicis	Extensor pollicis longus
Flexor pollicis brevis	
Abductor pollicis brevis	
Flexor pollicis longus	
Abductor pollicis longus	

METACARPOPHALANGEAL JOINT†

Flexion	Extension
Adductor pollicis	Extensor pollicis longus
Flexor pollicis brevis	Extensor pollicis brevis
Flexor pollicis longus	
Abductor pollicis brevis*	

INTERPHALANGEAL JOINT

Flexion	Extension
Flexor pollicis longus	Extensor pollicis longus
	Abductor pollicis brevis (due to attachment into extensor mechanism)*

*Secondary action
†Only one degree of freedom is considered for the metacarpophalangeal joint.

Palmar view

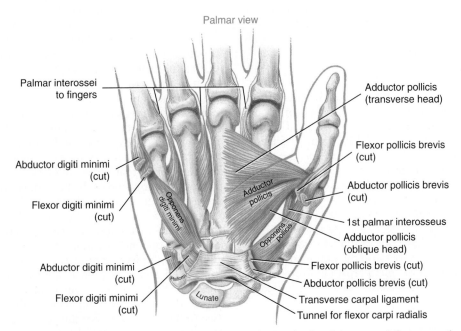

FIGURE 8-43. A palmar view of the deep muscles of the right hand. The abductor and flexor muscles of the thenar and hypothenar eminences have been cut away to expose the underlying opponens pollicis and opponens digiti minimi.

radial deviation. This activation is apparent by palpating the raised tendon of the flexor carpi ulnaris, located just proximal to the pisiform, during rapid and full extension of the thumb.

INTRINSIC MUSCLES OF THE HAND

The hand contains 20 intrinsic muscles. Despite their relatively small size, these muscles are essential to the fine control of the digits. Topographically, the intrinsic muscles are divided into four sets, as follows:
1. Muscles of the thenar eminence
   - Abductor pollicis brevis
   - Flexor pollicis brevis
   - Opponens pollicis
2. Muscles of the hypothenar eminence
   - Flexor digiti minimi
   - Abductor digiti minimi
   - Opponens digiti minimi
   - Palmaris brevis
3. Adductor pollicis
4. Lumbricals and interossei

Muscles of the Thenar Eminence
Anatomic Considerations
The *abductor pollicis brevis, flexor pollicis brevis, and opponens pollicis* make up the bulk of the thenar eminence (see Figure 8-34). The flexor pollicis brevis has two parts: a *superficial head*, which comprises most of the muscle, and a *deep head*, which consists of a small set of poorly defined fibers, often described as part of the oblique fibers of the adductor pollicis.[58,101] This chapter considers only the superficial head when discussing the flexor pollicis brevis. Deep to the abductor pollicis brevis is the opponens pollicis (Figure 8-43). All three thenar muscles have their proximal attachments on the transverse carpal ligament and adjacent carpal bones. Both the short abductor and flexor muscles have their distal attachments on the radial side of the base of the proximal phalanx. In addition, the abductor pollicis brevis attaches to the radial side of the extensor mechanism of the thumb; the flexor pollicis brevis frequently attaches to a sesamoid bone. The deeper opponens pollicis attaches distally to the entire radial border of the thumb metacarpal.

Functional Considerations
A primary responsibility of the muscles of the thenar eminence is to position the thumb in varying amounts of opposition, usually to facilitate grasping. As discussed earlier, opposition combines elements of CMC joint abduction, flexion, and medial rotation. Each muscle within the thenar eminence is a prime mover for at least one component of opposition, and an assistant for several others (see Box 8-1).[45,97]

The actions of the thenar muscles across the CMC joint become apparent when each muscle's line of force relative to a particular axis of rotation is viewed (Figure 8-44).[97] Note that the opponens pollicis has a line of force to *medially rotate* the thumb toward the fingers. Because the opponens pollicis has its distal attachment on the metacarpal (and proximal to the MCP joint), its entire contractile force is dedicated to controlling the CMC joint.

Implications of Median Nerve Injury
A severance of the median nerve paralyzes all three muscles of the thenar eminence: namely the opponens pollicis, flexor pollicis brevis, and abductor pollicis brevis. Consequently,

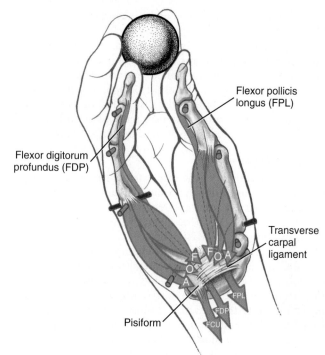

FIGURE 8-44. The actions of the thenar and hypothenar muscles are depicted during opposition of the thumb and small finger. (The axes of rotation for all flexion and extension movements are depicted in green. The axes of rotation for abduction and adduction movements at the metacarpophalangeal joint of the small finger and the carpometacarpal joint of the thumb are indicated in purple.) Other active muscles include the flexor pollicis longus and flexor digitorum profundus of the small finger. The flexor carpi ulnaris *(FCU)* stabilizes the pisiform bone for the abductor digiti minimi. *A*, abductor pollicis brevis and abductor digiti minimi; *F*, flexor pollicis brevis and flexor digiti minimi; *O*, opponens pollicis and opponens digiti minimi.

opposition of the thumb is essentially disabled. The thenar eminence region of the hand also becomes flat because of muscle atrophy. The functional loss of opposition, in conjunction with the anesthesia of the tips of the thumb and radial fingers, greatly reduces precision grip and other manipulative functions of the hand.

In addition to the important medial rotation function of the opponens pollicis, all three muscles of the thenar eminence independently perform the combined actions of *flexion and abduction* of the CMC joint. These kinematics are essential to lifting the thumb up and over the palm during opposition. Figure 8-45 compares these and other combined actions of the muscles that cross the CMC joint of the thumb. As noted by the location of the black dots, almost all the muscles have a combined action as a *flexor-abductor*, a *flexor-adductor*, an *extensor-adductor*, or an *extensor-abductor*. As indicated, the median nerve is the only source of innervation of the flexion-abduction quadrant of muscles. Although abduction of the thumb is still possible primarily because of the radial nerve–innervated abductor pollicis longus,[8] this action is usually overruled by the stronger remaining adduction torque potential of the ulnar nerve–innervated adductor pollicis muscle (see ADPo and ADPt). For this reason, persons with a median nerve injury are susceptible to an adduction contracture of the CMC joint of the thumb. As described earlier, an adduction bias to the thumb is certainly counterproductive to the natural kinematics of opposition.

Muscles of the Hypothenar Eminence
Anatomic Considerations

The muscles of the hypothenar eminence consist of the *flexor digiti minimi, abductor digiti minimi, opponens digiti minimi,* and *palmaris brevis* (see Figures 8-34 and 8-43). The abductor digiti minimi is the most superficial and medial of these muscles, occupying the extreme ulnar border of the hand. The relatively small flexor digiti minimi is located just lateral to, and often blended with, the abductor. Deep to these muscles is the opponens digiti minimi, the largest of the hypothenar muscles. The palmaris brevis is a thin and relatively insignificant muscle about the thickness of a postage stamp. It attaches between the transverse carpal ligament and an area of skin just distal to the pisiform bone (see Figure 8-34). The palmaris brevis raises the height of the hypothenar eminence, typically to assist with a deepening of the concavity of the palm.

The overall anatomic plan of the hypothenar muscles is similar to that of the muscles of the thenar eminence. The flexor digiti minimi and opponens digiti minimi both have their proximal attachments on the transverse carpal ligament and the hook of the hamate. The abductor digiti minimi has extensive proximal attachments from the pisohamate ligament, pisiform bone, and flexor carpi ulnaris tendon. During resisted or rapid abduction of the small finger, the flexor carpi ulnaris contracts to stabilize the attachment for the abductor digiti minimi. This effect can be verified by palpating the tendon of the flexor carpi ulnaris just proximal to the pisiform bone.

The abductor and flexor digiti minimi both have their distal attachments on the medial border of the base of the proximal phalanx of the small finger. Some fibers from the abductor also blend with the ulnar side of the extensor mechanism. The opponens digiti minimi has its distal attachment along the ulnar border of the fifth metacarpal, proximal to the MCP joint.

Functional Considerations

A common function of the hypothenar muscles is to raise and "cup" the ulnar border of the hand. This action deepens the distal transverse arch, and enhances digital contact with held objects (see Figure 8-44). When necessary, the abductor digiti minimi can spread the small finger for greater control of grasp. The opponens digiti minimi rotates, or opposes, the fifth metacarpal toward the middle digit. Contraction of the long finger flexors of the small finger, such as the flexor digitorum profundus, also contributes to raising the ulnar border of the hand. The actions of all the muscles that cross the joints of the small finger are listed in Box 8-2.

Injury to the ulnar nerve can completely paralyze the hypothenar muscles. The hypothenar eminence becomes flat owing to muscle atrophy. Raising and cupping the ulnar border of the hand is significantly reduced. Anesthesia over the entire small finger can contribute to a loss of dexterity.

Adductor Pollicis Muscle

The *adductor pollicis* is a two-headed muscle lying deep in the web space of the thumb, palmar to the second and third metacarpals (see Figure 8-43). The muscle has its proximal attachments on the most stable skeletal region of the hand. The thicker *oblique head* arises from the capitate bone, bases of the second and third metacarpals, and other adjacent connective tissues.[58] The thinner, triangular *transverse head* attaches on the palmar surface of the third metacarpal bone. Both heads join for a common distal attachment on the ulnar side of the base

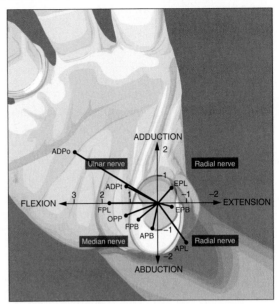

FIGURE 8-45. An illustration that associates the potential torque (strength) and combined actions of the muscles that cross the carpometacarpal *(CMC)* joint of the right thumb. The trapezium is outlined in light yellow at the base of the thumb. The black dots represent the location of each muscle relative to the two (primary) degrees of freedom of movement at the CMC joint: flexion-extension and adduction-abduction. With the exception of the flexor pollicis longus *(FPL)*, each muscle is classified as a flexor-abductor, a flexor-adductor, an extensor-adductor, or an extensor-abductor. Furthermore, the length of each line associated with each muscle is proportional to the maximum torque potential of the muscle, which considers *both* the muscle's moment arm and the cross-sectional area. The units used on the axes indicate torque in Nm. Observe that the muscles that fall within each of the four quadrants share the same source of innervation. *ADPo,* adductor pollicis, oblique head; *ADPt,* adductor pollicis, transverse head; *APB,* abductor pollicis brevis; *APL,* abductor pollicis longus; *EPB,* extensor pollicis brevis; *EPL,* extensor pollicis longus; *FPB,* flexor pollicis brevis; *FPL,* flexor pollicis longus; *OPP,* opponens pollicis. (The diagram is based on data originally plotted by Smutz WP, et al.[97] From Neumann DA, Bielefeld TB: The carpometacarpal joint of the thumb: stability, deformity, and therapeutic intervention, *J Orthop Sports Phys Ther* 33:386, 2003.)

of the proximal phalanx of the thumb; additional attachments include a sesamoid bone located near the MCP joint.

The adductor pollicis is a dominant muscle at the CMC joint, producing the greatest combination of flexion and adduction torque.[9] This important source of torque is applied to many activities, such as pinching an object between the thumb and index finger or closing a pair of scissors (Figure 8-46). The transverse head of the adductor pollicis uses a very long moment arm to generate both *flexion* (Figure 8-46, *A*) and *adduction* (Figure 8-46, *B*) torque at the base of the thumb. Although the transverse fibers have the greater leverage at the CMC joint, the thicker oblique head generates the greater flexion and adduction torque (compare ADPo and ADPt in Figure 8-45).[58,97]

Lumbricals and Interosseus Muscles

The *lumbricals* (from the Latin root *lumbricus,* earthworm) are four very slender muscles originating from the tendons of the flexor digitorum profundus (see Figures 8-33 and 8-34). Like the flexor digitorum profundus, the lumbricals have a dual source of innervation: the two lateral lumbricals by the median nerve, and the two medial lumbricals by the ulnar nerve.

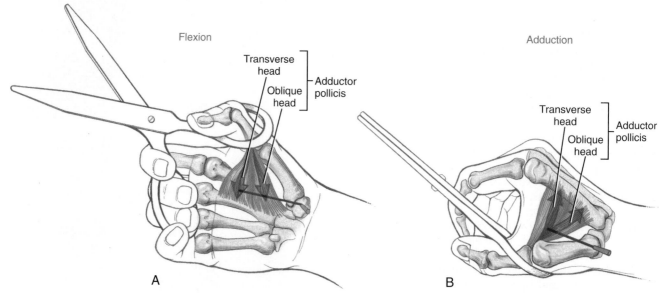

Flexion

Adduction

Transverse head

Oblique head

Adductor pollicis

Transverse head

Oblique head

Adductor pollicis

A

B

FIGURE 8-46. The biplanar action of the adductor pollicis muscle is illustrated using a pair of scissors for flexion (**A**) and adduction (**B**) at the thumb's carpometacarpal joint. In both **A** and **B**, the transverse head of the adductor pollicis produces a significant torque owing to its long moment arm about an anterior-posterior axis (*green,* **A**) and medial-lateral axis (*purple,* **B**). Both heads of the adductor pollicis are also strong flexors of the thumb's metacarpophalangeal joint.

BOX 8-2. Actions of Muscles That Cross the Joints of the Small Finger

CARPOMETACARPAL JOINT

Flexion and Opposition
Flexor digiti minimi
Opponens digiti minimi
Flexor digitorum superficialis and
    profundus
Palmaris brevis

Extension
Extensor digitorum
Extensor digiti minimi

METACARPOPHALANGEAL JOINT

Flexion
Flexor digiti minimi
Abductor digiti minimi
Lumbrical
Palmar interosseus
Flexor digitorum superficialis and
    profundus

Extension
Extensor digitorum
Extensor digiti minimi

Abduction
Abductor digiti minimi

Adduction
Palmar interosseus

PROXIMAL INTERPHALANGEAL JOINT

Flexion
Flexor digitorum superficialis and
    profundus

Extension
Extensor digitorum
Extensor digiti minimi
Lumbrical
Palmar interosseus

DISTAL INTERPHALANGEAL JOINT

Flexion
Flexor digitorum profundus

Extension
Extensor digitorum
Extensor digiti minimi
Lumbrical
Palmar interosseus

Palmar view

A₁ pulley at the metacarpophalangeal joint of the index finger

DISTAL

RADIAL

Tendon of flexor digitorum profundus   Tendon of flexor pollicis longus

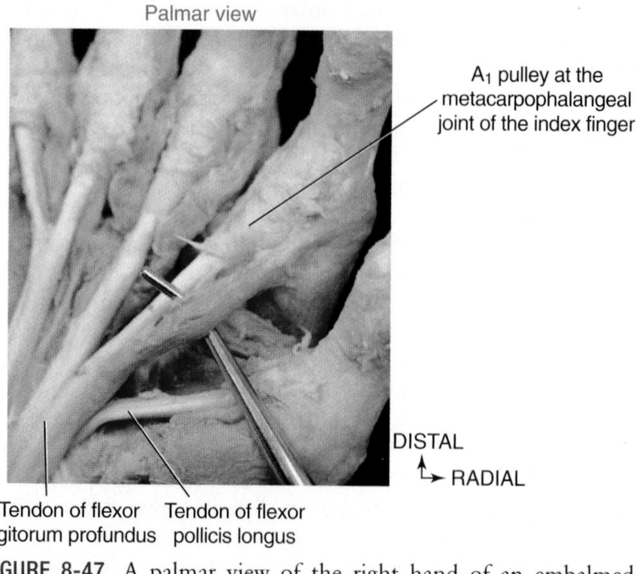

FIGURE 8-47. A palmar view of the right hand of an embalmed cadaver, highlighting the first lumbrical muscle. The probe is lifting the muscle belly of the first lumbrical from the underlying adductor pollicis muscle. The proximal attachment of the first lumbrical is shown arising from the tendon of the flexor digitorum profundus. The distal attachment of the first lumbrical can be seen blending with the oblique fibers of the extensor mechanism of the index finger.

All four lumbricals show marked variation in both size and attachments.[23,101] From their tendinous proximal attachments, the lumbricals course *palmar* to the deep transverse metacarpal ligament and then *radial* to the MCP joints (see Figure 8-41, first lumbrical). Distally, a typical lumbrical attaches to the adjacent lateral band of the extensor mechanism, most often via the oblique fibers of the dorsal hood (see close-up view of first lumbrical in Figure 8-47). This distal attachment enables the lumbricals to exert a proximal pull throughout the extensor mechanism.

The function of the lumbricals has been studied and debated for many years.[14,54,60,86,107] What is universally agreed on is that their contraction produces flexion at the MCP joints and extension at the PIP and DIP joints.[112] This seemingly paradoxic action is possible because the lumbricals pass *palmar* to the MCP joints but *dorsal* to the PIP and DIP joints (Figure 8-48).

Of all the intrinsic muscles of the hand, the lumbricals have the longest fiber length but the smallest cross-sectional area.[11,40,58] This anatomic design suggests that these muscles are capable of generating small amounts of force over a relatively long distance. Although a low force potential in a muscle generally suggests a limited role in controlling movement, this is not always the case. Muscles have other important kinesiologic functions besides producing force. The first lumbrical, for instance, possesses a very rich source of muscle spindles—sensory organs that closely monitor changes in the length of the muscle. The average spindle density of the first lumbrical is approximately three times greater than that of the interosseus muscles within the hand and eight times greater than that of the biceps brachii muscle.[81] This large density of muscle spindles in the lumbricals suggests an important role in providing sensory feedback during complex movements.[86,99] By also attaching to the tendons of the flexor digitorum profundus, perhaps the lumbricals are in position to help coordinate the interactions between the intrinsic and extrinsic muscles.

The *interosseus muscles* are named according to their general location between the metacarpal bones (see Figures 8-4 and 8-5). As with the lumbricals, variations in attachments and morphology are more the rule than the exception.[22,101] In general, the interossei act at the MCP joints to spread the digits apart (abduction) or bring them together (adduction).

The four *palmar interossei* of the hand are slender, typically single-headed muscles that occupy the palmar region of the interosseous spaces. The three palmar interossei to the fingers have their proximal attachments on the palmar surfaces and sides of the second, fourth, and fifth metacarpals (see Figure 8-43). The muscles' distal attachments vary but typically include the oblique fibers of the dorsal hood, and the sides of the bases of the proximal phalanges.[22] These muscles *adduct* the second, fourth, and fifth MCP joints toward the midline of the hand (Figure 8-49).[12] The palmar interosseus muscle to the thumb occupies the first palmar interosseous space. This deep muscle has its distal attachment on the ulnar side of the proximal phalanx of the thumb, and often attaches to a sesamoid bone at the MCP joint.[101] The first palmar interosseus is often small or partially formed and therefore is ignored in most biomechanical analysis. In theory, this muscle is positioned to help flex the MCP joint of the thumb, bringing the first metacarpal toward the midline of the hand.

The four *dorsal interossei* fill the dorsal sides of the interosseous spaces (see Figure 8-39). In contrast to the palmar interossei, the dorsal muscles typically have a bipennate shape. As a general rule, the dorsal interossei have distal attachments to the oblique fibers of the dorsal hood, as well as to the sides of the bases of the proximal phalanges. Some distal attachments may blend with more palmar aspects of the transverse fibers of the dorsal hood and the palmar plate.[22] The first dorsal interosseus (formerly *abductor indicis*) is the largest and most accessible for clinical inspection. With the index finger well stabilized, the first dorsal interosseus can assist the

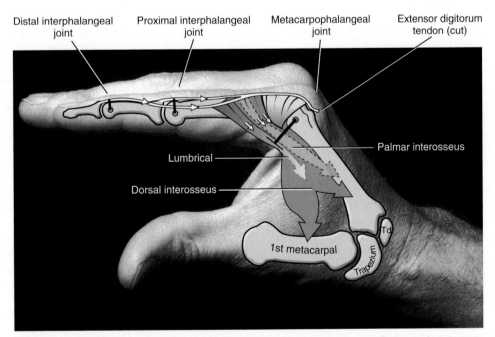

FIGURE 8-48. The combined actions of the lumbricals and interossei are shown as flexors at the metacarpophalangeal joint and extensors at the interphalangeal joints. The lumbrical is shown with the greatest moment arm for flexion at the metacarpophalangeal joint. The medial-lateral axis of rotation at each joint is shown as a small circle. Moment arms are depicted as thick black lines, originating at each axis of rotation. *Td*, trapezoid bone.

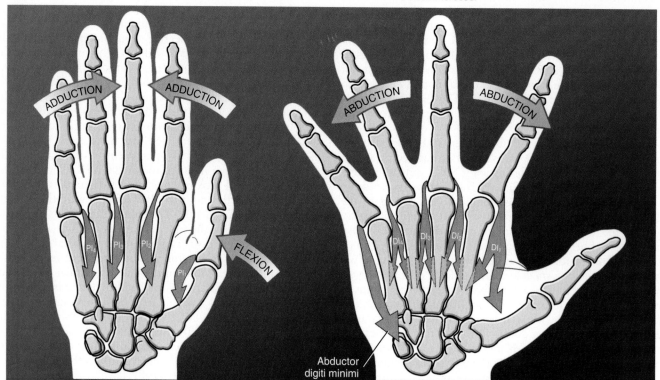

FIGURE 8-49. A palmar view of the frontal plane action of the palmar interossei (PI₁ to PI₄) and dorsal interossei (DI₁ to DI₄) at the metacarpophalangeal joints of the hand. The abductor digiti minimi is shown abducting the small finger.

adductor pollicis in *adducting* the thumb at the CMC joint. (This can be visualized by reversing the direction of the arrow of the first dorsal interosseus to the thumb in Figure 8-48.)

As a set, the dorsal interossei *abduct* the MCP joints of the index, middle, and ring fingers away from an imaginary reference line through the middle digit (see Figure 8-49). Abduction of the fifth MCP joint is performed by the abductor digiti minimi of the hypothenar group.

In addition to abducting and adducting the fingers, the interossei and abductor digiti minimi provide an important source of dynamic stability to the MCP joints. When the two hands shown in Figure 8-49 are visually superimposed, it is apparent that each MCP joint of the fingers is equipped with a pair of abducting and adducting muscles. The pairs act as dynamic collateral ligaments, providing strength to the MCP joints. Acting in pairs, this interosseus musculature also controls the extent of axial rotation permitted at the MCP joints.

To varying degrees, both palmar and dorsal interossei have a line of force that passes *palmar* to the MCP joints, especially when the MCP joints are flexed. The interossei, via their attachments into the extensor mechanism, pass *dorsal* to the IP joints of the fingers (see index finger in Figure 8-48). Like the lumbricals, therefore, contraction of the interossei flexes the MCP joints and extends the IP joints. The interossei produce greater flexion torques at the MCP joints than the lumbricals. Even though the lumbricals have the larger moment arm for this action, the overwhelmingly larger cross-section area of the interossei empowers them with the greater flexion torque potential. In contrast to the lumbricals, the interossei produce relatively larger forces but over a shorter contraction distance (Table 8-5).[40]

Interaction of the Extrinsic and Intrinsic Muscles of the Fingers

As described in Figure 8-48, simultaneous contraction of the intrinsic muscles of the fingers (lumbricals and interossei) produces a combined MCP joint flexion and IP joint extension. This position of the hand is referred to as the *intrinsic-plus position*. In contrast, simultaneous contraction of the *extrinsic muscles* of the fingers (extensor digitorum, flexor digitorum superficialis, and flexor digitorum profundus) produces MCP joint hyperextension and IP joint flexion: the *extrinsic-plus position*. The two opposite positions of the fingers are presented in Figure 8-50. A very important kinesiologic principle of the hand is that most functional or complex digital movements require a synergistic blending of these two opposite actions. This point is reinforced in the next sections.

The interaction between the extrinsic and intrinsic muscles of the hand can produce many combinations of movements used to perform a seemingly infinite number of functions. The following analysis, however, addresses the muscular interaction within a typical finger during two fundamental functions: *opening* and *closing of the hand*. The precise muscular interactions used to perform these actions is controversial and not completely understood, despite years of research and study based on anatomy, biomechanics, electromyography, and computer-simulated modeling.* Part of the obstacle in

---

*References 11, 14, 31, 43, 54, 56, 59, 60.

TABLE 8-5. Selected Anatomic and Functional Comparisons between the Lumbrical and Interosseus Muscles

	Lumbricals	Dorsal Interossei	Palmar Interossei
Innervation	Lateral: Median nerve Medial: Ulnar nerve	Ulnar nerve	Ulnar nerve
Primary distal attachments	Oblique fibers of the dorsal hood, and ultimately to the adjacent lateral band of the extensor mechanism	Oblique fibers of the dorsal hood (and ultimately to the adjacent lateral band), and to the side of the base of the proximal phalanx	Oblique fibers of the dorsal hood (and ultimately to the adjacent lateral band), and to the side of the base of the proximal phalanx
Contractile characteristics	Generate relatively small force over a relatively long distance	Generate relatively large force over a relatively short distance	Nondistinct
Primary actions	MCP joint flexion and PIP and DIP joint extension	*Abduction* of fingers; MCP joint flexion and PIP and DIP joint extension	*Adduction* of fingers; MCP joint flexion and PIP and DIP joint extension
Comments	Relatively large endowment of muscle spindles, suggesting an important source of sensory feedback to help guide movement	Distal attachments typically include bone and extensor mechanism Usually bipennate, with proximal attachments arising by two heads	Distal attachments typically include bone and extensor mechanism; usually single-headed muscles First palmar interosseus (to the thumb) assists with flexion of MCP joint

DIP, Distal interphalangeal; *MCP*, metacarpophalangeal; *PIP*, proximal interphalangeal.

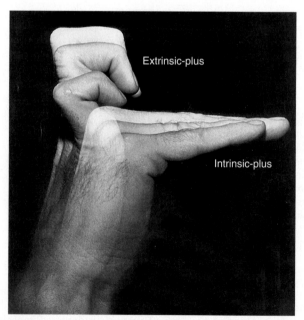

FIGURE 8-50. The extrinsic-plus and intrinsic-plus positions of the healthy hand.

understanding the muscular interactions is that similar movements can be performed by different combinations of muscles, both within and between persons.[42] Precise muscular interaction also depends on the speed or power of an activity, the skill of the performer, weight and shape of the manipulated object, and natural human variability. Of interest, much of what is known for certain has been learned by carefully observing the pathomechanical impairments of the hand that resulted from a disruption of the neuromusculoskeletal system.[9,49]

OPENING THE HAND: FINGER EXTENSION

Primary Muscular Activity

Opening the hand is often performed in preparation for grasp. The greatest resistance to complete extension of the fingers across the MCP and IP joints is usually not from gravity but from the viscoelastic resistance generated by the stretching of the extrinsic finger flexors, in particular the flexor digitorum profundus. The passive "recoil" force generated within this muscle is largely responsible for the partially flexed posture of a relaxed hand.

The primary extensors of the fingers are the *extensor digitorum* and the intrinsic muscles, specifically the lumbricals and interossei. In general, the lumbricals show a greater and more consistent level of electromyographic (EMG) activity than the interossei during finger extension.[60]

Figure 8-51, *A* shows the extensor digitorum exerting a force on the extensor mechanism, pulling the MCP joint toward extension. The intrinsic muscles of the fingers furnish both direct and indirect effects on the mechanics of extension of the IP joints (see Figure 8-51, *B* and *C*). The *direct effect* is provided by the proximal pull placed on the extensor mechanism; the *indirect effect* is provided by the production of a flexion torque at the MCP joint.[47] The flexion torque prevents the extensor digitorum from hyperextending the MCP joint—an action that prematurely dissipates most of its con-

Finger extension

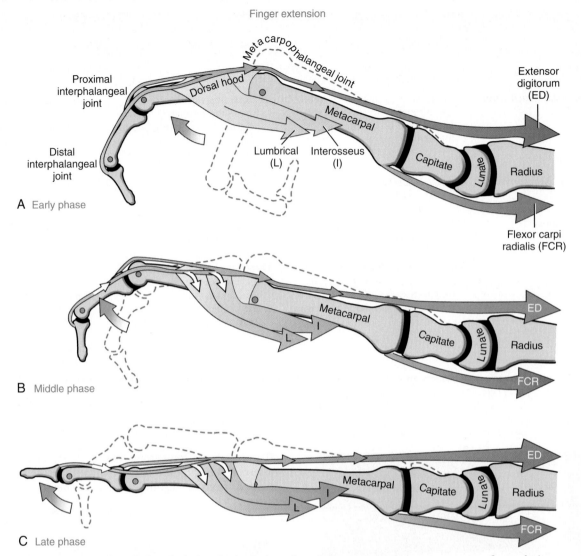

FIGURE 8-51. A lateral view depicting the intrinsic and extrinsic muscular interactions at one finger during *full extension*. The dashed outlines depict starting positions. **A,** Early phase: The extensor digitorum is shown extending primarily the metacarpophalangeal joint. **B,** Middle phase: The intrinsic muscles (lumbricals and interossei) assist the extensor digitorum with extension of the proximal and distal interphalangeal joints. The intrinsic muscles also produce a flexion torque at the metacarpophalangeal joint that prevents the extensor digitorum from hyperextending the metacarpophalangeal joint. **C,** Late phase: Muscle activation continues through full finger extension. Note the activation in the flexor carpi radialis to slightly flex the wrist. Observe the proximal migration of the dorsal hood between flexion and full extension. (The intensity of the red indicates the relative intensity of the muscle activity.)

tractile force. Only with the MCP joint blocked from being hyperextended can the extensor digitorum effectively tense the extensor mechanism sufficiently to completely extend the IP joints.

The extensor digitorum and intrinsic muscles of the fingers cooperate synergistically to extend the finger. Paradoxically, it is the *opposing* actions of the extensor digitorum and the intrinsic muscles across the MCP joint that allow them to synergistically extend the IP joints. This relationship is apparent on observation of a person with an *injury of the ulnar nerve* (Figure 8-52, *A*). Without active resistance from either of the intrinsic muscles of the medial two fingers, activation of the extensor digitorum causes a characteristic "clawing" of the

digits: the MCP joints hyperextend and the IP joints remain partially flexed. This is often called the "intrinsic-minus" posture because of the lack of intrinsic-innervated muscles. (This posture is functionally similar to the "extrinsic-plus" posture depicted in Figure 8-50.) Without the MCP joint flexion torque normally provided by the intrinsic muscles, the extensor digitorum functions *only* to hyperextend the MCP joints. This posture stretches the flexor digitorum profundus, thereby adding further resistance against extension of the IP joints. As shown in Figure 8-52, *B*, with manual application of a flexion torque across the MCP joint (i.e., a force normally furnished by the intrinsic muscles), contraction of the extensor digitorum is able to fully extend the IP joints.

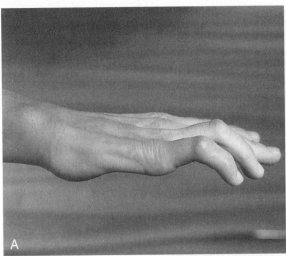 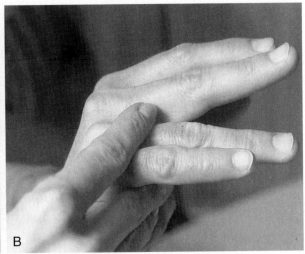

FIGURE 8-52. Attempts to extend the fingers with an ulnar nerve lesion and paralysis of the most intrinsic muscles of the fingers. **A,** The medial fingers show the "claw" position with metacarpophalangeal joints hyperextended and fingers partially flexed. Note the atrophy in the hypothenar eminence and interosseous spaces. **B,** By manually holding the metacarpophalangeal joints into flexion, the extensor digitorum, innervated by the radial nerve, is able to fully extend the interphalangeal joints.

SPECIAL FOCUS 8-7

Oblique Retinacular Ligaments: Transfer of Passive Extension Force from the Proximal Interphalangeal Joint to the Distal Interphalangeal Joint

As depicted in Figure 8-41, the oblique retinacular ligaments course from the palmar side of the PIP joint to the dorsal side of the distal interphalangeal (DIP) joint. Their oblique direction helps coordinate extension between the PIP and DIP joints.[32] The extensor digitorum and intrinsic muscles initiate extension of the PIP joint, which stretches the oblique retinacular ligament (Figure 8-53, steps 1 to 3). The passive force in the elongated oblique ligament is transferred distally, helping to *extend* the DIP joint (see Figure 8-53, step 4). The oblique retinacular ligament is sometimes called the "link ligament," suggesting its probable role in synchronizing extension at both joints.

The oblique retinacular ligament may become tight because of arthritis, trauma, or Dupuytren's contracture. *Dupuytren's contracture* is a condition of unknown cause involving a progressive thickening and shortening of the palmar and digital fascia of the hand.[61] The condition often results in a flexed posture of the fingers, especially on the medial side of the hand. The oblique retinacular ligament may also be involved, resulting in an exaggerated flexion contracture at the PIP joint. Attempts at passively extending a PIP joint with a tight oblique retinacular ligament often cause the DIP joint to passively extend.

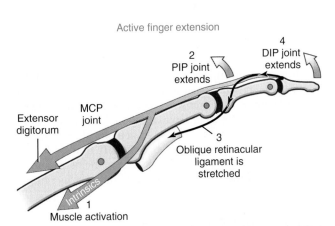

FIGURE 8-53. The transfer of passive force in the stretched oblique retinacular ligament during active extension of the finger. The numbered sequence (1 to 4) indicates the chronologic order of events.

Blocking the MCP joint from hyperextending also slackens the profundus tendon, thereby minimizing the muscle's passive resistance to extension of the IP joints. Preventing the MCP joints from hyperextending is one form of therapeutic intervention after paralysis of the intrinsic muscles of the

fingers. Therapists may fabricate a splint that limits extension of the MCP joints; surgeons may devise a muscular block against hyperextension by rerouting a tendon from a stronger, innervated muscle to the flexor side of the involved MCP joints.[33]

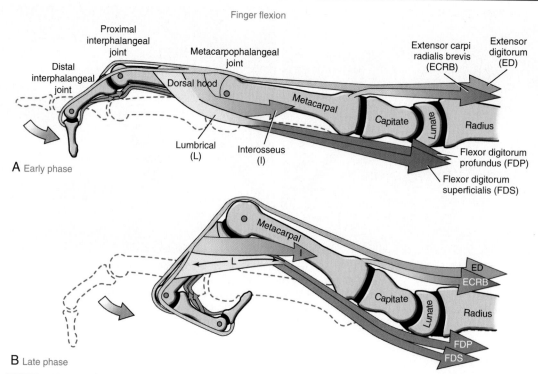

FIGURE 8-54. A side view depicting the intrinsic and extrinsic muscular interaction at one finger during a relatively "high-powered" finger *flexion*. The dashed outlines depict the starting positions. **A,** Early phase: The flexor digitorum profundus, flexor digitorum superficialis, and interosseus muscles actively flex the joints of the finger. The lumbrical is shown as being essentially inactive. **B,** Late phase: Muscle activation continues essentially unchanged through full flexion. The lumbrical remains essentially inactive but is stretched across both ends. The extensor carpi radialis brevis is shown extending the wrist slightly. The extensor digitorum helps decelerate flexion of the metacarpophalangeal joint. Note the distal migration of the dorsal hood between the early and late phases of flexion. (The intensity of the red indicates the relative intensity of the muscle activity.)

Function of Wrist Flexors during Finger Extension

Activation of the wrist flexor muscles normally accompanies active finger extension, especially when performed rapidly. Although this activity is depicted only in the flexor carpi radialis in Figure 8-51, other wrist flexors are also active. The wrist flexors offset the large extension potential of the extensor digitorum at the wrist. The wrist actually flexes slightly during rapid and complete finger extension. (Compare Figure 8-51, *A* with Figure 8-51, *C*.) Wrist flexion helps maintain optimal length of the extensor digitorum during active finger extension.

CLOSING THE HAND: FINGER FLEXION

Primary Muscle Action

The muscles used to close the hand depend in part on the specific joints that need to be flexed and on the force requirements of the action. Flexing the fingers against resistance or at relatively high speed requires activation of the *flexor digitorum profundus, flexor digitorum superficialis,* and, to a lesser extent, the *interosseus* muscles (Figure 8-54, *A*). Forces produced by the flexor digitorum profundus and superficialis flex all three joints of the fingers; the flexing finger pulls the extensor mechanism distally by several millimeters.

Although typically inactive while the hand is closing, the *lumbricals* may still passively assist with this action. Recall that

the lumbricals attach between the flexor digitorum profundus and the extensor mechanism. During active finger flexion, the lumbricals are stretched in a proximal direction owing to the contracting flexor digitorum profundus and at the same time are stretched in a distal direction owing to the distal migration of the extensor mechanism (see Figure 8-54, *B*, bidirectional arrow in lumbrical). Between full extension and full active flexion, a lumbrical must stretch an extraordinary distance.[86] The stretch generates a *passive flexion torque* across the MCP joint. Although small, this passive torque may supplement the *active flexion torque* produced by the interossei and, primarily, the extrinsic flexor musculature.[55]

Injury to the ulnar nerve can cause paralysis of most of the intrinsic muscles that act on the fingers. As a result, grasp is noticeably altered, especially in the sequencing of flexion across the joints. Normally, at least in the radial three fingers, the PIP and DIP joints flex first, followed closely in time by flexion at the MCP joints. With paralyzed intrinsic muscles, especially if overstretched by chronic hyperextension of the MCP joints, the initiation of flexion at the MCP joints appears delayed slightly. The resulting asynchronous flexion may interfere with the quality of grasp.

In contrast to making a relatively high-powered fist, making a relatively light or low-powered fist produces EMG activity almost exclusively from the flexor digitorum profundus. Because this muscle crosses all the joints of the fingers, its activation alone is minimally adequate to lightly close the fist. The flexor digitorum superficialis functions more as a reserve muscle, becoming active during a high-powered fist or when isolated PIP joint flexion is required.

The extensor digitorum shows consistent EMG activity while the hand is closing.[59] This activity reflects the muscle's role as an extension brake at the MCP joint. This important stabilization function allows the long finger flexors to shift their action distally to the PIP and DIP joints. Without coactivation of the extensor digitorum, the long finger flexors exhaust most of their flexion potential over the MCP joints, reducing their potential for more refined actions at the more distal joints.

Function of Wrist Extensors during Finger Flexion

Making a strong fist requires strong synergistic activation from the wrist extensor muscles (see Figure 8-54, extensor carpi radialis brevis). Wrist extensor activity can be verified by palpating the dorsum of the forearm while a fist is made. As explained in Chapter 7, the primary function of the wrist extensors, including the extensor digitorum, is to neutralize the strong wrist flexion tendency of the activated extrinsic finger flexor muscles (review Figure 7-25). While the hand is closing, wrist extension also helps maintain more optimal length of the extrinsic finger flexors. If the wrist extensors are paralyzed, attempts at making a fist result in a posture of wrist flexion *and* finger flexion. When combined with the increased passive tension in the overstretched extensor digitorum, the overshortened, activated finger flexors are incapable of producing an effective grip (see Figure 7-27).

HAND AS AN EFFECTOR ORGAN

The hand functions as the primary effector organ of the upper extremity for support, manipulation, and prehension. As a *support*, the hand can act in a nonspecific manner to brace or stabilize an object, often freeing the other hand for a more specific task. The hand may also be used as a simple platform to transfer or accept forces, such as when supporting the head when tired or to assist in standing from a seated position.

Functions of the Hand

- Support
- Manipulation:
  - Repetitive and blunt
  - Continuous and fluid
- Prehension used during grip and pinch:
  - Power grip
  - Precision grip
  - Power (key) pinch
  - Precision pinch
  - Hook grip

Perhaps the most varied function of the hand is its ability to *manipulate* objects. In a very general sense, the hand manipulates objects in two fundamental ways: digital motions may be *repetitive* and *blunt,* such as typing or scratching,

or, in contrast, *continuous* and *fluid,* in which the rate and intensity of motion are controlled, such as when writing or sewing. And, of course, many, if not most, types of digital manipulations combine both of these elements of movement.

Prehension describes the ability of the fingers and thumb to grasp or to seize, often for holding, securing, and picking up objects. Several terms have evolved over the years to describe the many forms of prehension.[52,73] Most forms of prehension can be described as a *grip* (or grasp), in which all digits are used, or as a *pinch,* in which primarily the thumb and index finger are used. Each form can be further classified based on the need for *power* (loosely defined as high force without regard to the exactness of the task) or *precision* (i.e., high level of exactness with low force). The specific classifications of prehension subsequently described are not intended to include *all* possible ways that the hand can be used. These definitions are nevertheless useful to establish a common reference for clinical communication.

Basically, most types of prehension activities fall into one of the following five types:

1. The *power grip* is used when stability and large forces are needed, without the need for precision. The shape of held objects tends to be spheric or cylindric. Using a hammer is a good example of a power grip (Figure 8-55, *A*). This activity requires strong forces from the finger flexors, especially from the fourth and fifth digits; intrinsic muscles of the fingers, especially the interossei; and the thumb adductor and flexor musculature. Wrist extensors are needed to stabilize the partially extended wrist.

2. The *precision grip* is used when control and/or delicate action is needed during prehension (see Figure 8-55, *B* and *C*). The thumb is usually held partially abducted, and the fingers are partially flexed. The precision grip uses the thumb and one or more of the digits to improve grip security or, if needed, to add variable amounts of force. The precision grip is modified to fit objects of varied sizes by altering the contour of the distal transverse arch of the hand (see Figure 8-55, *D* to *F*).

3. The *power (key) pinch* is used when large forces are needed to stabilize an object between the thumb and the lateral border of the index finger (see Figure 8-55, *G*). The power pinch is an extremely useful form of prehension, combining the force of the adductor pollicis and first dorsal interosseus with the dexterity and sensory acuity of the thumb and index finger.

4. The *precision pinch* is used to provide fine control to objects held between the thumb and index finger, without the need for high power. This type of pinch has many forms, such as the *tip-to-tip* or *pulp-to-pulp* method of holding an object (see Figure 8-55, *H* and *I,* respectively). The tip-to-tip pinch is used especially for tiny objects, when skill and precision are required. The pulp-to-pulp pinch provides greater surface area for contact with larger objects, thereby increasing prehensile security.

5. The *hook grip* is a form of prehension that does not involve the thumb. A hook grip is formed by the partially flexed PIP and DIP joints of the fingers. This grip is often used in a static manner for prolonged periods of time, such as holding a luggage strap (see Figure 8-55, *J*). The force of the hook grip is usually provided primarily by the flexor digitorum profundus.

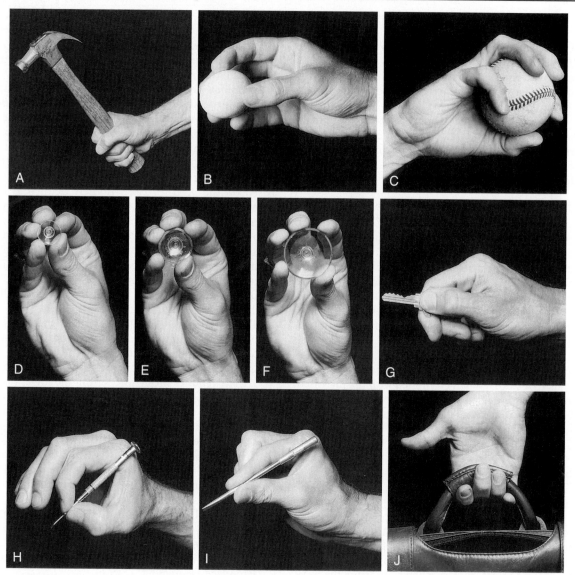

FIGURE 8-55. A normal hand is shown performing common types of prehension functions. **A,** Power grip. **B,** Precision grip to hold an egg. **C,** Precision grip to throw a baseball. **D** to **F,** Modifications of the precision grip by altering the concavity of the distal transverse arch. **G,** Power key pinch. **H,** Tip-to-tip prehension pinch. **I,** Pulp-to-pulp prehension pinch. **J,** Hook grip.

JOINT DEFORMITIES TYPICALLY CAUSED BY RHEUMATOID ARTHRITIS

One of the more destructive aspects of rheumatoid arthritis is chronic synovitis. Over time, synovitis tends to reduce the tensile strength of the periarticular connective tissues. Without the normal restraint provided by these tissues, forces from contact with the environment and, more significantly, muscle contraction can eventually destroy the mechanical integrity of a joint. The joint often becomes misaligned, unstable, and frequently deformed permanently. Knowledge of the pathomechanics of hand deformities associated with rheumatoid arthritis is a prerequisite for effective treatment. This holds true because so many traditional treatments for hand deformity address the mechanical cause of the problem.

Zigzag Deformity of the Thumb

Advanced rheumatoid arthritis often results in a zigzag deformity of the thumb. As defined in Chapter 7, a *zigzag deformity* results from the collapse of multiple interconnected joints in alternating directions. Although several combinations of deformity have been described,[3,71,102] one relatively common deformity involves CMC joint flexion and adduction, MCP joint hyperextension, and IP joint flexion (Figure 8-56).[5] In this example the collapse of the thumb starts with instability at the CMC joint. Ligaments that normally reinforce the medial (ulnar) side of the joint, such as the anterior oblique and ulnar collateral ligaments, can become weak and rupture because of the disease process. Subsequently the base of the thumb metacarpal dislocates off the radial or dorsal-radial

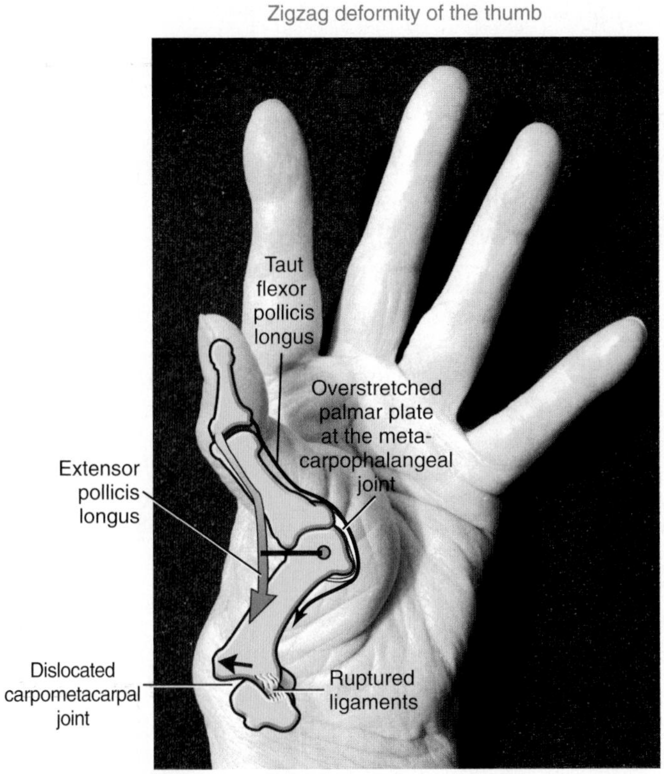

Zigzag deformity of the thumb

Taut
flexor
pollicis
longus

Overstretched
palmar plate
at the meta-
carpophalangeal
joint

Extensor
pollicis
longus

Dislocated
carpometacarpal
joint

Ruptured
ligaments

FIGURE 8-56. A palmar view showing the pathomechanics of a common zigzag deformity of the thumb caused by rheumatoid arthritis. The base of the thumb metacarpal dislocates in a general radial direction at the carpometacarpal joint *(arrow)*, initiating a series of events that lead to hyperextension at the metacarpophalangeal joint. The interphalangeal joint remains partially flexed because of the passive tension in the stretched and taut flexor pollicis longus.

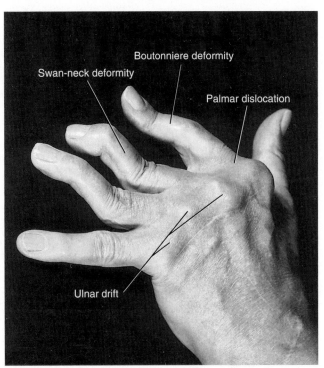

FIGURE 8-57. A hand showing the common deformities caused by severe rheumatoid arthritis. Particularly evident are the following: *palmar dislocation* of the metacarpophalangeal joint; *ulnar drift; swan-neck deformity;* and *boutonniere deformity.* See text for further details. (Courtesy of Teri Bielefeld, PT, CHT, Zablocki VA Hospital, Milwaukee, Wisconsin.)

edge of the trapezium (see arrow at base of first metacarpal in Figure 8-56). Altered moment arms of some of the muscles that cross the CMC joint may further contribute to this dislocation.[79] Once this dislocation occurs, the adductor and short flexor muscles, which are often in spasm, hold the thumb metacarpal rigidly against the palm. In time, rheumatoid disease may cause the muscles to become fibrotic and permanently shortened, maintaining the deformity at the CMC joint. In efforts to extend the rigid thumb out of the palm, a compensatory hyperextension deformity at the MCP joint often occurs.[3] A weakened and overstretched palmar plate at this joint offers little resistance to the extension forces produced by the extensor pollicis longus and brevis or contact forces produced during pinch. Eventual bowstringing of these tendons across the MCP joint increases their leverage as extensors, thereby further contributing to the hyperextension deformity. The IP joint tends to remain flexed as a result of the passive tension in the stretched flexor pollicis longus.

Clinical interventions for a zigzag deformity of the thumb depend on the specific mechanics of the collapse and the severity of the underlying rheumatoid disease. Nonsurgical intervention includes splinting to encourage more normal joint alignment, medicine to reduce chronic inflammation, and teaching patients ways to minimize stress on the joint.[76]

Surgery may be considered if more conservative intervention fails to slow the progression of the deformity.

Destruction of the Metacarpophalangeal Joints of the Finger

Advanced rheumatoid arthritis is often associated with deformities at the MCP joint of the fingers. The two most common deformities are *palmar dislocation* and *ulnar drift* (Figure 8-57). Although these two deformities typically occur together, they are discussed separately in the following sections.

PALMAR DISLOCATION OF THE METACARPOPHALANGEAL JOINT

When the fingers flex during grip, the tendons of the flexor digitorum superficialis and profundus are deflected palmarly across the MCP joint (Figure 8-58, *A*). This natural bend generates a bowstringing force in the palmar direction. As indicated in Figure 8-58, *A*, the bowstringing force is transferred through much of the MCP joint's periarticular connective tissue: from flexor A1 pulley, palmar plate, collateral ligaments, and, finally, to posterior tubercle of the metacarpal head. The greater the degree of flexion at the MCP joint, the greater the magnitude of the bowstringing force. In the healthy hand, this force is safely dissipated throughout the natural elasticity and strength of the tissues.

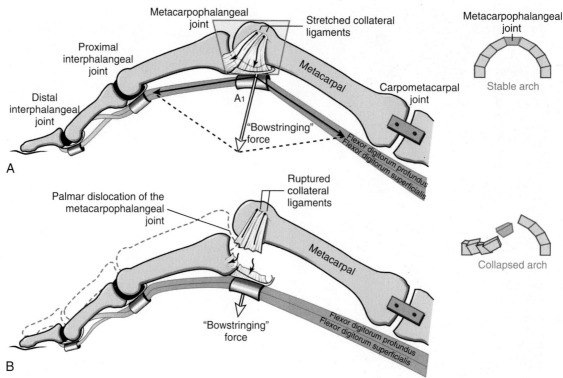

FIGURE 8-58. Pathomechanics of progressive palmar dislocation of the metacarpophalangeal joint of the finger. **A,** The bend in the flexor tendons across the metacarpophalangeal joint produces a palmar-directed, bowstringing force against the palmar plate, A_1 pulley, and collateral ligaments. In the healthy hand the passive tension in the stretched collateral ligaments adequately resists the palmar pull on the joint structures. **B,** In a finger with rheumatoid arthritis, the bowstringing force can rupture the weakened collateral ligaments. As a result, the proximal phalanx may eventually dislocate in a palmar direction.

In the hand with severe rheumatoid arthritis, the collateral ligaments may rupture because of the constant bowstringing force. In time, the proximal phalanx may translate excessively in a palmar direction, resulting in a completely dislocated MCP joint (see Figure 8-58, *B*). Palmar dislocation may collapse both the longitudinal and transverse arches of the hand, causing it to appear flat.

Patient education on ways to "protect" the MCP joint from further palmar dislocation is an important part of treatment.[7] Patients are instructed on how to perform functional activities that place limited demands on their finger flexor muscles.

ULNAR DRIFT

Ulnar "drift" deformity at the MCP joint consists of an excessive ulnar deviation and ulnar translation (slide) of the proximal phalanx. This deformity is common in advanced stages of rheumatoid arthritis and often occurs in conjunction with a palmar dislocation of the MCP joint (as indicated in Figure 8-57).

To fully understand the pathomechanics of ulnar drift, it is important to realize that all hands—healthy or otherwise—are constantly subjected to factors that favor an ulnar-deviated posture of the fingers.[7,27,105] These factors include gravity,

an asymmetric slope of the metacarpal heads, and the prevailing ulnar (medial) line of pull of the extrinsic flexor tendons as they pass the MCP joints. But perhaps the most influential factor stems from the relentless, ulnar-directed forces applied against the proximal phalanges of the radial fingers. These forces are produced by contact from hand-held objects and large "pinching" forces generated by the flexor muscles of the thumb. Figure 8-59, *A* shows these ulnar-directed forces pushing the index finger in an ulnar direction. The subsequent ulnar deviation of the MCP joint increases the ulnar deflection—or bend—in the extensor digitorum (ED) tendon as its crosses the dorsal side of the joint. The deflection creates a potentially destabilizing bowstringing force on the tendon. In the healthy hand, however, the transverse fibers of the dorsal hood and radial collateral ligament maintain the extensor tendon *over* the axis of rotation, thereby protecting the joint from drifting further into ulnar deviation.

The previous description reinforces the important role that healthy connective tissue plays in maintaining the stability of a joint. Often, in severe cases of rheumatoid arthritis, the radial transverse fibers of the dorsal hood rupture or overstretch, allowing the tendon of the extensor digitorum to slip toward the *ulnar* side of the joint's axis of rotation (see Figure 8-59, *B*). In this position, the force produced by the extensor digitorum acts with a moment arm that amplifies the ulnar deviated posture. This situation initiates a self-perpetuating

Pathomechanics associated with ulnar drift at the metacarpophalangeal joint

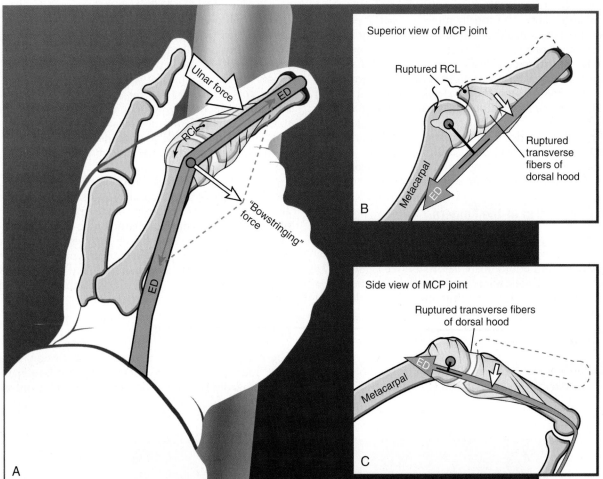

FIGURE 8-59. Pathomechanics associated with ulnar drift at the metacarpophalangeal *(MCP)* joint of the index finger. **A,** Ulnar-directed forces generated by the thumb produce a natural bowstringing force on the deflected tendon of the extensor digitorum *(ED)*. **B,** Superior view. In rheumatoid arthritis, rupture of the transverse fibers of the dorsal hood allows the extensor tendon to migrate ulnarly. **C,** Side view. Once unstable, the extensor digitorum tendon may also displace *palmar* to the MCP joint. In this case the displaced tendon creates a flexion torque at the MCP joint—often causing a palmar dislocation of the joint, in addition to the ulnar drift. The axis of rotation at each MCP joint is shown as a circle at the center of the metacarpal head. (In **B** and **C,** the moment arms are depicted as thick black lines originating at the axis of rotation.)

process: the greater the ulnar deviation, the greater the associated moment arm, and the greater the deforming ulnar deviation torque. In time, a weakened and overstretched radial collateral ligament may rupture, allowing the proximal phalanx to rotate and slide ulnarly, leading to complete joint dislocation. Persons with severe ulnar drift that affects multiple fingers are typically most concerned about appearance and the reduced function—especially related to pinch and power grip.

The pathomechanics of ulnar drift often involve a secondary destabilizing process at the MCP joints. In addition to ulnar migration, the tendon of the extensor digitorum may also slip palmarly into the natural "gullies" between the prominent metacarpal heads. This abnormal palmar position reduces the moment arm of the extensor digitorum for extending the MCP joint. As depicted in a side view in Figure 8-59, *C,* the extensor tendon may actually displace *palmar* to the medial-lateral axis of rotation. In this case the displaced tendon creates a flexion torque at the MCP joint. These

abnormal mechanics favor the palmar dislocation deformity previously described.

Treatment for ulnar drift typically includes normalizing the alignment of the joint and, when possible, minimizing the underlying mechanics that are responsible for the instability or deformity.[7] Common nonsurgical treatment includes using splints and specialized adaptive equipment and advising patients on how to minimize the deforming forces across the MCP joint.[66,77] Consider the strong ulnar deviation torque placed on the MCP joints of the right hand when the lid of a jar is tightened or a pitcher of water is held. This torque may, over time, predispose or accentuate ulnar drift. In general, patients are advised to avoid most heavy gripping and forceful key pinch activities, especially during the acute inflammation or painful stage of the rheumatoid arthritis.

Surgical intervention for excessive ulnar drift may include transferring the extensor digitorum tendon to the *radial* side of the MCP joint's anterior-posterior axis of rotation.[33] In more severe cases the damaged MCP joint may be replaced with a total joint arthoplasty. This usually provides relief of pain and restores some function, although the patient typically will not regain full range of motion. This surgery is often performed in conjunction with reconstruction of the joint's periarticular connective tissues. A fusion or arthroplasty of the wrist may also be indicated because the mechanics associated with a misaligned wrist can create potentially deforming forces on the MCP joint. Regardless of the specific surgery, proper post-surgical treatment is critical for successful rehabilitation.[7] This treatment is typically provided by certified hand therapists who have specialized in hand rehabilitation. A close working relationship is essential between the surgeon and the therapist.

Zigzag Deformities of the Fingers

Two classic zigzag deformities of the finger can occur, typically associated with advanced rheumatoid arthritis: swan-neck deformity and boutonniere deformity (see Figure 8-57). As noted in the previous photograph, both deformities often occur in conjunction with ulnar drift and palmar dislocation of the MCP joints.

SWAN-NECK DEFORMITY

Swan-neck deformity is characterized by hyperextension of the PIP joint with flexion at the DIP joint (see Figure 8-57, middle finger). The position of the MCP joint is variable. The intrinsic muscles in the hand affected by rheumatoid arthritis often become fibrotic and contracted. With weakened palmar plates at the PIP joint, the tension within the intrinsic muscles may eventually collapse the PIP joints into hyperextension (Figure 8-60, *A*). The hyperextended position of the PIP joint causes the lateral bands of the extensor mechanism to bow-string dorsally, *away* from the joint's axis of rotation. Bow-stringing increases the moment arm for the intrinsic muscles to extend the PIP joint, thereby accentuating the hyperextension deformity. The DIP joint tends to remain flexed because of the stretch placed on the tendon of the flexor digitorum profundus across the PIP joint.

As stated, swan-neck deformity is typically associated with the pathology of rheumatoid arthritis. The deformity may also develop, however, from acute trauma to the palmar plates, or from chronic spasticity or hypertonus of the intrinsic muscles of the hand, such as the lumbricals or interossei. Regardless of cause, treatment typically involves splinting to block hyperextension of the PIP joint, or surgery to repair the palmar plate or to implant a total joint arthroplasty.

BOUTONNIERE DEFORMITY

The *boutonniere deformity* is described as flexion of the PIP joint and hyperextension of the DIP joint (see Figure 8-57, index finger). (The term *boutonniere*—a French word meaning

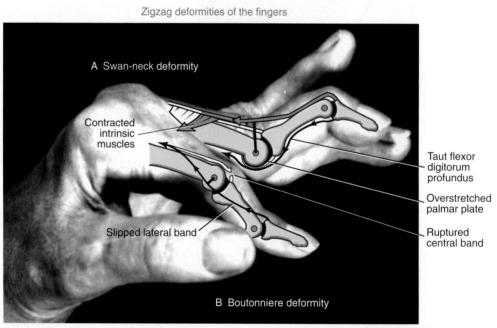

Zigzag deformities of the fingers

FIGURE 8-60. Two common zigzag deformities of the finger with severe rheumatoid arthritis. *A,* The middle finger shows the pathomechanics of the *swan-neck deformity.* The contracted intrinsic muscle—such as a lumbrical or second dorsal interosseus muscle (in red)—is creating an extension torque on the proximal interphalangeal (PIP) joint. Over time, the weakened palmar plate becomes overstretched, allowing the PIP joint to deform into severe hyperextension. The moment arm used by the extensor mechanism is shown as a short black line originating at the axis of rotation at the PIP joint. The distal interphalangeal (DIP) joint remains partially flexed because of the increased passive tension in the stretched flexor digitorum profundus tendon. *B,* The index finger depicts the pathomechanics of the *boutonniere deformity.* The central band has ruptured, causing the lateral bands to slip in a *palmar* direction relative to the PIP joint; thus the joint loses its only means of extension. The moment arm used by the slipped lateral bands is shown as a short black line originating at the axis of rotation at the PIP joint. The DIP joint remains hyperextended because of increased passive tension in the taut lateral bands.

SPECIAL FOCUS 8-8

Instability of the Metacarpophalangeal Joint: Additional Pathomechanics Associated with Instability of the Wrist

From a proximal to distal perspective, the wrist-and-hand unit consists of six major articulations. Such a long, continuous series of links is inherently mechanically unstable. Often, instability at a more proximal joint predisposes instability at a more distal joint: the so-called "zigzag" deformity. One classic zigzag deformity associated with the wrist and hand involves *ulnar drift of the metacarpophalangeal (MCP) joints* and *excessive radial deviation of the wrist.*

As a background to this discussion, recall that the potentially deforming ulnar-directed "bowstringing" force across the MCP joints is naturally minimized by the central alignment of the tendons of the extensor digitorum. This is illustrated in Figure 8-61, *A.* Instability of the wrist, however, can change the alignment between the extensor tendons and the MCP joints. As a possible sequela of either chronic inflammation or trauma, the entire carpus may shift (or translocate) in an ulnar direction (see Figure 8-61, *B*).[2] (These pathomechanics were described in Chapter 7.) The ulnar shift increases the moment arms of the radial deviator muscles of the wrist. Over time, therefore, the carpus and metacarpals may assume a more *radially rotated* position.[7] As depicted in Figure 8-61, *C,* the radially positioned metacarpals accentuate the ulnar bowstringing torque across the MCP joints. If the extensor mechanism cannot stabilize the tendons of the extensor digitorum, the tendons migrate ulnarly, gaining moment arm length (as shown on the index finger), which fuels the MCP joint's ulnar drift pathomechanics. Surgeons and therapists need to consider these pathomechanics as part of the assessment and treatment for ulnar drift.

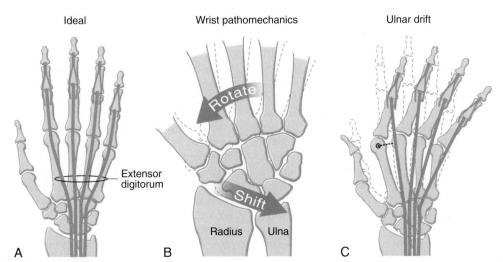

FIGURE 8-61. **A,** In the ideal or normal wrist, the tendons of the extensor digitorum are centrally maintained over or close to the dorsal side of the metacarpophalangeal (MCP) joints. **B,** Because of the natural *ulnar tilt* of the distal radius, compressive forces that cross a weakened wrist can eventually shift the carpus in an ulnar direction. The altered mechanics often cause the distal wrist and metacarpals to rotate in a radial direction. **C,** Pathomechanics of the wrist ultimately leading to excessive ulnar drift of the MCP joints. (See text for more explanation.) The axis of rotation and increased moment arm for ulnar deviation are depicted for the index finger. (From Bielefeld TB, Neumann DA: The unstable metacarpophalangeal joint in rheumatoid arthritis: anatomy, pathomechanics, and physical rehabilitation considerations, *J Orthop Sports Phys Ther* 35:502, 2005.)

buttonhole—describes the appearance of the head of the proximal phalanx as it slips through the "buttonhole" created by the displaced lateral bands.) The interphalangeal joints collapse essentially in a reciprocal pattern to that described for the swan-neck deformity. The primary cause of the boutonniere deformity is abnormal displacement of the bands of the extensor mechanism at the PIP joint and rupture of the central band, usually the result of chronic synovitis. The lateral bands slip toward the palmar side of the axis of rotation at the PIP joint (see Figure 8-60, *B*). Consequently, forces transferred across the slipped lateral bands (either from active or passive sources) cause *flexion* at the PIP joint instead of normal extension. Essentially, the PIP joint loses all sources of extension.

As depicted in Figure 8-60, the DIP joint in the boutonniere deformity remains hyperextended owing to the increased tension in the stretched lateral bands. The inability to flex the DIP joint interferes with the ease of picking up small objects, such as a coin from a table.

Early boutonniere deformity may be treated by splinting the PIP joint in extension. Surgery may be required to repair the central band and/or realign the lateral bands dorsal to the PIP joint. Sedentary patients with minimal deformity may gain some function and pain relief from a silicone implant at the PIP joint.

SYNOPSIS

The kinesiology of the hand is as fascinating as it is complex. On careful observation, it becomes clear that all of the 19 bones or 19 joints are morphologically different, and therefore each possesses a unique function.

The joints of the hand are organized into three sets of articulations: CMC, MCP, and IP. The CMC joints form the functional transition between the wrist and the hand. Located most proximally within the hand, these joints are fundamentally responsible for adjusting the curvature of the palm, from flat to deeply cup-shaped. The more peripheral CMC joints of the hand are particularly important in this regard because they allow the thumb to approach the tips of the other digits and they raise the ulnar border of the hand. In collaboration with the more stable second and third CMC joints, the peripheral joints allow the hand to securely hold a near-infinite number of irregularly curved shapes. Very specialized muscles, such as the opponens pollicis and opponens digiti minimi, are dedicated solely to controlling the first and fifth CMC joints. Trauma or disease involving these joints can deprive the hand of many postures that are unique to human prehension.

The relatively large MCP joints form the base of each digit. Each joint is stabilized by an elaborate set of periarticular connective tissues—a necessity, considering that each joint must support the weight of an entire set of phalanges. In addition, the MCP joints are subjected to particularly high loads as they function as the keystones for both the longitudinal and distal transverse arches of the hand. Specialized tissues like palmar plates and thickened collateral ligaments are required to stabilize these articulations while simultaneously permitting a relatively wide arc of movement. Trauma and disease, such as rheumatoid arthritis, can lead to instability of the MCP joints, which can disrupt the mechanical integrity of the entire hand.

Although the MCP joint of the thumb is limited primarily to flexion and extension, the MCP joints of the fingers move in two degrees of freedom. The combined motions of abduction and extension of the fingers, for example, maximize the breadth of the hand, which is especially useful for holding broad objects of varying curvatures. The fit of the object within the hand is further enhanced by the mobility profile expressed at the CMC joints, and by the passive, axial rotation permitted by the MCP joints.

The *IP joints* of the hand are located most distally within the upper extremity and therefore are most frequently in physical contact with surrounding objects. The distal pads of the digits, therefore, are soft in order to dampen contact forces; the distal digits also contain a very high density of sensory receptors, maximizing tactile sensitivity. Ironically, although the IP joints are most intimately involved with manipulation and grasp, they possess the most elementary kinematics of the digits. The IP joints flex and extend only; the other potential planes of motion are blocked by the bony fit of the joint and by periarticular connective tissues. The functional potential of the IP joints therefore is highly dependent on the more complex kinematics permitted in the more proximal joints of the hand.

Flexion range of motion is nevertheless extensive at the IP joints—from 70 degrees at the IP joint of the thumb to 120 degrees at the more ulnarly located proximal interphalangeal joints of the fingers. Such motion is needed to fully close the fist, hold a handbag, or otherwise maximize digital contact with objects. Full extension at these joints is equally important to open the hand in preparation for grasp.

Located most distally, the IP joints are most vulnerable to direct trauma, such as a lacerated tendon, or fracture within the joint. Such injury can significantly reduce functional mobility of the IP joints. Also, spastic paralysis from injury to the central nervous system can reduce the control over movement of the IP joints. Regardless of the cause, reduced control or loss of mobility of the IP joints can significantly minimize the functional potential of the hand.

The 29 muscles of the hand have been classified into extrinsic and intrinsic groups, primarily to facilitate anatomic organization. The muscular kinesiology, however, is based more on the functional interaction and synergy between the two groups. It is rare that an isolated contraction of an extrinsic or an intrinsic muscle causes a meaningful movement. A simple example supporting this premise is related to the kinesiology of extending the finger. One could assume that a muscle bearing the name *extensor digitorum* would independently perform this action. This is not the case; isolated contraction of the extensor digitorum only hyperextends the MCP joints, causing the proximal and distal IP joints to collapse into flexion. As described earlier in this chapter, simultaneous extension of all three joints of the fingers requires a coordinated interplay among the extensor digitorum *and* the intrinsic muscles, such as the lumbricals and interossei. More complex and rapid movements of the digits demands an even greater functional interdependence between the intrinsic and extrinsic muscles.

Valuable insights into the normal kinesiology of the hand can be discovered by carefully studying the pathomechanics after trauma, disease, or muscle paralysis. Typically the pathomechanics—and often resulting deformity—reflect the *loss* of a critical force once supplied by muscle or connective tissue. Restoring kinetic balance to the region is often a major component underlying surgical and therapeutic intervention for impairments of the hand. The hand surgeon, for example, may route the tendon of the extensor digitorum more radially over the MCP joints to overcompensate for an exaggerated "ulnar drift" posture; the therapist, for example, may devise a splint that prevents unwanted hyperextension of the MCP joints after paralysis of interosseus and lumbrical muscles—in essence, replacing the force otherwise produced by these now paralyzed muscles.

In closing, it is important to consider that the intent of most movements routinely performed throughout the upper limb relates indirectly or directly to optimizing prehension. Disease or injury that incapacitates the hand, therefore, significantly reduces the demands placed on the entire limb. This becomes apparent in a person with a severe hand injury who invariably develops some observable disuse muscle atrophy and restriction of movement as far proximally as the shoulder. This strong functional association between the hand and the entire upper limb should be considered during all clinical assessments of the upper limb.

ADDITIONAL CLINICAL CONNECTIONS

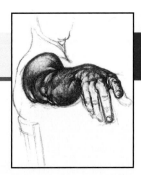

CLINICAL CONNECTION 8-1
"Tendon Transfer" Surgery to Restore Kinetic Balance and Function to the Partially Denervated Hand: a Look at Some Underlying Kinesiology

The median, ulnar, and radial nerves are all vulnerable to injury as they course throughout the upper limb. The nerves may be severely compressed or stretched, lacerated by fractured bone, or penetrated by foreign objects, including glass, knives, and bullets. These same nerves may also be involved in neuropathies. Injury or pathology involving these peripheral nerves can cause varying degrees of muscular paralysis, loss of sensation, and trophic changes in the skin.

The resulting impairments of a peripheral nerve injury or neuropathy can have devastating functional effects on the involved region of the body. Especially with peripheral nerve injuries, certain muscular actions of the wrist and hand may be completely lost. Furthermore, the skin in the associated region becomes vulnerable to injury because of the loss of sensation. Selective muscular paralysis results in a kinetic imbalance across the joint or joints, thereby increasing the likelihood of deformity. Consider, for example, a complete laceration of the median nerve at the level of the wrist. Paralysis of the muscles of the thenar eminence can completely disable the important movement of opposition of the thumb. Without therapeutic intervention, the thumb may also develop an adduction and lateral rotation contracture because of the unopposed pull of (1) the ulnar nerve–innervated adductor pollicis, and (2) the radial nerve–innervated extensor pollicis longus. Such a deformity is the antithesis of the position of opposition.

Injury to the major nerves of the upper limb often results in a predictable pattern of muscle paralysis, sensory loss, and potential deformity. (Neuroanatomic illustrations such as that contained in Appendix II, Part B can serve as useful guides for anticipating which muscles may be paralyzed after a nerve injury.) Regeneration of an injured nerve with return of motor and sensory function is physiologically possible; however, the extent of neuronal growth depends on several factors, including the continuity of the connective tissue sheath (endoneurial tube) that surrounds the individual axons. Crush and traction injuries that leave the endoneurial tube intact but destroy the axon have a better prognosis for regeneration.[96] After a complete laceration of the axon and endoneurial tube, surgical repair of the nerve is a necessary prerequisite for regeneration.[96] In ideal circumstances, a peripheral nerve can regenerate at a rate of about 1 mm/day (or about 1 inch/month). During this time, therapists often assume an important therapeutic role, including educat-

ing the patient about the medical condition, providing selected strengthening and stretching exercises, training to compensate for persistent muscular weakness, and splinting to reduce deformity and assist with or compensate for lost active motion.

In cases in which paralysis after nerve injury appears permanent, surgeons may perform a *"tendon transfer."*[92] This surgical procedure reroutes the tendon of an innervated muscle in such a manner that all or parts of the lost actions of the paralyzed muscle are restored. A tendon transfer surgery is particularly indicated when the paralysis significantly diminishes the performance of an important function—such as the loss of opposition of the thumb. A tendon transfer to restore opposition of the thumb is referred to as an *opponensplasty*. Although many types of opponensplasty techniques have been described, one common method involves surgically redirecting the tendon of the flexor digitorum superficialis (of the ring finger) to the thumb (Figure 8-62, *A*).[33] The natural split in the superficialis tendon is expanded and then the split tendon is sutured to both sides of the MCP joint of the thumb, at the point of attachment of the abductor pollicis brevis. In an attempt to mimic the line of force of the paralyzed thenar muscles, the transferred tendon is secured by a connective tissue pulley to the distal attachment of the flexor carpi ulnaris muscle. The restoration of abduction and medial rotation of the thumb is essential to the success of the operation (see Figure 8-62, *B*). Therapists must devise creative methods to train patients to use the transferred musculotendinous unit to accomplish its new action. Training is greatly enhanced if the patient has at least partial sensation in the involved digits and if the transferred muscle is a natural synergist to the paralyzed one.

Several different types of tendon transfer surgeries have been devised over the years for use after nerve injury in the distal upper extremity.[9,10,33] The specific choice of surgery depends on the location and extent of the nerve damage, the loss of function, the amount of residual sensation, and the passive range of motion of the involved joints. Equally important is the availability of a suitable musculotendinous unit for surgical transfer. Of particular interest to the surgeon is the transferred muscle's maximum *torque* potential. Because torque is the product of the muscle's force production and its internal moment arm, both variables need to be considered.

Continued

ADDITIONAL CLINICAL CONNECTIONS

CLINICAL CONNECTION 8-1
"Tendon Transfer" Surgery to Restore Kinetic Balance and Function to the Partially Denervated Hand: a Look at Some Underlying Kinesiology—cont'd

The relative force potential of a muscle that is considered for tendon transfer surgery can be estimated by its cross-sectional area. These data are published in the literature.[11,34,35] During surgery, it is very difficult to make a direct measurement of a transferred muscle's *moment arm* about a joint, for a given action. This variable of leverage, however, is very important. To optimize the functional results of the tendon transfer, it is often desirable that the surgeon closely match the transferred muscle's moment arm with that of the paralyzed one. As introduced in Chapter 1, two identical muscles with moment arms of different lengths will produce different kinetics and kinematics across a joint. For example, if a surgeon positions a muscle's tendon *too close* to the joint's axis of rotation, the reduced moment arm would minimize

the muscle's torque potential; the operation, therefore, may fail to match the muscle's strength to its functional demand. Alternatively, positioning the muscle's tendon *too far* from the joint's axis (i.e., creating an abnormally large moment arm) would create a situation in which a given amount of muscle shortening would produce a limited—and perhaps ineffective—amount of joint rotation.

Given the importance of knowing the transferred muscle's potential moment arm for an action, the late Dr. Paul Brand—a preeminent hand surgeon—devised a method to estimate this variable at the time of operation.[9] The power of this technique lies in its elegant simplicity: the geometric principle of a *radian*. As depicted by Figure 8-63, *A*, one radian (θ) is defined as the angle

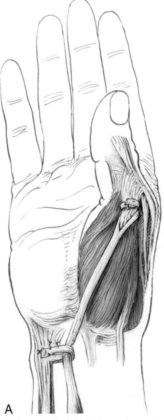

A

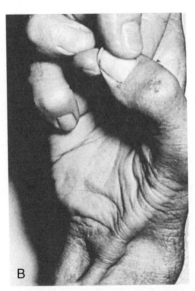

B

FIGURE 8-62. **A,** After an injury to the median nerve at the wrist, this relatively common type of opponensplasty intends to restore at least partial opposition of the thumb. The tendon of the flexor digitorum superficialis of the ring finger has been surgically rerouted to the MCP joint of the thumb. **B,** Photograph showing the results of opponensplasty. Observe the medial rotation and abduction of the thumb. The tendon of the flexor digitorum superficialis is evident under the skin. (From Hentz VR, Chase RA: *Hand surgery: a clinical atlas*, Philadelphia, 2001, Saunders.)

ADDITIONAL CLINICAL CONNECTIONS

CLINICAL CONNECTION 8-1
"Tendon Transfer" Surgery to Restore Kinetic Balance and Function to the Partially Denervated Hand: a Look at Some Underlying Kinesiology—cont'd

at the center of a circle that has an arc (s) equal to its radius (r): 1 radian equals 57.3 degrees. The concept of a radian can be extended to a rope rotating around a pulley, as shown in Figure 8-63, *B.* When the pulley is rotated 57.3 degrees, the rope that runs off the pulley (s) is equal to the radius of the pulley (r). Brand used the rope-and-pulley system as a model for a tendon and anatomic joint system, respectively; the radius of the pulley (r) is analogous to the internal moment arm of the muscle, and the rope is analogous to the excursion of its tendon. At the time of surgery, Brand estimated the internal moment arm of both the transferred tendon and the tendon of the paralyzed muscle by simply measuring the excursion of the tendons as the joint was passively rotated approximately 57 degrees (see Figure 8-63, *C*). *After 57 degrees of joint rotation, the resulting tendon excursion (labeled s) is equal to the internal moment arm (IMA) available to the muscle.* Brand sutured the transferred tendon in place when the moment arm approximated that of the tendon of the paralyzed muscle (or that established by normative data[9]). In cases in which

the moment arm of the transferred muscle was not acceptable, Brand attempted to reconcile the problem by redirecting the line of pull of the tendon or by selecting another one for use in the transfer.

Brand's use of the radian to estimate a muscle's internal moment arm assumes that the curvatures of the joint surfaces are perfect spheres. Because the surfaces of most joints of the hand are only approximately spheric, these estimates contain some error. Nevertheless, the error is likely small and clinically insignificant, especially when comparing moment arm lengths of the same joint within a given patient. The concept of using a radian to mathematically relate the excursion of a tendon to its moment arm remains a respected biomechanical technique.[29] The technique has been used with cadaver specimens to measure the natural change in moment arm length throughout the entire range of motion for most muscles of the hand.[47,97] Measurements have also quantified the degree to which an unstable joint alters the moment arm of the surrounding muscles.[79]

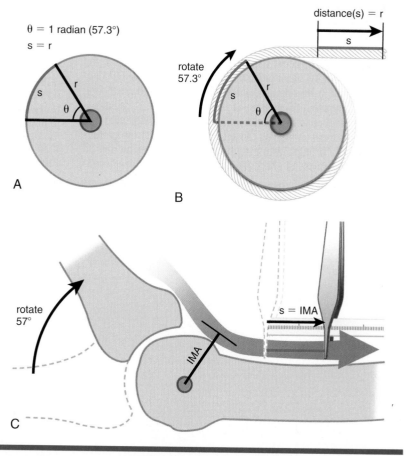

FIGURE 8-63. A, One radian (θ) equals 57.3 degrees. The arc of the circle *(s)* formed by a radian is equal to its radius *(r)*. (This relationship can also be stated mathematically: $\theta = s/r$.) **B,** The concept of the radian extended to a rope and rotating pulley. The radius of the pulley *(r)* equals s when θ = 1 radian (57.3 degrees). **C,** The concept of the radian applied to an anatomic joint, such as the MCP joint. The tendon excursion *(s)* resulting from approximately 57 degrees of joint rotation is the approximate length of the internal moment arm *(IMA)*.

ADDITIONAL CLINICAL CONNECTIONS

CLINICAL CONNECTION 8-2
Biomechanical Consequences of Lacerated or Incised Flexor Pulleys of the Hand

An important function of the flexor pulleys of the hand is to maintain a near constant moment arm length of the flexor tendons as they cross the joints of the fingers. If the pulleys are overstretched, lacerated, or torn, the force of the contracting muscle causes the tendon to bowstring away from the joint. Bowstringing of a tendon significantly increases its moment arm and, in turn, increases the mechanical advantage of the muscle at the joint. As described in Chapter 1, increasing a muscle's mechanical advantage has two effects on joint mechanics: (1) amplification of the torque produced per level muscle force, and (2) reduction of the angular rotation of the joint per linear distance of muscle contraction. The negative clinical implication of a torn, cut, or overstretched flexor pulley primarily involves the second factor. To illustrate this effect on grasping, assume that with intact A_2, A_3, and A_4 pulleys, the moment arm of the flexor digitorum profundus tendon is about 0.75 cm at the PIP joint (Figure 8-64, *A*). Based on the geometric principle of a *radian,* a muscle that shortens a length equal to its own moment arm at a joint will produce 1 radian (57 degrees) of joint rotation.[9] Accordingly, with intact pulleys, 1.5 cm of contraction of the flexor digitorum profundus with a 0.75-cm moment arm would theoretically produce 114 degrees (2 radians) of PIP joint flexion. This biomechanical situation is desirable because it allows a relatively small muscle contraction to produce a relative large rotation at the joint. A finger with a cut A_2 and A_3 pulley, as shown in Figure 8-64, *B,* could theoretically *double* the length of the moment arm of the flexor digitorum profundus across the PIP joint. Consequently, a muscle contraction of 1.5 cm would, in theory, produce only about 57 degrees of joint rotation (i.e., 1 radian)— *about half the motion produced with intact pulleys.* Assuming that the near maximal shortening range of the flexor digitorum profundus is 2 cm,[1] a finger with a ruptured pulley will not be able to flex fully, regardless of effort. Surgical correction is typically indicated for the more functionally important A_2 and A_4 pulleys of the fingers.[88]

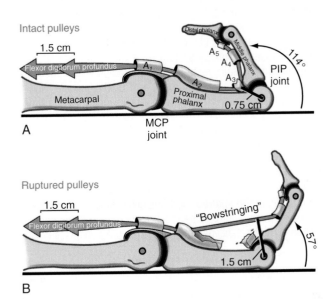

FIGURE 8-64. Pathomechanics of torn flexor pulleys. **A,** With intact pulleys, the moment arm of the flexor digitorum profundus (FDP) across the proximal interphalangeal (PIP) joint is about 0.75 cm. Theoretically, a 1.5-cm contraction of this muscle would cause about 114 degrees (or about 2 radians) of flexion at the PIP joint. **B,** A rupture of the A_2 and A_3 pulleys may increase the flexor moment arm of the FDP to 1.5 cm. A 1.5-cm contraction of the FDP would now produce only about 57 degrees of flexion of the PIP joints.

ADDITIONAL CLINICAL CONNECTIONS

CLINICAL CONNECTION 8-3
Muscular Biomechanics of a "Key Pinch": Highlighting the Demands Placed on the First Dorsal Interosseus Muscle

Pinching an object between the thumb and lateral side of the index finger is an important prehensile function. This function is often referred to as a "key pinch." An effective key pinch places especially large force demands on the first dorsal interosseus muscle. (This demand can be appreciated by palpating its prominent belly during the pinch, about 2.5 cm proximal to the lateral side of the metacarpophalangeal [MCP] joint of the index finger.) The first dorsal interosseus muscle must generate a strong enough *abduction* force at the MCP joint of the index finger to counteract the very potent *flexion* force produced by the many muscles of the thumb. The effect of these opposing muscular forces generates a pinch force between the index finger and thumb (indicated as F_T versus F_I in Figure 8-65). Flexion, the "strongest" of all thumb movements,[45] is driven primarily by the adductor pollicis, the flexor pollicis longus, and other muscles within the thenar eminence. As indicated in the figure, the internal moment arm used by the first dorsal interosseus to stabilize the MCP joint of the index finger is about 1 cm. Furthermore, the pinch force generated by the thumb (F_T) against the MCP joint of the index finger acts with an external moment arm of about 5 cm (compare IMA and EMA in Figure 8-65). This fivefold difference in leverage across the MCP joint requires that the first dorsal interosseus must produce a force about five times the pinching force applied by the thumb. Because many functional activities demand a pinch force that exceeds 45 N (10 lb), the first dorsal interosseus must be able to produce an abduction force of about 225 N (50 lb). To determine if this is physiologically possible, first consider that a skeletal muscle may produce a maximum force of about 28 N/cm^2 (40 lb/in^2). An average-sized first dorsal interosseus (with a cross-section area of about 3.8 cm^2)[19] would therefore be expected to produce about 106 N (24 lb) of force—only about half of that estimated earlier. It is clear, therefore, that a maximal-effort key pinch requires an additional source of abduction torque to assist the first dorsal interosseus in stabilizing the index finger. This is likely accomplished by the second dorsal interosseus, and possibly with the assistance of the radial-positioned lumbricals of the index and middle fingers.

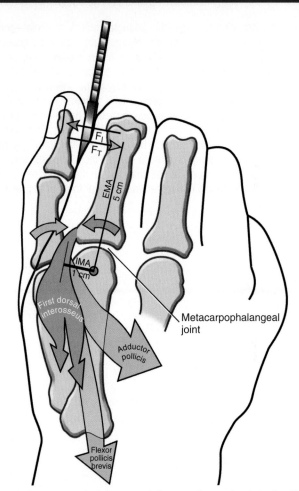

FIGURE 8-65. A dorsal view of the muscle mechanics of a "key pinch." Illustrated in lighter red, the adductor pollicis and flexor pollicis brevis are shown producing a pinch force through the thumb *(F_T)*. In dark red, the first dorsal interosseus is shown opposing the thumb's flexor force by producing a force through the index finger *(F_I)*. The external moment arm *(EMA)* at the metacarpophalangeal joint is 5 cm; the internal moment arm *(IMA)* at the metacarpophalangeal joint is 1 cm.

Continued

ADDITIONAL CLINICAL CONNECTIONS

CLINICAL CONNECTION 8-3
Muscular Biomechanics of a "Key Pinch": Highlighting the Demands Placed on the First Dorsal Interosseus Muscle—cont'd

With an ulnar nerve lesion, the adductor pollicis muscle—the dominant pinching muscle of the thumb—and all interosseus muscles may be paralyzed. Paralysis of these muscles typically decreases key pinch by almost 80%.[49] The region around the dorsal web space becomes hollow owing to atrophy in the previously mentioned muscles (Figure 8-66). A person with an ulnar nerve lesion often relies on the flexor pollicis longus (a median nerve–innervated muscle) to partially compensate for the loss of key pinch. This compensation is evident by the partially flexed interphalangeal (IP) joint of the thumb—known as *Froment's sign*. Pinch remains weak, however, primarily because of the inability of the paralyzed first dorsal interosseus muscle to counteract the flexor force of the flexor pollicis longus.

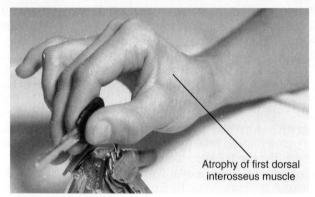

Atrophy of first dorsal interosseus muscle

FIGURE 8-66. A person with an ulnar nerve lesion attempting to perform a key pinch. Note the atrophy of the first dorsal interosseus muscle. The flexion at the interphalangeal joint of the thumb is an attempt to compensate for the paralysis of the adductor pollicis muscle.

REFERENCES

1. An KN, Ueba Y, Chao EY, et al: Tendon excursion and moment arm of index finger muscles, *J Biomech* 16:419-425, 1983.

2. Arimitsu S, Murase T, Hashimoto J, et al: A three-dimensional quantitative analysis of carpal deformity in rheumatoid wrists, *J Bone Joint Surg Br* 89:490-494, 2007.

3. Armbruster EJ, Tan V: Carpometacarpal joint disease: Addressing the metacarpophalangeal joint deformity, *Hand Clin* 24:295-299, 2008.

4. Batmanabane M, Malathi S: Movements at the carpometacarpal and metacarpophalangeal joints of the hand and their effect on the dimensions of the articular ends of the metacarpal bones, *Anat Rec* 213:102-110, 1985.

5. Belt E, Kaarela K, Lehtinen J, et al: When does subluxation of the first carpometacarpal joint cause swan-neck deformity of the thumb in rheumatoid arthritis: A 20-year follow-up study, *Clin Rheumatol* 17:135-138, 1998.

6. Bettinger PC, Linscheid RL, Berger RA, et al: An anatomic study of the stabilizing ligaments of the trapezium and trapeziometacarpal joint, *J Hand Surg [Am]* 24:786-798, 1999.

7. Bielefeld T, Neumann DA: The unstable metacarpophalangeal joint in rheumatoid arthritis: Anatomy, pathomechanics, and physical rehabilitation considerations, *J Orthop Sports Phys Ther* 35:502-520, 2005.

8. Boatright JR, Kiebzak GM: The effects of low median nerve block on thumb abduction strength, *J Hand Surg [Am]* 22:849-852, 1997.

9. Brand PW: *Clinical biomechanics of the hand*, St. Louis, 1985, Mosby.

10. Brand PW: The reconstruction of the hand in leprosy. 1952, *Clin Orthop Relat Res* 396:4-11, 2002.

11. Brand PW, Beach RB, Thompson DE: Relative tension and potential excursion of muscles in the forearm and hand, *J Hand Surg [Am]* 6:209-219, 1981.

12. Buford WL, Andersen CR: *Predicting moment arms in diarthrodial joints—3D computer simulation capability and muscle-tendon model validation.* Conference Proceedings. 2006; Annual International Conference of the IEEE Engineering in Medicine & Biology Society. 1:3407-3410, 2006.

13. Cheema TA, Cheema NI, Tayyab R, Firoozbakhsh K: Measurement of rotation of the first metacarpal during opposition using computed tomography, *J Hand Surg [Am]* 31:76-79, 2006.

14. Close JR, Kidd CC: The functions of the muscles of the thumb, the index, and long fingers. Synchronous recording of motions and action potentials of muscles, *J Bone Joint Surg Am* 51:1601-1620, 1969.

15. Cooney WP 3rd, Lucca MJ, Chao EY, Linscheid RL: The kinesiology of the thumb trapeziometacarpal joint, *J Bone Joint Surg Am* 63:1371-1381, 1981.

16. Cope JM, Berryman AC, Martin DL, Potts DD: Robusticity and osteoarthritis at the trapeziometacarpal joint in a Bronze Age population from Tell Abraq, United Arab Emirates, *Am J Phys Anthropol* 126:391-400, 2005.

17. Doyle JR, Blythe W: The finger flexor tendon sheath and pulleys: Anatomy and reconstruction. In *American academy of orthopaedic surgeons symposium on tendon surgery in the hand*, St. Louis, 1975, Mosby.

18. Dubousset JF: The Digital Joints. In Tubiana R, editor: *The hand*, Philadelphia, 1981, Saunders.

19. Dvir Z: Biomechanics of muscle. In Dvir Z, editor: *Clinical biomechanics*, Philadelphia, 2000, Churchill Livingstone.

20. Eaton RG, Littler JW: Ligament reconstruction for the painful thumb carpometacarpal joint, *J Bone Joint Surg Am* 55:1655-1666, 1973.

21. El Shennawy M, Nakamura K, Patterson RM, Viegas SF: Three-dimensional kinematic analysis of the second through fifth carpometacarpal joints, *J Hand Surg [Am]* 26:1030-1035, 2001.

22. Eladoumikdachi F, Valkov PL, Thomas J, Netscher DT: Anatomy of the intrinsic hand muscles revisited: part I. Interossei, *Plast Reconstr Surg* 110:1211-1224, 2002.

23. Eladoumikdachi F, Valkov PL, Thomas J, Netscher DT: Anatomy of the intrinsic hand muscles revisited: part II. Lumbricals, *Plast Reconstr Surg* 110:1225-1231, 2002.

24. Enoka RM: *Neuromechanics of human movement*, ed 3, Champaign, Ill, 2002, Human Kinetics.

25. Firoozbakhsh K, Yi IS, Moneim MS, Umada Y: A study of ulnar collateral ligament of the thumb metacarpophalangeal joint, *Clin Orthop Relat Res* 403:240-247, 2002.

26. Flatt AE: *The care of the rheumatoid hand*, ed 3, St. Louis, 1974, Mosby.

27. Flatt AE: Ulnar drift, *J Hand Ther* 9:282-292, 1996.

28. Fontana L, Neel S, Claise JM, et al: Osteoarthritis of the thumb carpometacarpal joint in women and occupational risk factors: A case-control study, *J Hand Surg [Am]* 32:459-465, 2007.

29. Goodman HJ, Choueka J: Biomechanics of the flexor tendons, *Hand Clin* 21:129-149, 2005.

30. Gray DJ, Gardner E: The innervation of the joints of the wrist and hand, *Anat Rec* 151:261-266, 1965.

31. Greenwald D, Shumway S, Allen C, Mass D: Dynamic analysis of profundus tendon function, *J Hand Surg [Am]* 19:626-635, 1994.

32. Hahn P, Krimmer H, Hradetzky A, Lanz U: Quantitative analysis of the linkage between the interphalangeal joints of the index finger. An in vivo study, *J Hand Surg [Br]* 20:696-699, 1995

33. Hentz VR, Chase RA: *Hand surgery: a clinical atlas*, Philadelphia, 2001, Saunders.

34. Holzbaur KR, Delp SL, Gold GE, Murray WM: Moment-generating capacity of upper limb muscles in healthy adults, *J Biomech* 40:2442-2449, 2007.

35. Holzbaur KR, Murray WM, Gold GE, Delp SL: Upper limb muscle volumes in adult subjects, *J Biomech* 40:742-749, 2007.

36. Hume MC, Gellman H, McKellop H, Brumfield RH Jr: Functional range of motion of the joints of the hand, *J Hand Surg [Am]* 15:240-243, 1990.

37. Imaeda T, An KN, Cooney WP 3rd, Linscheid R: Anatomy of trapeziometacarpal ligaments, *J Hand Surg [Am]* 18:226-231, 1993.

38. Imaeda T, Niebur G, Cooney WP 3rd, et al: Kinematics of the normal trapeziometacarpal joint, *J Orthop Res* 12:197-204, 1994.

39. Inman VT, Saunders JB: Referred pain from skeletal structures, *J Nerv Ment Dis* 99:660-667, 1944.

40. Jacobson MD, Raab R, Fazeli BM, et al: Architectural design of the human intrinsic hand muscles, *J Hand Surg [Am]* 17:804-809, 1992.

41. Jenkins M, Bamberger HB, Black L, Nowinski R: Thumb joint flexion. What is normal? *J Hand Surg [Br]* 23:796-797, 1998.

42. Johanson ME, Skinner SR, Lamoreux LW: Phasic relationships of the intrinsic and extrinsic thumb musculature, *Clin Orthop Relat Res* 322:120-130, 1996.

43. Kamper DG, George HT, Rymer WZ: Extrinsic flexor muscles generate concurrent flexion of all three finger joints, *J Biomech* 35:1581-1589, 2002.

44. Katarincic JA: Thumb kinematics and their relevance to function, *Hand Clin* 17:169-174, 2001.

45. Kaufman KR, An KN, Litchy WJ, et al: In-vivo function of the thumb muscles, *Clin Biomech (Bristol, Avon)* 14:141-150, 1999.

46. Keir PJ, Bach JM, Hudes M, Rempel DM: Guidelines for wrist posture based on carpal tunnel pressure thresholds, *Hum Factors* 49:88-99, 2007.

47. Koh S, Buford WL Jr, Andersen CR, Viegas SF: Intrinsic muscle contribution to the metacarpophalangeal joint flexion moment of the middle, ring, and small fingers, *J Hand Surg [Am]* 31:1111-1117, 2006.

48. Kovler M, Lundon K, McKee N, Agur A: The human first carpometacarpal joint: Osteoarthritic degeneration and 3-dimensional modeling, *J Hand Ther* 17:393-400, 2004.

49. Kozin SH, Porter S, Clark P, Thoder JJ: The contribution of the intrinsic muscles to grip and pinch strength, *J Hand Surg [Am]* 24:64-72, 1999.

50. Krishnan J, Chipchase L: Passive axial rotation of the metacarpophalangeal joint, *J Hand Surg [Br]* 22:270-273, 1997.

51. Kuczynski K: Carpometacarpal joint of the human thumb, *J Anat* 118:119-126, 1974.

52. Landsmeer JF: Power grip and precision handling, *Ann Rheum Dis* 21:164-170, 1962.

53. Leibovic SJ, Bowers WH: Anatomy of the proximal interphalangeal joint, *Hand Clin* 10:169-178, 1994.

54. Leijnse JN: Why the lumbrical muscle should not be bigger–a force model of the lumbrical in the unloaded human finger, *J Biomech* 30:1107-1114, 1997.

55. Leijnse JN, Kalker JJ: A two-dimensional kinematic model of the lumbrical in the human finger, *J Biomech* 28:237-249, 1995.

56. Leijnse JN, Spoor CW, Shatford R: The minimum number of muscles to control a chain of joints with and without tenodeses, arthrodeses, or braces–application to the human finger, *J Biomech* 38:2028-2036, 2005.

57. Li ZM, Tang J: Coordination of thumb joints during opposition, *J Biomech* 40:502-510, 2007.

58. Linscheid RL, An KN, Gross RM: Quantitative analysis of the intrinsic muscles of the hand, *Clin Anat* 4:265-284, 1991.

59. Long C: Intrinsic-extrinsic muscle control of the fingers. Electromyographic studies. *J Bone Joint Surg Am* 50:973-984, 1968.

60. Long C, Brown TD: Electromyographic kinesiology of the hand: Muscles moving the long finger, *J Bone Joint Surg Am* 46:1683-1706, 1964.

61. Loos B, Puschkin V, Horch RE: 50 years experience with Dupuytren's contracture in the Erlangen University Hospital–a retrospective analysis of 2919 operated hands from 1956 to 2006, *BMC Musculoskel Disorders* 8:60, 2007.

62. Loubert PV, Masterson TJ, Schroeder MS, Mazza AM: Proximity of collateral ligament origin to the axis of rotation of the proximal interphalangeal joint of the finger, *J Orthop Sports Phys Ther* 37:179-185, 2007.

63. MacConaill MA, Basmajian JV: *Muscles and movements: a basis for human kinesiology*, New York, 1977, Robert E. Krieger.

64. MacMoran JW, Brand PW: Bone loss in limbs with decreased or absent sensation: Ten year follow-up of the hands in leprosy, *Skeletal Radiol* 16:452-459, 1987.

65. Marklin RW, Simoneau GG, Monroe JF: Wrist and forearm posture from typing on split and vertically inclined computer keyboards, *Hum Factors* 41:559-569, 1999.

66. Masiero S, Boniolo A, Wassermann L, et al: Effects of an educational-behavioral joint protection program on people with moderate to severe rheumatoid arthritis: A randomized controlled trial, *Clin Rheumatol* 26:2043-2050, 2007.

67. Melvin JL: Therapist's management of osteoarthritis in the hand. In Mackin EJ, Callahan AD, Skriven TM, et al, editors: *Rehabilitation of the hand and upper extremity*, ed 5, St. Louis, 2005, Mosby.

68. Mo JH, Gelberman RH: Ligament reconstruction with trapezium retention arthroplasty for carpometacarpal arthritis, *J Hand Surg [Am]* 29:240-246, 2004.

69. Momose T, Nakatsuchi Y, Saitoh S: Contact area of the trapeziometacarpal joint, *J Hand Surg [Am]* 24:491-495, 1999.

70. Nakamura K, Patterson RM, Viegas SF: The ligament and skeletal anatomy of the second through fifth carpometacarpal joints and adjacent structures, *J Hand Surg [Am]* 26:1016-1029, 2001.

71. Nalebuff EA: Diagnosis, classification and management of rheumatoid thumb deformities, *Bull Hosp Jt Dis* 29:119-137, 1968.

72. Nanno M, Buford WL Jr, Patterson RM, et al: Three-dimensional analysis of the ligamentous attachments of the first carpometacarpal joint, *J Hand Surg [Am]* 31:1160-1170, 2006.

73. Napier JR: The prehensile movements of the human hand, *J Bone Joint Surg Br* 38:902-913, 1956.

74. Neto HS, Filho JM, Passini R Jr, Marques MJ: Number and size of motor units in thenar muscles, *Clin Anat* 17:308-311, 2004.

75. Neumann DA: *Observations from cineradiography analysis*, 2000, Unpublished work.

76. Neumann DA, Bielefeld T: The carpometacarpal joint of the thumb: Stability, deformity, and therapeutic intervention, *J Orthop Sports Phys Ther* 33:386-399, 2003.

77. Niedermann K, Forster A, Hammond A, et al: Development and validation of a German version of the joint protection behavior assessment in patients with rheumatoid arthritis, *Arthritis Rheum* 57:249-255, 2007.

78. Nilsson A, Liljensten E, Bergström C, Sollerman C: Results from a degradable TMC joint Spacer (Artelon) compared with tendon arthroplasty, *J Hand Surg [Am]* 30:380-389, 2005.

79. Omokawa S, Ryu J, Tang JB, et al: Trapeziometacarpal joint instability affects the moment arms of thumb motor tendons, *Clin Orthop Relat Res* 372:262-271, 2000.

80. Pagalidis T, Kuczynski K, Lamb DW: Ligamentous stability of the base of the thumb, *Hand* 13:29-36, 1981.

81. Peck D, Buxton DF, Nitz A: A comparison of spindle concentrations in large and small muscles acting in parallel combinations, *J Morphol* 180:243-252, 1984.

82. Pellegrini VD Jr: Osteoarthritis at the base of the thumb, *Orthop Clin North Am* 23:83-102, 1992.

83. Pellegrini VD Jr: Osteoarthritis of the trapeziometacarpal joint: The pathophysiology of articular cartilage degeneration. I. Anatomy and pathology of the aging joint, *J Hand Surg [Am]* 16:967-974, 1991.

84. Pellegrini VD Jr: Osteoarthritis of the trapeziometacarpal joint: The pathophysiology of articular cartilage degeneration. II. Articular wear patterns in the osteoarthritic joint, *J Hand Surg [Am]* 16:975-982, 1991.

85. Pellegrini VD Jr: Pathomechanics of the thumb trapeziometacarpal joint, *Hand Clin* 17:175-184, 2001.

86. Ranney D, Wells R: Lumbrical muscle function as revealed by a new and physiological approach, *Anat Rec* 222:110-114, 1988.

87. Rempel DM, Keir PJ, Bach JM: Effect of wrist posture on carpal tunnel pressure while typing, *J Orthop Res* 26:1269-1273, 2008.

88. Rispler D, Greenwald D, Shumway S, et al: Efficiency of the flexor tendon pulley system in human cadaver hands, *J Hand Surg [Am]* 21:444-450, 1996.

89. Rohrbough JT, Mudge MK, Schilling RC: Overuse injuries in the elite rock climber, *Med Sci Sports Exer* 32:1369-1372, 2000.

90. Roloff I, Schöffl VR, Vigouroux L, Quaine F: Biomechanical model for the determination of the forces acting on the finger pulley system, *J Biomech* 39:915-923, 2006.

91. Schulz CU, Anetzberger H, Pfahler M, et al: The relation between primary osteoarthritis of the trapeziometacarpal joint and supernumerary slips of the abductor pollicis longus tendon, *J Hand Surg [Br]* 27:238-241, 2002.

92. Schneider LW: Tendon transfers: An overview. In Mackin EJ, Callahan AD, Skirven TM, et al, editors: *Rehabilitation of the hand and upper extremity*, St Louis, 2002, Mosby.

93. Schweitzer TP, Rayan GM: The terminal tendon of the digital extensor mechanism: Part I, anatomic study, *J Hand Surg [Am]* 29:898-902, 2004.

94. Shaw SJ, Morris MA: The range of motion of the metacarpo-phalangeal joint of the thumb and its relationship to injury, *J Hand Surg [Br]* 17:164-166, 1992.

95. Simoneau GG, Marklin RW, Monroe JF: Wrist and forearm postures of users of conventional computer keyboards, *Hum Factors* 41:413-424, 1999.

96. Smith KL: Nerve response to injury and repair. In Mackin EJ, Callahan AD, Skirven TM, et al, editors: *Rehabilitation of the hand and upper extremity*, St Louis, 2002, Mosby.

97. Smutz WP, Kongsayreepong A, Hughes RE, et al: Mechanical advantage of the thumb muscles, *J Biomech* 31:565-570, 1998.

98. Sonne-Holm S, Jacobsen S: Osteoarthritis of the first carpometacarpal joint: A study of radiology and clinical epidemiology. Results from the Copenhagen Osteoarthritis Study, *Osteoarthritis Cartilage* 14:496-500, 2006.

99. Soukup T, Pedrosa-Domellöf F, Thornell LE: Intrafusal fiber type composition of muscle spindles in the first human lumbrical muscle, *Acta Neuropathol* 105:18-24, 2003.

100. Stack HG: Muscle function in the fingers, *J Bone Joint Surg Br* 44:899-902, 1962.

101. Standring S: *Gray's anatomy: the anatomical basis of clinical practice*, ed 40, St Louis, 2009, Elsevier.

102. Stein AB, Terrono AL: The rheumatoid thumb, *Hand Clin* 12:541-550, 1996.

103. Strong CL, Perry J: Function of the extensor pollicis longus and intrinsic muscle of the thumb, *J Am Phys Ther Assoc* 46:939-945, 1966.

104. Su FC, Chou YL, Yang CS, et al: Movement of finger joints induced by synergistic wrist motion, *Clin Biomech (Bristol, Avon)* 20:491-497, 2005.

105. Taguchi M, Zhao C, Zobitz ME, et al: Effect of finger ulnar deviation on gliding resistance of the flexor digitorum profundus tendon within the A1 and A2 pulley complex, *J Hand Surg [Am]* 31:113-117, 2006.

106. Taylor EJ, Desari K, D'Arcy JC, Bonnici AV: A comparison of fusion, trapeziectomy and silastic replacement for the treatment of osteoarthritis of the trapeziometacarpal joint, *J Hand Surg [Br]* 30:45-49, 2005.

107. Thomas DH, Long C: Biomechanical considerations of lumbricalis behavior in the human finger, *J Biomech* 1:107-115, 1968.

108. Ugbolue UC, Hsu WH, Goitz RJ, Li ZM: Tendon and nerve displacement at the wrist during finger movements, *Clin Biomech (Bristol, Avon)* 20:50-56, 2005.

109. Vigouroux L, Quaine F, Paclet F, et al: Middle and ring fingers are more exposed to pulley rupture than index and little during sport-climbing: A biomechanical explanation, *Clin Biomech (Bristol, Avon)* 23:562-570, 2008.

110. von Schroeder HP, Botte MJ: The dorsal aponeurosis, intrinsic, hypothenar, and thenar musculature of the hand, *Clin Orthop Relat Res* 383:97-107, 2001.

111. Wariyar B: Hansen's disease (leprosy), *Nebr Med J* 81:147-148, 1996.

112. Wells RP, Ranney DA: Lumbrical length changes in finger movement: A new method of study in fresh cadaver hands, *J Hand Surg [Am]* 11:574-577, 1986.

113. Williams EH, McCarthy E, Bickel KD: The histologic anatomy of the volar plate, *J Hand Surg [Am]* 23:805-810, 1998.

114. Xu L, Strauch RJ, Ateshian GA, et al: Topography of the osteoarthritic thumb carpometacarpal joint and its variations with regard to gender, age, site, and osteoarthritic stage, *J Hand Surg [Am]* 23:454-464, 1998.

115. Zancolli EA, Ziadenberg C, Zancolli E Jr: Biomechanics of the trapeziometacarpal joint, *Clin Orthop Relat Res* 220:14-26, 1987.

STUDY QUESTIONS

1 Compare the relative mobility permitted at the proximal and distal transverse arches of the hand.

2 List regions within the hand where you would most expect muscle atrophy after a longstanding (a) ulnar neuropathy and (b) median neuropathy.

3 The adductor pollicis is a forceful muscle requiring stable proximal bony attachments. After reviewing the muscle's proximal attachments, state whether this requirement has been met.

4 Which movements at the carpometacarpal joint of the thumb constitute opposition? Which muscles are most responsible for performing these individual movements?

5 Describe the path of the lumbrical muscle of the index finger, from its proximal to its distal attachment. Explain how this muscle can flex the metacarpophalangeal joint and simultaneously extend the interphalangeal joints.

6 Figure 8-42 shows the line of force of the extensor pollicis longus, extensor pollicis brevis, and abductor pollicis longus at the carpometacarpal joint. Of the three muscles, which (a) is capable of adduction, (b) is capable of abduction, and (c) has neither potential? Finally, which of these muscles can extend the carpometacarpal joint?

7 What is the role of the lumbricals and interossei in opening the hand (i.e., extending the fingers)?

8 Contrast the underlying pathomechanics in the swan-neck and boutonniere deformities.

9 Which of three intrinsic muscles illustrated in Figure 8-48 has the greatest moment arm for flexion of the metacarpophalangeal joint of the index finger?

10 Clinicians frequently splint the hand of a person with a fractured metacarpal bone in a position of the flexion of the metacarpophalangeal joint and near extension of the interphalangeal joint. What is the reason for doing this? Which muscle could eventually become tight (contracted) from this prolonged position?

11 A person with a damaged ulnar nerve at the level of the pisiform bone typically shows marked weakness of adduction of the carpometacarpal joint of the thumb. Why would this be? Which muscle could substitute for some of the loss of adduction at this joint?

12 How does the saddle-shaped joint structure of the carpometacarpal joint of the thumb influence the arthrokinematics of flexion and extension and abduction and adduction?

13 Rank the passive mobility of the carpometacarpal joints of the hand from least to most. What is the functional significance of this mobility pattern?

14 A patient shows marked weakness in the active movements of abduction and adduction of the fingers and in making a "key pinch." In addition, the patient shows atrophy of the muscles of the hypothenar eminence and decreased sensation over the ulnar border of the hand and distal forearm. Based on information displayed in Appendix II, Parts A through D, which spinal nerve roots are most likely associated with these impairments?

15 Assume a person has a completely lacerated flexor digitorum profundus (FDP) tendon of the ring finger at the level of the A_4 pulley. Furthermore, the person reports that attempts at making a fist result in *extension* rather than flexion of the distal interphalangeal joint of the ring finger. (This observation is often referred to by clinicians as "paradoxic extension.") Please offer a possible kinesiologic explanation for this phenomenon.

⊖ *Answers to the study questions can be found on the Evolve website.*

Reference Materials for Muscle Attachments and Innervation of the Upper Extremity

Part A: Spinal Nerve Root Innervation of the Muscles of the Upper Extremity

Muscle	C¹	C²	C³	C⁴	C⁵	C⁶	C⁷	C⁸	T¹
Serratus anterior					X	X	X	*X*	
Rhomboids, major and minor				*X*	X				
Subclavius					X	X			
Supraspinatus				*X*	X	X			
Infraspinatus					X	X			
Subscapularis					X	X	*X*		
Latissimus dorsi						X	X	X	
Teres major					*X*	X	*X*		
Pectoralis major (clavicular)					X	X			
Pectoralis major (sternocostal)						*X*	*X*	X	X
Pectoralis minor							*X*	X	*X*
Teres minor					X	X			
Deltoid					X	X			
Coracobrachialis						X	X		
Biceps					X	X			
Brachialis					X	X			
Triceps						*X*	X	X	*X*
Anconeus							X	X	
Brachioradialis					X	X			
Extensor carpi radialis longus and brevis					*X*	X	X	*X*	
Supinator					*X*	X			
Extensor digitorum						X	X	X	
Extensor digiti minimi						*X*	X	X	
Extensor carpi ulnaris						*X*	X	X	
Abductor pollicis longus						*X*	X	X	
Extensor pollicis brevis						*X*	X	X	
Extensor pollicis longus						*X*	X	X	
Extensor indicis						*X*	X	X	
Pronator teres						X	X		
Flexor carpi radialis						X	X	*X*	
Palmaris longus							X	X	*X*
Flexor digit. superficialis							X	X	X
Flexor digit. profundus I and II							*X*	X	X
Flexor pollicis longus							*X*	X	X
Pronator quadratus							*X*	X	X
Abductor pollicis brevis						*X*	*X*	X	*X*
Opponens pollicis						*X*	*X*	X	*X*
Flexor pollicis brevis						*X*	*X*	*X*	*X*
Lumbricals I and II							*X*	X	X
Flexor carpi ulnaris							*X*	X	*X*
Flexor digit. profundus III and IV							*X*	X	X
Palmaris brevis								X	X
Abductor digiti minimi								X	X
Opponens digiti minimi								X	X
Flexor digiti minimi								X	X
Palmar interossei								X	X
Dorsal interossei								X	X
Lumbricals III and IV								X	X
Adductor pollicis								X	X

Modified from Kendall FP, McCreary EK, Provance PG, et al: *Muscles: testing and function with posture and pain*, ed 5. Philadelphia, 2005, Lippincott Williams & Wilkins.
X, Minor-to-moderate distribution; **X**, major distribution.

Part B: Five Major Nerves and Their Motor Innervation Pattern throughout the Upper Extremity

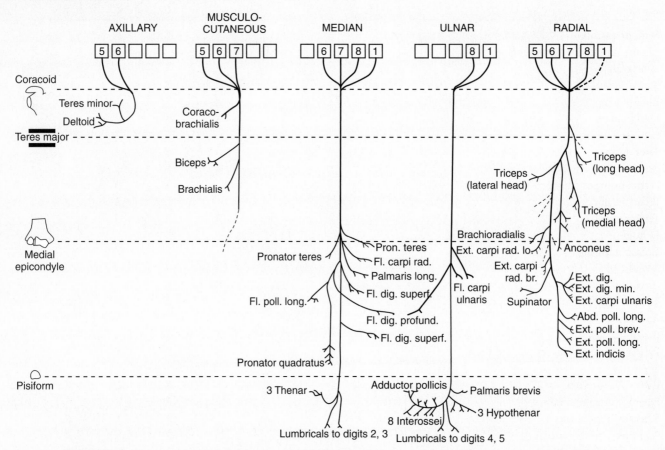

FIGURE II-1. Motor innervations of the upper extremity. (From Swanson AB, de Groot Swanson G: Principles and methods of impairment evaluation in the hand and upper extremity. In American Medical Association: *Guides to the evaluation of permanent impairment*, ed 4, Chicago, 1993, American Medical Association.)

Part C: Key Muscles for Testing the Function of Spinal Nerve Roots (C^5 to T^1)

The table shows the key muscles typically used to test the function of individual nerve roots of the brachial plexus (C^5-T^1). Reduced strength in a key muscle may indicate an injury to or pathologic process within the associated nerve root.

Key Muscles	Nerve Root	Sample Test Movements
Biceps brachii	C^5	Elbow flexion with forearm supinated
Middle deltoid	C^5	Shoulder abduction
Extensor carpi radialis longus	C^6	Wrist extension with radial deviation
Triceps brachii	C^7	Elbow extension
Extensor digitorum	C^7	Finger extension (metacarpophalangeal joint only)
Flexor digitorum profundus	C^8	Finger flexion (distal interphalangeal joint)
Dorsal and palmar interossei	T^1	Finger abduction and adduction

Part D: Dermatomes of the Upper Extremity

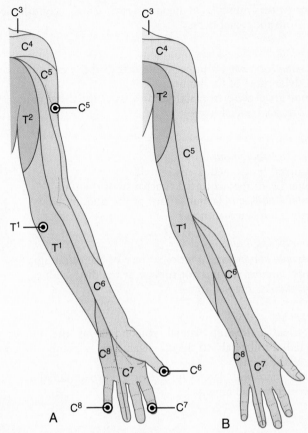

FIGURE II-2. Dermatomes of the upper limb. **A,** Anterior view of the left side. **B,** Posterior (dorsal) view of the right side. Bold dots indicate regions often used clinically to test each dermatome. Variations are common. C^7, seventh cervical nerve root; T^1, first thoracic nerve root; and so on. (Modified from Drake R, Vogl W, Mitchell A: Gray's Anatomy for Students. Philadelphia: Churchill Livingstone, 2005.)

Part E: Attachments and Innervation of the Muscles of the Upper Extremity

SHOULDER MUSCULATURE

Coracobrachialis
Proximal attachment: apex of the coracoid process by a common tendon with the short head of the biceps
Distal attachment: medial aspect of middle shaft of the humerus
Innervation: musculocutaneous nerve

Deltoid
Proximal attachments:
Anterior part: anterior surface of the lateral end of the clavicle
Middle part: superior surface of the lateral edge of the acromion
Posterior part: posterior border of the spine of the scapula
Distal attachment: deltoid tuberosity of the humerus
Innervation: axillary nerve

Infraspinatus
Proximal attachment: infraspinatous fossa
Distal attachment: middle facet of the greater tubercle of the humerus; part of the capsule of the glenohumeral joint
Innervation: suprascapular nerve

Latissimus Dorsi
Proximal attachments: posterior layer of the thoracolumbar fascia, spinous processes and supraspinous ligaments of the lower half of the thoracic vertebrae and all lumbar vertebrae, median sacral crest, posterior crest of the ilium, lower four ribs, small area near the inferior angle of the scapula, and muscular interdigitations from the obliquus external abdominis
Distal attachment: floor of the intertubercular groove of the humerus
Innervation: thoracodorsal (middle subscapular) nerve

Levator Scapula
Proximal attachments: transverse processes of C1 and C2 and posterior tubercles of transverse processes of C3 and C4
Distal attachment: medial border of the scapula between the superior angle and root of the spine
Innervation: ventral rami of spinal nerves (C^3-C^4) and the dorsal scapular nerve

Pectoralis Major
Proximal attachments:
Clavicular head: anterior margin of the medial one half of the clavicle
Sternocostal head: lateral margin of the manubrium and body of the sternum and cartilages of the first six or seven ribs; costal fibers blend with muscular slips from obliquus external abdominis
Distal attachment: crest of the greater tubercle of the humerus
Innervation: lateral and medial pectoral nerves

Pectoralis Minor
Proximal attachments: external surfaces of the third through the fifth ribs
Distal attachment: medial border of the coracoid process
Innervation: medial pectoral nerve

Rhomboid Major and Minor
Proximal attachments: ligamentous nuchae and spinous processes of C7 to T5
Distal attachment: medial border of scapula, from the root of the spine to the inferior angle
Innervation: dorsal scapular nerve

Serratus Anterior
Proximal attachments: external surface of the lateral region of the first to ninth ribs
Distal attachment: entire medial border of the scapula, with a concentration of fibers near the inferior angle
Innervation: long thoracic nerve

Subclavius
Proximal attachment: at the extreme anterior end of the first rib
Distal attachment: inferior middle third of the clavicle
Innervation: subclavian nerve

Subscapularis

Proximal attachment: subscapular fossa
Distal attachment: lesser tubercle of the humerus; part of the capsule of the glenohumeral joint
Innervation: upper and lower subscapular nerves

Supraspinatus

Proximal attachment: supraspinatus fossa
Distal attachment: upper facet of the greater tubercle of the humerus; part of the capsule of the glenohumeral joint
Innervation: suprascapular nerve

Teres Major

Proximal attachment: inferior angle of the scapula
Distal attachment: crest of the lesser tubercle of the humerus
Innervation: lower subscapular nerve

Teres Minor

Proximal attachment: posterior surface of the lateral border of the scapula
Distal attachment: lower facet of the greater tubercle of the humerus; part of the capsule of the glenohumeral joint
Innervation: axillary nerve

Trapezius

Proximal attachments (all parts): medial part of superior nuchal line and external occipital protuberance, ligamentum nuchae, spinous processes and supraspinous ligaments of the seventh cervical vertebra and all thoracic vertebrae
Distal attachments:
Upper part: posterior-superior edge of the lateral one third of the clavicle
Middle part: medial margin of the acromion and upper lip of the spine of the scapula
Lower part: medial end of the spine of the scapula, just lateral to the root
Innervation: primarily by the spinal accessory nerve (cranial nerve XI); secondary innervation directly from ventral rami of C^2-C^4

ELBOW AND FOREARM MUSCULATURE

Anconeus

Proximal attachment: posterior side of the lateral epicondyle of the humerus
Distal attachment: between the olecranon process and proximal surface of the posterior side of the ulna
Innervation: radial nerve

Biceps Brachii

Proximal attachments:
Long head: supraglenoid tubercle of the scapula
Short head: apex of the coracoid process of the scapula
Distal attachments: bicipital tuberosity of the radius; also to deep connective tissue within the forearm via the fibrous lacertus
Innervation: musculocutaneous nerve

Brachialis

Proximal attachment: distal aspect of the anterior surface of the humerus
Distal attachments: coronoid process and tuberosity on the proximal ulna
Innervation: musculocutaneous nerve (small contribution from the radial nerve)

Brachioradialis

Proximal attachment: upper two thirds of the lateral supracondylar ridge of the humerus
Distal attachment: near styloid process at the distal radius
Innervation: radial nerve

Pronator Teres

Proximal attachments:
Humeral head: medial epicondyle
Ulnar head: medial to the tuberosity of the ulna
Distal attachment: lateral surface of the middle radius
Innervation: median nerve

Pronator Quadratus

Proximal attachment: anterior surface of the distal ulna
Distal attachment: anterior surface of the distal radius
Innervation: median nerve

Supinator

Proximal attachments: lateral epicondyle of the humerus, radial collateral and annular ligaments, and supinator crest of the ulna
Distal attachment: lateral surface of the proximal radius
Innervation: radial nerve

Triceps Brachii

Proximal attachments:
Long head: infraglenoid tubercle of the scapula
Lateral head: posterior humerus, superior and lateral to the radial groove
Medial head: posterior humerus, inferior and medial to the radial groove
Distal attachment: olecranon process of the ulna
Innervation: radial nerve

WRIST MUSCULATURE

Extensor Carpi Radialis Brevis

Proximal attachment: common extensor-supinator tendon attaching to the lateral epicondyle of the humerus
Distal attachment: radial-posterior surface of the base of the third metacarpal
Innervation: radial nerve

Extensor Carpi Radialis Longus

Proximal attachments: common extensor-supinator tendon attaching to the lateral epicondyle of the humerus and the distal part of the lateral supracondylar ridge of the humerus
Distal attachment: radial-posterior surface of the base of the second metacarpal
Innervation: radial nerve

Extensor Carpi Ulnaris

Proximal attachments: common extensor-supinator tendon attaching to the lateral epicondyle of the humerus and the posterior border of the middle one third of the ulna

Distal attachment: posterior-ulnar surface of the base of the fifth metacarpal
Innervation: radial nerve

Flexor Carpi Radialis

Proximal attachment: common flexor-pronator tendon attaching to the medial epicondyle of the humerus
Distal attachments: palmar surface of the base of the second metacarpal and a small slip to the base of the third metacarpal
Innervation: median nerve

Flexor Carpi Ulnaris

Proximal attachments:
Humeral head: common flexor-pronator tendon attaching to the medial epicondyle of the humerus
Ulnar head: posterior border of the middle one third of the ulna
Distal attachments: pisiform bone, pisohamate and pisometacarpal ligaments, and palmar base of the fifth metacarpal bone
Innervation: ulnar nerve

Palmaris Longus

Proximal attachment: common flexor-pronator tendon attaching to the medial epicondyle of the humerus
Distal attachment: central part of the transverse carpal ligament and palmar aponeurosis of the hand
Innervation: median nerve

EXTRINSIC HAND MUSCULATURE

Abductor Pollicis Longus

Proximal attachments: posterior surface of the middle part of the radius and ulna, and adjacent interosseous membrane
Distal attachments: radial-dorsal surface of the base of the thumb metacarpal; occasional secondary attachments to the trapezium and thenar muscles
Innervation: radial nerve

Extensor Digitorum

Proximal attachment: common extensor-supinator tendon attaching to the lateral epicondyle of the humerus
Distal attachments: by four tendons, each to the base of the extensor mechanism and to the dorsal base of the proximal phalanx of the fingers
Innervation: radial nerve

Extensor Digiti Minimi

Proximal attachment: ulnar side of the belly of the extensor digitorum
Distal attachments: tendon usually divides, joining the ulnar side of the tendon of the extensor digitorum
Innervation: radial nerve

Extensor Indicis

Proximal attachments: posterior surface of the middle to distal part of the ulna and adjacent interosseous membrane
Distal attachment: tendon blends with the ulnar side of the index tendon of the extensor digitorum
Innervation: radial nerve

Extensor Pollicis Brevis

Proximal attachments: posterior surface of the middle to distal parts of the radius and adjacent interosseous membrane
Distal attachment: dorsal base of the proximal phalanx and extensor mechanism of the thumb
Innervation: radial nerve

Extensor Pollicis Longus

Proximal attachments: posterior surface of the middle part of the ulna and adjacent interosseous membrane
Distal attachment: dorsal base of the distal phalanx and extensor mechanism of the thumb
Innervation: radial nerve

Flexor Digitorum Profundus

Proximal attachments: proximal three fourths of the anterior and medial side of the ulna and adjacent interosseous membrane
Distal attachments: by four tendons, each to the palmar base of the distal phalanges of the fingers
Innervation:
Medial half: ulnar nerve
Lateral half: median nerve

Flexor Digitorum Superficialis

Proximal attachments:
Humeroulnar head: common flexor-pronator tendon attaching to the medial epicondyle of the humerus and the medial side of the coronoid process of the ulna
Radial head: oblique line just distal and lateral to the bicipital tuberosity
Distal attachments: by four tendons, each to the sides of the middle phalanges of the fingers
Innervation: median nerve

Flexor Pollicis Longus

Proximal attachments: middle part of the anterior surface of the radius and adjacent interosseous membrane
Distal attachment: palmar base of the distal phalanx of the thumb
Innervation: median nerve

INTRINSIC HAND MUSCULATURE

Abductor Digiti Minimi

Proximal attachments: pisohamate ligament, pisiform bone, and tendon of the flexor carpi ulnaris
Distal attachments: ulnar side of the base of the proximal phalanx of the little finger; also attaches into the extensor mechanism of the little finger
Innervation: ulnar nerve

Abductor Pollicis Brevis

Proximal attachments: transverse carpal ligament, palmar tubercles of the trapezium and scaphoid bones
Distal attachments: radial side of the base of the proximal phalanx of the thumb; also attaches into the extensor mechanism of the thumb
Innervation: median nerve

Adductor Pollicis

Proximal attachments:

Oblique head: capitate bone, base of the second and third metacarpal, and adjacent capsular ligaments of the carpometacarpal joints

Transverse head: palmar surface of the third metacarpal

Distal attachments: both heads attach on the ulnar side of the base of the proximal phalanx of the thumb and to the medial sesamoid bone at the metacarpophalangeal joint; also attaches into the extensor mechanism of the thumb

Innervation: ulnar nerve

Dorsal Interossei

Proximal attachments:

First: adjacent sides of the first (thumb) and second metacarpal

Second: adjacent sides of the second and third metacarpal

Third: adjacent sides of the third and fourth metacarpal

Fourth: adjacent sides of the fourth and fifth metacarpal

Distal attachments:

First: radial sides of the oblique fibers of the dorsal hood and base of the proximal phalanx of the index finger

Second: radial sides of the oblique fibers of the dorsal hood and base of the proximal phalanx of the middle finger

Third: ulnar sides of the oblique fibers of the dorsal hood and base of the proximal phalanx of the middle finger

Fourth: ulnar sides of the oblique fibers of the dorsal hood and base of the proximal phalanx of the ring finger

Innervation: ulnar nerve

Flexor Digiti Minimi

Proximal attachments: transverse carpal ligament and hook of the hamate

Distal attachment: ulnar side of the base of the proximal phalanx of the little finger

Innervation: ulnar nerve

Flexor Pollicis Brevis

Proximal attachments: transverse carpal ligament and palmar tubercle of the trapezium

Distal attachments: radial side of the base of the proximal phalanx of the thumb; also to the lateral sesamoid bone at the metacarpophalangeal joint

Innervation: median nerve

Lumbricals

Proximal attachments:

Medial two: adjacent sides of the flexor digitorum profundus tendons of the little, ring, and middle fingers

Lateral two: lateral sides of the flexor digitorum profundus tendons of the middle and index fingers

Distal attachment: lateral margin of the extensor mechanism via the oblique fibers of the dorsal hood

Innervation:

Medial two: ulnar nerve

Lateral two: median nerve

Opponens Digiti Minimi

Proximal attachments: transverse carpal ligament and hook of the hamate

Distal attachment: ulnar surface of the shaft of the fifth metacarpal

Innervation: ulnar nerve

Opponens Pollicis

Proximal attachments: transverse carpal ligament and palmar tubercle of the trapezium

Distal attachment: radial surface of the shaft of the thumb metacarpal

Innervation: median nerve

Palmaris Brevis

Proximal attachments: transverse carpal ligament and palmar fascia just distal and lateral to the pisiform bone

Distal attachment: skin on the ulnar border of the hand

Innervation: ulnar nerve

Palmar Interossei

Proximal attachments:

First: ulnar side of the thumb metacarpal

Second: ulnar side of the second metacarpal

Third: radial side of the fourth metacarpal

Fourth: radial side of the fifth metacarpal

Distal attachments:

First: ulnar side of the proximal phalanx of the thumb, blending with the adductor pollicis; also attaches to the medial sesamoid bone at the metacarpophalangeal joint

Second: ulnar sides of the oblique fibers of the dorsal hood and base of the proximal phalanx of the index finger

Third: radial sides of the oblique fibers of the dorsal hood and base of the proximal phalanx of the ring finger

Fourth: radial sides of the oblique fibers of the dorsal hood and base of the proximal phalanx of the small finger

Innervation: ulnar nerve

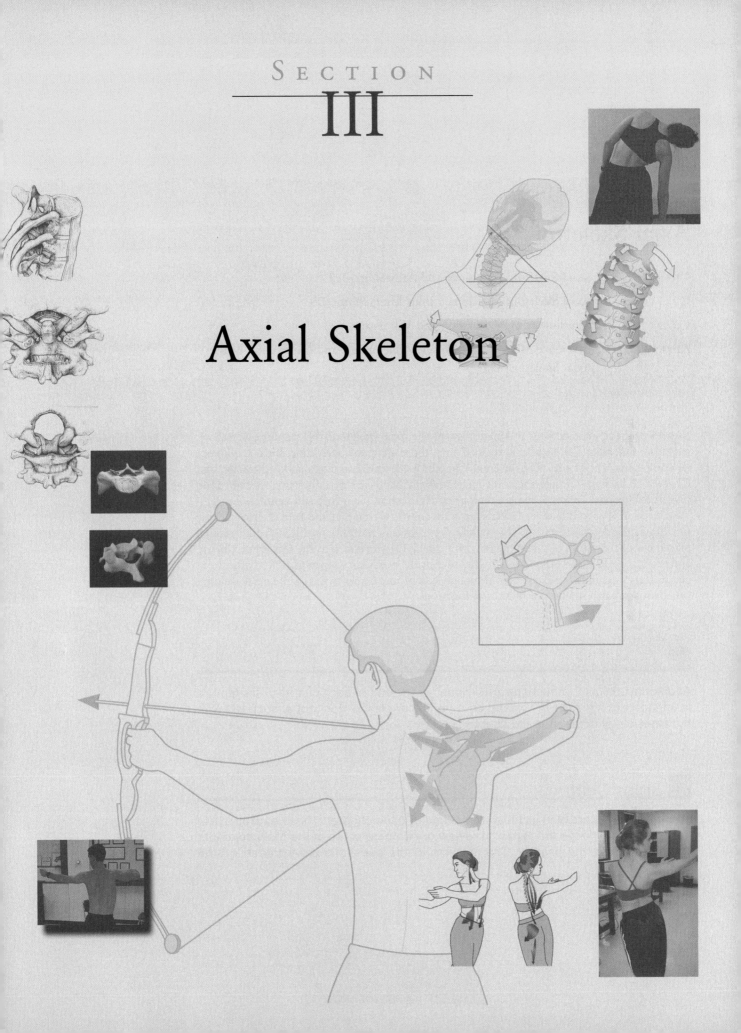

Axial Skeleton

Axial Skeleton

SECTION III focuses on the kinesiology of the axial skeleton: the cranium, vertebrae, sternum, and ribs. The section is divided into three chapters, each describing a different kinesiologic aspect of the axial skeleton. Chapter 9 presents osteology and arthrology, and Chapter 10 presents muscle and joint interactions. Chapter 11 describes two special topics related to the axial skeleton: the kinesiology of mastication (chewing) and ventilation.

Section III presents several overlapping functions that involve the axial skeleton. These functions include providing (1) "core stability" plus overall mobility to the body; (2) optimal placement of the senses of vision, hearing, and smell; (3) protection to the spinal cord, brain, and internal organs; and (4) bodily activities such as the mechanics of ventilation, mastication, childbirth, coughing, and defecation. Musculoskeletal impairments within the axial skeleton can cause limitation in any of these four functions.

▌ ADDITIONAL CLINICAL CONNECTIONS

Additional Clinical Connections are included at the end of each chapter. This feature is intended to highlight or expand on a particular clinical concept associated with the kinesiology covered in the chapter.

▌ STUDY QUESTIONS

Study Questions are also included at the end of each chapter. These questions are designed to challenge the reader to review or reinforce some of the main concepts contained within the chapter. The answers to the questions are included on the Evolve website ⊖.

Axial Skeleton: Osteology and Arthrology

DONALD A. NEUMANN, PT, PhD, FAPTA

The skeleton as a whole is divided into the axial skeleton and the appendicular skeleton. The *appendicular skeleton* consists of the bones of the extremities, including the clavicle, scapula, and pelvis; the *axial skeleton,* in contrast, consists of the cranium, vertebral column (spine), ribs, and sternum (Figure 9-1). As indicated in Figure 9-1, *A,* the axial and appendicular skeletons are joined by the sternoclavicular joints superiorly and the sacroiliac joints inferiorly.

The osteology and associated arthrology presented in this chapter focus primarily on the axial skeleton. This focus includes the craniocervical region, vertebral column, and sacroiliac joints, describing how these articulations provide stability, movement, and load transfer throughout the axial skeleton. Muscles play a large role in this function and are the primary focus of Chapter 10.

Disease, trauma, overuse, and normal aging can cause a host of neuromuscular and musculoskeletal problems involving the axial skeleton. Disorders of the vertebral column are often associated with neurologic impairment, primarily because of the close anatomic relationship between neural tissue (spinal cord and nerve roots) and connective tissue (vertebrae and associated ligaments, intervertebral discs, and synovial joints). A "slipped" or herniated disc, for example, can increase pressure on the adjacent neural tissues, resulting in local inflammation and also weakness, sensory disturbances, and reduced reflexes throughout the lower limb. To further complicate matters, certain movements and habitual postures of the vertebral column increase the likelihood of connective tissues impinging on neural tissues. An understanding of the detailed osteology and arthrology of the axial skeleton is crucial to an appreciation of the associated pathomechanics, as well as the rationale for many clinical tests and interventions.

Table 9-1 summarizes the terminology used to describe the relative location or region within the axial skeleton.

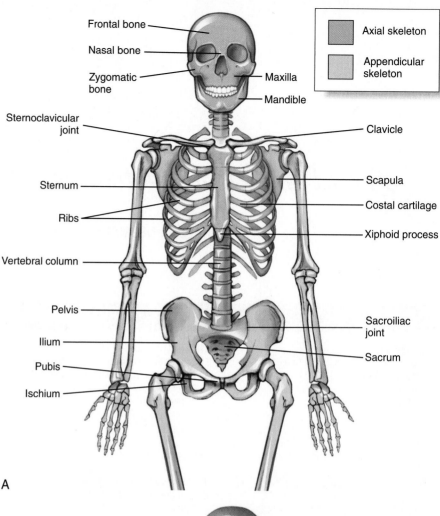

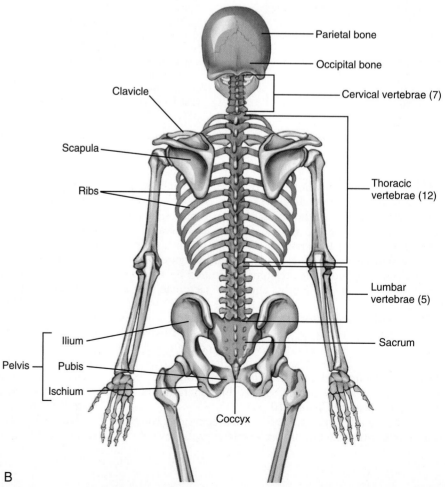

FIGURE 9-1. Human skeleton. **A,** Anterior view. **B,** Posterior view. The axial skeleton is highlighted in blue. (From Thibodeau GA, Patton KT: *Structure and function of the body*, ed 13, St Louis, 2008, Mosby.)

TABLE 9-1. **Terminology Describing Relative Location or Region within the Axial Skeleton**		
Term	**Synonym**	**Definition**
Posterior	Dorsal	Back of the body
Anterior	Ventral	Front of the body
Medial	None	Midline of the body
Lateral	None	Away from the midline of the body
Superior	Cranial	Head or top of the body
Inferior	Caudal (the "tail")	Tail, or the bottom of the body

The definitions assume a person is in the anatomic position.

OSTEOLOGY

Components within the Axial Skeleton

CRANIUM

The cranium encases and protects the brain and several essential sensory organs (eyes, ears, nose, and vestibular system). Of the many individual bones of the cranium, only the temporal and occipital bones are relevant to the material covered in Chapters 9 and 10.

Temporal and Occipital Bones

Each of the two *temporal* bones forms part of the lateral external surface of the skull, immediately surrounding and including the external acoustic meatus (Figure 9-2). The *mastoid process*, an easily palpable structure, is just posterior to the ear. This prominent process serves as an attachment for many muscles, such as the sternocleidomastoid.

The *occipital bone* forms much of the posterior base of the skull (Figure 9-3). The *external occipital protuberance* is a palpable midline point, serving as an attachment for the ligamentum nuchae and the medial part of the upper trapezius muscle. The *superior nuchal line* extends laterally from the

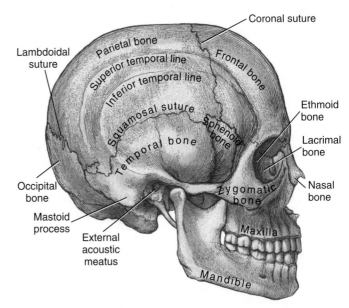

FIGURE 9-2. Lateral view of the skull.

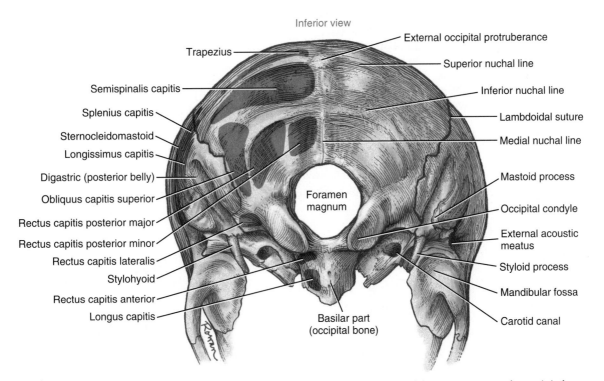

FIGURE 9-3. Inferior view of the occipital and temporal bones. The lambdoidal sutures separate the occipital bone medially, from the temporal bones laterally. Distal muscle attachments are indicated in gray, and proximal attachments are indicated in red.

external occipital protuberance to the base of the mastoid process of the temporal bone. This thin but distinct line marks the attachments of several extensor muscles of the head and neck, such as the trapezius and splenius capitis muscles. The *inferior nuchal line* marks the anterior edge of the attachment of the semispinalis capitis muscle.

Relevant Osteologic Features

Temporal Bone
- Mastoid process

Occipital Bone
- External occipital protuberance
- Superior nuchal line
- Inferior nuchal line
- Foramen magnum
- Occipital condyles
- Basilar part

The *foramen magnum* is a large circular hole located at the base of the occipital bone, serving as the passageway for the spinal cord. A pair of prominent *occipital condyles* projects from the anterior-lateral margins of the foramen magnum, forming the convex component of the atlanto-occipital joint. The *basilar part* of the occipital bone lies just anterior to the anterior rim of the foramen magnum.

VERTEBRAE: BUILDING BLOCKS OF THE SPINE

In addition to providing vertical stability throughout the trunk and neck, the vertebral column protects the spinal cord, ventral and dorsal nerve roots, and exiting spinal nerve roots (Figure 9-4). The relationship between the spinal cord and exiting nerve roots throughout the entire vertebral column is schematically shown in Figure III-1 in Appendix III, Part A.

The midthoracic vertebrae demonstrate many of the essential anatomic and functional characteristics of any given vertebra (Figure 9-5). As a general orientation, a given vertebra can be subdivided into three sections. Anteriorly is the large vertebral *body*–the primary weight-bearing component of a vertebra. Posteriorly are the transverse and spinous processes,

laminae, and articular processes, collectively referred to as *posterior elements* (also referred to as the "vertebral arch" or "neural arch"). The *pedicles*, the third section, act as bridges that connect the body with the posterior elements. Thick and strong, the pedicles transfer muscle forces applied to the posterior elements forward, for dispersion across the vertebral body and intervertebral discs. Table 9-2 provides greater details on the structure and function of the components of a typical midthoracic vertebra.

RIBS

Twelve pairs of ribs enclose the thoracic cavity, forming a protective cage for the cardiopulmonary organs. The posterior end of a typical rib has a *head*, a *neck*, and an *articular*

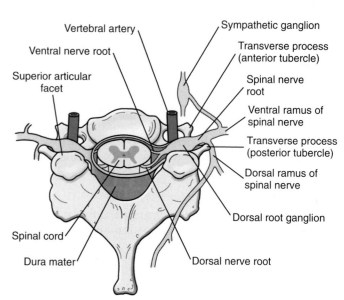

FIGURE 9-4. A cross-section of a spinal cord is shown. Note the relationship among the neural tissues, components of the cervical vertebra, and the vertebral artery. (Modified with permission from Magee DL: Orthopedic physical assessment, ed 3, Philadelphia, 1997, Saunders.)

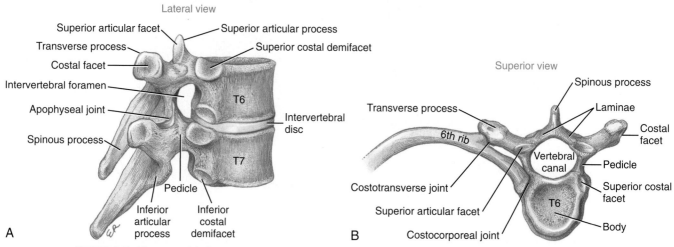

FIGURE 9-5. The essential characteristics of a vertebra. **A,** Lateral view of the sixth and seventh vertebrae (T6 and T7). **B,** Superior view of the sixth vertebra with right rib.

TABLE 9-2. Major Parts of a Midthoracic Vertebra

Part	Description	Primary Function
Body	Large cylindric mass of trabecular bone lined by a thin cortex of bone. The multidirectional trabecular core is lightweight while still offering excellent resistance against compression.	Primary weight-bearing structure of each vertebra.
Intervertebral disc	Thick ring of fibrocartilage between vertebral bodies of C2 and below.	Shock absorber and spacer throughout the vertebral column.
Interbody joint	A cartilaginous joint joint formed between the superior and inferior surfaces of an intervertebral disc and adjacent vertebral bodies.	Primary bond between vertebrae.
Pedicle	Short, thick dorsal projection of bone from the mid-to-superior part of the vertebral body.	Connects the vertebral body to the posterior elements of a vertebra.
Lamina	Thin vertical plate of bone connecting the base of the spinous process to each transverse process. (The term *laminae* refers to both right and left laminae.)	Protects the posterior aspect of the spinal cord.
Vertebral canal	Central canal located just posterior to the vertebral body. The canal is surrounded by the pedicles and laminae.	Houses and protects the spinal cord.
Intervertebral foramen	Lateral opening between adjacent vertebrae.	Passageway for spinal nerve roots exiting the vertebral canal.
Transverse process	Horizontal projection of bone from the junction of a lamina and a pedicle.	Attachments for muscles, ligaments, and ribs.
Costal facets (on body)	Rounded impressions formed on the lateral sides of the thoracic vertebral bodies. Most thoracic vertebral bodies have partial superior and inferior facets (called *demifacets*).	Attachment sites for the heads of ribs (costocorporeal joints).
Costal facets (on transverse process)	Oval facets located at the anterior tips of most thoracic transverse processes.	Attachment sites for the articular tubercle of ribs (costotransverse joints).
Spinous process	Dorsal midline projection of bone from the laminae.	Midline attachments for muscles and ligaments.
Superior and inferior articular processes, including articular facets and apophyseal joints	Paired vertical articular processes arising from the junction of a lamina and pedicle. Each process has smooth cartilage-lined articular facets. In general, superior articular facets face posteriorly, and inferior articular facets face anteriorly.	Superior and inferior articular facets form paired apophyseal joints. These synovial joints guide the direction and magnitude of intervertebral movement.

tubercle (Figure 9-6). The head and tubercle articulate with a thoracic vertebra, forming two synovial joints: costocorporeal (also called costo*vertebral*) and costotransverse, respectively (see Figure 9-5, *B*).[188] These joints anchor the posterior end of a rib to its corresponding vertebra. A typical *costocorporeal joint* connects the head of a rib to a pair of *costal demifacets* that span two adjacent vertebrae and the intervening intervertebral disc. A *costotransverse joint* connects the articular tubercle of a rib with a costal facet on the transverse process of a corresponding vertebra.

The anterior end of a rib consists of flattened hyaline cartilage. Ribs 1 through 10 attach either directly or indirectly to the sternum, thereby completing the thoracic rib cage anteriorly. The cartilage of ribs 1 to 7 attaches directly to the lateral border of the sternum via seven sternocostal joints (Figure 9-7). The cartilage of ribs 8 to 10 attaches to the sternum by fusing to the cartilage of the immediately superior rib. Ribs 11 and 12 do not attach to the sternum but are anchored by lateral abdominal muscles.

STERNUM

The sternum is slightly convex and rough anteriorly, and slightly concave and smooth posteriorly. The bone has three parts: the manubrium (Latin, meaning "handle"), the body, and the xiphoid process (from the Greek, "sword") (see Figure 9-7). Developmentally, the *manubrium* fuses with the body of the sternum at the *manubriosternal joint,* a cartilaginous (synarthrodial) articulation that often ossifies later in life.[188] Just lateral to the *jugular notch* of the manubrium are the *clavicular facets* of the *sternoclavicular joints.* Immediately inferior to the sternoclavicular joint is a *costal facet* that accepts the head of the first rib at the first *sternocostal joint.*

Osteologic Features of the Sternum
- Manubrium
- Jugular notch
- Clavicular facets for sternoclavicular joints
- Body
- Costal facets for sternocostal joints
- Xiphoid process

Intrasternal Joints
- Manubriosternal joint
- Xiphisternal joint

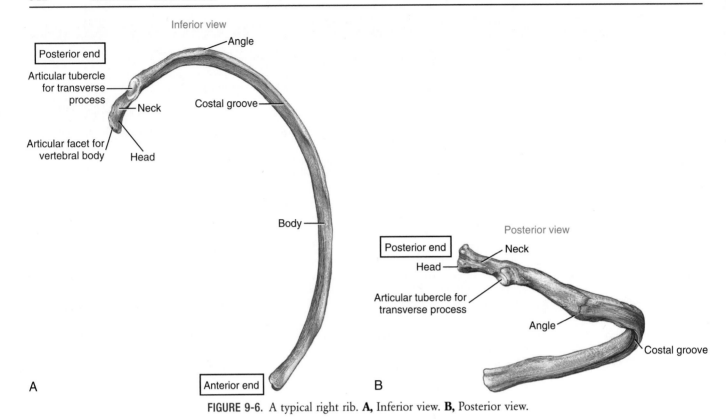

Inferior view

Posterior end

Articular tubercle
for transverse
process

Neck

Articular facet for
vertebral body

Head

Angle

Costal groove

Body

A   Anterior end

Posterior view

Posterior end

Neck

Head

Articular tubercle for
transverse process

Angle

Costal groove

B

FIGURE 9-6. A typical right rib. **A,** Inferior view. **B,** Posterior view.

The lateral edge of the body of the sternum is marked by a series of *costal facets* that accept the cartilages of ribs 2 to 7. The arthrology of the sternocostal joints is discussed in greater detail in Chapter 11, within the context of ventilation. The *xiphoid process* is attached to the inferior end of the body of the sternum by the *xiphisternal joint.* Like the manubriosternal joint, the xiphisternal joint is connected primarily by fibrocartilage. The xiphisternal joint often ossifies by 40 years of age.[188]

Vertebral Column as a Whole

The *vertebral (spinal) column* consists of the entire set of vertebrae. The word "trunk" is a general term that describes the body of a person, including the sternum, ribs, and pelvis but excluding the head, neck, and limbs.

The vertebral column usually consists of 33 vertebral bony *segments* divided into five regions. Normally there are seven *cervical,* twelve *thoracic,* five *lumbar,* five *sacral,* and four *coccygeal segments.* The sacral and coccygeal vertebrae are usually fused in the adult, forming individual sacral and coccygeal bones. Individual vertebrae are abbreviated alphanumerically; for example, C2 for the second cervical, T6 for the sixth thoracic, and L1 for the first lumbar. Each region of the vertebral column (e.g., cervical and lumbar) has a distinct morphology that reflects its specific function and movement potential. Vertebrae located at the cervicothoracic, thoracolumbar, and lumbosacral junctions often share characteristics that reflect the transition between major regions of the vertebral column. It is not uncommon, for example, for the transverse processes of C7 to have thoracic-like facets to accept a rib, or L5 may be "sacralized" (i.e., fused with the base of the sacrum).

NORMAL CURVATURES WITHIN THE VERTEBRAL COLUMN

The human vertebral column consists of a series of reciprocal curvatures within the sagittal plane (Figure 9-8, *A*). These natural curvatures contribute to "ideal" spinal posture while one is standing. The curvatures also define the *neutral position* of the different regions of the spine. In the neutral (anatomic) position, the cervical and lumbar regions are naturally convex anteriorly and concave posteriorly, exhibiting an alignment called *lordosis,* meaning to "bend backward." The degree of lordosis is usually less in the cervical region than in the lumbar region. The thoracic and sacrococcygeal regions, in contrast, exhibit a natural *kyphosis.* Kyphosis describes a curve that is concave anteriorly and convex posteriorly. The anterior concavity provides space for the organs within the thoracic and pelvic cavities.

The natural curvatures within the vertebral column are not fixed but are dynamic and change shape during movements and adjustment of posture. Further extension of the vertebral column accentuates the cervical and lumbar lordosis but reduces the thoracic kyphosis (see Figure 9-8, *B*). In contrast, flexion of the vertebral column decreases, or flattens, the cervical and lumbar lordosis but accentuates the thoracic kyphosis (see Figure 9-8, *C*). In contrast, the sacrococcygeal curvature is fixed, being concave anteriorly and convex posteriorly.

The embryonic vertebral column is kyphotic throughout its length. Lordosis in the cervical and lumbar regions occurs after birth, in association with motor maturation and the assumption of a more upright posture. In the cervical spine, extensor muscles pull on the head and neck as the prone-lying infant begins to observe the surroundings. More caudally, the

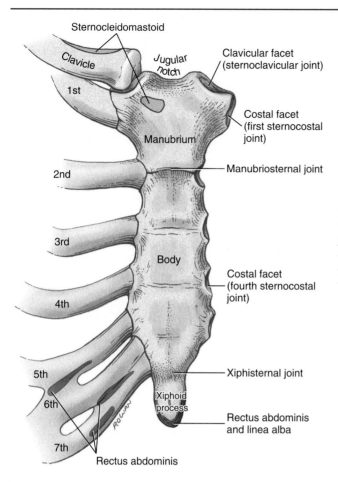

FIGURE 9-7. Anterior view of the sternum, part of the right clavicle, and the first seven ribs. The following articulations are seen: (1) intrasternal joints (manubriosternal and xiphisternal), (2) sternocostal joints, and (3) sternoclavicular joints. The attachment of the sternocleidomastoid muscle is indicated in red. The attachments of the rectus abdominis and linea alba are shown in gray.

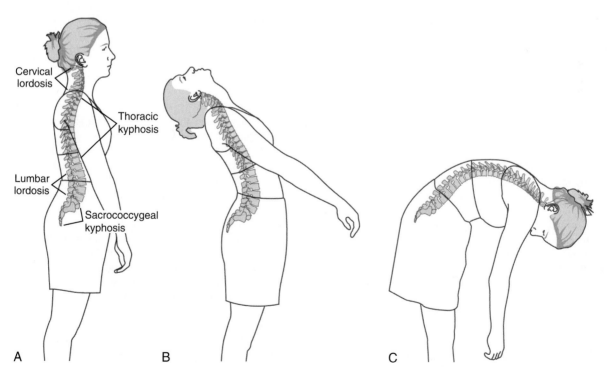

FIGURE 9-8. A side view shows the normal sagittal plane curvatures of the vertebral column. **A,** The neutral position while one is standing. **B,** Full extension of the vertebral column increases the cervical and lumbar lordosis but reduces (straightens) the thoracic kyphosis. **C,** Flexion of the vertebral column decreases the cervical and lumbar lordosis but increases the thoracic kyphosis.

developing hip flexor muscles pull inferiorly on the front of the pelvis as the infant starts walking. This muscular pull rotates (or tilts) the pelvis anteriorly relative to the hips, thereby positioning the lumbar spine into a relative lordosis. Once the child stands, the natural lordosis of the lumbar spine directs the body's line of gravity through or near the first lumbar vertebra (L1) and the base of the sacrum.

The sagittal plane curvatures within the vertebral column provide strength and resilience to the axial skeleton. A reciprocally curved vertebral column acts like an arch. Compression forces between vertebrae are partially shared by tension in stretched connective tissues and muscles located along the convex side of each curve. As is true with long bones such as the femur, the strength and stability of the vertebral column are derived, in part, from its ability to "give" slightly under a load, rather than to support large compression forces statically.

A potentially negative consequence of the natural spinal curvatures is the presence of shear forces at regions of transition between curves. Shear forces can cause premature loosening of surgical spinal fusions, especially those performed in the cervicothoracic and thoracolumbar regions.

LINE OF GRAVITY PASSING THROUGH THE BODY

Although highly variable, the line of gravity acting on a standing person with ideal posture passes near the mastoid process of the temporal bone, anterior to the second sacral vertebra, just posterior to the hip, and anterior to the knee and ankle (Figure 9-9). In the vertebral column, the line of gravity typically falls just to the concave side of the apex of each region's curvature. Ideal posture therefore allows gravity to produce a torque that helps maintain the optimal shape of the spinal curvatures. The external torque attributed to gravity is greatest at the apex of each region: C4 and C5, T6, and L3.

The image depicted in Figure 9-9 is more ideal than real because each person's posture is unique and transient. Factors that alter the spatial relationship between the line of gravity and the spinal curvatures include fat deposition, the specific shapes of the regional spinal curvatures, static posturing of the head and the limbs, muscle strength, connective tissue extensibility, and the position and magnitude of loads supported by the body. The particular orientation of the line of gravity relative to the axial skeleton has important biomechanical consequences on the stress placed on the region. For example, gravity passing posterior to the lumbar region produces a constant extension torque on the low back, facilitating natural lordosis. Alternatively, gravity passing anterior to the lumbar region produces a constant flexion torque. In both cases the external torque created by the line of gravity (and its associated external moment arm) must be neutralized by forces and torques produced actively by muscle and passively by connective tissues. In extreme postures, these forces may be high; if prolonged, they may lead to undesirable postural compensations as well as structural changes, often associated with pain.

Strictly anatomic factors can influence the unique shape of the spinal curves throughout the vertebral column; these include wedged-shaped intervertebral discs or vertebral bodies, spatial orientation of apophyseal (facet) joints, tension in ligaments, and the degree of natural muscle stiffness. The

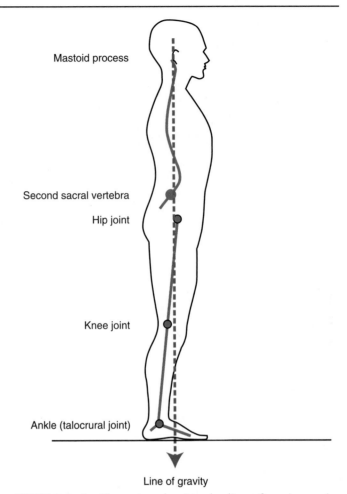

Mastoid process

Second sacral vertebra

Hip joint

Knee joint

Ankle (talocrural joint)

Line of gravity

FIGURE 9-9. An illustration showing the line of gravity passing through the body of a person standing with ideal posture. (Modified from Neumann DA: Arthrokinesiologic considerations for the aged adult. In Guccione AA, ed: *Geriatric physical therapy*, ed 2, Chicago, 2000, Mosby.)

intervertebral discs in the cervical and lower lumbar regions are slightly thicker anteriorly, for example, thereby favoring an anterior convexity in these regions.

The normal sagittal plane alignment of the vertebral column may be altered by disease, such as ankylosing spondylosis, poliomyelitis, spinal cord injury, muscular dystrophy, or osteoporosis and muscle weakness associated with advanced age. Often, relatively minor forms of abnormal or deviated postures occur in otherwise healthy persons. As illustrated in Figure 9-10, excessive lumbar lordosis may develop as compensation for excessive thoracic kyphosis and vice versa. The "swayback" posture shown in Figure 9-10, *C*, for example, describes a combined exaggerated lumbar lordosis and thoracic kyphosis. Often, other unexplainable postures exist such as the "rounded back" appearance in Figure 9-10, *E*. This posture shows a combined excessive thoracic kyphosis with reduced lumbar lordosis. Regardless of the cause or location of the postural deviation, the associated abnormal curvatures alter the spatial relation between the line of gravity and each spinal region. When severe, abnormal vertebral curvatures increase stress on muscles, ligaments, bones, discs, apophyseal joints, and exiting spinal nerve roots. Abnormal curves also

Ideal
posture   Common postural deviations

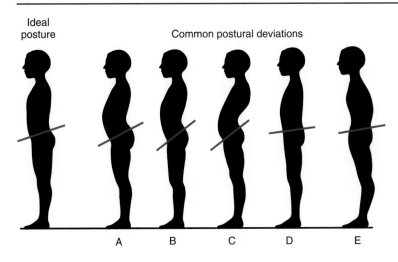

A   B   C   D   E

FIGURE 9-10. A drawing showing common postural deviations of the vertebral column and pelvis within the sagittal plane. All subjects in the figure are considered normal, from a neuromuscular perspective. The red line at each iliac crest indicates the varying degree of pelvic tilt (or lumbar lordosis). (Modified from McMorris RO: Faulty postures, *Pediatr Clin North Am* 8:217, 1961.)

change the volume of body cavities. An exaggerated thoracic kyphosis, for example, can significantly reduce the space for the lungs to expand during deep breathing.

LIGAMENTOUS SUPPORT OF THE VERTEBRAL COLUMN

The vertebral column is supported by an extensive set of ligaments. Spinal ligaments limit motion, help maintain natural spinal curvatures, and, by stabilizing the spine, protect the delicate spinal cord and spinal nerve roots. These ligaments, described in the following paragraphs and illustrated in Figure 9-11, all possess slightly different strengths and functions depending on their locations within the vertebral column.[85] The basic structure and generic function of each ligament are summarized in Table 9-3.

The *ligamentum flavum* originates on the anterior surface of one lamina and inserts on the posterior surface of the lamina below. Consisting of a series of paired ligaments, the ligamenta flava (plural) extend throughout the vertebral column, situated immediately posterior to the spinal cord. The ligamenta flava and adjacent laminae form the posterior wall of the vertebral canal.

Ligamentum flavum literally means "yellow ligament," reflecting its high content of light yellow elastic connective tissue. Histologically, the ligamentum flavum consists of about 80% elastin and 20% collagen.[223] The tissue's highly elastic nature is ideal for exerting a relatively constant, although modest, resistance throughout a wide range of flexion.[85] Measurements have shown that between the neutral position and full flexion, the ligamentum flavum experiences an approximately 35% increase in strain (elongation) (Figure 9-12).[139] Extreme and very forceful flexion beyond this length can ultimately lead to its rupture, possibly creating damaging compressive forces on the anterior side of the intervertebral disc.[4] The ligamenta flava are thickest in the lumbar region,[188] where the magnitude of intervertebral flexion is the largest of any region within the vertebral column.

The highly elastic nature of the ligamentum flavum is interesting from both a functional and a structural perspective. In addition to providing gradual resistance to the full range of flexion, its inherent elasticity also exerts a small but constant compression force between vertebrae, even in the neutral position.[23] The elasticity may prevent the ligament

from buckling inward during full extension. Such a buckling, or in-folding, might otherwise pinch and possibly injure the adjacent spinal cord.

The *interspinous ligaments* fill much of the space between adjacent spinous processes. The deeper, more elastin-rich fibers blend with the ligamenta flava; the more superficial fibers contain more collagen, and blend with the supraspinous ligaments.[223] The fiber direction and organization of the interspinous ligaments vary from region to region.[88] The interspinous ligaments in the lumbar region, for example, fan in an oblique posterior-cranial direction (see Figure 9-11, *A*). Fibers in this region are drawn taut only at the more extremes of flexion.

As evident by their name, the *supraspinous ligaments* attach between the tips of the spinous processes. As with the interspinous ligaments, these ligaments resist separation of adjacent spinous processes, thereby resisting flexion.[85] The ability to resist flexion is greatest in regions of the vertebral column where these structures are more robust and contain a greater proportion of collagen. Throughout the lumbar region, for example, the ligaments are not extensively developed; they are either sparse (especially between L4 and L5) or partially replaced by strands of thoracolumbar fascia or small musculotendinous fibers.[23,86,188] Not surprisingly, therefore, the supraspinous ligaments within the lumbar region are typically the first structures to rupture in extreme flexion.[5]

In the cervical region the supraspinous ligaments are very well developed and extend cranially as the *ligamentum nuchae.* This tough membrane consists of a bilaminar strip of fibroelastic tissue that attaches between the cervical spinous processes and external occipital protuberance.[188] Passive tension in a stretched ligamentum nuchae adds a small but useful means of support for the head and neck.[53] The ligamentum nuchae also provides a midline attachment for muscles, such as the trapezius and splenius capitis and cervicis. A prominent ligamentum nuchae accounts for some of the difficulty often encountered in palpating the spinous process in the mid to upper cervical region (Figure 9-13).

The *intertransverse ligaments* are poorly defined, thin or membranous structures that extend between adjacent transverse processes.[188] These tissues become taut in contralateral lateral flexion and, to a lesser degree, forward flexion.

The *anterior longitudinal ligament* is a long, strong, straplike structure attaching to the basilar part of the occipital bone

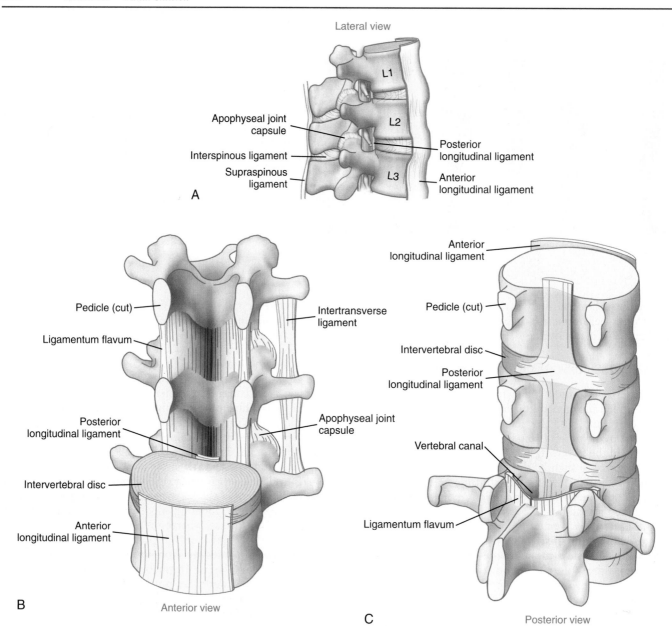

FIGURE 9-11. Primary ligaments that stabilize the vertebral column. **A,** Lateral overview of the first three lumbar vertebrae (L1 to L3). **B,** Anterior view of L1 to L3 vertebrae with the bodies of L1 and L2 removed by cutting through the pedicles. **C,** Posterior view of L1 to L3 vertebrae with the posterior elements of L1 and L2 removed by cutting through the pedicles. In **B** and **C,** the neural tissues have been removed from the vertebral canal.

and the entire length of the anterior surfaces of all vertebral bodies, including the sacrum. The deeper fibers blend with and reinforce the anterior sides of the intervertebral discs.[188] The anterior longitudinal ligament becomes taut in extension and slack in flexion.[85] In the cervical and lumbar regions, tension in the anterior longitudinal ligament helps limit the degree of natural lordosis. This ligament is narrow at its cranial end but widens as it courses caudally.

The *posterior longitudinal ligament* is a continuous band of connective tissue that attaches the entire length of the posterior surfaces of the vertebral bodies, between the axis (C2) and the sacrum. The posterior longitudinal ligament is located within the vertebral canal, immediately anterior to the spinal cord (see Figure 9-11, *A*). (It is important to note that the

posterior and anterior longitudinal ligaments are named according to their relationship to the *vertebral body,* not the spinal cord.) Throughout its length, the deeper fibers of the posterior longitudinal ligament blend with and reinforce the posterior side of the intervertebral discs.[188] Cranially, the posterior longitudinal ligament is a broad structure, narrowing as it descends toward the lumbar region. The slender lumbar portion limits its ability to restrain a posterior bulging (or herniated) disc. As with most ligaments of the vertebral column, the posterior longitudinal ligament becomes increasingly taut with flexion.[85]

Capsular ligaments of the apophyseal joints consist mostly of collagen fibers that attach along the rim of the facet surfaces (see Figure 9-11, *A*). As will be described in an upcoming

TABLE 9-3. Major Ligaments of the Vertebral Column

Name	Attachments	Function	Comment
Ligamentum flavum	Between the anterior surface of one lamina and the posterior surface of the lamina below	Limits flexion	Contains a high percentage of elastin. Lies immediately posterior to the spinal cord. Thickest in the lumbar region.
Supraspinous and interspinous ligaments	Between the adjacent spinous processes from C7 to the sacrum	Limit flexion	Ligamentum nuchae is the cervical and cranial extension of the supraspinous ligaments, providing a midline structure for muscle attachments, and support to the head.
Intertransverse ligaments	Between adjacent transverse processes	Limits contralateral lateral flexion and forward flexion	Few fibers exist in the cervical region. In the thoracic region, the ligaments are rounded and intertwined with local muscle. In the lumbar region, the ligaments are thin and membranous.
Anterior longitudinal ligament	Between the basilar part of the occipital bone and the entire length of the anterior surfaces of all vertebral bodies, including the sacrum	Limits extension or excessive lordosis in the cervical and lumbar regions. Reinforces the anterior sides of the intervertebral discs	Best developed in the lumbar spine. About twice the tensile strength as the posterior longitudinal ligament.
Posterior longitudinal ligament	Throughout the length of the posterior surfaces of all vertebral bodies, between the axis (C2) and the sacrum	Limits flexion. Reinforces the posterior sides of the intervertebral discs	Lies within the vertebral canal, just anterior to the spinal cord.
Capsules of the apophyseal joints	Margin of each apophyseal joint	Strengthen the apophyseal joints	Loose in the near-neutral position but become increasingly taut at the extremes of all other positions.

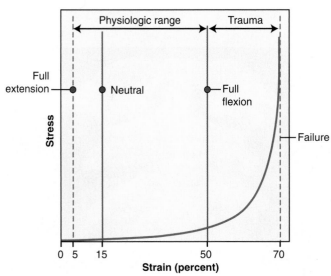

FIGURE 9-12. The stress-strain relationship of the ligamentum flavum is shown between full extension and the point of tissue failure beyond full normal-range flexion. Note that the ligament fails at a point 70% beyond its fully slackened length. (Data from Nachemson A, Evans J: Some mechanical properties of the third lumbar interlaminar ligament, *J Biomech* 1:211, 1968.)

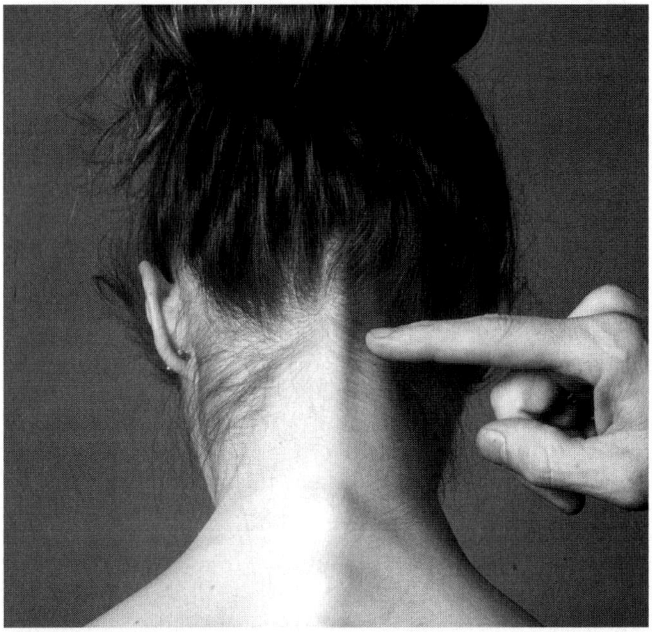

FIGURE 9-13. A prominent ligamentum nuchae in a thin healthy woman.

section on arthrology, apophyseal joints help interconnect and stabilize the intervertebral junctions. Equally important is their unique role in guiding the specific direction of intervertebral movement. Sensory mechanoreceptors embedded within the capsule likely provide muscles information to assist with this guidance.[36] The apophyseal joint capsules are reinforced by adjacent muscles (multifidus) and ligamenta flava, most notably in the lumbar region.[188]

The capsular ligaments of the apophyseal joints are strong, capable of supporting up to 1000 N (225 lb) of tension before failure.[48] The capsular ligaments are relatively loose (lax) in the neutral position but become increasingly taut as the joint approaches the extremes of all its movements. Passive tension is greatest in motions that create the largest translation or separation between joint surfaces. These kinematics are highly specific to the particular region of the vertebral column and will be revisited in subsequent sections of this chapter.

In closing, with the possible exception of the capsular ligaments of the apophyseal joints, knowledge of a ligament's location relative to the axis of rotation within a given intervertebral junction provides major insight into its primary functions. As will be further described in an upcoming section, the axis of rotation for intervertebral movement is near or through the region of the *vertebral body*. When sagittal plane movement is considered, for example, any ligament located posterior to the vertebral body is stretched during flexion. Conversely, any ligament located anterior to the vertebral body is stretched during extension. As noted by reviewing Figure 9-11, *A*, all ligaments except the anterior longitudinal ligament would become taut in flexion.

Regional Osteologic Features of the Vertebral Column

The adage that "function follows structure" is very applicable to the study of the vertebral column. Although all vertebrae have a common morphologic theme, each also has a specific shape that reflects its unique function. The following section, along with Table 9-4, highlights specific osteologic features of each region of the vertebral column.

CERVICAL REGION

The cervical vertebrae are the smallest and most mobile of all movable vertebrae. The high degree of mobility is essential to the large range of motion required by the head. Perhaps the most unique anatomic feature of the cervical vertebrae is the presence of *transverse foramina* located within the transverse processes (Figure 9-14). The important vertebral artery ascends through this foramen, coursing toward the foramen magnum to transport blood to the brain and spinal cord. In the neck, the vertebral artery is located immediately anterior to the exiting spinal nerve roots (see Figure 9-4).

The third through the sixth cervical vertebrae show nearly identical features and are therefore considered typical of this region. The upper two cervical vertebrae, the atlas (C1) and the axis (C2), and the seventh cervical vertebra (C7) are atypical for reasons described in a subsequent section.

Typical Cervical Vertebrae (C3 to C6)
C3 to C6 have small rectangular *bodies* made of a relatively dense and strong cortical shell.[199] The bodies are wider from side to side than front to back (Figures 9-14 and 9-15). The superior and inferior surfaces of the bodies are not as flat as those of most other vertebrae but are curved or notched. The superior surfaces are concave side to side, with raised lateral hooks called *uncinate processes* (*uncus* means "hook"). The inferior surfaces, in contrast, are concave anterior-posterior, with elongated anterior and posterior margins. When articulated, small, synovial-lined *uncovertebral joints* form between the uncinate process and adjacent part of the superior vertebra between C3 and C7. Uncovertebral joints are often called the

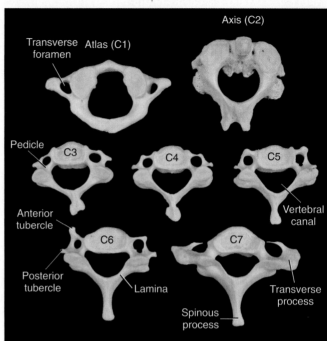

FIGURE 9-14. A superior view of seven cervical vertebrae.

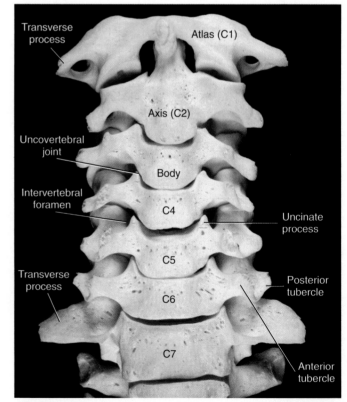

FIGURE 9-15. An anterior view of the cervical vertebral column.

TABLE 9-4. Osteologic Features of the Vertebral Column

	Body	Superior Articular Facets	Inferior Articular Facets	Spinous Processes	Vertebral Canal	Transverse Processes	Comments
Atlas (C1)	None	Concave, face generally superior	Flat to slightly concave, face generally inferior	None, replaced by a small posterior tubercle	Triangular, largest of cervical region	Largest of cervical region	Two large lateral masses, joined by anterior and posterior arches
Axis (C2)	Tall with a vertical projecting dens	Flat to slightly convex, face generally superior	Flat, face anterior and inferior	Largest of cervical region, bifid	Large and triangular	Form anterior and posterior tubercles	Large superior articular processes that support the atlas and cranium
C3-C6	Wider than deep; have uncinate processes	Flat, face posterior and superior	As above	Bifid	Large and triangular	End as anterior and posterior tubercles	Considered typical cervical vertebrae
C7	Wider than deep	As above	Transition to typical thoracic vertebrae	Large and prominent, easily palpable	Triangular	Thick and prominent, may have a large anterior tubercle forming an "extra rib"	Often called "vertebral prominens" because of large spinous process
T2-T9	Equal width and depth. Has costal demifacets for attachment of the heads of ribs 2 to 9	Flat, face mostly posterior	Flat, face mostly anterior	Long and pointed, slant inferiorly	Round, smaller than cervical	Project horizontally and slightly posterior, have costal facets for tubercles of ribs	Considered typical thoracic vertebrae
T1 and T10-T12	T1 has a full costal facet for rib 1 and a partial demifacet for rib 2. T10-T12 each has a full costal facet	As above	As above	As above	As above	T10-T12 may lack costal facets	Considered "atypical" thoracic vertebrae primarily because of manner of rib attachment
L1-L5	Wider than deep. L5 is slightly wedged (i.e., higher height anteriorly than posteriorly)	Slightly concave, face medial to posterior-medial	L1-L4 slightly convex, face lateral to anterior-lateral. L5: flat, faces anterior and slightly lateral	Stout and rectangular	Triangular, contains cauda equina	Slender, project laterally	Superior articular processes have mammillary bodies
Sacrum	Fused. Body of first sacral vertebra most evident	Flat, face posterior and slightly medial	None	None, replaced by multiple spinous tubercles	As above	None, replaced by multiple transverse tubercles	
Coccyx	Fusion of four rudimentary vertebrae	Rudimentary	Rudimentary	Rudimentary	Ends at the first coccyx	Rudimentary	

Cervical Osteophytes Causing Neurologic Symptoms in the Upper Extremity: One Possible Consequence of a Degenerated Intervertebral Disc

Fully hydrated and normal intervertebral discs naturally act as "spacers" between individual vertebrae. One benefit of this function is to partially unload the nearby *uncovertebral joints*. Lacking substantial articular cartilage, the relatively small uncovertebral joints are not designed to support large forces. Figure 9-16 illustrates how a healthy, full disc located between C3 and C4 creates a small protective gap between the adjacent C3-C4 uncovertebral joint. Figure 9-16 also shows how a degenerated and thinned disc between C4 and C5 increases the compression force at the C4-C5 uncovertebral joint. Over time, the increased compression can stimulate growth of an osteophyte ("bone spur"). The osteophyte is shown compressing elements of the C^5 spinal nerve root, which may, over time, lead to neurologic symptoms, including radiating (radicular) pain, muscle weakness, or altered sensations throughout the nerve's peripheral distribution, typically down the lateral aspect of the arm. In an indirect way, healthy intervertebral discs protect not only the surrounding bone, but also the nerve roots.

Anterior view

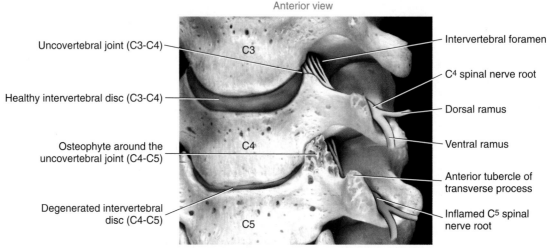

Uncovertebral joint (C3-C4)

C3

Healthy intervertebral disc (C3-C4)

Osteophyte around the uncovertebral joint (C4-C5)

C4

Degenerated intervertebral disc (C4-C5)

C5

Intervertebral foramen

C^4 spinal nerve root

Dorsal ramus

Ventral ramus

Anterior tubercle of transverse process

Inflamed C^5 spinal nerve root

FIGURE 9-16. A computer-enhanced image comparing the relative loading of the uncovertebral joints based on the health of the adjacent intervertebral discs. The osteophyte formed at the C4-C5 uncovertebral joint is shown to compress and inflame the exiting C^5 spinal nerve root.

"joints of Luschka," named after the person who first described them.[84] The exact function of uncovertebral joints is unclear, although they likely facilitate the kinematics of cervical motion. Clinically these joints become important when osteophytes form around their margins, often reducing the size of the adjacent intervertebral foramen. If large, these osteophytes may impinge on and irritate exiting cervical spinal nerve roots, thereby causing neurologic symptoms.

The *pedicles* of C3 to C6 are short and curved posterior-lateral (see Figure 9-14). Very thin *laminae* extend posterior-medially from each pedicle (Figure 9-17). The triangular *vertebral canal* is large in the cervical region in order to accommodate the thickening of the spinal cord associated with the formation of the cervical plexus and brachial plexus.

Within the C3 to C6 region, consecutive superior and inferior articular processes form a continuous articular "pillar," interrupted by apophyseal joints (Figure 9-18). The articular facets within each apophyseal joint are smooth and flat, with joint surfaces oriented midway between the frontal and horizontal planes. The *superior articular facets* face posterior and superior, whereas the *inferior articular facets* face anterior and inferior.

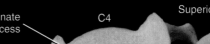

Posterior-lateral view

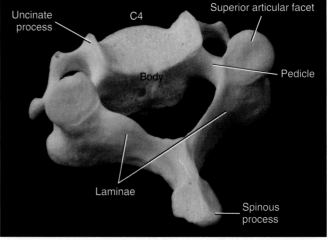

Uncinate process

C4

Superior articular facet

Body

Pedicle

Laminae

Spinous process

FIGURE 9-17. A posterior-lateral view of the fourth cervical vertebra.

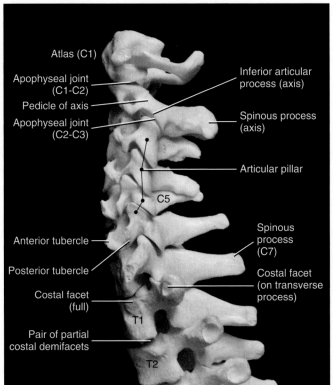

Lateral view

Atlas (C1)

Apophyseal joint
(C1-C2)

Pedicle of axis

Apophyseal joint
(C2-C3)

Inferior articular
process (axis)

Spinous process
(axis)

Articular pillar

C5

Anterior tubercle

Posterior tubercle

Spinous
process
(C7)

Costal facet
(on transverse
process)

Costal facet
(full)

T1

Pair of partial
costal demifacets

T2

FIGURE 9-18. A lateral view of the cervical vertebral column.

The *spinous processes* of C3 to C6 are short, with some processes being bifid (i.e., double) (see Figure 9-14, C3). The *transverse processes* are short lateral extensions that terminate as variably shaped *anterior* and *posterior tubercles*. The tubercles are unique to the cervical region, serving as attachments for muscles, such as the anterior scalene, levator scapulae, and splenius cervicis.

Atypical Cervical Vertebrae (C1, C2, and C7)

Atlas (C1)

As indicated by the name, the primary function of the atlas is to support the head. Possessing no body, pedicle, lamina, or spinous process, the atlas is essentially two large lateral masses joined by anterior and posterior arches (Figure 9-19, *A*). The short *anterior arch* has an *anterior tubercle* for attachment of the anterior longitudinal ligament. The much larger *posterior arch* forms nearly half the circumference of the entire atlantal ring. A small *posterior tubercle* marks the midline of the posterior arch. The lateral masses support the prominent superior articular processes, which in turn support the cranium.

The large and concave *superior articular facets* of the atlas generally face cranially, in a position to accept the large, convex occipital condyles. The *inferior articular facets* are generally flat to slightly concave. These facet surfaces generally face inferiorly, with their lateral edges sloped downward, approximately 20 degrees from the horizontal plane (see Figure 9-19, *B*). The atlas has large, palpable *transverse*

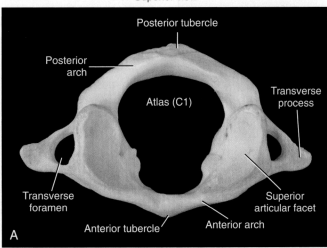

Superior view

Posterior tubercle

Posterior
arch

Atlas (C1)

Transverse
process

Transverse
foramen

Anterior tubercle

Superior
articular facet

Anterior arch

A

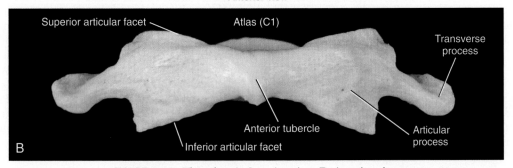

Anterior view

Superior articular facet

Atlas (C1)

Transverse
process

Anterior tubercle

Inferior articular facet

Articular
process

B

FIGURE 9-19. The atlas. **A,** Superior view. **B,** Anterior view.

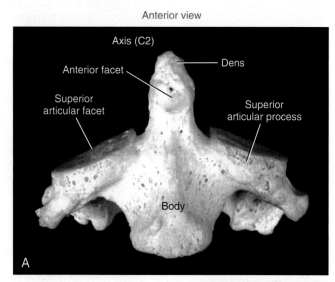

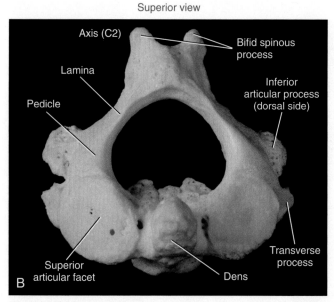

FIGURE 9-20. The axis. **A,** Anterior view. **B,** Superior view.

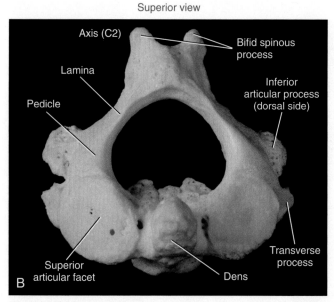

FIGURE 9-21. A superior view of the median atlanto-axial articulation.

processes, usually the most prominent of the cervical vertebrae. These transverse processes serve as attachment points for several small but important muscles that control fine movements of the cranium.

Axis (C2)

The axis has a large, tall *body* that serves as a base for the upwardly projecting *dens (odontoid process)* (Figure 9-20). Part of the elongated body is formed from remnants of the body of the atlas and the intervening disc. The dens provides a rigid vertical axis of rotation for the atlas and head (Figure 9-21). Projecting laterally from the body is a pair of superior articular processes (see Figure 9-20, *A*). These large processes have

slightly convex *superior articular facets* that are oriented about 20 degrees from the horizontal plane, matching the slope of the inferior articular facets of the atlas. Projecting from the prominent superior articular processes of the axis are a pair of stout *pedicles* and a pair of very short *transverse processes* (see Figure 9-20, *B*). A pair of inferior articular processes projects inferiorly from the pedicles, with *inferior articular facets* facing anteriorly and inferiorly (see Figure 9-18). The *spinous process* of the axis is bifid and very broad. The palpable spinous process serves as an attachment for many muscles, such as the semispinalis cervicis.

"Vertebra Prominens" (C7)

C7 is the largest of all cervical vertebrae, having many characteristics of thoracic vertebrae. C7 can have large *transverse processes,* as illustrated in Figure 9-15. A hypertrophic anterior tubercle on the transverse process may sprout an extra cervical rib, which may impinge on the brachial plexus. This vertebra also has a large *spinous process,* characteristic of other thoracic vertebrae (see Figure 9-18).

THORACIC REGION

Typical Thoracic Vertebrae (T2 to T9)

The second through the ninth thoracic vertebrae usually demonstrate similar features (see T6 and T7 in Figure 9-5). *Pedicles* are directed posteriorly from the body, making the vertebral canal narrower than in the cervical region. The large *transverse processes* project posterior-laterally, each containing a *costal facet* that articulates with the tubercle of the corresponding rib *(costotransverse joint)*. Short, thick *laminae* form a broad base for the downward-slanting *spinous processes.*

The superior and inferior articular facets in the thoracic region are oriented vertically with a slight forward pitch (Figure 9-22). The *superior articular facets* face generally posterior; the *inferior articular facets* face generally anterior. Once articulated, the superior and inferior facets form apophyseal joints, which are aligned relatively close to the frontal plane.

Each of the heads of ribs 2 through 9 typically articulates with a pair of *costal demifacets* that span one thoracic intervertebral junction (see pair of costal demifacets for the eighth rib in Figure 9-22). As described earlier, these articulations are called *costocorporeal joints.* A thoracic (intercostal) spinal nerve exits through a corresponding thoracic *intervertebral foramen,* located just anterior to the apophyseal joints.

Atypical Thoracic Vertebrae (T1 and T10 to T12)

The first and usually last three thoracic vertebrae are considered atypical mainly because of the particular manner of rib

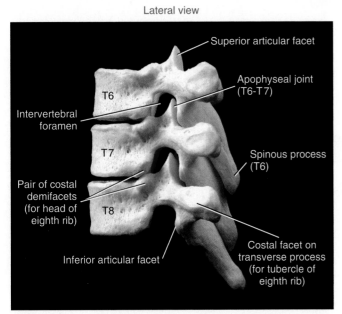

Lateral view

FIGURE 9-22. A lateral view of the sixth through eighth thoracic vertebrae.

attachment. T1 has a *full costal facet* superiorly that accepts the entire head of the first rib, and a *demifacet* inferiorly that accepts part of the head of the second rib (see Figure 9-18). The spinous process of T1 is especially elongated and often as prominent as the spinous process of C7. Although variable, the bodies of T10 through T12 may have a single, *full costal facet* for articulation with the heads of the tenth, eleventh, and twelfth ribs, respectively. T10 to T12 usually lack costotransverse joints.

LUMBAR REGION

Lumbar vertebrae have massive wide *bodies,* suitable for supporting the entire superimposed weight of the head, trunk, and arms (Figure 9-23). The total mass of the five lumbar vertebrae is approximately twice that of all seven cervical vertebrae.

For the most part, the lumbar vertebrae possess similar characteristics. *Laminae* and *pedicles* are short and thick, forming the posterior and lateral walls of the nearly triangular *vertebral canal. Transverse processes* project almost laterally; those associated with L1 to L4 are thin and tapered; however, the transverse processes of L5 are short, thick, and strong. *Spinous processes* are broad and rectangular, projecting horizontally from the junction of each lamina (Figure 9-24). This shape is strikingly different from the pointed, sloped spinous processes of the thoracic region. Short *mammillary processes* project from the posterior surfaces of each superior articular process. These structures serve as attachment sites for the multifidi muscles.

The articular facets of the lumbar vertebrae are oriented nearly vertically. The *superior articular facets* are moderately concave, facing medial to posterior-medial. As depicted in Figure 9-23, the superior facet surfaces in the upper lumbar region tend to be oriented closest with the sagittal plane, and the superior facet surfaces in the mid-to-lower lumbar region

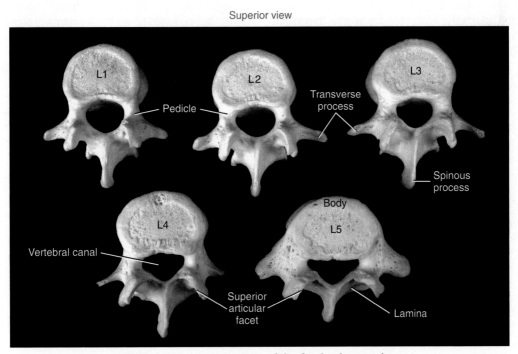

Superior view

FIGURE 9-23. A superior view of the five lumbar vertebrae.

Lateral view

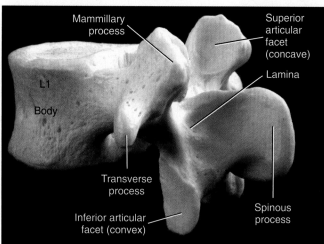

FIGURE 9-24. A lateral and slightly posterior view of the first lumbar vertebra.

are oriented approximately midway between the sagittal and frontal planes. The *inferior articular facets* are reciprocally matched to the shape and orientation of the superior articular facets. In general, the inferior articular facets are slightly convex, facing generally lateral to anterior-lateral (see Figure 9-24).

The inferior articular facets of L5 articulate with the superior articular facets of the sacrum. The resulting *L5-S1 apophyseal joints* are typically oriented much closer to the frontal plane than the other lumbar articulations. The L5-S1 apophyseal joints provide an important source of anterior-posterior stability to the lumbosacral junction.

SACRUM

The sacrum is a triangular bone with its base facing superiorly and apex inferiorly (Figure 9-26). An important function of the sacrum is to transmit the weight of the vertebral column to the pelvis. In childhood, each of five separate sacral vertebrae is joined by a cartilaginous membrane. By adulthood,

---

SPECIAL FOCUS 9-2

Developmental Anomalies of the Lumbar Apophyseal Joints

At birth the articular surfaces of the apophyseal joints within the lumbar spine are oriented very close to the frontal plane, similar to most thoracic apophyseal joints. Between birth and about 11 or 12 years of age, however, the orientation within all but the lower lumbar apophyseal joints gradually transforms to their final adult position biased slightly closer to the sagittal plane (Figure 9-25).[23,167] The slow structural transformation is governed by different rates of ossification within the articular processes. Bogduk describes the possibility that this transformation may be influenced by the developing upright posture of the child and the demands placed on certain muscles, such as the lumbar multifidi.[23] Although the apophyseal joints continue to grow throughout adolescence, their spatial orientation is essentially established before the teenage years.

Natural variations in the development of the lumbar apophyseal joints in childhood can create structural variations that persist into adulthood. Although variations can be extreme, most are relatively minor, such as a slight bilateral asymmetry between the right and left articular surfaces of the joints. (An example of this asymmetry is evident by comparing the superior articular facets of the lumbar vertebrae illustrated in Figure 9-23.) Slight bilateral asymmetries exist in about 20% to 30% of all adult lumbar vertebrae, although they are likely inconsequential.[23] In more extreme cases, however, the bilateral asymmetry could create uneven stress and instability throughout the intervertebral junctions.[47] Although evidence is mixed, the increased stress could potentially predispose a person to premature degeneration in the apophyseal joints or intervertebral discs.[63]

FIGURE 9-25. Graph showing the orientation of the articular surfaces of the lumbar apophyseal joints as a function of age. (From Bogduk N: *Clinical anatomy of the lumbar spine and sacrum*, ed 4, St Louis, 2005, Churchill Livingstone.)

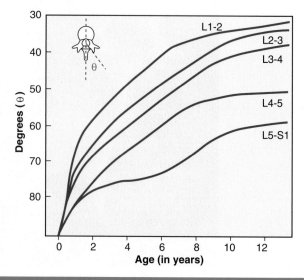

Anterior view

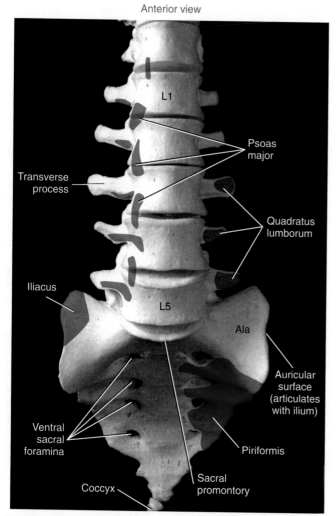

FIGURE 9-26. An anterior view of the lumbosacral region. Attachments of the piriformis, iliacus, and psoas major are indicated in red. Attachments of the quadratus lumborum are indicated in gray.

Posterior-lateral view

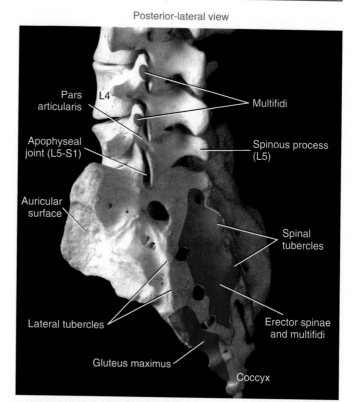

FIGURE 9-27. A posterior-lateral view of the lumbosacral region. Attachments of the multifidi, erector spinae, and gluteus maximus are indicated in red.

Superior view

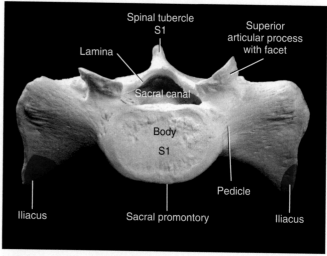

FIGURE 9-28. A superior view of the sacrum. Attachments of the iliacus muscles are indicated in red.

however, the sacrum has fused into a single bone, which still retains some anatomic features of generic vertebrae.

The anterior (pelvic) surface of the sacrum is smooth and concave, forming part of the posterior wall of the pelvic cavity (see Figure 9-26). Four paired *ventral (pelvic) sacral foramina* transmit the ventral rami of spinal nerve roots that form much of the sacral plexus. The dorsal surface of the sacrum is convex and rough due to the attachments of muscle and ligaments (Figure 9-27). Several *spinal and lateral tubercles* mark the remnants of fused spinous and transverse processes, respectively. Four paired *dorsal sacral foramina* transmit the dorsal rami of sacral spinal nerve roots.

The superior surface of the sacrum shows a clear representation of the *body* of the first sacral vertebra (Figure 9-28). The sharp anterior edge of the body of S1 is called the *sacral promontory*. The triangular *sacral canal* houses and protects the cauda equina. *Pedicles* are very thick, extending laterally as the *ala* (lateral wings) of the sacrum. Stout superior articular processes have *superior articular facets* that face generally posterior-medially. These facets articulate with the inferior facets of L5 to form L5-S1 apophyseal joints (see Figure 9-27). The large *auricular surface* articulates with the ilium, forming the sacro-

iliac joint. The sacrum narrows caudally to form its *apex*, a point of articulation with the coccyx.

COCCYX

The coccyx is a small triangular bone consisting of four fused vertebrae (see Figure 9-27). The base of the coccyx joins the apex of the sacrum at the *sacrococcygeal joint.* The joint has a fibrocartilaginous disc and is held together by several small ligaments. The sacrococcygeal joint usually fuses late in life. In youths, small *intercoccygeal joints* persist; however, these typically are fused in adults.[188]

SPECIAL FOCUS 9-3

Cauda Equina

At birth the spinal cord and vertebral column are nearly the same length. Thereafter, however, the vertebral column grows at a slightly faster rate than the spinal cord. As a consequence, in the adult the caudal end of the spinal cord terminates generally adjacent to the L1 vertebra. The lumbosacral spinal nerve roots therefore must travel a great distance caudally before reaching their corresponding intervertebral foramina (see Figure III-1 in Appendix III, Part A). As a group, the elongated nerves resemble a horse's tail, hence the term *cauda equina.*

The cauda equina is a set of peripheral nerves that are bathed in cerebrospinal fluid and located within the lumbosacral vertebral canal. Severe fracture or trauma in the lumbosacral region may damage the cauda equina but spare the spinal cord. Damage to the cauda equina may result in muscle paralysis and atrophy, altered sensation, and reduced reflexes. (Spasticity with exaggerated reflexes typically occurs with damage to the spinal cord.) The cauda equina is part of the peripheral nervous system (in contrast to the central nervous system). If severed, therefore, the nerves possess at least the physiologic potential for regeneration.

ARTHROLOGY

Typical Intervertebral Junction

The typical intervertebral junction has three functional components: (1) the transverse and spinous processes, (2) the apophyseal joints, and (3) an interbody joint (Figure 9-29). The *spinous* and *transverse processes* provide mechanical outriggers, or levers, that increase the mechanical leverage of muscles and ligaments. *Apophyseal joints* are primarily responsible for guiding intervertebral motion, much as railroad tracks guide the direction of a train. As will be emphasized, the geometry, height, and spatial orientation of the articular facets within the apophyseal joints greatly influence the prevailing direction of intervertebral motion.

Interbody joints connect an intervertebral disc with a pair of vertebral bodies. The primary function of these joints is to absorb and distribute loads across the vertebral column. Normally, at least in the lumbar region, the interbody joint accepts the overwhelming majority of weight that is borne through the intervertebral junction. As indicated in Figure 9-29, flexion of the spine shifts an even greater proportion of the superimposed body weight forward to the interbody joint. In addition, the interbody joints provide the greatest source of adhesion between vertebrae,[85] serve as the approximate axes of rotation, and function as deformable intervertebral spacers. As spacers, the intervertebral discs constitute about 25% of the total height of the vertebral column. The functional importance of the space created by a healthy intervertebral disc cannot be overstated. The greater the relative intervertebral space, the greater the ability of one vertebral body to "rock" forward and backward on another, for example. Without any disc space, the nearly flat bone-on-bone interface between two consecu-

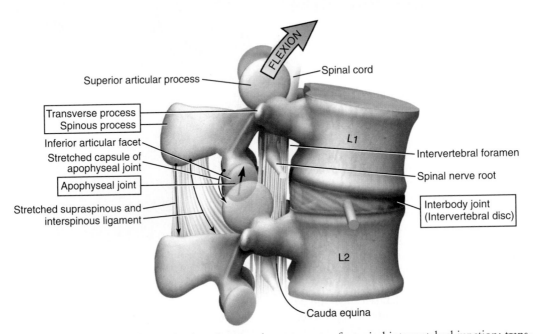

FIGURE 9-29. A model highlights the three functional components of a typical intervertebral junction: transverse and spinous processes, apophyseal joints, and interbody joint, including the intervertebral disc. The L1-L2 junction is shown flexing, guided by the sliding between the articular facet surfaces of the apophyseal joints *(black, thicker arrow).* The medial-lateral axis of rotation is shown through the interbody joint. The interspinous and supraspinous ligaments are shown stretched. Note the compression of the front of the intervertebral disc. Also note that the spinal cord terminates near the L1 vertebra and then forms the cauda equina.

tive bodies would block rotation in the sagittal and frontal planes—allowing only tipping or translation. Finally, the space created by the intervertebral discs provides adequate passage for the exiting spinal nerve roots.

Impairments involving the apophyseal or the interbody joints can result from trauma, cumulative stress, advanced age, disease, or combinations thereof. Regardless of cause, impairments involving these joints can lead to abnormal and painful kinematics, distorted posture, and mechanical impingement of neural tissues. Appreciating the spatial and physical relationships between the neurology, osteology, and arthrology of a typical intervertebral junction greatly enhances one's ability to understand and evaluate many of the approaches used to treat spinal-related pain and dysfunction.

TERMINOLOGY DESCRIBING MOVEMENT

With few important exceptions, movement within any given intervertebral junction is relatively small. When added across the entire vertebral column, however, these small movements can yield considerable angular rotation. The *osteokinematics* across the entire axial skeleton (which includes the vertebral column and cranium) are described as rotations within the three cardinal planes. Each plane, or degree of freedom, is associated with one axis of rotation, directed approximately through the body of the interbody joint (Figure 9-30).[174] By convention, movement throughout the vertebral column, including the head on the cervical spine, is described in a cranial-to-caudal fashion, with the direction of movement referenced by a point on the *anterior* side of the more cranial

(superior) vertebral segment. During C4-C5 axial rotation to the left, for example, a point on the anterior body of C4 rotates to the left, although the spinous process rotates to the right.

Arthrokinematics of intervertebral motion describe the relative movement *between* articular facet surfaces within the apophyseal joints. Most facet surfaces are flat or nearly flat, and terms such as *approximation, separation* (or *gapping*), and *sliding* adequately describe the arthrokinematics (Table 9-5).

STRUCTURE AND FUNCTION OF THE APOPHYSEAL JOINTS

The vertebral column contains 24 pairs of apophyseal joints. Each apophyseal joint is formed between opposing articular facet surfaces (Figure 9-31). Mechanically classified as *plane joints,* apophyseal joints are lined with articular cartilage and enclosed by a synovial-lined, well innervated capsule. Although exceptions and natural variations are common, the articular surfaces of most apophyseal joints are essentially flat. Slightly curved joint surfaces are present primarily in the upper cervical and throughout the lumbar regions.

The word *apophysis* means "outgrowth," emphasizing the protruding nature of the articular processes. Acting as mechanical barricades, the articular processes permit certain movements but block others. In general, the near–vertically oriented apophyseal joints within the lower thoracic, lumbar, and lumbosacral regions block excessive anterior translation of one vertebra on another. Functionally this is important because excessive anterior translation significantly compromises the volume of the vertebral canal—the space occupied by the spinal cord or passing spinal nerve roots.

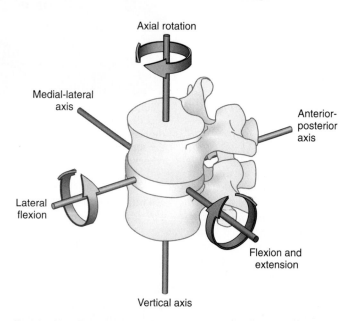

Terminology Describing the Osteokinematics of the Axial Skeleton

Common Terminology	Plane of Movement	Axis of Rotation	Other Terminology
Flexion and extension	Sagittal	Medial-lateral	Forward and backward bending
Lateral flexion to the right or left	Frontal	Anterior-posterior	Side bending to the right or left
Axial rotation to the right or left*	Horizontal	Vertical	Rotation, torsion

*Axial rotation of the spine is defined by the direction of movement of a point on the *anterior side* of the vertebral body.

FIGURE 9-30. Terminology describing the osteokinematics of the vertebral column; illustrated for a typical lumbar intervertebral junction.

TABLE 9-5. Terminology Describing the Arthrokinematics at the Apophyseal Joints

Terminology	Definition	Functional Example
Approximation of joint surfaces	An articular facet surface tends to move closer to its partner facet. Joint approximation is usually caused by a *compression* force.	Axial rotation between L1 and L2 typically causes an approximation (compression) of the contralateral apophyseal joint
Separation (gapping) between joint surfaces	An articular facet surface tends to move away from its partner facet. Joint separation is usually caused by a *distraction* force.	Therapeutic traction as a way to decompress or separate the apophyseal joints
Sliding (gliding) between joint surfaces	An articular facet translates in a linear or curvilinear direction relative to another articular facet. Sliding between joint surfaces is caused by a force directed tangential to the joint surfaces.	Flexion-extension of the mid to lower cervical spine

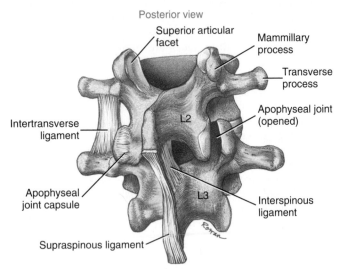

FIGURE 9-31. A posterior view of the second and third lumbar vertebrae. The capsule and associated ligaments of the right apophyseal joint are removed to show the vertical alignment of the joint surfaces. The top vertebra is rotated to the *right* to maximally expose the articular surfaces of the right apophyseal joint. Note the slight gapping within the right apophyseal joint.

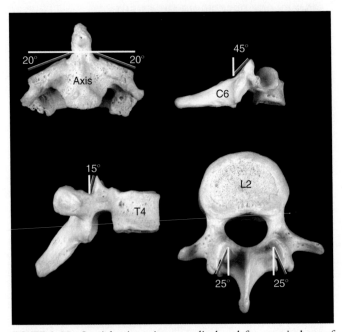

FIGURE 9-32. Spatial orientations are displayed for a typical set of superior articular facet surfaces (of apophyseal joints) from cervical, thoracic, and lumbar vertebrae. The red line indicates the plane of the superior articular facet, measured against a vertical or horizontal reference line.

The orientation of the plane of the facet surfaces within each joint strongly influences the kinematics at different regions across the vertebral column. As a general rule, *horizontal facet surfaces favor axial rotation*, whereas *vertical facet surfaces* (in either sagittal or frontal planes) *block axial rotation*. Most apophyseal joint surfaces, however, are oriented somewhere between the horizontal and vertical. Figure 9-32 shows the typical joint orientation for superior articular facets in the cervical, thoracic, and lumbar regions. The plane of the facet surfaces explains, in part, why axial rotation is far greater in the cervical region than in the lumbar region. Additional factors that influence the predominant motion at each spinal region include the sizes of the intervertebral discs (relative to the associated vertebral bodies), the overall shape of the vertebrae, local muscle actions, and attachments made by ribs or ligaments.

STRUCTURE AND FUNCTION OF THE INTERBODY JOINTS

From C2-C3 and L5-S1, 23 *interbody joints* can be found in the spinal column. Each interbody joint contains an intervertebral disc, vertebral endplates, and adjacent vertebral bodies.

Anatomically, this joint is classified as a cartilaginous *synarthrosis* (see Chapter 2).

Structural Considerations of the Lumbar Intervertebral Discs

Most of what is known about the structure and function of intervertebral discs is based on research performed in the lumbar region.[23] The research focus reflects the region's disproportionately high frequency of disc degeneration, especially in the lower vertebral segments.

A lumbar intervertebral disc consists of a central nucleus pulposus surrounded by an annulus fibrosus (Figure 9-33). The *nucleus pulposus* is a pulplike gel located in the mid-to-posterior part of the disc. In youth the nucleus pulposus within the lumbar discs consists of 70% to 90% water.[188] The hydrated nucleus allows the disc to function as a modified hydraulic shock absorption system, capable of continuously dissipating and transferring loads across consecutive vertebrae. The nucleus pulposus is thickened into a gel-like consistency by relatively large branching proteoglycans. Each

SPECIAL FOCUS 9-4

Intra-articular Structures Located within Apophyseal Joints

S mall and inconsistently formed accessory structures (inclusions) are typically found around the margins of apophyseal joints, most frequently described in the upper cervical and the lumbar regions.[23,129] In the lumbar spine, Bogduk describes two primary types of accessory structures: subcapsular fat pads and fibro-adipose meniscoids.[23] *Subcapsular fat pads* fill small crevices formed between the capsule and the underlying synovial membrane, typically at the superior and inferior margins of the joint. The subcapsular fat pads may extend outside the joint through very small crevices in the capsule. When fully formed, larger extracapsular fat pads within the lumbar region fill part of the space between the lamina and the overlying multifidi muscles.

Fibro-adipose meniscoids are another set of connective tissue found at the periphery of apophyseal joints. These structures range from thickenings or "pleats" of connective tissue variously placed along the internal surface of the joint capsule, to folds of synovium that encapsulate small fat pads, collagen fibers, and blood vessels. The larger fibro-adipose meniscoids can extend several millimeters into the apophyseal joint.[23]

The function of intra-articular inclusions within apophyseal joints is controversial. Some authors have described them as deformable spacers that help dissipate compression forces within the joint.[73,129] Others have speculated that the structures are designed to partially cover the articular cartilage that becomes exposed at the extremes of motion.[23] This transient coverage may protect and lubricate the exposed surfaces until the joint is returned to its neutral position. Although opinions vary, the intra-articular inclusions may have important clinical relevance. The larger fibro-adipose meniscoids in cervical regions may become impinged as the apophyseal joints forcefully hyperextend, such as during a cervical whiplash injury.[99] Meniscoids may proliferate after long-term immobilization and restrict spinal movement. Because these tissues are innervated, they may be a source of pain.[74]

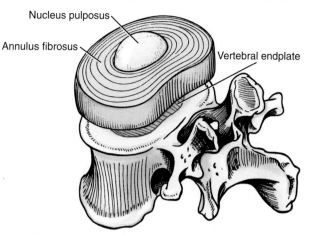

FIGURE 9-33. The intervertebral disc is shown lifted away from the underlying vertebral endplate. (Modified from Kapandji IA: *The physiology of joints,* vol 3, New York, 1974, Churchill Livingstone.)

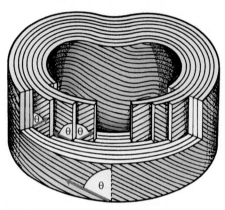

FIGURE 9-34. The detailed organization of the annulus fibrosus shown with the nucleus pulposus removed. Collagen fibers are arranged in multiple concentric layers, with fibers in every other layer running in identical directions. The orientation of each collagen fiber (depicted as θ) is about 65 degrees from the vertical. (Modified from Bogduk N: *Clinical anatomy of the lumbar spine,* ed 4, New York, 2005, Churchill Livingstone.)

proteoglycan is an aggregate of many water-binding glycosaminoglycans linked to core proteins (see Chapter 2).[6,66] Dispersed throughout the hydrated proteoglycan mixture are thin type II collagen fibers, elastin fibers, and other proteins. The collagen forms an infrastructure that helps support the proteoglycan network. Very small numbers of chondrocytes and fibrocytes are interspersed throughout the nucleus, ultimately responsible for the synthesis and regulation of the proteins and proteoglycans. In the very young, the nucleus pulposus contains a few chondrocytes that are remnants of the primitive notochord.[169,188]

The *annulus fibrosus* in the lumbar discs consists primarily of 15 to 25 concentric layers, or rings, of collagen fibers.[23] Like dough surrounding jelly in a doughnut, the collagen rings encase and physically entrap the liquid-based central nucleus. The annulus fibrosus contains material and cells similar to what is found in the nucleus pulposus, differing mainly in proportion. In the annulus, collagen makes up about 50% to 60% of the dry weight, as compared with only

15% to 20% in the nucleus pulposus.[23] Abundant elastin protein is interspersed in parallel to the rings of collagen, bestowing an element of circumferential elasticity to the annulus fibrosus.[225]

The outermost or peripheral layers of the annulus fibrosus consist primarily of type I and type II collagen.[35] This arrangement provides circumferential strength and flexibility to the disc, as well as a means to bond the annulus to the anterior and posterior longitudinal ligaments and to the adjacent rim of the vertebral bodies and endplates. (The outer layers of the annulus fibrosus contain the disc's only sensory nerves; see innervation of the disc, Chapter 10). The deeper, internal layers of the annulus contain less type I collagen and more water—gradually transforming into tissue with characteristics similar to those of the centrally located nucleus pulposus.[228]

Normally, compression forces acting on the disc increase the hydrostatic pressure within the water-logged nucleus pulposus. This rise in and containment of hydrostatic pressure ultimately absorb and evenly distribute loads across the entire intervertebral junction. Fully hydrated and pressurized discs protect not only the interbody joints, but also, indirectly, the apophyseal joints. A dehydrated and thinned disc places disproportionately greater compressive loads on the apophyseal joints. For this reason, some authorities claim that a degenerated disc leads to subsequent arthritis (or arthrosis) of the apophyseal joints.[97] Some authors, however, argue the opposite cause-and-effect relationship—that the loss of joint space within a degenerated apophyseal joints favors disc degeneration.[61] Both arguments are indeed valid.

The intervertebral discs are very important stabilizers of the spine. This stabilizing function is primarily a result of the structural configuration of the collagen fibers within the annulus fibrosus. As shown in Figure 9-34, most fibers are oriented in a rather precise geometric pattern. In the lumbar region, collagen rings are oriented, on average, about 65 degrees from the vertical, with fibers of adjacent layers traveling in opposite directions.[23,122] This structural arrangement offers significant resistance against intervertebral distraction (vertical separation), shear (sliding), and torsion (twisting).[85] If the embedded collagen fibers ran nearly vertically, the disc would most effectively resist distraction forces, but not sliding or torsion. In contrast, if all fibers ran nearly parallel to the top of the vertebral body, the disc would most effectively resist shear and torsion, but not distraction. The 65-degree angle likely represents a geometric compromise that permits tensile forces to be applied primarily against the most natural movements of the lumbar spine. Distraction forces are an inherent component of flexion, extension, and lateral flexion, occurring as one vertebral body tips slightly and thus separates from its neighbor. Shear and torsion forces are produced during virtually all movements of the vertebral column. Because of the alternating layering of the annulus, only collagen fibers oriented in the direction of the slide or twist become taut; fibers in every other layer slacken.

In contrast to the lumbar region, the annulus fibrosus in the cervical region does not have complete concentric rings that surround the nucleus.[130] When a cervical disc is viewed from above, the annulus has a near-crescent shape, thick along the anterior rim and progressively tapering to a very thin layer at the disc's lateral margins. Little or no annular fibers exist at the region of the uncovertebral joints. A small fissure (or cleft) typically extends horizontally inward from each uncovertebral joint, coursing to the deeper regions of the disc.[130] Although the function of the fissures is uncertain, they likely increase the freedom of movement within the cervical region. The posterior annulus is separate from the anterior and lateral regions; it is thin and oriented vertically, parallel with the adjacent posterior longitudinal ligament.[130]

Vertebral Endplates

The *vertebral endplates* in the adult are relatively thin cartilaginous caps of connective tissue that cover most of the superior and inferior surfaces of the vertebral bodies (see Figure 9-33). At birth the endplates are very thick, accounting for about 50% of the height of each intervertebral space. During childhood the endplates function as growth plates for the vertebrae; in the adult the endplates recede and occupy only about 5% of the height of each intervertebral space.[169]

The surface of the vertebral endplate that faces the disc is composed primarily of fibrocartilage, which binds directly and strongly to the collagen within the annulus fibrosus (Figure 9-35). This fibrocartilaginous bond forms the primary adhesion between consecutive vertebrae. In contrast, the surface of

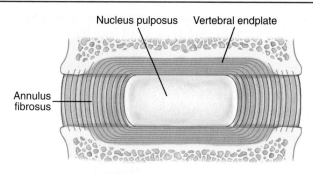

FIGURE 9-35. A vertical slice through the interbody joint shows the relative position of the vertebral endplates. (Modified from Bogduk N: *Clinical anatomy of the lumbar spine*, ed 4, New York, 2005, Churchill Livingstone.)

the endplate that faces the vertebral body is composed primarily of calcified cartilage that is weakly affixed to the bone. This endplate-bone interface is often described as the "weak link" within the interbody joint, often the first component of the interbody joint to fracture under high or repetitive compressive loading.[136] A perforated or fractured endplate can allow the proteoglycan gel to leak from the nucleus pulposus, causing structural disruption of the disc.[77,162] Such disruption has been shown to cause spinal instability.[227]

Only the outer, more peripheral rings of the annulus fibrosus contain blood vessels. For this reason, most of the disc has an inherently limited healing capacity. Essential nutrients, such as glucose and oxygen, must diffuse a great distance to reach the deeper cells that sustain the disc's low but essential metabolism. The source of these nutrients is in the blood vessels located in the more superficial annulus and, more substantially, blood stored in the adjacent vertebral bodies.[77] Most of these nutrients must diffuse across the vertebral endplate and through the disc's extracellular matrix, eventually reaching the cells residing deep in the disc.[62,165] These cells must receive nourishment to manufacture extracellular proteoglycans of the essential quantity and quality. Aged discs, for example, typically show reduced permeability and increased calcification of the vertebral endplates, which, in turn, reduce the flow of nutrients and oxygen into the disc.[25,169] This age-related process can inhibit cellular metabolism and synthesis of proteoglycans. Less proteoglycan content reduces the ability of the nucleus to attract and retain water, thereby limiting its ability to effectively absorb and transfer loads.[91]

Intervertebral Disc as a Hydrostatic Pressure Distributor

The vertebral column is the primary support structure for the trunk and upper body. While one stands upright for example, approximately 80% of the load supported by two adjoining lumbar vertebrae is carried through the interbody joint; the remaining 20% is carried by posterior elements, such as apophyseal joints and laminae.[5]

The intervertebral discs are uniquely designed as shock absorbers to protect the bone from excessive pressure that might result from body weight or strong muscle contraction. Compression forces push the endplates inward and toward the nucleus pulposus. Being filled mostly with water and therefore essentially incompressible, the young and healthy nucleus responds by deforming radially and outwardly against the annulus fibrosus (Figure 9-36, *A*). Radial deformation is

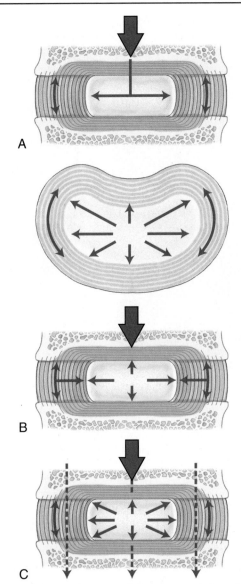

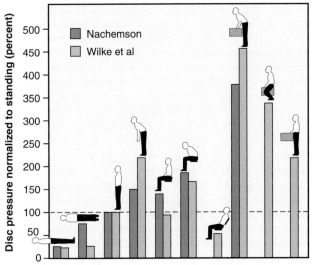

FIGURE 9-37. A comparison between data from two intradiscal pressure studies (see text). Each study measured in vivo pressures from a lumbar nucleus pulposus in a 70-kg subject during common postures and activities. The pressures are normalized to standing. (Modified from Wilke H-J, Neef P, Caimi M, et al: New in vivo measurements of pressures in the intervertebral disc in daily life, *Spine* 24:755, 1999.)

FIGURE 9-36. The mechanism of force transmission through an intervertebral disc. **A,** Compression force from body weight and muscle contraction *(straight arrows)* raises the hydrostatic pressure in the nucleus pulposus. In turn, the increased pressure elevates the tension in the annular fibrosus *(curved arrows)*. **B,** The increased tension in the annulus inhibits radial expansion of the nucleus. The rising nuclear pressure is also exerted upward and downward against the vertebral endplates. **C,** The pressure within the disc is evenly redistributed to several tissues as it is transmitted across the endplates to the adjacent vertebra. (Modified from Bogduk N: *Clinical anatomy of the lumbar spine*, ed 4, New York, 2005, Churchill Livingstone.)

resisted by the tension created within the stretched rings of collagen and elastin of the annulus fibrosus (see Figure 9-36, *B*). Pressure within the entire disc is thus uniformly elevated and transmitted evenly to the adjacent vertebra (see Figure 9-36, *C*). When the compressive force is removed from the endplates, the stretched elastin and collagen fibers return to their original preloaded length, ready for another compressive force. This mechanism allows compressive forces to be shared by multiple structures, thereby preventing a small spot of high pressure on any single tissue. Because it has viscoelastic properties, the intervertebral disc resists a fast or strongly applied compression more than a slow or light compression.[101] The disc therefore can be flexible at low loads and relatively rigid at high loads.

In Vivo Pressure Measurements from the Nucleus Pulposus

In vivo studies have confirmed that pressure within the nucleus pulposus in the lumbar region is relatively low at rest in the supine position.[13,140,219] Much larger disc pressures occur from activities that combine forward bending and the need for vigorous trunk muscle contraction. Intradiscal pressures can rise to surprisingly high levels and can produce transient changes in the shape of even the healthy disc. Sustained flexion in the lumbar spine, for example, can reduce the height of the disc slightly as water is slowly forced outward. Sustained and full lumbar *extension*, in contrast, reduces the pressure in the disc; this allows water to be reabsorbed into the disc, thus reinflating it to its natural level.

In vivo data on pressure within the disc during movement and changes in posture have greatly increased the understanding of ways to reduce injury to the disc. Data produced by two separate studies are compared in Figure 9-37.[138,219] Both studies reinforce three points: (1) disc pressures are large when one holds a load in front of the body, especially when bending forward; (2) lifting a load with knees flexed places less pressure on the lumbar disc than does lifting a load with the knees straight (the latter method typically generating more demands on the back muscles); and (3) sitting in a forward-slouched position produces greater disc pressure than sitting erect. These points serve as the theoretic basis for many educational programs designed for persons with disc degeneration, including disc herniation.

Diurnal Fluctuations in the Water Content within the Intervertebral Discs

When a healthy spine is unloaded, such as during bed rest, the pressure within the nucleus pulposus is relatively low.[138]

This relatively low pressure, combined with the hydrophilic nature of the nucleus pulposus, attracts water into the disc. As a result, the disc swells slightly when one is sleeping. When one is awake and upright, however, weight bearing produces compression forces across the vertebral endplates that push water out of the disc.[94] The natural cycle of swelling and contraction of the disc produces on average a 1% diurnal variation in overall body height.[201] The daily variation has a strong inverse relation to age. Karakida and colleagues used magnetic resonance imaging (MRI) to measure the variation in water content in the discs of a group of working persons between the ages of 23 and 56 years old, with no medical history of low-back pain.[100] Remarkably, significant diurnal variation in water content was found only in the discs of persons *younger than* 35 years of age. These findings are consistent with the fact that the water-retaining capacity of intervertebral discs naturally declines with increasing age.[6,14] The relative dehydration is caused by the parallel, age-related decline in the discs' proteoglycan content.[158,203]

A relatively dehydrated nucleus pulposus exerts less hydrostatic pressure when compressed.[23] Once relatively depressurized, the disc may bulge outward when compressed, similar to a "flat tire." The older, degenerated intervertebral disc is subsequently less able to uniformly cushion the vertebral body and endplates against compressive loads.[145] As a consequence, disc degeneration increases with age and affects most persons, to varying degrees, over 35 or 40 years of age.[78,100,158,164,206] A diagnosis of *disc degeneration* is most effectively made using MRI, typically based on a diminished signal intensity of the T2-weighted image (indicative of reduced water content), loss of distinction between the border of the annulus fibrosus and the nucleus pulposus, nuclear bulging, and loss of disc space.[78,100,157,164] The MRI scan in Figure 9-38 shows diminished signal intensity between L4-L5 and L5-S1 along with nuclear bulging. Furthermore, a degenerated disc may display circumferential, radial, and peripheral fissures (clefts) within the annulus.[78] According to Adams, these fissures can often be observed even in young adolescent persons.[6] Excessive degeneration may also be associated with complete depressurization of the nucleus in conjunction with delamination of the annular fibers and microfractures of the vertebral endplates.[78] In some cases the internal disruption of the annular fibers may lead to a herniation (prolapse) of the nucleus pulposus (typically posteriorly toward or into the spinal canal). Remarkably, a significant percentage of persons with observable signs of disc degeneration on MRI remain asymptomatic, *without* experiencing continued mechanical deterioration or loss of function.[95] The important topic of disc degeneration, including disc herniation, is described in more detail later in this chapter.

REGIONAL ANATOMY AND KINEMATICS ACROSS THE VERTEBRAL COLUMN

This section describes the anatomy and the kinematics throughout the various regions of the vertebral column. For each region, a maximum expected range of motion will be cited, assuming a starting, neutral position (Figure 9-39).[82,106,121] The reported range of motion in the literature is highly variable, reflecting differences in research design and differences resulting from the gender, age, and activity level of the subjects.[198] Data also vary for active and passive movements,

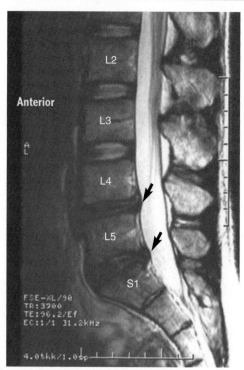

FIGURE 9-38. A midsagittal T2-weighted MRI scan of a 35-year-old man with a history of recurrent low-back pain that is provoked by prolonged or repeated lumbar flexion. Evidence of disc degeneration is indicated by a diminished (darker) signal intensity in the nuclear regions of L4-L5 and L5-S1. Posterior displacement or "bulging" of the disc is also noticeable at the L4-L5 and L5-S1 junctions *(arrows)*. (Image courtesy Paul F. Beattie PT, PhD.)

means used to stabilize the subject, and the tools used to measure the motion. Methods typically include the use of goniometers (manual, electrical, or fiberoptic), flexible rulers, or inclinometers or more sophisticated tools that employ three-dimensional MRI, planar and biplanar radiography, videofluoroscopy, ultrasonography, and computerized analysis using electromechanical, potentiometric, optical, or electromagnetic tracking systems.[*]

The connective tissues within the vertebral column play a major role in limiting and therefore defining the normal limits of motion across regions; selected examples are provided in Table 9-6. In cases of disease, trauma, or extended times of immobilization, these connective tissues may become abnormally stiff, thus interfering with normal kinematics. Understanding the structures' normal function is a prerequisite for the design of treatments aimed to increase intervertebral mobility.[85]

Introduction to Spinal Coupling

Movement performed within any given plane throughout the vertebral column is usually associated with an automatic, and usually imperceptible, movement in another plane. This kinematic phenomenon is called *spinal coupling*. Although spinal coupling can involve both rotation and translation, more clinical attention is paid to the rotational kinematics.

The mechanical explanations for the cause of most purported spinal coupling patterns are varied and typically

---

*References 19, 20, 108, 121, 197, 198, 222.

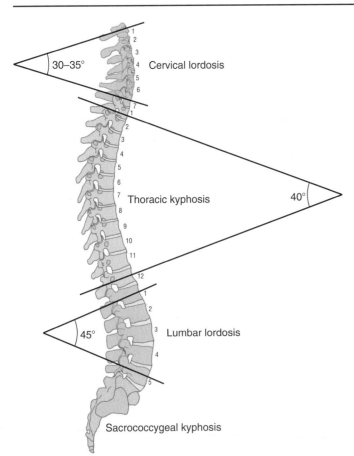

FIGURE 9-39. The normal sagittal plane curvatures across the regions of the vertebral column. The curvatures define the *neutral position* for each region, often referred to as "ideal" posture while standing.

TABLE 9-6. Selected Examples of Connective Tissues That May Limit Motions of the Vertebral Column

Motion of the Vertebral Column	Connective Tissues
Flexion	Ligamentum nuchae Interspinous and supraspinous ligaments Ligamentum flava Apophyseal joints* Posterior annulus fibrosus Posterior longitudinal ligament
Beyond neutral extension	Apophyseal joints Cervical viscera (esophagus and trachea) Anterior annulus fibrosus Anterior longitudinal ligament
Axial rotation	Annulus fibrosus Apophyseal joints Alar ligaments
Lateral flexion	Intertransverse ligaments Contralateral annulus fibrosus Apophyseal joints

*Depending on the movement, resistance generated by apophyseal joints may be caused by excessive approximation within the joint, increased tension within the capsule, or a combination of factors.

unclear. Explanations may include muscle action, articular facet alignment within apophyseal joints, preexisting posture, attachment of ribs, stiffness of connective tissues, and geometry of the physiologic curve itself.[42,58,111,135,182] The last explanation, rooted more in mechanics than biology, may be demonstrated by using a flexible rod as a model of the spine. Bend the rod about 30 to 40 degrees in one plane to mimic the natural lordosis or kyphosis of a particular region. While maintaining this curve, "laterally flex" the rod and note a slight automatic axial rotation. The biplanar bend placed on a flexible rod apparently creates unequal strains that are dissipated as torsion. This demonstration does not explain all coupling patterns observed clinically throughout the vertebral column, however.

Although some manual therapists incorporate spinal coupling into their assessment and treatment of spinal dysfunction, little consensus exists as to which coupling pattern is considered normal for a specific region.[42,111,182] One important exception is the relatively consistent coupling pattern that is naturally expressed between lateral flexion and rotation in the craniocervical region.[42,92] The specifics of this coupling pattern are described in detail in the section on kinematics of the craniocervical region.

Further study is needed to define a consistent spinal coupling pattern in the thoracic and lumbar regions. The motions of lateral flexion and axial rotation have indeed been shown to be coupled, although not consistently across multiple, controlled studies.[111,182] The inconsistency may reflect the natural variability of the phenomenon in these regions, as well as inadequate or different testing methodologies or conditions, dissimilar subject populations, or, more likely, a combination of these factors. Using a specific coupling pattern in the mid-to-lower thoracic and lumbar regions to direct a patient's evaluation and treatment should be done with caution and respect for its inconsistent and, at times, elusive nature.

Craniocervical Region

The terms "craniocervical region" and "neck" are used interchangeably. Both terms refer to the combined set of three articulations: *atlanto-occipital joint, atlanto-axial joint complex,* and *intracervical apophyseal joints* (C2 to C7). The overall organization used to present the regional anatomy and kinematics of the craniocervical region is outlined in Box 9-1. The upcoming section begins with an overview of the anatomy followed by a discussion of the kinematics, organized by plane of movement.

ANATOMY OF JOINTS

Atlanto-occipital Joint

The atlanto-occipital joints provide independent movement of the cranium relative to the atlas. The joints are formed by the protruding convex condyles of the occipital bone fitting into the reciprocally concave superior articular facets of the atlas (Figure 9-40). The congruent convex-concave relationship provides inherent structural stability to the articulation.

Anteriorly, the capsule of each atlanto-occipital joint blends with the *anterior atlanto-occipital membrane* (Figure 9-41). Posteriorly, the capsule is covered by a thin, broad *posterior atlanto-occipital membrane* (Figure 9-42). As depicted on the right side of Figure 9-42, the vertebral artery pierces the posterior atlanto-occipital membrane to enter the foramen magnum. This crucial artery supplies blood to the brain.

The concave-convex structure of the atlanto-occipital joints permits angular rotation in two degrees of freedom. The primary motions are flexion and extension. Lateral flexion is slight. Axial rotation is severely restricted and not considered as the third degree of freedom.

Atlanto-axial Joint Complex

The atlanto-axial joint complex has two articular components: a median joint and a pair of laterally positioned apophyseal joints. The median joint is formed by the dens of the axis (C2) projecting through an osseous-ligamentous ring created by the anterior arch of the atlas and the transverse ligament (Figure 9-43). Because the dens serves as a vertical axis for horizontal plane rotation of the atlas, the atlanto-axial joint is often described as a pivot joint.

The *median joint* within the atlanto-axial joint complex has two synovial cavities. The smaller, anterior cavity is formed between the anterior side of the dens and the posterior border of the anterior arch of the atlas (see Figure 9-43). A small anterior facet on the anterior side of the dens marks this articulation (see Figure 9-20, *A*). The much larger posterior cavity separates the posterior side of the dens and a cartilage-lined section of the *transverse ligament of the atlas*. This strong, 2-cm long ligament is essential to the horizontal plane stability of the atlanto-axial articulation.[33] Without its restraint, the atlas (and articulated cranium) can slip anteriorly relative to the axis, possibly damaging the spinal cord.[68,172]

The two *apophyseal joints* of the atlanto-axial joint are formed by the articulation of the inferior articular facets of the atlas with the superior facets of the axis (see exposed right joint in Figure 9-41). The surfaces of these apophyseal joints are generally flat and oriented close to the horizontal plane, a design that maximizes the freedom of axial rotation.

The atlanto-axial joint complex allows two degrees of freedom. About 50% of the total horizontal plane rotation within the craniocervical region occurs at the atlanto-axial joint complex. The second degree of freedom at this joint complex is flexion-extension. Lateral flexion is very limited and not considered a third degree of freedom.

Tectorial Membrane and the Alar Ligaments

A review of the anatomy of the atlanto-axial joint complex must include a brief description of the tectorial membrane and the alar ligaments, connective tissues that help connect

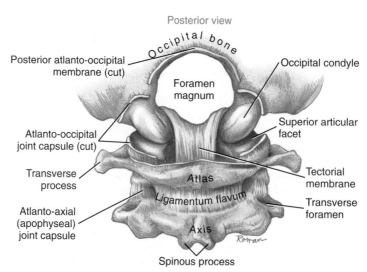

FIGURE 9-40. A posterior view of exposed atlanto-occipital joints. The cranium is rotated forward to expose the articular surfaces of the joints. Note the tectorial membrane as it crosses between the atlas and the cranium.

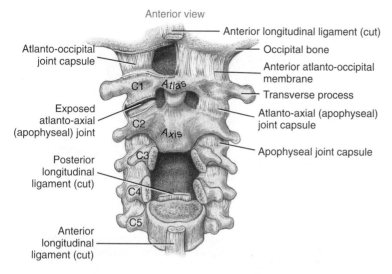

Anterior view

Atlanto-occipital joint capsule

Anterior longitudinal ligament (cut)

Occipital bone

Anterior atlanto-occipital membrane

C1   Atlas

Transverse process

Exposed atlanto-axial (apophyseal) joint

C2   Axis

Atlanto-axial (apophyseal) joint capsule

Apophyseal joint capsule

Posterior longitudinal ligament (cut)

C3

C4

Anterior longitudinal ligament (cut)

C5

FIGURE 9-41. An anterior view illustrates the connective tissues associated with the atlanto-occipital joint and the atlanto-axial joint complex. The right side of the atlanto-occipital membrane is removed to show the capsule of the atlanto-occipital joint. The capsule of the right atlanto-axial (apophyseal) joint is also removed to expose its articular surfaces. The spinal cord and the bodies of C3 and C4 are removed to show the orientation of the posterior longitudinal ligament.

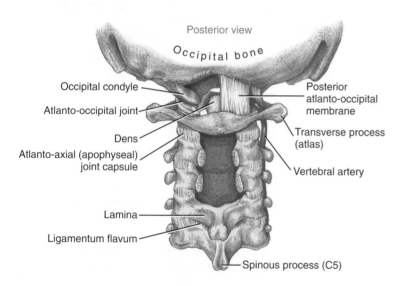

Posterior view

Occipital bone

Occipital condyle

Atlanto-occipital joint

Posterior atlanto-occipital membrane

Dens

Atlanto-axial (apophyseal) joint capsule

Transverse process (atlas)

Vertebral artery

Lamina

Ligamentum flavum

Spinous process (C5)

FIGURE 9-42. A posterior view illustrates the connective tissues associated with the atlanto-occipital joint and atlanto-axial joint complex. The left side of the posterior atlanto-occipital membrane and the underlying capsule of the atlanto-occipital joint are removed. The laminae and spinous processes of C2 and C3, the spinal cord, and the posterior longitudinal ligament and tectorial membrane are also removed to expose the posterior sides of the vertebral bodies and the dens.

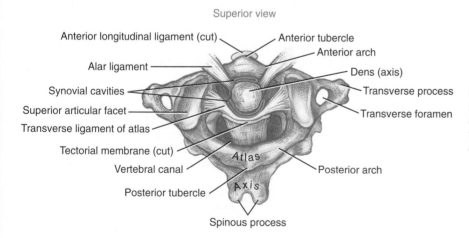

Superior view

Anterior longitudinal ligament (cut)

Anterior tubercle

Anterior arch

Alar ligament

Dens (axis)

Synovial cavities

Transverse process

Superior articular facet

Transverse foramen

Transverse ligament of atlas

Tectorial membrane (cut)

Vertebral canal

Atlas

Posterior arch

Axis

Posterior tubercle

Spinous process

FIGURE 9-43. A superior view of the dens and its structural relationship to the median atlanto-axial joint. The spinal cord is removed and the tectorial membrane is cut. Synovial membranes are in blue.

the cranium to the upper cervical spine. As discussed, the transverse ligament of the atlas makes firm contact with the posterior side of the dens (see Figure 9-43). Just posterior to the transverse ligament is a broad, firm sheet of connective tissue called the *tectorial membrane* (see Figure 9-40 and Figure 9-43). As a continuation of the posterior longitudinal liga-

ment, the tectorial membrane attaches to the basilar part of the occipital bone, just anterior to the rim of the foramen magnum.[188] There is limited published information on the function of the tectorial membrane. Based on attachments, however, the ligament likely provides generalized multidirectional stability to the craniocervical junction.

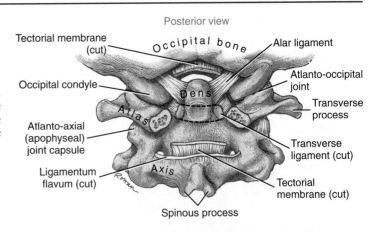

FIGURE 9-44. A posterior view of the atlanto-axial joint complex. The posterior arch of the atlas, tectorial membrane, and transverse ligament of the atlas are cut to expose the posterior side of the dens and the alar ligaments. The dashed lines indicate the removed segment of the transverse ligament of the atlas.

TABLE 9-7. Approximate Range of Motion for the Three Planes of Movement for the Joints of the Craniocervical Region

Joint or Region	Flexion and Extension (Sagittal Plane, Degrees)	Axial Rotation (Horizontal Plane, Degrees)	Lateral Flexion (Frontal Plane, Degrees)
Atlanto-occipital joint	Flexion: 5 Extension: 10 Total: 15	Negligible	About 5
Atlanto-axial joint complex	Flexion: 5 Extension: 10 Total: 15	35-40	Negligible
Intracervical region (C2-C7)	Flexion: 35-40 Extension: 55-60 Total: 90-100	30-35	30-35
Total across craniocervical region	Flexion: 45-50 Extension: 75-80 Total: 120-130	65-75	35-40

The horizontal and frontal plane motions are to one side only. Data are compiled from multiple sources (see text) and subject to large intersubject variations.

The *alar ligaments* are tough fibrous cords each about 1 cm in length with a thickness of a common pencil.[33,57] As shown in Figure 9-44, each ligament passes laterally and slightly upward from the apex of the dens to the medial sides of the occipital condyles. Clinically referred to as "check ligaments," the alar ligaments are respected for their ability to resist, or check, axial rotation of the head-and-atlas relative to the dens.[149] The pair of ligaments is loose in the neutral position but becomes increasingly taut during axial rotation; the ligament located contralateral to the side of the rotation exhibits slightly greater resistance to the movement.[45,57,172] In addition to limiting axial rotation, the alar ligaments also restrict the extremes of all other potential motions at the atlanto-occipital joint.

Intracervical Apophyseal Joints (C2 to C7)

The facet surfaces within apophyseal joints of C2 to C7 are orientated like shingles on a 45-degree sloped roof, approximately halfway between the frontal and horizontal planes (see Figure 9-18, C2-C3 articulation). This orientation enhances the freedom of movement in all three planes, a hallmark of cervical arthrology.

SAGITTAL PLANE KINEMATICS

The craniocervical region is the most mobile region within the entire vertebral column. Highly specialized joints facilitate precise positioning of the head, involving vision, hearing,

smell, and equilibrium. The individual joints within the craniocervical region normally interact in a highly coordinated manner. Table 9-7 lists typical ranges of motion contributed by each area of the craniocervical region.* Because of the large range and variability in the data presented in the literature, the actual values listed in this table are more useful for appreciating the *relative* kinematics among joints, and less as a strict objective guide for evaluating movement in patients.

Osteokinematics of Flexion and Extension

About 120 to 130 degrees of combined flexion and extension occur across the entire craniocervical region. From the neutral position of about 30 to 35 degrees of extension (resting lordosis), the craniocervical region *extends* some additional 75 to 80 degrees and *flexes* 45 to 50 degrees (Figures 9-45 and 9-46). Extension exceeds flexion throughout the craniocervical region, on average by a margin of just over 1.5 to 1.

In addition to muscles, connective tissues limit the extremes of craniocervical motion. For example, the ligamentum nuchae and interspinous ligaments provide significant restraint to the extremes of flexion, whereas the approximation of the apophyseal joints limits the extremes of extension.[163] Flexion is also limited by compression forces from the anterior margin of the annulus fibrosus, whereas extension is limited by the compression forces from the posterior margin of the annulus fibrosus. Additional tissues that limit or restrict

*References 20, 24, 58, 65, 147, 156, 197.

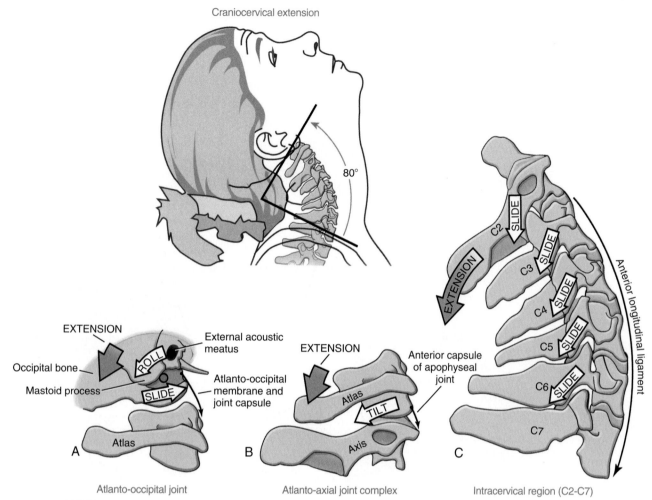

FIGURE 9-45. Kinematics of craniocervical extension. **A,** Atlanto-occipital joint. **B,** Atlanto-axial joint complex. **C,** Intracervical region (C2 to C7). Elongated and taut tissues are indicated by thin black arrows.

sagittal plane motion across the craniocervical region are listed in Table 9-6.

About 20% to 25% of the total sagittal plane motion at the craniocervical region occurs over the atlanto-occipital joint and atlanto-axial joint complex, and the remainder occurs over the apophyseal joints of C2 to C7.[147] The axis of rotation for flexion and extension is directed in a medial-lateral direction through each of the three joint regions: near the occipital condyles at the atlanto-occipital joint, the dens at the atlanto-axial joint complex, and the bodies or adjacent interbody joints of C2 to C7.[34,56]

The volume of the cervical vertebral canal is greatest in full flexion and least in full extension.[87] For this reason, a person with stenosis (narrowing) of the vertebral canal may be more vulnerable to spinal cord injury during hyperextension activities. Repeated episodes of hyperextension-related injuries may lead to cervical myelopathy (from the Greek root *myelo,* denoting spinal cord, and *pathos,* suffering) and related neurologic deficits.

Arthrokinematics of Flexion and Extension
Atlanto-occipital Joint
Like the rockers on a rocking chair, the convex occipital condyles *roll* backward in extension and forward in flexion within the concave superior articular facets of the atlas. Based on traditional convex-on-concave arthrokinematics, the condyles are expected to simultaneously *slide* slightly in the direction opposite to the roll (see Figure 9-45, *A* and Figure 9-46, *A*). Tension in articular capsules, associated atlanto-occipital membranes, and alar ligaments limits the extent of the arthrokinematics.

Atlanto-axial Joint Complex
Although the primary motion at the atlanto-axial joint complex is axial rotation, the joint structure allows about 15 degrees of total flexion and extension. Acting as a spacer between the cranium and axis, the ring-shaped atlas tilts forward during flexion and backward during extension (see Figure 9-45, *B* and Figure 9-46, *B*). The extent of the tilting is limited, in part, by contact between the transverse ligament of the atlas and dens (at full flexion) and anterior arch of the atlas and dens (at full extension).

Intracervical Articulations (C2 to C7)
Flexion and extension throughout the C2 to C7 vertebrae occur about an arc that follows the oblique plane set by the articular facets of the apophyseal joints. During *extension* the inferior articular facets of superior vertebrae slide *inferiorly* and *posteriorly,* relative to the superior articular facets of the inferior vertebrae (see Figure 9-45, *C*).

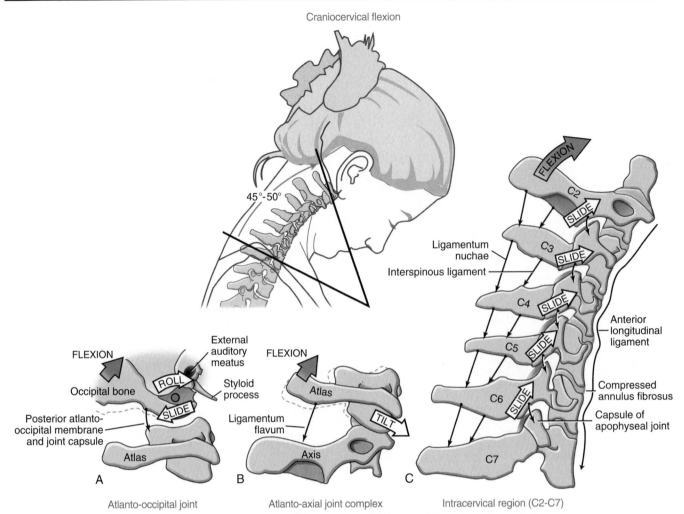

FIGURE 9-46. Kinematics of craniocervical flexion. **A,** Atlanto-occipital joint. **B,** Atlanto-axial joint complex. **C,** Intracervical region (C2 to C7). Note in **C** that flexion slackens the anterior longitudinal ligament and increases the space between the adjacent laminae and spinous processes. Elongated and taut tissues are indicated by thin black arrows; slackened tissue is indicated by a wavy black arrow.

These movements produce approximately 55 to 60 degrees of extension.

The neutral or slightly extended position of the cervical region maximizes the area of contact within the apophyseal joints. For this reason, this position is often considered the apophyseal joints' *close-packed position.* In fact, the neutral or slightly extended position is typically considered the close-packed position for *all* apophyseal joints across the vertebral column; moderate flexion is considered the joints' loose or open-packed position. (As described for most synovial joints in the body, the close-packed position is a unique position that increases the area of joint contact *and* increases the tension in the surrounding capsular ligaments. Because the capsular ligaments of apophyseal joints become increasingly tight on either side of the neutral or slightly extended position, these joints are an exception to this general rule.)

The arthrokinematics of *flexion* throughout the intracervical region occur in a reverse fashion to that described for extension. The inferior articular facets of the superior vertebrae slide *superiorly* and *anteriorly,* relative to the superior articular facets of the inferior vertebrae. As depicted in Figure 9-46, *C,* the sliding between the articular facets produces

approximately 35 to 40 degrees of flexion. Flexion stretches the capsule of the apophyseal joints and reduces the area of joint contact.

Overall, about 90 to 100 degrees of cervical flexion and extension occur as a result of the sliding within the cervical apophyseal joint surfaces. This extensive range of motion is in part a result of the relatively long and unobstructed arc of motion provided by the oblique plane of the facet surfaces. On average, about 15 degrees of sagittal plane motion occur at each intervertebral junction between C2-C3 and C7-T1. The largest sagittal plane angular displacement tends to occur at the C4-C5 or C5-C6 levels,[87,181] possibly accounting for the relatively high incidence of spondylosis and hyperflexion-related fractures at this level.

Osteokinematics of Protraction and Retraction

In addition to flexion and extension in the craniocervical region, the head can also translate forward (protraction) and backward (retraction) within the sagittal plane.[148] As indicated in Figure 9-47, from a neutral position, full range of protraction naturally exceeds full range of retraction by about 80% (6.23 cm versus 3.34 cm in the normal adult, respectively).[58]

Protraction   Retraction

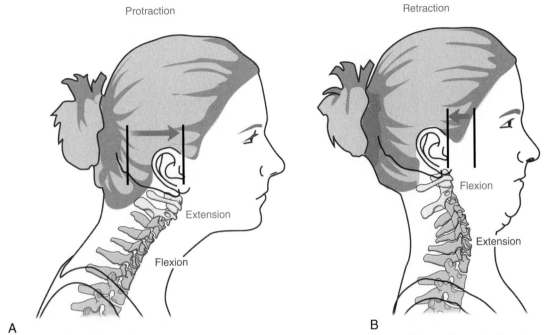

A   B

FIGURE 9-47. Protraction and retraction of the cranium. **A,** During protraction of the cranium, the lower-to-mid cervical spine flexes as the upper craniocervical region extends. **B,** During retraction of the cranium, in contrast, the lower-to-mid cervical spine extends as the upper craniocervical region flexes. Note the change in distance between the C1 and C2 spinous processes during the two movements.

The neutral position is about 35% *forward* from the fully retracted position.

Typically, *protraction* of the head flexes the lower-to-mid cervical spine and simultaneously extends the upper craniocervical region (see Figure 9-47, *A*). *Retraction* of the head, in contrast, extends or straightens the lower-to-mid cervical spine and simultaneously flexes the upper craniocervical region (see Figure 9-47, *B*). In both movements, *the lower-to-mid cervical spine follows the translation of the head.* Protraction and retraction of the head are physiologically normal and useful motions, often associated with enhancing vision. Prolonged periods of protraction, however, may lead to a chronic forward head posture, causing increased strain on the craniocervical extensor muscles.

HORIZONTAL PLANE KINEMATICS

Osteokinematics of Axial Rotation

Axial rotation of the head and neck is a very important function, intimately related to vision and hearing. The full range of craniocervical rotation is about 65 to 75 degrees but varies considerably with age.[197] Figure 9-48 shows a young person with about 80 degrees of active rotation to one side, for a total bilateral range of about 160 degrees. With an additional 160 to 170 degrees of total horizontal plane movement of the eyes, her bilateral visual field approaches 330 degrees, with little or no movement of the trunk.

About half the axial rotation of the craniocervical region occurs at the atlanto-axial joint complex, with the remaining throughout C2 to C7.[226] Rotation at the atlanto-occipital joint is restricted because of the deep-seated placement of the occipital condyles within the superior articular facets of the atlas.

Arthrokinematics of Axial Rotation
Atlanto-axial Joint Complex

The atlanto-axial joint complex is designed for maximal rotation within the horizontal plane. The design is most evident in the structure of the axis, with its vertical dens and near-horizontal superior articular facets (see Figure 9-32). The ring-shaped atlas and attached transverse ligament "twist" about the dens, producing about 35 to 40 degrees of axial rotation in each direction (see Figure 9-48, *A*). The generally flat inferior articular facets of the atlas slide in a curved path across the broad "shoulders" of the superior articular facets of the axis. Because of the limited axial rotation permitted at the atlanto-occipital joint, the cranium follows the rotation of the atlas nearly degree for degree. The axis of rotation for the head-and-atlas is provided by the vertically projected dens.

The extremes of axial rotation are limited primarily by contralaterally located alar ligaments, ligamentous tension in the apophyseal joints, and the many muscles that cross the craniocervical region (see Chapter 10). Full rotation stretches both vertebral arteries (see Figure 9-48, *A*).

Intracervical Articulations (C2 to C7)

Rotation throughout C2 to C7 is guided primarily by the spatial orientation of the facet surfaces within the apophyseal joints. The facet surfaces are oriented about 45 degrees between the horizontal and frontal planes (see Figure 9-32). The inferior facets slide *posteriorly* and *slightly inferiorly* on the same side as the rotation, and *anteriorly* and *slightly superiorly* on the side opposite the rotation (see Figure 9-48, *B*). Approximately 30 to 35 degrees of axial rotation occur to each side over the C2 to C7 region, nearly equal to that permitted at the atlanto-axial joint complex. Rotation is greatest in the more cranial vertebral segments.

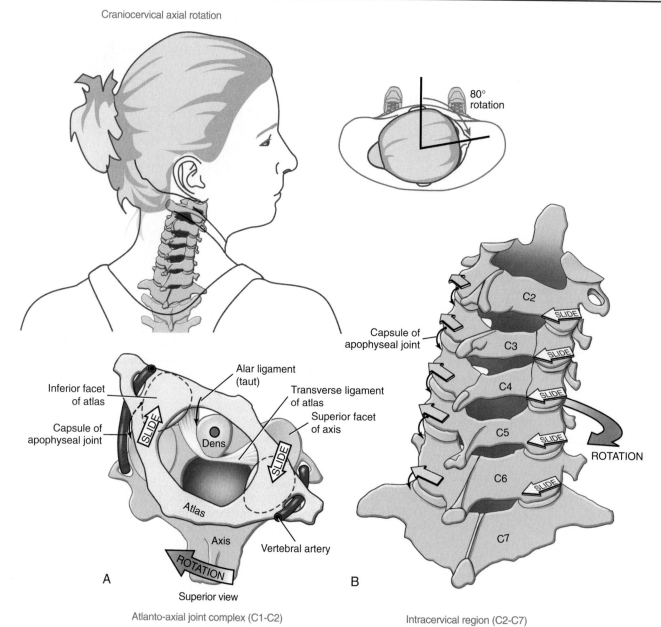

FIGURE 9-48. Kinematics of craniocervical axial rotation. **A,** Atlanto-axial joint complex. **B,** Intracervical region (C2 to C7).

FRONTAL PLANE KINEMATICS

Osteokinematics of Lateral Flexion

Approximately 35 to 40 degrees of lateral flexion are available to each side throughout the craniocervical region (Figure 9-49). The extremes of this movement can be demonstrated by attempting to touch the ear to the tip of the shoulder. Most of this movement occurs at the C2 to C7 region; however, about 5 degrees may occur at the atlanto-occipital joint. Lateral flexion at the atlanto-axial joint complex is negligible.

Arthrokinematics of Lateral Flexion
Atlanto-occipital Joint

A small amount of side-to-side *rolling* of the occipital condyles occurs over the superior articular facets of the atlas. Based on the convex-on-concave relationship of the joints,

the occipital condyles are expected to *slide* slightly in a direction opposite to the roll (see Figure 9-49, *A*).

Intracervical Articulations (C2 to C7)

The arthrokinematics of lateral flexion at the C2 to C7 vertebral segments are illustrated in Figure 9-49, *B*. The inferior articular facets on the side of the lateral flexion slide *inferiorly* and *slightly posteriorly*, and the inferior articular facets on the side opposite the lateral flexion slide *superiorly* and *slightly anteriorly*.

SPINAL COUPLING BETWEEN LATERAL FLEXION AND AXIAL ROTATION

The approximate 45-degree inclination of the articular facets of C2 to C7 dictates a mechanical *spinal coupling* between move-

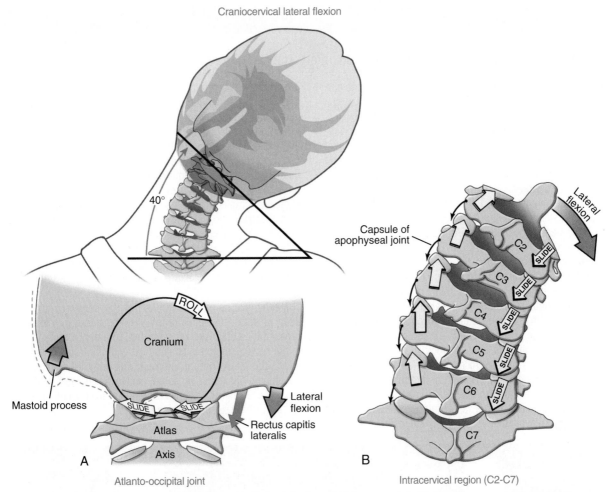

FIGURE 9-49. Kinematics of craniocervical lateral flexion. **A,** Atlanto-occipital joint. The rectus capitis lateralis is shown laterally flexing the joint. **B,** Intracervical region (C2 to C7). Note the ipsilateral coupling pattern between axial rotation and lateral flexion (see text for further details). Elongated and taut tissue is indicated by thin black arrows.

ments in the frontal and horizontal planes. Because an upper vertebra follows the plane of the articular facet of a lower vertebra, a component of lateral flexion and axial rotation occur simultaneously. For this reason, lateral flexion and axial rotation in the *mid-and-low* cervical region are mechanically coupled in an *ipsilateral fashion;* for example, lateral flexion to the right occurs with slight axial rotation to the right, and vice versa.[92]

The ipsilateral spinal coupling just described for the mid-to-lower craniocervical region is the most well accepted and least controversial coupling pattern of the entire vertebral column.[41] Although a few exceptions exist, this pattern has been documented using careful measurements, such as three-dimensional MRI. On casual visual observation, however, this coupling pattern is not so apparent. When asked, most persons appear to laterally flex the craniocervical region *without* an obligatory axial rotation of the face (or chin) to the side of the lateral flexion, or vice versa. The lack of a perceptible ipsilateral coupling is achieved by independent actions of either the atlanto-axial or atlanto-occipital joints. Consider, for instance, lateral flexion of C2 to C7 to the right. During this active motion, the atlanto-axial joint typically demonstrates a *contralateral* spinal coupling pattern by slightly rotating the atlas-and-cranium to the left, which conceals the fact that the C2 to C7 region actually rotated to the right.[92,93]

This compensatory action of the atlanto-axial joint minimizes the overall rotation of the head, which helps the eyes fixate on a stationary object during lateral flexion of the neck.

For reasons similar to those discussed in the previous paragraph, a compensatory contralateral coupling pattern usually also exists at the atlanto-occipital joints. This coupling minimizes any undesired lateral flexion of the head during axial rotation of the neck.[92,93] The contralateral coupling patterns expressed at both atlanto-axial and atlanto-occipital joints are controlled subconsciously by the actions of specialized muscles. This topic is addressed further in Chapter 10.

Thoracic Region

The thorax consists of a relatively rigid rib cage, formed by the ribs, thoracic vertebrae, and sternum. The rigidity of the region provides (1) a stable base for muscles to control the craniocervical region, (2) protection for the intrathoracic organs, and (3) a mechanical bellows for breathing (see Chapter 11).

ANATOMY OF THORACIC ARTICULAR STRUCTURES

The thoracic spine has 24 apophyseal joints, 12 on each side. Each joint possesses articular facets that face generally in the

SPECIAL FOCUS 9-5

Cervical Motion and Its Effect on the Diameter of the Intervertebral Foramina

Movement in the cervical region significantly affects the size of the intervertebral foramina. The difference in size can be large, especially during motions of flexion and extension.[104] This issue has important clinical implications because of the location of the exiting spinal nerve roots. Magnetic resonance imaging has shown that from a neutral position, 40 degrees of flexion *increases* the area of a cervical intervertebral foramen by 31%; extension to 30 degrees, in contrast, *decreases* the area by 20%.[137] The mechanical association between flexion and increased area in the C3-C4 intervertebral foramen can be appreciated by comparing the neutral position (Figure 9-50, *A*) with an extreme flexed position, shown in Figure 9-50, *B*. During flexion, an upward and forward slide of the inferior articular facet of C3 significantly widens the C3-C4 intervertebral foramen. Full flexion, therefore, allows greater room for passage of a spinal nerve root.

In addition to sagittal plane motion, the area of the intervertebral foramina also varies in size during lateral flexion and axial rotation. Lateral flexion increases the area within the contralateral intervertebral foramina—an obvious consequence after reviewing the arthrokinematics of this motion. Axial rotation also increases the area within the contralateral intervertebral foramina by as much as 20% after 40 degrees of craniocervical rotation.

The mechanics described thus far in this Special Focus have particular clinical relevance in cases of a stenosed (narrowed) intervertebral foramen, secondary to either an osteophyte or swelling of the connective tissue sheath surrounding the spinal nerve root. Compression against the spinal nerve root can result in *radiculopathy* (blocked transmission of motor or sensory nerve impulses) down the ipsilateral arm, usually in a path along the corresponding cervical dermatome. If the compression inflames the spinal nerve root, it may also precipitate *radicular* ("shooting") *pain* down a person's arm, usually initiated or exacerbated by excessive craniocervical motion. Consider, for example, a person with a severely stenosed intervertebral foramen on the right. A motion likely to compress the exiting nerve root would be full extension, especially if combined with the coupled motions of right lateral flexion and right axial rotation. This combination of movements may occur, for example, as a man shaves under his chin on the left side.

Mechanical or manual traction of the cervical region is often used in efforts to decompress a spinal nerve root that is compressed by a stenosed intervertebral foramen. Careful positioning of the cervical region in conjunction with the traction can in theory widen the intervertebral foramen. This may be accomplished by positioning the neck in some flexion, combined with tolerable amounts of lateral flexion and, usually, axial rotation *away from* the side of the suspected pathology.

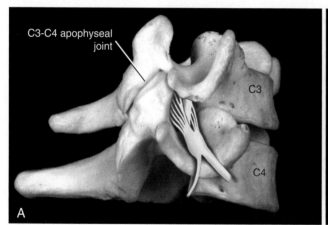
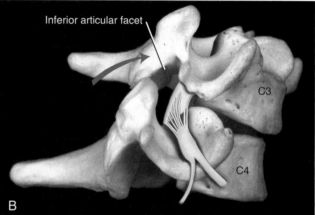

FIGURE 9-50. Illustration designed to show how full flexion between C3 and C4 affects the size of the intervertebral foramen. **A,** In the neutral position the facet surfaces within the apophyseal joint are in full contact. **B,** Maximum flexion is associated with an upward and forward movement of the inferior articular facet of C3. This "opening" of the apophyseal joint significantly increases the size of the intervertebral foramen, thereby providing greater room for passage of the C⁴ spinal nerve root. Note the reduced contact area within the flexed apophyseal joint.

frontal plane, with a mild forward slope that averages about 15 to 25 degrees from the vertical (see example of T4 in Figure 9-32).[124,150] The movement potential of these apophyseal joints is limited by the relative immobility of the adjacent costocorporeal and costotransverse joints. Indirectly, this pair of joints mechanically links most of the thoracic vertebrae anteriorly to the fixed sternum.

Most *costocorporeal joints* connect the head of a rib with a pair of costal demifacets on thoracic vertebral bodies and with the adjacent margin of an intervening intervertebral disc (Figure 9-51). The articular surfaces of the costocorporeal joints are slightly ovoid,[188] held together primarily by *capsular* and *radiate ligaments*.

Costotransverse joints connect the articular tubercle of most ribs to the costal facet on the transverse process of the corresponding thoracic vertebrae. An articular capsule surrounds this synovial joint. The extensive (nearly 2 cm long) *costotransverse ligament* firmly anchors the neck of a rib to the entire

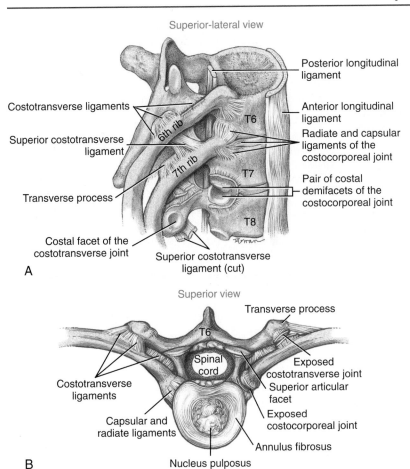

Superior-lateral view

Posterior longitudinal ligament

Costotransverse ligaments

Superior costotransverse ligament

6th rib

T6

Anterior longitudinal ligament

Radiate and capsular ligaments of the costocorporeal joint

7th rib

T7

Transverse process

Pair of costal demifacets of the costocorporeal joint

T8

Costal facet of the costotransverse joint

Superior costotransverse ligament (cut)

A

Superior view

Transverse process

T6

Spinal cord

Exposed costotransverse joint

Superior articular facet

Costotransverse ligaments

Exposed costocorporeal joint

Capsular and radiate ligaments

Annulus fibrosus

Nucleus pulposus

B

FIGURE 9-51. The costotransverse and costocorporeal joints of the midthoracic region. **A,** Superior-lateral view highlights the structure and connective tissues of the costotransverse and costocorporeal joints associated with the sixth through the eighth thoracic vertebrae. The eighth rib is removed to expose the costal facets of the associated costocorporeal and costotransverse joints. **B,** Superior view shows the capsule of the left costocorporeal and costotransverse joints cut to expose joint surfaces. Note the spatial relationships among the nucleus pulposus, annulus fibrosus, and spinal cord.

length of a corresponding transverse process (see Figure 9-51). In addition, each costotransverse joint is stabilized by a *superior costotransverse ligament*. This strong ligament attaches between the superior margin of the neck of one rib and the inferior margin of the transverse process of the vertebra located above (see Figure 9-51, *A*). Ribs 11 and 12 usually lack costotransverse joints.

Because the ribs attach to the thoracic vertebrae, the kinematics of the thorax and the costocorporeal and costotransverse joints must be mechanically related, although this topic has not been rigorously studied. This text focuses on the kinematics of the costocorporeal and costotransverse joints as they relate to ventilation in Chapter 11.

Key Anatomic Aspects of the Costocorporeal and Costotransverse Joints

Each Costocorporeal Joint
- Usually connects the head of rib with a pair of costal demifacets and the adjacent margin of an intervening intervertebral disc
- Is stabilized by radiate and capsular ligaments

Each Costotransverse Joint
- Usually connects the articular tubercle of a rib with the costal facet on the transverse process of a corresponding thoracic vertebra
- Is stabilized by the costotransverse and the superior costotransverse ligaments

---

With the exception of the sacroiliac joints, the thoracic region as a whole is normally the most mechanically stable portion of the vertebral column. Much of this inherent stability is afforded through attachments between the thoracic vertebrae and the rib cage. The constituents of the rib cage include the costocorporeal and costotransverse joints, ribs, sternocostal joints, and the sternum. In a study using cadavers, Watkins and colleagues showed that the rib cage (including the sternum) provides 20% to 40% of the total passive resistance against full thoracic motion.[215] This resistance, however, does not include additional factors that exist in the living, such as volitionally increasing intra-abdominal pressure (via a Valsalva maneuver) and activating intercostal and trunk muscles. Nevertheless, the presence of an intact and stable rib cage protects the thoracic spine, including the spinal cord. During a fall, for example, the impact to the thoracic spine is partially absorbed and dissipated by the rib cage and the associated muscles and connective tissues. Evidence for this can be found by the relatively high frequency of fractures of the sternum that occur in combination with thoracic spine injuries.[215]

KINEMATICS

When an adult is standing, the thoracic region typically exhibits about 40 to 45 degrees of natural kyphosis.[121] From the neutral position, motion occurs in all three planes. Although the range of motion at each thoracic intervertebral junction is relatively small, cumulative motion is considerable when expressed over the entire thoracic spine (Table 9-8). Few consistent and reliable data could be found in the literature that describe the three-dimensional kinematics in the thoracic region.[121] The values presented in Table 9-8, therefore, are based partially on visual observation.

The direction and extent of thoracic movement within any given plane are influenced by several factors, including the resting posture of the region, apophyseal joints, connections to the rib cage, and relative heights of the intervertebral discs. Compared with the cervical and lumbar regions, the thoracic region has by far the smallest disc-to-vertebral body height ratio. The relatively thin discs naturally limit the extent to which one vertebral body can rotate (or rock) on another before being blocked by bony compression, at least in the sagittal and frontal planes. Although this factor slightly reduces thoracic mobility, it adds another element of overall stability to the region.

Kinematics of Flexion and Extension

Approximately 30 to 40 degrees of flexion and 20 to 25 degrees of extension are available throughout the thoracic region. These kinematics are shown in context with flexion and extension over the entire thoracolumbar region in Figures 9-52 and 9-53, respectively. The extremes of *flexion* are limited

TABLE 9-8. **Approximate Range of Motion for the Three Planes of Movement for the Thoracic Region**

Flexion and Extension (Sagittal Plane, Degrees)	Axial Rotation (Horizontal Plane, Degrees)	Lateral Flexion (Frontal Plane, Degrees)
Flexion: 30-40 Extension: 20-25 Total: 50-65	30-35	25-30

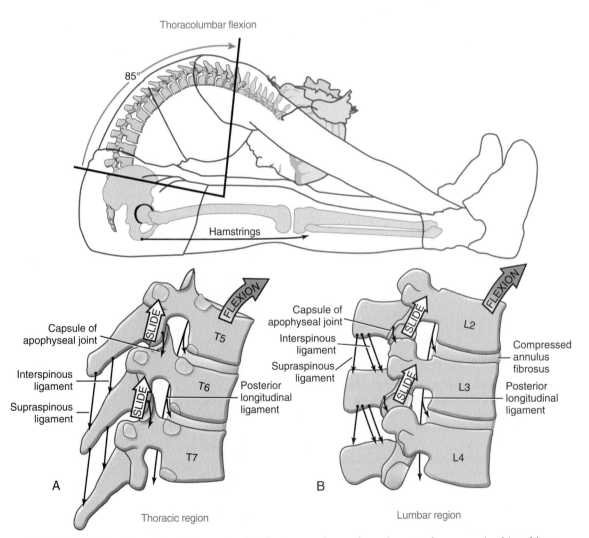

FIGURE 9-52. The kinematics of thoracolumbar flexion are shown through an 85-degree arc: in this subject, the sum of 35 degrees of thoracic flexion and 50 degrees of lumbar flexion. **A,** Kinematics at the thoracic region. **B,** Kinematics at the lumbar region. Elongated and taut tissues are indicated by thin black arrows.

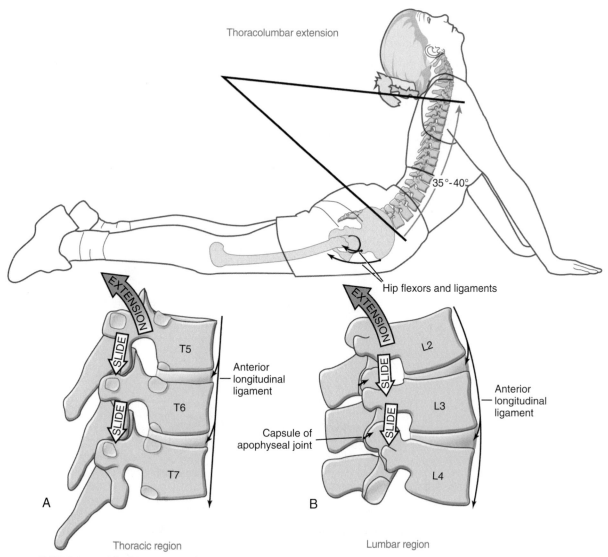

FIGURE 9-53. The kinematics of thoracolumbar extension are shown through an arc of 35 to 40 degrees: the sum of 20 to 25 degrees of thoracic extension and 15 degrees of lumbar extension. **A,** Kinematics at the thoracic region. **B,** Kinematics at the lumbar region. Elongated and taut tissue is indicated by thin black arrows.

by tension in connective tissues located posterior to the vertebral bodies, including the capsule of the apophyseal joints and supraspinous and posterior longitudinal ligaments. The extremes of *extension,* on the other hand, are limited by tension in the anterior longitudinal ligament and by potential impingement between laminae or between adjacent downward-sloping spinous processes, especially in the upper and middle thoracic vertebrae. The magnitude of thoracic flexion and extension is greater in the extreme caudal regions, in great part because of the "free-floating" most caudal ribs and the shift to a more sagittal plane orientation of the apophyseal joints.[124,182]

The arthrokinematics at the apophyseal joints in the thoracic spine are generally similar to those described for the C2 to C7 region. Subtle differences are related primarily to different shapes of the vertebrae, rib attachments, and different spatial orientations of the articular facets of apophyseal joints.

Flexion between T5 and T6, for example, occurs by a superior and slightly anterior sliding of the inferior facet surfaces of T5 on the superior facet surfaces of T6 (see Figure 9-52, *A*). The moderately forward-sloped articular surfaces of the apophyseal joints naturally facilitate flexion throughout the region. *Extension* occurs by a reverse process (see Figure 9-53, *A*).

Kinematics of Axial Rotation

Approximately 30 to 35 degrees of horizontal plane (axial) rotation occur to each side throughout the thoracic region. This motion is depicted in conjunction with axial rotation across the entire thoracolumbar region in Figure 9-54. Rotation between T6 and T7, for instance, occurs as the near–frontal plane–aligned inferior articular facets of T6 slide for a short distance against the similarly aligned superior articular facets of T7 (see Figure 9-54, *A*). The freedom of axial rotation

Thoracolumbar axial rotation

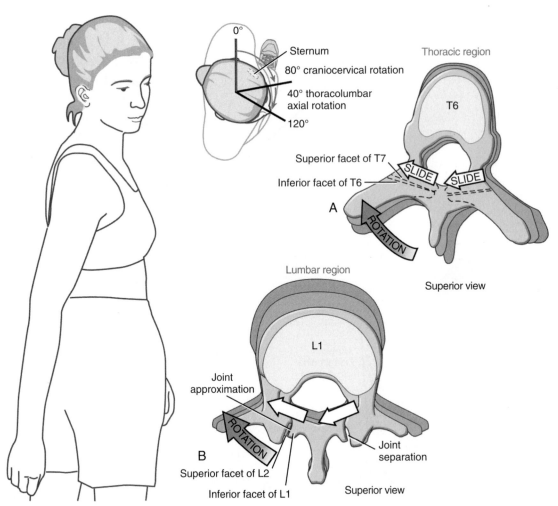

FIGURE 9-54. The kinematics of thoracolumbar axial rotation is depicted as the subject rotates her face 120 degrees to the right. The thoracolumbar axial rotation is shown through an approximate 40-degree arc: the sum of about 35 degrees of thoracic rotation and 5 degrees of lumbar rotation. **A,** Kinematics at the thoracic region. **B,** Kinematics at the lumbar region.

declines in lower regions of the thoracic spine. In this region, the apophyseal joints are slightly more vertically oriented as they shift to a more sagittal plane orientation.[124,182]

Kinematics of Lateral Flexion

The predominant frontal plane orientation of the thoracic facet surfaces suggests a relative freedom of lateral flexion. This potential for movement is never fully expressed, however, because of the stabilization provided by the attachments to the ribs. Lateral flexion in the thoracic region is illustrated in context with lateral flexion over the entire thoracolumbar region in Figure 9-55. Approximately 25 to 30 degrees of lateral flexion occur to each side in the thoracic region. As depicted in Figure 9-55, *A,* lateral flexion of T6 on T7 occurs as the inferior facet surface of T6 slides superiorly on the side contralateral to the lateral flexion and inferiorly on the side ipsilateral to the lateral flexion. Note that the ribs drop slightly on the side of the lateral flexion and rise slightly on the side opposite the lateral flexion.

Lumbar Region

ANATOMY OF THE ARTICULAR STRUCTURES

L1 to L4 Region

The facet surfaces of most lumbar apophyseal joints are oriented nearly vertically, with a moderate-to-strong sagittal plane bias (Figure 9-56). The orientation of the superior articular facet of L2, for example, is on average about 25 degrees from the sagittal plane (see Figure 9-32). This orientation favors sagittal plane motion at the expense of rotation in the horizontal plane.

L5-S1 Junction

As any typical intervertebral junction, the L5-S1 junction has an interbody joint anteriorly and a pair of apophyseal joints posteriorly. The facet surfaces of the L5-S1 apophyseal joints are usually oriented in a more frontal plane than those of other lumbar regions (see Figure 9-56).

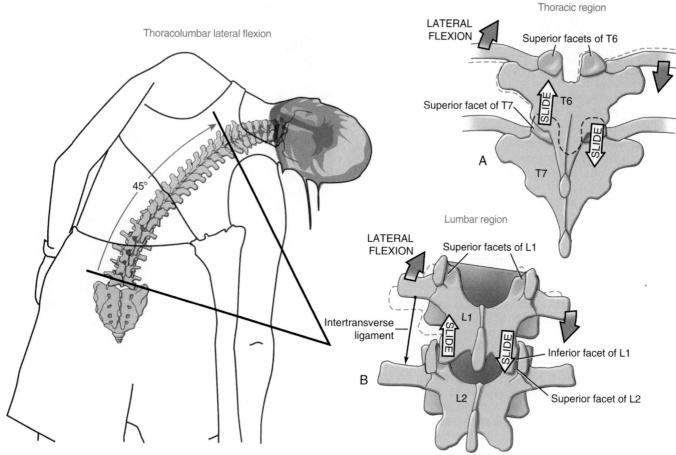

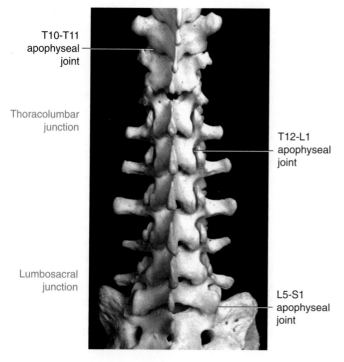

FIGURE 9-55. The kinematics of thoracolumbar lateral flexion are shown through an approximate 45-degree arc: the sum of 25 degrees of thoracic lateral flexion and 20 degrees of lumbar lateral flexion. **A,** Kinematics at the thoracic region. **B,** Kinematics at the lumbar region. Elongated and taut tissue is indicated by a thin black arrow.

FIGURE 9-56. A posterior view of the thoracolumbar and lumbosacral junctions. Note the transition in the orientation of the facet surfaces within the apophyseal joints at the two junctions. Also note that the bony specimen demonstrates a frontal plane bias at both L4-L5 and L5-S1 apophyseal joints. This variation is not uncommon.

Some Clinical Implications Regarding the Thoracolumbar Junction

At or near the thoracolumbar junction, the facet surfaces of the apophyseal joints change their orientation rather abruptly, from near-frontal to near-sagittal planes.[124] The exact point of this transition is variable, often starting one or two junctions cranialward, as shown in the specimen illustrated in Figure 9-56. This relative sharp frontal-to-sagittal plane transition in apophyseal joint orientation may create a sagittal plane hypermobility and instability in this region. This is evident in Figure 9-57 as a young boy with cerebral palsy attempts to support himself up on his knees. The lack of control and weakness of his trunk muscles allows the thoracolumbar junction to collapse into the plane of least bony resistance—in this case, into marked thoracolumbar hyperextension. This collapse creates a severe hyperlordosis in the region.

As a second clinical example, the aforementioned sharp frontal-to-sagittal plane transition in apophyseal joints may partially explain the relatively high incidence of traumatic paraplegia at the thoracolumbar junction. In certain high-impact accidents involving trunk flexion, the thorax, held relatively rigid by the rib cage, is free to violently flex as a unit over the upper lumbar region. A large flexion torque delivered to the thorax may concentrate an excessive hyperflexion stress at the point of transition. If severe enough, the stress may fracture or dislocate the bony elements and possibly injure the caudal end of the spinal cord or the cauda equina. Surgical fixation devices implanted to immobilize an unstable thoracolumbar junction are particularly susceptible to stress failure, compared with devices implanted in other regions of the vertebral column.

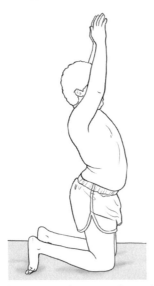

FIGURE 9-57. Illustration of a young boy with cerebral palsy with weak and poor control of his trunk muscles. Note the excessive hyperextension in the region of the thoracolumbar junction. (Courtesy Lois Bly, PT, MA.)

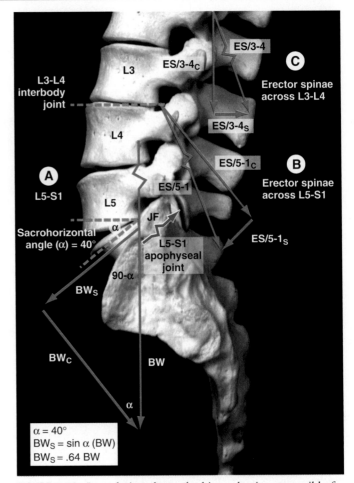

$$\alpha = 40°$$
$$BW_S = \sin \alpha \, (BW)$$
$$BW_S = .64 \, BW$$

FIGURE 9-58. Lateral view shows the biomechanics responsible for the shear forces at the interbody joints of L5-S1 and middle lumbar region (L3-L4). **A,** The sacrohorizontal angle (α) at L5-S1 is the angle between the horizontal plane and the superior surface of the sacrum. BW (body weight) is the weight of the body located above the sacrum. BW_C is the force of body weight directed perpendicular to the superior surface of the sacrum. BW_S is the shear force of body weight directed parallel to the superior surface of the sacrum. The joint force *(JF)* at the L5-S1 apophyseal joint is shown as a short blue arrow. **B,** The force vector of the active erector spinae is shown as it crosses L5-S1 (ES/5-1). ES/5-1$_C$ is the force of the muscle directed perpendicular to the superior surface of the sacrum. ES/5-1$_S$ is the shear force of the muscle directed parallel to the superior surface of the sacrum. **C,** The force vector of the erector spinae is shown as it crosses L3-L4 (ES/3-4). ES/3-4$_C$ is the compression force of the muscle directed perpendicular to the superior surface of L4. ES/3-4$_S$ is the shear force of the muscle directed parallel to the superior surface of L4. See text for further details. (Created with the assistance of Guy Simoneau, PT, PhD.)

The base (top) of the sacrum is naturally inclined anteriorly and inferiorly, forming an approximate 40-degree *sacrohorizontal angle* when one is standing (Figure 9-58, *A*).[106] Given this angle, the resultant force resulting from body weight (BW) creates an *anterior* shear force (BW_S), and a compressive force (BW_C) acting perpendicular to the superior surface of the sacrum. The magnitude of the anterior shear is equal to the product of BW times the sine of the sacrohorizontal angle. A typical sacrohorizontal angle of 40 degrees produces an anterior shear force at the L5-S1 junction equal to 64% of superimposed BW. Increasing the degree of lumbar lordosis enlarges the sacrohorizontal angle, which in effect increases the anterior shear at the L5-S1 junction. If the sacrohorizontal angle were increased to 55 degrees, for example, the anterior shear force would increase to 82% of superimposed BW. During standing or sitting, lumbar lordosis can be increased by this amount by anterior tilting of the pelvis (see Figure 9-63, *A*). (Tilting the pelvis is defined as a short-arc sagittal plane rotation of the pelvis relative to both femoral heads. The direction of the tilt is indicated by the direction of rotation of the iliac crests.)

Several structures resist the natural anterior shearing force produced at the L5-S1 junction. The wide and strong *anterior longitudinal ligament* crosses anterior to the L5-S1 junction. The *iliolumbar ligament* arises from the inferior aspect of the transverse processes of L4-L5 and adjacent fibers of the quadratus lumborum muscle. The ligament attaches inferiorly to the ilium, just anterior to the sacroiliac joint, and to the upper-lateral aspect of the sacrum (see Figure 9-70). Bilaterally, the iliolumbar ligaments provide a firm anchor between the naturally stout transverse processes of L5 and the underlying ilium and sacrum.[23,72,224]

In addition to the aforementioned connective tissues, the wide, sturdy articular facets of the L5-S1 apophyseal joints provide bony stabilization to the L5-S1 junction. The near–frontal plane inclination of the facet surfaces is ideal for resisting the anterior shear at this region. This resistance creates a compression force within the L5-S1 apophyseal joints (see blue force vector in Figure 9-58, *A*, labeled JF). Without adequate stabilization, the lower end of the lumbar region can slip forward relative to the sacrum.[76] This abnormal, potentially serious condition is known as *anterior spondylolisthesis*.

SPECIAL FOCUS 9-7

Anterior Spondylolisthesis at L5-S1

*A*nterior spondylolisthesis is a general term that describes an anterior slipping or displacement of one vertebra relative to another. This condition often occurs at the L5-S1 junction, as illustrated in Figure 9-59. The term *spondylolisthesis* is derived from the Greek *spondylo,* meaning vertebra, and *listhesis,* meaning to slip. This condition may be acquired after excessive stress or pathology, or it may be congenital.[207] Most often, an anterior spondylolisthesis in the lower lumbar region is associated with a bilateral fracture (or deficit) through the *pars articularis,* a section of a lumbar vertebra midway between the superior and inferior articular processes (see Figure 9-27). The acquired form of anterior spondylolisthesis at L5 and S1 may be progressive, in some cases caused by repetitive physical activities that involve hyperextension of the region. Severe cases of anterior spondylolisthesis may damage the cauda equina, as this bundle of nerves passes by the L5-S1 junction.

As described for Figure 9-58, *A,* increased lumbar lordosis increases the normal sacrohorizontal angle, thereby increasing the anterior shear force between L5 and S1. Exercises or other actions that create a forceful hyperextension of the lower lumbar spine are therefore contraindicated for persons with anterior spondylolisthesis, especially if the condition is unstable or progressive.[207] As shown in Figure 9-58, *B,* the force vector of the erector spinae muscle that crosses L5-S1 (ES/5-1) creates an anterior shear force (ES/5-1$_S$) parallel to the superior body of the sacrum. The direction of this shear is a function of the orientation of the adjacent erector spinae fibers and the 40-degree sacrohorizontal angle. In theory, a greater muscular force increases the anterior shear at the L5-S1 junction, especially if the muscle activation exaggerates the lordosis.

The anterior-directed shear forces produced by the lumbar erector spinae occur primarily at the L5-S1 junction and not, as a rule, throughout the entire lumbar region.[102] As indicated in Figure 9-58, *C,* in normal posture the superior surfaces of the bodies of the middle lumbar vertebrae are typically positioned in a more horizontal orientation. The erector spinae muscle fibers that cross this region more likely produce a *posterior* shear across the lumbar interbody joints (see Figure 9-58, *C,* ES/3-4$_S$).[125] This muscle-produced shear may be physiologically useful, offering resistance to the anterior shear that may be produced during bending and lifting loads in front of the body.

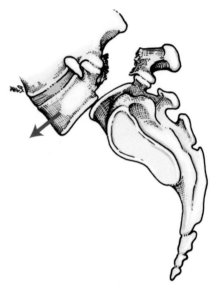

FIGURE 9-59. Severe anterior spondylolisthesis at the L5-S1 junction, after a fracture of the pars articularis. (See text for more details.) (Modified from Canale ST, Beaty JH: *Campbell's operative orthopedics,* ed 11, St Louis, 2008, Mosby.)

TABLE 9-9. Approximate Range of Motion for the Three Planes of Movement for the Lumbar Region

Flexion and Extension (Sagittal Plane, Degrees)	Axial Rotation (Horizontal Plane, Degrees)	Lateral Flexion (Frontal Plane, Degrees)
Flexion: 40-50 Extension: 15-20 Total: 55-70	5-7	20

BOX 9-2. Order of the Subtopics Involving the Sagittal Plane Kinematics at the Lumbar Region

Flexion of the lumbar spine
Extension of the lumbar spine
Lumbopelvic rhythm during trunk flexion and extension
  • Variations of lumbopelvic rhythms during *trunk flexion* from a standing position: a kinematic analysis
  • Lumbopelvic rhythm during *trunk extension* from a forward bent position: a muscular analysis
Effect of pelvic tilting on the kinematics of the lumbar spine
  • Kinesiologic correlations between anterior pelvic tilt and increased lumbar lordosis
  • Kinesiologic correlations between posterior pelvic tilt and decreased lumbar lordosis

KINEMATICS

While a healthy adult is standing, the lumbar spine typically exhibits about 40 to 50 degrees of lordosis,[23,106] although a wide variation exists. From this neutral position, the lumbar spine can move in three degrees of freedom. Data on the range of lumbar motion are highly variable; typical values are listed in Table 9-9.* The following sections focus on the kinematics of each plane of motion within the lumbar region.

Sagittal Plane Kinematics: Flexion and Extension

Although data vary considerably across studies and populations, about 40 to 50 degrees of flexion and 15 to 20 degrees of extension occur at the lumbar spine.[144,152,153,198,213] The total 55- to 70-degree arc of sagittal plane motion is substantial, considering it occurs across only five intervertebral junctions. This predominance of sagittal plane motion is largely a result of the prevailing sagittal plane orientation of the facet surfaces of the lumbar apophyseal joints.

Many important and common activities of daily living involve flexion and extension of the midsection of the body, including the hips. Consider, for example, bending forward to touch the ground, ascending steep steps, or getting out of an automobile or a young child transitioning between crawling and sitting. All these activities involve a kinematic interaction among the trunk, lumbar spine, and the pelvis on femurs (hips). As described later in this chapter, this kinematic interaction exists as far cranially as the craniocervical region.

The following section of the chapter focuses on several subtopics within the broad topic of sagittal plane kinematics of the lumbar spine. Box 9-2 lists the order of these subtopics.

Flexion of the Lumbar Region

Figure 9-52, *B* shows the kinematics of flexion of the lumbar region in context with flexion of the trunk and hips. Pelvic-on-femoral (hip) flexion increases the passive tension in the stretched hamstring muscles. With the lower end of the vertebral column fixed by the sacroiliac joints, continued flexion of the middle and upper lumbar region reverses the natural lordosis in the low back.

During flexion between L2 and L3, for example, the inferior articular facets of L2 slide superiorly and anteriorly, relative to the superior facets of L3. As a consequence, compression

forces from body weight are transferred *away from* the apophyseal joints (which normally support about 20% of the total spinal load in erect standing) and *toward* the discs and vertebral bodies.[5,174] The compressed anterior aspects of the discs and stretched posterior ligaments support more of the total load as the trunk is progressively flexed. In extreme flexion the fully stretched articular capsules of the apophyseal joints restrain further forward migration of the superior vertebra.[194]

The extreme flexed position significantly reduces the contact area within the apophyseal joints. Paradoxically, although a fully flexed lumbar spine reduces the total load on a given apophyseal joint, it is possible that the *contact pressure* (force per unit area) may actually increase because of the reduced surface area to distribute the load. The absolute increase in contact pressure may or may not be excessive, however, depending on the total magnitude of the forces that are acting on the flexed joint. The presence of strong trunk muscle activation in a flexed position can drive contact pressures very high. Exceedingly high pressure can damage the flexed apophyseal joints, especially if sustained over a prolonged period or if the articular surfaces are abnormally shaped.

The degree of flexion of the lumbar spine significantly affects the diameter of each intervertebral foramen and the potential deformation of the nucleus pulposus. Relative to a neutral position, full flexion increases the diameter of the intervertebral foramen by 19%.[90] Lumbar flexion therefore may be used therapeutically as a way to temporarily reduce the pressure on a lumbar spinal nerve root that is impinged on by an obstructed foramen.[173] In certain circumstances, however, this potential therapeutic advantage may be associated with a potential therapeutic disadvantage. For example, excessive or prolonged flexion of the lumbar region generates increased compression force on the anterior side of the disc, ultimately deforming the gel-like nucleus pulposus in a posterior direction.* In the healthy spine the magnitude of the posterior deformation is small and usually of no consequence. Actual migration of the disc is normally resisted by increased tension in the stretched posterior side of the annulus fibrosus. A disc with a weak, cracked, or distended posterior annulus may, however, experience a posterior migration (or oozing) of the

---
*References 81, 105, 121, 144, 152, 153, 198, 213.

*References 3, 9, 27, 64, 67, 176, 200.

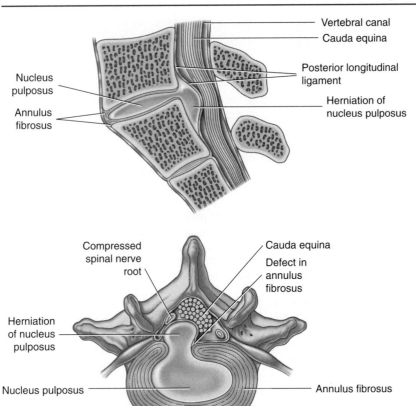

Nucleus
pulposus

Annulus
fibrosus

Vertebral canal

Cauda equina

Posterior longitudinal
ligament

Herniation of
nucleus pulposus

Compressed
spinal nerve
root

Herniation
of nucleus
pulposus

Nucleus pulposus

Cauda equina

Defect in
annulus
fibrosus

Annulus fibrosus

FIGURE 9-60. Two views of a full herniated nucleus pulposus in the lumbar region. (From Standring S: *Gray's anatomy*, ed 40, New York, 2009, Churchill Livingstone.)

nucleus pulposus. In some cases the nuclear material may impinge against the spinal cord or nerve roots (Figure 9-60). This potentially painful impairment is frequently referred to as a *herniated* or *prolapsed disc*, or more formally a *herniated nucleus pulposus*. Persons with a herniated disc may experience pain or altered sensation, muscle weakness, and reduced reflexes in the lower extremity, consistent with the specific motor and sensory distribution of the impinged nerve root.

Extension of the Lumbar Region

Extension of the lumbar region is essentially the reverse kinematics of flexion, and it increases the natural lordosis (see Figure 9-53). When lumbar extension is combined with full hip extension, the increased passive tension in the stretched flexor muscles and capsular ligaments of the hip promotes lumbar lordosis by generating an anteriorly tilting force on the pelvis. Extension between L2 and L3, for example, occurs as the inferior articular facets of L2 slide inferiorly and slightly posteriorly relative to the superior facets of L3.

From a flexed position, moving into the neutral or slightly extended position increases the contact area within the apophyseal joints, at a time when these joints are typically accepting a greater percentage of body weight.[174,179] This situation may help limit the contact pressure within the joints. This protective scenario does not apply, however, to the physiologic *extremes* of lumbar extension. In full lumbar hyperextension, the tips of the inferior articular facets (of a top vertebra) slide inferiorly beyond the joint surface of the superior articular facets of the vertebra below. Contact pres-

sures can therefore be very high in the hyperextended lumbar spine as the relatively "sharp" tips of the inferior articular facet contact the adjacent lamina region. For this reason, a chronic posture of lumbar hyperlordosis can place large and potentially damaging stress on the apophyseal joints and adjacent regions. Furthermore, hyperextension of the lumbar spine can compress the interspinous ligaments, possibly creating a source of low-back pain.[85]

As with flexion, extension of the lumbar spine significantly affects the diameter of the intervertebral foramina and the potential for deforming the nucleus pulposus.[9,67,176] Relative to the neutral position, full lumbar extension reduces the diameter of the intervertebral foramina by 11%.[90] For this reason a person with nerve root impingement caused by a stenosed intervertebral foramen should limit activities that involve hyperextension, especially if they cause weakness or altered sensations in the extremities. Full extension, however, tends to deform the nucleus pulposus in an *anterior* direction,[64,200] thereby potentially limiting the more typical posterior migration of the nucleus.[9,18] Full sustained lumbar extension has been shown to reduce pressure within the disc[138,175] and in some cases to reduce the contact pressure between the displaced nuclear material and the neural tissues. Evidence of the latter is often described as "centralization" of symptoms, meaning that the pain or altered sensation (formerly perceived in the lower extremities because of nerve root impingement) migrates *toward* the low back.[55,217] Centralization therefore suggests reduced contact pressure between the displaced nuclear material and a nerve root. The reduced contact pres-

More about the Herniated Nucleus Pulposus

The formal name for a herniated or prolapsed disc is a *herniated nucleus pulposus.* Herniations typically involve a posterior-lateral or posterior migration of the nucleus pulposus toward the very sensitive neural tissues (i.e., the spinal cord, cauda equina, ventral or dorsal nerve roots, or exiting spinal nerve roots). Not all herniated discs are as remarkable as that illustrated in Figure 9-60.[95] In relatively mild cases the displaced nucleus migrates posteriorly but remains well within the confines of the annulus fibrosus. More moderate cases, however, may progress to a point at which the nuclear material, although still remaining within the posterior annulus, *bulges* or *protrudes* beyond the circumference of the posterior rim of the vertebral body. In more severe cases this nuclear material completely herniates through the annular wall (or posterior longitudinal ligament) and *extrudes* into the epidural space (depicted in Figure 9-60). The extruded nuclear material may contain fragments of the degenerated annulus and vertebral endplates.[220] In some cases the extruded material may become lodged in the epidural space—frequently referred to as *sequestration* of the herniated disc. Extruded or sequestered herniations may have a better prognosis than a protruded or bulging disc. Once displaced into the spinal canal, the herniated nucleus attracts macrophages that can assist with resorption of the displaced material.[95]

Disc-related pain may result from the degenerated disc itself or from consequences of a herniated nucleus pulposus. Pain associated with a degenerated disc may be from damage to the innervated periphery of the posterior annulus fibrosus, posterior longitudinal ligament, or vertebral endplates. Perhaps more serious, however, is the pain and radiculopathy caused by the herniated disc compressing the neural tissues within the spinal canal (as seen in Figure 9-60). In both scenarios, pain increases when the local tissues are inflamed.[116] Compressed and inflamed nerves within the spinal canal or intervertebral foramina typically produce pain and altered sensations that are topographically associated with the dermatomes in the lower extremities. The symptoms are often referred to as "sciatica" because of the strong likelihood that the herniated disc affects nerve roots associated with the sciatic nerve (L^4-S^3). Although pain may be a large component of a herniated nucleus pulposus, it is not a universal consequence of the pathlogy.[26]

Posterior disc herniation in the lumbar region typically involves two often interrelated mechanisms. The first involves a large, sudden compression or shear force delivered against an otherwise relatively healthy lumbar spine. This mechanism of injury may be associated with a single traumatic event, such as extremely strenuous coughing or vomiting[154] or the lifting of a very large load. A second and much more common mechanism involves a series of lower-magnitude forces delivered against the lumbar spine over the course of several years, most often involving *preexisting disc degeneration.*[63,214] A degenerated disc may possess radial clefts (or fissures) that serve as a path of least resistance for the migration of the nuclear material.

Repetitive or chronic flexion of the lumbar spine increases the vulnerability of a posterior or posterior-lateral disc herniation. Flexion stretches and thins the posterior side of the annulus while the nuclear gel is forced posteriorly, often under high hydrostatic pressure. These pressures increase during strenuous lifting or bending activities that require strong activation of trunk muscles.[138,175] With sufficiently high hydrostatic pressure, the nuclear gel can create or find a preexisting fissure in the posterior annulus.

Lumbar flexion combined with a twisting motion (i.e., axial rotation combined with lateral flexion) further increases the vulnerability of a posterior or posterior-lateral disc herniation.[175,200] When the spine is rotated, only half the posterior fibers of the annulus are taut, reducing its resistance to the approaching nuclear gel. Computer modeling and cadaveric research have also shown that combined axial rotation and lateral flexion concentrate large circumferential tensions in the annular fibers located within the posterior-lateral quadrant of the disc.[175,200] Over time, this region is more prone to develop fissures or cracks, thereby providing little resistance to the encroaching nuclear material.

It has been argued that a severely degenerated (and dehydrated) disc seldom experiences the classic herniated nucleus pulposus.[29] Apparently, a dehydrated nucleus is too dry and not under sufficient hydrostatic pressure to flow through the annulus. Although exceptions certainly exist, the classic herniated nucleus pulposus tends to occur more frequently in persons under the age of about 40 years old, at a time when the nucleus is still able to retain a relatively large volume of water. Furthermore, the chance of experiencing a herniated disc tends to be greater in the morning, when the nucleus contains its greatest daily water content.[15,118]

Mechanical or Structural Factors That Favor a Herniated Nucleus Pulposus in the Lumbar Spine

1. Preexisting disc degeneration with radial fissures, cracks, or tears in the posterior annulus that allow a path for the flow of nuclear material
2. Sufficiently hydrated nucleus capable of exerting high intradiscal pressure
3. Inability of the posterior annulus to resist pressure from the migrating nucleus
4. Sustained or repetitive loading applied over a flexed and rotated spine

---

sure after sustained full extension may occur because the nuclear material is pushed forward and away from the neural tissues, because the neural tissues are pulled posteriorly and away from the nuclear material, or both. Emphasizing lumbar extension exercises and postures as a way to reduce radiating pain and radiculopathy from a posterior herniated nucleus pulposus was popularized by Robin McKenzie, and such exercises are well known as "McKenzie exercises."[127] Therapeutic approaches that emphasize sustained active and passive extension have been shown to offer varying degrees of relief of symptoms and improvement of function in persons with a known posterior or posterior-lateral disc herniation.[30,38] This one approach, however, is likely not beneficial for everyone with chronic low-back pain.[119]

Lumbopelvic Rhythm during Trunk Flexion and Extension

In conjunction with the hip joints, the lumbar spine provides the major flexion and extension pivot point for the human body as a whole. Consider, in this respect, activities such as forward and backward bending of the trunk, climbing a steep hill, and lifting objects from the ground. The kinematic relationship between the lumbar spine and hip joints during such sagittal plane movements has been referred to as *lumbopelvic rhythm.* (A loose analogy of this concept exists for the shoulder and was described as *scapulohumeral rhythm* in Chapter 5.) Paying attention to the lumbopelvic rhythm in persons with painful or labored movements may provide clues for detecting abnormal muscle and joint interactions within the region.[110,134,180,196] These clues may provide insight into effective treatment for the underlying pathomechanics.

Variations of Lumbopelvic Rhythms during *Trunk Flexion* from a Standing Position: a Kinematic Analysis. Consider the common action of bending forward toward the ground while keeping the knees nearly straight. This motion in the healthy adult has been measured as a combination of about 40 degrees of lumbar flexion performed nearly simultane-ously with about 70 degrees of hip (pelvic-on-femoral) flexion (Figure 9-61, *A*).[60] Although other kinematic strategies are likely, those which deviate significantly from this pattern may help distinguish pathology or impairments affecting the lower spine from those affecting the hip joints.

Figure 9-61, *B* and *C* shows abnormal lumbopelvic rhythms associated with marked restriction in mobility at the hip joints *(B)* or lumbar region *(C)*. In both *B* and *C*, the amount of overall trunk flexion is reduced. If greater trunk flexion is required, the hip joints or lumbar region may mutually compensate for the other's limited mobility. This situation may increase the stress on the compensating region. As depicted in Figure 9-61, *B*, with *limited hip flexion* from, for example, restricted hamstring extensibility, bending the trunk toward the floor requires greater flexion in the lumbar and lower thoracic spinal regions. Eventually, exaggerated flexion may overstretch and subsequently weaken the posterior connective tissues within the region (including the thoracolumbar fascia), thereby reducing the ability of these tissues to limit further flexion. A chronic posture of increased flexion of the lumbar spine places a disproportionally larger compressive load on the intervertebral discs, theoretically increasing their likelihood for degeneration.

Figure 9-61, *C* demonstrates a kinematic scenario where *flexion of the lumbar spine is limited.* Reaching toward the floor

Variations of lumbopelvic rhythms during trunk flexion: A kinematic analysis

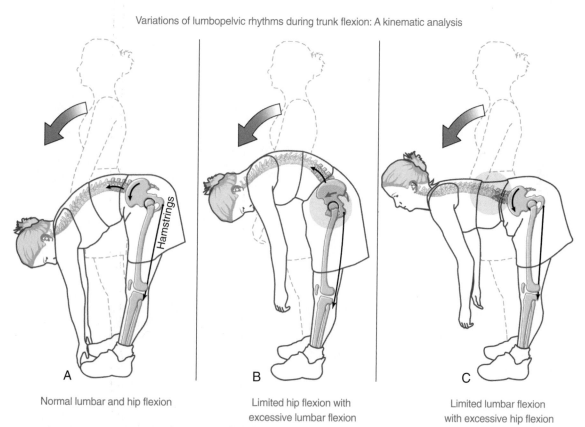

A	B	C
Normal lumbar and hip flexion	Limited hip flexion with excessive lumbar flexion	Limited lumbar flexion with excessive hip flexion

FIGURE 9-61. Three different lumbopelvic rhythms used to flex the trunk forward and toward the floor with knees held straight. **A,** A normal kinematic strategy used to flex the trunk from a standing position, incorporating a near simultaneous 40 degrees of flexion of the lumbar spine and 70 degrees of hip (pelvic-on-femoral) flexion. **B,** With limited flexion in the hips (for example, from tight hamstrings), greater flexion is required of the lumbar and lower thoracic spine. **C,** With limited lumbar mobility, greater flexion is required of the hip joints. In **B** and **C,** the red shaded circles and red arrows indicate regions of restricted mobility.

Lumbopelvic rhythm during trunk extension: A Muscular analysis

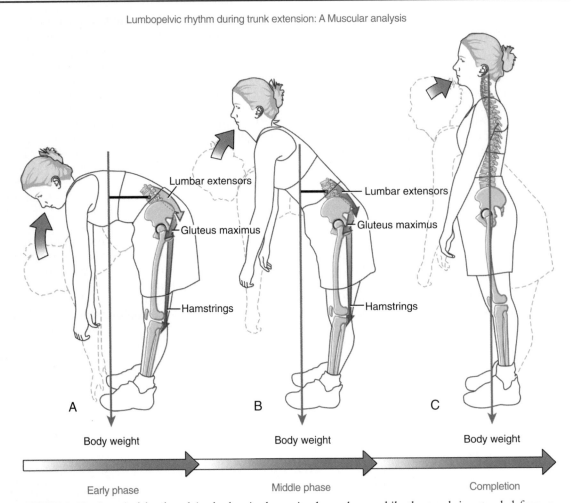

FIGURE 9-62. A typical lumbopelvic rhythm is shown in three phases while the trunk is extended from a forward bent position. The motion is conveniently divided into three chronologic phases (**A** to **C**). In each phase the axis of rotation for the trunk extension is arbitrarily placed through the body of L3. **A,** In the *early phase,* trunk extension occurs to a greater extent through extension of the hips (pelvis on femurs), under strong activation of hip extensor muscles (gluteus maximus and hamstrings). **B,** In the *middle phase,* trunk extension occurs to a greater degree by extension of the lumbar spine, requiring increased activation from lumbar extensor muscles. **C,** At the *completion* of the event, muscle activity typically ceases once the line of force from body weight falls posterior to the hips. The external moment arm used by body weight is depicted as a solid black line. The greater intensity of red indicates relatively greater intensity of muscle activation.

requires disproportionally greater flexion of the hips, thereby creating greater demands on the hip extensor muscles. As a consequence, the hip joints are subjected to greater compression loads. In persons with healthy hips, this relatively low-level increase in compression force is usually well tolerated. In a person with a preexisting hip condition (such as osteoarthritis or hip instability), however, the increased compression force may be painful and possibly accelerate a degenerative process.

Lumbopelvic Rhythm during *Trunk Extension* from a Forward Bent Position: a Muscular Analysis. The typical lumbopelvic rhythm used to extend the trunk from a forward bent position is depicted in a series of consecutive phases in Figure 9-62, *A* to *C*. Extension of the trunk with knees

extended is often initiated by extension of the hip joints (see Figure 9-62, *A*). This is usually followed after a short delay by extension of the lumbar spine (see Figure 9-62, *B* to *C*).[141] This short delay in lumbar extension places greater extension torque demands on the powerful hip extensor muscles (such as the hamstrings and gluteus maximus) at the time when the external flexion torque on the lumbar region is greatest (see external moment arm depicted as a dark black line in Figure 9-62, *A*). This may be a beneficial strategy to naturally protect the low-back muscles and joints from large forces. In this scenario, the demand on the lumbar extensor muscles increases only *after* the trunk has been sufficiently raised and the external moment arm, relative to body weight, has been minimized (see Figure 9-62, *B*). Persons with low-back pain or existing degenerative conditions may purposely further

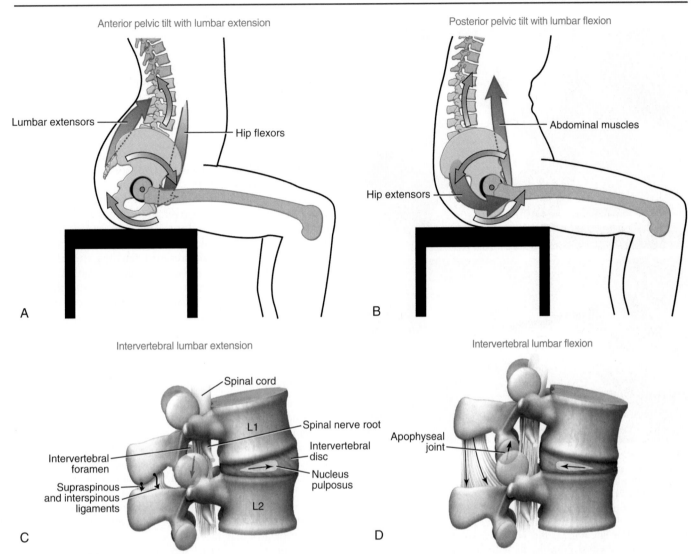

FIGURE 9-63. Anterior and posterior tilting of the pelvis and its effect on the kinematics of the lumbar spine. **A** and **C,** *Anterior pelvic tilt* extends the lumbar spine and increases the lordosis. This action tends to shift the nucleus pulposus anteriorly and reduces the diameter of the intervertebral foramen. **B** and **D,** *Posterior pelvic tilt* flexes the lumbar spine and decreases the lordosis. This action tends to shift the nucleus pulposus posteriorly and increases the diameter of the intervertebral foramen. Muscle activity is shown in red.

delay strong activation of the lumbar extensor muscles until the trunk is nearly vertical. Once standing fully upright, hip and back muscles are typically relatively inactive, as long as the force vector resulting from body weight falls posterior to the hip joints (see Figure 9-62, *C*).

Effect of Pelvic Tilting on the Kinematics of the Lumbar Spine
Flexion and extension of the lumbar spine typically occur by one of two fundamentally different movement strategies. The first strategy is often used to maximally displace the upper trunk and upper extremities relative to the thighs, such as when lifting or reaching. This strategy, depicted in Figures 9-61, *A* and 9-62, combines near maximal flexion and extension of the lumbar spine with a wide arc of pelvic-on-femoral (hip) and trunk motion. A second, more subtle movement strategy involves a relatively *short-arc* forward or backward tilt (or rotation) *of the pelvis,* with the trunk remaining nearly stationary. As depicted in Figure 9-63, *A* to *D*, an anterior

pelvic tilt accentuates lumbar lordosis, whereas a posterior pelvic tilt reduces lumbar lordosis.[112] The extremes of these postures can significantly alter the diameter of the lumbar vertebral canal and intervertebral foramina and create a pressure gradient that may deform or push the nucleus pulposus slightly—in a direction *away from* the compressed side of the disc.

The axis of rotation for pelvic tilting is in a medial-lateral direction through both hip joints. This mechanical association strongly links the (pelvic-on-femoral) movement of the hip joints with that of the lumbar spine. This relationship is discussed further in the next section and again in Chapter 12.

Kinesiologic Correlations between Anterior Pelvic Tilt and Increased Lumbar Lordosis. Active anterior pelvic tilt is caused by contraction of the hip flexor and back extensor muscles (see Figure 9-63, *A*). Strengthening and increasing the

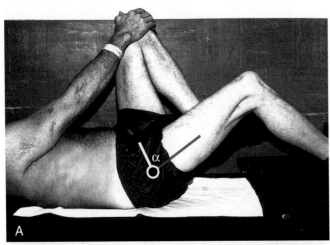

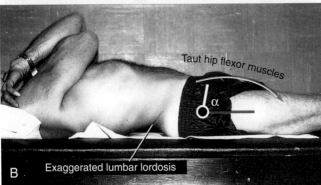

Taut hip flexor muscles

α

B   Exaggerated lumbar lordosis

FIGURE 9-64. The relationship between taut hip flexor muscles, excessive anterior pelvic tilt, and exaggerated lumbar lordosis in a person with marked right hip osteoarthritis. The medial-lateral axis of rotation of the hip is shown as an open white circle. **A,** A right hip flexion contracture is shown by the angle (α) formed between the femur *(red line)* and a *white line* representing the iliac crest of the pelvis. The left normal hip is held flexed to keep the pelvis as posteriorly tilted as possible. **B,** With both legs allowed to lie against the mat, tension created in the taut and shortened right hip flexors tilts the pelvis anteriorly, exaggerating the lumbar lordosis. The increased lordosis is evident by the hollow in the low-back region. The hip flexion contracture is still present but is masked by the anteriorly tilted position of the pelvis. (Photograph from the archives of the late Mary Pat Murray, PT, PhD, FAPTA, Marquette University.)

postural control of these muscles, in theory, favors a more lordotic posture of the lumbar spine.[173] Whether a person can subconsciously adopt and maintain a newly learned pelvic posture over an extended period is uncertain. Nevertheless, maintaining the natural lordotic posture in the lumbar spine is a fundamental principle espoused by McKenzie for some persons with a posteriorly herniated nucleus pulposus.[127]

The lumbar region may demonstrate greatly exaggerated lordosis that is physiologically undesirable. This could be caused by muscle weakness, such as weakness of the hip extensor and abdominal muscles in a child with severe muscular dystrophy. The pathomechanics of exaggerated lumbar lordosis often involve a hip flexion contracture with increased passive tension (tightness) in the hip flexor muscles (Figure

9-64).[75] As described earlier in this chapter, possible negative consequences of exaggerated lordosis include increased compression within the lumbar apophyseal joints or increased contact pressure between posterior elements of lumbar vertebrae.[179] Furthermore, exaggerated lumbar lordosis is associated with an increased anterior shear force at the lumbosacral junction and, in some persons, possibly favoring the development of an anterior spondylolisthesis.

Kinesiologic Correlations between Posterior Pelvic Tilt and Decreased Lumbar Lordosis. Active posterior pelvic tilt is produced by contraction of the hip extensor and abdominal muscles (see Figure 9-63, *B*). Strengthening and increasing the patient's conscious control over these muscles theoretically favor a reduced lumbar lordosis. This concept was the trademark of the once popular "Williams flexion exercises," a therapeutic approach that stressed stretching the hip flexor and low-back extensor muscles while strengthening the abdominal and hip extensor muscles.[221] In principle, these exercises were considered most appropriate for persons with low-back pain caused by excessive lumbar lordosis. As previously described, exaggerated lumbar lordosis increases the sacrohorizontal angle, which may predispose a person to an anterior spondylolisthesis of the lower lumbar region.

Horizontal Plane Kinematics: Axial Rotation

Only about 5 to 7 degrees of horizontal plane rotation occur to each side throughout the lumbar region.[151,198] Clinical measurements often exceed this amount, likely because of extraneous motion at the hip joint (pelvis rotating on the femur) and the lower thoracic region.[144] The 5 to 7 degrees of rotation are shown in context with the rotation of the thoracolumbar region in Figure 9-54, *B*. Axial rotation between L1 and L2 to the right, for instance, occurs as the left inferior articular facet of L1 approximates or compresses against the left superior articular facet of L2. Simultaneously, the right inferior articular facet of L1 separates (distracts) slightly from the right superior articular facet of L2.

The limited amount of axial rotation permitted within the lumbar region is remarkable. Just over 1 degree of unilateral axial rotation has been measured at the L3-L4 intervertebral junction.[189] The relatively strong sagittal plane orientation of the lumbar apophyseal joints physically restrict axial rotation. As indicated in Figure 9-54, *B*, the apophyseal joints located contralateral to the side of the rotation compress (or approximate), thereby blocking further movement. Much of the actual rotation is accompanied by compression of the articular cartilage within the contralateral apophyseal joint. (Recall that the direction of rotation of any part of the axial skeleton is based on a point on the *anterior* side of the region, not the spinous process.) Axial rotation is also restricted by tension created in the stretched annulus fibrosus.[107] In theory, an axial rotation of 3 degrees at any lumbar intervertebral junction would damage the articular facet surfaces and tear the collagen fibers in the annulus fibrosus.[23] Most normal physiologic movements remain safely under this potentially damaging limit.

The natural bony resistance to axial rotation in the lumbar region provides vertical stability throughout the lower end of the vertebral column. The well-developed lumbar multifidi muscles and relatively rigid sacroiliac joints reinforce this stability.

SPECIAL FOCUS 9-9

Using Knowledge of Kinesiology to Help Guide Treatment of Chronic Low-Back Pain: a Selected Example

There are many nonsurgical, therapeutic approaches for treating persons with chronic low-back pain. One reason for the many differing approaches is the frequent lack of understanding of the exact mechanical dysfunction, pathology, and underlying cause of the pain. Pain in the low back can stem from multiple anatomic sources, including muscle, bone, superficial regions of the intervertebral disc, spinal nerve root or spinal cord impingement, ligament, dura mater, fascia, or apophyseal and sacroiliac joints. Treatment approaches also vary based on the formal training, clinical experience, and theoretic and philosophical background of the clinician. Some clinicians direct their nonsurgical treatment for low-back pain based primarily on pathoanatomic or mechanical-based models. Others, however, rely more on classifying, or subgrouping, their patients based on clusters of examination findings that have been shown to favorably respond to a given therapeutic approach.[30,39,71,195]

A thorough discussion of the various physical therapy approaches to chronic low-back pain is not within the scope of this chapter.

In short, however, approaches include training to improve the strength and control of muscles, selective activation and stretching of muscles and connective tissues to optimize vertebral movement and alignment,[161] advice on modifying posture or design of the workplace, mobilization and manipulation,[10] traction, soft-tissue massage, and physical modalities (e.g., heat, electrical stimulation, and therapeutic ultrasound). Many approaches associated with the treatment (as well as diagnosis) of low-back pain involve movement of the lumbar region. For this reason the clinician must understand the associated kinesiology. To highlight one example of this point, consider the marked and usually contrasting biomechanical effects that are associated with flexion and extension of the lumbar intervertebral junctions (Table 9-10). The contrasting biomechanics can give important clues as far as the source of pain or mechanical dysfunction, and ultimately the most effective treatment.

TABLE 9-10. Some Contrasting Kinesiologic Effects of Lumbar Flexion and Extension

Structure	Effect of Flexion	Effect of Extension
Nucleus pulposus	Deformed or pushed posteriorly	Deformed or pushed anteriorly
Annulus fibrosus	Posterior side stretched	Anterior side stretched
Apophyseal joint	Capsule stretched Minimizes articular contact area Articular loading decreased	Capsule slackened (neutral extension only) Maximizes articular contact area (neutral extension only) Articular loading increased
Intervertebral foramen	Widened	Narrowed
Posterior longitudinal ligament	Increased tension (elongated)	Decreased tension (slackened)
Ligamentum flavum	Increased tension (elongated)	Decreased tension (slackened)
Interspinous ligament	Increased tension (elongated)	Decreased tension (slackened)
Supraspinous ligament	Increased tension (elongated)	Decreased tension (slackened)
Anterior longitudinal ligament	Decreased tension (slackened)	Increased tension (elongated)
Spinal cord	Increased tension (elongated)	Decreased tension (slackened)

Frontal Plane Kinematics: Lateral Flexion

About 20 degrees of lateral flexion occur to each side in the lumbar region.[151,198,213] Except for differences in orientation and structure of the apophyseal joints, the arthrokinematics of lateral flexion are nearly the same in the lumbar region as in the thoracic region. Ligaments on the side opposite the lateral flexion limit the motion (see Figure 9-55, *B*). Normally the nucleus pulposus deforms slightly away from the direction of the movement, or, stated differently, toward the convex side of the bend.[200]

Sitting Posture and Its Effect on Alignment within the Lumbar and Craniocervical Regions

For many persons a great deal of time is spent sitting—at work, at school, at home, or in a vehicle. The posture of the pelvis during sitting can have a substantial influence on the spinal alignment throughout the vertebral column. The topic of

sitting posture therefore has important therapeutic implications on the treatment and prevention of problems throughout the axial skeleton. The following discussion highlights the effects of *sagittal plane* posturing of the pelvis, specifically as it affects the lumbar and craniocervical regions.

Consider the classic contrast made between "poor" and "ideal" sitting postures (Figure 9-65). In the poor or slouched posture depicted in Figure 9-65, *A*, the pelvis is posteriorly tilted with a relatively flexed (flattened) lumbar spine. Eventually this posture may lead to adaptive shortening in connective tissues and muscles, ultimately perpetuating the undesirable posture.

A slouched sitting posture increases the external moment arm between the line of force of the upper body and lumbar vertebrae (see red line in Figure 9-65, *A*). This situation places greater demands on tissues that normally resist flexion of the lower trunk, including the intervertebral discs. As explained

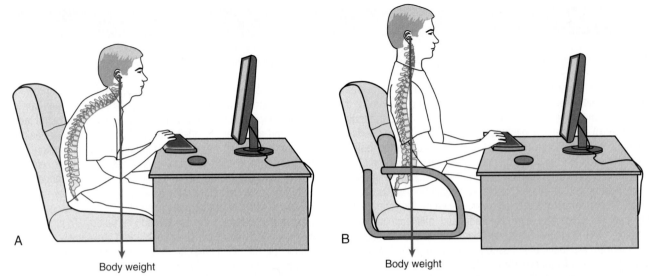

Body weight

Body weight

FIGURE 9-65. Sitting posture and its effects on the alignment of the lumbar and craniocervical regions. **A,** With a slouched sitting posture, the lumbar spine flexes, which reduces its normal lordosis. As a consequence, the head tends to assume a forward (protracted) posture (see text). **B,** With an ideal sitting posture, possibly aided with a low-back cushion, the lumbar spine assumes a more normal lordosis, which facilitates a more desirable "chin-in" (retracted) position of the head. The line of gravity resulting from body weight is shown in red.

earlier in this chapter, in vivo pressure measurements typically demonstrate larger pressures within the lumbar discs in slouched sitting compared with erect sitting.[219] Even in healthy persons, the increased pressures from the slouched sitting position can deform the nucleus pulposus posteriorly slightly, especially in the L4-L5 and L5-S1 regions.[9] A habitually slouched sitting posture may, in time, overstretch and thus weaken the posterior annulus fibrosus, reducing its ability to block a posteriorly protruding nucleus pulposus. This biomechanical scenario may be related to the pathogenesis of a significant number of cases of nonspecific low-back pain.[9] The position of the pelvis and lumbar spine during sitting strongly influences the posture of the axial skeleton as far cranially as the craniocervical region.[128] On average, the flat posture of the low back is associated with a more protracted position of the craniocervical region (i.e., a "forward head" posture) (see Figure 9-65, *A*).[22] Sitting with the lumbar spine flexed tips the thoracic and lower cervical regions forward slightly, toward flexion. In order to maintain a horizontal visual gaze—such as that typically required to view a computer monitor—the *upper* craniocervical region must compensate by extending slightly. Over time, this posture may result in adaptive shortening in the small posterior suboccipital muscles (see Chapter 10) and posterior ligaments and membranes associated with the atlanto-axial and atlanto-occipital joints. As depicted in Figure 9-65, *B,* the ideal sitting posture that includes the natural lordosis (and increased anterior pelvic tilt) extends the lumbar spine. The change in posture at the base (caudal aspect) of the spine has an optimizing influence on the adjacent more cranial segments. The more upright and extended thoracic spine facilitates a more retracted (extended) base of the cervical spine, yielding a more desirable "chin-in" position. Because the base of the cervical spine is more extended, the upper craniocervical region tends to flex slightly to a more neutral posture.

The ideal sitting posture depicted in Figure 9-65, *B* is difficult for many persons to maintain, especially for several hours at a time. Fatigue often develops in the lumbar extensor muscles. A prolonged, slouched sitting posture may thus be an unavoidable occupational hazard, at least some of the time. In addition to the possible negative effects of a chronically flexed lumbar region, the slouched sitting posture may also increase the muscular stress at the base of the cervical spine. The forward-head posture increases the external flexion torque on the cervical column as a whole, necessitating greater force production from the extensor muscles and local connective tissues. Sitting posture may be improved by a combination of awareness; strengthening and stretching the appropriate muscles; eyeglasses if needed; and ergonomically designed seating, which includes adequate lumbar support.

SUMMARY OF THE KINEMATICS WITHIN THE VERTEBRAL COLUMN

With the visual aid of Figure 9-66, the following points summarize several kinematic themes of the vertebral column.

1. The *cervical spine* permits relatively large amounts of motion in all three planes. Most notable is the high degree of axial rotation permitted at the atlanto-axial joint. Ample range of motion is necessary to maximize the movement of the head—the site of hearing, sight, smell, and equilibrium.

2. The *thoracic spine* permits a relatively constant amount of lateral flexion. This kinematic feature reflects the general frontal plane orientation of the apophyseal joints combined with the stabilizing effect of the ribs. The thoracic spine supports and protects the thorax and its enclosed organs. As described in Chapter 11, an important function of the thorax is to provide a mechanical bellows for ventilation.

3. The *thoracolumbar spine,* from a cranial-to-caudal direction, permits increasing amounts of flexion and extension at the expense of axial rotation. This feature reflects, among

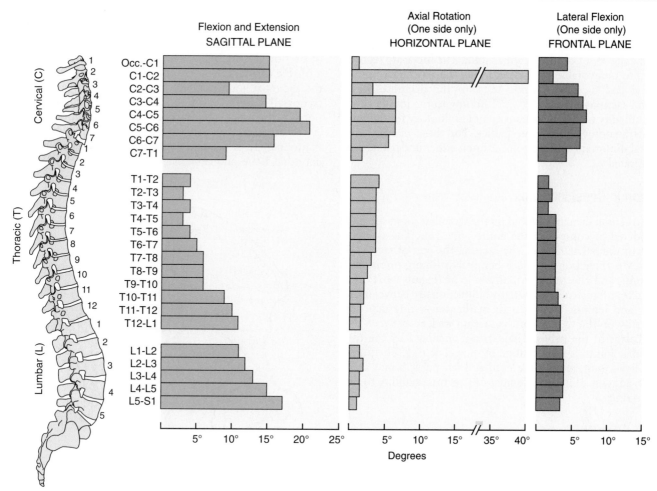

FIGURE 9-66. A graph summarizing the overall maximal range of motion (in degrees) allowed across three planes, throughout the cervical, thoracic, and lumbar regions. Data represent a compilation of several sources indicated in the text. (Styled after White AA, Panjabi MM: Kinematics of the spine. In White AA, Panjabi MM, eds: *Clinical biomechanics of the spine*, Philadelphia, 1990, Lippincott.)

other things, the progressive transformation of the orientation of the apophyseal joints, from the horizontal and frontal planes in the cervical-thoracic junction to the near-sagittal plane in the lumbar region. The prevailing near-sagittal plane and vertical orientation of the lumbar region naturally favor flexion and extension but restrict axial rotation.

4. The *lumbar spine,* in combination with flexion and extension of the hips, forms the primary pivot point for sagittal plane motion of the entire trunk.

SACROILIAC JOINTS

The sacroiliac joints mark the transition between the caudal end of the axial skeleton and the lower appendicular skeleton (review Figure 9-1). The analogous articulations at the cranial end of the axial skeleton are the sternoclavicular joints of the shoulder complex. Both the sternoclavicular and sacroiliac joints possess unique structural characteristics that satisfy their unique functions. The saddle-shaped sternoclavicular joint is designed primarily for extensive triplanar mobility, a definite necessity for providing wide placement of the hands

in space. In contrast, the large, tight-fitting sacroiliac joint is designed primarily for stability, ensuring effective transfer of potentially large loads between the vertebral column, the lower extremities, and ultimately the ground.

Although difficult to accurately diagnose, sacroiliac joints are believed to be the source of pain in about 15% to 30% of persons with chronic low-back pain.[21,40,120] Pain may be secondary to injury to the joint or to the surrounding periarticular connective tissues. Injury may be the result of obvious trauma, such as falling directly onto the region, unexpectedly stepping into a hole or off a steep step, or a difficult childbirth. Injury may also be caused by repetitive, unilateral or unidirectional torsions applied to the pelvis and low back, such as during figure skating or in other sports that demand frequent kicking or high-velocity throwing. Finally, the sacroiliac joint may be injured from joint stress caused by postural abnormalities. Examples include pelvic asymmetry resulting from misaligned ilia or uneven leg lengths, excessive lumbar lordosis, or scoliosis.[40,70] More often, however, the mechanism of injury or pathology underlying a painful sacroiliac joint is not readily apparent. If pain persists that cannot be attributed to pathology involving the sacroiliac joint, a through medical evaluation is needed to rule out other conditions, such as a herniated disc or even more serious pathology.

Much remains to be learned about the clinical evaluation and management of the sacroiliac joint. The literature reports mixed to unfavorable reviews regarding the accuracy of most clinical and medical imaging tests for the diagnoses of a painful sacroiliac joint.[40,69,80,109,168] Adding to the joint's clinical ambiguity is the lack of consistent terminology for describing its anatomy and biomechanics. For these reasons, the clinical importance of this joint is often either understated or exaggerated.

Anatomic Considerations

The structural demands placed on the sacroiliac joints are best considered in context of the entire *pelvic ring.* The components of the pelvic ring are the sacrum, the pair of sacroiliac joints, the three bones of each hemipelvis (ilium, pubis, and ischium), and the pubic symphysis joint (Figure 9-67). The pelvic ring transfers body weight bidirectionally between the trunk and femurs. The strength of the pelvic ring depends primarily on the tight fit of the sacrum wedged between the two halves of the pelvis. The sacrum, anchored by the two sacroiliac joints, is the keystone of the pelvic ring. The pubic symphysis joint, joining the right and left pubic bones anteriorly, adds an additional element of structural stability to the pelvic ring.

JOINT STRUCTURE

The sacroiliac joint is located just anterior to the posterior-superior iliac spine of the ilium. Structurally the joint consists of a relatively rigid articulation between the auricular surface (from Latin *auricle,* meaning little ear) of the sacrum and the matching auricular surface of the ilium. The articular surface of the joint has a semicircular, boomerang shape,

with the open angle of the boomerang facing posteriorly (Figure 9-68).

In childhood the sacroiliac joint has all the characteristics of a synovial joint, being relatively mobile and surrounded by a pliable capsule. Between puberty and adulthood, however, the sacroiliac joint gradually transforms from a diarthrodial (synovial) joint to a modified synarthrodial joint.[188] Most notably, the articular surfaces change from smooth to rough. A mature sacroiliac joint possesses numerous, reciprocally contoured elevations and depressions, etched within the subchondral bone and articular cartilage (Figure 9-69).[212] With

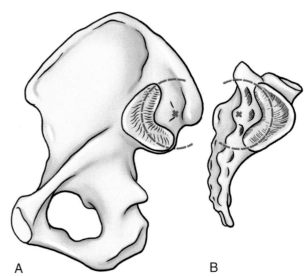

A   **B**

FIGURE 9-68. The exposed auricular surfaces of the right sacroiliac joint are shown. **A,** Iliac surface. **B,** Sacral surface. (Modified from Kapandji IA: *The physiology of joints,* vol 3, New York, 1974, Churchill Livingstone.)

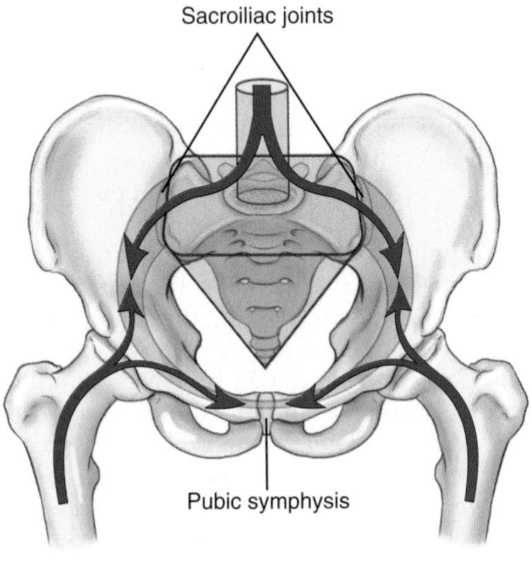

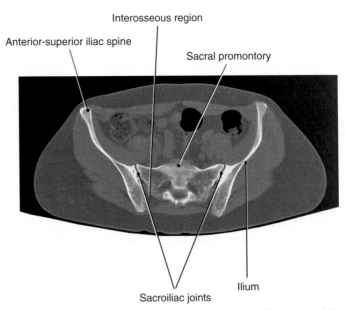

FIGURE 9-67. The components of the pelvic ring. The arrows show the direction of body weight force as it is transferred between the pelvic ring, trunk, and femurs. The keystone of the pelvic ring is the sacrum, which is wedged between the two ilia and secured bilaterally by the sacroiliac joints. (Redrawn after Kapandji IA: *The physiology of joints,* vol 3, New York, 1974, Churchill Livingstone.)

FIGURE 9-69. A horizontal cross-sectional computed tomographic scan at the level of the sacroiliac joints. Note the irregular articular surfaces. (From Kelley LL, Petersen CM: *Sectional anatomy for imaging professionals,* ed 2, St Louis, 2006, Mosby.)

ageing, the joint capsule becomes increasingly fibrotic, less pliable, and less mobile. The presence of osteophytes and structural defects in and around the joint is common in the fourth and fifth decades, or even younger.[178] Some ligaments within the joint have been shown to ossify by the sixth decade.[171] By the eighth decade, the hyaline cartilage thins and deteriorates, and in about 10% of the population the joint may completely ossify and fuse—far more often in men than in women.[51] The stiffer and less mobile aged joint, coupled with decreased bone density, partially explains the increased risk of sacral fractures in the elderly. Anthropologists routinely use the degenerative condition of the sacroiliac joint as a method to determine the approximate age of a specimen.

The rather dramatic changes in the articular structure of the sacroiliac joints between birth and old age are in some ways similar to those of joints that develop osteoarthrosis. For unexplained reasons, degenerative-like changes occur more often on the iliac side of the joint.[98] It is likely that these typically asymptomatic degenerative changes are not pathologic, in the strict sense of the word, but rather a structural remodeling to accommodate to the increased loading associated with physical maturation. The subchondral bone and articular cartilage naturally develop rough and irregular surfaces to optimally resist excessive movements between the sacrum and ilium.[212] The reason why the joint continues to degenerate and stiffen throughout life is unclear. As with all joints, however, the sacroiliac joint may develop a pathologic-based osteoarthritis at any age, often associated with ankylosing spondylitis.

LIGAMENTS

The sacroiliac joint is reinforced primarily by an extensive and thick set of ligaments. The primary stabilizers are the anterior sacroiliac, iliolumbar, interosseous, and posterior sacroiliac ligaments.[188] The sacrotuberous and sacrospinous ligaments offer a secondary source of stability.

Ligaments That Stabilize the Sacroiliac Joint
Primary
• Anterior sacroiliac
• Iliolumbar
• Interosseous
• Short and long posterior sacroiliac
Secondary
• Sacrotuberous
• Sacrospinous

The *anterior sacroiliac ligament* is a thickening of the anterior and inferior regions of the capsule (Figure 9-70). The *iliolumbar ligament,* described earlier as an important stabilizer of the lumbosacral joint, blends with parts of the anterior sacroiliac ligament. Both of the aforementioned ligaments reinforce the anterior side of the sacroiliac joint.[160]

The *interosseous ligament* consists of a set of very strong and short fibers that fills most of the relatively wide gap that naturally exists along the posterior and superior margins of the joint. (This gap, evident in Figure 9-69, has been referred to as the "interosseous region" of the sacroiliac joint.[171]) The interosseus ligament has been partially exposed in Figure 9-70 by removing part of the left side of the sacrum and other local ligaments. The interosseous ligament strongly and rigidly binds the sacrum with the ilium, in a manner similar to the syndesmotic distal tibiofibular joint.

Short and long *posterior sacroiliac ligaments* further reinforce the posterior side of the sacroiliac joint (Figure 9-71). The extensive but relatively thin set of *short posterior sacroiliac ligaments* originates along the posterior-lateral side of the sacrum. The ligaments run superiorly and laterally to insert on the ilium, near the iliac tuberosity and the posterior-superior iliac spine. Many of these fibers blend with the deeper interosseous ligament. Fibers of the well-developed *long posterior sacro-*

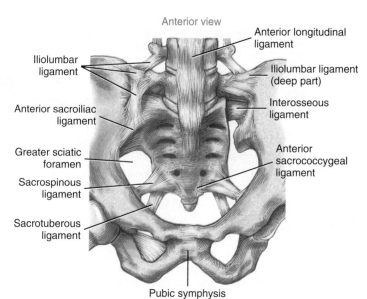

Anterior view

Iliolumbar ligament

Anterior longitudinal ligament

Iliolumbar ligament (deep part)

Anterior sacroiliac ligament

Interosseous ligament

Greater sciatic foramen

Anterior sacrococcygeal ligament

Sacrospinous ligament

Sacrotuberous ligament

Pubic symphysis

FIGURE 9-70. An anterior view of the lumbosacral region and pelvis shows the major ligaments in the region, especially those of the sacroiliac joint. On the specimen's left side, part of the sacrum, superficial parts of the iliolumbar ligament, and the anterior sacroiliac ligament are removed to expose the auricular surface of the ilium and deeper interosseous ligament.

iliac ligament originate in the regions of the third and fourth sacral segments and then course toward an attachment on the posterior-superior iliac spine of the ilium. Many fibers of the posterior sacroiliac ligament blend with the sacrotuberous ligament.

Although the sacrotuberous and sacrospinous ligaments do not actually cross the sacroiliac joint, they nevertheless assist indirectly with its stabilization (see Figure 9-71). The *sacrotuberous ligament* is large, arising from the posterior-superior iliac spine, lateral sacrum, and coccyx, attaching

distally to the ischial tuberosity. The distal attachment blends with the tendon of the biceps femoris (lateral hamstring) muscle. The *sacrospinous ligament* is located deep to the sacrotuberous ligament, arising from the lateral margin of the caudal end of the sacrum and coccyx, attaching distally to the ischial spine.

INNERVATION

The sacroiliac joints are innervated by sensory nerves and therefore are capable of relaying pain to the nervous system.[126,209] What is not clear in the literature, however, is the exact spinal source of the innervation. Anatomic reviews on the subject consistently include the dorsal rami of L^5-S^3 spinal nerve roots, and less often the ventral rami of L^4-S^2.[69,70]

Persons with a painful sacroiliac joint often report symptoms in the ipsilateral lower lumbar and medial buttock area (often near the posterior-superior iliac spine). Although less consistently, pain or hyperesthesia may also be experienced throughout the lower extremity.[183]

THORACOLUMBAR FASCIA

The thoracolumbar fascia plays an important functional role in the mechanical stability of the low back, including the sacroiliac joint.[211] This fascia is most extensive in the lumbar region, where it is organized into anterior, middle, and posterior layers. Three layers of the thoracolumbar fascia partially surround and compartmentalize the posterior muscles of the lower back, as illustrated in Figure 9-72.

The *anterior and middle layers* of the thoracolumbar fascia are named according to their position relative to the quadratus lumborum muscle. Both layers are anchored medially to the transverse processes of the lumbar vertebrae and inferiorly to the iliac crests. The *posterior layer* of the thoracolumbar fascia covers the posterior surface of the erector spinae and, more superficially, the latissimus dorsi muscle. This layer of the thoracolumbar fascia attaches to the spinous processes of all lumbar vertebrae and the sacrum, and to the ilium near the posterior-superior iliac spines. These attachments provide

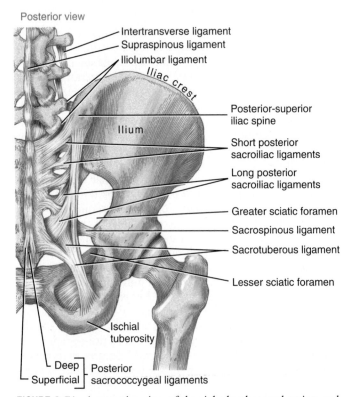

Posterior view

- Intertransverse ligament
- Supraspinous ligament
- Iliolumbar ligament
- Iliac crest
- Ilium
- Posterior-superior iliac spine
- Short posterior sacroiliac ligaments
- Long posterior sacroiliac ligaments
- Greater sciatic foramen
- Sacrospinous ligament
- Sacrotuberous ligament
- Lesser sciatic foramen
- Ischial tuberosity
- Deep ⎱ Posterior
- Superficial ⎰ sacrococcygeal ligaments

FIGURE 9-71. A posterior view of the right lumbosacral region and pelvis shows the major ligaments that reinforce the sacroiliac joint.

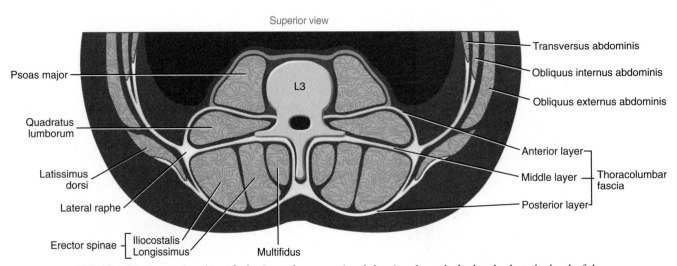

Superior view

- Psoas major
- Quadratus lumborum
- Latissimus dorsi
- Lateral raphe
- Erector spinae ⎱ Iliocostalis / Longissimus
- Multifidus
- L3
- Transversus abdominis
- Obliquus internus abdominis
- Obliquus externus abdominis
- Anterior layer ⎱
- Middle layer ⎰ Thoracolumbar fascia
- Posterior layer ⎰

FIGURE 9-72. A superior view of a horizontal cross-sectional drawing through the low back at the level of the third lumbar vertebra. The anterior, middle, and posterior layers of the thoracolumbar fascia are shown surrounding various muscle groups.

mechanical stability to the sacroiliac joint. Stability is enhanced by attachments of the gluteus maximus and latissimus dorsi.

The posterior and middle layers of the thoracolumbar fascia fuse at their lateral margins, forming a *lateral raphe*. This tissue blends with fascia of the transversus abdominis and, to a lesser extent, with the obliquus internus abdominis (internal oblique) muscle. The functional significance of these muscular attachments is addressed in greater detail in Chapter 10.

Kinematics

Relatively small and poorly defined rotational and translational movements occur at the sacroiliac joint, most notably in the near-sagittal plane. Although difficult to measure, the magnitude of these movements in the adult has been reported to be from 1 to 4 degrees for rotation, and 1 to 2 mm for translation.[59,103,191] Movements at the sacroiliac joint likely occur as a combination of compression of the articular cartilage and slight movement between joint surfaces. The kinematics of the sacroiliac joints do not appear well coordinated with specific movements of the trunk or lower extremity.

Several terms and axes of rotation have been proposed to describe the motion at the sacroiliac joints.[8,23,59] Although no terminology completely describes the complex rotational and translational movements, two terms, nevertheless, are typically used for this purpose: *nutation* and *counternutation*. They describe movements limited to the near-sagittal plane, around a near–medial-lateral axis of rotation that traverses the interosseous ligament (Figure 9-73). *Nutation* (meaning to nod) is defined as the relative *anterior tilt* of the base (top) of the sacrum relative to the ilium. *Counternutation* is a reverse motion defined as the relative *posterior tilt* of the base of the sacrum relative to the ilium. (Note the term *relative* used in the above definitions.) As depicted in Figure 9-73, nutation and counternutation can occur by sacral-on-iliac rotation (as previously defined), by iliac-on-sacral rotation, or by both motions performed simultaneously.

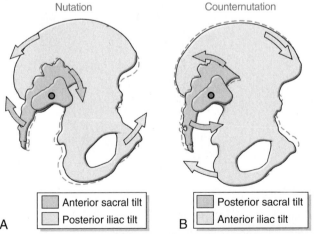

Nutation   Counternutation

| Anterior sacral tilt | Posterior sacral tilt |
| Posterior iliac tilt | Anterior iliac tilt |

A   B

FIGURE 9-73. The kinematics at the sacroiliac joints. **A,** Nutation. **B,** Counternutation. (See text for definitions.) Sacral rotations are indicated by darker shade of tan, iliac rotations are indicated by the lighter shade of tan. The axis of rotation for sagittal plane movement is indicated by the small green circle.

Terms Describing Motion at the Sacroiliac Joint
- *Nutation* occurs by anterior sacral-on-iliac rotation, posterior iliac-on-sacral rotation, or both motions performed simultaneously.
- *Counternutation* occurs by posterior sacral-on-iliac rotation, anterior iliac-on-sacral rotation, or both motions performed simultaneously.

FUNCTIONAL CONSIDERATIONS

The sacroiliac joints perform two functions: (1) a stress relief mechanism within the pelvic ring and (2) a stable means for load transfer between the axial skeleton and lower limbs.

Stress Relief

The movements at the sacroiliac joints, although slight, permit an important element of stress relief within the entire pelvic ring. This stress relief is especially important during walking and running and, in women, during childbirth.

During walking, the reciprocal flexion and extension pattern of the lower limbs causes each side of the pelvis to rotate slightly out of phase with the other. At normal speed of walking, the heel of the advancing lower limb strikes the ground as the toes of the opposite limb are still in contact with the ground. At this instant, tension in the hip muscles and ligaments generates oppositely directed torsions on the right and left iliac crests. The torsions are most notable in the sagittal plane, as nutation and counternutation, but also in the horizontal planes. Intrapelvic torsions are amplified with increased walking speed. Although slight, movements at each sacroiliac joint during walking help dissipate damaging stress that would otherwise occur in the pelvic ring if it were a solid and continuous structure. The pubic symphysis joint has a similar role in relieving stress throughout the pelvic ring.

Movement of the sacroiliac joints increases during labor and delivery.[32] A significant increase in joint laxity occurs during the last trimester of pregnancy and is especially notable in women during their second pregnancy as compared with the first. Increased nutation during childbirth rotates the lower part of the sacrum posteriorly, thereby increasing the size of the pelvic outlet and favoring the passage of the infant. The articular surfaces of the sacroiliac joints are smoother in women, presenting less resistance to these slight physiologic motions.

Sacroiliac joint pain is not uncommon in women during pregnancy. The combination of weight gain, increased lumbar lordosis, and hormone-induced laxity of ligaments may stress the sacroiliac joints and surrounding capsule.

Stability during Load Transfer: Mechanics of Generating a Nutation Torque at the Sacroiliac Joints

The plane of the articular surfaces of the sacroiliac joint is largely vertical. This orientation renders the joint vulnerable to vertical slipping, especially when subjected to large forces. Nutation at the sacroiliac joints increases the compression and shear forces between joint surfaces, thereby increasing articular stability.[212] For this reason, the close-packed position of the sacroiliac joint is considered to be in full nutation. Forces that create a nutation torque therefore help stabilize the sacroiliac joints. Torques are created by gravity, stretched ligaments, and muscle activation.

Nutation torque increases the stability at the sacroiliac joints. This torque is produced by three forces:
• Gravity
• Passive tension from stretched ligaments
• Muscle activation

Stabilizing Effect of Gravity

The downward force of gravity resulting from body weight passes through the lumbar vertebrae, usually just anterior to an imaginary line connecting the midpoints of the two sacroiliac joints. At the same time, the femoral heads produce an upward directed compression force through the acetabula. Each of these two forces acts with a separate moment arm to create a *nutation torque* about the sacroiliac joints (Figure 9-74, *A*). The torque resulting from body weight rotates the *sacrum* anteriorly relative to the ilium, whereas the torque resulting from hip compression force rotates the *ilium* posteriorly relative to the sacrum. This nutation torque "locks" the joints by increasing the friction between the rough and reciprocally contoured articular surfaces.[186,212] This locking mechanism relies primarily on gravity and congruity of the joint surfaces rather than extra-articular structures such as ligaments and muscles.

Stabilizing Effect of Ligaments and Muscles

As described previously, the first line of stability of the sacroiliac joints is created through a nutation torque created through the actions of gravity and weight bearing through the pelvis. Stability is adequate for activities that involve relatively low, static loading between the pelvis and the vertebral column, such as sitting and standing. For larger and more dynamic loading, however, the sacroiliac joints are reinforced by ligaments and muscles. As described in Figure 9-74, *B*,

nutation torque stretches many of the connective tissues at the sacroiliac joint, such as the sacrotuberous and interosseous ligaments. Increased tension in these ligaments further compresses the surfaces of the sacroiliac joints, thereby adding to their transarticular stability.[23]

In addition to ligaments, several trunk and hip muscles reinforce and stabilize the sacroiliac joints (Box 9-3). Such myogenic stability is necessary during activities such as lifting, load carrying, or running. The stabilizing action of many of these muscles is based on their attachments to the thoracolumbar fascia and to the sacrospinous and sacrotuberous ligaments.[185,210] Contractile forces from muscles listed in Box 9-3 can stabilize the sacroiliac joints by (1) generating active compression forces against the articular surfaces, (2) increasing magnitude of nutation torque and subsequently engaging an active locking mechanism, (3) pulling on connective tissues that reinforce the joints, and (4) any combination of these effects. As one example, consider the muscular interaction depicted in Figure 9-74, *C*. Contraction of the erector

---

BOX 9-3. Muscles That Reinforce and Stabilize the Sacroiliac Joint

Erector spinae
Lumbar multifidi
Abdominal muscles
  • Rectus abdominis
  • Obliquus abdominis internus and externus
  • Transversus abdominis
Hip extensor muscles (such as biceps femoris and gluteus maximus)
Latissimus dorsi
Iliacus and piriformis

The stabilizing effects of nutation torque

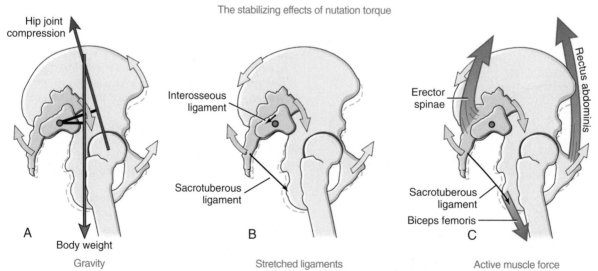

FIGURE 9-74. Nutation torque increases the stability at the sacroiliac joints. **A,** Two forces resulting primarily from gravity from body weight *(red downward-directed arrow)* and hip joint compression *(brown upward-directed arrow)* generate a nutation torque at the sacroiliac joints. Each force has a moment arm *(black line)* that acts from the axis of rotation *(green circle at joint)*. **B,** The nutation torque stretches the interosseous and sacrotuberous ligaments, ultimately compressing and stabilizing the sacroiliac joints. **C,** Muscle contraction *(red)* creates an active nutation torque across the sacroiliac joints. Note the biceps femoris transmitting tension through the sacrotuberous ligament.

spinae muscle rotates the sacrum anteriorly, whereas contraction of the rectus abdominis and biceps femoris (one of the hamstring muscles) rotates the ilium posteriorly, two elements that produce nutation torque. Through direct attachments, the biceps femoris increases the tension within the sacrotuberous ligament. The muscular interaction explains, in part, why strengthening of many of the muscles listed in Box 9-3 is recommended for treatment of an unstable sacroiliac joint.[205] Furthermore, increased strength or control of muscles such as the latissimus dorsi and gluteus maximus, erector spinae, internal oblique, and transversus abdominis muscles provides stability to the sacroiliac joints via their connections into the thoracolumbar fascia. The more horizontally disposed muscles, such as the internal oblique and especially the transversus abdominis, also provide joint stability by compressing the ilia inward toward the sacrum. Finally, the iliacus (part of the iliopsoas) and piriformis muscles, by attaching directly into the capsule or margins of the sacroiliac joints (review Figure 9-26), also provide a secondary source of stability to the sacroiliac articulation.[184] Without adequate stabilization, the sacroiliac joints may become more easily malaligned or hypermobile—two factors that can potentially stress the joint and contribute to a painful condition.

SYNOPSIS

The bony components of the axial skeleton include the cranium, vertebral column, sternum, and ribs. Of these four components, the vertebral column is most aptly designed to accept the loads produced by body weight and activated muscle. The absorption and distribution of these loads are a prime function of the intervertebral discs. The strength and compliance of the vertebral column is governed by ligaments and muscles, acting in conjunction with the normal, reciprocally shaped curvatures of the spine.

Each vertebra within a given vertebral region has a unique shape. Consider, for example, the contrasting shapes between the axis (C2) and L4; their very different morphology contrasts the different functional demands imposed on the two ends of the vertebral column. The axis, with its vertically projecting dens, is a central pivot point for the wide range of axial rotation allowed by the head and neck. The body of L4, in contrast, is designed to support large superimposed loads.

The typical intervertebral junction has three important elements: transverse and spinal processes for attachments of muscles and ligaments, interbody joints for intervertebral adhesion and shock absorption, and finally the apophyseal joints for partially guiding the relative kinematics of each region. This third element is particularly important in understanding the kinematics throughout the axial skeleton. Remarkably, much of the characteristic motion allowed within each region of the vertebral column is dictated by the spatial orientation of apophyseal joints. Consider, most cranially, the geometric disposition of the apophyseal joints within the cervical region. The articular surfaces are oriented nearly horizontally at the atlanto-axial joint and at nearly 45 degrees between the horizontal and frontal planes throughout the remainder of the cervical region. This specific geometry bestows the craniocervical region with the greatest potential for three-dimensional movement of any region in the vertebral column—a necessity considering the location of the sources of many special senses within the head.

Although the 12 pairs of apophyseal joints within the thoracic region are oriented close to the frontal plane, the expected freedom of lateral flexion is limited because of the splinting action of the ribs. Relative rigidity within the thoracic cage is a requirement for the mechanics of ventilation and for protection of the heart and lungs.

The near–sagittal plane orientation of middle and upper apophyseal joints within the lumbar region allows ample flexion and extension of the lower end of the vertebral column while simultaneously resisting horizontal plane rotation. The combined sagittal plane motion provided by the lumbar spine and the pelvis (relative to the hip joints) provides an important flexion and extension hinging point for the entire body. The "lumbopelvic rhythm" expressed in this region amplifies the forward reach of the upper extremities and hands, important for bending down to pick objects off the floor or reaching upward to a high shelf.

The relative frontal plane bias of the apophyseal joints of the L5-S1 junction provides important restraint to potentially damaging anterior shear force created between the caudal end of the lumbar spine and the base of the sacrum. This forward shear increases with increased lumbar lordosis, often performed in conjunction with an excessive anterior tilt of the pelvis relative to the femoral heads.

The most caudal articulations of the axial skeleton are the sacroiliac joints. These joints provide a relatively rigid junction for the transmission of large forces between the end of the axial spine and the lower extremities. These relatively large joints are naturally well stabilized, although they must permit small movements that help open the birth canal, and dissipate stress within the pelvic ring while walking and running.

When optimally aligned and supported by healthy connective tissues and muscles, the vertebral column and craniocervical region satisfy a seemingly paradoxic need for mobility and vertical stability to the body as a whole. The important role of muscle in providing vertical stability to the axial skeleton is a recurring theme throughout Chapter 10. An abnormally aligned axial skeleton can exaggerate the deforming potential of gravity and active muscles, which can cause excessive and often damaging stress to bone, discs, ligaments, and the neural tissues. The rationale for many treatments for impairments of the axial skeleton is based on optimizing ideal posture throughout the body.

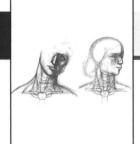

ADDITIONAL CLINICAL CONNECTIONS

CLINICAL CONNECTION 9-1
Degenerative Disc Disease: Interactions between Mechanical and Biologic Factors

As described throughout this chapter, disc degeneration is associated with several pathologic conditions of the spine. Many of these conditions are directly or indirectly related to the reduced shock absorption quality of a degenerated disc. The ability of intervertebral discs to optimally absorb and redistribute loads starts to decline at a relatively (and surprisingly) young age. As a consequence, disc degeneration may start as early as the second decade and affects most persons by their third and fourth decades of life.[78,100,133] Although the data vary considerably, studies report that 30% to 70% of all adults have at least some detectable signs of disc degeneration on magnetic resonance imaging[187,214]; however, most persons are asymptomatic and report no loss of function. Disc degeneration, at least in its modest form, is therefore considered a natural part of the ageing process. The development of more severe disc degeneration associated with marked pain is *not,* however, considered a normal part of aging. Disc degeneration associated with marked pain, and its associated functional limitations, should more appropriately be called *degenerative disc disease.*

Degenerative disc disease is a major medical and economic problem, accounting for up to 90% of all adult spinal surgeries in the United States.[11] Researchers strive to understand and improve the treatment for persons with degenerative disc disease; however, its epidemiology and etiology are complicated and multifactorial.[16] Epidemiologic research is hampered by unclear operational definitions of the disease, in addition to the fact that so many adults with significant disc degeneration remain asymptomatic.[6,78] Furthermore, it is difficult to distinguish which elements of disc degeneration occur naturally with ageing (and associated wear and tear) and which are strictly pathologic.[157]

Much of the research on the pathogenesis of degenerative disc disease focuses on mechanical and biologic factors.[6,89,158,177] *Mechanical factors* are the most intuitive and easiest to understand. There is little doubt that excessive mechanical loading of a disc can initiate the process of disc degeneration, especially if the discs are excessively dehydrated or have been previously injured. Ensuing mechanical instability of the intervertebral junction may create higher stresses and biochemical changes within the disc, thereby continuing the cycle of stress-induced degeneration.[116,227]

The fact that mechanical overload may initiate the process of disc degeneration in some persons and not others is a mystery.[6] Other risk factors besides mechanical overload obviously contrib-

ute to the pathogenesis. The strongest risk factor for degenerative disc disease is related to genetic inheritance.[16] Secondary risk factors include advanced age, poor disc nutrition (which may implicate smoking), occupation, anthropometrics (i.e., body size and proportion), and long-term exposure to total body vibration.* Except for genetics, several of the aforementioned factors may need to be present together to significantly increase the risk for developing degenerative disc disease.

Possible Risk Factors for Degenerative Disc Disease
- Genetics (primary)
- Advanced age
- Poor disc nutrition
- Occupation (physical work history)
- Anthropometrics (i.e., body size and proportion)
- Long-term exposure to total body vibration

Although excessive forces delivered to a partially dehydrated disc may help explain the *initiation* of degenerative disc disease, it cannot explain the large intersubject variations in pain and inflammation or rate of disease progression. Significant evidence suggests that the severity and progression of disc disease is strongly associated with the body's *biologic response* to the degenerative process.[6,89,158,177] Following tears of the annulus fibrosus, for example, vascularized granulation tissue invades the injured region (a phenomenon referred to as *neovascularization*), apparently as a normal component of inflammatory healing.[155] Afferent neurons transmitting pain (nociceptors) also invade the vascularized granulation tissue, even in areas where nerves and blood vessels normally do not exist.[44,96] In addition, mast cells, macrophages, enzymes, and a host of *cytokines* (proteins and peptides that mediate and regulate specific cellular functions, such as tissue growth and inflammation) have been found within the granulation tissue.[155,177] Through a very complicated and only partially understood process, the cytokines indirectly stimulate growth and sensitivity of the nociceptors, as well as increase the inflammation in the region.[1,29,158,216] In some persons this inflammatory response may prolong and amplify the pain (referred to as *peripheral sensitization*). This process may also promote the release of more

---

*References 7, 16, 79, 132, 146, 208.

ADDITIONAL CLINICAL CONNECTIONS

CLINICAL CONNECTION 9-1
Degenerative Disc Disease: Interactions between Mechanical and Biologic Factors—cont'd

proinflammatory cytokines, which stimulate additional nociceptors in the annulus as well as the adjacent spinal canal and nerve sheaths surrounding the spinal nerve roots.[23] As a result, pain that originated as a torn annulus may also be expressed clinically as radiating pain down the course of the associated dermatome of the lower extremity. This process may help explain why a relatively nonstressful movement of the back in a person with degenerated discs may produce a heightened pain response, involving both the back and the lower extremity.[29,193]

The chondrocytes and fibroblasts located within the intervertebral discs are able to detect minute physical characteristics of the surrounding physical environment, such as tension, compression, osmotic pressure, and nuclear hydrostatic pressure.[89,116,166,177,202] Excessive compression on the disc, for example, has been experimentally shown to produce cell-mediated responses that include excessive release of proteinases, cytokines, and nitric oxide.[158] These substances can alter the biosynthesis and distribution of the extracellular matrix, including proteoglycans and collagen.[12,89] In a degenerating disc, this process produces a structurally and functionally inferior matrix, which is less able to safely absorb or distribute loads. Left unregulated, this process may accelerate the degenerative process. If normally regulated, however, this process may remodel the structure of disc, allowing it to better tolerate varying loads throughout one's lifetime. Figure 9-75 summarizes

**Mechanical and Biologic Interactions
That May Be Associated with Degenerative Disc Disease**

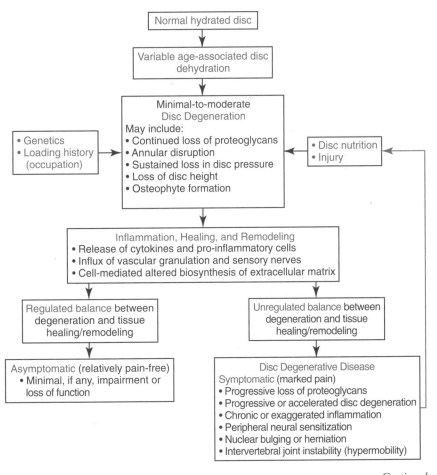

FIGURE 9-75. A series of mechanical and biologic interactions that may be associated with degenerative disc disease. The red arrow indicates possible feedback loops that may perpetuate the disease process. See text for further details.

Continued

ADDITIONAL CLINICAL CONNECTIONS

CLINICAL CONNECTION 9-1
Degenerative Disc Disease: Interactions between Mechanical Factors and Biologic Factors—cont'd

one possible set of mechanical and biologic interactions that may be involved in the development of degenerative disc disease.

In an attempt to improve the understanding of the multifactorial processes underlying degenerative disc disease, Adams and Roughley proposed the following definition: "The process of disc degeneration is an aberrant, cell mediated response to progressive structural failure."[6] This definition succinctly incorporates the interactions between mechanical and biologic factors described previously and serves as a model for clinical research. Beattie and colleagues, for example, have raised the hypothesis that controlled loading and unloading of the spine through therapeutic efforts,

such as traction, graded muscle contractions, joint manipulations, and repeated movements, may in some way improve the hydration of a moderately degenerated disc.[17] Perhaps greater hydration can improve the mechanical properties and biochemical environment within the damaged disc, thereby reducing the vicious cycle of inflammation and further degeneration. Such a hypothesis requires integrated research among the various clinical and research scientists who study the pathogenesis and treatment of degenerative disc disease. Ultimately, understanding more about this interaction will hopefully lead to improved patient care.

ADDITIONAL CLINICAL CONNECTIONS

CLINICAL CONNECTION 9-2
Scoliosis and Hyperkyphosis: Classic Examples of Structural Deformity Involving the Thoracic Spine

Maintaining the spine in normal alignment throughout life requires a delicate balance between intrinsic forces, governed by muscles and osseous-ligamentous structures, and extrinsic forces, governed by gravity. When the balance fails, deformity occurs. Herniated discs and nerve root impingements are relatively uncommon in the thoracic spine. This may be a result of, in part, the relatively low intervertebral mobility and high stability provided by the rib cage. Postural abnormalities, deformity, or malalignment, however, occur relatively frequently in the thoracic region. The thoracic spine, constituting about half the entire length of the vertebral column, is particularly vulnerable to the effects of asymmetric or exaggerated forces created by gravity, muscle, or connective tissue. Scoliosis and hyperkyphosis are classic examples of significant deformity involving the thoracic spine and are thus featured in this two-part Additional Clinical Connection.

PART I: SCOLIOSIS Scoliosis (from the Greek, meaning curvature) is a deformity of the vertebral column characterized by abnormal curvatures *in all three planes*—most notably, however, in the frontal and horizontal (Figure 9-76, *A*).[2,114] The deformity most often involves the thoracic spine; however, other regions of the spine are often affected (as apparent in the figure). Scoliosis is typically defined as either functional or structural. *Functional scoliosis* can be corrected by an active shift in posture, whereas *structural scoliosis* is a fixed deformity that cannot be corrected fully by an active shift in posture.

Approximately 80% of all cases of structural scoliosis are termed *idiopathic,* meaning the condition has no apparent biologic or mechanical cause.[204,218] For unknown reasons, progressive idiopathic scoliosis affects adolescent females four times as often as males, especially those experiencing a rapid growth spurt.[114,123] Overall, approximately 2% to 3% of the adolescent population aged 10 to 16 years exhibits a lateral (frontal plane) curvature that exceeds 10 degrees.[114]

Several theories have attempted to explain the cause of adolescent idiopathic scoliosis, including natural, subtle differences in bilateral symmetry of the body, uneven growth or abnormal histologic structure of connective tissues (such as the vertebral endplates, intertransverse ligaments, and annulus fibrosus), asymmetry in paraspinal muscle activation, and asymmetry in spinal loading leading to abnormal vertebral growth and remodeling of the intervertebral discs.* Genetics may also play a role in this condition.[31]

Approximately 20% of cases of structural scoliosis are caused by neuromuscular or muscular pathology, trauma, or congenital

abnormalities. Examples of pathology include poliomyelitis, muscular dystrophy, spinal cord injury, and cerebral palsy. In these cases the scoliosis is typically initiated by an asymmetry of muscular forces acting on the vertebral column.

Typically, scoliosis is described by the location, direction, and number of fixed frontal plane curvatures (lateral bends) within the vertebral column. The most common pattern of scoliosis consists of a single lateral curve with an apex in the T7-T9 region.[43] Other patterns may involve a secondary or compensatory curve, most often in the thoracolumbar or lumbar regions. The direction of the primary lateral curve is defined by the side of the convexity of the lateral deformity. The magnitude of the lateral curvature is typically measured on a radiograph by drawing the *Cobb angle* (Figure 9-77). Because the thoracic vertebrae are most often involved with scoliosis, asymmetry of the rib cage is common. The ribs on the side of the thoracic concavity are pulled together, and the ribs on the side of the convexity are spread apart. The degree of torsion, or horizontal plane deformity, can be measured on an anterior-posterior radiograph by noting the rotated position of the vertebral pedicles.

The deformity in structural scoliosis typically has a remarkably fixed *contralateral* spinal coupling pattern involving lateral flexion and axial rotation.[204] The spinous processes of the involved vertebrae are typically rotated in the horizontal plane, toward the side of the concavity of the fixed thoracic curvature. The ribs therefore are forced to follow the horizontal plane rotation of the thoracic vertebrae. This explains why the *rib hump* is typically on the convex side of the frontal plane curvature (see Figure 9-76, *A*). The exact mechanism responsible for the fixed contralateral coupling pattern is not well understood.

Several factors are considered when deciding on the method of treating adolescent idiopathic scoliosis, including the magnitude of the frontal plane curve, the degree of progression, the cosmetic appearance of the deformity, and, particularly important, whether the child is in a growth spurt. In general, the larger the frontal plane curve and the younger the skeletal maturation of the child, the greater the likelihood of significant progression of the deformity.[114] Treatment options often include careful observation for progression of the scoliosis, physical therapy, bracing, and surgery. (Figure 9-76, *B* shows the clinical and radiographic views of a young girl after anterior spinal fusion and placement of instrumentation.) Five- through 20-year follow-up studies indicate that bracing and surgery can control or partially correct the curves in adolescent idiopathic scoliosis.[49,50,54,114,115] The objective of bracing is to prevent a small curve from progressing to a large one. The objective of surgery is to stabilize the curve and provide partial correction. Surgery, however, is not without an inherent risk to the

*References 31, 37, 170, 190, 204, 225.

Continued

ADDITIONAL CLINICAL CONNECTIONS

CLINICAL CONNECTION 9-2
Scoliosis and Hyperkyphosis: Classic Examples of Structural Deformity Involving the Thoracic Spine—cont'd

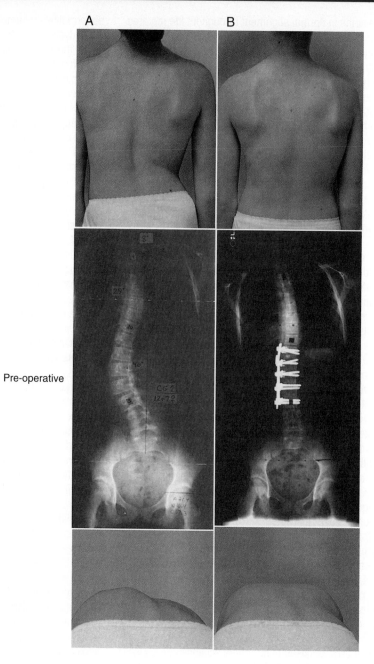

A

B

Pre-operative

Postoperative

FIGURE 9-76. Illustration of a 12-year-old, skeletally immature girl with structural scoliosis. **A,** Preoperative photographs and radiograph show the primary frontal plane curve in the thoracolumbar region. The lateral bend is 46 degrees, with its convexity (apex) to the girl's left side. The bottom photograph shows the girl bent forward at the waist, displaying the horizontal plane component of the scoliosis, or "rib hump," on the subject's left side. **B,** Postoperative photographs and radiograph of the same girl after an anterior spinal fusion and placement of instrumentation. Note the correction of the rib hump in the accompanying bottom photograph. (From Lenke LG: CD *Horizon Legacy Spinal System anterior dual-rod surgical technique manual*, Memphis, 2002, Medtronic Sofamor Danek.)

ADDITIONAL CLINICAL CONNECTIONS

CLINICAL CONNECTION 9-2
Scoliosis and Hyperkyphosis: Classic Examples of Structural Deformity Involving the Thoracic Spine—cont'd

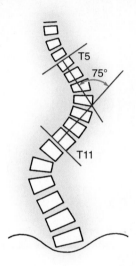

FIGURE 9-77. A *Cobb angle* measures the degree of lateral bend in a spinal curvature associated with scoliosis. In this example the thoracic spine shows a Cobb angle of 75 degrees, with the apex of the curve at the T4-T5 junction. The Cobb angle is measured from a radiograph showing an anterior-posterior view. (From Canale ST, Beaty JH: *Campbell's operative orthopaedics*, ed 11, Philadelphia, 2008, Mosby.)

child. A very general guideline is used by some physicians to help decide between bracing and surgery options. Children with a thoracic Cobb angle of about 40 degrees or less are stronger candidates for bracing; children with a Cobb angle greater than about 50 degrees, however, are stronger candidates for surgery. Children with a Cobb angle between 40 and 50 degrees are considered to be in a "gray area" as to which is the more effective treatment. It is important to realize that the aforementioned guidelines are very general and vary based on other factors, such as the child's skeletal maturity, degree of curve progression, cosmetic appearance, and presence of multiple curves. The presence of a significantly reduced thoracic kyphosis (or actual lordosis) warrants stronger consideration for surgery, based on the likely ineffectiveness of bracing and the potential compromise in pulmonary function.[114]

PART II: HYPERKYPHOSIS OF THE THORACIC REGION
On average, about 40 to 45 degrees of natural kyphosis exist while one is standing at ease.[106,121] In some persons,

however, *excessive thoracic kyphosis* (formally termed *hyperkyphosis*) may develop and cause functional limitations.[192] Hyperkyphosis may occur as a consequence of trauma and related spinal instability, abnormal growth and development of vertebrae, severe degenerative disc disease, or marked osteoporosis and subsequent vertebral fractures—typically associated with advanced ageing.[46,131] A modest increase in thoracic kyphosis and associated loss in body height is a normal aspect of reaching advanced age and is usually not debilitating.

The two most common conditions associated with progressive thoracic kyphosis are Scheuermann's kyphosis and osteoporosis. *Scheuermann's kyphosis,* or "juvenile kyphosis," is the most common cause of thoracic hyperkyphosis in adolescence. Although the cause of the condition is unknown, it is characterized primarily by the abnormal growth rate of different parts of the vertebrae, resulting in excessive anterior wedging of the thoracic and upper lumbar vertebral bodies. This condition appears to have a significant genetic predisposition, with a reported incidence of 1% to 8% of the general population.[117] The developing hyperkyphosis is rigid and cannot be volitionally reversed. Bracing may be effective in reducing the progression of the deformity in modest cases; surgery, however, may be warranted in severe cases that do not respond to conservative treatment.[113]

Osteoporosis of the spine and associated compression fractures may lead to the genesis and ultimate progression of thoracic hyperkyphosis often seen in elderly women.[52] Osteoporosis is a chronic metabolic bone disease that affects primarily postmenopausal women; this condition is not a normal part of aging. Multiple vertebral fractures resulting from osteoporosis may lead to reduced height of the anterior sides of vertebral bodies, thereby promoting the progression of the excessive thoracic kyphosis. One such scenario is demonstrated by analyzing the postures depicted in Figure 9-78, *A* to *C*,[142] each modeled after actual radiographs of live subjects. In the ideal spinal posture, the line of force from body weight falls slightly to the concave side of the apex of the normal cervical and thoracic curvatures (see Figure 9-78, *A*). Gravity therefore can act with an external moment arm that favors normal thoracic and cervical curvatures. The ideal posture shown in Figure 9-78, *A* creates a small cervical extension torque and small thoracic flexion torque. In the thoracic spine the tendency to collapse further into kyphosis is normally resisted, in part, by compression forces between the anterior sides of the interbody joints. Vertebrae weakened from osteoporosis may be unable to resist the anterior compression forces.[159] Over time, the compression forces may produce excessive anterior wedging of the vertebral bodies, thereby accentuating the slow collapse into hyperkyphosis.

Continued

ADDITIONAL CLINICAL CONNECTIONS

CLINICAL CONNECTION 9-2
Scoliosis and Hyperkyphosis: Classic Examples of Structural Deformity Involving the Thoracic Spine—cont'd

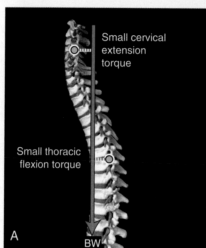

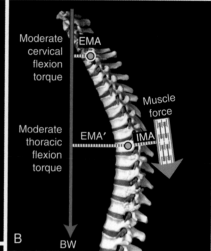

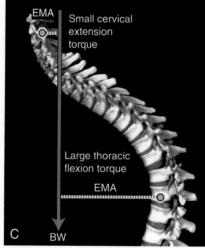

FIGURE 9-78. Lateral views show the biomechanical relationships between the line of gravity from body weight (BW) and varying degrees of thoracic kyphosis. In each of the three models, the axes of rotation are depicted as the near midpoint of the thoracic and cervical regions *(green circles)*. **A,** In a person with ideal standing posture and normal thoracic kyphosis, body weight creates a small cervical extension torque and a small thoracic flexion torque. The external moment arms used by body weight are shown as dashed red lines. **B,** In a person with moderate thoracic hyperkyphosis, body weight creates a moderate cervical and thoracic flexion torque (*EMA'*, external moment arm at midthoracic spine; *EMA*, external moment arm at midcervical spine; *IMA*, internal moment arm for trunk extensor muscle force). **C,** In a person with severe thoracic hyperkyphosis, body weight causes a small cervical extension torque and a large thoracic flexion torque. Skeletal models are based on lateral radiographs of actual standing persons.

Furthermore, if significant disc degeneration and dehydration of the nucleus are present, the hyperkyphotic posture may further compress the anterior side of the discs.[157] At this point a pathologic deforming process has been well initiated (see Figure 9-78, *B*). The increased flexed posture shifts the line of force resulting from body weight farther anteriorly, thus increasing the length of the external moment arm (EMA') and the magnitude of the flexed kyphotic posture.[28] As a result, both thoracic and cervical spine regions may be subjected to a moderate flexion torque (see Figure 9-78, *B*). Increased extensor muscle and posterior ligamentous tension is needed to hold the trunk, neck, and head upright. The increased force passing through the interbody joints can create compression

fractures in the vertebral bodies along with the formation of osteophytes. At this point, the vicious cycle is well established.

The magnitude of compression force exerted between vertebrae of a hyperkyphotic thoracic spine can be surprisingly large. The amount of compression force associated with the posture depicted in Figure 9-78, *B* can be estimated by assuming a condition of static equilibrium within the sagittal plane: the product of body weight (BW) force and the external moment arm (EMA') equals the product of the muscle force times the internal moment arm (IMA). Assuming that the EMA is about twice the length of the IMA, rotary equilibrium in the sagittal plane requires a muscle force of twice body weight. Assume that a 180-lb person (1 lb = 4.448 newtons) has about

ADDITIONAL CLINICAL CONNECTIONS

CLINICAL CONNECTION 9-2
Scoliosis and Hyperkyphosis: Classic Examples of Structural Deformity Involving the Thoracic Spine—cont'd

60% of body weight (108 lb) located above the midthoracic region. An extensor muscle force of approximately 216 lb (2×108 lb) is needed to hold the flexed posture. When considering superimposed body weight, a total of about 324 lb of compression force (216 lb of muscle force plus 108 lb of body weight) is exerted on a midthoracic interbody joint. Applying this same biomechanical solution to the ideal posture shown in Figure 9-78, *A* yields a 50% *reduction* in total interbody joint compression force. This reduction is based on the ideal posture having an external moment arm approximately half the length of the internal moment arm. Although this simple mathematic model is not absolutely accurate and does not consider dynamic aspects of movement, it emphasizes how posture can have a profound effect on the forces produced across an interbody joint.[83]

The thoracic posture shown in Figure 9-78, *B* may progress, in extreme cases, to that shown in Figure 9-78, *C*, once commonly referred to as a "widow's hump." As shown, the line of force from body weight has produced a small upper cervical extension torque and a large thoracic flexion torque. Note that despite the large thoracic kyphosis, the person can extend her upper craniocervical region enough to maintain a horizontal visual gaze. The main point of Figure 9-78, *C*, however, is to appreciate the biomechanical impact that a large external flexion torque can have on the progression of severe thoracic hyperkyphosis. Such severe hyperkyphosis has been shown to reduce the inspiratory and vital capacity of the lungs,[46] as well as to increase the risk of falling because of a reduced sense of balance. The hyperkyphosis may even further progress with a continued history of multiple compression fractures, untreated osteoporosis, progressive degenerative disc disease, and weakening of the trunk extensor muscles.[131] Muscle weakness may be the result of reduced activity as well as an altered length-tension relationship within the overstretched trunk extensor muscles.[28,143]

Treatment of excessive thoracic kyphosis depends strongly on the severity of the deformity, age, and health of the person. Options may include pharmacologic agents to reduce osteoporosis, surgery, and physical therapy—including postural education, taping and orthosis, and balance training if applicable.[28]

REFERENCES

1. Abe Y, Akeda K, An HS, et al: Proinflammatory cytokines stimulate the expression of nerve growth factor by human intervertebral disc cells, *Spine* 32:635-642, 2007.
2. Adam CJ, Askin GN, Pearcy MJ: Gravity-induced torque and intravertebral rotation in idiopathic scoliosis, *Spine* 33:E30-E37, 2008.
3. Adams MA, Hutton WC: Gradual disc prolapse, *Spine* 10:524-531, 1985.
4. Adams MA, Hutton WC: Prolapsed intervertebral disc. A hyperflexion injury 1981 Volvo Award in Basic Science, *Spine* 7:184-191, 1982.
5. Adams MA, Hutton WC, Stott JR: The resistance to flexion of the lumbar intervertebral joint, *Spine* 5:245-253, 1980.
6. Adams MA, Roughley PJ: What is intervertebral disc degeneration, and what causes it? *Spine* 31:2151-2161, 2006.
7. Ala-Kokko L: Genetic risk factors for lumbar disc disease (review), *Ann Med* 34:42-47, 2002.
8. Alderink GL: The sacroiliac joint: review of anatomy, mechanics and function, *J Orthop Sports Phys Ther* 13:71-84, 1991.
9. Alexander LA, Hancock E, Agouris I, et al: The response of the nucleus pulposus of the lumbar intervertebral discs to functionally loaded positions, *Spine* 32:1508-1512, 2007.
10. American Physical Therapy Association: Guide to Physical Therapist Practice. Second Edition. American Physical Therapy Association, *Phys Ther* 81:9-746, 2001.
11. An HS, Anderson PA, Haughton VM, et al: Introduction: disc degeneration: summary, *Spine* 29:2677-2678, 2004.
12. An HS, Masuda K: Relevance of in vitro and in vivo models for intervertebral disc degeneration, *J Bone Joint Surg Am* 88(Suppl 2):88-94, 2006.
13. Andersson GB, Ortengren R, Nachemson A: Intradiskal pressure, intra-abdominal pressure and myoelectric back muscle activity related to posture and loading, *Clin Orthop Relat Res* 129:156-164, 1977.
14. Antoniou J, Steffen T, Nelson F, et al: The human lumbar intervertebral disc: evidence for changes in the biosynthesis and denaturation of the extracellular matrix with growth, maturation, ageing, and degeneration, *J Clin Invest* 98:996-1003, 1996.
15. Awad JN, Moskovich R: Lumbar disc herniations: surgical versus nonsurgical treatment, *Clin Orthop Relat Res* 443:183-197, 2006.
16. Battie MC, Videman T: Lumbar disc degeneration: epidemiology and genetics, *J Bone Joint Surg Am* 88(Suppl 2):3-9, 2006.
17. Beattie PF: Current understanding of lumbar intervertebral disc degeneration: a review with emphasis upon etiology, pathophysiology, and lumbar magnetic resonance imaging findings, *J Orthop Sports Phys Ther* 38:329-340, 2008.
18. Beattie PF, Brooks WM, Rothstein JM, et al: Effect of lordosis on the position of the nucleus pulposus in supine subjects. A study using magnetic resonance imaging, *Spine* 19:2096-2102, 1994.
19. Bell JA, Stigant M: Development of a fibre optic goniometer system to measure lumbar and hip movement to detect activities and their lumbar postures, *J Med Eng Technol* 31:361-366, 2007.
20. Bergman GJ, Knoester B, Assink N, et al: Variation in the cervical range of motion over time measured by the "flock of birds" electromagnetic tracking system, *Spine* 30:650-654, 2005.
21. Bernard TN Jr, Kirkaldy-Willis WH: Recognizing specific characteristics of nonspecific low back pain, *Clin Orthop Relat Res* 217:266-280, 1987.
22. Black KM, McClure P, Polansky M: The influence of different sitting positions on cervical and lumbar posture, *Spine* 21:65-70, 1996.
23. Bogduk N: *Clinical anatomy of the lumbar spine and sacrum*, 4th ed, New York, 2005, Churchill Livingstone.
24. Bogduk N, Mercer S: Biomechanics of the cervical spine. I: Normal kinematics, *Clin Biomech (Bristol, Avon)* 15:633-648, 2000.
25. Boos N, Weissbach S, Rohrbach H, et al: Classification of age-related changes in lumbar intervertebral discs: 2002 Volvo Award in basic science, *Spine* 27:2631-2644, 2002.
26. Borenstein DG, O'Mara JW Jr, Boden SD, et al: The value of magnetic resonance imaging of the lumbar spine to predict low-back pain in asymptomatic subjects: a seven-year follow-up study, *J Bone Joint Surg Am* 83:1306-1311, 2001.
27. Brault JS, Driscoll DM, Laakso LL, et al: Quantification of lumbar intradiscal deformation during flexion and extension, by mathematical analysis of magnetic resonance imaging pixel intensity profiles, *Spine* 22:2066-2072, 1997.
28. Briggs AM, van Dieën JH, Wrigley TV, et al: Thoracic kyphosis affects spinal loads and trunk muscle force, *Phys Ther* 87:595-607, 2007.
29. Brisby H: Pathology and possible mechanisms of nervous system response to disc degeneration, *J Bone Joint Surg Am* 88(Suppl 2):68-71, 2006.
30. Browder DA, Childs JD, Cleland JA, Fritz JM: Effectiveness of an extension-oriented treatment approach in a subgroup of subjects with low back pain: a randomized clinical trial, *Phys Ther* 87:1608-1618, 2007.
31. Burwell RG, Freeman BJ, Dangerfield PH, et al: Etiologic theories of idiopathic scoliosis: enantiomorph disorder concept of bilateral symmetry, physeally-created growth conflicts and possible prevention, *Stud Health Technol Inform* 123:391-397, 2006.
32. Calguneri M, Bird HA, Wright V: Changes in joint laxity occurring during pregnancy, *Ann Rheum Dis* 41:126-128, 1982.
33. Cattrysse E, Barbero M, Kool P, et al: 3D morphometry of the transverse and alar ligaments in the occipito-atlanto-axial complex: an in vitro analysis, *Clin Anat* 20:892-898, 2007.
34. Chancey VC, Ottaviano D, Myers BS, Nightingale RW: A kinematic and anthropometric study of the upper cervical spine and the occipital condyles, *J Biomech* 40:1953-1959, 2007.
35. Chelberg MK, Banks GM, Geiger DF, Oegema TR Jr: Identification of heterogeneous cell populations in normal human intervertebral disc, *J Anat* 186:43-53, 1995.
36. Chen C, Lu Y, Kallakuri S, et al: Distribution of A-delta and C-fiber receptors in the cervical facet joint capsule and their response to stretch, *J Bone Joint Surg Am* 88:1807-1816, 2006.
37. Cheung J, Veldhuizen AG, Halberts JP, et al: Geometric and electromyographic assessments in the evaluation of curve progression in idiopathic scoliosis, *Spine* 31:322-329, 2006.
38. Choi G, Raiturker PP, Kim MJ, et al: The effect of early isolated lumbar extension exercise program for patients with herniated disc undergoing lumbar discectomy, *Neurosurgery* 57:764-772, 2005.
39. Cleland JA, Fritz JM, Whitman JM, Heath R: Predictors of short-term outcome in people with a clinical diagnosis of cervical radiculopathy, *Phys Ther* 87:1619-1632, 2007.
40. Cohen SP: Sacroiliac joint pain: a comprehensive review of anatomy, diagnosis, and treatment, *Anesth Analg* 101:1440-1453, 2005.
41. Cook C, Hegedus E, Showalter C, Sizer PS Jr: Coupling behavior of the cervical spine: a systematic review of the literature, *J Manipulative Physiol Ther* 29:570-575, 2006.
42. Cook C, Showalter C: A survey on the importance of lumbar coupling biomechanics in physiotherapy practice, *Man Ther* 9:164-172, 2004.
43. Coonrad RW, Murrell GA, Motley G, et al: A logical coronal pattern classification of 2,000 consecutive idiopathic scoliosis cases based on the scoliosis research society-defined apical vertebra, *Spine* 23:1380-1391, 1998.
44. Coppes MH, Marani E, Thomeer RT, Groen GJ: Innervation of "painful" lumbar discs, *Spine* 22:2342-2349, 1997.
45. Crisco JJ III, Panjabi MM, Dvorak J: A model of the alar ligaments of the upper cervical spine in axial rotation, *J Biomech* 24:607-614, 1991.
46. Culham EG, Jimenez HA, King CE: Thoracic kyphosis, rib mobility, and lung volumes in normal women and women with osteoporosis, *Spine* 19:1250-1255, 1994.
47. Cyron BM, Hutton WC: Articular tropism and stability of the lumbar spine, *Spine* 5:168-172, 1980.
48. Cyron BM, Hutton WC: The tensile strength of the capsular ligaments of the apophyseal joints, *J Anat* 132(Pt 1):145-150, 1981.
49. Danielsson AJ, Hasserius R, Ohlin A, Nachemson AL: A prospective study of brace treatment versus observation alone in adolescent idiopathic scoliosis: a follow-up mean of 16 years after maturity, *Spine* 32:2198-2207, 2007.
50. Danielsson AJ, Nachemson AL: Radiologic findings and curve progression 22 years after treatment for adolescent idiopathic scoliosis: comparison of brace and surgical treatment with matching control group of straight individuals, *Spine* 26:516-525, 2001.
51. Dar G, Peleg S, Masharawi Y, et al: Sacroiliac joint bridging: demographical and anatomical aspects, *Spine* 30:E429-E432, 2005.
52. De Smet AA, Robinson RG, Johnson BE, Lukert BP: Spinal compression fractures in osteoporotic women: patterns and relationship to hyperkyphosis, *Radiology* 166:497-500, 1988.
53. Dempster WT: *Space Requirements for the Seated Operator. WADC-TR-55-159*, Dayton, 1955, Wright Patterson Air Force Base.
54. Dolan LA, Weinstein SL: Surgical rates after observation and bracing for adolescent idiopathic scoliosis: an evidence-based review, *Spine* 32:S91-S100, 2007.
55. Donelson R, Aprill C, Medcalf R, Grant W: A prospective study of centralization of lumbar and referred pain. A predictor of symptomatic discs and anular competence, *Spine* 22:1115-1122, 1997.

56. Dvorak J, Panjabi MM, Novotny JE, Antinnes JA: In vivo flexion/extension of the normal cervical spine, *J Orthop Res* 9:828-834, 1991.

57. Dvorak J, Schneider E, Saldinger P, Rahn B: Biomechanics of the craniocervical region: the alar and transverse ligaments, *J Orthop Res* 6:452-461, 1988.

58. Edmondston SJ, Henne SE, Loh W, Ostvold E: Influence of craniocervical posture on three-dimensional motion of the cervical spine, *Man Ther* 10:44-51, 2005.

59. Egund N, Olsson TH, Schmid H, Selvik G: Movements in the sacroiliac joints demonstrated with roentgen stereophotogrammetry, *Acta Radiol Diagn (Stockh)* 19:833-846, 1978.

60. Esola MA, McClure PW, Fitzgerald GK, Siegler S: Analysis of lumbar spine and hip motion during forward bending in subjects with and without a history of low back pain, *Spine* 21:71-78, 1996.

61. Eubanks JD, Lee MJ, Cassinelli E, Ahn NU: Does lumbar facet arthrosis precede disc degeneration? A postmortem study, *Clin Orthop Relat Res* 464:184-189, 2007.

62. Fagan A, Moore R, Vernon RB, et al: ISSLS prize winner: The innervation of the intervertebral disc: a quantitative analysis, *Spine* 28:2570-2576, 2003.

63. Farfan HF, Huberdeau RM, Dubow HI: Lumbar intervertebral disc degeneration: the influence of geometrical features on the pattern of disc degeneration—a post mortem study, *J Bone Joint Surg Am* 54:492-510, 1972.

64. Fazey PJ, Song S, Mønsås S, et al: An MRI investigation of intervertebral disc deformation in response to torsion, *Clin Biomech (Bristol, Avon)* 21:538-542, 2006.

65. Feipel V, Rondelet B, Le PJ, Rooze M: Normal global motion of the cervical spine: an electrogoniometric study, *Clin Biomech (Bristol, Avon)* 14:462-470, 1999.

66. Feng H, Danfelter M, Strömqvist B, Heinegård D: Extracellular matrix in disc degeneration, *J Bone Joint Surg Am* 88(Suppl 2):25-29, 2006.

67. Fennell AJ, Jones AP, Hukins DW: Migration of the nucleus pulposus within the intervertebral disc during flexion and extension of the spine, *Spine* 21:2753-2757, 1996.

68. Fielding JW, Cochran GB, Lawsing JF 3rd, Hohl M: Tears of the transverse ligament of the atlas. A clinical and biomechanical study, *J Bone Joint Surg Am* 56:1683-1691, 1974.

69. Foley BS, Buschbacher RM: Sacroiliac joint pain: anatomy, biomechanics, diagnosis, and treatment, *Am J Phys Med Rehabil* 85:997-1006, 2006.

70. Forst SL, Wheeler MT, Fortin JD, Vilensky JA: The sacroiliac joint: anatomy, physiology and clinical significance, *Pain Physician* 9:61-67, 2006.

71. Fritz JM, Lindsay W, Matheson JW, et al: Is there a subgroup of patients with low back pain likely to benefit from mechanical traction? Results of a randomized clinical trial and subgrouping analysis, *Spine* 32:E793-E800, 2007.

72. Fujiwara A, Tamai K, Yoshida H, et al: Anatomy of the iliolumbar ligament, *Clin Orthop Relat Res* 167-172, 2000.

73. Giles LG: Human lumbar zygapophyseal joint inferior recess synovial folds: a light microscope examination, *Anat Rec* 220:117-124, 1988.

74. Giles LG, Taylor JR: Human zygapophyseal joint capsule and synovial fold innervation, *Br J Rheumatol* 26:93-98, 1987.

75. Glard Y, Launay F, Viehweger E, et al: Hip flexion contracture and lumbar spine lordosis in myelomeningocele, *J Pediatr Orthop* 25:476-478, 2005.

76. Grobler LJ, Robertson PA, Novotny JE, Pope MH: Etiology of spondylolisthesis. Assessment of the role played by lumbar facet joint morphology, *Spine* 18:80-91, 1993.

77. Grunhagen T, Wilde G, Soukane DM, et al: Nutrient supply and intervertebral disc metabolism. *J Bone Joint Surg Am* 88(Suppl 2):30-35, 2006.

78. Haefeli M, Kalberer F, Saegesser D, et al: The course of macroscopic degeneration in the human lumbar intervertebral disc, *Spine* 31:1522-1531, 2006.

79. Hangai M, Kaneoka K, Kuno S, et al: Factors associated with lumbar intervertebral disc degeneration in the elderly, *Spine J* 8:732-740, 2008.

80. Hansen HC, Kenzie-Brown AM, Cohen SP, et al: Sacroiliac joint interventions: a systematic review, *Pain Physician* 10:165-184, 2007.

81. Hansen L, de Zee M, Rasmussen J, et al: Anatomy and biomechanics of the back muscles in the lumbar spine with reference to biomechanical modeling, *Spine* 31:1888-1899, 2006.

82. Harrison DD, Janik TJ, Troyanovich SJ, Holland B: Comparisons of lordotic cervical spine curvatures to a theoretical ideal model of the static sagittal cervical spine, *Spine* 21:667-675, 1996.

83. Harrison DE, Colloca CJ, Harrison DD, et al: Anterior thoracic posture increases thoracolumbar disc loading, *Eur Spine J* 14:234-242, 2005.

84. Hayashi K, Yabuki T: Origin of the uncus and of Luschka's joint in the cervical spine, *J Bone Joint Surg Am* 67:788-791, 1985.

85. Heuer F, Schmidt H, Klezl Z, et al: Stepwise reduction of functional spinal structures increase range of motion and change lordosis angle, *J Biomech* 40:271-280, 2007.

86. Heylings DJ: Supraspinous and interspinous ligaments of the human lumbar spine, *J Anat* 125:127-131, 1978.

87. Holmes A, Han ZH, Dang GT, et al: Changes in cervical canal spinal volume during in vitro flexion-extension, *Spine* 21:1313-1319, 1996.

88. Hukins DW, Kirby MC, Sikoryn TA, et al: Comparison of structure, mechanical properties, and functions of lumbar spinal ligaments, *Spine* 15:787-795, 1990.

89. Iatridis JC, MaClean JJ, Roughley PJ, Alini M: Effects of mechanical loading on intervertebral disc metabolism in vivo, *J Bone Joint Surg Am* 88(Suppl 2):41-46, 2006.

90. Inufusa A, An HS, Lim TH, et al: Anatomic changes of the spinal canal and intervertebral foramen associated with flexion-extension movement, *Spine* 21:2412-2420, 1996.

91. Ishihara H, Urban JP: Effects of low oxygen concentrations and metabolic inhibitors on proteoglycan and protein synthesis rates in the intervertebral disc, *J Orthop Res* 17:829-835, 1999.

92. Ishii T, Mukai Y, Hosono N, et al: Kinematics of the cervical spine in lateral bending: in vivo three-dimensional analysis, *Spine* 31:155-160, 2006.

93. Ishii T, Mukai Y, Hosono N, et al: Kinematics of the subaxial cervical spine in rotation in vivo three-dimensional analysis, *Spine* 29:2826-2831, 2004.

94. Jenkins JP, Hickey DS, Zhu XP, et al: MR imaging of the intervertebral disc: a quantitative study, *Br J Radiol* 58:705-709, 1985.

95. Jensen MC, Brant-Zawadzki MN, Obuchowski N, et al: Magnetic resonance imaging of the lumbar spine in people without back pain, *N Engl J Med* 331:69-73, 1994.

96. Johnson WE, Evans H, Menage J, et al: Immunohistochemical detection of Schwann cells in innervated and vascularized human intervertebral discs, *Spine* 26:2550-2557, 2001.

97. Kalichman L, Hunter DJ: Lumbar facet joint osteoarthritis: a review, *Semin Arthritis Rheum* 37:69-80, 2007.

98. Kampen WU, Tillmann B: Age-related changes in the articular cartilage of human sacroiliac joint, *Anat Embryol (Berl)* 198:505-513, 1998.

99. Kaneoka K, Ono K, Inami S, Hayashi K: Motion analysis of cervical vertebrae during whiplash loading, *Spine* 24:763-769, 1999.

100. Karakida O, Ueda H, Ueda M, Miyasaka T: Diurnal T2 value changes in the lumbar intervertebral discs, *Clin Radiol* 58:389-392, 2003.

101. Keller TS, Spengler DM, Hansson TH: Mechanical behavior of the human lumbar spine. I: Creep analysis during static compressive loading, *J Orthop Res* 5:467-478, 1987.

102. Kingma I, Staudenmann D, van Dieen JH: Trunk muscle activation and associated lumbar spine joint shear forces under different levels of external forward force applied to the trunk, *J Electromyogr Kinesiol* 17:14-24, 2007.

103. Kissling RO, Jacob HA: The mobility of the sacroiliac joint in healthy subjects, *Bull Hosp Jt Dis* 54:158-164, 1996.

104. Kitagawa T, Fujiwara A, Kobayashi N, et al: Morphologic changes in the cervical neural foramen due to flexion and extension: in vivo imaging study, *Spine* 29:2821-2825, 2004.

105. Kondratek M, Krauss J, Stiller C, Olson R: Normative values for active lumbar range of motion in children, *Pediatr Phys Ther* 19:236-244, 2007.

106. Korovessis PG, Stamatakis MV, Baikousis AG: Reciprocal angulation of vertebral bodies in the sagittal plane in an asymptomatic Greek population, *Spine* 23:700-704, 1998.

107. Krismer M, Haid C, Rabl W: The contribution of anulus fibers to torque resistance, *Spine* 21:2551-2557, 1996.

108. Kulig K, Landel R, Powers CM: Assessment of lumbar spine kinematics using dynamic MRI: a proposed mechanism of sagittal plane motion induced by manual posterior-to-anterior mobilization, *J Orthop Sports Phys Ther* 34:57-64, 2004.

109. Laslett M, Aprill CN, McDonald B, Young SB: Diagnosis of sacroiliac joint pain: validity of individual provocation tests and composites of tests, *Man Ther* 10:207-218, 2005.

110. Lee RY, Wong TK: Relationship between the movements of the lumbar spine and hip, *Hum Mov Sci* 21:481-494, 2002.

111. Legaspi O, Edmond SL: Does the evidence support the existence of lumbar spine coupled motion? A critical review of the literature, *J Orthop Sports Phys Ther* 37:169-178, 2007.

112. Levine D, Whittle MW: The effects of pelvic movement on lumbar lordosis in the standing position, *J Orthop Sports Phys Ther* 24:130-135, 1996.

113. Lonner BS, Newton P, Betz R, et al: Operative management of Scheuermann's kyphosis in 78 patients: radiographic outcomes, complications, and technique, *Spine* 32:2644-2652, 2007.

114. Lonstein JE: Scoliosis: surgical versus nonsurgical treatment, *Clin Orthop Relat Res* 443:248-259, 2006.

115. Lonstein JE, Winter RB: The Milwaukee brace for the treatment of adolescent idiopathic scoliosis. A review of one thousand and twenty patients, *J Bone Joint Surg Am* 76:1207-1221, 1994.

116. Lotz JC, Ulrich JA: Innervation, inflammation, and hypermobility may characterize pathologic disc degeneration: review of animal model data, *J Bone Joint Surg Am* 88(Suppl 2):76-82, 2006.

117. Lowe TG, Line BG: Evidence based medicine: analysis of Scheuermann kyphosis, *Spine* 32:S115-S119, 2007.

118. Lu YM, Hutton WC, Gharpuray VM: Do bending, twisting, and diurnal fluid changes in the disc affect the propensity to prolapse? A viscoelastic finite element model, *Spine* 21:2570-2579, 1996.

119. Machado LA, de Souza MS, Ferreira PH, Ferreira ML: The McKenzie method for low back pain: a systematic review of the literature with a meta-analysis approach, *Spine* 31:E254-E262, 2006.

120. Maigne JY, Aivaliklis A, Pfefer F: Results of sacroiliac joint double block and value of sacroiliac pain provocation tests in 54 patients with low back pain, *Spine* 21:1889-1892, 1996.

121. Mannion AF, Knecht K, Balaban G, et al: A new skin-surface device for measuring the curvature and global and segmental ranges of motion of the spine: reliability of measurements and comparison with data reviewed from the literature, *Eur Spine J* 13:122-136, 2004.

122. Marchand F, Ahmed AM: Investigation of the laminate structure of lumbar disc anulus fibrosus, *Spine* 15:402-410, 1990.

123. Marks M, Petcharaporn M, Betz RR, et al: Outcomes of surgical treatment in male versus female adolescent idiopathic scoliosis patients, *Spine* 32:544-549, 2007.

124. Masharawi Y, Rothschild B, Dar G, et al: Facet orientation in the thoracolumbar spine: three-dimensional anatomic and biomechanical analysis, *Spine* 29:1755-1763, 2004.

125. McGill SM, Hughson RL, Parks K: Changes in lumbar lordosis modify the role of the extensor muscles, *Clin Biomech (Bristol, Avon)* 15:777-780, 2000.

126. McGrath MC, Zhang M: Lateral branches of dorsal sacral nerve plexus and the long posterior sacroiliac ligament, *Surg Radiol Anat* 27:327-330, 2005.

127. McKenzie RA: *The lumbar spine: mechanical diagnosis and therapy*, Waikanae, New Zealand, 1981, Spinal Publications.

128. McLean L: The effect of postural correction on muscle activation amplitudes recorded from the cervicobrachial region, *J Electromyogr Kinesiol* 15:527-535, 2005.

129. Mercer S, Bogduk N: Intra-articular inclusions of the cervical synovial joints, *Br J Rheumatol* 32:705-710, 1993.

130. Mercer S, Bogduk N: The ligaments and annulus fibrosus of human adult cervical intervertebral discs, *Spine* 24:619-626, 1999.

131. Mika A, Unnithan VB, Mika P: Differences in thoracic kyphosis and in back muscle strength in women with bone loss due to osteoporosis, *Spine* 30:241-246, 2005.

132. Mikkonen P, Leino-Arjas P, Remes J, et al: Is smoking a risk factor for low back pain in adolescents? A prospective cohort study, *Spine* 33:527-532, 2008.

133. Miller JA, Schmatz C, Schultz AB: Lumbar disc degeneration: correlation with age, sex, and spine level in 600 autopsy specimens, *Spine* 13:173-178, 1988.

134. Milosavljevic S, Pal P, Bain D, Johnson G: Kinematic and temporal interactions of the lumbar spine and hip during trunk extension in healthy male subjects, *Eur Spine J* 17:122-128, 2008.

135. Miyasaka K, Ohmori K, Suzuki K, Inoue H: Radiographic analysis of lumbar motion in relation to lumbosacral stability. Investigation of moderate and maximum motion, *Spine* 25:732-737, 2000.

136. Moore RJ: The vertebral endplate: disc degeneration, disc regeneration, *Eur Spine J* 15(Suppl 3):S333-S337, 2006.

137. Muhle C, Resnick D, Ahn JM, et al: In vivo changes in the neuroforaminal size at flexion-extension and axial rotation of the cervical spine in healthy persons examined using kinematic magnetic resonance imaging, *Spine* 26:E287-E293, 2001.

138. Nachemson A: Lumbar intradiscal pressure. Experimental studies on post-mortem material, *Acta Orthop Scand Suppl* 43:1-104, 1960.

139. Nachemson A: Some mechanical properties of the third lumbar interlaminar ligament (ligamentum flavum), *J Biomech* 1:211-220, 1968.

140. Nachemson A: The load on lumbar disks in different positions of the body, *Clin Orthop Relat Res* 45:107-122, 1966.

141. Nelson JM, Walmsley RP, Stevenson JM: Relative lumbar and pelvic motion during loaded spinal flexion/extension, *Spine* 20:199-204, 1995.

142. Neumann DA: Arthrokinesiologic considerations for the aged adult. In: Guccione AA, editor: *Geriatric physical therapy*, ed 2, Chicago, 2000, Mosby.

143. Neumann DA, Soderberg GL, Cook TM: Electromyographic analysis of hip abductor musculature in healthy right-handed persons, *Phys Ther* 69:431-440, 1989.

144. Ng JK, Kippers V, Richardson CA, Parnianpour M: Range of motion and lordosis of the lumbar spine: reliability of measurement and normative values, *Spine* 26:53-60, 2001.

145. Niosi CA, Oxland TR: Degenerative mechanics of the lumbar spine, *Spine J* 4:202S-208S, 2004.

146. Oda H, Matsuzaki H, Tokuhashi Y, et al: Degeneration of intervertebral discs due to smoking: experimental assessment in a rat-smoking model, *J Orthop Sci* 9:135-141, 2004.

147. Ordway NR, Seymour R, Donelson RG, et al: Cervical sagittal range-of-motion analysis using three methods. Cervical range-of-motion device, 3space, and radiography, *Spine* 22:501-508, 1997.

148. Ordway NR, Seymour RJ, Donelson RG, et al: Cervical flexion, extension, protrusion, and retraction. A radiographic segmental analysis, *Spine* 24:240-247, 1999.

149. Panjabi M, Dvorak J, Crisco JJ 3rd, et al: Effects of alar ligament transection on upper cervical spine rotation, *J Orthop Res* 9:584-593, 1991.

150. Panjabi MM, Oxland T, Takata K, et al: Articular facets of the human spine. Quantitative three-dimensional anatomy, *Spine* 18:1298-1310, 1993.

151. Pearcy M, Portek I, Shepherd J: The effect of low-back pain on lumbar spinal movements measured by three-dimensional x-ray analysis, *Spine* 10:150-153, 1985.

152. Pearcy M, Portek I, Shepherd J: Three-dimensional x-ray analysis of normal movement in the lumbar spine, *Spine* 9:294-297, 1984.

153. Pearcy MJ, Tibrewal SB: Axial rotation and lateral bending in the normal lumbar spine measured by three-dimensional radiography, *Spine* 9:582-587, 1984.

154. Pecha MD: Herniated nucleus pulposus as a result of emesis in a 20-yr-old man, *Am J Phys Med Rehabil* 83:327-330, 2004.

155. Peng B, Hao J, Hou S, et al: Possible pathogenesis of painful intervertebral disc degeneration, *Spine* 31:560-566, 2006.

156. Penning L: Normal movements of the cervical spine, *AJR Am J Roentgenol* 130:317-326, 1978.

157. Pfirrmann CW, Metzdorf A, Elfering A, et al: Effect of aging and degeneration on disc volume and shape: a quantitative study in asymptomatic volunteers, *J Orthop Res* 24:1086-1094, 2006.

158. Podichetty VK: The aging spine: the role of inflammatory mediators in intervertebral disc degeneration, *Cell Mol Biol (Noisy-le-grand)* 53:4-18, 2007.

159. Pollintine P, Dolan P, Tobias JH, Adams MA: Intervertebral disc degeneration can lead to "stress-shielding" of the anterior vertebral body: a cause of osteoporotic vertebral fracture? *Spine* 29:774-782, 2004.

160. Pool-Goudzwaard A, Hoek vD, Mulder P, et al: The iliolumbar ligament: its influence on stability of the sacroiliac joint, *Clin Biomech (Bristol, Avon)* 18:99-105, 2003.

161. Powers CM, Beneck GJ, Kulig K, et al: Effects of a single session of posterior-to-anterior spinal mobilization and press-up exercise on pain response and lumbar spine extension in people with nonspecific low back pain, *Phys Ther* 88:485-493, 2008.

162. Przybyla A, Pollintine P, Bedzinski R, Adams MA: Outer annulus tears have less effect than endplate fracture on stress distributions inside intervertebral discs: relevance to disc degeneration, *Clin Biomech (Bristol, Avon)* 21:1013-1019, 2006.

163. Przybyla AS, Skrzypiec D, Pollintine P, et al: Strength of the cervical spine in compression and bending, *Spine* 32:1612-1620, 2007.

164. Pye SR, Reid DM, Smith R, et al: Radiographic features of lumbar disc degeneration and self-reported back pain, *J Rheumatol* 31:753-758, 2004.

165. Rajasekaran S, Babu JN, Arun R, et al: ISSLS prize winner: A study of diffusion in human lumbar discs: a serial magnetic resonance imaging study documenting the influence of the endplate on diffusion in normal and degenerate discs, *Spine* 29:2654-2667, 2004.

166. Rannou F, Richette P, Benallaoua M, et al: Cyclic tensile stretch modulates proteoglycan production by intervertebral disc annulus fibrosus

cells through production of nitrite oxide, *J Cell Biochem* 90:148-157, 2003.

167. Reichmann S: The postnatal development of form and orientation of the lumbar intervertebral joint surfaces, *Z Anat Entwicklungsgesch* 133:102-123, 1971.

168. Riddle DL, Freburger JK: Evaluation of the presence of sacroiliac joint region dysfunction using a combination of tests: a multicenter intertester reliability study, *Phys Ther* 82:772-781, 2002.

169. Roberts S, Evans H, Trivedi J, Menage J: Histology and pathology of the human intervertebral disc, *J Bone Joint Surg Am* 88(Suppl 2):10-14, 2006.

170. Roberts S, Menage J, Eisenstein SM: The cartilage end-plate and intervertebral disc in scoliosis: calcification and other sequelae, *J Orthop Res* 11:747-757, 1993.

171. Rosatelli AL, Agur AM, Chhaya S: Anatomy of the interosseous region of the sacroiliac joint, *J Orthop Sports Phys Ther* 36:200-208, 2006.

172. Saldinger P, Dvorak J, Rahn BA, Perren SM: Histology of the alar and transverse ligaments, *Spine* 15:257-261, 1990.

173. Scannell JP, McGill SM: Lumbar posture—should it, and can it, be modified? A study of passive tissue stiffness and lumbar position during activities of daily living, *Phys Ther* 83:907-917, 2003.

174. Schmidt H, Heuer F, Claes L, Wilke HJ: The relation between the instantaneous center of rotation and facet joint forces—A finite element analysis, *Clin Biomech (Bristol, Avon)* 23:270-278, 2008.

175. Schmidt H, Kettler A, Heuer F, et al: Intradiscal pressure, shear strain, and fiber strain in the intervertebral disc under combined loading, *Spine* 32:748-755, 2007.

176. Schnebel BE, Simmons JW, Chowning J, Davidson R: A digitizing technique for the study of movement of intradiscal dye in response to flexion and extension of the lumbar spine, *Spine* 13:309-312, 1988.

177. Setton LA, Chen J: Mechanobiology of the intervertebral disc and relevance to disc degeneration, *J Bone Joint Surg Am* 88(Suppl 2):52-57, 2006.

178. Shibata Y, Shirai Y, Miyamoto M: The aging process in the sacroiliac joint: helical computed tomography analysis, *J Orthop Sci* 7:12-18, 2002.

179. Shirazi-Adl A, Drouin G: Load-bearing role of facets in a lumbar segment under sagittal plane loadings, *J Biomech* 20:601-613, 1987.

180. Shum GL, Crosbie J, Lee RY: Movement coordination of the lumbar spine and hip during a picking up activity in low back pain subjects, *Eur Spine J* 16:749-758, 2007.

181. Simpson AK, Biswas D, Emerson JW, et al: Quantifying the effects of age, gender, degeneration, and adjacent level degeneration on cervical spine range of motion using multivariate analyses, *Spine* 33:183-186, 2008.

182. Sizer PS Jr, Brismee JM, Cook C: Coupling behavior of the thoracic spine: a systematic review of the literature, *J Manipulative Physiol Ther* 30:390-399, 2007.

183. Slipman CW, Jackson HB, Lipetz JS, et al: Sacroiliac joint pain referral zones, *Arch Phys Med Rehabil* 81:334-338, 2000.

184. Snijders CJ, Hermans PF, Kleinrensink GJ: Functional aspects of cross-legged sitting with special attention to piriformis muscles and sacroiliac joints, *Clin Biomech (Bristol, Avon)* 21:116-121, 2006.

185. Snijders CJ, Ribbers MT, de Bakker HV, et al: EMG recordings of abdominal and back muscles in various standing postures: validation of a biomechanical model on sacroiliac joint stability, *J Electromyogr Kinesiol* 8:205-214, 1998.

186. Snijders CJ, Vleeming A, Stoeckart R: Transfer of lumbosacral load to iliac bones and legs. Part 1: Biomechanics of self-bracing of the sacroiliac joints and its significance for treatment and exercise, *Clin Biomech (Bristol, Avon)* 8:285-294, 1993.

187. Stadnik TW, Lee RR, Coen HL, et al: Annular tears and disk herniation: prevalence and contrast enhancement on MR images in the absence of low back pain or sciatica, *Radiology* 206:49-55, 1998.

188. Standring S: *Gray's anatomy: the anatomical basis of clinical practice*, ed 40, St Louis, 2009, Elsevier.

189. Steffen T, Rubin RK, Baramki HG, et al: A new technique for measuring lumbar segmental motion in vivo. Method, accuracy, and preliminary results, *Spine* 22:156-166, 1997.

190. Stokes IA, Gardner-Morse M: Muscle activation strategies and symmetry of spinal loading in the lumbar spine with scoliosis, *Spine* 29:2103-2107, 2004.

191. Sturesson B, Selvik G, Uden A: Movements of the sacroiliac joints. A roentgen stereophotogrammetric analysis, *Spine* 14:162-165, 1989.

192. Takahashi T, Ishida K, Hirose D, et al: Trunk deformity is associated with a reduction in outdoor activities of daily living and life satisfaction in community-dwelling older people, *Osteoporos Int* 16:273-279, 2005.

193. Takebayashi T, Cavanaugh JM, Kallakuri S, et al: Sympathetic afferent units from lumbar intervertebral discs, *J Bone Joint Surg Br* 88:554-557, 2006.

194. Taylor JR, Twomey LT: Age changes in lumbar zygapophyseal joints. Observations on structure and function, *Spine* 11:739-745, 1986.

195. Teyhen DS, Flynn TW, Childs JD, Abraham LD: Arthrokinematics in a subgroup of patients likely to benefit from a lumbar stabilization exercise program, *Phys Ther* 87:313-325, 2007.

196. Thomas JS, Gibson GE: Coordination and timing of spine and hip joints during full body reaching tasks, *Hum Mov Sci* 26:124-140, 2007.

197. Tousignant M, Smeesters C, Breton AM, et al: Criterion validity study of the cervical range of motion (CROM) device for rotational range of motion on healthy adults, *J Orthop Sports Phys Ther* 36:242-248, 2006.

198. Troke M, Moore AP, Maillardet FJ, Cheek E: A normative database of lumbar spine ranges of motion, *Man Ther* 10:198-206, 2005.

199. Truumees E, Demetropoulos CK, Yang KH, Herkowitz HN: Failure of human cervical endplates: a cadaveric experimental model, *Spine* 28:2204-2208, 2003.

200. Tsantrizos A, Ito K, Aebi M, Steffen T: Internal strains in healthy and degenerated lumbar intervertebral discs, *Spine* 30:2129-2137, 2005.

201. Tyrrell AR, Reilly T, Troup JD: Circadian variation in stature and the effects of spinal loading, *Spine* 10:161-164, 1985.

202. Urban JP: The role of the physicochemical environment in determining disc cell behaviour, *Biochem Soc Trans* 30:858-864, 2002.

203. Urban JP, McMullin JF: Swelling pressure of the lumbar intervertebral discs: influence of age, spinal level, composition, and degeneration, *Spine* 13:179-187, 1988.

204. Van der Plaats A, Veldhuizen AG, Verkerke GJ: Numerical simulation of asymmetrically altered growth as initiation mechanism of scoliosis, *Ann Biomed Eng* 35:1206-1215, 2007.

205. van Wingerden JP, Vleeming A, Buyruk HM, Raissadat K: Stabilization of the sacroiliac joint in vivo: verification of muscular contribution to force closure of the pelvis, *Eur Spine J* 13:199-205, 2004.

206. Vernon-Roberts B, Moore RJ, Fraser RD: The natural history of age-related disc degeneration: the pathology and sequelae of tears, *Spine* 32:2797-2804, 2007.

207. Vibert BT, Sliva CD, Herkowitz HN: Treatment of instability and spondylolisthesis: surgical versus nonsurgical treatment, *Clin Orthop Relat Res* 443:222-227, 2006.

208. Videman T, Levalahti E, Battie MC: The effects of anthropometrics, lifting strength, and physical activities in disc degeneration, *Spine* 32:1406-1413, 2007.

209. Vilensky JA, O'Connor BL, Fortin JD, et al: Histologic analysis of neural elements in the human sacroiliac joint, *Spine* 27:1202-1207, 2002.

210. Vleeming A, Pool-Goudzwaard AL, Hammudoghlu D, et al: The function of the long dorsal sacroiliac ligament: its implication for understanding low back pain, *Spine* 21:556-562, 1996.

211. Vleeming A, Pool-Goudzwaard AL, Stoeckart R, et al: The posterior layer of the thoracolumbar fascia. Its function in load transfer from spine to legs, *Spine* 20:753-758, 1995.

212. Vleeming A, Volkers AC, Snijders CJ, Stoeckart R: Relation between form and function in the sacroiliac joint. Part II: Biomechanical aspects, *Spine* 15:133-136, 1990.

213. Waddell G, Somerville D, Henderson I, Newton M: Objective clinical evaluation of physical impairment in chronic low back pain (see comment), *Spine* 17:617-628, 1992.

214. Waris E, Eskelin M, Hermunen H, et al: Disc degeneration in low back pain: a 17-year follow-up study using magnetic resonance imaging, *Spine* 32:681-684, 2007.

215. Watkins R 4th, Watkins R 3rd, Williams L, et al: Stability provided by the sternum and rib cage in the thoracic spine, *Spine* 30:1283-1286, 2005.

216. Weiler C, Nerlich AG, Bachmeier BE, Boos N: Expression and distribution of tumor necrosis factor alpha in human lumbar intervertebral discs: a study in surgical specimen and autopsy controls, *Spine* 30:44-53, 2005.

217. Werneke MW, Hart DL, Resnik L, et al: Centralization: prevalence and effect on treatment outcomes using a standardized operational definition and measurement method, *J Orthop Sports Phys Ther* 38:116-125, 2008.

218. White AA III, Panjabi MM: The clinical biomechanics of scoliosis, *Clin Orthop Relat Res* 100-112, 1976.

219. Wilke HJ, Neef P, Caimi M, et al: New in vivo measurements of pressures in the intervertebral disc in daily life, *Spine* 24:755-762, 1999.

220. Willburger RE, Ehiosun UK, Kuhnen C, et al: Clinical symptoms in lumbar disc herniations and their correlation to the histological composition of the extruded disc material, *Spine* 29:1655-1661, 2004.
221. Williams PC: Examination and conservative treatment for disk lesions of the lower spine, *Clin Orthop Relat Res* 5:28-40, 1955.
222. Wong KW, Luk KD, Leong JC, et al: Continuous dynamic spinal motion analysis, *Spine* 31:414-419, 2006.
223. Yahia LH, Garzon S, Strykowski H, Rivard CH: Ultrastructure of the human interspinous ligament and ligamentum flavum. A preliminary study, *Spine* 15:262-268, 1990.
224. Yamamoto I, Panjabi MM, Oxland TR, Crisco JJ: The role of the iliolumbar ligament in the lumbosacral junction, *Spine* 15:1138-1141, 1990.
225. Yu J, Fairbank JC, Roberts S, Urban JP: The elastic fiber network of the anulus fibrosus of the normal and scoliotic human intervertebral disc, *Spine* 30:1815-1820, 2005.
226. Zhang QH, Teo EC, Ng HW, Lee VS: Finite element analysis of moment-rotation relationships for human cervical spine, *J Biomech* 39:189-193, 2006.
227. Zhao F, Pollintine P, Hole BD, et al: Discogenic origins of spinal instability, *Spine* 30:2621-2630, 2005.
228. Zifchock RA, Davis I, Hillstrom H, Song J: The effect of gender, age, and lateral dominance on arch height and arch stiffness, *Foot Ankle Int* 27:367-372, 2006.

STUDY QUESTIONS

1 Describe the osteokinematics at the craniocervical region during cranial *protraction* (from a fully retracted position). Which tissues, if normal, would become relatively slackened in a position of full protraction?

2 How could the natural elasticity of the ligamentum flavum protect the interbody joint against excessive and potentially damaging compression forces?

3 Based on moment arm length alone, which connective tissue most effectively limits flexion torque within the thoracolumbar region?

4 Are the intertransverse ligaments between L3 and L4 positioned to limit sagittal plane rotation? If so, which motion?

5 Describe the arthrokinematics at the apophyseal joints between L2 and L3 during full axial rotation to the right.

6 From an anterior to posterior direction, list, in order, the connective tissues that exist at the atlanto-axial joint. Start anteriorly with the anterior arch of the atlas, and finish posteriorly at the tips of the spinous processes. Be sure to include the dens and transverse ligament of the atlas in your answer.

7 Define *nutation* and *counternutation* at the sacroiliac joint.

8 Persons with a history of posterior herniated disc are usually advised against lifting a large load held in front the body, especially with a flexed lumbar spine. How would you justify this advice?

9 Describe the articulations between the sixth rib and the midthoracic spine.

10 Explain how a severely degenerated disc can lead to osteophyte formation in the midcervical spine.

11 Assume the subject depicted in Figure 9-10, *C* has increased lumbar lordosis primarily as a result of tightened (shortened) hip flexor muscles. Describe the possible negative kinesiologic or biomechanical consequences that may result within the lumbar and lumbosacral regions.

12 Describe the mechanical role of the annulus fibrosis in distributing compression forces across the interbody joint.

13 With the visual aid of Figure III-1 (in Appendix III, Part A), explain why a posterior herniated disc between the bodies of L4 and L5 can compress the L^4 spinal nerve root, but possibly L^5 and all sacral nerve roots as well.

14 Describe the general transition in spatial orientation of the articular surfaces of the apophyseal joints, starting with the atlanto-axial joint and finishing with the lumbosacral junction. Explain how this transition influences the predominant kinematics across the various regions. Include in your answer the kinematics associated with the most often expressed spinal coupling pattern within the mid and lower craniocervical region.

15 Describe arthrokinematics at the apophyseal joints between C4 and C5 during full extension.

Answers to the study questions can be found on the Evolve website.

C H A P T E R

10

Axial Skeleton: Muscle and Joint Interactions

DONALD A. NEUMANN, PT, PhD, FAPTA

CHAPTER AT A GLANCE

O steologic and arthrologic components of the axial skeleton are presented in Chapter 9. Chapter 10 focuses on the many muscle and joint interactions occurring within the axial skeleton. The muscles control posture and stabilize the axial skeleton, protect the spinal cord and internal organs, produce torques required for movement of the body as a whole, and, lastly, furnish fine mobility to the head and neck for optimal placement of the eyes, ears, and nose. Muscles associated with ventilation and mastication (chewing) are presented in Chapter 11.

The anatomic structure of the muscles within the axial skeleton varies considerably in length, shape, fiber direction, cross-sectional area, and leverage across the underlying joints. Such variability reflects the diverse demands placed on the musculature, from manually lifting and transporting heavy objects to producing subtle motions of the head for accenting a lively conversation.

Muscles within the axial skeleton cross multiple regions of the body. The trapezius muscle, for example, attaches to the clavicle and the scapula within the appendicular skeleton and to the vertebral column and the cranium within the axial skeleton. Protective guarding because of an inflamed upper trapezius can therefore affect the quality of motion throughout the upper extremity and craniocervical region.

The primary aim of this chapter is to elucidate the structure and function of the muscles within the axial skeleton. This information is essential to the evaluation and treatment of a wide range of musculoskeletal impairments, such as postural malalignment, deformity, or instability; muscle injury, spasm, excessive stiffness, or weakness; and generalized neck and back pain.

INNERVATION OF THE MUSCLES AND JOINTS WITHIN THE TRUNK AND CRANIOCERVICAL REGIONS

An understanding of the organization of the innervation of the craniocervical and trunk muscles begins with an appreciation of the formation of a typical *spinal nerve root* (Figure 10-1). Each spinal nerve root is formed by the union of ventral and dorsal *nerve roots*: the *ventral nerve roots* contain primarily "outgoing" (efferent) axons that supply motor commands to muscles and other effector organs associated with the autonomic system. The *dorsal nerve roots* contain primarily "incoming" (afferent) dendrites, with the cell body of the neuron located in an adjacent *dorsal root ganglion*. Sensory neurons transmit information to the spinal cord from the muscles, joints, skin, and other organs associated with the autonomic nervous system.

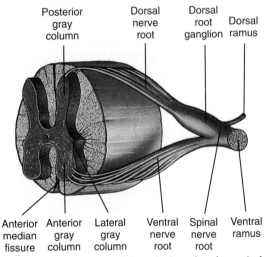

Posterior gray column   Dorsal nerve root   Dorsal root ganglion   Dorsal ramus

Anterior median fissure   Anterior gray column   Lateral gray column   Ventral nerve root   Spinal nerve root   Ventral ramus

FIGURE 10-1. A cross-section of the spinal cord and a typical spinal nerve root are illustrated. Multiple *ventral and dorsal nerve roots*, flowing from and to the gray matter of the spinal cord, respectively, fuse into a single *spinal nerve root*. The enlarged dorsal root ganglion contains the cell bodies of the afferent (sensory) neurons. The spinal nerve root immediately divides into a relatively small dorsal ramus and a much larger ventral ramus. (Modified from Standring S: *Gray's anatomy: the anatomical basis of clinical practice*, ed 40, St Louis, 2009, Elsevier.)

FIGURE 10-2. A cross-sectional view of an unspecified region of the thoracic trunk, highlighting a typical spinal nerve root and the path of its ventral and dorsal rami. The ventral ramus is shown forming an intercostal nerve, which innervates muscles in the anterior-lateral trunk, such as the intercostal and abdominal muscles. The dorsal ramus is shown innervating trunk extensor muscles, such as the erector spinae and multifidi. Although not depicted, the ventral and dorsal rami also contain sensory fibers that innervate ligaments and other connective tissues. (Modified from Standring S: *Gray's anatomy: the anatomical basis of clinical practice*, ed 40, St Louis, 2009, Elsevier.)

Near or within the intervertebral foramen, the ventral and dorsal nerve roots join to form a *spinal nerve root.* (Spinal nerve roots are often described as "mixed," emphasizing the point that they contain *both sensory and motor fibers*.) The spinal nerve root thickens owing to the merging of the motor and sensory neurons and the presence of the dorsal root ganglion.

The vertebral column contains 31 pairs of spinal nerve roots: 8 cervical, 12 thoracic, 5 lumbar, 5 sacral, and 1 coccygeal. The abbreviations *C, T, L,* and *S* with the appropriate superscript number designate each spinal nerve root—for example, C^5 and T^6. The cervical region has seven vertebrae but eight cervical nerve roots. The suboccipital nerve (C^1) leaves the spinal cord between the occipital bone and posterior arch of the atlas (C1). The C^8 spinal nerve root exits the spinal cord between the seventh cervical vertebra and the first thoracic vertebra. Spinal nerve roots T^1 and below exit the spinal cord just inferior or caudal to their respective vertebral bodies.

Once a spinal nerve root exits its intervertebral foramen, it immediately divides into a *ventral and dorsal ramus* (the Latin word *ramus* means "path") (see Figure 10-1). Depending on location, the ventral ramus forms nerves that innervate, in general, the muscles, joints, and skin of the *anterior-lateral trunk and neck, and the extremities*. The dorsal ramus, in contrast, forms nerves that innervate, in general, the muscles, joints, and skin of the *posterior trunk and neck*. This anatomic organization is depicted generically by the illustration in Figure 10-2.

Ventral Ramus Innervation

Throughout the vertebral column, each ventral ramus of a spinal nerve root either forms a plexus or continues as an individual named nerve.

PLEXUS

A plexus is an intermingling of ventral rami that form peripheral nerves, such as the radial, phrenic, or sciatic nerve. The four major plexuses, excluding the small coccygeal plexus, are formed by ventral rami: cervical (C^1-C^4), brachial (C^5-T^1), lumbar (T^{12}-L^4), and sacral (L^4-S^4). Most of the nerves that flow from the brachial, lumbar, and sacral plexuses innervate structures associated with the limbs, or, more precisely, the appendicular skeleton. Most nerves that flow from the cervical plexus, however, innervate structures associated with the axial skeleton.

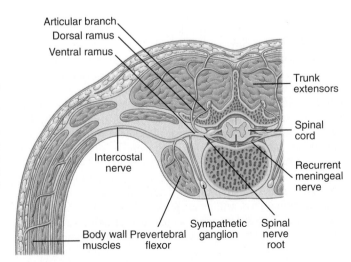

Articular branch
Dorsal ramus
Ventral ramus

Trunk extensors

Spinal cord

Recurrent meningeal nerve

Intercostal nerve

Body wall muscles   Prevertebral flexor   Sympathetic ganglion   Spinal nerve root

INDIVIDUAL NAMED NERVES

Many of the ventral rami within the trunk and craniocervical regions do not join a plexus; rather, they remain as individual named nerves. Each of these nerves typically innervates only a part or a segment of a muscle or connective tissue. This is why, for instance, many muscles that extend across a large part of the axial skeleton possess multiple levels of segmental innervation. The two most recognized sets of individual segmental nerves derived from the ventral rami are the intercostal (thoracic) and the recurrent meningeal nerves (see Figure 10-2).

Intercostal Nerves (T^1 to T^{12})

Each of the 12 ventral rami of the thoracic spinal nerve roots forms an *intercostal nerve,* innervating an intercostal dermatome and the set of intercostal muscles that share the same intercostal space. (Refer to dermatome chart in Appendix III, Part B, Figure III-2.) The T^1 ventral ramus forms the first intercostal nerve and part of the lower trunk of the brachial plexus. The ventral rami of T^7-T^{12} also innervate the muscles of the anterior-lateral trunk (i.e., the "abdominal" muscles). The T^{12} ventral ramus forms the last intercostal (subcostal) nerve and part of the L^1 ventral ramus of the lumbar plexus.

Recurrent Meningeal Nerves

A single recurrent meningeal (sinuvertebral) nerve branches off the extreme proximal aspect of each ventral ramus. After its bifurcation, the recurrent meningeal nerve courses back into the intervertebral foramen (hence the name "recurrent" [see Figure 10-2]). As a set, these often very small nerves provide sensory and sympathetic nerve supply to the meninges that surround the spinal cord, and to connective tissues associated with the interbody joints.[23] Most notably, the recurrent meningeal nerve supplies sensation to the posterior longitudinal ligament and adjacent areas of the superficial part of the annulus fibrosus. Sensory nerves innervating the anterior longitudinal ligament reach the spinal cord via small branches from nearby ventral rami and adjacent sympathetic connections.[23]

Dorsal Ramus Innervation

A dorsal ramus branches from every spinal nerve root, innervating structures in the posterior trunk usually in a highly segmental fashion. With the exception of the C^1 and C^2 dorsal rami, which are discussed separately, all dorsal rami are smaller than their ventral rami counterparts (see Figure 10-2). In general, dorsal rami course a relatively short distance posteriorly (dorsally) before innervating selected adjacent muscles and connective tissues on the back of the trunk (Box 10-1).

The dorsal ramus of C^1 ("suboccipital" nerve) is primarily a motor nerve, innervating the suboccipital muscles. The dorsal ramus of C^2 is the largest of the cervical dorsal rami, innervating local muscles as well as contributing to the formation of the greater occipital nerve (C^2 and C^3)—a sensory nerve to the posterior and superior scalp region.

TRUNK AND CRANIOCERVICAL REGIONS

The muscles of the axial skeleton are organized into two broad and partially overlapping areas: the *trunk* and the *craniocervical region* (Table 10-1). The muscles within each area are further organized into sets, based more specifically on their location.

> **BOX 10-1. Structures Innervated by Dorsal Rami of Spinal Nerve Roots (C^1-S^5)**
>
> **MUSCLES**
> * Deep layer of muscles of the posterior trunk
> * Muscles of the posterior craniocervical region
>
> **SKIN**
> * Dermatome (sensory) distribution across most of the posterior trunk
>
> **JOINTS**
> * Ligaments attaching to the posterior side of the vertebrae
> * Capsule of the apophyseal joints
> * Dorsal ligaments of the sacroiliac joints

The muscles within each area of the body are presented in two sections, the first covering anatomy and individual muscle actions, and the second covering examples of the functional interactions among related muscles. Throughout this chapter, the reader is encouraged to consult Chapter 9 for a review of the pertinent osteology related to the attachments of muscles. Appendix III, Part C should be consulted for a summary of more detailed muscular anatomy and innervation of the muscles of the axial skeleton.

Before beginning the description of the muscles of the trunk, the following fundamental topics will be reviewed, many of which are specifically related to the kinesiology of the axial skeleton.

Production of Internal Torque

By convention, the "strength" of a muscle action within the axial skeleton is expressed as an *internal torque,* defined for the sagittal, frontal, and horizontal planes. Within each plane, the maximal internal torque potential is equal to the product of (1) the muscle force generated parallel to a given plane, and (2) the length of the internal moment arm available to the muscle (Figure 10-3).

The spatial orientation of a muscle's line of force determines its effectiveness for producing a torque for a particular action. Consider, for example, the obliquus externus abdominis muscle producing a force across the lateral thorax, with a line of force oriented about 30 degrees from the vertical (Figure 10-4). The muscle's resultant force vector can be trigonometrically partitioned into unequal vertical and horizontal force components. The vertical force component—about 86% of the muscle's maximal force—is available for producing lateral flexion or flexion torques. The horizontal force component—about 50% of the muscle's maximal force—is available for producing an axial rotation torque. (This estimation is based on the cosine and sine of 30 degrees, respectively.) For any muscle of the axial skeleton to contribute *all* its force potential toward axial rotation, its overall line of force must be directed solely in the horizontal plane. For a muscle to contribute *all* its force potential toward either lateral flexion or flexion-extension, its overall line of force must be directed vertically. (Realize, though, that a vertically oriented muscle cannot produce any axial rotation because it lacks the moment arm required to produce a torque in the horizontal plane. As described in Chapter 1, a muscle force is *incapable* of producing a torque within a given plane if it either *parallels* or *pierces* the associated axis of rotation.)

The lines of force of muscles that control movement of the axial skeleton have a spatial orientation that varies over a wide

TABLE 10-1. Anatomic Organization of the Muscles of the Axial Skeleton*

Anatomic Region	Set	Muscles
Muscles of the trunk	Set 1: Muscles of the posterior trunk ("back" muscles)	**Superficial Layer** Trapezius, latissimus dorsi, rhomboids, levator scapula, serratus anterior
		Intermediate Layer† Serratus posterior superior Serratus posterior inferior
		Deep Layer Three groups: 1. Erector spinae group (spinalis, longissimus, iliocostalis) 2. Transversospinal group (semispinalis muscles, multifidi, rotators) 3. Short segmental group (interspinalis muscles, intertransversarius muscles)
	Set 2: Muscles of the anterior-lateral trunk ("abdominal" muscles)	Rectus abdominis Obliquus internus abdominis Obliquus externus abdominis Transversus abdominis
	Set 3: Additional muscles	Iliopsoas Quadratus lumborum
Muscles of the craniocervical region	Set 1: Muscles of the anterior-lateral craniocervical region	Sternocleidomastoid Scalenus anterior Scalenus medius Scalenus posterior Longus colli Longus capitis Rectus capitis anterior Rectus capitis lateralis
	Set 2: Muscles of the posterior craniocervical region	**Superficial Group** Splenius cervicis Splenius capitis
		Deep Group ("Suboccipital" Muscles) Rectus capitis posterior major Rectus capitis posterior minor Obliquus capitis superior Obliquus capitis inferior

*A muscle is classified as belonging to the "trunk" or "craniocervical region" based on the location of most of its attachments.
†These muscles are discussed in Chapter 11.

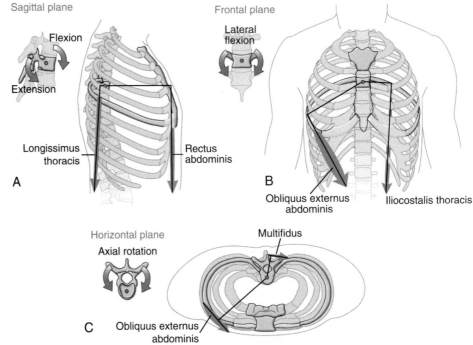

FIGURE 10-3. Selected muscles of the trunk are shown producing an internal torque within each of the three cardinal planes. The internal torque is equal to the product of the muscle force *(red arrows)* within a given plane and its internal moment arm *(black lines from each axis of rotation).* The body of T6 is chosen as the representative axis of rotation *(small open circle).* In each case the strength of a muscle action is determined by the distance and spatial orientation of the muscle's line of force relative to the axis of rotation.

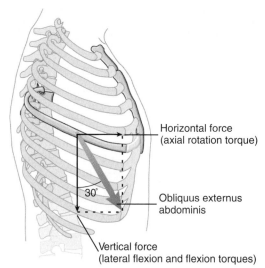

Horizontal force
(axial rotation torque)

30°

Obliquus externus
abdominis

Vertical force
(lateral flexion and flexion torques)

FIGURE 10-4. The line of force of the obliquus externus abdominis muscle is shown directed in the sagittal plane, with a spatial orientation about 30 degrees from the vertical. The resultant muscle force vector *(red)* is trigonometrically partitioned into a vertical force for the production of lateral flexion and flexion torques, and a horizontal force for the production of axial rotation torque.

spatial spectrum, from nearly vertical to nearly horizontal. This fact is important with regard to a muscle or muscle group's torque potential for a given action. For instance, because more of the total muscle mass of the trunk is biased vertically than horizontally, maximal efforts usually produce greater frontal and sagittal plane torques than horizontal plane torques.[145]

Special Considerations for the Study of Muscle Actions within the Axial Skeleton

To understand the actions of muscles located within the axial skeleton, it is necessary to first consider the muscle during both unilateral and bilateral activations. *Bilateral activation* usually produces pure flexion or extension of the axial skeleton. Any potential for lateral flexion or axial rotation is neutralized by opposing forces in contralateral muscles. *Unilateral activation,* in contrast, tends to produce flexion or extension of the axial skeleton, with some combination of lateral flexion and contralateral or ipsilateral axial rotation. (The term *lateral flexion* of the axial skeleton implies "ipsilateral" lateral flexion and therefore is not so specified throughout this chapter.)

The action of a muscle within the axial skeleton depends, in part, on the relative degree of fixation, or stabilization, of the attachments of the muscle. As an example, consider the effect of a contraction of a member of the erector spinae group—a muscle that attaches to both the thorax and pelvis. With the pelvis stabilized, the muscle can extend the thorax; with the thorax stabilized, the muscle can anteriorly rotate (tilt) the pelvis. (Both of these motions occur in the sagittal plane.) If the thorax and pelvis are both free to move, the muscle can simultaneously extend the thorax *and* anteriorly tilt the pelvis. Unless otherwise stated, it is assumed that the superior (cranial) end of a muscle is less constrained and therefore freer to move than its inferior or caudal counterpart.

Depending on body position, gravity may assist or resist movements of the axial skeleton. Slowly flexing the head from the anatomic (standing) position, for example, is normally controlled by eccentric activation of the neck extensor muscles. Gravity, in this case, is the prime "flexor" of the head, whereas the extensor muscles control the speed and extent of the action. Rapidly flexing the head, however, requires a burst of concentric activation from the neck flexor muscles, because the desired speed of the motion may be greater than that produced by action of gravity alone. Unless otherwise stated, it is assumed that the action of a muscle is performed via a concentric contraction, rotating a body segment against gravity or against some other form of external resistance.

Muscles of the Trunk: Anatomy and Their Individual Actions

The following section describes the relationships between the anatomy and the actions of the muscles of the trunk. Musculature is divided into three sets: (1) muscles of the *posterior trunk,* (2) muscles of the *anterior-lateral trunk,* and (3) *additional muscles* (see Table 10-1).

SET 1: MUSCLES OF THE POSTERIOR TRUNK ("BACK" MUSCLES)

The muscles of the posterior trunk are organized into three layers: superficial, intermediate, and deep (see Table 10-1).

Muscles in the Superficial and Intermediate Layers of the Back

The muscles in the *superficial layer* of the back are presented in the study of the shoulder (see Chapter 5). They include the trapezius, latissimus dorsi, rhomboids, levator scapula, and serratus anterior. The trapezius and latissimus dorsi are most superficial, followed by the deeper rhomboids and levator scapula. The serratus anterior muscle is located more laterally on the thorax.

In general, bilateral activation of the muscles of the superficial layer extends the adjacent region of the axial skeleton. Unilateral activation, however, laterally flexes and, in most cases, axially rotates the region. The right middle trapezius, for example, assists with right lateral flexion and left axial rotation of the upper thoracic region.

The muscles included in the *intermediate layer* of the back are the serratus posterior superior and the serratus posterior inferior. They are located just deep to the rhomboids and latissimus dorsi. The serratus posterior superior and inferior are thin muscles that contribute little to the movement or stability of the trunk. Their function is more likely related to the mechanics of ventilation and therefore is described in Chapter 11.

Muscles within the superficial and intermediate layers of the back are often referred to as "extrinsic" because, from an embryologic perspective, they were originally associated with the front "limb buds" and only later in their development migrated dorsally to their final position on the back. Although muscles such as the levator scapula, rhomboids, and serratus anterior are located within the back, technically they belong with upper limb muscles. All extrinsic muscles of the back are therefore innervated by ventral rami of spinal nerves (i.e., the brachial plexus or intercostal nerves).

Muscles in the Deep Layer of the Back

Muscles in the deep layer of the back are the (1) erector spinae group, (2) transversospinal group, and (3) short segmental

Muscles of the Superficial Layer of the Back: an Example of Muscles "Sharing" Actions between the Axial and Appendicular Skeletons

Chapter 5 describes the actions of the muscles of the superficial layer of the back, based on their ability to rotate the appendicular skeleton (i.e., humerus, scapula, or clavicle) toward a fixed axial skeleton (i.e., head, sternum, vertebral column, or ribs). The same muscles, however, are equally capable of performing the "reverse" action (i.e., rotating segments of the axial skeleton toward the fixed appendicular skeleton). This muscular action is demonstrated by highlighting the functions of the trapezius and rhomboids during use of a bow and arrow. As indicated in Figure 10-5, several muscles produce a force needed to stabilize the position of the scapula and abducted arm. Forces produced in the upper trapezius, middle trapezius, and rhomboids simultaneously rotate the cervical and upper thoracic spine to the left, indicated by the bidirectional arrows.[23,82] This "contralateral" axial rotation effect is shown for C6 in the inset within Figure 10-5. As the muscle pulls the spinous process of C6 to the *right,* the anterior side of the vertebra is rotated to the *left.* The trapezius and rhomboids also stabilize the scapula against the pull of the posterior deltoid, long head of the triceps, and serratus anterior. The shared actions of these muscles demonstrate the inherent efficiency of the musculoskeletal system. In this example, a few muscles accomplish multiple actions across both the axial and appendicular skeletons.

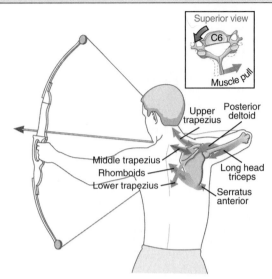

FIGURE 10-5. The actions of several muscles of the right shoulder and upper trunk are shown as an archer uses a bow and arrow. The upper trapezius, middle trapezius, and rhomboids demonstrate the dual action of (1) rotating the cervical and upper thoracic spine *to the left* (see inset) and (2) stabilizing the position of the right scapula relative to the thorax. The bidirectional arrows indicate the muscles simultaneously rotating the spinous process toward the scapula and stabilizing the scapula against the pull of the long head of the triceps, posterior deltoid, and serratus anterior.

TABLE 10-2. Muscles in the Deep Layer of the Back

Group (and Relative Depth)	Individual Muscles	General Fiber Direction	Comments
Erector spinae (superficial)	Iliocostalis lumborum	Cranial and lateral	Most effective leverage for lateral flexion
	Iliocostalis thoracis	Vertical	
	Iliocostalis cervicis	Cranial and medial	
	Longissimus thoracis	Vertical	Most developed of erector spinae group
	Longissimus cervicis	Cranial and medial	
	Longissimus capitis	Cranial and lateral	
	Spinalis thoracis	Vertical	Poorly defined, the spinalis capitis usually fuses with the semispinalis capitis
	Spinalis cervicis	Vertical	
	Spinalis capitis	Vertical	
Transversospinal (intermediate)	**Semispinalis**		
	Semispinalis thoracis	Cranial and medial	Cross six to eight intervertebral junctions
	Semispinalis cervicis	Cranial and medial	
	Semispinalis capitis	Vertical	
	Multifidi	Cranial and medial	Cross two to four intervertebral junctions
	Rotatores		
	Rotator brevis	Horizontal	Rotator brevis crosses just one intervertebral junction; rotator longus crosses two
	Rotator longus	Cranial and medial	Rotatores are most developed in thoracic region
Short segmental (deep)	Interspinalis	Vertical	Both muscles cross one intervertebral junction and are most developed in the cervical region
	Intertransversarius	Vertical	Interspinalis muscles are mixed with the interspinous ligaments

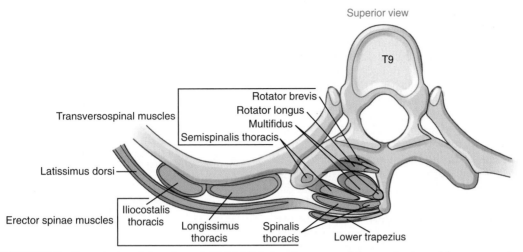

FIGURE 10-6. Cross-sectional view through T9 highlighting the topographic organization of the erector spinae and the transversospinal group of muscles. The short segmental group of muscles is not shown.

group (Table 10-2). The anatomic organization of the erector spinae and transversospinal groups is illustrated in Figure 10-6.

In general, from superficial to deep, the fibers of the muscles in the deep layer become progressively shorter and more angulated. A muscle within the more superficial erector spinae group may extend virtually the entire length of the vertebral column. In contrast, each muscle within the deeper, short segmental group crosses only one intervertebral junction.

Although a few exceptions prevail, muscles in the deep layer of the back are innervated segmentally through the dorsal rami of spinal nerves.[132] A particularly long muscle within the erector spinae group, for instance, is innervated by multiple dorsal rami throughout the spinal cord. A shorter muscle such as one multifidus, however, is innervated by a single dorsal ramus.[100]

Embryologically, and unlike the muscles in the extremities and anterior-lateral trunk, the muscles in the deep layer of the back have retained their original location dorsal to the neuraxis. For this reason these muscles have also been called "intrinsic" or "native" muscles of the back. As a general rule, most intrinsic muscles of the back are innervated by dorsal rami of adjacent spinal nerves.

Erector Spinae Group

The erector spinae are an extensive and rather poorly defined group of muscles that run on both sides of the vertebral column, roughly within one hand's width from the spinous processes (Figure 10-7). Most are located deep to the posterior layer of thoracolumbar fascia (see Chapter 9) and the muscles in the intermediate and superficial layers of the back. The erector spinae consist of the *spinalis, longissimus,* and *iliocostalis* muscles. Each muscle is further subdivided topographically into three regions, producing a total of nine named muscles (see Table 10-2). Individual muscles overlap and vary greatly in size and length.[23]

The bulk of the erector spinae muscles have a common attachment on a broad and thick *common tendon,* located in the region of the sacrum (see Figure 10-7). This common tendon anchors the erector spinae to many locations (Box 10-2). From this common tendon arise three poorly organized vertical columns of muscle: the spinalis, longissimus, and iliocostalis.[132] The general muscle attachments are described in the following sections; more specific attachments can be found in Appendix III, Part C.

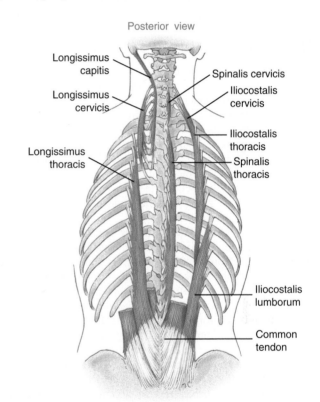

FIGURE 10-7. The muscles of the erector spinae group. For clarity, the left iliocostalis, left spinalis, and right longissimus muscles are cut just superior to the common tendon. (Modified from Luttgens K, Hamilton N: *Kinesiology: scientific basis of human motion,* ed 9, Madison, Wis, 1997, Brown and Benchmark.)

BOX 10-2. Attachments Made by the Common Tendon of the Erector Spinae
• Median sacral crests
• Spinous processes and supraspinous ligaments in the lower thoracic and entire lumbar region
• Iliac crests
• Sacrotuberous and sacroiliac ligaments
• Gluteus maximus
• Multifidi

Spinalis Muscles. Spinalis muscles include the *spinalis thoracis*, *spinalis cervicis*, and *spinalis capitis*. In general, this small and often indistinct (or missing) column of muscle arises from the upper part of the common tendon. The muscle ascends by attaching to adjacent spinous processes of most thoracic vertebrae or, in the cervical region, the ligamentum nuchae. The spinalis capitis, if present, often blends with the semispinalis capitis.[132]

Longissimus Muscles. The longissimus muscles include the longissimus thoracis, longissimus cervicis, and longissimus capitis. As a set, these muscles form the largest and most developed column of the erector spinae group. The fibers of the *longissimus thoracic* muscles fan cranially from the common tendon, attaching primarily to the posterior end of most ribs. In the neck, the *longissimus cervicis* angles slightly medially before attaching to the posterior tubercle of the transverse processes of the cervical vertebrae (see Figure 10-7). The *longissimus capitis*, in contrast, courses slightly laterally and attaches to the posterior margin of the mastoid process of the temporal bone. The slightly more oblique angulation of the superior portion of the longissimus capitis and cervicis suggests that these muscles assist with *ipsilateral* axial rotation of the craniocervical region.

Iliocostalis Muscles. The iliocostalis muscles include the iliocostalis lumborum, iliocostalis thoracis, and iliocostalis cervicis. This group occupies the most lateral column of the erector spinae. The *iliocostalis lumborum* arises from the common tendon and courses upward and slightly outward to attach lateral to the angle of the lower ribs. The *iliocostalis thoracis* continues vertically to attach just lateral to the angle of the middle and upper ribs. From this point, the *iliocostalis cervicis* continues cranially and slightly medially to attach to posterior tubercles of the transverse processes of the midcervical vertebrae, along with the longissimus cervicis.

Summary. The erector spinae muscles cross a considerable distance throughout the axial skeleton. This anatomic feature suggests a design more suited for control of gross movements across a large part of axial skeleton (such as extending the trunk while rising from a low chair) rather than finer movements at selected intervertebral junctions.[15] *Bilateral contraction* of the erector spinae as a group extends the trunk, neck, or head (Figure 10-8).[47] The muscles' relatively large cross-sectional areas enable them to generate large extension torque across the axial spine, such as for lifting or carrying heavy objects.[37]

By attaching to the sacrum and to the pelvis, the erector spinae can anteriorly tilt the pelvis, thereby accentuating the lumbar lordosis. (Pelvic tilt describes a sagittal plane rotation of the pelvis around the hip joints. The direction of the tilt is indicated by the rotation direction of the iliac crests.) As depicted in Figure 10-8, *A*, the anterior pelvic tilt is accentuated by the increased tension in stretched hip flexor muscles, such as the iliacus.

Contracting unilaterally, the more laterally disposed iliocostalis muscles are the most effective lateral flexors of the erector spinae group. The cranial or cervical components of the longissimus and iliocostalis muscles assist with ipsilateral axial rotation, especially when the head and neck are fully and contralaterally rotated. The iliocostalis lumborum assists slightly with ipsilateral axial rotation.

Transversospinal Muscles

Located immediately deep to the erector spinae muscles is the transversospinal muscle group: the *semispinalis, multifidi,* and *rotatores* (Figures 10-9 and 10-10). Semispinalis muscles are

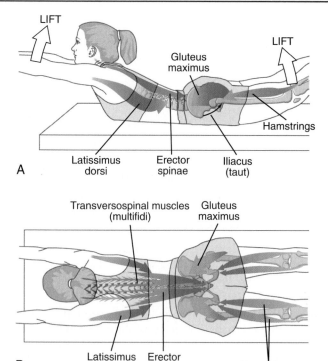

FIGURE 10-8. Muscle activation patterns of a healthy person during extension of the trunk and head. The upper and lower extremities are also being lifted away from the supporting surface. **A,** Side view. **B,** Top view. Note in **A** that the stretched iliacus muscle contributes to the anterior-tilted position of the pelvis.

located superficially; the multifidi, intermediately; and the rotatores, deeply.

The name *transversospinal* refers to the general attachments of most of the muscles (i.e., from the transverse processes of one vertebra to the spinous processes of a more superiorly located vertebra). With a few exceptions, these attachments align most muscle fibers in a cranial-and-medial direction. Many of the muscles within the transversospinal group are morphologically similar, varying primarily in length and in the number of intervertebral junctions that each muscle crosses (Figure 10-11). Although somewhat oversimplified, this concept can greatly assist in learning the overall anatomy and actions of these muscles.

Semispinalis Muscles. The semispinalis muscles consist of the semispinalis thoracis, semispinalis cervicis, and semispinalis capitis (see Figure 10-9). In general, each muscle, or main set of fibers within each muscle, crosses six to eight intervertebral junctions. The *semispinalis thoracis* consists of many thin muscle fasciculi, interconnected by long tendons. Muscle fibers attach from transverse processes of T6 to T10 to spinous processes of C6 to T4. The *semispinalis cervicis*, much thicker and more developed than the semispinalis thoracis, attaches from upper thoracic transverse processes to spinous processes of C2 to C5. Muscle fibers that attach to the prominent spinous process of the axis (C2) are particularly well developed, serving as important stabilizers for the suboccipital muscles (described ahead).

The *semispinalis capitis* lies deep to the splenius and trapezius muscles. The muscle arises primarily from upper thoracic transverse processes. The muscle thickens superiorly as it attaches to a relatively large region on the occipital bone, filling much of the area between the superior and inferior nuchal lines (see Figure 9-3).

Posterior view

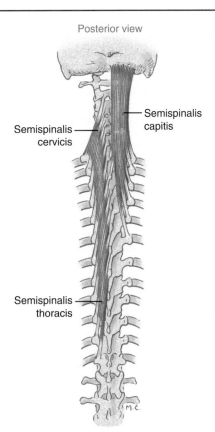

Semispinalis
cervicis

Semispinalis
capitis

Semispinalis
thoracis

FIGURE 10-9. A posterior view shows the more superficial semispinalis muscles within the transversospinal group. For clarity, only the left semispinalis cervicis, left semispinalis thoracis, and right semispinalis capitis are included. (Modified from Luttgens K, Hamilton N: *Kinesiology: scientific basis of human motion*, ed 9, Madison, Wis, 1997, Brown and Benchmark.)

Posterior view

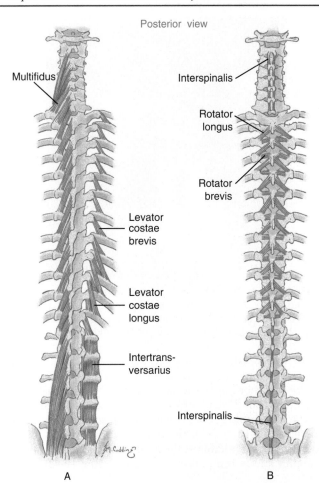

Multifidus

Interspinalis

Rotator
longus

Rotator
brevis

Levator
costae
brevis

Levator
costae
longus

Intertrans-
versarius

Interspinalis

A

B

FIGURE 10-10. A posterior view shows the deeper muscles within the transversospinal group (multifidi on entire left side of **A;** rotatores bilaterally in **B**). The muscles within the short segmental group (intertransversarius and interspinalis) are depicted in **A** and **B,** respectively. Note that intertransversarius muscles are shown for the right side of the lumbar region only. The levator costarum muscles are involved with ventilation and are discussed in Chapter 11. (Modified from Luttgens K, Hamilton N: *Kinesiology: scientific basis of human motion*, ed 9, Madison, Wis, 1997, Brown and Benchmark.)

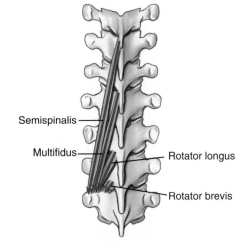

Semispinalis

Multifidus

Rotator longus

Rotator brevis

Muscle group	Relative length and depth	Average number of crossed intervertebral junctions
Semispinalis	Long; superficial	6-8
Multifidi	Intermediate	2-4
Rotatores	Short; deep	1-2

FIGURE 10-11. Simplified depiction of the spatial orientation of muscles within the left transversospinal muscle group. Additional information is listed in tabular format. (Note that the muscles illustrated normally exist bilaterally, throughout the entire cranial-caudal aspect of the vertebral column; their unilateral location in the figure is simplified for the sake of clarity.)

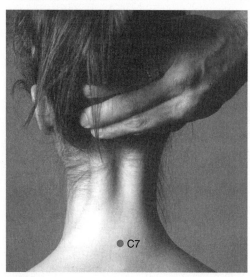

FIGURE 10-12. A thin, healthy 22-year-old woman demonstrates the contours of the activated right and left semispinalis capitis muscles. Manual resistance is applied against a strong extension effort of the head. The dot indicates the spinous process of the C7 vertebra.

The semispinalis cervicis and capitis are the largest muscles that cross the posterior side of the neck. Their large size and near-vertical fiber direction account for the fact that these muscles provide 35% to 40% of the total extension torque of the craniocervical region.[145] Right and left semispinalis capitis muscles are readily palpable as thick and round cords on either side of the midline of the upper neck, especially evident in infants and in thin, muscular adults (Figure 10-12).

Multifidi. Multifidi are situated just deep to the semispinalis muscles. The plural "multifidi" indicates a collection of multiple fibers, rather than a set of individual muscles. All multifidi share a similar fiber direction and length, extending between the posterior sacrum and the axis (C2).[6,23,132] In general, the multifidi originate from the transverse process of one vertebra and insert on the spinous process of a vertebra located two to four intervertebral junctions above (see Figure 10-10, *A*).

Multifidi are thickest and most developed in the lumbosacral region (see multiple attachments listed in Box 10-3).[100] The overlapping fibers of the multifidi fill much of the concave space formed between the spinous and transverse processes. The multifidi provide an excellent source of extension torque and associated stability to the base of the spine. Excessive force in the lumbar multifidi—from either active contraction or protective spasm—may be expressed clinically as an exaggerated lordosis.

Rotatores. The rotatores are the deepest of the transversospinal group of muscles. Like the multifidi, the rotatores consist of a large set of individual muscle fibers. Although the rotatores exist throughout the entire vertebral column, they are best developed in the thoracic region (see Figure 10-10, *B*).[132] Each fiber attaches between the transverse process of one vertebra and the lamina and base of the spinous process of a vertebra located one or two intervertebral junctions above. By definition, the *rotator brevis* spans one intervertebral junction, and the *rotator longus* spans two intervertebral junctions.

Summary. On average, the transversospinal muscles cross fewer intervertebral junctions than the erector spinae group. This

---

BOX 10-3. Multiple Attachments of the Multifidi throughout the Lumbosacral Region

INFERIOR ATTACHMENTS
- Mammillary processes of lumbar vertebrae
- Lumbosacral ligaments
- Deeper part of the common tendon of the erector spinae
- Posterior surface of the sacrum
- Posterior-superior iliac spine of pelvis
- Capsule of apophyseal joints

SUPERIOR ATTACHMENTS
- Lumbar spinous processes

---

feature suggests that, in general, the transversospinal muscles favor a design for producing relatively fine controlled movements and stabilizing forces across the axial skeleton.[15,22]

Contracting bilaterally, the transversospinal muscles extend the axial skeleton (see Figure 10-8, *B*). Increased extension torque exaggerates the cervical and lumbar lordosis and decreases the thoracic kyphosis. The size and thickness of the transversospinal muscles are greatest at either end of the axial skeleton. *Cranially,* the semispinalis cervicis and capitis are very well-developed extensors of the craniocervical region; *caudally,* the multifidi are very well-developed extensors of the lower lumbar region, accounting for two thirds of the muscular-based stability in this region.[154]

Contracting unilaterally, the transversospinal muscles laterally flex the spine; however, their leverage for this action is limited because of their close proximity to the vertebral column. The more obliquely oriented transversospinal muscles assist with *contralateral* axial rotation. From a relatively fixed transverse process, contraction of a single left multifidus or rotator longus, for example, can rotate a superiorly located spinous process toward the left and, as a result, rotate the anterior side of the vertebra to the right. Compared with all the trunk muscles, however, the transversospinal muscles are secondary axial rotators. The leverage for this rotation is relatively poor because of the muscle's proximity to the vertebral column. (Compare the multifidi with the obliquus abdominis externus, for example, in Figure 10-3, *C*). Furthermore, the prevailing line of force of most transversospinal muscle fibers is directed more vertically than horizontally, thereby providing a greater force potential for extension than for axial rotation.

Short Segmental Group of Muscles

The short segmental group of muscles consists of the *interspinalis* and the *intertransversarius muscles* (see Figure 10-10). (The plural "interspinales and intertransversarii" is often used to describe all the members within the entire set of these muscles.) They lie deep to the transversospinal group of muscles. The name "short segmental" refers to the extremely short length and highly segmented organization of the muscles. Each individual interspinalis or intertransversarius muscle crosses just one intervertebral junction. These muscles are most developed in the cervical region, where fine control of the head and neck is so critical.[132]

Each pair of interspinalis muscles is located on both sides of, and often blends with, the corresponding interspinous ligament. The interspinales have a relatively favorable leverage and optimal fiber direction for producing extension torque. The magnitude of this torque, however, is relatively small considering the muscles' small size and therefore low force potential.

Each right and left pair of intertransversarius muscles is located between adjacent transverse processes. The anatomy of the intertransversarii as a group is more complex than that of the interspinales.[132] In the cervical region, for example, each intertransversarius muscle is divided into small anterior and posterior muscles, between which pass the ventral rami of spinal nerves.

Unilateral contraction of the intertransversarii as a group laterally flexes the vertebral column. Although the magnitude of the lateral flexion torque is relatively small compared with that of other muscle groups, the torque likely provides an important source of intervertebral stability.

Summary. The highly segmented nature of the interspinalis and intertransversarius muscles is ideal for fine motor control of the axial skeleton. Because these unisegmental muscles possess a relatively high density of muscle spindles, they likely provide the nervous system (and therefore other muscles) a rich source of sensory feedback, especially in the craniocervical region.[23]

SET 2: MUSCLES OF THE ANTERIOR-LATERAL TRUNK ("ABDOMINAL" MUSCLES)

The muscles of the anterior-lateral trunk include the rectus abdominis, obliquus externus abdominis, obliquus internus abdominis, and transversus abdominis (Figure 10-13). As a group, these muscles are often collectively referred to as the "abdominal" muscles. The rectus abdominis is a long strap-like muscle located on both sides of the midline of the body. The obliquus externus abdominis, obliquus internus abdominis, and transversus abdominis—the lateral abdominals—are wide and flat, layered superficial to deep, across the anterior-lateral aspects of the abdomen.

The abdominal muscles have several important physiologic functions, including supporting and protecting abdominal viscera and increasing intrathoracic and intra-abdominal pressures. As will be further described in Chapter 11, increasing the pressures in these cavities assists with functions such as forced expiration of air from the lungs, coughing, defecation, and child birth. This chapter focuses more on the kinesiologic functions of the abdominal muscles.

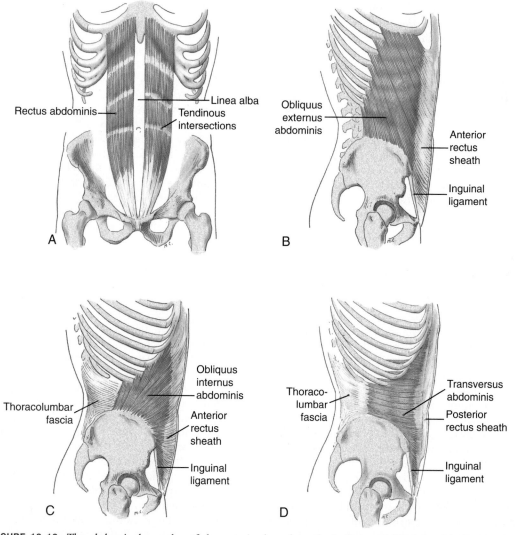

FIGURE 10-13. The abdominal muscles of the anterior-lateral trunk. **A,** Rectus abdominis with the anterior rectus sheath removed. **B,** Obliquus externus abdominis. **C,** Obliquus internus abdominis, deep to the obliquus externus abdominis. **D,** Transversus abdominis, deep to other abdominal muscles. (Modified from Luttgens K, Hamilton N: *Kinesiology: scientific basis of human motion,* ed 9, Madison, Wis, 1997, Brown and Benchmark.)

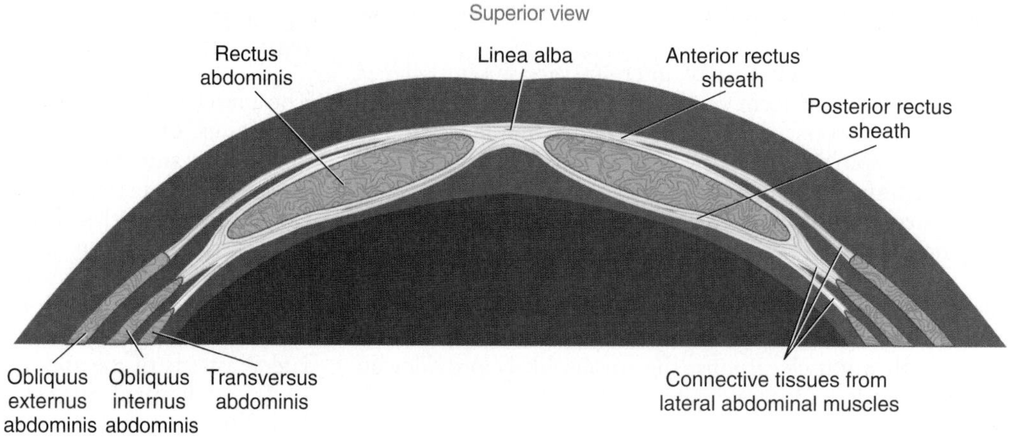

Superior view

Rectus
abdominis   Linea alba   Anterior rectus
                                                sheath

                                                    Posterior rectus
                                                        sheath

FIGURE 10-14. Horizontal cross-sectional view of the anterior abdominal wall shown at the approximate level of the third lumbar vertebra.

Obliquus   Obliquus   Transversus   Connective tissues from
externus   internus   abdominis   lateral abdominal muscles
abdominis   abdominis

Formation of the Rectus Sheaths and Linea Alba

The obliquus externus abdominis, obliquus internus abdominis, and transversus abdominis muscles from the right and left sides of the body fuse at the midline of the abdomen through a blending of connective tissues. Each muscle contributes a thin bilaminar sheet of connective tissue that ultimately forms the *anterior and posterior rectus sheaths.* As depicted in Figure 10-14, the anterior rectus sheath is formed from connective tissues from the obliquus externus abdominis and the obliquus internus abdominis muscles. The posterior rectus sheath is formed from connective tissues from the obliquus internus abdominis and transversus abdominis. Both sheaths surround the vertically oriented rectus abdominis muscle and continue medially to fuse with identical connective tissues from the other side of the abdomen. The connective tissues thicken and crisscross as they traverse the midline, forming the *linea alba* (the Latin word *linea* means "line," and *albus,* "white"). The linea alba runs longitudinally between the xiphoid process and pubic symphysis and pubic crest.

The crisscross arrangement of the fibers within the linea alba adds strength to the abdominal wall, much like the laminated structure of plywood. The linea alba also mechanically links the right and left lateral abdominal muscles, providing an effective way to transfer muscular force across the midline of the body.

Anatomy of the Abdominal Muscles

The *rectus abdominis* muscle consists of right and left halves, separated by the linea alba. Each half of the muscle runs longitudinally, widening as it ascends within an open sleeve formed between the anterior and posterior rectus sheaths. The muscle is intersected and reinforced by three fibrous bands, known as *tendinous intersections.* These bands blend with the anterior rectus sheath. The rectus abdominis arises from the region on and surrounding the crest of the pubis, and it attaches superiorly on the xiphoid process and cartilages of the fifth through seventh ribs.

The anatomic organization of the obliquus externus abdominis, obliquus internus abdominis, and transversus abdominis muscles is different from that of the rectus abdominis. As a group, the more laterally placed muscles originate laterally or posterior-laterally on the trunk and run in a different direction toward the midline, eventually blending with the linea alba and contralateral rectus sheaths (Table 10-3).

The *obliquus externus abdominis* (informally referred to as the "external oblique") is the largest and most superficial of the lateral abdominal muscles. The external oblique muscle travels

in an inferior-and-medial direction, similar to the direction of the hands placed diagonally in front pockets of pants. The *obliquus internus abdominis* (or less formally the "internal oblique") is located immediately deep to the external oblique muscle, forming the second layer of the lateral abdominals. Fibers originate from the iliac crest and, to a varying degree, blend with the adjacent thoracolumbar fascia. From this lateral attachment point, the fibers course in a cranial-and-medial direction toward the linea alba and lower ribs. As evident in Figure 10-13, *C,* the inferior attachments of the internal oblique muscle extend to the inguinal ligament. The average fiber direction of the internal oblique muscle is nearly perpendicular to the average fiber direction of the overlying external oblique muscle.

The *transversus abdominis* is the deepest of the abdominal muscles. The muscle is also known as the "corset muscle," reflecting its role in compressing the abdomen as well as stabilizing the lower back through attachments into the thoracolumbar fascia.[132] Of all the abdominal muscles, the transversus abdominis has the most extensive and consistent attachments into the thoracolumbar fascia,[136] followed closely by the internal oblique muscle.

Actions of the Abdominal Muscles

Bilateral action of the rectus abdominis and oblique abdominal muscles reduces the distance between the xiphoid process and the pubic symphysis. Depending on which body segment is the most stable, bilateral contraction of these abdominal muscles flexes the thorax and upper lumbar spine, posteriorly tilts the pelvis, or both. Figure 10-15 depicts a diagonally performed sit-up maneuver that places a relatively large demand on the oblique abdominal muscles. During a standard sagittal plane sit-up, however, the opposing axial rotation and lateral flexion tendencies of the various abdominal muscles are neutralized by opposing right and left muscles.

As described in Chapter 9, the axes of rotation for all motions of the vertebral column are located in the region of the interbody joints. The relative posterior placement of the axes relative to the trunk equips the abdominal muscles, most notably the rectus abdominis, with very favorable leverage for generating trunk flexion torque (Figure 10-16). Note in Figure 10-16 that, with the exception of the psoas major, all muscles have a moment arm to produce torques in *both* sagittal and frontal planes.

Contracting unilaterally, the abdominal muscles laterally flex the trunk. The external and internal obliques are particularly effective in this action owing to their relatively favorable

TABLE 10-3. Attachments and Individual Actions of the Lateral Abdominal Muscles

Muscle	Lateral Attachments	Midline Attachments	Actions on the Trunk
Obliquus externus abdominis	Lateral side of ribs 4-12	Iliac crest, linea alba, and contralateral rectus sheaths	*Bilaterally:* flexion of the trunk and posterior tilt of the pelvis *Unilaterally:* lateral flexion and contralateral rotation of the trunk
Obliquus internus abdominis	Iliac crest, inguinal ligament, and thoracolumbar fascia	Ribs 9-12, linea alba, and contralateral rectus sheaths	*Bilaterally:* as above, plus increases tension in the thoracolumbar fascia *Unilaterally:* lateral flexion and ipsilateral rotation of the trunk
Transversus abdominis	Iliac crest, thoracolumbar fascia, inner surface of the cartilages of ribs 6-12, and the inguinal ligament	Linea alba and contralateral rectus sheaths	*Bilaterally:* stabilization of attachment sites for other abdominal muscles; compression of the abdominal cavity; increases tension in the thoracolumbar fascia

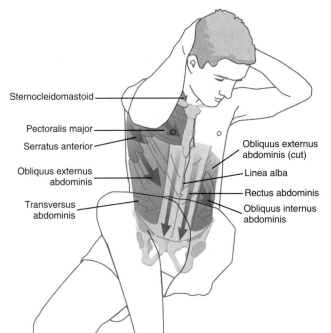

FIGURE 10-15. Typical muscle activation pattern of a healthy person performing a diagonal sit-up maneuver that incorporates trunk flexion and axial rotation to the left. During this action, the right external oblique muscle acts synergistically with the left internal oblique muscle. Note the simultaneous bilateral activation of the rectus abdominis and the deeper transversus abdominis.

FIGURE 10-16. Horizontal cross-sectional view through several muscles of the trunk at the approximate level of the third lumbar vertebra *(L3)*. The potential of muscles to produce a torque in both sagittal and frontal planes is shown. The anterior-posterior *(AP)* axis of rotation *(red)* and medial-lateral *(ML)* axis of rotation *(black)* intersect in the center of the third lumbar vertebra. Muscles located anterior and posterior to the medial-lateral axis have the potential to flex and extend the trunk, respectively; muscles located right and left to the anterior-posterior axis have the potential to laterally flex the trunk to right and left, respectively.

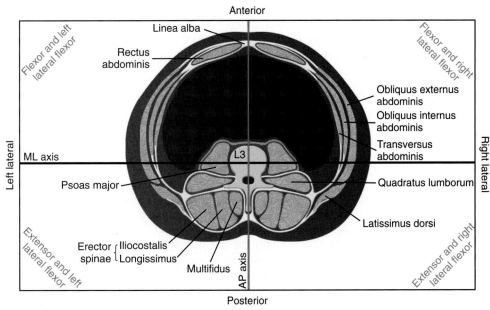

Role of Trunk Extensors as "Rotational Synergists" to the Oblique Abdominal Muscles

The external and internal oblique muscles are the primary axial rotators of the trunk. Secondary axial rotators include the ipsilateral latissimus dorsi, the more oblique components of the ipsilateral iliocostalis lumborum, and the contralateral transversospinal muscles. These secondary axial rotators are also effective extensors of the trunk. During a strong axial rotation movement, these extensor muscles are able to offset or neutralize *the potent trunk flexion potential of the oblique abdominal muscles.*[98,154] Without this neutralizing action, a strenuous action of axial rotation would automatically be combined with flexion of the trunk. The aforementioned extensor muscles resist the flexion tendency of the oblique abdominal muscles, but also contribute slightly to the axial rotation torque.

The multifidi muscles provide a particularly important element of extension stability to the lumbar region during axial rotation.[128,156] Pathology involving the apophyseal joints or discs in the lumbar region may be associated with weakness, fatigue, or reflexive inhibition of these muscles. Without adequate activation from the multifidi during axial rotation, the partially unopposed oblique muscles would, in theory, create a subtle and undesirable flexion bias to the base of the spine.

---

leverage (i.e., long moment arms) (see Figure 10-16) and, as a pair, relatively large cross-sectional area. The combined cross-sectional area of the external and internal obliques at the level of the L4-L5 junction is almost twice that of the rectus abdominis muscle.[106]

Lateral flexion of the trunk often involves activation of both trunk flexor and extensor muscles. For example, lateral flexion against resistance to the right demands a contraction from the right external and internal oblique, right erector spinae, and right transversospinal muscles. Coactivation amplifies the total frontal torque while simultaneously stabilizing the trunk within the sagittal plane.[12]

By far, the internal and external oblique muscles are the most effective axial rotators of the trunk.[7,12,73,141] The external oblique muscle is a contralateral rotator, and the internal oblique muscle is an ipsilateral rotator. The strong axial rotation potential of these muscles reflects their relatively large cross-sectional area and favorable leverage (see Figure 10-3, *C* for long moment arm length of the obliquus externus abdominis). During active axial rotation in a particular direction, the external oblique muscle on one side functions synergistically with the internal oblique on the other side.[141] This functional synergy produces a diagonal line of force that crosses the midline through the muscles' mutual attachment into the linea alba (see Figure 10-15). Contraction of the two muscles therefore reduces the distance between one shoulder and the contralateral iliac crest.

Several electromyographic (EMG) studies using intramuscular (fine-wire) electrodes demonstrate some degree of bilateral activation of the *transversus abdominis* during axial rotation.[38,82,141] It has been shown that during axial rotation the middle and lower fibers of the transversus abdominis coactivate at slightly different times than the upper fibers.[141] Although the exact role of the transversus abdominis during axial rotation is uncertain,

the muscle appears to function more as a *stabilizer* for the oblique abdominal muscles than a torque generator of axial rotation. Bilateral activation of the transversus abdominis can stabilize the ribs, linea alba, and thoracolumbar fascia—areas that serve as attachments for the internal or external oblique muscles.

The torque demands placed on the axial rotators of the trunk vary considerably based on the nature of an activity and position of the body.[12] Torque demands are relatively large during high-power axial rotations, such as sprinting, wrestling, and throwing a discus or javelin. The demands may be very low, however, during activities that involve slow twisting of the trunk while in an upright position, such as during walking over level surfaces.

Axial rotation performed primarily within the horizontal plane places little to no gravity-induced external torque on the rotator muscles. The muscles' primary resistance, in this case, is caused by the inertia of the trunk and the passive tension created by stretching antagonist muscles.

Comparing Trunk Flexor versus Trunk Extensor Peak Torque
In the healthy adult, on average, the magnitude of a maximal-effort trunk flexion torque is typically *less than* maximal-effort trunk extension torque. Although data vary based on gender, age, history of back pain, and angular velocity of the testing device, the *flexor-to-extensor torque ratios* determined isometrically for the trunk and craniocervical regions are between 0.45 and 0.77.[20,80,114,145] Although the trunk flexor muscles normally possess greater leverage for sagittal plane torque (see Figure 10-16), the trunk extensor muscles possess greater mass and, equally important, greater overall vertical orientation of muscle fibers.[95,106] The typically greater torque potential of the trunk extensor muscles reflects the muscles' predominant role in counteracting gravity, either for the maintenance of upright posture or for carrying loads in front of the body.

SET 3: ADDITIONAL MUSCLES (ILIOPSOAS AND QUADRATUS LUMBORUM)

Although the iliopsoas and quadratus lumborum are not anatomically considered muscles of the trunk, they are strongly associated with the kinesiology of the region.

Iliopsoas

The iliopsoas is a large muscle consisting of two parts: the iliacus and the psoas major (see Figure 12-27). As are most hip flexors, the iliopsoas is innervated by the femoral nerve, a large branch from the lumbar plexus. The iliacus has a proximal attachment on the iliac fossa and lateral sacrum, just anterior and superior to the sacroiliac joint. The psoas major attaches proximally to the transverse processes of T12 to L5, including the intervertebral discs. The two muscles fuse distal to the inguinal ligament and typically attach as a single tendon to the lesser trochanter of the femur.

The iliopsoas is a long muscle, exerting a potent kinetic influence across the trunk, lumbar spine, lumbosacral junction, and hip joints. Crossing anterior to the hip, it is a dominant flexor, drawing the femur toward the pelvis or the pelvis toward the femur. In the latter movement, the iliopsoas can anteriorly tilt the pelvis, a motion that increases the lordosis of the lumbar region (review in Figure 9-63, *A*). With muscular assistance from the abdominal muscles, a strong bilateral contraction of the iliopsoas can also rotate the pelvis *and* superimposed trunk over fixed femurs. Based on this ability,

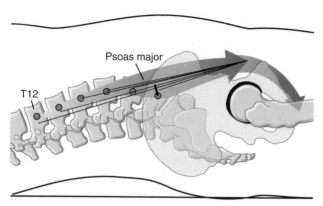

FIGURE 10-17. A lateral view of the psoas major highlights its multiple lines of force relative to the medial-lateral axes of rotation within the T12-L5 and L5-S1 segments. Note that the lines of force pass near or through the axes, with the exception of L5-S1. The flexion moment arm of the psoas major at L5-S1 is shown as the short black line.

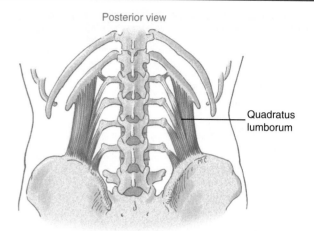

FIGURE 10-18. A posterior view of the quadratus lumborum muscles. (Modified from Luttgens K, Hamilton N: *Kinesiology: scientific basis of human motion*, ed 9, Madison, Wis, 1997, Brown and Benchmark.)

the iliopsoas is as much a respected trunk flexor as a hip flexor. This discussion resumes later in the chapter.

Function of the Psoas Major at the Lumbosacral Region

In the anatomic position the psoas major demonstrates leverage for lateral flexion of the lumbar spine (see Figure 10-16).[95] Little, if any, leverage exists for axial rotation.

The flexor and extensor capacity of the psoas major differs throughout the lumbosacral region. Across the L5-S1 junction, the psoas major has an approximate 2-cm moment arm for flexion (Figure 10-17).[107] The psoas major is therefore an effective flexor of the lower end of the lumbar spine relative to the sacrum. Progressing superiorly toward L1, however, the line of force of the psoas major gradually shifts slightly *posterior,* falling either through or just posterior to the multiple medial-lateral axes of rotation (see cross-section at L3 in Figure 10-16). The muscle's location reduces or eliminates its flexor or extensor capacity. The psoas major therefore is neither a dominant flexor nor extensor of the lumbar region, but rather a dominant vertical stabilizer of the region.[57,127] (The term "vertical stabilizer" describes a muscular function of stabilizing a region of the axial skeleton in a near-vertical position while maintaining its natural physiologic curve.) Because of the lack of effective leverage in the lumbar region, the psoas major has a minimal role in directly influencing the degree of lordosis.[127] The iliopsoas, however (as all hip flexor muscles), can indirectly increase the lordotic posture of the lumbar spine by tilting the pelvis anteriorly across the hip joints.

Actions of the Iliopsoas

Iliacus
- Predominant hip flexor, both femur-on-pelvis and pelvis-on-femur

Psoas Major
- Predominant hip flexor, both femur-on-pelvis and pelvis-on-femur
- Lateral flexor of the lumbar region
- Flexor of the lower lumbar spine relative to the sacrum
- Vertical stabilizer of the lumbar spine

Quadratus Lumborum

Anatomically, the quadratus lumborum is considered a muscle of the posterior abdominal wall. The muscle attaches inferiorly

to the iliolumbar ligament and iliac crest and superiorly to the twelfth rib and the tips of the stout transverse processes of L1 to L4 (Figure 10-18). The relative thickness of the muscle is evident by viewing Figure 10-16. The quadratus lumborum is innervated by the ventral rami of spinal nerves T^{12}-L^3.

Contracting *bilaterally,* the quadratus lumborum is an extensor of the lumbar region. Its action is based on the line of force passing about 3.5 cm posterior to the medial-lateral axis of rotation at L3.[107]

Contracting *unilaterally,* the quadratus lumborum has very favorable leverage as a lateral flexor of the lumbar region.[57] The axial rotation potential of the quadratus lumborum, however, is minimal.

Clinically, the quadratus lumborum is often called a "hip hiker" when its role in walking is being described, especially for persons with paraplegia at or below the L^1 neurologic level. By elevating (hiking) one side of the pelvis, the quadratus lumborum raises the lower limb to clear the foot from the ground during the swing phase of brace-assisted ambulation.

Actions of the Quadratus Lumborum

Acting Bilaterally
- Extension of the lumbar region
- Vertical stabilization of the lumbar spine, including the lumbosacral junction

Acting Unilaterally
- Lateral flexion of the lumbar region
- Elevation of one side of the pelvis ("hip hiking")

The psoas major and the quadratus lumborum run nearly vertically on both sides of the lumbar vertebrae (see Figure 10-16). A strong bilateral contraction of these muscles affords excellent vertical stability throughout the lumbar spine, including the L5-S1 junction. Theoretically, exercises that increase the volitional control and conditioning of these muscles may benefit a person with pain related to instability of the lumbar region.

Muscles of the Trunk: Functional Interactions among Muscles

Thus far in this chapter, the discussion of the muscles of the trunk has focused primarily on their anatomy and, for the

TABLE 10-4. Actions of Most Muscles of the Trunk

Muscle	Flexion	Extension	Lateral Flexion	Axial Rotation*
Trapezius	—	XX	XX	XX (CL)
Spinalis muscles (as a group)	—	XX	X	—
Longissimus thoracis	—	XXX	XX	—
Longissimus cervicis	—	XXX	XX	XX (IL)
Longissimus capitis	—	XXX	XX	XX (IL)
Iliocostalis lumborum	—	XXX	XXX	X (IL)
Iliocostalis thoracis	—	XXX	XXX	—
Iliocostalis cervicis	—	XXX	XXX	XX (IL)
Semispinalis thoracis	—	XXX	X	X (CL)
Semispinalis cervicis	—	XXX	X	X (CL)
Semispinalis capitis	—	XXX	X	—
Multifidi	—	XXX	X	XX (CL)
Rotatores	—	XX	X	XX (CL)
Interspinalis muscles	—	XX	—	—
Intertransversarius muscles	—	X	XX	—
Rectus abdominis	XXX	—	XX	—
Obliquus externus abdominis	XXX	—	XXX	XXX (CL)
Obliquus internus abdominis	XXX	—	XXX	XXX (IL)
Transversus abdominis†	—	—	—	—
Psoas major	X	X	XX	—
Quadratus lumborum	—	XX	XX	—

*CL, contralateral rotation; IL, ipsilateral rotation.

†Acts primarily to increase intra-abdominal pressure and, via attachments to the thoracolumbar fascia, to stabilize the lumbar region. Also stabilizes the attachment sites for the other lateral abdominal muscles.

Unless otherwise stated, the actions describe movement of the muscle's superior or lateral aspect relative to its fixed inferior or medial aspect. The actions are assumed to occur from the anatomic position, against an external resistance. A muscle's relative potential to move or stabilize a region is assigned X (minimal), XX (moderate), or XXX (maximum), based on moment arm (leverage), cross-sectional area, and fiber direction; — indicates no effective or conclusive action.

most part, individual actions (Table 10-4). The upcoming discussion pays more attention to the functional interactions *among* the muscles or muscle groups. Two themes are explored: (1) muscular-based stability of the trunk, and (2) muscular kinesiology of performing a standard sit-up movement. The second interaction exemplifies a classic kinesiologic relationship between the trunk and hip muscles.

MUSCULAR-BASED STABILITY OF THE TRUNK

Active muscle force provides the primary mechanism for stabilizing the axial skeleton, including the trunk.[12,28,84,148] Although ligaments and other connective tissues provide a secondary source of this stability, only muscles can adjust both the magnitude and timing of their forces.

Muscular-based stability of the trunk is often referred to as "core stability." Such stability ensures a near-static posture of the trunk even under the influence of destabilizing external forces.[16] Consider, for example, the wave of muscular activation experienced throughout the trunk when one attempts to stand or sit upright in an accelerating bus or train. Normally, trunk muscles are able to subconsciously stabilize the position of the trunk relative to the surrounding environment and, equally important, to stabilize the individual spinal segments within the axial skeleton. Ideally, a stable trunk optimizes postural alignment and limits excessive, and potentially stressful, micromotions between intervertebral junctions. Finally, stability of the trunk also establishes a firm base for muscles to move the limbs.

This chapter partitions the muscular stabilizers of the trunk into two groups. *Intrinsic muscular stabilizers* include the relatively short, deep, and segmented muscles that attach primarily *within* the region of the vertebral column. *Extrinsic muscular stabilizers*, in contrast, include relatively long muscles that attach, either partially or totally, to structures *outside* the region of the vertebral column, such as the cranium, pelvis, ribs, and lower extremities.

Intrinsic Muscular Stabilizers of the Trunk

The intrinsic muscular stabilizers of the trunk include the *transversospinal* and *short segmental* groups of muscles. These deep and relatively short muscles are depicted in a highly diagrammatic fashion in Figure 10-19, *A*. In general, these muscles stabilize the spine by controlling the precise alignment and stiffness among a relatively few intervertebral junctions at a time. The relative high density of muscle spindles residing in many of these segmental muscles enhances their fine-tuning ability.[113]

Intrinsic Muscular Stabilizers of the Trunk

- Transversospinal group
  - Semispinalis muscles
  - Multifidi
  - Rotatores
- Short segmental group
  - Interspinalis muscles
  - Intertransversarius muscles

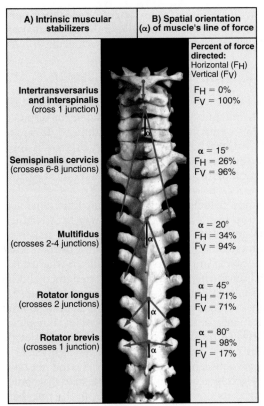

A) Intrinsic muscular stabilizers	B) Spatial orientation (α) of muscle's line of force
	Percent of force directed: Horizontal (F_H) Vertical (F_V)
Intertransversarius and interspinalis (cross 1 junction)	$F_H = 0\%$ $F_V = 100\%$
Semispinalis cervicis (crosses 6-8 junctions)	$\alpha = 15°$ $F_H = 26\%$ $F_V = 96\%$
Multifidus (crosses 2-4 junctions)	$\alpha = 20°$ $F_H = 34\%$ $F_V = 94\%$
Rotator longus (crosses 2 junctions)	$\alpha = 45°$ $F_H = 71\%$ $F_V = 71\%$
Rotator brevis (crosses 1 junction)	$\alpha = 80°$ $F_H = 98\%$ $F_V = 17\%$

FIGURE 10-19. Diagrammatic representation of the spatial orientation of the lines of force of the intrinsic muscular stabilizers. *A,* The lines of force of muscles are shown within the frontal plane. *B,* The spatial orientation of the lines of force of each muscle is indicated by the angle (α) formed relative to the vertical position. The percentage of muscle force directed vertically is equal to the cosine of α; the percentage of muscle force directed horizontally is equal to the sine of α. Assuming adequate leverage, the vertically directed muscle forces produce extension and lateral flexion, and the more horizontally directed muscle forces produce axial rotation. Note that the muscles illustrated exist throughout the entire vertebral column; their location in the figure is simplified for the sake of clarity.

As indicated in Figure 10-19, *B,* the spatial orientation of each muscle's line of force (depicted by α) produces a unique stabilization effect on the vertebral column. Vertically running interspinalis and intertransversarius muscles produce 100% of their force in the vertical direction (F_V). In contrast, the near-horizontally oriented rotator brevis muscle produces close to 100% of its force in the horizontal direction (F_H). All of the remaining muscles produce forces that are directed diagonally, at some angle between 0 and 90 degrees. The muscles act as an array of bilaterally matched guy wires, specifically aligned to compress as well as control the shear between intervertebral junctions. In addition to effectively securing both vertical and horizontal stability, collectively these muscles exert extension, lateral flexion, and axial rotation torques across the entire vertebral column. Without such fine muscle control, the multi-segmented vertebral column becomes very vulnerable to exaggerated spinal curvature, excessive interspinal mobility, and, in some cases, painful instability.

Extrinsic Muscular Stabilizers of the Trunk

The primary extrinsic muscular stabilizers of the trunk include the abdominal muscles, erector spinae, quadratus lumborum,

psoas major, and the hip muscles (by connecting the lumbo-pelvic region with the lower extremities). These relatively long and often thick muscles stabilize the trunk by creating a strong and semirigid link between the cranium, vertebral column, pelvis, and lower extremities.[28] Because many of these muscles cross a broad region of the body or trunk, they likely provide relatively coarse control over trunk stability. In addition, because many of these muscles possess a sizable cross-sectional area and leverage, they are, as a group, also important torque generators for the trunk and adjacent hip joints.[22]

> **Extrinsic Muscular Stabilizers of the Trunk**
> - Muscles of the anterior-lateral trunk ("abdominals")
>   - Rectus abdominis
>   - Obliquus externus abdominis
>   - Obliquus internus abdominis
>   - Transversus abdominis
> - Erector spinae
> - Quadratus lumborum
> - Psoas major
> - Hip muscles that connect the lumbopelvic regions with the lower extremity

---

External forces applied against the upper trunk can produce substantial destabilizing leverage against the more caudal or inferior regions of the axial skeleton. The stabilization function of the extrinsic muscles is therefore particularly important in the lower trunk. Chronic instability at the base of the spine can lead to postural malalignment throughout the entire vertebral column, as well as predispose to local impairments such as spondylolisthesis or degeneration of the lumbar apophyseal, interbody, and sacroiliac joints.

To further illustrate the potential role of the extrinsic stabilizers, Figure 10-20 shows a person activating his external muscular stabilizers in response to an impending external perturbation. Note the concentration of muscular activity in the lower region of the trunk. Activation of the psoas major, quadratus lumborum, erector spinae, and abdominal muscles provides substantial stability to the lumbopelvic regions, in all three planes. Strong activation of abdominal muscles also helps to increase intra-abdominal pressure—a mechanism believed to exert a stabilizing effect throughout the lumbar region.[67] The horizontally disposed transversus abdominis, in particular, creates a circumferential splinting effect across the entire low back region, including the sacroiliac joints.

Activation of the abdominal muscles also helps stabilize the pelvis against the pull of extensor muscles such as the erector spinae, quadratus lumborum, and gluteus maximus. With the pelvis and caudal end of the spine well stabilized, forces that have an impact on the trunk are effectively transferred across the sacroiliac joints, through the hips, and ultimately through the lower extremities. Strengthening exercises designed to increase the stability of the low back and lower trunk regions ideally should include activities that challenge both the trunk and the hip muscles, in all three planes of motion.

In closing, it should be pointed out that although the external and internal muscular stabilizers have been presented separately, in reality there is a large overlap and redundancy in their functions. This may be appreciated by mentally superimposing the muscular arrows depicted in both Figures 10-19 and 10-20. In ideal health, all muscles of the trunk contribute to the stabilization of the trunk, in both static and dynamic conditions.[28,36,135,147,148]

The specific strategy used by any single muscle differs, however, based on factors such as its depth, morphology, spatial orientation, and skeletal or connective tissue attachments.

PERFORMING A STANDARD SIT-UP MOVEMENT

Most functional activities require a concurrent activation of both the trunk and hip muscles. Consider, for instance, the combined movements of the trunk and hips while one swings a baseball bat, reaches toward the floor, or shovels snow. To introduce this important synergistic relationship, the following discussion focuses on the muscular actions of performing a standard *sit-up* movement.

In addition to being a very important functional activity, the full sit-up is often performed as a way to strengthen the abdominal muscles. The common goal of the resistive exercise is to increase the strength and control of these muscles, often as a way to improve overall stability of the trunk. In a very broad sense, the strategies used to strengthen abdominal muscles usually fall into one of four categories (Figure 10-21). In column 1 of Figure 10-21, the abdominal muscles contract to produce an isometric force to maintain a *near-constant distance* between the xiphoid process and the anterior pelvis. In columns 2 to 4, the abdominal muscles contract to *reduce* the distance between the xiphoid process and the anterior pelvis. (By acting eccentrically, the same muscles could also be challenged to slowly resist an *increase* in distance between these two regions of the body.) Of the examples illustrated in Figure 10-21, perhaps the most traditional exercise, at least historically, is the standard sit-up, depicted in column 3.[48]

A full sit-up performed in a bent-knee position can be divided into two phases. The trunk flexion phase terminates when both scapulae are raised off the mat (Figure 10-22, *A*). The later hip flexion phase involves an additional 70 to 90 degrees of combined lumbar flexion and pelvic-on-femoral (hip) flexion (see Figure 10-22, *B*).

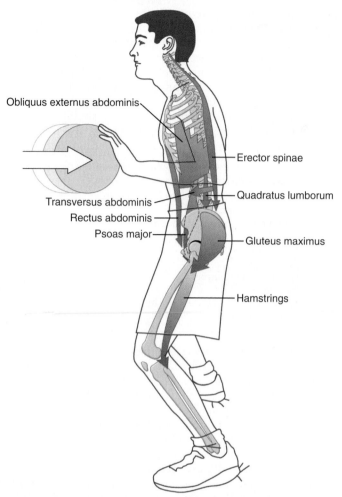

Obliquus externus abdominis

Erector spinae

Quadratus lumborum

Transversus abdominis

Rectus abdominis

Psoas major

Gluteus maximus

Hamstrings

FIGURE 10-20. A typical activation pattern for a sample of external muscular stabilizers.

#1 Isometric activity	#2 Rotating the trunk toward the stationary pelvis	#3 Rotating the trunk and pelvis toward the stationary legs	#4 Rotating the pelvis (and/or legs) toward the stationary trunk
Pictured example: 1. Keeping the trunk rigid while maintaining "all fours" position, then progressing to raising one arm and the contralateral leg. **Other examples:** 2. Balancing the trunk upright while seated on a relatively unstable object, such as a large inflatable ball. 3. Holding a rigid trunk while maintaining a "military style" push-up. 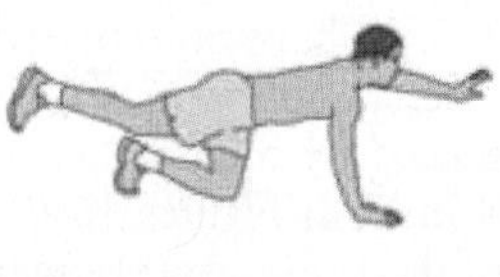	**Pictured example:** 1. Partial sit-ups ("crunches"), with or without a footstool. **Other examples:** 2. As above, but incorporate diagonal plane movements of the trunk, or alter body position relative to vertical. 3. Lateral trunk curls. 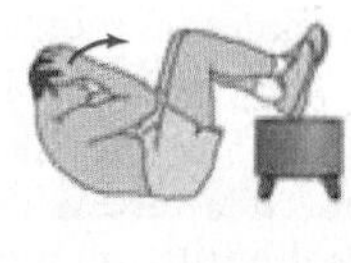	**Pictured example:** 1. Traditional sit-up. **Other examples:** 2. As above, but incorporate diagonal plane movements, or alter body position relative to vertical. 3. As in #1, but alter arm position and/or hold weights to vary external torque. 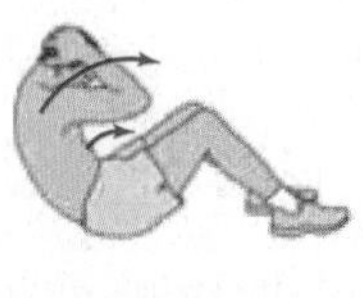	**Pictured example:** 1. Antigravity or other methods of resisted hip flexion. **Other examples:** 2. As above, but incorporate diagonal plane movements. 3. Straight leg raises while supine or in other positions relative to vertical. 4. Posterior pelvic tilt while supine. 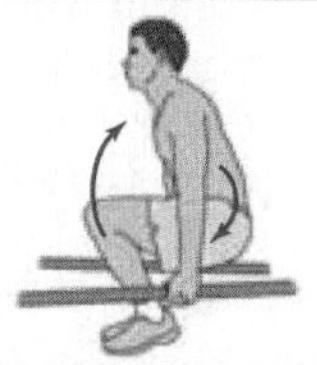

FIGURE 10-21. Four strategies typically used to perform abdominal strengthening exercises. Pictured examples are illustrated across the bottom row.

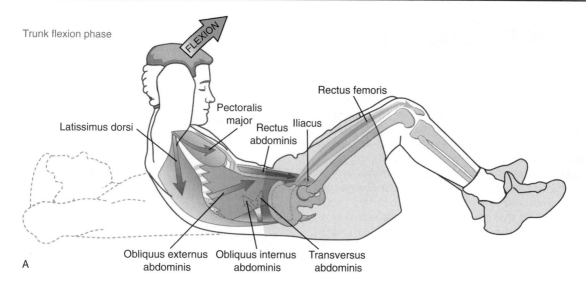

Trunk flexion phase

Latissimus dorsi

Pectoralis major

Rectus abdominis

Iliacus

Rectus femoris

Obliquus externus abdominis

Obliquus internus abdominis

Transversus abdominis

A

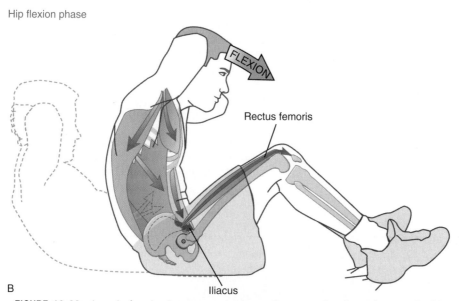

Hip flexion phase

Rectus femoris

Iliacus

B

FIGURE 10-22. A typical activation pattern is shown for a sample of muscles, as a healthy person performs a standard full *sit-up*. The intensity of the red color is related to the assumed intensity of the muscle activation. The full sit-up is divided into two phases: the trunk flexion phase, followed by the hip flexion phase. **A,** The *trunk flexion phase* of the sit-up involves strong activation of the abdominal muscles, especially the rectus abdominis. **B,** The *hip flexion phase* of the sit-up involves continued activation of the abdominal muscles but, more important, also the hip flexor muscles. Note in **B** the large pelvic-on-femoral contribution to the sit-up maneuver.

As depicted in Figure 10-22, *A,* the *trunk flexion phase* is driven primarily by contraction of the abdominal muscles, most notably the rectus abdominis.[8,48] Contraction of these muscles flexes the thoracolumbar spine and tilts (rotates) the pelvis posteriorly, thereby flattening the lumbar spine. The EMG level of the hip flexor muscles is relatively low during the trunk flexion phase, regardless of the position of the hips and knees.[8,48] Partially flexing the hips before performing the exercise releases passive tension in the hip flexor muscles while simultaneously increasing the passive tension in the gluteus maximus. These combined effects may assist the abdominal muscles in maintaining a posteriorly tilted pelvis.

Finally, as illustrated in Figure 10-22, *A,* the latissimus dorsi, by passing anterior to the upper thoracic spine, may assist in flexing this region of the thorax; the sternal head of the pectoralis major may assist in advancing the upper extremities toward the pelvis.

During the *hip flexion phase* of the sit-up, the pelvis and trunk rotate toward the femurs. The hip flexion phase is marked by stronger active contraction of the hip flexor muscles.[48] Although any hip flexor muscle can assist with this action, Figure 10-22, *B* shows the iliacus and rectus femoris as the active participants. Relative levels of EMG from the iliacus, sartorius, and rectus femoris are significantly greater when the legs are actively held fixed to the supporting surface.[8] The axis of rotation during the hip flexion phase of the full sit-up shifts toward the hip joints. Depending on technique, the abdominal muscles may continue to contract strongly or remain isometrically active. Their activation, however, does not contribute to hip (pelvic-on-femoral) flexion; rather, these muscles hold the flexed thoracolumbar region firmly against the rotating pelvis.

Persons with moderately weakened abdominal muscles typically display a characteristic posture when attempting to

Comparing the Abdominal "Crunch" Exercise with the Standard Full Sit-up

The early, trunk flexion phase of the full sit-up (depicted in Figure 10-22, *A*) is similar in many respects to the popular, and often recommended, "crunch" exercise for strengthening the abdominal muscles. Both the crunch and the full sit-up place significant and clinically challenging demands on the abdominal muscles as a whole.[56] Differences exist, however, as the crunch places relatively greater demands on the rectus abdominis, whereas the full sit-up places relatively greater demands on the oblique musculature. Furthermore, when compared with a full (bent-knee) sit-up, the crunch exercise (as depicted in Figure 10-22, *A*) places only marginal demands on the hip flexor muscles. Perhaps the most clinically significant difference in the two exercises is the fact that the crunch exercise involves only marginal amounts of flexion in the lumbar spine, reported to be only 3 degrees.[120] This is strikingly less than the lumbar flexion that accompanies a full (bent-knee) sit-up. The flexion of the lumbar spine during the full-sit up can create greater pressure on the discs (see Chapter 9). The crunch exercise therefore may be more appropriate than the full sit-up in persons with a history of disc pathology. This precaution appears prudent, especially considering that the crunch exercise still places significant demands on the abdominal muscles.

perform a full sit-up. Throughout the attempt, the hip flexor muscles dominate the activity. As a result there is minimal thoracolumbar flexion and excessive and "early" pelvic-on-femoral (hip) flexion. The dominating contraction of the hip flexor muscles exaggerates the lumbar lordosis, especially during the initiation of the maneuver.[86]

Muscles of the Craniocervical Region: Anatomy and Their Individual Actions

The following sections describe the anatomy and individual actions of the muscles that act exclusively within the craniocervical region. Musculature is divided into two sets: (1) muscles of the *anterior-lateral* craniocervical region and (2) muscles of the *posterior* craniocervical region (review Table 10-1).

Figure 10-23 serves as an introduction to the potential actions of many muscles in the craniocervical region. The illustration depicts selected muscles as flexors or extensors, or right or left lateral flexors, depending on their attachment relative to the axes of rotation through the atlanto-occipital joints. Although Figure 10-23 describes the muscle actions at the atlanto-occipital joint only, the relative position of the muscles provides a useful guide for an understanding of the actions at other joints within the craniocervical region. This figure is referenced throughout the upcoming sections.

SET 1: MUSCLES OF THE ANTERIOR-LATERAL CRANIOCERVICAL REGION

The muscles of the anterior-lateral craniocervical region are listed in Box 10-4. With the exception of the sternocleido-mastoid, which is innervated primarily by the spinal accessory

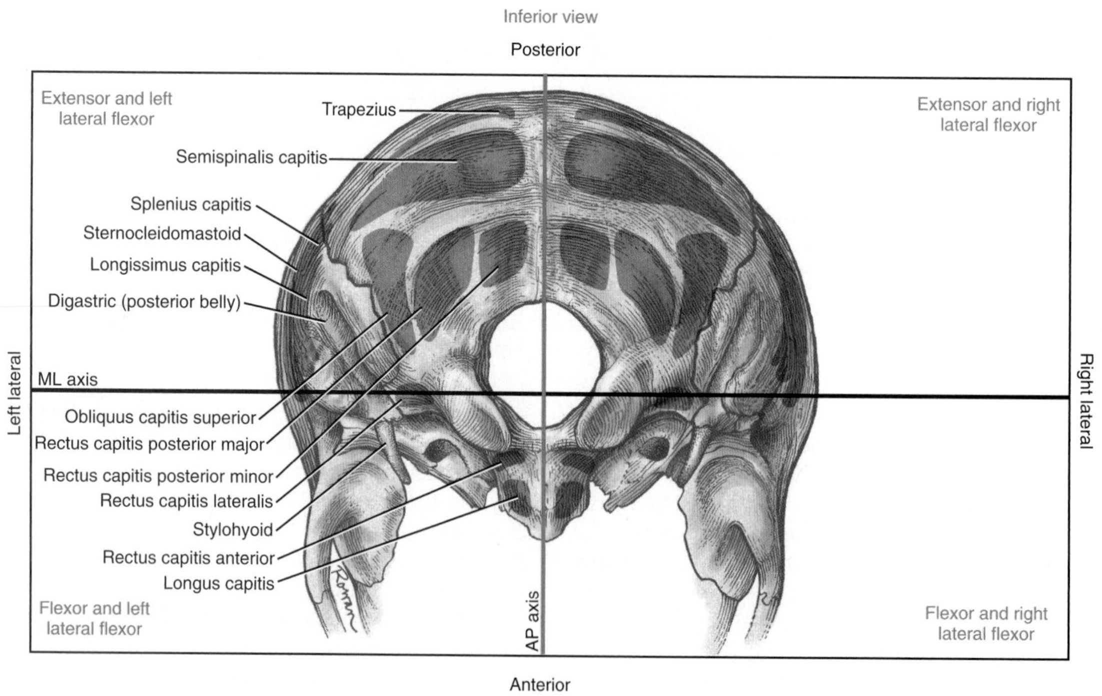

Inferior view

Posterior

Extensor and left lateral flexor

Extensor and right lateral flexor

Trapezius

Semispinalis capitis

Splenius capitis

Sternocleidomastoid

Longissimus capitis

Digastric (posterior belly)

Left lateral

ML axis

Right lateral

Obliquus capitis superior

Rectus capitis posterior major

Rectus capitis posterior minor

Rectus capitis lateralis

Stylohyoid

Rectus capitis anterior

Longus capitis

Flexor and left lateral flexor

AP axis

Flexor and right lateral flexor

Anterior

FIGURE 10-23. The potential action of muscles that attach to the inferior surface of the occipital and temporal bones is highlighted. The actions of the muscles across the atlanto-occipital joint are based on their location relative to the medial-lateral *(ML) (black)* and anterior-posterior *(AP) (red)* axis of rotation at the level of the occipital condyles. Note that the actions of most muscles fit into one of four quadrants. (Distal muscle attachments are indicated in gray, and proximal attachments are indicated in red.)

nerve (cranial nerve XI), the muscles in this region are innervated by small unnamed nerves that branch from the ventral rami of the cervical plexus.

Sternocleidomastoid

The sternocleidomastoid is typically a prominent muscle located superficially on the anterior aspect of the neck. Inferiorly the muscle attaches by two heads: the medial (sternal) and lateral (clavicular) (Figure 10-24). From this attachment, the muscle ascends obliquely across the neck to attach to the cranium, specifically between the mastoid process of the temporal bone and the lateral half of the superior nuchae line.

Acting unilaterally, the sternocleidomastoid is a lateral flexor and contralateral axial rotator of the craniocervical region. Contracting bilaterally, a pair of sternocleidomastoid muscles can flex *or* extend the craniocervical region depending on the specific area. Evident from a lateral view of a neutral cervical spine, the line of force of the right sternocleidomastoid is directed across the neck in an oblique fashion (see Figure 10-24, inset). Below approximately C3, the sternocleidomastoid crosses *anterior* to the medial-lateral axes of rotation; above C3, however, the sternocleidomastoid

crosses just *posterior* to the medial-lateral axes of rotation.[145] Acting together, the sternocleidomastoid muscles provide a strong *flexion* torque to the mid-to-lower cervical spine and a minimal *extension* torque to the upper cervical spine, including the atlanto-axial and atlanto-occipital joints.

Computer models predict that the sagittal plane torque potential of the different regions of the sternocleidomastoid is strongly affected by the initial posture of the craniocervical region.[145] Primarily because of moment arm changes, the position of flexion of the mid-to-lower cervical spine, for example, nearly doubles the muscle's flexion torque potential in this region. This becomes especially relevant in persons with an established marked forward head posture, referred to as protraction of craniocervical region in Chapter 9 (see Figure 9-47, *A*). Because this posture has greater flexion at the mid-to-lower cervical region, it may perpetuate the biomechanics that cause the forward head posture.

Scalenes

The scalene muscles attach between the tubercles of the transverse processes of the middle to lower cervical vertebrae and the first two ribs (Figure 10-25). (As a side note, the Latin or Greek root of the word *scalene* refers to a triangle with three unequal sides.) The specific attachments of these muscles are listed in Appendix III, Part C. The brachial plexus courses between the scalene anterior and scalene medius. Hypertrophy, spasm, or excessive stiffness of these muscles can compress the brachial plexus and cause motor and sensory disturbances in the upper extremity.

The function of the scalene muscles depends on which skeletal attachments are most fixed. With the cervical spine well stabilized, the scalene muscles raise the ribs to assist with inspiration during breathing. Alternatively, with the first two ribs well stabilized, contraction of the scalene muscles moves the cervical spine.

Contracting unilaterally, the scalene muscles laterally flex the cervical spine.[29] Their axial rotation potential is likely limited because the muscle's line of force nearly pierces the vertical

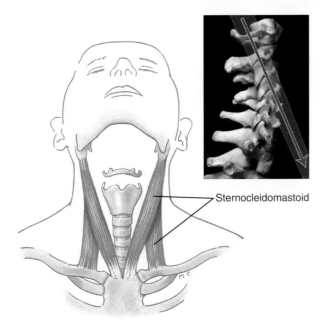

FIGURE 10-24. An anterior view of the sternocleidomastoid muscles. The inset shows a lateral view of the oblique orientation of the sternocleidomastoid muscle *(arrow)* as it crosses the craniocervical region. (Modified from Luttgens K, Hamilton N: *Kinesiology: scientific basis of human motion*, ed 9, Madison, Wis, 1997, Brown and Benchmark.)

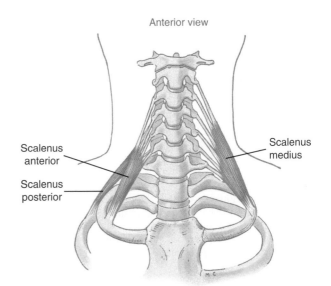

Anterior view

Scalenus anterior

Scalenus posterior

Scalenus medius

FIGURE 10-25. An anterior view of the right scalenus posterior and scalenus anterior, and the left scalenus medius. (Modified from Luttgens K, Hamilton N: *Kinesiology: scientific basis of human motion*, ed 9, Madison, Wis, 1997, Brown and Benchmark.)

axis of rotation. This topic remains controversial, however, with little scientific backing.[39,65,83,86,122] The only rigorous study found on this subject concluded that the scalenes have a modest (5-degree) *ipsilateral* rotation function, at least when activated from the anatomic position.[32] This conclusion, however, is difficult to confirm based on casual inspection of a human skeletal model, especially for the scalenus anterior. Further clarification is needed on the axial rotation function of the three scalene muscles. Their axial rotation function is likely highly dependent on the posture of the region and, even more important, on the starting position from which the muscles contract. It appears that an important function of the scalene muscles is their ability to *return* the craniocervical region to its near-neutral position from a fully rotated position. This more global and perhaps primary function may be overlooked when the neutral position is used as a starting point to analyze the muscles' action.

Contracting bilaterally, the scalenus anterior and scalenus medius appear to have a limited moment arm to flex the cervical spine, particularly in the lower regions. The muscles' bilateral activity is most likely related to ventilation (as described previously) and providing stability to the cervical region. The cervical attachments of all three scalene muscles split into several individual fasciculi (see Figure 10-25). Like a system of guy wires that stabilize a large antenna, the scalene muscles provide excellent bilateral and vertical stability to the middle and lower cervical spine. Fine control of the upper craniocervical region is more the responsibility of the shorter, more specialized muscles, such as the rectus capitis anterior and the suboccipital muscles (discussed ahead).

Longus Colli and Longus Capitis

The longus colli and longus capitis are located deep to the cervical viscera (trachea and esophagus), on both sides of the cervical column (Figure 10-26). These muscles function as a *dynamic anterior longitudinal ligament,* providing an important element of vertical stability to the region.[49,87]

The *longus colli* consists of multiple fascicles that closely adhere to the anterior surfaces of the upper three thoracic and all cervical vertebrae. This segmented muscle ascends the cervical region through multiple attachments between the vertebral bodies, anterior tubercles of transverse processes, and anterior arch of the atlas. The longus colli is the only muscle that attaches in its entirety to the anterior surface of the vertebral column. Compared with the scalene and sterno-cleidomastoid muscles, the longus colli is a relatively thin muscle. The more anterior fibers of the longus colli flex the cervical region. The more lateral fibers act in conjunction with the scalene muscles to vertically stabilize the region.

The *longus capitis* arises from the anterior tubercles of the transverse processes of the mid-to-lower cervical vertebrae and inserts into the basilar part of the occipital bone (see Figure 10-23). The primary action of the longus capitis is to flex and stabilize the upper craniocervical region. Lateral flexion is a secondary action.

Rectus Capitis Anterior and Rectus Capitis Lateralis

The rectus capitis anterior and rectus capitis lateralis are two short muscles that arise from the elongated transverse processes of the atlas (C1) and insert on the inferior surface of the occipital bone (see Figure 10-26). The rectus capitis lateralis attaches laterally to the occipital condyle; the rectus capitis anterior, the smaller of the recti, attaches immediately anterior to the occipital condyle (see Figure 10-23).

The actions of the rectus capitis anterior and lateralis muscles are limited to the atlanto-occipital joint; each muscle controls one of the joint's two degrees of freedom (see Chapter 9). The rectus capitis anterior is a flexor, and the rectus capitis lateralis is a lateral flexor.

SET 2: MUSCLES OF THE POSTERIOR CRANIOCERVICAL REGION

The muscles of the posterior craniocervical region are listed in Box 10-5. They are innervated by dorsi rami of cervical spinal nerves.

> ### BOX 10-5. Muscles of the Posterior Craniocervical Region
>
> - Splenius muscles
>   - Splenius cervicis
>   - Splenius capitis
> - Suboccipital muscles
>   - Rectus capitis posterior major
>   - Rectus capitis posterior minor
>   - Obliquus capitis superior
>   - Obliquus capitis inferior

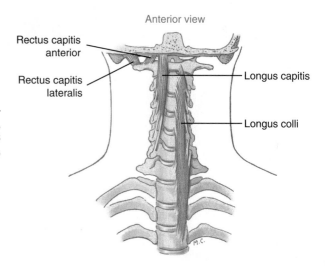

FIGURE 10-26. An anterior view of the deep muscles in the neck. The following muscles are shown: right longus capitis, right rectus capitis anterior, right rectus capitis lateralis, and left longus colli. (Modified from Luttgens K, Hamilton N: *Kinesiology: scientific basis of human motion*, ed 9, Madison, Wis, 1997, Brown and Benchmark.)

SPECIAL FOCUS 10-4

Soft-Tissue Whiplash Injury

The soft tissues of the cervical spine are particularly vulnerable to injury from a whiplash event associated with an automobile accident. Whiplash associated with cervical hyperextension generally creates greater strain on soft tissues than does whiplash associated with cervical hyperflexion.[133] Hyperextension occurs over a relatively large range of motion and therefore severely strains the craniocervical flexor muscles, cervical viscera, and other anteriorly located connective tissues, as well as excessively compressing the apophyseal joints and posterior elements of the cervical spine (Figure 10-27, *A*). In contrast, the maximum extent of flexion is partially blocked by the chin striking the chest (see Figure 10-27, *B*). Ideally, head restraints located within most automobiles help limit the extent of hyperextension and reduce injury from a collision.

Hyperextension injuries tend to occur more often from rear-end impact automobile collisions. Careful measurements of human replicas and cadaver material show that immediately on contact the craniocervical region sharply *retracts,* followed by a more prolonged hyperextension.[93,117] The brief retraction phase is usually completed *before* the cranium hits the head restraint. The *anterior longitudinal ligament* within the mid and lower cervical spine is particularly vulnerable to injury during this unprotected phase of the whiplash event.

The *alar ligaments* are particularly vulnerable to injury during the prolonged hyperextension phase of a rear-end collision, especially when the head is rotated at the time of the collision.[44] Rotation of the head stretches the alar ligaments, which places them closer to their point of mechanical failure.

In addition, research has shown that the severe hyperextension associated with whiplash places excessive strain on flexor muscles, in particular the longus colli and longus capitis.[108] In one study, a 56% strain (elongation) was measured in the longus colli—a level that can cause tissue damage. Often a person with a hyperextension injury shows a correlating pattern of marked tenderness and protective spasm in the region of the longus colli. Excessive strain in other muscles (such as the sternocleidomastoid and scalenus anterior) and the cervical viscera may also cause tenderness. Spasm in the longus colli tends to produce a relatively straight cervical spine, lacking the normal lordosis. Persons with a strained and painful longus colli often have difficulty shrugging their shoulders—an action produced primarily by the upper trapezius. When the longus colli and other flexors are too painful to fully contract, the upper trapezius muscle loses its stable cervical attachment and therefore becomes an ineffective elevator of the shoulder girdle. This clinical scenario is an excellent example of the interdependence of muscle function, in which one muscle's action depends on the stabilization force of another.

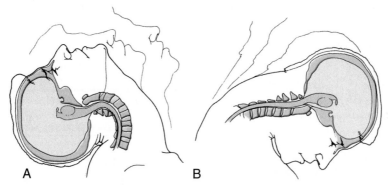

FIGURE 10-27. During whiplash injuries, cervical hyperextension **(A)** typically exceeds cervical flexion **(B).** As a result, the anterior structures of the cervical region are more vulnerable to strain injury. (From Porterfield JA, DeRosa C: *Mechanical neck pain: perspectives in functional anatomy,* Philadelphia, 1995, Saunders.)

Splenius Cervicis and Capitis

The splenius cervicis and capitis muscles are a long and thin pair of muscles, named by their resemblance to a bandage (from the Greek *splenion,* bandage) (Figure 10-28). As a pair, the splenius muscles arise from the inferior half of the ligamentum nuchae and spinous processes of C7 to T6, just deep to the trapezius muscles. The *splenius capitis* attaches just posterior and deep to the sternocleidomastoid (see Figure 10-23). The *splenius cervicis* attaches to the posterior tubercles of the transverse processes of C1 to C3. Much of this cervical attachment is shared by the levator scapula muscle.

Contracting unilaterally, the splenius muscles perform lateral flexion and ipsilateral axial rotation of the head and cervical spine. Contracting bilaterally, the splenius muscles extend the upper craniocervical region.

Suboccipital Muscles

The suboccipital muscles consist of four paired muscles located very deep in the neck, immediately superficial to the atlanto-occipital and atlanto-axial joints (Figure 10-29). These relatively short but thick muscles attach among the atlas, axis, and occipital bone. (Their specific muscular attachments are listed in Appendix III, Part C.)

The suboccipital muscles are not easily palpable. They lie deep to the upper trapezius, splenius group, and semispinalis capitis muscles (see Figure 10-23). In conjunction with the rectus capitis anterior and lateralis, the suboccipital muscles are dedicated to providing precise control over the atlanto-occipital and atlanto-axial joints. This level of control is essential for optimal positioning of the eyes, ears, and nose. As indicated in Figure 10-30, each suboccipital muscle (plus each

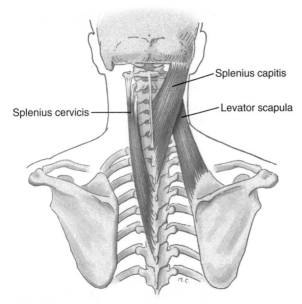

FIGURE 10-28. A posterior view of the left splenius cervicis, right splenius capitis, and right levator scapula. Although not visible, the cervical attachments of the levator scapula are similar to the cervical attachments of the splenius cervicis. (Modified from Luttgens K, Hamilton N: *Kinesiology: scientific basis of human motion*, ed 9, Madison, Wis, 1997, Brown and Benchmark.)

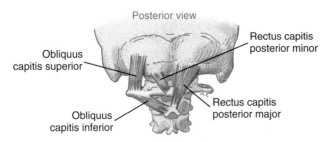

FIGURE 10-29. A posterior view of the suboccipital muscles. The left obliquus capitis superior, left obliquus capitis inferior, left rectus capitis posterior minor, and right rectus capitis posterior major are shown. (Modified from Luttgens K, Hamilton N: *Kinesiology: scientific basis of human motion*, ed 9, Madison, Wis, 1997, Brown and Benchmark.)

short rectus muscle) has a unique level of control and dominance over the joints of the upper craniocervical region.

Muscles of the Craniocervical Region: Functional Interactions among Muscles That Cross the Craniocervical Region

Nearly 30 pairs of muscles cross the craniocervical region. These include the muscles that act exclusively within the craniocervical region (Figure 10-30 and Table 10-5), plus those classified as muscles of the posterior trunk that cross the craniocervical region (e.g., trapezius and longissimus capitis).

This section highlights the functional interactions among the muscles that cross the craniocervical regions during two activities: (1) stabilizing the craniocervical region and (2) producing the movements of the head and neck that optimize the function of visual, auditory, and olfactory systems. Although many other functional interactions exist for these muscles, the

two activities provide a format for describing key kinesiologic principles involved in this important region of the body.

STABILIZING THE CRANIOCERVICAL REGION

The muscles that cross the craniocervical region comprise much of the bulk of the neck, especially in the regions lateral and posterior to the cervical vertebrae. When strongly activated, this mass of muscle serves to protect the cervical viscera and blood vessels, intervertebral discs, apophyseal joints, and neural tissues.[87]

Resistive or so-called "stabilization" exercises are often performed by athletes involved in contact sports as a means to hypertrophy this musculature. Hypertrophy alone, however, may not necessarily prevent neck injury. Data on the biomechanics of whiplash injury, for example, suggest that the time required to react to an impending injury and generate a substantial stabilizing force may exceed the time

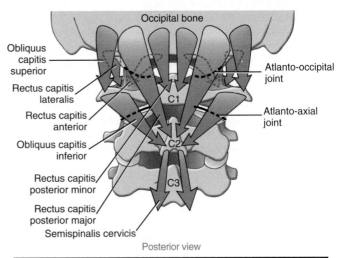

MUSCLES	ATLANTO-OCCIPITAL JOINT			ATLANTO-AXIAL JOINT		
	FLEXION	EXTENSION	LATERAL FLEXION	FLEXION	EXTENSION	AXIAL ROTATION*
Rectus capitis anterior	XX	–	X	–	–	–
Rectus capitis lateralis	–	–	XX	–	–	–
Rectus capitis posterior major	–	XXX	XX	–	XXX	XX(IL)
Rectus capitis posterior minor	–	XX	X	–	–	–
Obliquus capitis inferior	–	–	–	–	XX	XXX(IL)
Obliquus capitis superior	–	XXX	XXX	–	–	–

*CL = contralateral rotation, IL = ipsilateral rotation

FIGURE 10-30. A posterior view depicts the lines of force of muscles relative to the underlying atlanto-occipital and atlanto-axial joints. Each of these joints allows two primary degrees of freedom. Note that the attachment of the semispinalis cervicis muscle provides a stable base for the rectus capitis posterior major and the obliquus capitis inferior, two of the larger and more dominant suboccipital muscles. The chart summarizes the actions of the muscles at the atlanto-occipital and atlanto-axial joints. A muscle's relative potential to perform a movement is assigned one of three scores: X, minimal; XX, moderate; and XXX, maximum. The dash indicates no effective torque production.

TABLE 10-5. Actions of Selected Muscles Located within the Craniocervical Region

Muscle	Flexion	Extension	Lateral Flexion	Axial Rotation
Sternocleidomastoid	XXX	X*	XXX	XXX (CL)
Scalenus anterior	XX	—	XXX	—
Scalenus medius	X	—	XXX	—
Scalenus posterior	—	—	XX	—
Longus colli	XX	—	X	—
Longus capitis	XX	—	X	—
Splenius capitis	—	XXX	XX	XXX (IL)
Splenius cervicis	—	XXX	XX	XXX (IL)

*Upper parts of sternocleidomastoid extend the upper cervical region, atlanto-axial joint, and atlanto-occipital joint.

CL, Contralateral rotation; *IL,* ipsilateral rotation.

The actions are assumed to occur from the anatomic position, against an external resistance. A muscle's relative potential to move or stabilize a region is scored as X (minimal), XX (moderate), or XXX (maximum) based on moment arm (leverage), cross-sectional area, and fiber direction; — indicates no effective or conclusive action.

SPECIAL FOCUS 10-5

Specialized Muscles That Control the Atlanto-axial and Atlanto-occipital Joints: an Example of Fine-Tuning of Cervical Spinal Coupling

The specialized muscles listed in Figure 10-30 exert fine control over the movements of the upper craniocervical region. One benefit of this control is related to the spinal coupling pattern typically expressed within the cervical region. As described in Chapter 9, an ipsilateral spinal coupling pattern exists in the mid-and-lower cervical region between the motions of axial rotation and lateral flexion. Axial rotation, resulting primarily from the orientation of the facet surfaces within the apophyseal joints, is mechanically associated with slight ipsilateral lateral flexion, and vice versa. The expression of this coupling pattern can be obscured, however, by the action of the specialized muscles that control the atlanto-occipital and atlanto-axial joints. Consider, for example, right axial rotation of the craniocervical region. In order for a level horizontal visual gaze to be maintained throughout axial rotation, the left rectus capitis lateralis, for instance, produces a slight left lateral flexion torque to the head. This muscular action offsets the tendency of the head to laterally flex to the right with the rest of the cervical region during the right axial rotation. Similarly, right lateral flexion of the mid-to-lower cervical region (which is coupled with slight right axial rotation) may be accompanied by a slight offsetting left axial rotation torque applied to the head by the obliquus capitis inferior muscle. In both examples, the muscular actions allow the head and eyes to more precisely visually fix on an object.

of the whiplash event.[44] For this reason, athletes need to anticipate a potentially harmful situation and contract the neck musculature *before* impact. The timing of muscle contraction appears as important to protecting the neck as the magnitude of the muscle force.

In addition to protecting the neck, forces produced by muscles provide the primary source of vertical stability to the craniocervical region. The "critical load" of the cervical spine (i.e., maximum compressive load that the neck, unsupported by muscle, can sustain before buckling) is between 10.5 and 40 N (between 2.4 and 9 lb). Remarkably, this is less than the actual weight of the head.[116,118] A coordinated interaction of craniocervical muscles generates forces that are, on average, directed nearly *through* the instantaneous axis of rotation at each intervertebral junction. By passing through or close to these multiple axes, the forces compress the vertebral segments together, thereby stabilizing them without buckling. The magnitude of these compression forces generated across the craniocervical region is quite high—nearly three times the weight of the head during the low-level muscle activation required to just balance the head during upright standing, and up to 23 times the weight of the head (or 1.7 times body weight) during maximal-effort muscle activation.[109,118]

Much of the muscular stabilization of the craniocervical region is accomplished by the relatively short, segmented muscles such as the multifidi, rotatores, longus colli and capitis, and interspinalis muscles. With relatively short fibers and multiple bony attachments, these muscles exert a fine, coordinated control of the stability in the region.[25] This stability is augmented by other longer and typically thicker muscles, including the scalenes, sternocleidomastoid, levator scapula, semispinalis capitis and cervicis, and trapezius. When needed, these muscles form an extensive and strong guy-wire system that ensures vertical stability, most notably in frontal and sagittal planes. Figure 10-31, *A* highlights a sample of muscles that act as guy wires to maintain ideal anterior-posterior alignment throughout the craniocervical region. Ideally, the co-contraction of flexor and extensor muscles counterbalances, and as a consequence vertically stabilizes the region. Note that the muscles depicted in Figure 10-31, *A* are anchored inferiorly to several different structures: the sternum, clavicle, ribs, scapula, and vertebral column. These bony structures themselves must be stabilized by other muscles, such as the lower trapezius and subclavius, to secure the scapula and clavicle, respectively.

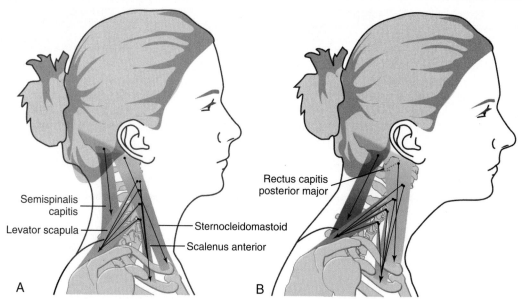

FIGURE 10-31. A, Four muscles are acting as guy wires to maintain ideal posture within the craniocervical region. **B,** Mechanics associated with a chronic forward head posture as discussed in Special Focus 10-6. The protracted position of the craniocervical region places greater stress on the levator scapula and semispinalis capitis muscles. The rectus capitis posterior major—one of the suboccipital muscles—is shown actively extending the upper craniocervical region. The highly active and stressed muscles are depicted in brighter red.

SPECIAL FOCUS 10-6

Muscular Imbalance Associated with Chronic Forward Head Posture

The ideal posture shown in Figure 10-31, *A* depicts an optimally balanced craniocervical "guy-wire" system. Excessive muscular tension in any of the muscles, however, can disrupt the vertical stability of the region. One such disruption is a chronic forward head posture, involving excessive protraction of the craniocervical region (see Figure 10-31, *B*). Habitual forward head posture can occur for at least two different reasons. First, severe hyperextension of the neck can injure anterior muscles, such as the sternocleidomastoid, longus colli, and scalenus anterior. As a result, chronic spasm in the excessively strained muscles translates the head forward, resulting in excessive flexion, especially at the cervicothoracic junction. A clinical sign often associated with forward head posturing is a realignment of the sternocleidomastoid within the sagittal plane. The cranial end of the muscle, normally aligned posterior to the sternoclavicular joint, shifts anteriorly with the head to a position directly above the sternoclavicular joint (compare Figure 10-31, *A* with *B*).

A second cause of a chronic forward head posture may be related to a progressive shortening of several anterior neck muscles. One such scenario involves purposely protracting the craniocervical region to improve visual contact with objects manipulated in front of the body. This activity is typical when viewing a computer screen or a television. This position, if adopted for an extended period, may alter the functional resting length of the muscles, eventually transforming the forward posture into a person's "natural" posture.

Regardless of the factors that predispose a person to a chronic forward head posture, the posture itself stresses extensor muscles, such as the levator scapula and semispinalis capitis (see Figure 10-31, *B*).[108] A suboccipital muscle, such as the rectus capitis posterior major, may become fatigued as a result of its prolonged extension activity required to "level" the head and eyes. Over time, increased muscular stress throughout the entire craniocervical region can lead to localized and painful muscle spasms, or "trigger points," common in the levator scapula and suboccipital muscles. This condition is often associated with headaches and radiating pain into the scalp and temporomandibular joints. The key to most treatment for chronic forward head posture is to restore optimal craniocervical posture,[49] accomplished through improved postural awareness, ergonomic workplace design, therapeutic exercise, motor relearning, or specific manual therapy techniques.*

---

*References 15, 16, 23, 78, 123, 148.

PRODUCING EXTENSIVE AND WELL-COORDINATED MOVEMENTS OF THE HEAD AND NECK: OPTIMIZING THE PLACEMENT OF THE EYES, EARS, AND NOSE

The craniocervical region allows the greatest triplanar mobility of any region of the axial skeleton. Ample movement is essential for optimal spatial orientation of the eyes, ears, and nose. Although all planes of motion are equally important in this regard, the following section highlights movement within the horizontal plane.

Figure 10-32 illustrates a total body movement that exhibits a sample of the muscular interactions used to maximize the extent of right axial rotation of the craniocervical region. Note that full axial rotation of the craniocervical region provides the

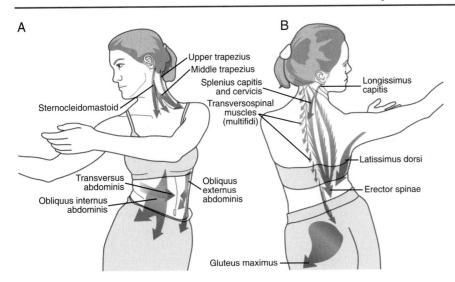

FIGURE 10-32. A typical activation pattern of selected muscles of the craniocervical region, trunk, and hip as a healthy person rotates the entire body to the right within the horizontal plane. **A,** Anterior view. **B,** Posterior view.

eyes with well over 180 degrees of visual scanning. As depicted, rotation to the right is driven by simultaneous activation of the left sternocleidomastoid and left trapezius (see Figure 10-32, *A*); right splenius capitis and cervicis; right upper erector spinae, such as the longissimus capitis; and left transversospinal muscles, such as the multifidi (see Figure 10-32, *B*). Although not depicted, several suboccipital muscles (namely the right rectus capitis posterior major and right obliquus capitis inferior) are actively controlling atlanto-axial joint rotation.

Activation of the muscles listed provides the required rotational power and control to the head and neck, as well as simultaneously stabilizing the craniocervical region in both the frontal and sagittal planes. For example, the extension potential provided by the splenius capitis and cervicis, trapezius, and upper erector spinae is balanced by the flexion potential of the sternocleidomastoid. Furthermore, the left lateral flexion potential of the left sternocleidomastoid and left trapezius is balanced by the right lateral flexion potential of the right splenius capitis and cervicis.

Full axial rotation of the craniocervical region requires muscular interactions that extend into the trunk and lower extremities. Consider, for example, the activation of the right and left oblique abdominal muscles (see Figure 10-32, *A*). They provide much of the torque needed to rotate the thoracic region, which serves as a structural foundation for the craniocervical region. Furthermore, as suggested by Figure 10-32, *B*, the erector spinae and transversospinal muscles are active throughout the posterior trunk to offset the potent trunk flexion tendency of the oblique abdominal muscles. The latissimus dorsi is an ipsilateral rotator of the trunk when the glenohumeral joint is well stabilized by other muscles.[12] The left gluteus maximus is shown actively rotating the pelvis and attached lumbosacral region to the right, relative to the fixed left femur.

SELECTED BIOMECHANICAL ISSUES OF LIFTING: A FOCUS ON REDUCING BACK INJURY

Lifting heavy objects can generate large compression, tension, and shear forces throughout the body, most notably across the lumbopelvic regions. At some critical level, forces acting on a region may exceed the structural tolerance of the local muscles, ligaments and capsules, and apophyseal and inter-

body joints. Lifting is a leading risk factor associated with low-back pain in the United States and is especially related to occupation.[50,52,74,85] Disability associated with low-back pain is a significant problem, in terms of both cost and suffering. An estimated 30% of the workforce in the United States regularly handles materials in a potentially harmful manner, including by lifting.[112]

This topic of the biomechanics of lifting describes (1) *why* the low-back region is vulnerable to lifting-related injury and (2) *how* the forces in the low-back region may be minimized in order to reduce the chance of injury.

Muscular Mechanics of Extension of the Low Back during Lifting

The forces generated by the extensor muscles of the posterior trunk during lifting are transferred either directly or indirectly to the joints and connective tissues (tendons, ligaments, fascia, discs) within the low back. The following sections therefore focus on the role of the muscles during lifting, and how forces produced by muscles may be modified to reduce the stress on the structures in the low-back region.

ESTIMATING THE MAGNITUDE OF FORCE IMPOSED ON THE LOW BACK DURING LIFTING

Considerable research has been undertaken to quantify the relative demands placed on the various structures in the low back during lifting or performance of other strenuous activities.[3,11,30,125,153] This research helps clinicians and members of governmental agencies develop safety guidelines and limits for lifting, especially in the workplace.* Of particular interest with regard to lifting injury are the variables of peak force (or torque) produced by muscles; tension developed within stretched ligaments; and compression and shear forces developed against the intervertebral discs and apophyseal joints. Measurement of these variables is typically not made directly but estimated through sophisticated mathematic or computer-based models. A simple but less accurate method of estimating forces imposed on the low back uses calculations based on the assumption of static equilibrium.

---

*References 12, 31, 42, 74, 94, 101, 150.

The following section presents the steps used in making these calculations in order to estimate the approximate compression force on the L2 vertebra while a load is lifted in the sagittal plane. Although this example provides a limited amount of information on a rather complex biomechanical event, it does yield valuable insight into the relationship between the force produced by the muscle and the compression force imposed on a representative structure within the low back.

Figure 10-33 (top box) shows the data required to make an approximate estimate of the compression force against the L2 vertebra during lifting. The subject is depicted midway through a vertical lift of a moderately heavy load, weighing 25% of his body weight. The axis of rotation for the sagittal plane motion is oriented in the medial-lateral direction, arbitrary set at L2 (see Figure 10-33, open circle). Estimating the compression force is a two-step process; each step assumes a condition of static rotary and linear equilibrium.

Step 1 solves for extensor muscle force by assuming that the sum of the internal and external torques within the sagittal plane is equal to zero (Σ Torques = 0). Note that two external torques are described: one resulting from the external load (EL) and one resulting from the subject's body weight (BW) located above L2. The extensor muscle force (MF) is defined as the MF generated on the posterior (extensor) side of the axis of rotation. If the back extensor muscles are assumed to have an average internal moment arm of 5 cm, the extensor muscles must produce at least 2512 N (565.1 lb) of force to lift the load.

Step 2 estimates the compressive reaction force (RF) imposed on the L2 vertebra during lifting. (This *reaction force* implies that the L2 vertebra must "push" back against the other downward acting forces.) A rough estimate of this force can be made by assuming static linear equilibrium. (For the sake of simplicity, the calculations assume that muscle force [MF] acts totally in the vertical direction and is therefore parallel with body weight and the external load forces.) The RF vector (see Figure 10-33) is also assumed to be equal in magnitude but opposite in direction to the sum of MF, BW, and EL.

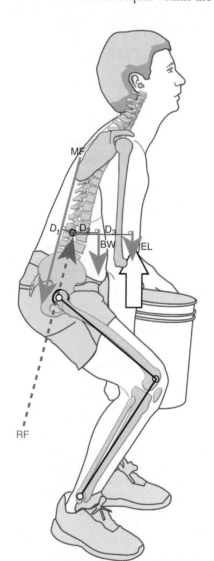

Data for Calculations:

- Internal moment arm (D_1) = **5 cm**
- Total body weight = **800 N** (about 180 lbs)
- Body weight (BW) above L2 = 65% of total body weight, or about **520 N**
- External moment arm used by BW (D_2) = **13 cm**
- External load (EL) = 25% of total body weight = **200 N** (about 45 lbs)
- External moment arm used by EL (D_3) = **29 cm**

Step 1: Estimate Muscle Force (MF)
By Assuming Σ Torques = 0
Internal torque = External torque
$(MF \times D_1) = (BW \times D_2 + EL \times D_3)$
$(MF \times 0.05 \text{ m}) = (520 \text{ N} \times 0.13 \text{ m}) + (200 \text{ N} \times 0.29 \text{ m})$
$MF = \dfrac{125.6 \text{ Nm}}{0.05 \text{ m}}$
MF = 2512 N (about 565.1 lbs)

Step 2: Estimate Compression Reaction Force (RF) on L2
By Assuming Σ Forces = 0
Upward directed forces = Downward directed forces
RF = MF + BW + EL
RF = (2512 N) + (520 N) + (200 N)
RF = 3232 N (726. 6 lbs); directed upward

FIGURE 10-33. The steps used to estimate the approximate compressive reaction force *(RF)* on the L2 vertebra while a load is lifted. The biomechanics are limited to the sagittal plane, around an axis of rotation arbitrarily set at L2 *(green circle)*. The mathematic solutions assume a condition of static equilibrium. All abbreviations are defined in the boxes. (To simplify the mathematics, the calculations assume that all forces are acting in a vertical direction. This assumption introduces modest error in the results. All moment arm directions are designated as positive.)

The solution to this example suggests that a compression force of approximately 3232 N (over 725 lb) is exerted on L2 while an external load weighing 200 N (about 45 lb) is lifted. To put this magnitude of force into practical perspective, consider the following two points. First, the National Institute of Occupational Safety and Health (NIOSH) has set guidelines to protect workers from excessive loads on the lumbar region caused by lifting and handling materials. NIOSH has recommended an upper safe limit of 3400 N (764 lb) of compression force on the L5-S1 junction.[1,151] Second, the maximal load-carrying capacity of the lumbar spine is estimated to be 6400 N (1439 lb),[76] almost twice the maximal safe force recommended by NIOSH. The limit of 6400 N of force applies to a 40-year-old man; this limit decreases by 1000 N each subsequent decade. These force values are very general guidelines that may not always apply to all persons in all lifting situations.

The static model very likely underestimates the actual compressive force on the L2 vertebra for the following two reasons. First, the model accounts for muscle force produced by the back extensors only. Other muscles, especially those with near-vertical fiber orientation such as the rectus abdominis and the psoas major, certainly add to the muscular-based compression on the lumbar spine. Second, the model assumes static equilibrium, thereby ignoring the additional forces needed to accelerate the body and load upward. A rapid lift requires greater muscle force and imposes greater compression and shear on the joints and connective tissues in the low back. For this reason, it is usually recommended that a person lift loads slowly and smoothly, a condition not always practical in all settings.

WAYS TO REDUCE THE FORCE DEMANDS ON THE BACK MUSCLES DURING LIFTING

The calculations performed in Step 2 of Figure 10-33 show that muscle force (MF) is, by far, the most influential variable for determining the magnitude of the compressive (reaction) force on the lumbar spine. Proportional reductions in muscle force, therefore, have the greatest effect on reducing the overall compression force on the structures in the low back.

An important factor responsible for the large forces in the low-back muscles during lifting is the disparity in the length of the associated internal and external moment arms. The internal moment arm (D_1) depicted in Figure 10-33 is assumed to be 5 cm. The extensor muscles are therefore at a sizable mechanical *disadvantage* and must produce a force many times larger than the weight of the load being lifted. As previously demonstrated, lifting an external load weighing 25% of one's body weight produces a compression force on L2 of four times one's body weight!

Therapeutic and educational programs are often designed to reduce the likelihood of back injury by minimizing the need for very large extensor muscle forces during lifting. In theory, this can be accomplished in four ways. *First,* reduce the rate of lifting. As previously stated, reducing lifting velocity proportionately decreases the amount of back extensor muscle force.

Second, reduce the weight of the external load. Although this point is obvious, it is not always possible.

Third, reduce the length of the external moment arm of the external load. This is likely the most effective and practical method of decreasing compressive reaction forces on the low back.[23] As demonstrated in Figure 10-33, ideally a load should be lifted from between the knees, thereby minimizing the

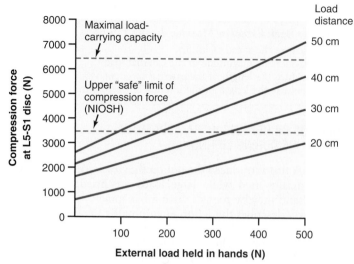

FIGURE 10-34. Graph shows the predicted compression force at the L5-S1 disc as a function of load size and the distance the loads are held in front of the body (1 lb = 4.448 N). The two red horizontal lines indicate (1) the maximal load-carrying capacity of the lumbar region before structural failure and (2) the upper safe limits of compression force on the lumbar spine as determined by the National Institute of Occupational Safety and Health. (Plot modified from Chaffin DB, Andersson GBJ: *Occupational biomechanics,* ed 2, New York, 1991, John Wiley & Sons.)

distance between the load and the lumbar region. Based on the calculations, this ideal method of lifting produced a compression force on the lumbar region that remained close to the upper limits of safety proposed by NIOSH. Lifting the same load with a *longer* external moment arm may create very large and potentially dangerous compression forces on the low back. Figure 10-34 shows a plot of predicted compression (reaction) forces on the L5-S1 disc as a function of both load size and distance between the load and the front of the chest.[31] Although perhaps an extreme and unrealistic example, the plot predicts that holding an external load weighing 200 N (45 lb) 50 cm in front of the body creates about 4500 N of compression force, greatly exceeding the upper safe limit of 3400 N.

In everyday life, lifting an object from between the knees or in a similar manner is not always practical. Consider the act of sliding a large patient toward the head of a hospital bed. The inability to reduce the distance between the patient's center of mass (located anterior to S2) and the lifter can dramatically compromise the safety of the lifter.

Fourth, increase the *internal* moment arm available to the low-back extensor muscles. A larger internal moment arm for extension allows a given extension torque to be generated with less muscle force. As stated, less muscle force typically equates to less force on the vertebral elements. Increased lumbar lordosis does indeed increase the internal moment arm available to the lumbar erector spinae muscles.[10,140] Lifting with an accentuated lumbar lordosis, however, is not always possible or desirable. Lifting a very heavy load off the floor, for example, typically requires a flexed lumbar spine, which decreases the extensor muscles' moment arm.[81] (Biomechanically, this situation would require greater muscle force per given extensor torque.) Even if possible, maintaining an exaggerated lumbar lordosis may have the negative consequences of generating excessive compression loads on the apophyseal joints and other posterior elements of the spine.

> **Four Ways to Reduce the Amount of Force Required of the Back Extensor Muscles during Lifting**
> * Reduce the speed of lifting.
> * Reduce the magnitude of the external load.
> * Reduce the length of the external moment arm.
> * Increase the length of the internal moment arm.

ROLE OF INCREASING INTRA-ABDOMINAL PRESSURE DURING LIFTING

Bartelink first introduced the notion that the Valsalva maneuver, typically used while large loads are lifted, may help unload and thereby protect the lumbar spine.[17] The Valsalva maneuver describes the action of voluntarily increasing intraabdominal pressure by vigorous contraction of the abdominal muscles against a closed glottis. The Valsalva maneuver creates a rigid column of high pressure within the abdomen that pushes upward against the diaphragm, anteriorly against the deeper abdominal muscles (transversus abdominis and internal oblique), posteriorly against the lumbar spine, and downward against the pelvic floor muscles. With this column acting as an inflated "intra-abdominal balloon," Bartelink proposed that performing the Valsalva maneuver while lifting would create an *extension* torque on the lumbar spine, thereby reducing the demands on the lumbar extensor muscles and ultimately lowering the muscular-based compression forces on the lumbar spine.

Although the notion of strongly increasing intra-abdominal pressure as a way to *reduce* compression forces on the spine is intriguing, studies have generally refuted the overall biomechanical validity of the concept.[10,13,105,111] Although evidence exists that the Valsalva maneuver does indeed generate a modest lumbar extension torque,[67] the strong activation of the abdominal muscles actually creates a net *increase* in compression forces on the lumbar spine. Because all abdominal muscles (except the transversus abdominis) are strong flexors of the trunk and lumbar spine, their strong activation requires even greater counterbalancing forces from the antagonistic extensor muscles. The resulting increased activation of virtually *all* the trunk muscles creates an overall increase in muscle-based compression forces on the lumbar spine.[11]

Most persons, however, likely benefit from the Valsalva maneuver while lifting. In a healthy person without low back pathology, the resulting increased compression force on the lumbar spine can be a useful and relatively safe source of stability to the region. A strong contraction of the abdominal muscles also provides an important bracing effect to the lumbopelvic region, which is helpful in resisting unwanted torsions created by the asymmetric lifting of external loads.[38,55] Forces produced by the transversus abdominis may be particularly effective in stabilizing the lumbopelvic region during lifting, for at least two reasons. First, the transversus abdominis has extensive attachments into the thoracolumbar fascia. Forces produced by muscle activation generate a circumferential corset effect around the entire low-back region. Second, by acting primarily in the transverse direction, the transversus abdominis can increase intra-abdominal pressure *without* creating a concurrent flexion torque or an increase in vertical compression force on the lumbar spine.[11,90] The transverse fibers of the internal oblique muscles are able to assist transversus abdominis with these aforementioned functions.

ADDITIONAL SOURCES OF EXTENSION TORQUE USED FOR LIFTING

The maximal force-generating capacity of the low-back extensor muscles in a typical young adult is estimated to be approximately 4000 N (900 lb).[23] If an average internal moment arm of 5 cm is assumed, this muscle group is then expected to produce about *200 Nm* of trunk extension torque (i.e., 4000 N × 0.05 m). What is perplexing, however, is the fact that maximal-effort lifting likely requires extensor torques that may greatly *exceed* 200 Nm. For instance, the person depicted lifting the load in Figure 10-33 would have exceeded his theoretic 200-Nm strength limit if the external load were increased to about 80% of his body weight. Although this is a considerable weight, it is not unusual for a person to successfully lift much greater loads, such as those regularly encountered by heavy labor workers and by competitive "power lifters." In attempts to explain this apparent discrepancy, two secondary sources of extension torque are proposed: (1) passive tension generated from stretching the posterior ligamentous system, and (2) muscular-generated tension transferred through the thoracolumbar fascia.

Passive Tension Generation from Stretching the Posterior Ligamentous System

When stretched, healthy ligaments and fascia exhibit some degree of natural elasticity. This feature allows connective tissue to temporarily store a small part of the force that initially causes the elongation. Bending forward in preparation for lifting progressively elongates several connective tissues in the lumbar region, and presumably the passive tension developed in these tissues can assist with an extension torque.[10,45] These connective tissues, collectively known as the *posterior ligamentous system*, include the posterior longitudinal ligament, ligamentum flavum, apophyseal joint capsule, interspinous ligament, and posterior layer of the thoracolumbar fascia.[53]

In theory, about 72 Nm of total passive extensor torque are produced by maximally stretching the posterior ligamentous system (Table 10-6).[23] Adding this passive torque to the hypothetic 200 Nm of active torque yields a total of 272 Nm of extension torque available for lifting. A fully engaged (stretched) posterior ligamentous system can therefore generate about 25% of the total extension torque for lifting. Note, however, that this 25% passive torque reserve is available only after the lumbar spine is maximally flexed, which in reality is rare during lifting. Even some competitive power lifters, who appear to lift with a fully rounded low back, avoid the extremes of flexion.[34] It is generally believed that maximum or near-maximum flexion of the lumbar spine should be avoided during lifting.[23,104] The lumbar region should be held in a near-neutral position.[104] This position favors a near-maximal contact area within the apophyseal joints, which may help reduce articular stress. Furthermore, maintaining the neutral position during lifting may align the local extensor muscles to be most effective at resisting anterior shear.[102]

Although the neutral position of the lumbar spine while lifting may reduce the chance of injury to the low back, it engages only a small portion of the total passive torque reserve available to assist with extension. Most of the extension torque must therefore be generated by active muscle contraction.[121] It is important, therefore, that the extensor muscles be strong enough to meet the potentially large demands placed on the low back by heavy lifting. Adequate strength in the lumbar

TABLE 10-6. Maximal Passive Extensor Torque Produced by Stretched Connective Tissues in the Lumbar Region

Connective Tissue	Average Maximum Tension (N)*	Extensor Moment Arm (m)†	Maximal Passive Extensor Torque (Nm)‡
Posterior longitudinal ligament	90	0.02	1.8
Ligamentum flava	244	0.03	7.3
Capsule of apophyseal joints	680	0.04	27.2
Interspinous ligament	107	0.05	5.4
Posterior layer of thoracolumbar fascia, including supraspinous ligaments and the aponeurosis covering the erector spinae muscles	500	0.06	30.0
Total			71.7

Data from Bogduk N, Twomey L: *Clinical anatomy of the lumbar spine*, ed 4, New York, 2005, Churchill Livingstone.

*Average maximum tension is the tension within each stretched tissue at the point of rupture.

†*Extensor moment arm* is the perpendicular distance between the attachment sites of the ligaments and the medial-lateral axis of rotation within a representative lumbar vertebra.

‡*Maximal passive extensor torque* is estimated by the product of maximum tension (force) and extensor muscle moment arm.

multifidi is particularly critical in this regard.[21,47,57] Without adequate strength in these muscles, the lumbar spine may be pulled into excessive flexion by the external torque imposed by the large load. Excessive flexion in the lumbar region while loads are lifted is generally *not* considered a safe lifting technique.

Muscular-Generated Tension Transferred through the Thoracolumbar Fascia

The thoracolumbar fascia is thickest and most extensively developed in the lumbar region (see Figure 9-72). Much of the tissue attaches to the lumbar spine, sacrum, and pelvis in a position well *posterior* to the axis of rotation at the lumbar region. Theoretically, therefore, passive tension within stretched thoracolumbar fascia can produce an extension torque in the lumbar region and thus augment the torque created by the low-back musculature.

In order for the thoracolumbar fascia to generate useful tension, it must be first stretched and rendered taut. This can occur in two ways. First, the fascia is stretched simply when one bends forward and flexes the lumbar spine in preparation for lifting. Second, the fascia is stretched by active contraction of muscles that attach directly into the thoracolumbar fascia. The prevailing horizontal fiber direction of most of the thoracolumbar fascia, however, limits the amount of extension torque that can be produced at the lumbar spine.[24] Theoretically, the force transferred to the thoracolumbar fascia by contraction of the transversus abdominis and internal oblique may contribute 6 Nm of extensor torque across the lumbar spine (compared with the approximately 200 Nm of active torque generated by the low-back extensor muscles[99]). Although the actual extension torque is small, the tension transferred through the thoracolumbar fascia provides an additional element of stabilization to the region.

The latissimus dorsi and gluteus maximus may also indirectly contribute to lumbar extension torque via their extensive attachments to the thoracolumbar fascia. Both are active during lifting, but for different reasons (Figure 10-35). The gluteus maximus stabilizes and controls the hips. The latissimus dorsi helps transfer the external load being lifted from the arms to the trunk. In addition to attaching into the thoracolumbar fascia, the latissimus dorsi attaches into the posterior aspect of the pelvis, sacrum, and spine. Based on these attachments and its relative moment arm for producing

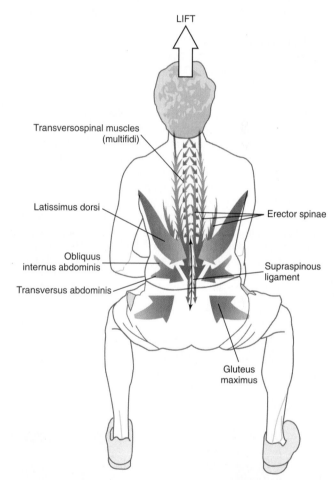

FIGURE 10-35. A posterior view of a typical activation pattern of selected muscles as a healthy person lifts a load with the hands. The supraspinous ligament is shown elongated and subjected to increased tension.

lumbar extension (see Figure 10-16), the latissimus dorsi has all the attributes of a respected extensor of the low back. The oblique fiber direction of the muscle as it ascends the trunk can also provide torsional stability to the axial skeleton, especially when bilaterally active. This stability may be especially useful when large loads are handled in an asymmetric fashion.

SPECIAL FOCUS 10-7

Two Contrasting Lifting Techniques: the Stoop versus the Squat Lift

The stoop lift and the squat lift represent the biomechanical extremes of a broad continuum of possible lifting strategies (Figure 10-36). Understanding some of the biomechanic and physiologic differences between these methods of lifting may provide insight into the advantages or disadvantages of other, more common lifting strategies.

The *stoop lift* is performed primarily by extending the hips and lumbar region while the knees remain slightly flexed (see Figure 10-36, *A*). This lifting strategy is associated with greater flexion of the low back, especially at the initiation of the lift. By necessity, the stoop lift creates a long external moment arm between the trunk (and load) and the low back. The greater external torque requires greater extension forces from the low-back and trunk extensor muscles. In combination with a markedly flexed lumbar spine, the stoop lift can create large and possibly damaging compression and shear forces on the discs.

The *squat lift,* in contrast, typically begins with near maximally flexed knees (see Figure 10-36, *B*). The knees and hips extend during the lift, powered by the quadriceps and hip extensor muscles. Depending on the physical characteristics of the load and the initial depth of the squat, the lumbar region may remain extended; in a neutral position, or partially flexed throughout the lift. Perhaps the greatest advantage of the squat lift is that it typically allows the load to be raised more naturally from between the knees. The squat lift can, in theory, reduce the external moment arm of the load and trunk and, as a consequence, diminish the extensor torque demands on the muscles of the back.

The squat lift is most often advocated as the safer of the two techniques in terms of producing less stress on the low back and therefore preventing back injuries.[18] Little overwhelming direct proof, however, can be found to support this strongly held clinical belief.[10,23,143] As with many espoused clinical principles, the advantage of one particular concept or technique is often at least partially offset by a disadvantage. This holds true for the apparent advantage of the squat lift over the stoop lift. Although the squat lift may reduce the demands on the extensor muscles and other tissues in the low back, it usually creates greater demands on the knees.[129] The extreme degree of initial knee flexion associated with the full squat places high force demands on the quadriceps muscles to extend the knees. The forces impose very large pressures across the tibiofemoral and patellofemoral joints. Healthy persons may tolerate high pressures at these joints without negative consequences; however, someone with painful or arthritic knees may not. The adage that lifting with the legs "spares the back and spoils the knees" does, therefore, have some validity.

Another factor to consider when comparing the benefits of the squat lift over the stoop lift is the total work required to lift the load. The mechanical work performed during lifting is equal to the weight of the body and the load multiplied by the vertical displacement of the body and the load. The stoop lift is 23% to 34% more metabolically "efficient" than the squat lift in terms of work performed per level of oxygen consumption.[152] The squat lift requires greater work because a greater proportion of the total body mass must be moved through space.

Rather than performing a squat lift or a stoop lift, in reality most people choose an individualized or freestyle lifting technique. A freestyle technique allows the lifter to combine some of the benefits of the squat lift with the more metabolically efficient stoop lift. Workers have reported a higher self-perceived maximal safe limit when allowed to lift with a freestyle technique rather than with a set technique.[134]

The "stoop" lift   **The "squat" lift**

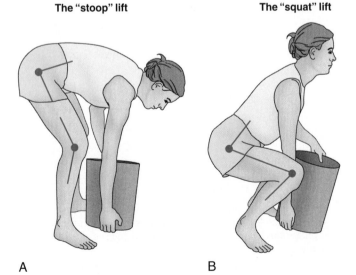

A   B

FIGURE 10-36. Two contrasting styles of lifting. **A,** The initiation of the stoop lift. **B,** The initiation of the squat lift. The axes of rotation are shown at the hip and knee joints.

TABLE 10-7. Factors Considered to Contribute to Safe Lifting Techniques

Consideration	Rationale	Comment
A lifted load should be as light as practical, and held as close to the body as possible.	Minimizes the external torque of the load, thereby minimizing the force demands on the back muscles.	Lifting an external load from between the knees is an effective way to reduce the load's external moment arm, although not always practical to implement.
Lift with the lumbar spine as close as possible to its neutral (lordotic) position (i.e., avoid *extremes* of flexion and extension).	Vigorous contraction of the back extensor muscles with the lumbar spine *maximally flexed* may damage the intervertebral discs. In contrast, vigorous contraction of the back extensor muscles with the lumbar spine *maximally extended* may damage the apophyseal joints.	Lifting with limited flexion or extension in the lumbar spine may be acceptable for some persons, depending on the health and experience of the lifter. Varying amounts of flexion or extension each have biomechanical advantages. • Lifting with the lumbar spine in *minimal-to-moderate flexion* increases the passive tension generated by the posterior ligamentous system, possibly reducing the force demands on extensor muscles. • Lifting with the lumbar spine *near complete extension* may augment the moment arm for some of the extensor muscles while the apophyseal joints remain in or near their close-packed position.
When lifting, fully use the hip and knee extensor muscles to minimize the force demands on the low-back muscles.	Very large forces produced by low-back extensor muscles can injure the muscles themselves, intervertebral discs, vertebral endplates, or apophyseal joints.	A person with hip or knee arthritis may be unable to effectively use the muscles in the legs to assist the back muscles. The squat lift may encourage the use of the leg muscles but also increases the overall work demands on the body.
Minimize the vertical and horizontal distance that a load must be lifted.	Minimizing the distance that the load is moved reduces the total work of the lift, thereby reducing fatigue; minimizing the distance that the load is moved reduces the extremes of movement in the low back and lower extremities.	Using handles or an adjustable-height platform may be helpful.
Avoid twisting when lifting.	Torsional forces applied to vertebrae can predispose the person to intervertebral disc injury.	A properly designed work environment can reduce the need for twisting during lifting.
Lift as slowly and smoothly as conditions allow.	A slow and smooth lift reduces the peak force generated in muscles and connective tissues.	
Lift with a moderately wide and slightly staggered base of support provided by the legs.	A relatively wide base of support affords greater overall stability of the body, thereby reducing the chance of a fall or slip.	
When possible, use the assistance of a mechanical device or additional people to lift something.	Using assistance in lifting can reduce the demand on the back of the primary lifter.	Using a mechanical hoist (Hoyer lift) or a "two-man" transfer may be prudent in many settings.

Summary of Factors That Likely Contribute to Safe Lifting

The lifting technique used in Figure 10-33 illustrates two fundamental features that likely contribute to safe lifting technique: (1) the lumbar spine is held in a neutral lordotic position, and (2) the load is lifted from between the knees. The rationales for these and other factors considered to contribute to safe lifting are listed in Table 10-7. Other, more general considerations include (1) knowing one's physical limits, (2) thinking the lift through before the event, and (3) within practical and health limits, remaining in optimal physical and cardiovascular condition.

SYNOPSIS

In the broad view, the muscles of the trunk and craniocervical regions have at least three interrelated functions: movement, stabilization, and assisting with activities such as ventilation, chewing and swallowing, defecation, and childbirth. This chapter focuses primarily on movement and stabilization.

Ultimately, muscles that control movement of the trunk and craniocervical regions do so either by contracting or by resisting elongation by a more dominating force. The specificity of such control can be greatly enhanced by the muscles' unique anatomic characteristics, such as shape, size, fiber orientation, and innervation. Consider, for example, the very short and vertical rectus capitis lateralis muscle in the upper craniocervical region. Contraction of this muscle is designed to make small and precise adjustments to the atlanto-occipital joint, perhaps to help track an object as it crosses the visual field. Such an action is primarily reflexive in nature and linked to neural centers that help coordinate vision and associated righting and postural reactions of the head and neck. The nervous system likely provides ample neural connections between the rectus capitis lateralis and a host of other structures, including other craniocervical muscles, apophyseal joints, and vestibular-and-ocular apparatus. Injury to the small and deep muscles of the craniocervical region may potentially disrupt this stream of neurologic signaling. In cases of reduced craniocervical proprioception, movements may become slightly uncoordinated and subsequently place higher than normal stress on the local joints. This stress may prolong pain after an injury, as is often the case with whiplash trauma.

In contrast to small muscles, such as the rectus capitis lateralis, consider the much larger internal oblique abdominis that courses obliquely across the middle and lower abdomen. This muscle extends between the linea alba anteriorly and the thoracolumbar fascia posteriorly. During a 100-meter sprint, for example, this muscle is repetitively strongly activated as it accelerates and decelerates rotation of the trunk. The highly segmental innervation of this muscle may allow a more sequential activation across the whole muscle, perhaps facilitating a "wave" of contractile force that is transmitted throughout the abdomen and low back. During the strong activation of the abdominal muscles during sprinting, the diaphragm muscle must contract and descend against a very high intra-abdominal pressure. This topic is further explored in the next chapter.

In addition to generating forces required for movement, the muscles of the trunk and craniocervical regions also have the primary responsibility of stabilizing the axial spine. This stability must occur in three dimensions, across multiple segments, and for an infinite number of both anticipated and unexpected environmental situations. Consider, for example, the need to stabilize the trunk before landing from a jump or while attempting to stand upright on a rocking boat. One primary benefit of this stabilization is to protect the joints, discs, and ligaments within the axial spine and, perhaps more important, the delicate spinal cord and exiting spinal nerve roots.

Muscular stabilization can be provided simply through large muscle bulk. This is particularly evident at the craniocervical and lumbosacral regions, where the cross-sectional areas of the paravertebral muscles are the largest. At the lumbosacral region, for example, the vertebral column is closely surrounded by thick, oblique-to–vertically oriented muscles, such as the psoas major, quadratus lumborum, multifidi, and lower erector spinae.

Other, more complex methods of muscular stability exist across the axial spine, much of which is "preprogrammed" within the nervous system. For instance, certain trunk muscles subconsciously contract slightly before active movements of the upper limbs, especially when performed rapidly. This preparatory activity helps stabilize the trunk against unwanted reactive movements that may, over time, damage the spine. Furthermore, during lower extremity movements, the activation of trunk muscles is essential to stabilize and fixate the proximal attachments of several muscles that cross the hips and knees. The importance of this muscular stabilization is often evident in persons with weakened abdominal muscles secondary to pathology, such as a child with muscular dystrophy. In this case a strong contraction of the hip flexor muscles, for example, produces an excessive and undesired anterior tilting of the pelvis relative to the hip joints. This position of the pelvis, in turn, creates an exaggerated lordosis of the lumbar spine. Over time, this abnormal posture may increase the wear on the apophyseal joints and increase anterior shearing across the lumbosacral junction.

In closing, patients with injury and disease involving the axial spine often demonstrate a complicated set of musculoskeletal symptoms, typically affecting their ability to move freely and comfortably and to limit the stress placed on their vertebral and neural tissues. The complexity and often uncertainty of the underlying pathomechanics in these conditions partially accounts for the many different treatment and rehabilitation options used to treat the associated disorders, especially those that involve chronic pain. The degree of uncertainty can be minimized only by continued and focused clinical and laboratory research in this area.

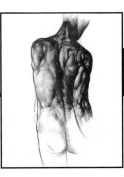

ADDITIONAL CLINICAL CONNECTIONS

CLINICAL CONNECTION 10-1
A Closer Look at the Spinal Stabilizing Functions of Selected Abdominal Muscles and the Lumbar Multifidi

The following discussion highlights examples of spinal stabilization functions performed by the abdominal muscles (most notably the transversus abdominis and internal oblique) and the multifidi. These muscles are featured primarily because of the large body of research that has focused on their ability (or lack thereof) to stabilize the lumbopelvic region of the trunk (which includes the lumbar spine, lumbosacral junction, and sacroiliac joints).[4,142] The topic of lumbopelvic muscular stabilization has attracted the attention of researchers and clinicians primarily because of the high incidence of instability and stress-related degeneration in this region.

ABDOMINAL MUSCLES: Much of what is known about the kinesiology of the muscular stabilizers of the lumbopelvic region is based on electromyographic (EMG) research, often with the use of fine-wire (needle) electrodes. One common methodology used in this research involves the recording of the order in which various trunk muscles respond to expected or unexpected whole-body perturbations. As an example, Figure 10-37, *A* shows the onset of the EMG responses of a selected set of abdominal muscles as a healthy, pain-free person rapidly flexes his arm after a visual stimulus.[142] The top EMG signal (depicted in red) is from a shoulder flexor—the anterior deltoid—and the remaining EMG signals are from the *external oblique,* the middle and lower regions of the *internal oblique,* and the upper, middle, and lower regions of the *transversus abdominis.* All muscles recorded from this one subject responded at slightly different times (indicated by vertical arrows) relative to the initiation of the deltoid's EMG signal (red dashed line). Figure 10-37, *B* shows the overall data from the experiment, based on 11 healthy subjects.[72]

As previously discovered through research in this area, the lower and middle fibers of the transversus abdominis and internal oblique muscles consistently activate *before* the activation of the deltoid muscle.[141] This anticipatory muscle response is believed to be a subconscious, feedforward mechanism employed by the

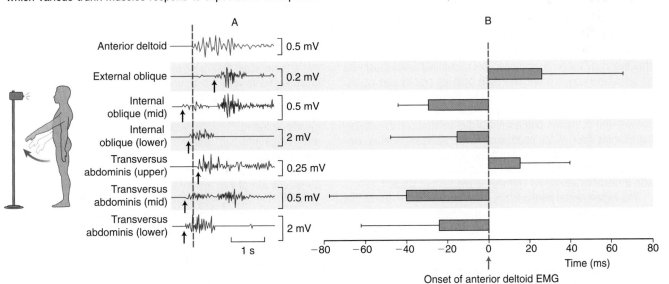

FIGURE 10-37. A, The electromyographic (EMG) responses are shown from selected abdominal muscles as a healthy person rapidly flexes his arm after a visual stimulus. The different onset times of EMG signals from the abdominal muscles *(vertical dark arrows)* are compared with the onset of the EMG signal from the anterior deltoid *(red),* a shoulder flexor muscle. **B,** The overall results of the experiment are shown, averaged across 110 trials in 11 healthy subjects. (Data redrawn from Urquhart DM, Hodges PW, Story IH: Postural activity of the abdominal muscles varies between regions of these muscles and between body positions, *Gait Posture* 22:295, 2005.)

Continued

ADDITIONAL CLINICAL CONNECTIONS

CLINICAL CONNECTION 10-1
A Closer Look at the Spinal Stabilizing Functions of Selected Abdominal Muscles and the Lumbar Multifidi–cont'd

nervous system to minimize reactive countermovements of the trunk.[142] Although subtle and not completely understood, this anticipatory muscular response may help protect the lumbopelvic region from potentially damaging shear forces.[5]

It is interesting that multiple regions of the transversus abdominis and internal oblique activate at different times in response to the rapidly elevated arm. It is as though the different regions within these muscles respond as distinct anatomic entities. Although separated by only a very short time period, the sequential muscular responses provide insight into the complex stabilizing functions of these muscles. Consider, in this regard, the following proposed functions for each of the three regions of the transversus abdominis.[124,131,142] Contraction of the *upper fibers* of the transversus abdominis may help stabilize the rib cage and linea alba. The *lower fibers* are believed to compress and thereby help stabilize the sacroiliac joints.[68] Contraction of the *middle fibers* of the transversus abdominis transfers tension directly to the lumbar spinous processes and sacrum by connections into the thoracolumbar fascia (see Chapter 9). This action is part of the "corset" effect described earlier in this chapter for this muscle.

Furthermore, bilateral contraction of the *middle fibers* of the transversus abdominis is particularly effective (along with other abdominal muscles) at compressing the abdominal cavity and thereby increasing intra-abdominal pressure (described earlier as the Valsalva maneuver). Evidence exists that the rise in intra-abdominal pressure not only exerts a modest extension torque on the lumbar spine, but also stabilizes the region.[67,68] For the most effective stabilization, the cylinder-like abdominal cavity must also be simultaneously compressed from both its cranial and caudal ends. This is normally accomplished by concurrent activation and descent of the diaphragm muscle—the roof of the abdominal cavity—and activation and ascent of the pelvic floor muscles—the ultimate floor of the abdominal cavity. Although sparse, evidence does exist from both animal and human subjects that these muscular interactions do indeed occur in a coordinated manner, with a resulting increased stiffness in the lumbar spine.[70]

The experimental methodology illustrated in Figure 10-37 has also been used to study the sequential activation of the abdominal muscles in response to rapidly flexing the *lower* limb.[72] Consistently, the abdominal muscles (including the rectus abdominis) respond *before* the activation of the hip flexor muscles. It is interesting that the transversus abdominis and internal oblique are consistently the first of the trunk muscles to respond, on average 50 to 100 msec before the hip flexor muscles. This activation pattern of the abdominal muscles, as a group, reflects their need to stabilize the lower trunk during the leg movement, as well as to fixate the lumbopelvic region against the pull of the contracting hip flexor muscles. The transversus abdominis and the oblique abdominal muscles also respond before rapid active hip *abduction* and *extension* movements as well. These abdominal muscles appear "dedicated" to stabilizing the lower trunk, regardless of the direction of the forces produced by the contracting hip musculature.

Hodges and colleagues used a similar experimental protocol to study the sequential muscle activation in persons with chronic low back pain.[71,110,123] Remarkably, this research showed a consistent, short delay in the onset of EMG signals from the transversus abdominis—the activation of this muscle occurring most often *after* the activation of the prime movers of the rapid limb motion. Whether a short delay in abdominal muscle activation can create sufficient reactive stress in the lumbopelvic region to ultimately cause low-back pain is not known, although it is an intriguing question. Cadaveric studies have indeed shown that axial rotation of as little as 2 to 3 degrees per intervertebral lumbar junction can potentially injure the apophyseal and interbody joints (see Chapter 9). A single "unprotected" stress event may not be significant; however, multiple events that accumulate over many years may predispose the region to injury.

LUMBAR MULTIFIDI: Research has shown that in addition to the transversus abdominis and internal oblique muscles, the *lumbar multifidi* are consistently recruited early in healthy persons in response to various perturbations imposed against the body.[27,57,88,89,154] The multifidi are extremely capable stabilizers of the lumbar spine, especially in the lower segments.[21,149] The muscles' regional extensor strength is augmented by their relatively large size; they account for about one third of the total cross-sectional area of all deep paraspinal muscles at the L4 level.[23,98] In addition to their thickness, the multifidi also have a highly segmented morphology and innervation and are rich with muscle spindles.[103,123,154] These anatomic features favor precise and, when needed, authoritative control over intersegmental lumbar stability.*

The lumbar multifidi have consistently shown preferential and persistent atrophy in persons with acute or chronic low-back pain.[63,96] This finding is noteworthy, considering the muscles' proposed importance in stabilizing the lumbar region. The amount of atrophy in the lumbar multifidi is striking; a 30% reduction in cross-sectional area has been reported,[64] in some cases within days of the onset of the painful symptoms.[66] The reason for preferential atrophy in these muscles is uncertain. Evidence suggests several explanations, however, ranging from denervation after nerve root injury to reflexive neural inhibition after trauma to the disc or capsule of the apophyseal joints.[21]

---

*References 21, 40, 62, 66, 75, 91.

ADDITIONAL CLINICAL CONNECTIONS

Marked and persisting atrophy of the lumbar multifidi has also been demonstrated in *pain-free* healthy subjects who were subjected to 8 weeks of strict bed rest.[16,123] Of particular interest was the response of a subgroup of the subjects who, while remaining on strict bed rest, were allowed to exercise twice daily (performing resistive exercise in conjunction with receiving whole-body vibration). These subjects demonstrated statistically less multifidi atrophy, and the atrophy did not persist as long as in the inactive, control group of subjects. It appears that the lumbar multifidi are particularly sensitive to musculoskeletal pathology in the lumbar region, as well as reduced weight bearing through the axial skeleton. Regardless of the underlying mechanism, it is reasonable to assume that marked and prolonged atrophy of these muscles reduces the mechanical stability of the lumbar spine, potentially leaving it vulnerable to stress-related injury. For this reason, exercises designed for the treatment of persons with low-back pain often incorporate specific exercises to strengthen the lumbar multifidi.[14,47,63]

ADDITIONAL CLINICAL CONNECTIONS

CLINICAL CONNECTION 10-2
Therapeutic Exercise as a Way to Improve Lumbopelvic Stability: a Brief Overview

A significant percentage of the stress-related musculoskeletal pathology of the trunk occurs at the lumbopelvic region. This region includes the lumbar spine, lumbosacral junction, and the sacroiliac joints. The term *lumbopelvic instability* has evolved to describe a painful, usually nonspecific, condition that is associated with hypermobility at one or more of the articulated segments.[156] The amount of hypermobility may be slight and difficult to quantify through routine clinical assessment. This condition, nevertheless, is believed capable of generating excessive stress on spinal-related structures, including the interbody, apophyseal joint and sacroiliac joints, spinal ligaments, and neural tissues. Persons often seek medical attention when pain occurs with movement in the region. The clinical picture of this condition is often complicated by the uncertainty regarding whether lumbopelvic instability is the *cause* or the *effect* of other impairments in the low back, such as degenerative disc disease.*

Weakness, fatigue, or the inability to specifically control the timing or magnitude of forces produced by the trunk muscles has long been suspected as a potential cause, or at least an associated factor, in the pathogenesis of lumbopelvic instability. For this reason, specific muscular-based exercises are often considered an essential component of conservative treatment for this condition. It is beyond the scope of this chapter to describe the details or varying effectiveness of the many types of exercises designed to improve muscular-based lumbopelvic stability; this information can be found in other sources.† The following box, however, lists four themes that tend to be emphasized with this therapeutic approach. It is important to note that exercises of any kind may not be appropriate in cases of specific *structural* instability of the lumbopelvic region (such as acute or significant spondylolisthesis), acute disc herniation, or any conditions involving marked pain or deteriorating neurologic symptoms.

---

*References 16, 19, 51, 58, 92, 97, 123.

---

†References 4, 61, 67, 69, 138, 146.

The following four themes tend to be emphasized when designing exercises to improve the muscular-based stability of the lumbopelvic region.

1. Train persons how to *selectively activate deeper stabilizers* of the trunk, most notably the lumbar multifidi, transversus abdominis, and internal oblique. Activation of these muscles appears particularly important for establishing a baseline stability of the lumbopelvic region, especially in advance of unexpected or sudden movements of the trunk or extremities.[71,72,123] The literature suggests that some persons with low-back pain have difficulty selectively activating these muscles, especially while maintaining a neutral position of the lumbar spine.[61] As a part of the initial treatment, some clinicians attempt to instruct persons to "draw in" (or hollow) the abdomen, an action performed almost exclusively by bilateral contraction of the transversus abdominis and internal oblique.[26,59,60,115,144] Teaching subjects to selectively activate these deeper muscles can be enhanced by using feedback supplied by rehabilitation real-time ultrasound imaging.[16,60,123,137] Once a subject has learned to selectively activate these muscles, the next step is to maintain the activation during the performance of other abdominal exercises or during activities of daily living——a concept referred to as "core awareness."[28,35,36,138,148] Such awareness needs to be maintained as more challenging resistive exercises are applied to the other important stabilizing muscles of the trunk and lower extremities.[130]

2. Design resistive exercises that *challenge a wide range* of muscles of the trunk. Optimal stability of the trunk is based on an interaction of both the intrinsic and extrinsic muscular stabilizers.[15,47] Lumbopelvic stability, in particular, requires activation from deeper segmental muscles, but also from the transversus abdominis and more superficial muscles such as the quadratus lumborum, psoas major, rectus abdominis, and oblique abdominals.

3. Design resistive exercises that favor an increase not only in muscle strength (i.e., peak force production) but also in *muscle endurance*. During most routine activities, only modest levels of muscle force are required to establish a baseline of core stability of the lumbopelvic region.[102] Although this level of muscular effort may be relatively low, it typically must be sustained over several hours. Injuries to the spine likely occur more often if the surrounding muscles are fatigued.

4. Provide exercises that challenge *postural control, equilibrium, and positional awareness of the body as a whole*.[46] Some persons with chronic low-back pain have shown reduced proprioception (position sense) of the lumbopelvic region and reduced standing balance, compared with healthy controls. Whether these deficits are related to each other and to the cause of low-back pain is not known. Some authors assert that the deficits may be related to delayed muscle reaction times coupled with impaired neuromuscular feedback.[48]

ADDITIONAL CLINICAL CONNECTIONS

CLINICAL CONNECTION 10-3
Torticollis and Sleeping Position: Is There a Link?

Torticollis (from the Latin *tortus,* twisted, + *collum,* neck) or "wryneck" typically describes a pathologic condition of chronic shortening of the sternocleidomastoid muscle. The condition, generally identified in the young child or infant, may be congenital or acquired. A child or infant with torticollis typically has an asymmetric craniocervical posture that reflects the primary actions of the tightened muscle. The child illustrated in Figure 10-38 has a tight left sternocleidomastoid (see arrow), with a corresponding posture of slight left lateral flexion combined with right axial rotation of his craniocervical region.

The incidence of torticollis is 0.4% to 3.9% of newborn infants in the United States.[32,43] The range of these estimates reflects different methods for detecting the condition. The underlying cause of torticollis most often involves muscle tissue, although it may involve nonmuscular systems. The far more common muscular-based torticollis usually involves fibrous growths within the sternocleidomastoid—a condition termed *idiopathic muscular fibrosis.*[43] Although the exact cause of this condition is unknown, it is frequently associated with a difficult childbirth labor, breech delivery, or intrauterine malpositioning or crowding.[32] The more serious, non–muscular-based torticollis involves pathology associated with the nervous system (including vision) or the skeletal system (typically associated with cervical dysplasia).[43]

Approximately one third of infants with torticollis also develop *plagiocephaly.*[43] This condition is an abnormal molding and subsequent distortion in the shape of a young infant's naturally soft cranium. The distorted shape is typically caused by the infant's head resting in a single prolonged position against another surface. Some authors believe that an infant with an *existing* torticollis may develop a secondary plagiocephaly (involving the posterior-lateral cranium) before or shortly after birth, as a result of the prolonged and concentrated contact against the infant's rotated cranium. Alternately, other authors assert that an infant born *free of* torticollis may eventually develop plagiocephaly with a secondary torticollis simply because of a favored rotated position of the head while the infant sleeps in a supine position.[2] Once developed, the positional plagiocephaly strongly reinforces the established asymmetric (rotated) head position adapted for sleeping. The constant rotated position of the head produces a chronic slackening of the contralateral sternocleidomastoid, which eventually develops into a contracture and the classic expression of torticollis. According to deChalain, many infants who develop torticollis after plagiocephaly do not have fibrotic changes in the tightened sternocleidomastoid muscle; the deformity develops purely as a consequence of muscle tightness caused by the abnormal craniocervical positioning.[43,155]

The notion that plagiocephaly can, in some cases, lead to a positional torticollis was reinforced by a series of events that occurred in the 1990s. Within this decade, the American Academy of Pediatrics published recommendations that healthy infants be placed in a supine position for sleeping as a way to reduce the incidence of sudden infant death syndrome (SIDS).[155] The so-called "*back*-to-sleep" recommendation had a dramatic effect on the sleeping pattern of many infants in the United States. The incidence of infants positioned prone for sleep decreased by 66% from 1992 to 1996.[9,139] Although a direct cause-and-effect relationship cannot be unequivocally stated, the rate of SIDS declined approximately 38% during this same time period.[43] The remarkable and simultaneous decline in the incidence of SIDS nevertheless strongly reinforced the fundamental premise of the "back-to-sleep" campaign. Subsequent evidence strongly suggests that the increased frequency of supine-only sleeping has also led to an increase in the incidence of positional plagiocephaly, most notably affecting the posterior-lateral cranium.[79] Furthermore, additional data show that the dramatic increase in positional plagiocephaly has led to a parallel increase in positional torticollis.[119]

Without a doubt, the huge and life-saving success of the "back-to-sleep" campaign of the 1990s far outweighs the poten-

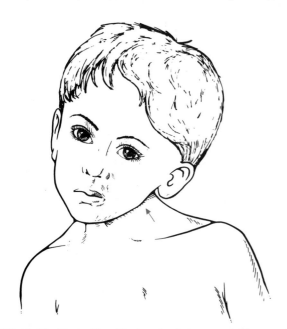

FIGURE 10-38. Torticollis affecting the left sternocleidomastoid of a young boy *(arrow).* Note the posture of slight left lateral flexion combined with right axial rotation of his craniocervical region. (From Herring JA: *Tachdjian's pediatric orthopaedics,* ed 3, Philadelphia, 2002, Saunders.)

Continued

ADDITIONAL CLINICAL CONNECTIONS

CLINICAL CONNECTION 10-3
Torticollis and Sleeping Position: Is There a Link?—cont'd

tial negative consequence caused by the increased incidence of plagiocephaly and secondary torticollis. Efforts are ongoing to minimize the incidence of the latter two conditions. Clinicians have advised parents or guardians to alternate the head position of the supine-positioned infant.[41,54,77,126] Clinicians also advocate that parents or guardians set aside short periods of supervised and interactive "prone-play" (or "tummy time") with the infant, while still strictly adhering to the "back-to-sleep" principle.[33] Encouraging more prone-lying while infants are awake will very likely

reduce the likelihood of developing the plagiocephaly (and secondary torticollis), and may also facilitate the infant's natural motor development.[33]

Regardless of the exact cause of torticollis, parents or guardians of a child with torticollis need to be instructed in how to stretch the tight muscle and how to position and handle the child to promote elongation of the involved muscle. In severe cases of contracture, the muscle may be surgically released.

REFERENCES

1. National Institute for Occupational Safety and Health (NIOSH): Work Practices Guide for Manual Lifting, Report No. 81-122, Cincinnati, Ohio, NIOSH 1992.
2. American Academy of Pediatrics Task Force on Infant Positioning and SIDS: Positioning and sudden infant death syndrome (SIDS): update, *Pediatrics* 98:1216-1218, 1996.
3. Adams MA, Dolan P: A technique for quantifying the bending moment acting on the lumbar spine in vivo, *J Biomech* 24:117-126, 1991.
4. Akuthota V, Ferreiro A, Moore T, Fredericson M: Core stability exercise principles, *Curr Sports Med Rep* 7:39-44, 2008.
5. Allison GT, Morris SL, Lay B: Feedforward responses of transversus abdominis are directionally specific and act asymmetrically: implications for core stability theories, *J Orthop Sports Phys Ther* 38:228-237, 2008.
6. Anderson JS, Hsu AW, Vasavada AN: Morphology, architecture, and biomechanics of human cervical multifidus, *Spine* 30:E86-E91, 2005.
7. Andersson EA, Grundstrom H, Thorstensson A: Diverging intramuscular activity patterns in back and abdominal muscles during trunk rotation, *Spine* 27:E152-E160, 2002.
8. Andersson EA, Nilsson J, Ma Z, Thorstensson A: Abdominal and hip flexor muscle activation during various training exercises, *Eur J Appl Physiol Occup Physiol* 75:115-123, 1997.
9. Argenta LC, David LR, Wilson JA, Bell WO: An increase in infant cranial deformity with supine sleeping position, *J Craniofac Surg* 7:5-11, 1996.
10. Arjmand N, Shirazi-Adl A: Biomechanics of changes in lumbar posture in static lifting, *Spine* 30:2637-2648, 2005.
11. Arjmand N, Shirazi-Adl A: Role of intra-abdominal pressure in the unloading and stabilization of the human spine during static lifting tasks, *Eur Spine J* 15:1265-1275, 2006.
12. Arjmand N, Shirazi-Adl A, Parnianpour M: Trunk biomechanics during maximum isometric axial torque exertions in upright standing, *Clin Biomech (Bristol, Avon)* 23:969-978, 2008.
13. Aspden RM: Intra-abdominal pressure and its role in spinal mechanics, *Clin Biomech (Bristol, Avon)* 2:168-174, 1987.
14. Ballock RT, Song KM: The prevalence of nonmuscular causes of torticollis in children, *J Pediatr Orthop* 16:500-504, 1996.
15. Barr KP, Griggs M, Cadby T: Lumbar stabilization: core concepts and current literature, Part 1, *Am J Phys Med Rehabil* 84:473-480, 2005.
16. Barr KP, Griggs M, Cadby T: Lumbar stabilization: a review of core concepts and current literature, Part 2, *Am J Phys Med Rehabil* 86:72-80, 2007.
17. Bartelink DL: The role of abdominal pressure in relieving the pressure on the lumbar intervertebral discs, *J Bone Joint Surg Br* 39:718-725, 1957.
18. Bazrgari B, Shirazi-Adl A, Arjmand N: Analysis of squat and stoop dynamic liftings: muscle forces and internal spinal loads, *Eur Spine J* 16:687-699, 2007.
19. Beattie PF: Current understanding of lumbar intervertebral disc degeneration: a review with emphasis upon etiology, pathophysiology, and lumbar magnetic resonance imaging findings, *J Orthop Sports Phys Ther* 38:329-340, 2008.
20. Beimborn DS, Morrissey MC: A review of the literature related to trunk muscle performance, *Spine* 13:655-660, 1988.
21. Belavý DL, Hides JA, Wilson SJ, et al: Resistive simulated weightbearing exercise with whole body vibration reduces lumbar spine deconditioning in bed-rest, *Spine* 33:E121-E131, 2008.
22. Bergmark A: Stability of the lumbar spine. A study in mechanical engineering, *Acta Orthop Scand Suppl* 230:1-54, 1989.
23. Bogduk N: *Clinical Anatomy of the Lumbar Spine and Sacrum*, ed 4, New York, 2005, Churchill Livingstone.
24. Bogduk N, Macintosh JE: The applied anatomy of the thoracolumbar fascia, *Spine* 9:164-170, 1984.
25. Boyd-Clark LC, Briggs CA, Galea MP: Muscle spindle distribution, morphology, and density in longus colli and multifidus muscles of the cervical spine, *Spine* 27:694-701, 2002.
26. Brenner AK, Gill NW, Buscema CJ, Kiesel K: Improved activation of lumbar multifidus following spinal manipulation: a case report applying rehabilitative ultrasound imaging, *J Orthop Sports Phys Ther* 37:613-619, 2007.
27. Briggs AM, Greig AM, Bennell KL, Hodges PW: Paraspinal muscle control in people with osteoporotic vertebral fracture, *Eur Spine J* 16:1137-1144, 2007.
28. Brown SH, Vera-Garcia FJ, McGill SM: Effects of abdominal muscle coactivation on the externally preloaded trunk: variations in motor control and its effect on spine stability, *Spine* 31:E387-E393, 2006.
29. Buford JA, Yoder SM, Heiss DG, Chidley JV: Actions of the scalene muscles for rotation of the cervical spine in macaque and human, *J Orthop Sports Phys Ther* 32:488-496, 2002.
30. Butler HL, Hubley-Kozey CL, Kozey JW: Changes in trunk muscle activation and lumbar-pelvic position associated with abdominal hollowing and reach during a simulated manual material handling task, *Ergonomics* 50:410-425, 2007.
31. Chaffin DB, Andersson GBJ: *Occupational Biomechanics*, 2nd ed, New York, 1991, John Wiley and Sons.
32. Chen MM, Chang HC, Hsieh CF, et al: Predictive model for congenital muscular torticollis: analysis of 1021 infants with sonography, *Arch Phys Med Rehabil* 86:2199-2203, 2005.
33. Cheng JC, Wong MW, Tang SP, et al: Clinical determinants of the outcome of manual stretching in the treatment of congenital muscular torticollis in infants. A prospective study of eight hundred and twenty-one cases, *J Bone Joint Surg Am* 83:679-687, 2001.
34. Cholewicki J, McGill SM: Lumbar posterior ligament involvement during extremely heavy lifts estimated from fluoroscopic measurements, *J Biomech* 25:17-28, 1992.
35. Cholewicki J, Reeves NP: All abdominal muscles must be considered when evaluating the intra-abdominal pressure contribution to trunk extensor moment and spinal loading, *J Biomech* 37:953-954, 2004.
36. Cholewicki J, VanVliet JJ: Relative contribution of trunk muscles to the stability of the lumbar spine during isometric exertions, *Clin Biomech (Bristol, Avon)* 17:99-105, 2002.
37. Cook TM, Neumann DA: The effects of load placement on the EMG activity of the low back muscles during load carrying by men and women, *Ergonomics* 30:1413-1423, 1987.
38. Cresswell AG, Grundstrom H, Thorstensson A: Observations on intra-abdominal pressure and patterns of abdominal intra-muscular activity in man, *Acta Physiol Scand* 144:409-418, 1992.
39. Cutter N: *Handbook of Manual Muscle Testing*, St Louis, 1999, McGraw-Hill.
40. Danneels LA, Vanderstraeten GG, Cambier DC, et al: CT imaging of trunk muscles in chronic low back pain patients and healthy control subjects, *Eur Spine J* 9:266-272, 2000.
41. Davis BE, Moon RY, Sachs HC, Ottolini MC: Effects of sleep position on infant motor development, *Pediatrics* 102:1135-1140, 1998.
42. Dawson AP, McLennan SN, Schiller SD, et al: Interventions to prevent back pain and back injury in nurses: a systematic review, *Occup Environ Med* 64:642-650, 2007.
43. de Chalain TM, Park S: Torticollis associated with positional plagiocephaly: a growing epidemic, *J Craniofac Surg* 16:411-418, 2005.
44. Deng YC, Goldsmith W: Response of a human head/neck/upper-torso replica to dynamic loading–I. Physical model, *J Biomech* 20:471-486, 1987.
45. Dolan P, Mannion AF, Adams MA: Passive tissues help the back muscles to generate extensor moments during lifting, *J Biomech* 27:1077-1085, 1994.
46. Ebenbichler GR, Oddsson LI, Kollmitzer J, Erim Z: Sensory-motor control of the lower back: implications for rehabilitation, *Med Sci Sport Exerc* 33:1889-1898, 2001.
47. Ekstrom RA, Osborn RW, Hauer PL: Surface electromyographic analysis of the low back muscles during rehabilitation exercises, *J Orthop Sports Phys Ther* 38:736-745, 2008.
48. Escamilla RF, Babb E, DeWitt R et al: Electromyographic analysis of traditional and nontraditional abdominal exercises: implications for rehabilitation and training, *Phys Ther* 86:656-671, 2006.
49. Falla D, Jull G, Russell T, et al: Effect of neck exercise on sitting posture in patients with chronic neck pain, *Phys Ther* 87:408-417, 2007.
50. Ferguson SA, Marras WS: A literature review of low back disorder surveillance measures and risk factors, *Clin Biomech (Bristol, Avon)* 12:211-226, 1997.
51. Ferreira PH, Ferreira ML, Maher CG, et al: Specific stabilisation exercise for spinal and pelvic pain: a systematic review, *Aust J Physiother* 52:79-88, 2006.
52. Fujishiro K, Weaver JL, Heaney CA, et al: The effect of ergonomic interventions in healthcare facilities on musculoskeletal disorders, *Am J Ind Med* 48:338-347, 2005.
53. Gracovetsky S, Farfan HF, Lamy C: The mechanism of the lumbar spine, *Spine* 6:249-262, 1981.

54. Graham JM Jr: Tummy time is important, *Clin Pediatr* 45:119-121, 2006.

55. Grenier SG, McGill SM: Quantification of lumbar stability by using 2 different abdominal activation strategies, *Arch Phys Med Rehabil* 88: 54-62, 2007.

56. Halpern AA, Bleck EE: Sit-up exercises: an electromyographic study, *Clin Orthop Relat Res* 145:172-178, 1979.

57. Hansen L, de ZM, Rasmussen J, et al: Anatomy and biomechanics of the back muscles in the lumbar spine with reference to biomechanical modeling, *Spine* 31:1888-1899, 2006.

58. Hayden JA, van Tulder MW, Malmivaara A, Koes BW: Exercise therapy for treatment of non-specific low back pain, *Cochrane Database Syst Rev* 20;(3):CD000335, 2005 Jul.

59. Henry SM, Teyhen DS: Ultrasound imaging as a feedback tool in the rehabilitation of trunk muscle dysfunction for people with low back pain, *J Orthop Sports Phys Ther* 37:627-634, 2007.

60. Herbert WJ, Heiss DG, Basso DM: Influence of feedback schedule in motor performance and learning of a lumbar multifidus muscle task using rehabilitative ultrasound imaging: a randomized clinical trial, *Phys Ther* 88:261-269, 2008.

61. Hides J, Wilson S, Stanton W, et al: An MRI investigation into the function of the transversus abdominis muscle during "drawing-in" of the abdominal wall, *Spine* 31:E175-E178, 2006.

62. Hides JA, Richardson CA, Jull GA: Multifidus muscle recovery is not automatic after resolution of acute, first-episode low back pain, *Spine* 21:2763-2769, 1996.

63. Hides JA, Stanton WR, McMahon S, et al: Effect of stabilization training on multifidus muscle cross-sectional area among young elite cricketers with low back pain, *J Orthop Sports Phys Ther* 38:101-108, 2008.

64. Hides JA, Stokes MJ, Saide M, et al: Evidence of lumbar multifidus muscle wasting ipsilateral to symptoms in patients with acute/subacute low back pain, *Spine* 19:165-172, 1994.

65. Hislop HJ, Montgomery J: *Daniel's and Worthingham's Muscle Testing*, 6th ed, Philadelphia, 1995, Saunders.

66. Hodges P, Holm AK, Hansson T, Holm S: Rapid atrophy of the lumbar multifidus follows experimental disc or nerve root injury, *Spine* 31:2926-2933, 2006.

67. Hodges P, Kaigle HA, Holm S, et al: Intervertebral stiffness of the spine is increased by evoked contraction of transversus abdominis and the diaphragm: in vivo porcine studies, *Spine* 28:2594-2601, 2003.

68. Hodges PW, Cresswell AG, Daggfeldt K, Thorstensson A: In vivo measurement of the effect of intra-abdominal pressure on the human spine, *J Biomech* 34:347-353, 2001.

69. Hodges PW, Cresswell AG, Thorstensson A: Perturbed upper limb movements cause short-latency postural responses in trunk muscles, *Exp Brain Res* 138:243-250, 2001.

70. Hodges PW, Richardson CA: Contraction of the abdominal muscles associated with movement of the lower limb, *Phys Ther* 77:132-142, 1997.

71. Hodges PW, Richardson CA: Feedforward contraction of transversus abdominis is not influenced by the direction of arm movement, *Exp Brain Res* 114:362-370, 1997.

72. Hodges PW, Richardson CA: Inefficient muscular stabilization of the lumbar spine associated with low back pain. A motor control evaluation of transversus abdominis, *Spine* 21:2640-2650, 1996.

73. Hoek van Dijke GA, Snijders CJ, Stoeckart R, Stam HJ: A biomechanical model on muscle forces in the transfer of spinal load to the pelvis and legs, *J Biomech* 32:927-933, 1999.

74. Hoogendoorn WE, Bongers PM, de Vet HC, et al: Flexion and rotation of the trunk and lifting at work are risk factors for low back pain: results of a prospective cohort study, *Spine* 25:3087-3092, 2000.

75. Hyun JK, Lee JY, Lee SJ, Jeon JY: Asymmetric atrophy of multifidus muscle in patients with unilateral lumbosacral radiculopathy, *Spine* 32:E598-E602, 2007.

76. Jager M, Luttmann A: The load on the lumbar spine during asymmetrical bi-manual materials handling, *Ergonomics* 35:783-805, 1992.

77. Jantz JW, Blosser CD, Fruechting LA: A motor milestone change noted with a change in sleep position, *Arch Pediatr Adolesc Med* 151:565-568, 1997.

78. Johnston V, Jull G, Souvlis T, Jimmieson NL: Neck movement and muscle activity characteristics in female office workers with neck pain, *Spine* 33:555-563, 2008.

79. Jones MW: The other side of "back to sleep." *Neonatal Netw* 22:49-53, 2003.

80. Jordan A, Mehlsen J, Bülow PM, et al: Maximal isometric strength of the cervical musculature in 100 healthy volunteers, *Spine* 24:1343-1348, 1999.

81. Jorgensen MJ, Marras WS, Gupta P, Waters TR: Effect of torso flexion on the lumbar torso extensor muscle sagittal plane moment arms, *Spine* 3:363-369, 2003.

82. Juker D, McGill S, Kropf P, Steffen T: Quantitative intramuscular myoelectric activity of lumbar portions of psoas and the abdominal wall during a wide variety of tasks, *Med Sci Sports Exerc* 30:301-310, 1998.

83. Kapandji IA: *The physiology of the joints*, 5 ed, Edinburgh, 1982, Churchill Livingstone.

84. Kavcic N, Grenier S, McGill SM: Determining the stabilizing role of individual torso muscles during rehabilitation exercises, *Spine* 29:1254-1265, 2004.

85. Kelsey JL: The epidemiology of diseases of the hip: a review of the literature, *Int J Epidemiol* 6:269-280, 1977.

86. Kendall FP, McCreary AK, Provance PG: *Muscles: Testing and function*, 4th ed, Baltimore, 1993, Williams & Wilkins.

87. Kettler A, Hartwig E, Schultheiss M, et al: Mechanically simulated muscle forces strongly stabilize intact and injured upper cervical spine specimens, *J Biomech* 35:339-346, 2002.

88. Kiefer A, Shirazi-Adl A, Parnianpour M: Stability of the human spine in neutral postures, *Eur Spine J* 6:45-53, 1997.

89. Kiefer A, Shirazi-Adl A, Parnianpour M: Synergy of the human spine in neutral postures, *Eur Spine J* 7:471-479, 1998.

90. Kingma I, Faber GS, Suwarganda EK, et al: Effect of a stiff lifting belt on spine compression during lifting, *Spine* 31:E833-E839, 2006.

91. Kjaer P, Bendix T, Sorensen JS, et al: Are MRI-defined fat infiltrations in the multifidus muscles associated with low back pain? *BMC Medicine* 5:2, 2007.

92. Koumantakis GA, Watson PJ, Oldham JA: Trunk muscle stabilization training plus general exercise versus general exercise only: randomized controlled trial of patients with recurrent low back pain, *Phys Ther* 85:209-225, 2005.

93. Krakenes J, Kaale BR: Magnetic resonance imaging assessment of craniovertebral ligaments and membranes after whiplash trauma, *Spine* 31:2820-2826, 2006.

94. Kuijer W, Dijkstra PU, Brouwer S, et al: Safe lifting in patients with chronic low back pain: comparing FCE lifting task and NIOSH lifting guideline, *J Occup Rehabil* 16:579-589, 2006.

95. Kumar, S: Moment arms of spinal musculature determined from CT scans, *Clin Biomech (Bristol, Avon)* 3:137-144, 1988.

96. Laasonen EM: Atrophy of sacrospinal muscle groups in patients with chronic, diffusely radiating lumbar back pain, *Neuroradiology* 26:9-13, 1984.

97. Liddle SD, Baxter GD, Gracey JH: Exercise and chronic low back pain: what works? *Pain* 107:176-190, 2004.

98. Macintosh JE, Bogduk, N: The biomechanics of the lumbar multifidus, *Clin Biomech (Bristol, Avon)* 1:205-213, 1986.

99. Macintosh JE, Bogduk N, Gracovetsky S: The biomechanics of the thoracolumbar fascia, *Clin Biomech (Bristol, Avon)* 2:78-83, 1987.

100. Macintosh JE, Valenica F, Bogduk N: The morphology of the human lumbar multifidus, *Clin Biomech* 1:196-204, 1986.

101. Martimo KP, Verbeek J, Karppinen J, et al: Manual material handling advice and assistive devices for preventing and treating back pain in workers. *Cochrane Database Syst Rev* 3:CD005958, 2007.

102. McGill SM: Biomechanics of the thoracolumbar spine. In Dvir Z, editor: *Clinical biomechanics*, Philadelphia, 2000, Churchill Livingstone.

103. McGill SM: Kinetic potential of the lumbar trunk musculature about three orthogonal orthopaedic axes in extreme postures, *Spine* 16:809-815, 1991.

104. McGill SM, Hughson RL, Parks K: Changes in lumbar lordosis modify the role of the extensor muscles, *Clin Biomech (Bristol, Avon)* 15:777-780, 2000.

105. McGill SM, Norman RW: Reassessment of the role of intra-abdominal pressure in spinal compression, *Ergonomics* 30:1565-1588, 1987.

106. McGill SM, Patt N, Norman RW: Measurement of the trunk musculature of active males using CT scan radiography: implications for force and moment generating capacity about the L4/L5 joint, *J Biomech* 21:329-341, 1988.

107. McGill SM, Santaguida L, Stevens J: Measurement of the trunk musculature from T5 to L5 using MRI scans of 15 young males corrected for muscle fibre orientation, *Clin Biomech (Bristol, Avon)* 8:171-178, 1993.

108. McLean L: The effect of postural correction on muscle activation amplitudes recorded from the cervicobrachial region, *J Electromyogr Kinesiol* 15:527-535, 2005.

109. Moroney SP, Schultz AB, Miller JA: Analysis and measurement of neck loads, *J Orthop Res* 6:713-720, 1988.

110. Moseley GL, Hodges PW, Gandevia SC: External perturbation of the trunk in standing humans differentially activates components of the medial back muscles, *J Physiol* 547:581-587, 2003.

111. Nachemson AL, Andersson BJ, Schultz AB: Valsalva maneuver biomechanics. Effects on lumbar trunk loads of elevated intraabdominal pressures, *Spine* 11:476-479, 1986.

112. National Institute for Occupational Safety and Health (NIOSH): The National Occupational Exposure Survey. Report No. 89-103. 1989. Cincinnati, NIOSH, 1989.

113. Nitz AJ, Peck D: Comparison of muscle spindle concentrations in large and small human epaxial muscles acting in parallel combinations, *Am Surg* 52:273-277, 1986.

114. Nordin M, Kahanovitz N, Verderame R, et al: Normal trunk muscle strength and endurance in women and the effect of exercises and electrical stimulation. Part 1: Normal endurance and trunk muscle strength in 101 women, *Spine* 12:105-111, 1987.

115. Oh JS, Cynn HS, Won JH, et al: Effects of performing an abdominal drawing-in maneuver during prone hip extension exercises on hip and back extensor muscle activity and amount of anterior pelvic tilt, *J Orthop Sports Phys Ther* 37:320-324, 2007.

116. Panjabi MM, Cholewicki J, Nibu K, et al: Critical load of the human cervical spine: an in vitro experimental study, *Clin Biomech (Bristol, Avon)* 13:11-17, 1998.

117. Panjabi MM, Ivancic PC, Maak TG, et al: Multiplanar cervical spine injury due to head-turned rear impact, *Spine* 31:420-429, 2006.

118. Patwardhan AG, Havey RM, Ghanayem AJ, et al: Load-carrying capacity of the human cervical spine in compression is increased under a follower load, *Spine* 25:1548-1554, 2000.

119. Persing J, James H, Swanson J, et al: Prevention and management of positional skull deformities in infants. American Academy of Pediatrics Committee on Practice and Ambulatory Medicine, Section on Plastic Surgery and Section on Neurological Surgery, *Pediatrics* 112:199-202, 2003.

120. Porterfield JA, DeRosa C: *Mechanical low back pain: perspectives in functional anatomy*, Philadelphia, 1998, Saunders.

121. Potvin JR, McGill SM, Norman RW: Trunk muscle and lumbar ligament contributions to dynamic lifts with varying degrees of trunk flexion, *Spine* 16:1099-1107, 1991.

122. Reese NB: *Muscle and sensory testing*, Philadelphia, 1999, Saunders.

123. Richardson C, Hodges PW, Hides JA: *Therapeutic exercise for lumbopelvic stabilization*, ed 2, St. Louis, 2004, Churchill Livingstone.

124. Richardson CA, Snijders CJ, Hides JA, et al: The relation between the transversus abdominis muscles, sacroiliac joint mechanics, and low back pain, *Spine* 27:399-405, 2002.

125. Rohlmann A, Graichen F, Bergmann G: Loads on an internal spinal fixation device during physical therapy, *Phys Ther* 82:44-52, 2002.

126. Saeed NR, Wall SA, Dhariwal DK: Management of positional plagiocephaly, *Arch Dis Child* 93:82-84, 2008.

127. Santaguida PL, McGill SM: The psoas major muscle: a three-dimensional geometric study, *J Biomech* 28:339-345, 1995.

128. Sato H, Kikuchi S: The natural history of radiographic instability of the lumbar spine, *Spine* 18:2075-2079, 1993.

129. Schipplein OD, Trafimow JH, Andersson GB, Andriacchi TP: Relationship between moments at the L5/S1 level, hip and knee joint when lifting, *J Biomech* 23:907-912, 1990.

130. Smith CE, Nyland J, Caudill P, et al: Dynamic trunk stabilization: a conceptual back injury prevention program for volleyball athletes, *J Orthop Sports Phys Ther* 38:703-720, 2008.

131. Snijders CJ, Ribbers MT, de Bakker HV, et al: EMG recordings of abdominal and back muscles in various standing postures: validation of a biomechanical model on sacroiliac joint stability, *J Electromyogr Kinesiol* 8:205-214, 1998.

132. Standring S: *Gray's anatomy: the anatomical basis of clinical practice*, ed 40, St Louis, 2009, Elsevier.

133. Stemper BD, Yoganandan N, Pintar FA, Rao RD: Anterior longitudinal ligament injuries in whiplash may lead to cervical instability, *Med Eng Phys* 28:515-524, 2006.

134. Stevenson J, Bryant T, Greenhorn D, et al: The effect of lifting protocol on comparisons with isoinertial lifting performance, *Ergonomics* 33:1455-1469, 1990.

135. Tarnanen SP, Ylinen JJ, Siekkinen KM, et al: Effect of isometric upper-extremity exercises on the activation of core stabilizing muscles, *Arch Phys Med Rehabil* 89:513-521, 2008.

136. Tesh KM, Dunn JS, Evans JH: The abdominal muscles and vertebral stability, *Spine* 12:501-508, 1987.

137. Teyhen DS, Gill NW, Whittaker JL, et al: Rehabilitative ultrasound imaging of the abdominal muscles, *J Orthop Sports Phys Ther* 37:450-466, 2007.

138. Teyhen DS, Rieger JL, Westrick RB, et al: Changes in deep abdominal muscle thickness during common trunk-strengthening exercises using ultrasound imaging, *J Orthop Sports Phys Ther* 38:596-605, 2008.

139. Turk AE, McCarthy JG, Thorne CH, Wisoff JH: The "back to sleep campaign" and deformational plagiocephaly: is there cause for concern? *J Craniofac Surg* 7:12-18, 1996.

140. Tveit P, Daggfeldt K, Hetland S, Thorstensson A: Erector spinae lever arm length variations with changes in spinal curvature, *Spine* 19:199-204, 1994.

141. Urquhart DM, Hodges PW: Differential activity of regions of transversus abdominis during trunk rotation, *Eur Spine J* 14:393-400, 2005.

142. Urquhart DM, Hodges PW, Story IH: Postural activity of the abdominal muscles varies between regions of these muscles and between body positions, *Gait Posture* 22:295-301, 2005.

143. van Dieen JH, Hoozemans MJ, Toussaint HM: Stoop or squat: a review of biomechanical studies on lifting technique, *Clin Biomech (Bristol, Avon)* 14:685-696, 1999.

144. Van K, Hides JA, Richardson CA: The use of real-time ultrasound imaging for biofeedback of lumbar multifidus muscle contraction in healthy subjects, *J Orthop Sports Phys Ther* 36:920-925, 2006.

145. Vasavada AN, Li S, Delp SL: Influence of muscle morphometry and moment arms on the moment-generating capacity of human neck muscles, *Spine* 23:412-422, 1998.

146. Vasseljen O, Dahl HH, Mork PJ, Torp HG: Muscle activity onset in the lumbar multifidus muscle recorded simultaneously by ultrasound imaging and intramuscular electromyography, *Clin Biomech (Bristol, Avon)* 21:905-913, 2006.

147. Vera-Garcia FJ, Brown SH, Gray JR, McGill SM: Effects of different levels of torso coactivation on trunk muscular and kinematic responses to posteriorly applied sudden loads, *Clin Biomech (Bristol, Avon)* 21:443-455, 2006.

148. Vera-Garcia FJ, Elvira JL, Brown SH, McGill SM: Effects of abdominal stabilization maneuvers on the control of spine motion and stability against sudden trunk perturbations, *J Electromyogr Kinesiol* 17:556-567, 2007.

149. Ward SR, Kim CW, Eng CM, et al: Architectural analysis and intraoperative measurements demonstrate the unique design of the multifidus muscle for lumbar spine stability, *J Bone Joint Surg Am* 91:176-185, 2009.

150. Waters TR, Lu ML, Occhipinti E: New procedure for assessing sequential manual lifting jobs using the revised NIOSH lifting equation, *Ergonomics* 50:1761-1770, 2007.

151. Waters TR, Putz-Anderson V, Garg A, Fine LJ: Revised NIOSH equation for the design and evaluation of manual lifting tasks, *Ergonomics* 36:749-776, 1993.

152. Welbergen E, Kemper HC, Knibbe JJ, et al: Efficiency and effectiveness of stoop and squat lifting at different frequencies, *Ergonomics* 34:613-624, 1991.

153. Wilke HJ, Rohlmann A, Neller S, et al: ISSLS prize winner: A novel approach to determine trunk muscle forces during flexion and extension—a comparison of data from an in vitro experiment and in vivo measurements, *Spine* 28:2585-2593, 2003.

154. Wilke HJ, Wolf S, Claes LE, et al: Stability increase of the lumbar spine with different muscle groups. A biomechanical in vitro study, *Spine* 20:192-198, 1995.

155. Willinger M, Hoffman HJ, Wu KT, et al: Factors associated with the transition to nonprone sleep positions of infants in the United States: the National Infant Sleep Position Study, *JAMA* 280:329-335, 1998.

156. Zhao F, Pollintine P, Hole BD, et al: Discogenic origins of spinal instability, *Spine* 30:2621-2630, 2005.

STUDY QUESTIONS

1 Describe the most likely craniocervical posture resulting from (a) unilateral and (b) bilateral spasm (or shortening) in the sternocleidomastoid muscle(s).

2 Why are the superficial and intermediate muscles of the posterior back classified as "extrinsic" muscles? Describe how the specific innervation of these muscles is associated with this classification.

3 List structures that receive sensory innervation from the recurrent meningeal nerve. What nerves provide sensory innervation to the capsule of the apophyseal joints?

4 Justify why an isolated strong contraction of the semispinalis thoracis would likely produce *contralateral* axial rotation, whereas a strong isolated contraction of the longissimus cervicis or capitis would likely produce *ipsilateral* axial rotation. Use Figures 10-7 and 10-9 as a reference for answering this question.

5 Assume a person has a complete spinal cord injury at the level of T8. Based on your knowledge of muscle innervation, predict which muscles of the trunk would be unaffected and which would be partially or completely paralyzed. Consider only the abdominal muscles, multifidi, and erector spinae in your response.

6 List three muscles that attach to *anterior* tubercles and three that attach to *posterior* tubercles of transverse processes of cervical vertebrae. What important structure passes between these muscle attachments?

7 As a group, the trunk extensor muscles produce greater maximal-effort torque than the trunk flexor muscles (abdominals). Cite two factors that can account for this difference in strength.

8 Which of the major trunk muscles would experience the most significant stretch (elongation) after a motion of full trunk extension, right lateral flexion, and right axial rotation?

9 Based on Figure 10-16, which muscle has the greatest moment arm for (a) flexion and (b) lateral flexion at L3?

10 Describe how an overshortened (contracted) iliacus muscle can cause an increased lumbar lordosis while a person is standing. What effect could this posture have on the stress at the lumbosacral junction?

11 At the level of the third lumbar vertebra, which connective tissues form the anterior rectus sheath (of the abdominal wall)?

12 What is the primary difference between a dorsal ramus of a spinal nerve root and a dorsal nerve root?

13 Using Figure 10-23 as a reference, which muscle, based solely on its size, would theoretically produce the greatest extension force across the atlanto-occipital joints?

14 Describe the similarities and differences in the structure of the multifidi and the semispinales muscles.

15 As indicated in Figure 10-30, why is the axial rotation function of the rectus capitis posterior major muscle limited to the atlanto-axial joint only?

⊖ *Answers to the study questions can be found on the Evolve website.*

CHAPTER

11

Kinesiology of Mastication and Ventilation

DONALD A. NEUMANN, PT, PhD, FAPTA

CHAPTER AT A GLANCE

PART 1: MASTICATION

Mastication is the process of chewing, tearing, and grinding food with the teeth. This process involves an interaction among the central nervous system and muscles of mastication, the teeth, the tongue, and the pair of temporomandibular joints (TMJs). The joints form the pivot point between the lower jaw (mandible) and the base of the cranium. The TMJ is one of the most continuously used joints in the body, not only during mastication, but also during swallowing and speaking. The first part of this chapter focuses on the kinesiology of the TMJs during mastication.

OSTEOLOGY AND TEETH

Regional Surface Anatomy

Figure 11-1 highlights some of the surface anatomy associated with the TMJ. The *mandibular condyle* fits within the mandibular fossa of the temporal bone. The condyle can be palpated just anterior to the *external auditory meatus* (i.e., the opening into the ear). The cranial attachment of the temporalis muscle fills a broad, slightly concave region of the skull known as the *temporal fossa*. The temporal, parietal, frontal, sphenoid, and zygomatic bones all contribute to the temporal fossa.

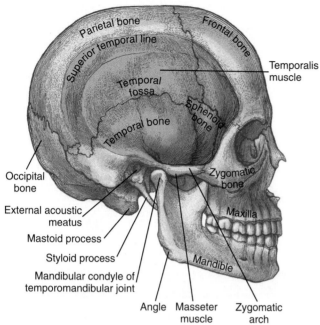

FIGURE 11-1. Lateral view of the skull with emphasis on bony landmarks associated with the temporomandibular joint. The proximal attachments of the temporalis and masseter muscles are indicated in red.

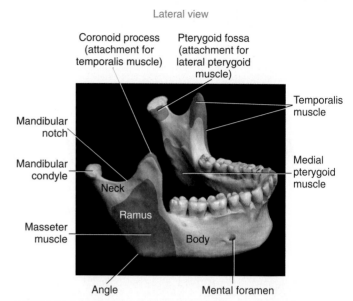

FIGURE 11-2. Lateral view of the mandible. Distal attachments of muscles are shown.

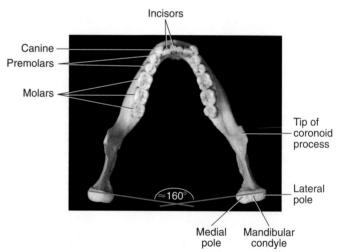

FIGURE 11-3. The mandible as viewed from above. The names of the permanent teeth are indicated. The long (side-to-side) axis through each mandibular condyle intersects at an approximate 160-degree angle.

Additional surface anatomy associated with the TMJ includes the *mastoid process* of the temporal bone, the *angle of the mandible,* and the *zygomatic arch.* The zygomatic arch is formed by the union of the zygomatic process of the temporal bone and the temporal process of the zygomatic bone.

Individual Bones

The mandible, maxillae, temporal, zygomatic, sphenoid, and hyoid bones are all related to the structure or function of the TMJ.

MANDIBLE

The mandible is the largest of the facial bones (see Figure 11-1). It is a very mobile bone, suspended from the cranium by the muscles, ligaments, and capsule of the TMJ. Muscles of mastication attach either directly or indirectly to the mandible. Muscle contraction positions the teeth embedded within the mandible firmly against the teeth embedded within the fixed maxillae.

Relevant Osteologic Features of the Mandible
- Body
- Ramus
- Angle
- Coronoid process
- Condyle
- Notch
- Neck
- Pterygoid fossa

The two main parts of the mandible are the body and the two rami (Figure 11-2). The *body,* the horizontal portion of the bone, accepts the lower 16 adult teeth (Figure 11-3). The *rami* of the mandible project vertically from the posterior aspect of the body (see Figure 11-2). Each ramus has an external and internal surface and four borders. The posterior and inferior borders of the ramus join at the readily palpable *angle* of the mandible. The masseter and medial pterygoid muscles—two powerful muscles of mastication—share similar attachments in the region of the angle of the mandible.

At the superior end of the ramus are the coronoid process, mandibular condyle, and mandibular notch. The *coronoid process* is a triangular projection of thin bone that extends upward from the anterior border of the ramus. This process is the primary inferior attachment of the temporalis muscle. The mandibular *condyle* extends upward from the posterior border of the ramus. The condyle forms the convex bony component of the TMJ. Extending between the coronoid process and mandibular condyle is the mandibular *notch*. The mandibular *neck* is a slightly constricted region located immediately below the condyle. The lateral pterygoid muscle attaches to the anterior-medial surface of the mandibular neck, within a depression called the *pterygoid fossa* (Figures 11-2 and 11-4).

MAXILLA

The right and left maxillae fuse to form a single maxilla, or upper jaw. The maxilla is fixed within the skull through rigid articulations to adjacent bones (see Figure 11-1). The maxillae extend superiorly, forming the floor of the nasal cavity and the orbit of the eyes. The lower horizontal portions of the maxillae accept the upper teeth.

TEMPORAL BONE

Two temporal bones exist—one on each side of the cranium. The *mandibular fossa* forms the bony concavity of the TMJ, highlighted in a side view in the lower part of Figure 11-5. The highest point of the fossa is the *dome*, often very thin and membranous (see main illustration in Figure 11-5). The fossa is bound anteriorly by the *articular eminence* and poste-

---

> **Relevant Osteologic Features of the Temporal Bone**
> - Mandibular fossa
> - Dome
> - Articular eminence
> - Postglenoid tubercle
> - Styloid process
> - Zygomatic process

riorly by the *postglenoid tubercle* and the tympanic part of the temporal bone. On full opening of the mouth, the condyles of the mandible slide anteriorly and inferiorly across the pair of sloped articular eminences.

The *styloid process* is a long slender extension of bone that protrudes from the inferior aspect of the temporal bone (see Figure 11-1). The pointed process serves as an attachment for the stylomandibular ligament (to be discussed further) and three small muscles (styloglossus, stylohyoid, and stylopharyngeus). The *zygomatic process* of the temporal bone forms the posterior half of the zygomatic arch (see main illustration in Figure 11-5).

ZYGOMATIC BONE

The right and left zygomatic bones constitute the major part of the cheeks and the lateral orbits of the eyes (see Figure 11-1). The *temporal process* of a zygomatic bone contributes the anterior half of the zygomatic arch (see Figure 11-5). A large part of the masseter muscle attaches to the zygomatic bone and the adjacent zygomatic arch.

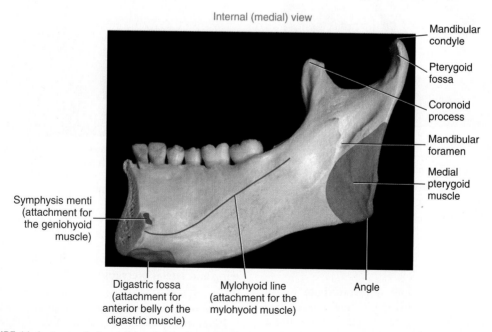

Internal (medial) view

Mandibular condyle
Pterygoid fossa
Coronoid process
Mandibular foramen
Medial pterygoid muscle

Symphysis menti (attachment for the geniohyoid muscle)

Digastric fossa (attachment for anterior belly of the digastric muscle)

Mylohyoid line (attachment for the mylohyoid muscle)

Angle

FIGURE 11-4. Internal view of the right side of the mandible. The bone is bisected in the near sagittal plane. The attachments of the mylohyoid and geniohyoid muscles are indicated in red; the attachments of the anterior belly of the digastric and medial pterygoid muscles are indicated in gray. Note the one missing third molar ("wisdom tooth").

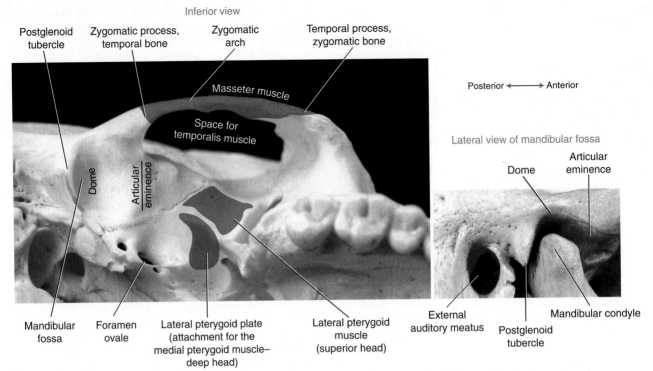

FIGURE 11-5. Main photograph: Inferior view of the skull highlighting the right mandibular fossa, lateral pterygoid plate, and zygomatic arch. The proximal attachments of the masseter, medial pterygoid (deep head), and lateral pterygoid (superior head) muscles are shown in red. Small photograph at right shows a close-up, lateral perspective of the mandibular fossa and adjacent bony features. This disc is not present.

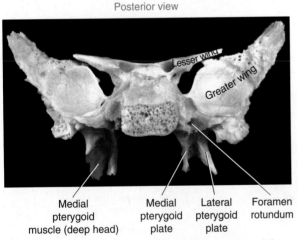

FIGURE 11-6. Posterior view of a sphenoid bone removed from the cranium. The proximal attachment of the medial pterygoid muscle (deep head) is indicated in red.

FIGURE 11-7. Lateral view of the right side of the cranium with a section of the zygomatic arch removed. The greater wing and lateral side of the lateral pterygoid plate are visible. Note the attachments in red for the pterygoid muscles.

SPHENOID BONE

Although the sphenoid bone does not contribute to the structure of the TMJ, it does provide proximal attachments for the medial and lateral pterygoid muscles. When articulated within the cranium, the sphenoid bone lies transversely across the base of the skull. The relevant osteologic features of the sphenoid bone are its *greater wing, medial pterygoid plate,* and *lateral pterygoid plate* (Figure 11-6). When a section of the

zygomatic arch is removed, the lateral surfaces of the greater wing and lateral pterygoid plate are revealed (Figure 11-7).

Relevant Osteologic Features of the Sphenoid Bone
- Greater wing
- Medial pterygoid plate
- Lateral pterygoid plate

TABLE 11-1.	**Permanent Teeth**		
Names	**Functions**	**Numbers**	**Structural Characteristics**
Incisors	Cut food	Maxillary, 4 Mandibular, 4	Sharp edges
Canines	Tear food	Maxillary, 2 Mandibular, 2	Longest permanent teeth; crown has a single cusp
Premolars	Crush food	Maxillary, 4 Mandibular, 4	Crown has two cusps (bicuspid); lower second premolars may have three cusps
Molars	Grind food into small particles for swallowing	Maxillary, 6 Mandibular, 6	Crown has four or five cusps

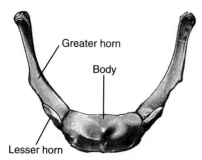

FIGURE 11-8. Superior view of the hyoid bone, located at the base of the throat. (From Standring S: *Gray's anatomy: the anatomical basis of clinical practice*, ed 39, St Louis, 2005, Elsevier.)

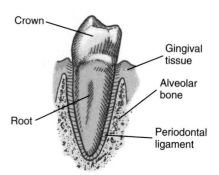

FIGURE 11-9. The tooth and its periodontal supportive structures. The width of the periodontal ligaments is greatly exaggerated for illustrative purposes. (From Okeson JP: *Management of temporomandibular disorders and occlusion*, ed 6, Chicago, 2005, Mosby.)

HYOID BONE

The hyoid is a U-shaped bone that can be palpated at the base of the throat, just anterior to the body of the third cervical vertebra (Figure 11-8). The *body* of the hyoid is convex anteriorly. The bilateral *greater horns* form its slightly curved sides. The hyoid is suspended primarily by a bilateral pair of stylohyoid ligaments. Several muscles involved with moving of the tongue, swallowing, and speaking attach to the hyoid bone (see Figure 11-21).

Teeth

The maxillae and mandible each contain 16 permanent teeth (see Figure 11-3 for names of lower teeth). The structure of each tooth reflects its function in mastication (Table 11-1).

Each tooth has two basic parts: crown and root (Figure 11-9). Normally the *crown* is covered with enamel and is located above the gingiva (gum). The *root* of each tooth is embedded in alveolar bone. The *periodontal ligaments* help attach the roots of the teeth within their sockets.

Cusps are conical elevations that arise on the surface of a tooth. *Maximal intercuspation* describes the position of the mandible when the cusps of the opposing teeth are in maximal contact. The term is frequently used interchangeably with *centric relation*, especially in describing the relative position of the articular surfaces within the TMJ. The relaxed *postural position* of the mandible allows a slight "freeway space" (interocclusal clearance) between the upper and lower teeth. Normally the teeth make contact (occlude) only during chewing and swallowing.

ARTHROLOGY OF THE TEMPOROMANDIBULAR JOINT

The temporomandibular joint (TMJ) is a loosely fitting articulation formed between the mandibular condyle and the mandibular fossa of the temporal bone (see Figures 11-1 and 11-5). It is a synovial joint that permits a wide range of rotation as well as translation. An *articular disc* cushions the potentially large and repetitive forces inherent to mastication. The disc separates the joint into two synovial joint cavities (Figure 11-10). The *inferior joint cavity* is between the inferior aspect of the disc and the mandibular condyle. The larger *superior joint cavity* is between the superior surface of the disc and the segment of bone formed by the mandibular fossa and the articular eminence.

Although the right and left TMJs function together, each retains its ability to function relatively independently. Mastication is typically performed asymmetrically, with one side of the mandible exerting a greater biting force than the other. The dominant side is often referred to as the "working" side, whereas the nondominant side is referred to as the "balancing" side.[24] Different demands are placed on the muscles and joints of the working and balancing sides.

Osseous Structure

MANDIBULAR CONDYLE

The mandibular condyle is flattened from front to back, with its medial-lateral length twice as long as its anterior-posterior

Lateral view

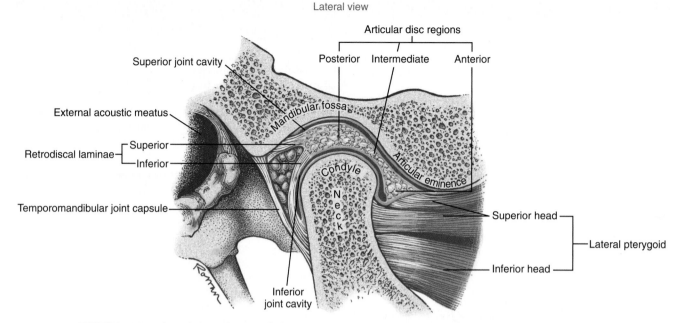

FIGURE 11-10. A lateral view of a sagittal plane cross-section through a normal right temporomandibular joint. The mandible is in a position of maximal intercuspation, with the disc in its ideal position relative to the condyle and the temporal bone.

length (see Figure 11-3). The condyle is generally convex, possessing short projections known as *medial* and *lateral poles.* The medial pole is more prominent than the lateral. While the mouth is opening and closing, the outside edge of the lateral pole can be palpated as a point under the skin just anterior to the external auditory meatus.

The articular surface of the mandibular condyle is lined with a thin but dense layer of *fibrocartilage.* This tissue absorbs forces associated with mastication better than hyaline cartilage, and it has a superior reparative process.[65] Both of these functions are important, given the extraordinary demands placed on the TMJ.

MANDIBULAR FOSSA

The mandibular fossa of the temporal bone is divided into two surfaces: articular and nonarticular. The *articular surface* of the fossa is formed by the articular eminence, occupying the sloped anterior wall of the fossa (see Figures 11-5 and 11-10). This thick and smooth load-bearing surface is lined with a thick layer of fibrocartilage. Full opening of the mouth requires that each condyle slide forward across the articular eminence. The slope of the articular eminence is, on average, 55 degrees from the horizontal plane.[29] The magnitude of the slope partially determines the kinematic path of the condyle during opening and closing of the mouth.

The *nonarticular surface* of the mandibular fossa consists of a very thin layer of bone and fibrocartilage that occupies much of the superior (dome) and posterior walls of the fossa (see Figure 11-5). This thin region is not an adequate load-bearing surface. A large upward force applied to the chin can fracture this region of the fossa, possibly even sending bone fragments into the cranium.

Articular Disc

The articular disc within the TMJ consists primarily of dense fibrocartilage that, with the exception of its periphery, lacks a blood supply and sensory innervation. The histology of this tissue is generally similar to that of other load-bearing intra-articular discs of the body, such as the disc within the distal radio-ulnar joint and the meniscus of the knee. The fibrocartilage in the TMJ is flexible but firm owing to its high collagen content. The entire periphery of the disc attaches to the surrounding capsule of the joint.

The disc is divided into three regions: posterior, intermediate, and anterior (see Figure 11-10). The shape of each region allows the disc to accommodate to the varying contours of the condyle and the fossa. The *posterior region* of the disc is convex superiorly and concave inferiorly. The concavity accepts most of the condyle, much like a ball-and-socket joint. The extreme posterior region attaches to the loosely organized *retrodiscal laminae,* containing collagen and elastin fibers. Connections made by the laminae anchor the disc posteriorly to bone. A meshwork of fat, blood vessels, and sensory nerves fills the space between the superior and inferior laminae.

The *posterior region* of the articular disc attaches to the following:
- Collagen-rich *inferior retrodiscal lamina,* which in turn attaches to the periphery of the superior neck of the mandible along with the capsule of the TMJ
- Elastin-rich *superior retrodiscal lamina,* which in turn attaches to the tympanic plate of the temporal bone just posterior to the mandibular fossa

The *intermediate region* of the disc is concave inferiorly and generally flat superiorly. The *anterior region* is nearly flat inferiorly and slightly concave superiorly to accommodate the convexity of the articular eminence. The anterior region of the disc attaches to several tissues.

The *anterior region* of the articular disc attaches to the following:
- Periphery of the superior neck of the mandible, along with the anterior capsule of the TMJ
- Tendon of the superior head of the lateral pterygoid muscle
- Temporal bone just anterior to the articular eminence

The thickness of the disc varies between its anterior and posterior regions. The thinnest intermediate region is only 1 mm thick.[36] The anterior and posterior regions, however, are about two to three times thicker. The disc is constricted at its intermediate region.[55] The constriction, flanked by the adjacent thicker anterior and posterior regions, forms a dimple on the disc's inferior surface. In maximal intercuspation, the dimpled intermediate region of the disc should fit between the anterior-superior edge of the condyle and the articular eminence of the fossa. The disc position protects the condyle as it slides forward across the articular eminence during the later phase of opening the mouth widely.

The articular disc maximizes the congruency within the TMJ to reduce contact pressure. The disc also adds stability to the joint and helps guide the condyle of the mandible during movement. In the healthy TMJ, the disc slides with the translating condyle. Movement is governed by intra-articular pressure, by muscle forces, and by collateral ligaments that attach the periphery of the disc to the condyle.

Capsular and Ligamentous Structures

FIBROUS CAPSULE

The TMJ and disc are surrounded by a loose *fibrous capsule*. The internal surfaces of the capsule are lined with a synovial membrane. Superiorly the capsule attaches to the rim of the mandibular fossa, as far anterior as the articular eminence. Inferiorly the capsule attaches to the periphery of the articular disc and to the superior neck of the mandible. Anteriorly the capsule and part of the anterior edge of disc attach to the tendon of the superior head of the lateral pterygoid muscle (see Figure 11-10).

The capsule of the TMJ provides significant support to the articulation. Medially and laterally the capsule is relatively firm, providing stability to the joint during lateral movements such as those produced during chewing. Anteriorly and posteriorly, however, the capsule is relatively lax, allowing the condyle and disc to translate forward when the mouth is opened.

LATERAL LIGAMENT

The primary ligament reinforcing the TMJ is the *lateral (temporomandibular) ligament* (Figure 11-11, *A*). The lateral ligament has been described as a combination of horizontal and oblique fibers (see Figure 11-11, *B*).[71] The more superficial

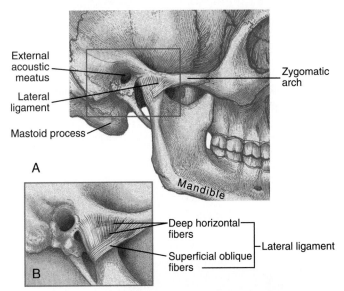

FIGURE 11-11. **A,** The lateral ligament of the temporomandibular joint. **B,** The lateral ligament's main fibers: oblique and horizontal.

oblique fibers course in an anterior-superior direction, from the posterior neck of the mandible to the lateral margins of the articular eminence and zygomatic arch. The deeper *horizontal fibers* share similar temporal attachments. They course horizontally and posteriorly to attach into the lateral pole of the mandibular condyle.

The primary function of the lateral ligament is to stabilize the lateral side of the capsule. Tears or excessive elongation of the lateral ligament may cause the disc to migrate medially by an unopposed pull of the superior head of the lateral pterygoid muscle. As described in the discussion of arthrokinematics, the oblique fibers of the lateral ligament have a special function in guiding the movement of the condyle during opening of the mouth.[55]

ACCESSORY LIGAMENTS

The *stylomandibular* and *sphenomandibular ligaments* are the accessory ligaments of the TMJ. Both are located medial to the joint capsule (Figure 11-12). The ligaments help suspend the mandible from the cranium and likely have only a limited dynamic role in mastication.

Supporting Connective Tissues within the Temporomandibular Joint
- Articular disc
- Fibrous capsule
- Lateral temporomandibular joint ligament
- Sphenomandibular ligament
- Stylomandibular ligament

Osteokinematics

The osteokinematics of the mandible are most often described as protrusion and retrusion, lateral excursion, and depression and elevation (Figures 11-13 to 11-15). All of these move-

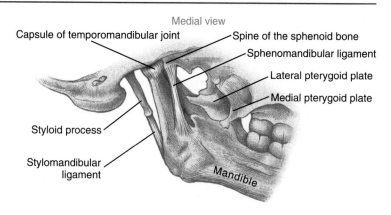

FIGURE 11-12. A medial view of the temporomandibular joint capsule shows the stylomandibular and sphenomandibular ligaments.

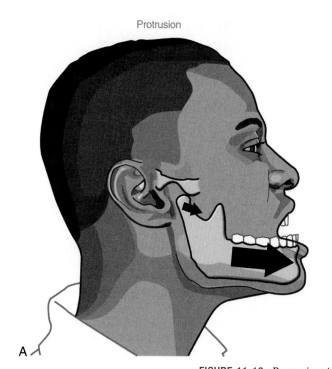

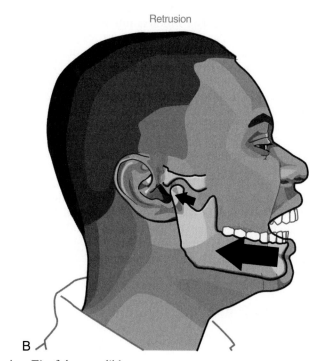

FIGURE 11-13. Protrusion **(A)** and retrusion **(B)** of the mandible.

ments occur to varying degrees during mastication. For a more detailed analysis of mandibular movements, the reader is encouraged to consult the classic work by Posselt,[61] thoroughly summarized by Okeson.[55]

PROTRUSION AND RETRUSION

Protrusion of the mandible occurs as it translates *anteriorly* without significant rotation (see Figure 11-13, *A*). Protrusion is an important component of the mouth's opening maximally. *Retrusion* of the mandible occurs in the reverse direction (see Figure 11-13, *B*). Retrusion provides an important component of closing the widely opened and protruded mouth.

LATERAL EXCURSION

Lateral excursion of the mandible occurs primarily as a side-to-side translation (see Figure 11-14, *A*). The direction (right or

left) of active lateral excursion can be described as either contralateral or ipsilateral to the side of the primary muscle action. In the adult, an average of 11 mm (about ½ inch) of maximal unilateral excursion is considered normal.[74] Lateral excursion of the mandible is usually combined with other relatively slight translations and rotations. Normally the specific path of movement is guided by the shape of the mandibular fossa and position of the articular disc.

DEPRESSION AND ELEVATION

Depression of the mandible causes the mouth to *open*, a fundamental component of chewing (see Figure 11-15, *A*). Maximal opening of the mouth typically occurs during actions such as yawning and singing. In the adult the mouth can be opened an average of 50 mm as measured between the incisal edges of the upper and lower front teeth.[2,35,74] The interincisal opening is typically large enough to fit three adult "knuckles" (proximal interphalangeal joints). Typical mastica-

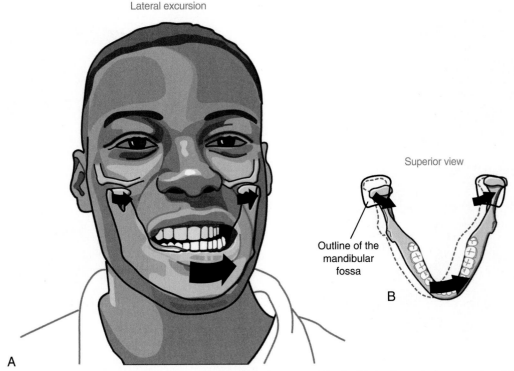

Lateral excursion

Superior view

Outline of the mandibular fossa

A

B

FIGURE 11-14. Lateral excursion of the mandible **(A)** shown combined with horizontal plane rotation **(B).**

tion, however, requires an average maximal opening of 18 mm—about 36% of maximum (sufficient to accept one adult knuckle). Being unable to fit two knuckles between the edges of the upper and lower incisors is usually considered abnormal in the average sized adult. *Elevation* of the mandible *closes* the mouth—an action used to grind food during mastication (see Figure 11-15, *B*).

Arthrokinematics

Movement of the mandible typically involves bilateral action of the TMJs. Abnormal function in one joint naturally interferes with the function of the other. Depending on the osteokinematics, the arthrokinematics of the TMJ normally involve both rotation and translation. In general, during *rotational movement* the mandibular condyle rolls relative to the inferior surface of the disc, and during *translational movement* the mandibular condyle *and* disc slide essentially together. The disc usually moves in the direction of the translating condyle.

PROTRUSION AND RETRUSION

During protrusion and retrusion the mandibular condyle and disc translate anteriorly and posteriorly, respectively, relative to the fossa (see Figure 11-13). The condyle and disc follow the downward slope of the articular eminence. The mandible slides slightly downward during protrusion and upward during retrusion. The path of movement varies depending on the degree of opening of the mouth.

LATERAL EXCURSION

Lateral excursion involves primarily a side-to-side translation of the condyle and disc within the fossa. Slight multiplanar rotations are typically combined with lateral excursion.[55] Figure 11-14, *B*, shows an example of lateral excursion combined with slight horizontal plane rotation. The left condyle forms a pivot point within the fossa as the right condyle rotates slightly anteriorly and medially.

DEPRESSION AND ELEVATION

Opening and closing of the mouth occur by depression and elevation of the mandible, respectively. During these movements, each TMJ experiences a combination of rotation *and* translation among the mandibular condyle, articular disc, and fossa. No other joint in the body experiences such a large proportion of translation and rotation. Because rotation and translation occur simultaneously, the axis of rotation is constantly moving. In the ideal case the movements within both TMJs result in a maximal range of mouth opening with a minimal stress placed on the articular surfaces.

The arthrokinematics of opening the mouth are depicted for an early and a late phase in Figure 11-16. The *early phase,* constituting the first 35% to 50% of the range of motion, involves primarily *rotation* of the mandible relative to the cranium.[66,88] As depicted in Figure 11-16, *A*, the condyle rolls posteriorly within the concave inferior surface of the disc. (The direction of the roll is described relative to the rotation of a point on the ramus of the mandible.) The rolling motion

Depression

Elevation

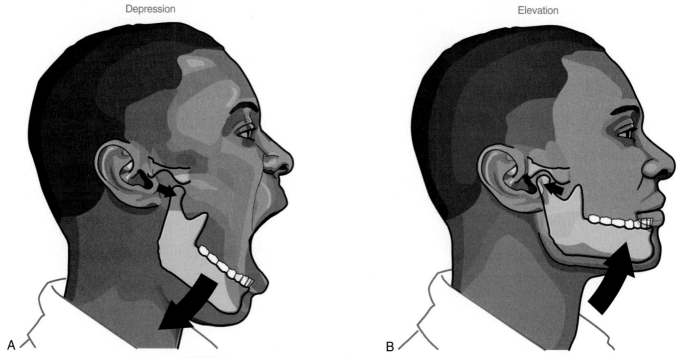

FIGURE 11-15. Depression **(A)** and elevation **(B)** of the mandible.

Opening the mouth

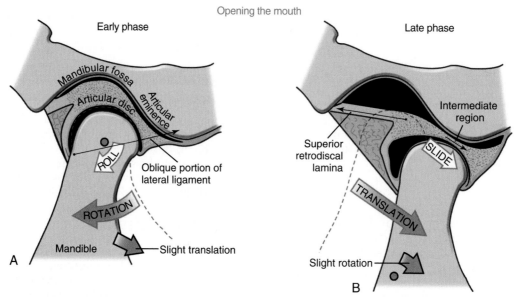

FIGURE 11-16. Arthrokinematics of opening the mouth, illustrated for the right temporomandibular joint only: early phase **(A)** and late phase **(B)**.

swings the body of the mandible inferiorly and posteriorly. The axis of rotation is not fixed but migrates within the vicinity of the condyles.[24,60]

The rolling motion of the condyle stretches the oblique portion of the lateral ligament. The increased tension in the ligament helps to initiate the late phase of the mouth's opening.[5,71]

The *late phase* of opening the mouth consists of the final 50% to 65% of the total range of motion. This phase is marked by a gradual transition from primary rotation to primary translation. The transition can be readily appreciated by palpating the condyle of the mandible during the full opening of the mouth. During the translation the condyle *and* disc slide together in a forward and inferior direction against the slope of the articular eminence (see Figure 11-16, *B*). At the end of opening, the axis of rotation shifts inferiorly. The exact point of the axis is difficult to define because it depends on the person's unique rotation-to-translation ratio. At the later phase of opening, the axis is usually below the neck of the mandible.[24]

Full opening of the mouth maximally stretches and pulls the disc anteriorly. The extent of the forward translation (protrusion) is limited, in part, by tension in the stretched, elastic superior retrodiscal lamina. The intermediate region of the disc translates forward while remaining between the superior aspect of the condyle and the articular eminence. This placement of the disc maximizes joint congruency and reduces intra-articular stress.

The arthrokinematics of *closing the mouth* occur in the reverse order of that described for opening. When the mouth is fully opened and prepared to close, tension in the superior retrodiscal lamina starts to retract the disc, initiating the early translational phase of closing. The later phase is dominated by rotation of the condyle within the concavity of the disc, terminated when contact is made between the upper and lower teeth.

MUSCLE AND JOINT INTERACTION

Innervation of the Muscles and Joints

The muscles of mastication and their innervation are listed in Table 11-2. Based primarily on size, the muscles of mastication are divided into two groups: primary and secondary. The primary muscles are the masseter, temporalis, medial pterygoid, and lateral pterygoid. The secondary muscles are much smaller. The primary muscles of mastication are innervated by the mandibular nerve, a division of the *trigeminal nerve* (cranial nerve V). This nerve exits the skull via the foramen ovale, which is just medial and slightly anterior to the mandibular fossa (see Figure 11-5).

The central part of the disc within the TMJ lacks sensory innervation. The periphery of the disc, capsule, lateral ligament, and retrodiscal tissues, however, possess pain fibers and mechanoreceptors.[75,87] In addition, mechanoreceptors and sensory nerves from oral mucosa, periodontal ligaments, and muscles provide the nervous system with a rich source of proprioception. This sensory information helps protect the soft oral tissues, such as the tongue and cheeks, from trauma caused by the teeth during chewing or speaking. Furthermore, the sensation helps coordinate the neuromuscular reflexes that synchronize the functional interaction among the muscles of the TMJ and in the craniocervical region. The sensory innervation from the TMJ is carried through two branches of the mandibular nerve: auriculotemporal and masseteric.[75]

Muscular Anatomy and Function

PRIMARY MUSCLES OF MASTICATION

The primary muscles of mastication are the masseter, temporalis, medial pterygoid, and lateral pterygoid. Refer to Appendix III, Part C for a summary of muscle attachments.

Masseter

The masseter is a thick, strong muscle, easily palpable just above the angle of the mandible (Figure 11-17, *A*). The muscle, as a whole, originates from the zygomatic arch and zygomatic bone (see Figures 11-1 and 11-5) and inserts inferiorly on the external surface of the ramus of the mandible (see Figure 11-2).

The masseter has superficial and deep heads (see Figure 11-17, *A*). The fibers of the larger, more *superficial head* travel inferiorly and posteriorly, attaching inferiorly near the angle of the mandible. The fibers from the smaller *deep head* attach inferiorly to the upper region of the ramus of the mandible, close to the base of the coronoid process.

The actions of both heads of the masseter are essentially the same. Bilateral contraction *elevates* the mandible to bring the teeth into contact during mastication.[55,75] The line of force of the muscle is nearly perpendicular to the biting surface of the molars. The primary function of the masseter, therefore, is to develop large forces between the molars for effective grinding and crushing of food. Bilateral action of the masseters also *protrudes* the mandible slightly. Unilateral contraction of the masseter, however, causes slight *ipsilateral excursion* of the mandible. Such an action may occur during a lateral grinding motion while chewing (Figure 11-18). The multiple actions of the masseter are necessary for effective mastication.

Temporalis

The temporalis is a flat, fan-shaped muscle that fills much of the concavity of the temporal fossa of the skull (see Figure 11-17, *B*). From its cranial attachment, the muscle forms a

Muscles	Innervation
Primary Muscles	
Masseter	Branch of the mandibular nerve, a division of cranial nerve V
Temporalis	Branch of the mandibular nerve, a division of cranial nerve V
Medial pterygoid	Branch of the mandibular nerve, a division of cranial nerve V
Lateral pterygoid	Branch of the mandibular nerve, a division of cranial nerve V
Secondary Muscles	
Suprahyoid Group	
Digastric (posterior belly)	Facial nerve (cranial nerve VII)
Digastric (anterior belly)	Inferior alveolar nerve (branch of the mandibular nerve, a division of cranial nerve V)
Geniohyoid	C^1 via the hypoglossal nerve (cranial nerve XII)
Mylohyoid	Inferior alveolar nerve (branch of the mandibular nerve, a division of cranial nerve V)
Stylohyoid	Facial nerve (cranial nerve VII)
Infrahyoid Group	
Omohyoid	Ventral rami of C^1-C^3
Sternohyoid	Ventral rami of C^1-C^3
Sternothyroid	Ventral rami of C^1-C^3
Thyrohyoid	Ventral rami of C^1 (via cranial nerve XII)

TABLE 11-2. Primary and Secondary Muscles of Mastication and Their Innervation

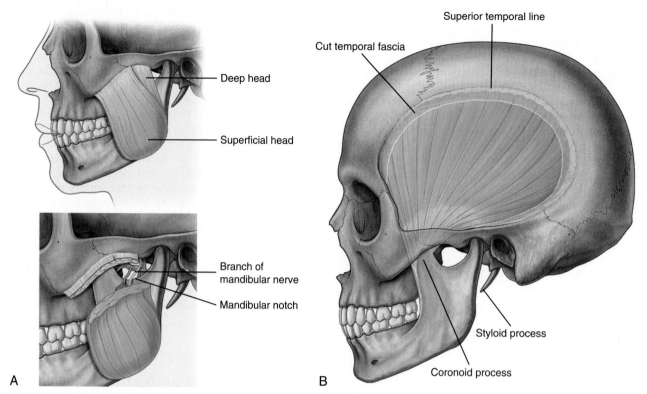

FIGURE 11-17. Illustration highlighting the left masseter (intact and cut specimens) **(A)** and left temporalis **(B)** muscles. (From Drake RL, Vogl W, Mitchell AWM: *Gray's anatomy for students*, St Louis, 2005, Churchill Livingstone.)

broad tendon that narrows distally as it passes through a space formed between the zygomatic arch and the lateral side of the skull (see Figure 11-5). The muscle attaches distally to the coronoid process and to the anterior edge and medial surface of the ramus of the mandible (see Figure 11-2). Bilateral contractions of the temporalis muscles *elevate the mandible.* The more oblique posterior fibers *elevate and retrude* the mandible.[55]

Similar to the masseter, the temporalis courses slightly medially as its approaches its distal attachment. Unilateral contraction of the temporalis, therefore, as when chewing in a side-to-side manner, causes slight *ipsilateral excursion* of the mandible (see Figure 11-18).

Medial Pterygoid

The medial pterygoid muscle arises from two heads (Figure 11-19, *A*). The much larger *deep head* attaches on the medial surface of the lateral pterygoid plate of the sphenoid bone (see Figures 11-5 and 11-6). The smaller *superficial head* attaches to a region of the posterior side of the maxilla, just above the third molar (see Figure 11-7).[75] Both heads course nearly parallel with the masseter muscle and attach on the internal surface of the ramus, near the angle of the mandible (see Figures 11-2 and 11-4).

The actions of the two heads of the medial pterygoid are essentially identical. Acting bilaterally, the medial pterygoid *elevates* and, to a limited extent, *protrudes* the mandible. Because of the oblique line of force of the muscle relative to the frontal plane, a unilateral contraction of the medial pterygoid produces a very effective *contralateral excursion* of the mandible (see Figure 11-18).

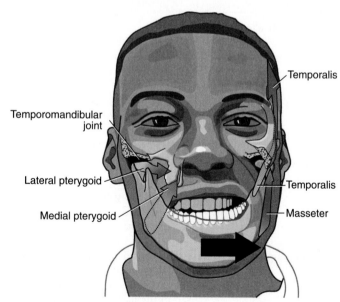

FIGURE 11-18. Frontal plane view shows the muscular interaction during *left lateral excursion* of the mandible. This action may occur during a side-to-side grinding motion while chewing. The muscles producing the movement are indicated in red.

Lateral Pterygoid

The lateral pterygoid muscle is generally described as a bipennate muscle with two distinct heads (see Figure 11-19, *B*).[20,52,55,75] The *superior head* arises from the greater wing of the sphenoid bone (see Figures 11-5 and 11-7). The considerably larger *infe-*

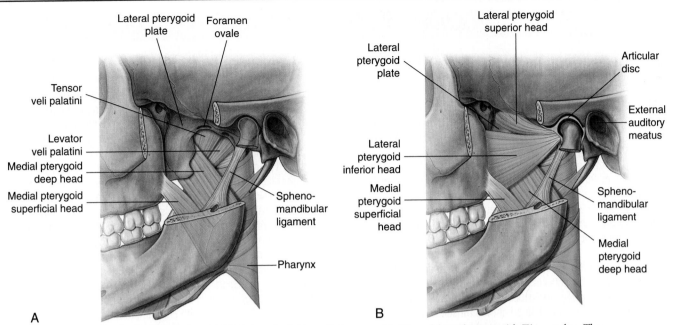

FIGURE 11-19. Illustration highlighting the left medial pterygoid **(A)** and lateral pterygoid **(B)** muscles. The mandible and zygomatic arch have been cut for better exposure of the pterygoid muscles. (From Drake RL, Vogl W, Mitchell AWM: *Gray's anatomy for students*, St Louis, 2005, Churchill Livingstone.)

rior head arises from the lateral surface of the lateral pterygoid plate and adjoining region of the maxilla (see Figure 11-7).

As a whole, the lateral pterygoid muscle traverses nearly horizontally to insert into (1) the neck of the mandible and the pterygoid fossa, (2) the articular disc, and (3) the capsule of the TMJ (review Figure 11-10).* Although the subject continues to be debated,[9] many sources state that about 65% of the fibers of the *superior head* attach into the pterygoid fossa (see Figure 11-2), whereas the remaining fibers attach into the medial wall of the capsule and part of the medial side of the articular disc. The *inferior head* attaches within the pterygoid fossa and adjacent neck of the mandible.

The precise action and role of the two heads of the lateral pterygoid muscle during mastication is controversial and not completely understood.[52,53,82] The lack of understanding partially reflects the muscle's deep location and subsequent technical challenge to electromyographic study.[20] Most authors, however, agree that unilateral contraction of both heads of the lateral pterygoid produces *contralateral excursion* of the mandible (see Figure 11-18). Unilateral muscle contraction also rotates the ipsilateral condyle anterior-medially within the horizontal plane. Usually a given right or left lateral pterygoid muscle contracts synergistically with other muscles during mastication. For example, as depicted in Figure 11-18, a biting motion that involves left lateral excursion is controlled by the right lateral and medial pterygoid muscles and by the left masseter and temporalis.

Bilateral contraction of both heads of the lateral pterygoid muscle produces a strong *protrusion* of the mandible.[42] As fully described in the discussion of muscular control of opening and closing of the mouth, the two heads of the lateral pterygoid muscles are active at different phases of opening and closing of the mouth. (For this and other mor-

phologic considerations, some authors have argued that the two heads of the lateral pterygoid are actually separate muscles.[20]) Most sources suggest that the *inferior head* is the primary depressor of the mandible, especially during resisted opening of the mouth.[44,52,55,59] The *superior head*, in contrast, helps control the tension within the disc and its position during resisted closure of the jaw.[44,52] This action is especially important during resisted, unilateral closure of the jaw, such as when biting down on a hard piece of candy.

SECONDARY MUSCLES OF MASTICATION

The suprahyoid and infrahyoid muscles are considered secondary muscles of mastication (Figure 11-21). These muscles are listed in Table 11-2. Forces produced by these muscles are transferred either directly or indirectly to the mandible. The *suprahyoid muscles* attach between the base of the cranium, hyoid bone, and mandible; the *infrahyoid muscles* attach superiorly to the hyoid and inferiorly to the thyroid cartilage, sternum, and scapula. The mandibular attachments of three of the suprahyoid muscles—anterior belly of the digastric, geniohyoid, and mylohyoid—are shown in Figure 11-4. Appendix III, Part C includes the attachments of the suprahyoid and infrahyoid muscles.

With the hyoid bone stabilized by sufficient activation of the infrahyoid muscles, the suprahyoid muscles can assist with depression of the mandible and thereby opening of the mouth.[8] The suprahyoid and infrahyoid muscles are also involved in speech, tongue movement, and swallowing and in controlling of boluses of food before swallowing.

SUMMARY OF INDIVIDUAL MUSCLE ACTION

Table 11-3 provides a summary of the individual actions of the muscles of mastication.

---

*References 9, 20, 55, 75, 82, 83.

Functional Interactions between the Masseter and Medial Pterygoid Muscles

The medial pterygoid and masseter muscles form a *functional sling* around the angle of the mandible (Figure 11-20). Simultaneous contractions of these muscles can exert a powerful biting force that is directed through the jaw and ultimately between the upper and lower molars. The maximal bite force in this region averages about 422 N (95 lb) in the adult, twice that generated between the incisors.[42]

Acting on the internal and external sides of the mandible, the masseter and medial pterygoid also produce an important side-to-side force between the upper and lower molars. As shown in Figure 11-18, simultaneous contraction of the right medial pterygoid and left masseter produces left lateral deviation. Contraction of these muscles in this synergistic fashion can produce a very effective shear force between the molars and food, on both sides of the mouth. The combined muscular action is very effective at grinding and crushing food before swallowing.

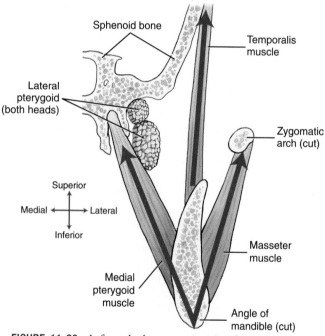

FIGURE 11-20. A frontal plane, cross-sectional perspective of the cranium is shown through the mid region of the zygomatic arch. This cross-sectional perspective includes the primary muscles of mastication (left side only). The lines of force are indicated for the primary muscles that close the mouth: masseter, temporalis, and medial pterygoid. Note the functional sling formed around the angle of the mandible by the masseter and medial pterygoid muscles.

MUSCULAR CONTROL OF OPENING AND CLOSING OF THE MOUTH

Opening the Mouth

Opening the mouth is performed primarily through contraction of the *inferior head of the lateral pterygoid* and the *suprahyoid*

Internal Derangement of the Disc

Mechanical dysfunction of the temporomandibular joint (TMJ) often causes painful, labored, and reduced movements of the jaw. One relatively common dysfunction involves an abnormal position of the disc relative to the condyle and fossa, an impairment referred to as *internal derangement of the disc*.[81] The derangement can be caused by pathology, trauma, or other conditions within the joint, including altered disc shape, abnormal slope of the articular eminence, overstretched capsule, or loss of elasticity within the superior retrodiscal lamina.[29] In addition, internal derangement of the disc may be associated with hyperactivity of muscle, most notably the *superior head of the lateral pterygoid.* Based on the line of pull and attachments of these muscle fibers, excessive activation can pull the disc in an anterior and medial direction relative to the joint.[42,82,83] The cause of the hyperactivity in this muscle is not known for certain, but it can be associated with chronic emotional stress and parafunctional habits, such as excessive tooth grinding or clenching of the teeth.[20] Once the disc is abnormally positioned, it is vulnerable to potentially large and damaging stress.[55,58]

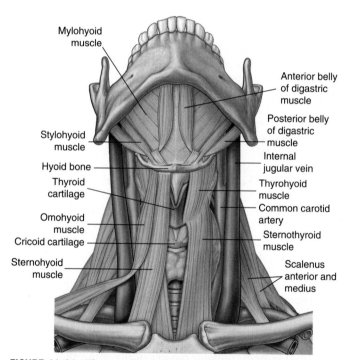

FIGURE 11-21. The suprahyoid and infrahyoid muscles are shown, attaching to the hyoid bone. The geniohyoid is deep to the mylohyoid and not visible. (From Drake RL, Vogl W, Mitchell AWM: *Gray's anatomy for students,* St Louis, 2005, Churchill Livingstone.)

group of muscles. This action is depicted in Figure 11-22, *A* as the mouth opens in preparation to bite on a grape. The inferior head of the lateral pterygoid is primarily responsible for the forward translation (protrusion) of the mandibular condyle. This muscle is also involved in a force-couple with the contracting suprahyoid muscles. The force-couple rotates

TABLE 11-3. Actions of the Muscles of Mastication

Muscle	Elevation (Closing of the Mouth)	Depression (Opening of the Mouth)	Lateral Excursion	Protrusion	Retrusion
Masseter	XXX	–	X (IL)	X	–
Medial pterygoid	XXX	–	XXX (CL)	X	–
Lateral pterygoid (superior head)	*	–	XXX (CL)	XXX	–
Lateral pterygoid (inferior head)	–	XXX	XXX (CL)	XXX	
Temporalis	XXX	–	X (IL)	–	XXX (posterior fibers)
Suprahyoid muscle group	–	XXX	–	–	X†

CL, contralateral excursion; *IL*, ipsilateral excursion.
*Stabilizes or adjusts the position of the articular disc.
†By direct action of the geniohyoid, mylohyoid, and digastric (anterior belly) only.
A muscle's relative potential to move the mandible is assigned one of three scores: X = minimal, XX = moderate, and XXX = maximum. A dash indicates no effective muscular action.

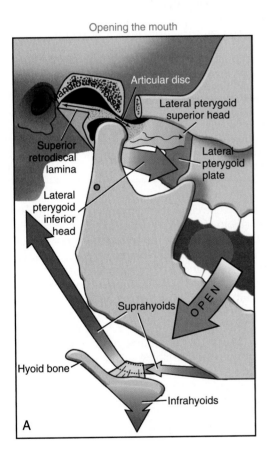

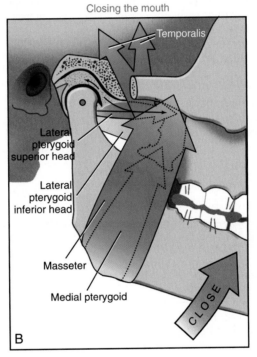

FIGURE 11-22. The muscle and joint interaction during opening (**A**) and closing (**B**) of the mouth. The relative degree of muscle activation is indicated by the different intensities of red. In **B**, the superior head of the lateral pterygoid muscle is shown eccentrically active. The locations of the axes of rotation (shown as small green circles in **A** and **B**) are estimates only.

the mandible around its axis of rotation, shown as a green opened circle below the neck of the mandible. Although mandibular rotation is minimal during the late phase of opening the mouth, it does facilitate the extremes of this action. Gravity also assists with opening the mouth.

As described previously, the disc and condyle slide forward as a unit during the late phase of opening of the mouth. The disc is stretched and pulled anteriorly by (1) the translating condyle, and (2) increased intra-articular pressure created by activation of the inferior head of the lateral pterygoid. Although the superior head of the lateral pterygoid attaches directly to the disc, most of the literature indicates that it is relatively inactive while the mouth is opening.

Closing the Mouth

Closing the mouth against resistance is performed primarily by contraction of the *masseter, medial pterygoid,* and *temporalis muscles* (see Figure 11-22, *B*). These muscles all have a very favorable moment arm (leverage) for this action. The more oblique posterior fibers of the temporalis muscle also *retrude* the mandible. This action translates the mandible in a posterior-superior direction, helping to reseat the condyle within the fossa.

Although the muscular action is not completely understood or agreed on, the *superior head* of the lateral pterygoid is likely active eccentrically during closing of the mouth. The activation tends to be greatest on the "working" side of the mandible (i.e., that side most involved with chewing).[55] Eccentric activation exerts a forward tension on the disc and neck of the mandible (see Figure 11-22, *B*). The tension helps to stabilize and optimally position the disc between the condyle and articular eminence. The muscle activation also helps balance the strong retrusion force generated by the posterior fibers of the temporalis.

TEMPOROMANDIBULAR DISORDERS

The term *temporomandibular disorders* (TMDs) is broad and often vague and refers to a number of clinical problems that involve the masticatory system.[81] TMDs are typically associated with impairments involving the muscles, the joint, or both.[63,78] In addition to pain during movement, the signs and symptoms of TMDs include joint sounds ("popping"), reduced molar bite forces, reduced range in opening of the mouth, headaches, joint locking, and referred pain to the face and scalp.* Many factors are associated with the causes of TMD, including stress or other emotional disturbances, daily oral parafunctional habits (e.g., grinding of teeth, repetitive biting of the lip or tongue), asymmetric muscle activity, sleep bruxism, chronic forward head posturing, or sensitization of the central nervous system. Although most cases are self-limiting, a small percentage may progress to osteoarthritis, which can lead to significant degenerative changes within the joint, remodeling of bone, and a marked loss of function.[41,68]

No single mechanical or physiologic explanation can account for the myriad symptoms associated with TMD.[34,67]

SPECIAL FOCUS 11-3

The Special Role of the Superior Head of the Lateral Pterygoid in Adjusting Disc Position

The specific position of the disc relative to the condyle during biting is strongly influenced by the type of resistance created by the objects being chewed. While the mouth is closing against a relatively low bite resistance, such as on a grape as depicted in Figure 11-22, *B*, the thin intermediate region of the disc is typically in its ideal position between the condyle and articular eminence. During the application of a large, asymmetric bite force, however, the position of the disc may need to be adjusted. Unilaterally biting on a hard piece of candy between the molars, for example, momentarily reduces the intra-articular pressure within the ipsilateral temporomandibular joint. Until the candy is crushed, it acts as a "spacer" between the upper and lower jaw, which reduces joint contact. During this event, a forceful *concentric contraction* of the superior head of the lateral pterygoid muscle can protrude the disc forward, thereby sliding its thicker, posterior region between the condyle and articular eminence. The thicker surface increases the congruency within the joint, helping to stabilize it against the uneven forces applied to the mandible as a whole.

The pathomechanics involved with a particular disorder may stem from increased joint stress from abnormal anatomy or dentition; internal derangement of the disc; or trauma, such as a fall, blow to the face, or cervical whiplash injury. Other predisposing factors may include chronic overloading of the joint and rheumatic disease.[25,41] Often, however, the exact cause of TMDs is unknown.

The treatment for TMDs is mixed and depends primarily on the nature of the underlying problem. The multiple symptoms associated with TMDs often require collaborative treatments from a team of clinicians, which may include dentists, physicians, physical therapists, and psychologists.[11,27,39,55,56] The more common conservative treatments for TMDs are listed in the box.

Common Conservative Treatments for Temporomandibular Disorders

Therapeutic exercise
Biofeedback, relaxation techniques, stress management
Cold or heat
Patient education (postural correction)
Manual therapy
Ultrasound, iontophoresis, phonophoresis
Transcutaneous electrical nerve stimulation
Behavioral modification
Pharmacotherapy
Intra-articular injections (local anesthetics or corticosteroids)
Occlusal therapy (altering tooth structure or jaw position)
Intra-oral appliances (splints)

Discussing the relative clinical effectiveness of the different conservative treatments for TMDs is not in the scope of this chapter. Briefly, however, it is worth noting that a few clinical studies have reported that therapeutic exercise, manual therapy, splint therapy, and patient education can reduce pain and improve range of jaw motion in persons with TMDs.[10,27,41,48] Not all studies concur with these findings, however.[48,49,76] The conflicting results as to the effectiveness of treatment for TMDs result from, in part, the design of the research studies. Many of the studies have not optimally controlled for confounding variables, such as dissimilar treatment interventions or use of subjects with widely varying severities of pathology.

Surgical intervention is relatively rare for persons with TMDs and usually is performed only when the pain is so great or motion so limited that the quality of life is significantly reduced. In addition to arthrocentesis, surgery may involve arthroscopy to inspect the joint and remove adhesions, condylotomy to realign the condyle relative to the disc, arthrotomy (open joint procedures such as disc repositioning and discectomy), and TMJ replacement.[21] Surgery is usually ineffective if performed without other more conservative interventions.

SYNOPSIS

Part 1 of this chapter presents the kinesiology of the temporomandibular joint (TMJ). The pair of joints is physically engaged literally thousands of times per day, not only during mastication, but also during swallowing, speaking, singing,

---

*References 3, 33, 35, 68, 72, 81.

and other nonspecific, subconscious activities. These activities invariably produce compression and shear forces on the joints' articular surfaces and periarticular connective tissues. Forces range from being very small–for instance, during swallowing–to perhaps hundreds of newtons–for instance, during vigorous chewing of food. These forces originate primarily from the actions of muscles. Muscles interact synergistically to open and close the mouth as well as to move the mandible in side-to-side and front-to-back fashions–actions that very effectively crush and grind food before it is swallowed.

In addition to producing large and multidirectional forces, the TMJs must allow extensive motion of the mandible, from just a few millimeters during whispering, to perhaps 5 cm of depression during biting of a large apple. The unique functional demands placed on the TMJs are reflected by the joints' distinctive structure. The joint is loosely articulated to allow both rotation and translation of the mandibular condyle. This combined "sliding-and-hinge joint" increases the potential excursion of the mandible. As a way to protect the joint from potentially large and repetitive forces, the bony articular surfaces are lined with a layer of fibrocartilage and are partially covered by a thick intra-articular disc. The primary functions of the disc are to guide the arthrokinematics, stabilize the joint, and, perhaps most important, reduce stress on the joint's articular surfaces.

During movement of the mandible the disc is constantly repositioned to optimally reduce contact stress–especially between the mandibular condyle and sloped articular eminence of the mandibular fossa. The positioning of the disc is guided by a combination of forces, including passive tension from stretched capsule and retrodiscal laminae, compression from the mandibular condyle, and active forces from the superior head of the lateral pterygoid muscle. In some persons the disc becomes temporally or permanently displaced, no longer able to protect the joint from potentially damaging stress. In more severe and chronic cases, internal derangement of the disc may lead to very painful and reduced motion of the mandible, often associated with chronic inflammation and degeneration of periarticular connective tissue.

Other painful chronic conditions exist at the TMJ, even when the disc is well aligned. Such conditions are often perplexing and difficult to treat. Treatment approaches vary considerably across disciplines. Regardless of approach, clinicians are challenged with understanding the complicated anatomy and kinesiology of the TMJ. This knowledge is the first step toward appreciating the varied clinical manifestations of temporomandibular disorders, as well as understanding the rationale for most conservative and surgical treatment interventions.

PART 2: VENTILATION

Ventilation is the mechanical process by which air is inhaled and exhaled through the lungs and airways. This rhythmic process occurs 12 to 20 times per minute at rest and is essential to the maintenance of life. This chapter now focuses on the kinesiology of ventilation.

Ventilation allows for the exchange of oxygen and carbon dioxide between the alveoli of the lungs and the blood. This exchange is essential to oxidative metabolism within muscle fibers. The process converts chemical energy stored in ATP into the mechanical energy needed to move and stabilize the joints of the body.

The relative intensity of ventilation can be described as "quiet" or "forced." In the healthy population, *quiet ventilation* occurs during relatively sedentary activities that have low metabolic demands. In contrast, *forced ventilation* occurs during strenuous activities that require rapid and voluminous exchange of air, such as exercising, or in the presence of some respiratory diseases. A wide and continuous range of ventilation intensity exists between quiet and forced ventilation.

Figure 11-23 shows the lung volumes and capacities in the normal adult. As depicted, the *total lung capacity* is about 5.5 to 6 L of air. *Vital capacity*, normally about 4500 mL, is the maximum volume of air that can be exhaled after a maximal inhalation. *Tidal volume* is the volume of air moved in and out of the lungs during each ventilation cycle. At rest, tidal volume is about 0.5 L, approximately 10% of vital capacity.

Ventilation is driven by a combination of active and passive forces that alter the volume within the expandable thorax. The change in intrathoracic volume causes a change in air pressure as described by *Boyle's law*. This law states that, given a fixed temperature and mass, the *volume* and *pressure* of a gas, such as air, are inversely proportional. Increasing the volume within the chamber of a piston, for example, lowers the pressure of the contained air. Because air flows spontaneously from high to low pressure, the relatively high air pressure outside the piston forces air into an opening at the top of the piston. In other words, the negative pressure created within the piston sucks air into its chamber (Figure 11-24, *A*). This analogy between the thorax and the piston can be very helpful in understanding the mechanics of ventilation. As will be described, much of the physics of human ventilation is based on the inverse relationship between volume and pressure of a gas.

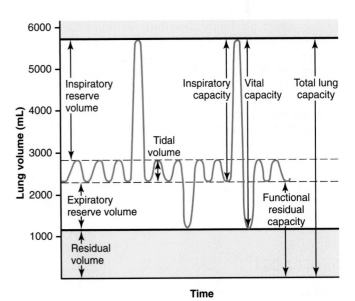

FIGURE 11-23. The lung volumes and capacities in the normal adult. Lung capacity is the sum of two or more volumes. (From Guyton AC, Hall JE: *Textbook of medical physiology*, ed 10, Philadelphia, 2000, Saunders.)

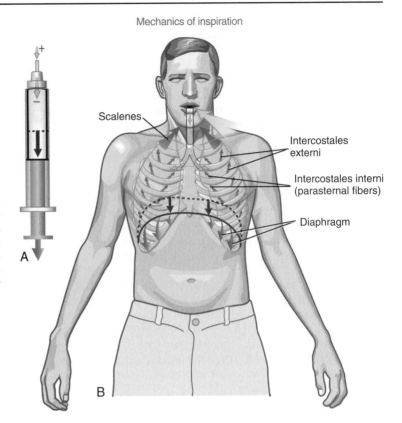

FIGURE 11-24. The muscular mechanics of inspiration. **A,** Using an expanding piston and air to show an analogy using Boyle's law. Increasing the volume within a piston reduces the air pressure within the chamber of the piston. The negative air pressure creates suction that draws the outside, higher-pressure air into the piston through an aperture at the top of the piston. **B,** A healthy adult shows how contraction of the primary muscles of inspiration (diaphragm, scalenes, and intercostales) increases intrathoracic volume, which in turn expands the lungs and reduces alveolar pressure. The negative alveolar pressure draws air into the lungs. The descent of the diaphragm is indicated by the pair of thick, purple, vertical arrows.

During *inspiration* the intrathoracic volume is increased by contraction of the muscles that attach to the ribs and sternum (see Figure 11-24, *B*). As the thorax expands, the pressure within the interpleural space, which is already negative, is further reduced, creating a suction that expands the lungs. The resulting expansion of the lungs reduces alveolar pressure below atmospheric pressure, ultimately drawing air from the atmosphere to the lungs.

Expiration is the process of expiring (exhaling) air from the lungs into the environment. In accord with the analogy to the piston previously described, *decreasing* the volume within the chamber of a piston *increases* the pressure on the contained air, forcing it outward. Expiration in the human occurs by a similar process. Reducing the intrathoracic volume increases the alveolar pressure, thereby driving air from the alveoli, out of the lungs, and to the atmosphere.

In healthy persons, *quiet expiration* is primarily a passive process that does not depend on muscle activation. When the muscles of inspiration relax after contraction, the intrathoracic volume is naturally decreased by the elastic recoil of lungs, thorax, and connective tissues of stretched inspiratory muscles. *Forced expiration,* such as that required to cough or blow out a candle, requires the active force produced by expiratory muscles, such as the abdominals.

ARTHROLOGY

Thorax

The thorax, or rib cage, is a closed system that functions as a mechanical bellows for ventilation. The internal aspect of the thorax is sealed from the outside by several structures

> **BOX 11-1. Tissues That Seal the Thorax**
>
> **POSTERIOR-LATERALLY**
> • Thoracic vertebrae
> • Ribs
> • Intercostal muscles and membrane
>
> **ANTERIORLY**
> • Costal cartilages
> • Sternum
> • Intercostal muscles and membranes
>
> **SUPERIORLY**
> • Upper ribs and clavicles
> • Cervical fascia that surrounds the esophagus and trachea
> • Cervical muscles
>
> **INFERIORLY**
> • Diaphragm muscle

(Box 11-1). Although this chapter focuses on the thorax as a mechanical bellows, the thorax also protects cardiopulmonary organs and large vessels; serves as a structural base for the cervical spine; and provides a site for attachment of muscles that either directly or indirectly act on the head, neck, and extremities.

Articulations within the Thorax

The thorax changes shape during ventilation by varying amounts of movement of the manubriosternal joint and five additional sets of articulations.

STERNOCOSTAL JOINTS

Bilaterally the anterior cartilaginous ends of the first seven ribs articulate with the lateral sides of the sternum. In a broad sense, these articulations are referred to as *sternocostal joints* (see Figure 11-25). Because of the intervening cartilage between the bones of the ribs and the sternum, however, each sternocostal joint is structurally divided into costochondral and chondrosternal junctions.

The *costochondral junctions* represent the transition between the bone and cartilage of the anterior ends of each rib. No capsule or ligament reinforces these junctions. The periosteum of the ribs gradually transforms into the perichondrium of the cartilage. Costochondral junctions permit very little movement.

The *chondrosternal junctions* are formed between the medial ends of the cartilage of the ribs and the small concave costal facets on the sternum. The first chondrosternal junction is a synarthrosis, providing a relatively stiff connection with the sternum.[75] The second through the seventh joints, however, are synovial in nature, permitting slight gliding motions. Fibrocartilaginous discs are sometimes present, especially in the lower joints, where cavities are frequently absent. Each synovial joint is surrounded by a capsule that is strengthened by *radiate ligaments*.

INTERCHONDRAL JOINTS

The opposed borders of the cartilages of ribs 5 through 10 form small, synovial-lined *interchondral joints,* strengthened by *interchondral ligaments* (see Figure 11-25). Ribs 11 and 12 do not attach anteriorly to the sternum.

COSTOCORPOREAL AND COSTOTRANSVERSE JOINTS

The posterior end of the ribs attaches to the vertebral column via the costocorporeal (costovertebral) and costotransverse joints. The *costocorporeal joints* connect the heads of each of the 12 ribs to the corresponding sides of the bodies of the thoracic vertebrae. The *costotransverse joints* connect the articular tubercles of ribs 1 to 10 to the transverse processes of the corresponding thoracic vertebrae. Ribs 11 and 12 usually lack costotransverse joints. The anatomy and ligamentous structures of these joints are described and illustrated in Chapter 9 (see Figure 9-51).

THORACIC INTERVERTEBRAL JOINTS

Movement within the thoracic vertebral column occurs primarily at the interbody and apophyseal joints within the region. It is likely that forced ventilation is associated with modest movement at these joints, although this topic has not been thoroughly investigated. The structure and function of these joints is described in Chapter 9.

Changes in Intrathoracic Volume during Ventilation

VERTICAL CHANGES

During inspiration the vertical diameter of the thorax is increased primarily by contraction and subsequent lowering of the dome of the diaphragm muscle (see Figure 11-24, *B*).

Articulations within the Thorax
- Manubriosternal joint
- Sternocostal joints (including the costochondral and chondrosternal junctions)
- Interchondral joints
- Costocorporeal joints
- Costotransverse joints
- Thoracic intervertebral joints

MANUBRIOSTERNAL JOINT

The manubrium fuses with the body of the sternum at the *manubriosternal joint* (Figure 11-25). This fibrocartilaginous articulation is classified as a synarthrosis, similar to the structure of the pubic symphysis. A partial disc fills the cavity of the manubriosternal joint, completely ossifying late in life. Before ossification, the joint may contribute modestly to expansion of the thorax.

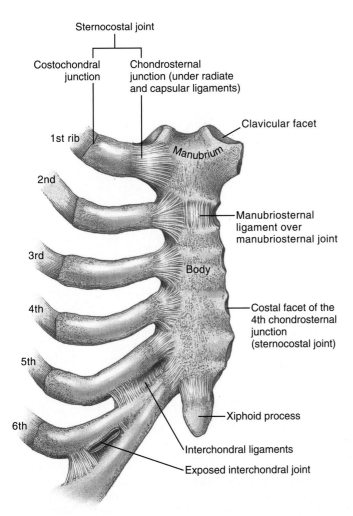

FIGURE 11-25. Anterior view of part of the thoracic wall highlights the manubriosternal joint, sternocostal joints (with costochondral and chondrosternal junctions), and interchondral joints. The ribs are removed on the left side to expose the costal facets.

During quiet expiration the diaphragm relaxes, allowing the dome to recoil upward to its resting position.

ANTERIOR-POSTERIOR AND MEDIAL-LATERAL CHANGES

Elevation and depression of the ribs and sternum produce changes in the anterior-posterior and medial-lateral diameters of the thorax. To varying degrees, all articulations within the thorax contribute to these changes in diameter.

During *inspiration* the shaft of the ribs elevates in a path generally perpendicular to the axis of rotation that courses between the costotransverse and costocorporeal joints (Figure 11-26). The downward sloped shaft of the ribs rotates upward and outward, increasing the intrathoracic volume in both anterior-posterior and medial-lateral diameters. A slight rotation of the posterior joints produces a relatively large displacement of the shaft of the ribs. This mechanism is somewhat similar to the rotation of a bucket handle. During *forced inspiration* the movement of the ribs is combined with slight extension throughout the thoracic spine.

The specific path of movement of a given rib depends partially on its unique shape and on the spatial orientation of the axis of rotation that runs through the costotransverse

and costocorporeal joints. In the *upper six ribs* the axis is displaced horizontally approximately 25 to 35 degrees from the frontal plane; in the *lower six ribs* the axis is displaced horizontally approximately 35 to 45 degrees from the frontal plane. (The anatomic specimen used to illustrate Figure 11-26, *A* shows an approximate 35-degree horizontal displacement from the frontal plane.) This slight difference in angulations causes the upper ribs to elevate slightly more in the anterior direction, thereby facilitating the forward and upward movement of the sternum.

The elevating ribs and sternum create slight bending and twisting movements within the pliable cartilages associated with the joints of the thorax. As depicted in Figure 11-26, *B*, torsion created in the twisted cartilage within a sternocostal joint stores a component of the energy used to elevate the ribs. The energy is partially recaptured during expiration, as the rib cage recoils to its relatively constricted state.

During *expiration* the muscles of inspiration relax, allowing the ribs and the sternum to return to their preinspiration position. The lowering of the body of the ribs combined with the inferior and posterior movements of the sternum decreases the anterior-posterior and medial-lateral diameters of the thorax. During *forced expiration* the movement of the

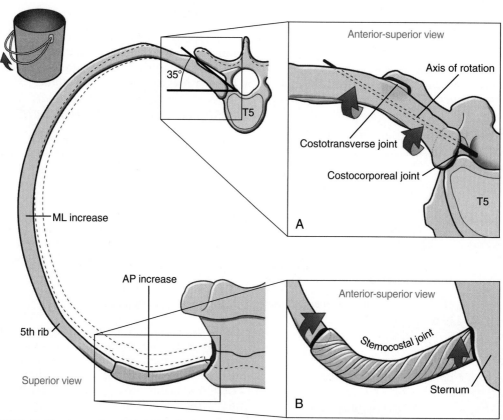

FIGURE 11-26. A top view of the fifth rib shows the "bucket-handle" mechanism of elevation of the ribs during inspiration. The ghosted outline of the rib indicates its position before inspiration. Elevation of the rib increases both the anterior-posterior *(AP)* and medial-lateral *(ML)* diameters of the thorax. The rib connects to the vertebral column via the costotransverse and costocorporeal joints **(A)** and to the sternum via the sternocostal joint **(B)**. During elevation, the neck of the rib moves around an axis of rotation that courses between the costotransverse and costocorporeal joints. The elevating rib creates a twist or torsion in the cartilage associated with the sternocostal joint.

Factors That Can Oppose Expansion of the Thorax

The work performed by the muscles of inspiration must overcome the natural elastic recoil of the lung tissue and connective tissues that comprise the thorax. Additional work is performed to overcome the resistance of the inspired air as it passes through the extensive airways. The amount of air that reaches the alveoli depends on the reduced alveolar pressure, which is determined in part by the net effect of muscle contraction and the mechanical properties that oppose thoracic expansion.

Several factors can significantly oppose expansion of the thorax. Advanced age, for example, is associated with *increased stiffness* (reduced compliance) of the joints and connective tissues that make up the rib cage.[23] The lung tissue, however, loses elastic recoil and becomes *more compliant* with advanced age.[90] (Compliance, in this context, is a measure of the extensibility of the lungs produced by a given drop in transpulmonary pressure.) The *net* compliance of the total respiratory system (thorax and lungs) decreases with advanced age.[89] A greater reduction in pressure is therefore required to inspire a given volume of air. In effect, muscles have to work harder during inspiration. This partially explains why reaching advanced age is typically associated with a slight decrease in tidal volume and a slight increase in respiratory frequency.

Diseases or abnormal postures can also oppose thoracic expansion. Rheumatoid arthritis, for example, can increase the stiffness of the cartilage of the sternocostal joints, thereby resisting an increase in intrathoracic volume. Severe scoliosis or kyphosis may also physically limit the expansion of the thorax.[79]

Common Measurements Used to Determine the Functions of the Ventilatory Muscles

- Muscle morphology such as mass, cross-sectional area, line of force relative to ribs
- Fiber type
- Ventilatory pressures, including changes in pleural pressure per unit of normalized muscle force
- Electromyography from human and animal sources
- Fluoroscopic, ultrasonic, and magnetic resonance imaging
- Effects of nerve stimulation

In addition, clinical observations of the effects of muscle paralysis after spinal cord injury have helped tremendously in the understanding of the normal function of the ventilatory muscles.[32,51,77]

As will be described, any muscle that attaches to the thorax can potentially assist with the mechanics of ventilation. More specifically, a muscle that *increases* intrathoracic volume is a muscle of *inspiration;* a muscle that *decreases* intrathoracic volume is a muscle of *expiration.* The detailed anatomy and innervation of the muscles of ventilation are found throughout Appendix III, Part C, in particular in the section on muscles related primarily to ventilation.

Muscles of Quiet Inspiration

The muscles of quiet inspiration are the diaphragm, scalenes, and intercostales (review Figure 11-24). These muscles are considered primary because they are typically active during all work intensities. Active contraction of the diaphragm muscle is dedicated totally toward the mechanics of inspiration. The intercostales and the scalene muscles, however, also stabilize and rotate parts of the axial skeleton. The mode of action and innervation of the primary muscles of inspiration are summarized in Table 11-4.

DIAPHRAGM MUSCLE

The *diaphragm* is a dome-shaped, thin, musculotendinous sheet of tissue that separates the thoracic cavity from the abdominal cavity. Its convex upper surface is the floor of the thoracic cavity, and its concave lower surface is the roof of the abdominal cavity.

The diaphragm has three parts based on bony attachments: the *costal part* arises from the upper margins of the lower six ribs; the relatively small and variable *sternal part* arises from the posterior side of the xiphoid process; and the thicker *crural part* is attached to the bodies of the upper three lumbar vertebrae through two distinct tendinous attachments known as the *right* and *left crus.* The crural part of the diaphragm contains the longest and most vertically oriented fibers.

The three sets of peripheral attachments of the diaphragm converge to form a *central tendon* at the upper dome of the muscle. Each half of the diaphragm receives its innervation via the phrenic nerve, with nerve roots originating from spinal nerve roots C^3-C^5, but primarily C^4.

Because of the position of the liver within the abdomen, the right side of the resting diaphragm lies slightly higher than the left. During quiet inspiration, the dome of the diaphragm drops about 1.5 cm. During forced inspiration the

---

ribs is accompanied by slight flexion throughout the thoracic spine.

MUSCULAR ACTIONS DURING VENTILATION

The kinesiology of ventilation is very complex and can involve a very large number of muscular interactions, spread across the entire axial skeleton. Such a robust system is needed to precisely control the many different intensities of ventilation, including related activities such as laughing, yawning, holding one's breath while swimming, sighing, and sniffing. Furthermore, with the exception of the diaphragm muscle, all other muscles of ventilation are frequently simultaneously involved with the control of movement and stability of the trunk and craniocervical regions and, indirectly, the upper and lower extremities.

A great deal is still to be learned about the specific functions of the muscles of ventilation. Some methods used to study this topic are listed in the box.*

---

*References 7, 12, 15, 37, 50, 70, 73, 77, 80.

TABLE 11-4. Primary Muscles of Inspiration

Muscle	Mode of Action	Innervation	Location of Illustrations
Diaphragm	*Primary:* The dome of the contracting diaphragm lowers and flattens during inspiration. This movement increases the vertical diameter of the thorax. *Secondary:* The descent of the diaphragm is resisted by the abdomen, which in turn stabilizes the position of the dome of the diaphragm. Further diaphragmatic contraction can *elevate* the lower ribs.	Phrenic nerve (C^3-C^5)	Chapter 11 (Figure 11-27)
Scalenes	The scalene anterior, medius, and posterior increase intrathoracic volume by elevating the ribs and the sternum.	Ventral rami of spinal nerve roots (C^3-C^7)	Chapter 10
Intercostales	The parasternal fibers of intercostales interni and the intercostales externi increase intrathoracic volume by elevating the ribs. During inspiration, all intercostales stabilize the intercostal spaces to prevent an inward collapse of the thoracic wall.	Intercostal nerves (T^2-T^{12})	Chapter 11 (Figure 11-28)

diaphragm flattens and may drop as far as 6 to 10 cm.[75] At maximum inspiration the right side descends to the level of the body of T11; the left side descends to the level of the body of T12.

The diaphragm is the most important muscle of inspiration, performing 60% to 80% of the work of the ventilatory process.[1,62] The muscle's predominant role in inspiration is largely a result of its ability to increase intrathoracic volume in *all* three diameters: vertical, medial-lateral, and anterior-posterior. A given level of muscle contraction therefore yields a relatively large drop in intrathoracic pressure.

The diaphragm is the first muscle to be activated by the nervous system during an inspiratory effort.[70] With the lower ribs stabilized, the initial contraction of the diaphragm causes a lowering and flattening of its dome (Figure 11-27). This lowering piston action substantially increases the *vertical diameter* of the thorax. This action is the primary method by which the diaphragm increases intrathoracic volume. An additional increase in volume requires resistance from within the abdomen. The descent of the diaphragm into the abdominal cavity is resisted by an increase in intra-abdominal pressure; by compressed abdominal contents; and by passive tension in stretched abdominal muscles, such as the transversus abdominis. At some point this abdominal resistance stabilizes the position of the dome of the diaphragm, allowing its continued contraction to *elevate* the lower six ribs. The elevation can be visualized by reversing the direction of the arrowheads in Figure 11-27. As described earlier, elevation of the ribs expands the thorax in the anterior-posterior and medial-lateral diameters.

SCALENE MUSCLES

The *scalenus anterior, medius,* and *posterior* muscles attach between the cervical spine and the upper two ribs (see Chapter 10). If the cervical spine is assumed to be well stabilized, bilateral contraction of the muscles increases intrathoracic volume by elevating the upper ribs and attached sternum. The scalene muscles are active, along with the diaphragm, during every inspiration cycle.[13,38,70]

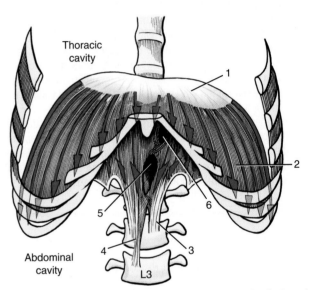

FIGURE 11-27. The action of the diaphragm muscle during the initiation phase of inspiration. *1,* Central tendon; *2,* muscle fibers (costal part); *3,* left crus; *4,* right crus; *5,* opening for the aorta; *6,* opening for the esophagus. (Modified from Kapandji IA: *The physiology of joints,* vol 3, New York, 1974, Churchill Livingstone.)

INTERCOSTALES MUSCLES

Anatomy

The *intercostales* are a thin, three-layer set of muscles that occupy the intercostal spaces. Each set of intercostal muscles within a given intercostal space is innervated by an adjacent intercostal nerve (Figure 11-28).

The *intercostales externi* are most superficial, analogous in depth and fiber direction to the obliquus abdominis externus of the trunk (see Chapter 10). There are 11 per side, and each intercostalis externus arises from the lower border of a rib and inserts on the upper border of the rib below (see Figure 11-28, inset). Fibers travel obliquely between ribs in an inferior and medial direction. The intercostales externi are most developed laterally. Anteriorly, within the region of the sternocos-

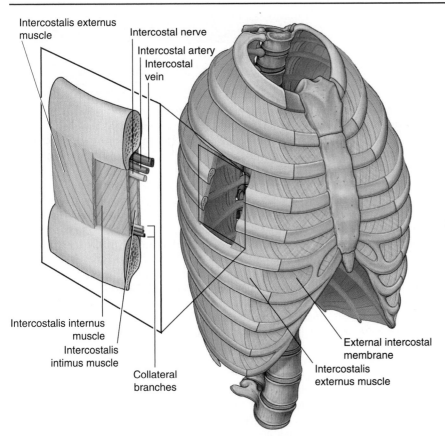

FIGURE 11-28. Illustration showing the three layers of intercostales muscles. (From Drake RL, Vogl W, Mitchell AWM: *Gray's anatomy for students,* St Louis, 2005, Churchill Livingstone.)

tal joints, the intercostales externi are replaced by a thin external intercostal membrane.

The *intercostales interni* are deep to the externi and are analogous in depth and fiber direction to the obliquus abdominis internus of the trunk. There are also 11 per side, with each muscle occupying one intercostal space, in a manner similar to that in the intercostales externi. A major difference, however, is that the fibers of the intercostales interni travel perpendicular to the fibers of the intercostales externi (see Figure 11-28, inset). The intercostales interni are most developed anteriorly within the region of the sternocostal joints; posteriorly, the muscles terminate as the internal intercostal membrane.

Primarily because of differences in function, recent research literature typically refers to the intercostales interni as two different sets of muscle fibers: the *parasternal intercostals,* occupying the region of the sternocostal joints, and the *interosseous intercostals,* occupying the more lateral and posterior-lateral intercostal spaces.[15] This terminology will be used in subsequent discussions.

Finally, the *intercostales intimi* are the deepest and least developed of the intercostales. Often referred to as the "innermost intercostals," these muscles run parallel and deep to the intercostales interni (see Figure 11-28, inset). Fibers of the intercostales intimi located near the angle of the ribs (often designated as *subcostales* muscles) may cross one or two intercostal spaces. The intercostales intimi are most developed in the lower thorax. The actions of these deep and relatively inaccessible muscles have not been extensively studied. It is tempting to speculate, however, that they have actions similar to those of the adjacent intercostales interni.[75]

Function of the Intercostales Externi and Interni Muscles

The intercostales externi and interni muscles are often informally referred to as the "external and internal intercostals," respectively. The specific actions of the intercostal muscles during ventilation are not completely understood and are controversial.[15] The disagreement on this subject is traced back to the teachings of Galen (circa 130-200 AD), Leonardo da Vinci (1452-1519), and Vesalius (1514-1564).[15] In more recent times the conventional teaching on this topic is that the external intercostals muscles drive *inspiration,* and the internal intercostals drive *forced expiration.*[75] To a large extent these functions are based on the contrasting lines of force (fiber direction) of the muscles relative to the axis of rotation through the posterior end of the ribs. In theory, isolated contraction of an external intercostal muscle has greater leverage to elevate the lower rib than to depress the upper. Conversely, an isolated contraction of an internal intercostal muscle has greater leverage to depress the upper rib than to elevate the lower.[15]

Although the proposed relatively simple reciprocal actions of the external and internal intercostals have generally been supported through EMG and other methods of research, the overall muscular kinesiology is far more complicated.* De Troyer and colleagues provide a compelling argument that the action of any given intercostal muscle is influenced not only by its fiber direction and line of pull but also, perhaps more important, by factors associated with the specific region where the muscle resides.[15] These regional-specific factors

---

*References 4, 12, 28, 37, 43, 64, 86.

include the local muscles' force- and torque-generating capability (based on cross-sectional areas and moment arm lengths, respectively), curvature of the ribs, stabilizing influence of other muscles, and most important, differing intensities of neural drive.[14,15,28]

Although the specific actions of the intercostal muscles are variable and not completely understood, the following summary statements reflect the most consistent results from animal and human research.

- The *external intercostal muscles* are primary muscles of *inspiration*.[14,70] The effectiveness of this action is greatest in the dorsal and upper (cranial) regions of the thorax and diminishes in a ventral-to-caudal direction.[14,86]
- The *parasternal fibers of the internal intercostal muscles* are primary muscles of *inspiration*.[70] The effectiveness of this action, however, diminishes in a cranial-to-caudal direction.[16,86]
- The *interosseous fibers of the internal intercostal muscles* are primary muscles of *forced expiration*.[5] The effectiveness of this action persists throughout the thorax.

In addition to functioning as muscles of inspiration or expiration, the lateral set of intercostal muscles (both external and internal) show considerable activation during axial rotation of the trunk. In a similar manner as the "oblique abdominals" (see Chapter 10), the *external* intercostals are most active during contralateral trunk rotation, and the more *internal* intercostals are most active during ipsilateral trunk rotation.[64] The relative contribution of these muscles to the overall biomechanics of axial rotation of the trunk is uncertain.

In addition to expanding the intrathoracic volume during inspiration, contraction of the external and parasternal intercostal muscles also adds a degree of rigidity to the rib cage.[4,14,28] Although often overlooked, this stabilizing function is a very important component of ventilation.[6] With the assistance of the scalene muscles, the splinting action on the ribs prevents the thoracic wall from being partially sucked inward by the reduced intrathoracic pressure caused by contraction of the diaphragm.

As the intercostal muscles contract to stiffen the thoracic cage during inspiration, muscles located in the pharyngeal region also contract slightly to stiffen and dilate the upper airway. One of the main upper airway dilator muscles is the *genioglossus*, a dominant extrinsic muscle of the tongue.[75] The neural control of this muscle during breathing has been extensively studied, primarily because of its possible role in obstructive sleep apnea.[4,69]

Muscles of Forced Inspiration

Forced inspiration requires additional muscles to assist the primary muscles of inspiration. As a group, the additional muscles are referred to as *muscles of forced inspiration,* or *accessory muscles of inspiration.* Table 11-5 lists a sample of several muscles of forced inspiration, including their mode of action. Each muscle has a line of action that can directly or indirectly increase intrathoracic volume. Most muscles listed in Table 11-5 are illustrated elsewhere in this textbook. The serratus posterior superior and serratus posterior inferior are illustrated in Figure 11-29.

The muscles of forced inspiration are typically used in healthy persons to increase the rate and volume of inspired

---

S P E C I A L   F O C U S   1 1 - 5

"Paradoxic Breathing" after Cervical Spinal Cord Injury

In the healthy person, ventilation typically involves a characteristic pattern of movement between the thorax and abdomen. During inspiration the thorax expands outwardly owing to the elevation of the ribs. The abdomen may protrude slightly because of the anterior displacement of the abdominal viscera, compressed by the descending diaphragm.

A complete cervical spinal cord injury below the C4 vertebra typically does not paralyze the diaphragm because its innervation is primarily from the C^4 spinal nerve root. The intercostal and abdominal muscles are, however, typically totally paralyzed. The person with this level of spinal cord injury often displays a "paradoxic breathing" pattern. The pathomechanics of this breathing pattern provide insight into the important functional interactions among the diaphragm, intercostals, and abdominal muscles during inspiration.

Without the splinting action of the intercostal muscles across the intercostal spaces, the lowering of the dome of the diaphragm creates an internal suction within the chest that constricts the upper thorax, especially in its anterior-posterior diameter.[22,84] The term *paradoxic breathing* describes the constriction, rather than the normal expansion, of the rib cage during inspiration. The constriction of the thorax can reduce the vital capacity of a person with an acute cervical spinal cord injury. In the healthy adult, vital capacity is about 4500 mL (review Figure 11-23). About 3000 mL of this inspired volume is accounted for by contraction and full descent of the diaphragm. The vital capacity of a person immediately after a C^4 spinal cord injury may fall as low as 300 mL. Although the diaphragm may be operating at near-normal capacity, the constricting (rather than the normally expanding) thorax limits the inhalation of 2700 mL of air. Several weeks after a spinal injury, however, the atonic (flaccid) intercostals typically become more rigid. The increased muscle tone can act as a splint to the thoracic wall, as evidenced by the fact that vital capacity in an average-size adult with an injury at C^4 or below often returns to near 3000 mL.

In addition to the constriction of the upper thorax during inspiration, a person with an acute cervical spinal cord injury often displays marked *forward protrusion* of the abdomen during inspiration. The atonic and paralyzed abdominal muscles offer little resistance to the forward migration of the abdominal contents. Without this resistance, the contracting diaphragm loses its effectiveness to expand the middle and lower ribs. These pathomechanics also contribute to the loss of vital capacity after a cervical spinal cord injury.

While seated, a person with an acute cervical spinal cord injury may benefit from an elastic abdominal binder. In the seated position the dome of the diaphragm rests lower than in the supine position. An abdominal binder can offer beneficial resistance to the descent of the diaphragm until the anticipated return of firmness in the muscles that support the anterior abdominal wall.[30]

TABLE 11-5. A Sample of Muscles of Forced Inspiration

Muscle	Mode of Action	Innervation	Location of Illustrations
Serratus posterior superior	Increases intrathoracic volume by elevating the upper ribs.	Intercostal nerves (T^2-T^5)	Chapter 11 (Figure 11-29)
Serratus posterior inferior	Stabilizes the lower ribs for initial contraction of the diaphragm.	Intercostal nerves (T^9-T^{12})	Chapter 11 (Figure 11-29)
Levator costarum (longus and brevis)	Increase intrathoracic volume by elevating the ribs.	Dorsi rami of adjacent thoracic spinal nerve roots (C^7-T^{11})	Chapter 10
Sternocleidomastoid	Increases intrathoracic volume by elevating the sternum and upper ribs.	Primary source: spinal accessory nerve (cranial nerve XI)	Chapter 10
Latissimus dorsi	Increases intrathoracic volume by elevating the lower ribs; requires the arms to be fixed.	Thoracodorsal nerve (C^6-C^8)	Chapter 5
Iliocostalis thoracis and cervicis (erector spinae)	Increase intrathoracic volume by extending the trunk.	Adjacent dorsal rami of spinal nerve roots	Chapter 10
Pectoralis minor	Increases intrathoracic volume by elevating the upper ribs; requires activation from muscles such as trapezius and levator scapulae to stabilize the scapula.	Medial pectoral nerve (C^8-T^1)	Chapter 5
Pectoralis major (sternocostal head)	Increases intrathoracic volume by elevating the middle ribs and sternum; requires the arms to be fixed. Greater flexion or abduction of the shoulders increases the vertical line of force of the muscle fibers relative to the muscle's thoracic attachments; this strategy increases the effectiveness of this muscle in increasing intrathoracic volume.	Medial pectoral nerve (C^8-T^1)	Chapter 5
Quadratus lumborum	Stabilizes the lower ribs for contraction of the diaphragm during early forced inspiration.	Ventral rami of spinal nerve roots (T^{12}-L^3)	Chapter 10

air. These muscles may also be recruited at rest to help compensate for the weakness, fatigue, or otherwise reduced function of one or more of the primary muscles of inspiration, such as the diaphragm.

Muscles of Forced Expiration

Quiet expiration is normally a passive process, driven primarily by the elastic recoil of the thorax, lungs, and relaxing diaphragm. In the healthy lungs this passive process is sufficient to exhale the approximately 500 mL of air normally released with quiet expiration.

During forced expiration, active muscle contraction is required to rapidly reduce intrathoracic volume. *Muscles of forced expiration* include the four abdominal muscles, the transversus thoracis, and the interosseous fibers of the intercostales interni (Figure 11-30). The mode of action of the muscles of forced expiration is summarized in Table 11-6.

ABDOMINAL MUSCLES

The "abdominal" muscles include the rectus abdominis, obliquus externus abdominis, obliquus internus abdominis,

and transversus abdominis (see Chapter 10). Contraction of these muscles has a direct and indirect effect on forced expiration. By acting directly, contraction of the abdominal muscles flexes the thorax and depresses the ribs and sternum. These actions rapidly and forcefully reduce intrathoracic volume, such as when coughing, sneezing, or vigorously exhaling to the limits of the expiratory reserve volume. When acting indirectly, contraction of the abdominal muscles—especially the transversus abdominis—increases intra-abdominal pressure and compresses the abdominal viscera. The increased pressure can forcefully push the relaxed diaphragm upward, well into the thoracic cavity (see Figure 11-30). In this manner, active contraction of the abdominal muscles takes advantage of the parachute-shaped diaphragm to help expel air from the thorax. As described in Chapter 10, the increased intra-abdominal pressure is also used during activities involving the Valsalva maneuver, including defecation, childbirth, and lifting of loads or stabilization of the lumbar spine.

Although the abdominal muscles are described here as muscles of forced expiration, their contraction also enhances inspiration. As the diaphragm is forced upward at maximal expiration, it is stretched to an optimal point on its length-tension curve. As a consequence, the muscle is more

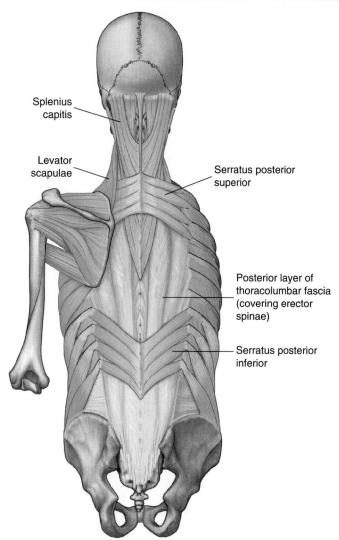

prepared to initiate a forceful contraction at the next inspiration cycle.

TRANSVERSUS THORACIS AND INTERCOSTALES INTERNI

The transversus thoracis (also referred to as the *triangularis sterni*) is a muscle of forced expiration.[16,17] The muscle is located on the internal side of the thorax, running horizon-

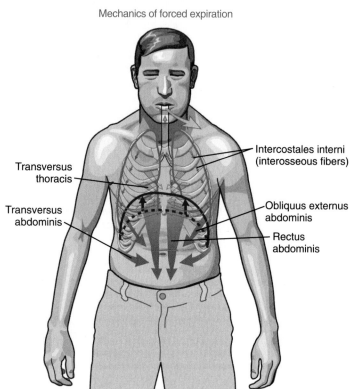

FIGURE 11-29. Illustration highlighting the serratus posterior superior and serratus posterior inferior muscles. These muscles are located within the intermediate layer of the posterior trunk muscles. (From Drake RL, Vogl W, Mitchell AWM: *Gray's anatomy for students,* St Louis, 2005, Churchill Livingstone.)

FIGURE 11-30. Muscle activation during forced expiration. Contraction of "abdominal" muscles, transversus thoracis, and intercostales interni (interosseous fibers) increases intrathoracic and intra-abdominal pressures. The passive recoil of the diaphragm is indicated by the pair of thick, purple, vertical arrows.

TABLE 11-6. **Muscles of Forced Expiration**			
Muscle	**Mode of Action**	**Innervation**	**Location of Illustrations**

Abdominal muscles:
  Rectus abdominis
  Obliquus externus abdominis
  Obliquus internus abdominis
  Transversus abdominis
	1. Decrease intrathoracic volume by flexing the trunk and depressing the ribs.
	2. Compress the abdominal wall and contents, which increases intra-abdominal pressure; as a result, the relaxed diaphragm is pushed upward, decreasing intrathoracic volume.
		Intercostal nerves (T^7-L^1)	Chapter 10

Transversus thoracis	Decreases intrathoracic volume by depressing the ribs.	Adjacent intercostal nerves	Chapter 11 (Figure 11-31)
Intercostales interni (interosseous fibers)	The interosseous fibers of the intercostales interni decrease intrathoracic volume by depressing the ribs.	Intercostal nerves (T^2-T^{12})	Chapter 11 (Figure 11-28)

tally and obliquely superiorly between the lower third of the sternum and the sternocostal joints of the adjacent four or five ribs (Figure 11-31). The muscle's neural activation is synchronized with the abdominal muscles and interosseous fibers of the internal intercostals during forced expiration.[15,17]

SPECIAL FOCUS 11-6

Important Physiologic Functions of the Abdominal Muscles

Forceful expiration is driven primarily by contraction of the abdominal muscles. These muscles are strongly involved in several physiologic functions, including singing, laughing, coughing, and adequately responding to a "gag" reflex when one is choking. The latter two functions are particularly vital to health and safety. Coughing or vigorously "clearing the throat" is a natural way to remove secretions from the bronchial tree, thereby reducing the likelihood of lung infection. A strong contraction of the abdominal muscles is also used to dislodge objects lodged in the trachea.

Persons with weakened or completely paralyzed abdominal muscles must learn alternative methods of coughing or have others "manually" assist with this function. Consider, for example, a person with a complete spinal cord lesion at the T^4 level. Because of the innervation of the abdominal muscles (ventral rami of T^7-L^1), this person would likely have completely paralyzed abdominal muscles. Persons with paralyzed or very weakened abdominal muscles must exercise extra caution to prevent choking.

Internal view

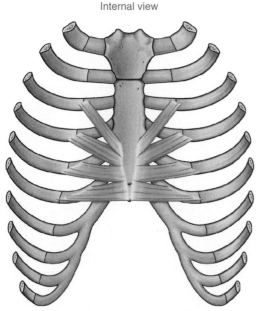

FIGURE 11-31. An internal view of the anterior thoracic wall shows the transversus thoracis muscle. (From Drake RL, Vogl W, Mitchell AWM: *Gray's anatomy for students*, St Louis, 2005, Churchill Livingstone.)

SYNOPSIS

Simply stated, the purpose of ventilation is to produce the intrathoracic pressure gradient that results in bulk flow of air in and out of the lungs. This air flow allows for the exchange of oxygen and carbon dioxide gas within the lungs. This process sustains oxidative cellular respiration, which among other things makes available the energy required for human movement. Part 2 of this chapter focuses almost exclusively on the muscle and joint interactions that drive the mechanics of ventilation.

Four phases of ventilation were studied: quiet inspiration, forced inspiration, quiet expiration, and forced expiration. In each phase but quiet expiration, muscle contraction provides the primary mechanism that changes the volume within the flexible thorax. Based on Boyle's law, changing intrathoracic volume has an inverse relationship on the contained intrathoracic pressure. Because air spontaneously flows away from high pressure and toward low pressure, a muscle force that increases intrathoracic volume will assist with inspiration. Conversely, a muscle force that reduces intrathoracic volume will assist in expiration.

Passive tension created within stretched connective tissues embedded within muscle, ligaments, and the cartilage of the sternocostal joints also has an important role in ventilation, specifically expiration. Once stretched after inspiration, these connective tissues exhibit "elastic recoil" that assists with forcing air out of the lungs.

Pathology, trauma, prolonged inactivity, and, in some persons, advanced age can significantly affect the mechanics of ventilation. Consider, for example, the effects of abnormal muscle function. An extreme example is a complete spinal cord injury above C^4, causing paralysis or at least marked weakness of most primary muscles of ventilation, most notably the diaphragm. Without sufficient force from the diaphragm muscle, attempts to expand the thorax during inspiration may generate only small or no change in intrathoracic pressure. As a result, inspiration draws in negligible amounts of air to the lungs, perhaps insufficient to sustain life without medical intervention. Typically, such intervention is furnished through a mechanical ventilator, an electrically powered device that forces pressurized air into the lungs (via a tracheotomy) at a preset volume, flow rate, humidity, and concentration of oxygen.

Another example of abnormal muscle function affecting ventilation may occur in some persons with cerebral palsy. Although the person may have full innervation of their muscles, the muscles may exhibit excessive tone. Hypertonicity of the abdominal muscles, for example, may result in a sustained increase in intra-abdominal pressure, resisting the descent of the diaphragm during inspiration. If the diaphragm cannot overcome the resistance, the likely reduced vital capacity may limit the physical endurance of the person in other activities, including locomotion. This scenario may be particularly relevant if the person's ability to walk is already labored by increased tone, weakness, or poor control of muscles in the lower extremity.

In addition to abnormal functioning of muscle, pathology affecting the skeletal and other connective tissue systems of the thorax can also affect the mechanics of ventilation. Consider, for example, moderate-to-severe scoliosis, posttraumatic thoracic kyphosis, or ankylosing spondylitis. All these conditions can oppose thoracic expansion and therefore reduce vital capacity. Often, a secondary effect of these conditions is reduced exercise tolerance and subsequent difficulty in maintaining a healthy level of aerobic fitness. Therapeutic interventions for these persons must, when feasible, incorporate creative strategies that appropriately challenge the cardiopulmonary system while simultaneously respecting the limitations imposed by the primary pathology.

ADDITIONAL CLINICAL CONNECTIONS

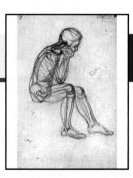

CLINICAL CONNECTION 11-1
The Influence of Posture on the Potential Stress on the Temporomandibular Joint

Based on muscular anatomy, it is likely that posture of the head can influence the resting posture of the mandible.[31,47,54] Consider, for example, the chronic forward head posture described previously in Chapters 9 and 10. The person depicted in Figure 11-32 shows a variant of this posture. Observe that the protracted (forward) head is combined with a flexed upper thoracic and lower cervical spine and with an extended upper craniocervical region. This posture stretches infrahyoid muscles, such as the sternohyoid

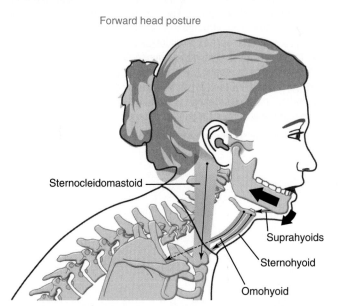

FIGURE 11-32. A forward head posture shows one mechanism by which passive tension in selected suprahyoid and infrahyoid muscles alters the resting posture of the mandible. The mandible is pulled inferiorly and posteriorly, changing the position of the condyle within the temporomandibular joint.

and omohyoid, which can create an inferior and posterior pull on the hyoid bone. The traction is transferred to the mandible through suprahyoid muscles such as the anterior belly of the digastric. As a result, the mandible is pulled in a direction of retrusion and depression. Because of the attachment of the omohyoid to the scapula, poor posture of the shoulder girdle (i.e., an excessively depressed, downwardly rotated, or protracted scapulothoracic joint) can place additional stretch on this muscle and therefore additional pull on the mandible.

Altering the resting posture of the mandible changes the position of its condyle within the mandibular fossa of the temporal bone. A posteriorly displaced condyle could, in theory, compress the delicate retrodiscal tissues, creating inflammation and muscle spasm. Spasm in the lateral pterygoid muscle may be a natural protective mechanism to *protrude* the mandible away from the compressed retrodiscal tissues. Chronic spasm within this muscle may, however, abnormally position the disc *anterior and medial* to the condyle. This situation may predispose a person to a condition of internal derangement of the disc. Although the data suggest an association between abnormal craniocervical posture and disorders of the temporomandibular joint (TMJ),[40] it is difficult to find supporting literature that unequivocally proves such a cause-and-effect relationship.

One underlying concept espoused in the preceding discussion is that the kinesiology of one part of the axial skeleton affects another. Usually this kinesiologic interrelationship is positive in the sense that it optimizes the ease and physiologic efficiency of movement. Abnormal posture, however, can negatively affect this relationship. As described earlier, abnormal scapulothoracic posture affects mandibular posture, and ultimately increases the stress on the TMJ. This premise should reinforce the clinically held notion that an evaluation of a person with a temporomandibular disorder should include a thorough analysis of the posture of the trunk as a whole, from lumbar spine to craniocervical region.

ADDITIONAL CLINICAL CONNECTIONS

CLINICAL CONNECTION 11-2
Chronic Obstructive Pulmonary Disease: Altered Muscle Mechanics

Chronic obstructive pulmonary disease (COPD) is a disorder that typically incorporates three components: (1) chronic bronchitis, (2) emphysema, and (3) asthma. Symptoms include chronic inflammation and narrowing of the bronchioles, chronic cough, and mucus-filled airways, with overdistension and destruction of the alveoli. A significant complication of COPD is the loss of elastic recoil within the lungs and collapsed bronchioles. As a result, air remains trapped in the lungs at the end of quiet or forced expiration. In advanced cases the thorax remains in a chronic state of relative inflation, regardless of the actual phase of ventilation. This complication is called *hyperinflation of the lungs.*[19,26] The thorax of a person with COPD, therefore, often develops a "barrel-shaped" appearance, describing a fixed expansion of the chest and rib cage, primarily in anterior-posterior directions.

The excessive air in the lungs at the end of expiration can alter the position and geometry of the muscles of inspiration, especially the diaphragm. In severe cases the diaphragm remains relatively low in the thorax, with a flattened dome. This change in position and shape can alter the muscle's *resting length* and *line of force.*[45] Operating at a chronically shortened length reduces the muscle's efficiency—often measured as the ratio of power output per level of muscle activation.[4,26,46] Furthermore, the lowered position can redirect the line of force of the costal fibers to a more horizontal orientation (review Figure 11-27). As a consequence, the muscle loses some of its effectiveness in elevating the ribs.[85] At a low enough position, the line of force of the muscle can paradoxically draw the lower ribs *inward* toward the midline of the body, thereby inhibiting lateral expansion of the ribs. These factors can significantly reduce the effectiveness of the diaphragm to fill the lungs during inspiration.

Because of the compromised function of the diaphragm and the increased resistance to airflow in the narrowed bronchioles, persons with advanced COPD often overuse certain muscles during quiet inspiration. Muscles such as the scalenes[18] and other accessory muscles of inspiration (such as sternocleidomastoid and erector spinae) appear to be overactive in phase with inspiration, even at relatively low levels of exertion. Often, a person with COPD may stand or walk with the body partially bent over while placing one or both arms on a stable object, such as the back of a chair, grocery cart, or walker. This strategy stabilizes the distal attachments of arm muscles, such as the sternocostal head of the pectoralis major and latissimus dorsi. As a consequence, these muscles can assist with inspiration by elevating the sternum and ribs. Although this method increases the number of muscles available to assist with inspiration, it also increases the workload of standing and walking, often starting a vicious circle of increased fatigue and dyspnea.

REFERENCES

1. Aliverti A, Cala SJ, Duranti R, et al: Human respiratory muscle actions and control during exercise, *J Appl Physiol* 83:1256–1269, 1997.
2. Baltali E, Zhao KD, Koff MF, et al: A method for quantifying condylar motion in patients with osteoarthritis using an electromagnetic tracking device and computed tomography imaging, *J Oral Maxillofac Surg* 66:848–857, 2008.
3. Buescher JJ: Temporomandibular joint disorders, *Am Fam Physician* 76:1477–1482, 2007.
4. Butler JE: Drive to the human respiratory muscles, *Respir Physiol Neurobiol* 159:115–126, 2007.
5. Butler JE, Gandevia SC: The output from human inspiratory motoneurone pools, *J Physiol* 586:1257–1264, 2008.
6. Butler JE, McKenzie DK, Gandevia SC: Discharge frequencies of single motor units in human diaphragm and parasternal muscles in lying and standing, *J Appl Physiol* 90:147–154, 2001.
7. Cala SJ, Kenyon CM, Lee A, et al: Respiratory ultrasonography of human parasternal intercostal muscle in vivo, *Ultrasound Med Biol* 24:313–326, 1998.
8. Castro HA, Resende LA, Bérzin F, König B: Electromyographic analysis of superior belly of the omohyoid muscle and anterior belly of the digastric muscle in mandibular movements, *Electromyogr Clin Neurophysiol* 38:443–447, 1998.
9. Christo JE, Bennett S, Wilkinson TM, Townsend GC: Discal attachments of the human temporomandibular joint, *Aust Dent J* 50:152–160, 2005.
10. Cleland J, Palmer J: Effectiveness of manual physical therapy, therapeutic exercise, and patient education on bilateral disc displacement without reduction- of the temporomandibular joint: a single-case design, *J Orthop Sports Phys Ther* 34:535–548, 2004.
11. Cooper BC, Kleinberg I: Establishment of a temporomandibular physiological state with neuromuscular orthosis treatment affects reduction of TMD symptoms in 313 patients, *Cranio* 26:104–117, 2008.
12. De Troyer A: Relationship between neural drive and mechanical effect in the respiratory system, *Adv Exp Med Biol* 508:507–514, 2002.
13. De Troyer A, Estenne M: Functional anatomy of the respiratory muscles, *Clin Chest Med* 9:175–193, 1988.
14. De Troyer A, Gorman RB, Gandevia SC: Distribution of inspiratory drive to the external intercostal muscles in humans, *J Physiol* 546:943–954, 2003.
15. De Troyer A, Kirkwood PA, Wilson TA: Respiratory action of the intercostal muscles, *Physiol Rev* 85:717–756, 2005.
16. De Troyer A, Legrand A, Gevenois PA, Wilson TA: Mechanical advantage of the human parasternal intercostal and triangularis sterni muscles, *J Physiol* 513:915–925, 1998.
17. De Troyer A, Ninane V, Gilmartin JJ, et al: Triangularis sterni muscle use in supine humans, *J Appl Physiol* 62:919–925, 1987.
18. De Troyer A, Peche R, Yernault JC, Estenne M: Neck muscle activity in patients with severe chronic obstructive pulmonary disease, *Am J Respir Crit Care Med* 150:41–47, 1994.
19. Decramer M: Hyperinflation and respiratory muscle interaction, *Eur Respir J* 10:934–941, 1997.
20. Desmons S, Graux F, Atassi M, et al: The lateral pterygoid muscle, a heterogeneous unit implicated in temporomandibular disorder: a literature review, *Cranio* 25:283–291, 2007.
21. Dolwick MF: Temporomandibular joint surgery for internal derangement, *Dent Clin North Am* 51:195–208, 2007.
22. Estenne M, DeTroyer A: Relationship between respiratory muscle electromyogram and rib cage motion in tetraplegia, *Am Rev Respir Dis* 132:53–59, 1985.
23. Estenne M, Yernault JC, De TA: Rib cage and diaphragm-abdomen compliance in humans: effects of age and posture, *J Appl Physiol* 59:1842–1848, 1985.
24. Ferrario VF, Sforza C, Miani A Jr, et al: Open-close movements in the human temporomandibular joint: does a pure rotation around the intercondylar hinge axis exist? *J Oral Rehabil* 23:401–408, 1996.
25. Fink M, Tschernitschek H, Stiesch-Scholz M: Asymptomatic cervical spine dysfunction (CSD) in patients with internal derangement of the temporomandibular joint, *Cranio* 20:192–197, 2002.
26. Finucane KE, Panizza JA, Singh B: Efficiency of the normal human diaphragm with hyperinflation, *J Appl Physiol* 99:1402–1411, 2005.
27. Furto ES, Cleland JA, Whitman JM, Olson KA: Manual physical therapy interventions and exercise for patients with temporomandibular disorders, *Cranio* 24:283–291, 2006.
28. Gandevia SC, Hudson AL, Gorman RB, et al: Spatial distribution of inspiratory drive to the parasternal intercostal muscles in humans, *J Physiol* 573:263–275, 2006.
29. Gokalp H, Turkkahraman H, Bzeizi N: Correlation between eminence steepness and condyle disc movements in temporomandibular joints with internal derangements on magnetic resonance imaging, *Eur J Orthod* 23:579–584, 2001.
30. Goldman JM, Rose LS, Williams SJ, et al: Effect of abdominal binders on breathing in tetraplegic patients, *Thorax* 41:940–945, 1986.
31. Goldstein DF, Kraus SL, Williams WB, et al: Influence of cervical posture on mandibular movement, *J Prosthet Dent* 52:421–426, 1984.
32. Gollee H, Hunt KJ, Allan DB, et al: A control system for automatic electrical stimulation of abdominal muscles to assist respiratory function in tetraplegia, *Med Eng Phys* 29:799–807, 2007.
33. Graff-Radford SB: Temporomandibular disorders and other causes of facial pain, *Curr Pain Headache Rep* 11:75–81, 2007.
34. Guarda-Nardini L, Manfredini D, Ferronato G: Temporomandibular joint total replacement prosthesis: current knowledge and considerations for the future, *Int J Oral Maxillofac Surg* 37:103–110, 2008.
35. Hansdottir R, Bakke M: Joint tenderness, jaw opening, chewing velocity, and bite force in patients with temporomandibular joint pain and matched healthy control subjects, *J Orofac Pain* 18:108–113, 2004.
36. Hansson T, Oberg T, Carlsson GE, Kopp S: Thickness of the soft tissue layers and the articular disk in the temporomandibular joint, *Acta Odontol Scand* 35:77–83, 1977.
37. Hawkes EZ, Nowicky AV, McConnell AK: Diaphragm and intercostal surface EMG and muscle performance after acute inspiratory muscle loading, *Respir Physiol Neurobiol* 155:213–219, 2007.
38. Hudson AL, Gandevia SC, Butler JE: The effect of lung volume on the co-ordinated recruitment of scalene and sternomastoid muscles in humans, *J Physiol* 584:261–270, 2007.
39. Iglarsh ZA, Snyder-Mackler L: Temporomandibular joint and the cervical spine. In Richardson JV, Iglarsh ZA, editors: *Clinical orthopaedic physical therapy*, Philadelphia, 1994, Saunders.
40. Ioi H, Matsumoto R, Nishioka M, et al: Relationship of TMJ osteoarthritis/osteoarthrosis to head posture and dentofacial morphology, *Orthod Craniofac Res* 11:8–16, 2008.
41. Ismail F, Demling A, Hessling K, et al: Short-term efficacy of physical therapy compared to splint therapy in treatment of arthrogenous TMD: *J Oral Rehabil* 34:807–813, 2007.
42. Lafreniere CM, Lamontagne M, el-Sawy R: The role of the lateral pterygoid muscles in TMJ disorders during static conditions, *Cranio* 15:38–52, 1997.
43. Le Bars P, Duron B: Are the external and internal intercostal muscles synergist or antagonist in the cat? *Neurosci Lett* 51:383–386, 1984.
44. Mahan PE, Wilkinson TM, Gibbs CH, et al: Superior and inferior bellies of the lateral pterygoid muscle EMG activity at basic jaw positions, *J Prosthet Dent* 50:710–718, 1983.
45. Marchand E, Decramer M: Respiratory muscle function and drive in chronic obstructive pulmonary disease, *Clin Chest Med* 21:679–692, 2000.
46. McKenzie DK, Gorman RB, Tolman J, et al: Estimation of diaphragm length in patients with severe chronic obstructive pulmonary disease, *Respir Physiol* 123:225–234, 2000.
47. McLean L: The effect of postural correction on muscle activation amplitudes recorded from the cervicobrachial region, *J Electromyogr Kinesiol* 15:527–535, 2005.
48. McNeely ML, Armijo OS, Magee DJ: A systematic review of the effectiveness of physical therapy interventions for temporomandibular disorders, *Phys Ther* 86:710–725, 2006.
49. Minakuchi H, Kuboki T, Matsuka Y, et al: Randomized controlled evaluation of non-surgical treatments for temporomandibular joint anterior disk displacement without reduction, *J Dent Res* 80:924–928, 2001.
50. Mizuno M: Human respiratory muscles: fibre morphology and capillary supply, *Eur Respir J* 4:587–601, 1991.
51. Morgan MD, Gourlay AR, Silver JR, et al: Contribution of the rib cage to breathing in tetraplegia, *Thorax* 40:613–617, 1985.
52. Murray GM, Bhutada M, Peck CC, et al: The human lateral pterygoid muscle, *Arch Oral Biol* 52:377–380, 2007.
53. Murray GM, Phanachet I, Uchida S, Whittle T: The role of the human lateral pterygoid muscle in the control of horizontal jaw movements, *J Orofac Pain* 15:279–292, 2001.
54. Nicolakis P, Erdogmus B, Kopf A, et al: Exercise therapy for craniomandibular disorders, *Arch Phys Med Rehabil* 81:1137–1142, 2000.

55. Okeson JP: *Management of temporomandibular disorders and occlusion*, ed 6. St. Louis, 2005, Mosby.

56. Orlando B, Manfredini D, Salvetti G, Bosco M: Evaluation of the effectiveness of biobehavioral therapy in the treatment of temporomandibular disorders: a literature review, *Behav Med* 33:101–118, 2007.

57. Osborn JW: The temporomandibular ligament and the articular eminence as constraints during jaw opening, *J Oral Rehabil* 16:323–333, 1989.

58. Perez del PA, Doblare M: Finite element analysis of the temporomandibular joint during lateral excursions of the mandible, *J Biomech* 39:2153–2163, 2006.

59. Phanachet I, Whittle T, Wanigaratne K, Murray GM: Functional properties of single motor units in the inferior head of human lateral pterygoid muscle: task firing rates, *J Neurophysiol* 88:751–760, 2002.

60. Piehslinger E, Celar AG, Celar RM, Slavicek R: Computerized axiography: principles and methods, *Cranio* 9:344–355, 1991.

61. Posselt U: Movement areas of the mandible, *J Prosthet Dent* 7:375–385, 1957.

62. Ratnovsky A, Elad D: Anatomical model of the human trunk for analysis of respiratory muscles mechanics, *Respir Physiol Neurobiol* 148:245–262, 2005.

63. Ries LG, Alves MC, Berzin F: Asymmetric activation of temporalis, masseter, and sternocleidomastoid muscles in temporomandibular disorder patients, *Cranio* 26:59–64, 2008.

64. Rimmer KP, Ford GT, Whitelaw WA: Interaction between postural and respiratory control of human intercostal muscles, *J Appl Physiol* 79:1556–1561, 1995.

65. Robinson PD: Articular cartilage of the temporomandibular joint: can it regenerate? *Ann R Coll Surg Engl* 75:231–236, 1993.

66. Rocabado M: Arthrokinematics of the temporomandibular joint, *Dent Clin North Am* 27:573–594, 1983.

67. Rollman GB, Gillespie JM: The role of psychosocial factors in temporomandibular disorders, *Curr Rev Pain* 4:71–81, 2000.

68. Rutkiewicz T, Könönen M, Suominen-Taipale L, et al: Occurrence of clinical signs of temporomandibular disorders in adult Finns, *J Orofac Pain* 20:208–217, 2006.

69. Saboisky JP, Butler JE, Fogel RB, et al: Tonic and phasic respiratory drives to human genioglossus motoneurons during breathing, *J Neurophysiol* 95:2213–2221, 2006.

70. Saboisky JP, Gorman RB, De Troyer A, et al: Differential activation among five human inspiratory motoneuron pools during tidal breathing, *J Appl Physiol* 102:772–780, 2007.

71. Sato H, Strom D, Carlsson GE: Controversies on anatomy and function of the ligaments associated with the temporomandibular joint: a literature survey, *J Orofac Pain* 9:308–316, 1995.

72. Schiffman EL, Fricton JR, Haley DP, Shapiro BL: The prevalence and treatment needs of subjects with temporomandibular disorders, *J Am Dent Assoc* 120:295–303, 1990.

73. Singh B, Panizza JA, Finucane KE: Breath-by-breath measurement of the volume displaced by diaphragm motion, *J Appl Physiol* 94:1084–1091, 2003.

74. Sinn DP, de Assis EA, Throckmorton GS: Mandibular excursions and maximum bite forces in patients with temporomandibular joint disorders, *J Oral Maxillofac Surg* 54:671–679, 1996.

75. Standring S: *Gray's anatomy: the anatomical basis of clinical practice*, ed 40, St Louis, 2009, Elsevier.

76. Stiesch-Scholz M, Fink M, Tschernitschek H, Rossbach A: Medical and physical therapy of temporomandibular joint disk displacement without reduction [see comment], *Cranio* 20:85–90, 2002.

77. Strakowski JA, Pease WS, Johnson EW: Phrenic nerve stimulation in the evaluation of ventilator-dependent individuals with C4- and C5-level spinal cord injury, *Am J Phys Med Rehabil* 86:153–157, 2007.

78. Suvinen TI, Kemppainen P: Review of clinical EMG studies related to muscle and occlusal factors in healthy and TMD subjects, *J Oral Rehabil* 34:631–644, 2007.

79. Takahashi S, Suzuki N, Asazuma T, et al: Factors of thoracic cage deformity that affect pulmonary function in adolescent idiopathic thoracic scoliosis, *Spine* 32:106–112, 2007.

80. Takazakura R, Takahashi M, Nitta N, Murata K: Diaphragmatic motion in the sitting and supine positions: healthy subject study using a vertically open magnetic resonance system, *J Magn Res Imaging* 19:605–609, 2004.

81. Tanaka E, Detamore MS, Mercuri LG: Degenerative disorders of the temporomandibular joint: etiology, diagnosis, and treatment, *J Dent Res* 87:296–307, 2008.

82. Tanaka E, Hirose M, Inubushi T, et al: Effect of hyperactivity of the lateral pterygoid muscle on the temporomandibular joint disk, *J Biomech Eng* 129:890–897, 2007.

83. Taskaya-Yilmaz N, Ceylan G, Incesu L, Muglali M: A possible etiology of the internal derangement of the temporomandibular joint based on the MRI observations of the lateral pterygoid muscle, *Surg Radiol Anat* 27:19–24, 2005.

84. Urmey W, Loring S, Mead J, et al: Upper and lower rib cage deformation during breathing in quadriplegics, *J Appl Physiol* 60:618–622, 1986.

85. Vassilakopoulos T, Zakynthinos S, Roussos C: Respiratory muscles and weaning failure, *Eur Respir J* 9:2383–2400, 1996.

86. Wilson TA, Legrand A, Gevenois PA, De Troyer A: Respiratory effects of the external and internal intercostal muscles in humans, *J Physiol* 530:319–330, 2001.

87. Wink CS, St OM, Zimny ML: Neural elements in the human temporomandibular articular disc, *J Oral Maxillofac Surg* 50:334–337, 1992.

88. Yustin DC, Rieger MR, McGuckin RS, Connelly ME: Determination of the existence of hinge movements of the temporomandibular joint during normal opening by Cine-MRI and computer digital addition, *J Prosthodont* 2:190–195, 1993.

89. Zaugg M, Lucchinetti E: Respiratory function in the elderly, *Anesthesiol Clin North Am* 18:47–58, 2000.

90. Zeleznik J: Normative aging of the respiratory system, *Clin Geriatr Med* 19:1–18, 2003.

STUDY QUESTIONS

PART 1: MASTICATION

1 Explain the mechanism by which the *intermediate region* of the articular disc within the temporomandibular joint (TMJ) protects the joint throughout the late phase of opening the mouth.

2 Compare the distal attachments of the medial and lateral pterygoid muscles. Which attachments form a "functional sling" with the masseter muscle?

3 Explain how, in theory, an overly depressed scapulothoracic joint could predispose internal derangement of the articular disc of the TMJ.

4 Compare the differences in structure and functional demands normally placed on articular and nonarticular parts of the mandibular fossa.

5 Describe the functional role of the oblique fibers of the lateral ligament of the TMJ in opening the mouth.

6 Explain the function of the temporalis muscles in closing the mouth.

7 Describe the synergistic relationship between the masseter and contralateral medial pterygoid muscle during the production of shearing (grinding) force between the molars.

8 Using Figure 11-22 as a guide, describe the specific function of the lateral pterygoid muscle during opening and closing of the mouth.

9 Describe how the inferior head of the lateral pterygoid muscle and the suprahyoid muscles act synergistically during a rapid opening of the mouth.

10 List the bones that make up temporal fossa of the cranium.

PART 2: VENTILATION

11 Describe the function of the diaphragm muscle during inspiration, and explain why it is considered the most important muscle of ventilation.

12 Explain how the sternocostal head of the pectoralis major could function as an effective muscle of forced inspiration.

13 How could a chronically lowered (flattened) diaphragm muscle negatively affect the mechanics of ventilation?

14 List the articulations that most likely affect the anterior-posterior and medial-lateral dimensions of the thorax during ventilation.

15 What structures seal the inferior and superior poles of the thoracic cavity?

16 Explain how the normal "tone" within the "abdominal" muscles contributes to the mechanics of inspiration.

17 How does paralysis of the intercostal muscles in a person with quadriplegia contribute to the pathomechanics of "paradoxic breathing"?

18 Describe the changes in intrathoracic and intra-abdominal pressure during forced expiration.

19 List factors explaining why quiet expiration is considered a "passive" process.

20 List the muscles most likely rendered fully paralyzed after a complete spinal cord lesion at the bony level of T4.

⊖ *Answers to the study questions can be found on the Evolve website.*

Reference Materials for Muscle Attachments and Innervation of the Axial Skeleton

Part A: Formation of the Cauda Equina

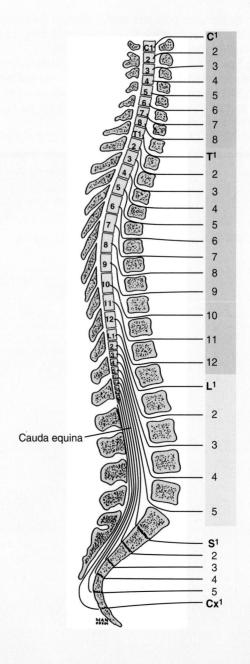

Cauda equina

FIGURE III-1. The anatomic relationship of the spinal cord and spinal nerve roots to the bony elements of the vertebral column. The spinal cord is shown in yellow, and spinal nerve roots are shown in black. The intervertebral foramina through which the spinal nerve roots pass are shown in multiple colors on the right. In the adult the spinal cord is shorter than the vertebral column. The lumbar and sacral nerve roots must therefore travel a considerable distance before each reaches its corresponding intervertebral foramen. These spinal nerve roots coursing through the vertebral canal of the lumbar and sacral vertebrae are called the *cauda equina*. Note that the spinal cord terminates at the L1-L2 intervertebral foramen, cranial to the cauda equina. (From Haymaker W, Woodhall B: *Peripheral nerve injuries,* ed 2, Philadelphia, 1995, Saunders.)

Part B: Thoracic Dermatomes of the Trunk

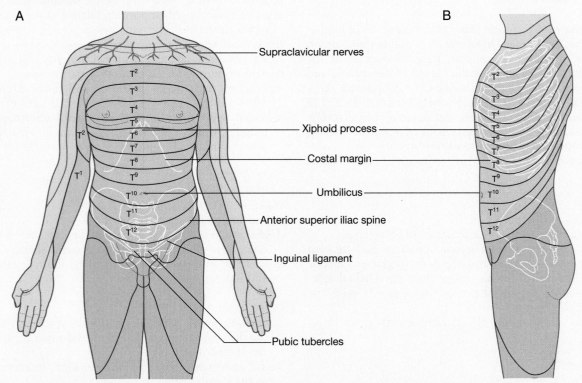

FIGURE III-2. The thoracic dermatomes of the trunk. **A,** Anterior view. **B,** Lateral view. T^1, first thoracic nerve root, and so on. (From Drake R, Vogl W, Mitchell A: *Gray's anatomy for students,* Philadelphia, 2005, Churchill Livingstone.)

Part C: Attachments and Innervation of the Muscles of the Axial Skeleton

MUSCLES OF THE TRUNK

Set 1: Muscles of The Posterior Trunk

See Appendix II for attachments and innervations of the muscles in the superficial layer of the posterior trunk (trapezius, latissimus dorsi, serratus anterior, and so forth).

Erector Spinae Group (Iliocostalis, Longissimus, and Spinalis Muscles)

Iliocostalis Lumborum
Inferior attachment: common tendon*
Superior attachments: angle of ribs 6 to 12

Iliocostalis Thoracis
Inferior attachments: angle of ribs 6 to 12
Superior attachments: angle of ribs 1 to 6

Iliocostalis Cervicis
Inferior attachments: angle of ribs 3 to 7
Superior attachments: posterior tubercles of the transverse processes of C4 to C6

---

*The broad common tendon connects the inferior end of most of the erector spinae to the base of the axial skeleton. The specific attachments of the tendon include the sacrum, spinous processes and supraspinous ligaments in the lower thoracic and entire lumbar region, iliac crests, sacrotuberous and sacroiliac ligaments, gluteus maximus, and multifidi muscles.

Longissimus Thoracis
Inferior attachment: common tendon
Superior attachments: tubercle and angle of ribs 3 to 12; transverse processes of T1 to T12

Longissimus Cervicis
Inferior attachments: transverse processes of T1 to T4
Superior attachments: posterior tubercles of the transverse processes of C2 to C6

Longissimus Capitis
Inferior attachments: transverse processes of T1 to T5 and articular processes of C4 to C7
Superior attachments: posterior margin of the mastoid process of the temporal bone

Spinalis Thoracis
Inferior attachment: common tendon
Superior attachments: spinous processes of most thoracic vertebrae

Spinalis Cervicis
Inferior attachments: ligamentum nuchae and spinous processes of C7 to T1
Superior attachments: spinous process of C2

Spinalis Capitis (Blends with Semispinalis Capitis)
Innervation to the erector spinae: dorsal rami of adjacent spinal nerve roots (C^3-L^5)

Transversospinal Group (Multifidi, Rotatores, and Semispinalis Muscles)

Multifidi
Inferior attachments (lumbar): mammillary processes of lumbar vertebrae, lumbosacral ligaments, deep part of the common tendon of the erector spinae, posterior surface of the sacrum, posterior-superior iliac spine of the pelvis, and capsule of the lumbar and lumbosacral apophyseal joints
Inferior attachments (thoracic): transverse processes of T1 to T12
Inferior attachments (cervical): articular processes of C3 to C7
Superior attachments: spinous processes of vertebrae located two to four intervertebral junctions superior
Innervation: dorsal rami of adjacent spinal nerve roots (C^4-S^3)

Rotatores: Longus and Brevis
Inferior attachments: transverse processes of all vertebrae
Superior attachments: base of spinous processes and adjacent laminae of vertebrae located one or two segments superior
    Note: The rotator longus crosses two intervertebral junctions; the more horizontal rotator brevis crosses only one intervertebral junction.
Innervation: dorsal rami of adjacent spinal nerve roots (C^4-L^4)

Semispinalis Thoracis
Inferior attachments: transverse processes of T6 to T10
Superior attachments: spinous processes of C6 to T4

Semispinalis Cervicis
Inferior attachments: transverse processes of T1 to T6
Superior attachments: spinous processes of C2 to C5, primarily C2

Semispinalis Capitis
Inferior attachments: transverse processes of C7 to T7 and articular processes of C4 to C6
Superior attachments: between the superior and inferior nuchal lines of the occipital bone
Innervation to the semispinalis muscles: dorsal rami of adjacent spinal nerve roots (C^1-T^6)

Short Segmental Group (Interspinalis and Intertransversarius Muscles)

Interspinalis Muscles
These paired muscles attach regularly between adjacent spinous processes within the cervical vertebrae (except C1 and C2) and the lumbar vertebrae. In the thoracic spine, the interspinalis muscles exist only at the extreme upper and lower regions.
Innervation: dorsal rami of adjacent spinal nerve roots (C^3-L^5)

Intertransversarius Muscles
These paired right and left muscles attach between adjacent transverse processes of all cervical, lower thoracic, and lumbar vertebrae. In the cervical region, the intertransversarius muscles are subdivided into small anterior and posterior muscles, indicating their position relative to the anterior and posterior tubercles of the transverse processes, respectively. In the lumbar region the intertransversarus muscles are subdivided into small lateral and medial muscles, indicating their relative position between the transverse processes.
Innervation: the anterior, posterior, and lateral intertransversarus muscles are innervated by ventral rami of adjacent spinal nerve roots (C^3-L^5); the medial intertransversarus muscles, within the lumbar region, are innervated by the dorsal rami of adjacent spinal nerve roots (L^1-L^5)

Set 2: Muscles of the Anterior-lateral Trunk: "Abdominal" Muscles

Obliquus Externus Abdominis
Lateral attachments: lateral side of ribs 4 to 12
Medial attachments: anterior half of the outer lip of the iliac crest, linea alba, and contralateral rectus sheath
Innervation: intercostal nerves (T^8-T^{12}), iliohypogastric (L^1), and ilioinguinal (L^1) nerves

Obliquus Internus Abdominis
Lateral attachments: anterior two thirds of the middle lip of the iliac crest, inguinal ligament, and often from the thoracolumbar fascia
Medial attachments: ribs 9 to 12, linea alba, and contralateral rectus sheath
Innervation: intercostal (T^8-T^{12}), iliohypogastric (L^1), and ilioinguinal (L^1) nerves

Rectus Abdominis
Superior attachments: xiphoid process and cartilages of ribs 5 to 7
Inferior attachments: crest of pubis and adjacent ligaments supporting the pubic symphysis joint
Innervation: intercostal nerves (T^7-T^{12})

Transversus Abdominis
Lateral attachments: anterior two thirds of the inner lip of the iliac crest, thoracolumbar fascia, inner surface of the cartilages of ribs 6 to 12, and inguinal ligament
Medial attachments: linea alba and contralateral rectus sheath
Innervation: intercostal (T^7-T^{12}), iliohypogastric (L^1), and ilioinguinal (L^1) nerves

MUSCLES OF THE CRANIOCERVICAL REGION

Set 1: Muscles of the Anterior-lateral Craniocervical Region

Longus Capitis
Inferior attachments: anterior tubercles of transverse processes of C3 to C6
Superior attachment: inferior surface of the basilar part of the occipital bone, immediately anterior to the attachment of the rectus capitis anterior
Innervation: ventral rami of spinal nerve roots C^1-C^3

Longus Colli
Superior Oblique Portion
Inferior attachments: anterior tubercles of transverse processes of C3 to C5
Superior attachment: tubercle on anterior arch of C1

Vertical Portion

Inferior attachments: anterior surface of the bodies of C5 to T3

Superior attachments: anterior surface of the bodies of C2 to C4

Inferior Oblique Portion

Inferior attachments: anterior surface of the bodies of T1 to T3

Superior attachments: anterior tubercles of transverse processes of C5 to C6

Innervation: ventral rami of adjacent spinal nerve roots (C^2-C^8)

Rectus Capitis Anterior

Inferior attachment: anterior surface of the transverse process of C1

Superior attachment: inferior surface of the basilar part of the occipital bone immediately anterior to the occipital condyle

Innervation: ventral rami of spinal nerve roots C^1-C^2

Rectus Capitis Lateralis

Inferior attachment: superior surface of the transverse process of C1

Superior attachment: inferior surface of the occipital bone immediately lateral to the occipital condyle

Innervation: ventral rami of spinal nerve roots C^1-C^2

Scalenes

Scalenus Anterior

Superior attachments: anterior tubercles of the transverse processes of C3 to C6

Inferior attachment: inner border of first rib

Scalenus Medius

Superior attachments: posterior tubercles of the transverse processes of C2 to C7

Inferior attachment: upper border of the first rib, posterior to the attachment of the scalenus anterior

Scalenus Posterior

Superior attachments: posterior tubercles of the transverse processes of C5 to C7

Inferior attachment: external surface of the second rib

Innervation to the scalene muscles: ventral rami of adjacent spinal nerve roots (C^3-C^7)

Sternocleidomastoid

Inferior attachments: sternal head, anterior surface of the upper aspect of the manubrium of the sternum; clavicular head; posterior-superior surface of the medial one third of the clavicle

Superior attachments: lateral surface of the mastoid process of the temporal bone and lateral one half of the superior nuchal line of the occipital bone

Innervation: spinal accessory nerve (cranial nerve XI); a secondary source of innervation is through the ventral rami of nerve roots from the mid and upper cervical plexus, which may carry sensory (proprioceptive) information

Set 2: Muscles of the Posterior Craniocervical Region

Splenius Capitis

Inferior attachments: inferior half of the ligamentum nuchae and spinous processes of C7 to T4

Superior attachments: mastoid process of the temporal bone and the lateral one third of the superior nuchal line of the occipital bone

Innervation: dorsal rami of spinal nerve roots C^2-C^8

Splenius Cervicis

Inferior attachments: spinous processes of T3 to T6

Superior attachments: posterior tubercles of the transverse processes of C1 to C3

Innervation: dorsal rami of spinal nerve roots C^2-C^8

Suboccipital Muscles

Obliquus Capitis Inferior

Inferior attachment: apex of the spinous process of C2

Superior attachment: inferior margin of the transverse process of C1

Obliquus Capitis Superior

Inferior attachment: superior margin of the transverse process of C1

Superior attachments: between the lateral end of the inferior and superior nuchal lines

Rectus Capitis Posterior Major

Inferior attachment: spinous process of C2

Superior attachment: immediately anterior and medial to the lateral end of the inferior nuchal line

Rectus Capitis Posterior Minor

Inferior attachment: tubercle on the posterior arch of C1

Superior attachment: immediately anterior to the medial end of the inferior nuchal line, just posterior to the foramen magnum

Innervation to suboccipital muscles: suboccipital nerve (dorsal ramus of spinal nerve root C^1)

MISCELLANEOUS: QUADRATUS LUMBORUM

Quadratus Lumborum

Inferior attachments: iliolumbar ligament and crest of the ilium

Superior attachments: rib 12 and tips of the transverse processes of the L1 to L4

Innervation: ventral ramus of spinal nerve roots T^{12}-L^3

PRIMARY MUSCLES OF MASTICATION

Masseter: Combined Superficial and Deep Heads

Proximal attachments: lateral-inferior surfaces of the zygomatic bone and inferior surfaces of the zygomatic arch

Distal attachment: external surface of the mandible, between the angle and just below the coronoid process

Innervation: branch of the mandibular nerve, a division of cranial nerve V

Temporalis

Proximal attachments: temporal fossa and deep surfaces of temporal fascia

Distal attachments: apex and medial surfaces of the coronoid process of the mandible and the entire anterior edge of the ramus of the mandible

Innervation: branch of the mandibular nerve, a division of cranial nerve V

Medial Pterygoid: Combined Superficial and Deep Heads

Proximal attachments: medial surface of the lateral pterygoid plate; small area on the posterior-lateral maxilla, just above the socket for the third molar

Distal attachment: internal surface of the mandible between the angle and mandibular foramen

Innervation: branch of the mandibular nerve, a division of cranial nerve V

Lateral Pterygoid (Superior Head)

Proximal attachment: greater wing of the sphenoid bone

Distal attachments: medial wall of the capsule of the temporomandibular joint (TMJ), medial side of the articular disc, and pterygoid fossa of the mandible

Lateral Pterygoid (Inferior Head)

Proximal attachments: lateral side of the lateral pterygoid plate and adjoining region of the maxilla

Distal attachments: pterygoid fossa and adjacent neck of the mandible

Innervation: branch of the mandibular nerve, a division of cranial nerve V

SUPRAHYOID MUSCLES

Digastric: Posterior Belly

Proximal attachment: mastoid notch of the temporal bone

Distal attachment: facial sling attached to the lateral aspect of the hyoid bone

Innervation: facial nerve (cranial nerve VII)

Digastric: Anterior Belly

Proximal attachment: fascial sling attached to the lateral aspect of the hyoid bone

Distal attachment: base of the mandible near its midline (digastric fossa)

Innervation: inferior alveolar nerve (branch of the mandibular nerve, a division of cranial nerve V)

Geniohyoid

Proximal attachment: small region at the midline of the anterior aspect of the mandible's internal surface (symphysis menti)

Distal attachment: body of the hyoid bone

Innervation: C^1 via the hypoglossal nerve (cranial nerve XII)

Mylohyoid

Proximal attachment: the internal surface of the mandible, bilaterally on the mylohyoid line

Distal attachment: body of the hyoid bone

Innervation: inferior alveolar nerve (branch of the mandibular nerve, a division of cranial nerve V)

Stylohyoid

Proximal attachment: base of the styloid process of the temporal bone

Distal attachment: anterior edge of the greater horn of the hyoid bone

Innervation: facial nerve (cranial nerve VII)

INFRAHYOID MUSCLES

Omohyoid

Inferior attachment: upper border of the scapula near the scapular notch

Superior attachment: body of the hyoid bone

Innervation: ventral rami of spinal nerve roots C^1-C^3

Sternohyoid

Inferior attachments: posterior surface of the medial end of the clavicle, superior-posterior part of the manubrium sternum, and posterior sternoclavicular ligament

Superior attachment: body of the hyoid bone

Innervation: ventral rami of spinal nerve roots C^1-C^3

Sternothyroid

Inferior attachments: posterior part of the manubrium of the sternum and the cartilage of the first rib

Superior attachment: thyroid cartilage

Innervation: ventral rami of spinal nerve roots C^1-C^3

Thyrohyoid

Inferior attachment: thyroid cartilage

Superior attachment: junction of the body and greater horn of the hyoid bone

Innervation: ventral ramus of spinal nerve root C^1 (via cranial nerve XII)

MUSCLES RELATED PRIMARILY TO VENTILATION

Diaphragm

Inferior Attachments

Costal part: inner surfaces of the cartilages and adjacent bony regions of ribs 6 to 12

Sternal part: posterior side of the xiphoid process

Crural (lumbar) part: (1) two aponeurotic arches covering the external surfaces of the quadratus lumborum and psoas major muscles; (2) right and left crus, originating from the bodies of L1 to 3 and their intervertebral discs

Superior Attachment

Central tendon near the center of the dome of the muscle

Innervation: phrenic nerve (C^3-C^5)

Intercostales Externi

Attachments: Eleven per side; each muscle arises from the lower border of a rib and inserts on the upper border of the rib below. Fibers are the most superficial of the intercostales muscles, running in an inferior and medial direction. Fibers are most *developed laterally.*

Intercostales Interni

Attachments: Eleven per side; each muscle arises from the lower border of a rib and inserts on the upper border of the rib below. Fibers run in a plane immediately deep to the intercostales externi. Fibers of the intercostales interni run in an inferior and slightly lateral direction, nearly perpendicular to the direction of the intercostales externi. Fibers of the intercostales interni are most developed adjacent to the sternum, parasternally.

Intercostales Intimi

Attachments: Each muscle arises from the lower border of a rib near its angle and inserts on the upper border of the second or third rib below. Fibers run parallel and deep to the intercostales interni. Fibers of the intercostales intimi located near the angle of the ribs, often called *subcostales,* may cross two intercostal spaces. The intercostales intimi are most developed in the lower thorax.

Innervation to the intercostales: intercostal nerves (T^2-T^{12})

Levatores Costarum (Longus and Brevis)

Superior attachments: ends of the transverse processes of C7 to T11

Inferior attachments: external surfaces of ribs, between the tubercle and angle. Muscles may attach to the rib immediately inferior to its superior attachment (levatores costarum brevis), or, most notably in the lower segments, to the rib two segments inferior to its superior attachment (levatores costarum longus)

Innervation: dorsal rami of adjacent thoracic spinal nerve roots (C^7-T^{11})

Serratus Posterior Inferior

Superior attachments: posterior surfaces of ribs 9 to 12, near their angles

Inferior attachments: spinous processes and supraspinous ligaments of T11 to L3

Innervation: intercostal nerves (T^9-T^{12})

Serratus Posterior Superior

Superior attachments: spinous processes of C6 to T3, including supraspinous ligaments and ligamentum nuchae

Inferior attachments: posterior surfaces of ribs 2 to 5, near their angles

Innervation: intercostal nerves (T^2-T^5)

Transversus Thoracis

Inferior (medial) attachments: inner surfaces of the lower third of the body of the sternum and adjacent surfaces of the xiphoid process

Superior (lateral) attachments: internal surfaces of the sternocostal joints associated with the second (or third) through the sixth ribs

Innervation: adjacent intercostal nerves

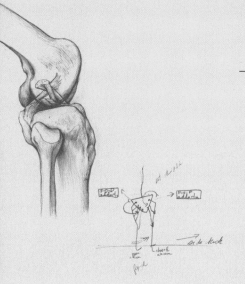

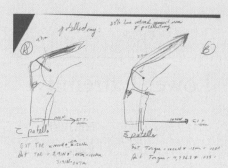

Section

IV

Lower Extremity

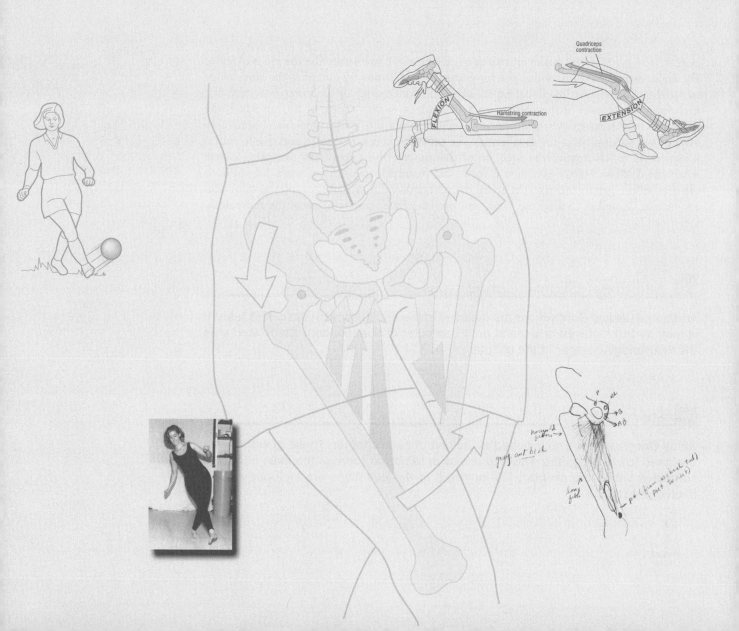

Section IV

Lower Extremity

SECTION IV is divided into four chapters. Chapters 12 to 14 describe the kinesiology of the major articular regions within the lower extremity; Chapter 15 describes the kinesiology of walking, an ultimate functional expression of the kinesiology of the lower extremity. For each limb, about 60% of the walking cycle is involved in the "stance phase," in which the distal end of the extremity is fixed to the ground. During the "swing phase"—the remaining 40% of the walking cycle—the distal end of the extremity is unconstrained and free to move. Chapters 12 to 14 describe the function of the muscles and joints from two perspectives: when the distal end of the extremity is fixed, and when it is free. An understanding of both types of actions greatly increases the ability to appreciate the beauty and complexity of human movement, as well as to diagnose, treat, and prevent related impairments of the musculoskeletal system.

Additional Clinical Connections

Additional Clinical Connections are included at the end of each chapter. This feature is intended to highlight or expand on a particular clinical concept associated with the kinesiology covered in the chapter.

Study Questions

Study Questions are also included at the end of each chapter. These questions are designed to challenge the reader to review or reinforce some of the main concepts contained within the chapter. The answers to the questions are included on the Evolve website.⊝

CHAPTER 12

Hip

DONALD A. NEUMANN, PT, PhD, FAPTA

The hip is the articulation between the large spherical head of the femur and the deep socket provided by the acetabulum of the pelvis (Figure 12-1). Because of the joints' central location within the body, the logical question arises: do the hips serve as "base" joints for the lower extremities, or basilar joints for the entire superimposed pelvis and trunk? As this chapter unfolds, it will become clear that the hips serve *both* roles. For this reason the hips play a dominant kinesiologic role in movements across a large part of the body. Pathology or trauma affecting the hips typically causes a wide range of functional limitations, including difficulty in walking, dressing, driving a car, lifting and carrying loads, and climbing stairs.

The hip joint has many anatomic features that are well suited for stability during standing, walking, and running. The femoral head is stabilized by a deep socket that is surrounded and sealed by an extensive set of connective tissues. Many large and forceful muscles generate the necessary torques needed to accelerate the body upward and forward, or decelerate the body in a controlled fashion. Weakness in these muscles can have a profound impact on the mobility and stability of the body as a whole.

Hip disease and injury are relatively common, particularly in the very young and in the elderly. An abnormally formed hip in an infant may be prone to dislocation. The hip in the aged adult is vulnerable to degenerative joint disease. Increased osteoporosis coupled with increased risk of falling also predisposes the elderly to a higher incidence of hip fracture.

This chapter describes the structure of the hip, its associated capsule and ligaments, and the actions of the surrounding musculature. This information is the basis for treatment and diagnosis of musculoskeletal problems in this important region of the body.

OSTEOLOGY

Innominate

Each *innominate* (from the Latin *innominatum*, meaning nameless) is the union of three bones: the *ilium, pubis,* and *ischium* (see Figures 12-1 and 12-2). The right and left innominates connect with each other anteriorly at the pubic symphysis and posteriorly at the sacrum. These connections form a

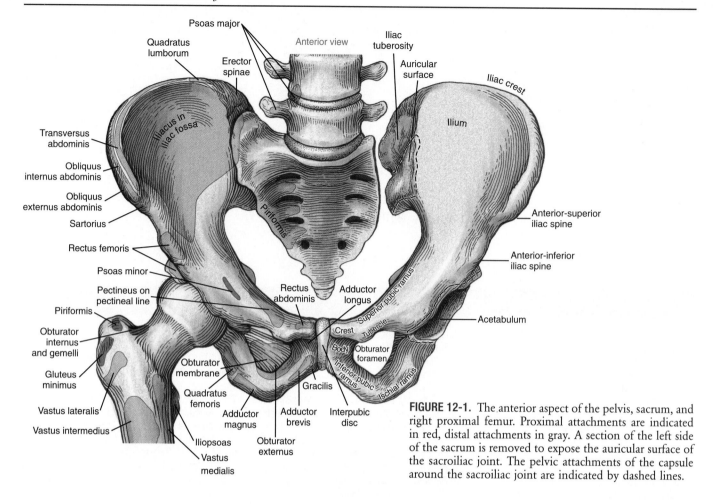

Psoas major
Quadratus lumborum
Erector spinae
Anterior view
Iliac tuberosity
Auricular surface
Iliac crest
Transversus abdominis
Iliacus in iliac fossa
Ilium
Obliquus internus abdominis
Obliquus externus abdominis
Sartorius
Rectus femoris
Psoas minor
Pectineus on pectineal line
Piriformis
Obturator internus and gemelli
Gluteus minimus
Vastus lateralis
Vastus intermedius
Piriformis
Rectus abdominis
Adductor longus
Superior pubic ramus
Crest
Tubercle
Body
Obturator foramen
Inferior pubic ramus
Ischial ramus
Anterior-superior iliac spine
Anterior-inferior iliac spine
Acetabulum
Obturator membrane
Quadratus femoris
Adductor magnus
Adductor brevis
Obturator externus
Gracilis
Interpubic disc
Iliopsoas
Vastus medialis

FIGURE 12-1. The anterior aspect of the pelvis, sacrum, and right proximal femur. Proximal attachments are indicated in red, distal attachments in gray. A section of the left side of the sacrum is removed to expose the auricular surface of the sacroiliac joint. The pelvic attachments of the capsule around the sacroiliac joint are indicated by dashed lines.

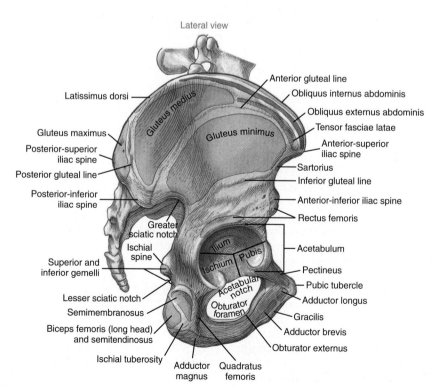

Lateral view
Latissimus dorsi
Gluteus medius
Gluteus maximus
Posterior-superior iliac spine
Posterior gluteal line
Posterior-inferior iliac spine
Greater sciatic notch
Ischial spine
Superior and inferior gemelli
Lesser sciatic notch
Semimembranosus
Biceps femoris (long head) and semitendinosus
Ischial tuberosity
Adductor magnus
Quadratus femoris
Anterior gluteal line
Obliquus internus abdominis
Obliquus externus abdominis
Tensor fasciae latae
Anterior-superior iliac spine
Sartorius
Inferior gluteal line
Anterior-inferior iliac spine
Rectus femoris
Ilium
Pubis
Ischium
Acetabulum
Pectineus
Pubic tubercle
Adductor longus
Gracilis
Adductor brevis
Obturator externus
Gluteus minimus
Acetabular notch
Obturator foramen

FIGURE 12-2. A lateral view of the right innominate bone. Proximal attachments of muscle are indicated in red, distal attachments in gray.

complete osteoligamentous ring, referred to as the *pelvis* (from the Latin, meaning basin or bowl). The pelvis is associated with three important and very different functions. First, the pelvis serves as a common attachment point for many large muscles of the lower extremity and the trunk. The pelvis also transmits the weight of the upper body and trunk either to the ischial tuberosities during sitting or to the lower extremities during standing and walking. Last, with the aid of the muscles and connective tissues of the pelvic floor, the pelvis supports the organs involved with bowel, bladder, and reproductive functions.

The external surface of the pelvis has three striking features. The large fan-shaped *wing* (or *ala*) of the ilium forms the superior half of the innominate. Just below the wing is the deep, cup-shaped *acetabulum*. Just inferior and slightly medial to the acetabulum is the *obturator foramen*—the largest foramen in the body. This foramen is covered by an *obturator membrane* (see Figure 12-1).

While a person stands, the pelvis is normally oriented so that when viewed laterally a vertical line passes between the anterior-superior iliac spine and the pubic tubercle (see Figure 12-2).

ILIUM

The external surface of the ilium is marked by rather faint *posterior, anterior,* and *inferior gluteal lines* (see Figure 12-2). These lines help to identify attachment sites of the gluteal muscles. At the most anterior extent of the ilium is the easily palpable *anterior-superior iliac spine* (see Figures 12-1 and 12-2). Below this spine is the *anterior-inferior iliac spine.* The prominent *iliac crest,* the most superior rim of the ilium, continues

posteriorly and ends at the *posterior-superior iliac spine* (Figure 12-3). The soft tissue superficial to the posterior-superior iliac spine is often marked by a dimple in the skin. The less prominent *posterior-inferior iliac spine* marks the superior rim of the *greater sciatic notch.* The opening of this notch is converted to the *greater sciatic foramen* by the *sacrotuberous* and *sacrospinous ligaments.*

The internal aspect of the ilium has three notable features (see Figure 12-1). Anteriorly, the smooth concave *iliac fossa* is filled by the iliacus muscle. Posteriorly, the *auricular surface* articulates with the sacrum at the sacroiliac joint. Just posterior to the auricular surface is the large, rough *iliac tuberosity,* which marks the attachments of sacroiliac ligaments.

Osteologic Features of the Ilium

External Surface
- Posterior, anterior, and inferior gluteal lines
- Anterior-superior iliac spine
- Anterior-inferior iliac spine
- Iliac crest
- Posterior-superior iliac spine
- Posterior-inferior iliac spine
- Greater sciatic notch
- Greater sciatic foramen
- Sacrotuberous and sacrospinous ligaments

Internal Surface
- Iliac fossa
- Auricular surface
- Iliac tuberosity

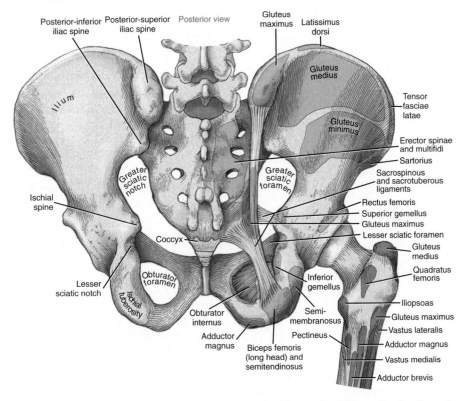

FIGURE 12-3. The posterior aspect of the pelvis, sacrum, and right proximal femur. Proximal attachments of muscles are indicated in red, distal attachments in gray.

Osteologic Features of the Pubis
- Superior pubic ramus
- Body
- Crest
- Pectineal line
- Pubic tubercle
- Pubic symphysis joint and disc
- Inferior pubic ramus

PUBIS

The *superior pubic ramus* extends anteriorly from the anterior wall of the acetabulum to the large flattened *body* of the pubis (see Figure 12-1). The upper border of the body of the pubis is the pubic *crest*, serving as an attachment for the rectus abdominus muscle. On the upper surface of the superior ramus is the *pectineal line,* marking the attachment of the pectineus muscle. The *pubic tubercle* projects anteriorly from the superior pubic ramus, serving as an attachment for the inguinal ligament. The *inferior pubic ramus* extends from the body of the pubis posteriorly to the junction of the ischium.

The two pubic bones articulate in the midline by way of the *pubic symphysis joint* (see Figure 12-1). This relatively immobile joint is typically classified as a synarthrosis. Hyaline cartilage lines the opposing surfaces of the articulation; the surfaces are not completely flat but possess small raised ridges, likely designed to resist shear.[160] The joint is firmly bound by a fibrocartilaginous *interpubic disc* and ligaments. The interpubic disc is strengthened by an interlacing of collagen fibers, combined with distal attachments made by the rectus abdominis muscles.[160] Up to 2 mm of translation and very slight rotation occur at the pubic symphysis joint.[168] The pubic symphysis provides stress relief throughout the anterior ring of the pelvis during walking and, in women, during childbirth.

Symphysis pubis dysfunction can occur in some women during pregnancy or just after birth. This painful condition is associated with increased instability in the symphysis pubis caused by the physiologic relaxation of the joint's supporting ligaments.[89]

ISCHIUM

The sharp *ischial spine* projects from the posterior side of the ischium, just inferior to the greater sciatic notch (see Figure 12-3). The *lesser sciatic notch* is located just inferior to the spine. The *sacrotuberous* and *sacrospinous ligaments* convert the lesser sciatic notch into a *lesser sciatic foramen.*

Projecting posteriorly and inferiorly from the acetabulum is the large, stout *ischial tuberosity* (see Figure 12-3). This palpable structure serves as the proximal attachment for many muscles of the lower extremity, most notably the hamstrings and part of the adductor magnus. The *ischial ramus* extends anteriorly from the ischial tuberosity, ending at the junction with the inferior pubic ramus (see Figure 12-1).

ACETABULUM

Located just above the obturator foramen is the large cup-shaped acetabulum (see Figure 12-2). The acetabulum forms the socket of the hip. All three bones of the pelvis contribute to the formation of the acetabulum: the ilium and ischium contribute about 75%, and the pubis contributes the remain-

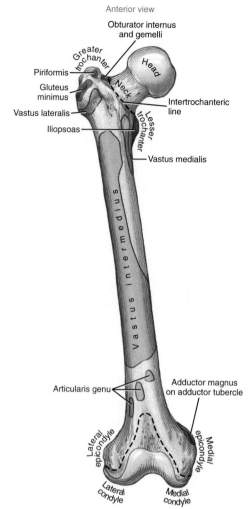

Anterior view

FIGURE 12-4. The anterior aspect of the right femur. Proximal attachments of muscles are indicated in red, distal attachments in gray. The femoral attachments of the hip joint capsule and the knee joint capsule are indicated by dashed lines.

Osteologic Features of the Ischium
- Ischial spine
- Lesser sciatic notch
- Lesser sciatic foramen
- Ischial tuberosity
- Ischial ramus

ing approximately 25%. The specific features of the acetabulum are discussed in the section on arthrology.

Femur

The femur is the longest and strongest bone of the human body (Figure 12-4). Its shape and robust stature reflect the powerful action of muscles and contribute to the long stride length during walking. At its proximal end, the femoral *head* projects medially and slightly anteriorly for an articulation with the acetabulum. The femoral *neck* connects the femoral head to the shaft. The neck serves to displace the proximal shaft of the femur laterally away from the joint, thereby reducing the likelihood of bony impingement against the pelvis. Distal to the neck, the shaft of the femur courses slightly medially, effectively placing the knees and feet closer to the midline of the body.

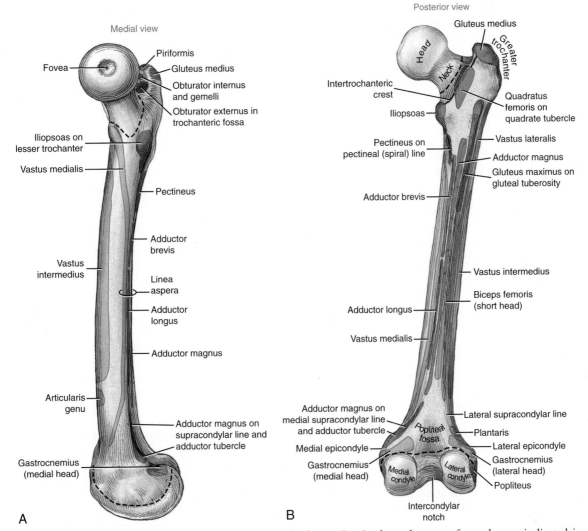

Medial view

Fovea
Piriformis
Gluteus medius
Obturator internus and gemelli
Obturator externus in trochanteric fossa
Iliopsoas on lesser trochanter
Vastus medialis
Pectineus
Adductor brevis
Vastus intermedius
Linea aspera
Adductor longus
Adductor magnus
Articularis genu
Adductor magnus on supracondylar line and adductor tubercle
Gastrocnemius (medial head)

A

Posterior view

Gluteus medius
Head
Greater trochanter
Neck
Intertrochanteric crest
Quadratus femoris on quadrate tubercle
Iliopsoas
Vastus lateralis
Pectineus on pectineal (spiral) line
Adductor magnus
Gluteus maximus on gluteal tuberosity
Adductor brevis
Vastus intermedius
Biceps femoris (short head)
Adductor longus
Vastus medialis
Adductor magnus on medial supracondylar line and adductor tubercle
Lateral supracondylar line
Popliteal fossa
Plantaris
Medial epicondyle
Lateral epicondyle
Gastrocnemius (medial head)
Medial condyle
Lateral condyle
Gastrocnemius (lateral head)
Popliteus
Intercondylar notch

B

FIGURE 12-5. The medial **(A)** and posterior **(B)** surfaces of the right femur. Proximal attachments of muscles are indicated in red, distal attachments in gray. The femoral attachments of the hip joint capsule and the knee joint capsule are indicated by dashed lines.

Osteologic Features of the Femur
- Femoral head
- Femoral neck
- Intertrochanteric line
- Greater trochanter
- Trochanteric fossa
- Intertrochanteric crest
- Quadrate tubercle
- Lesser trochanter
- Linea aspera
- Pectineal (spiral) line
- Gluteal tuberosity
- Lateral and medial supracondylar lines
- Adductor tubercle

The shaft of the femur displays a slight anterior convexity (Figure 12-5, *A*). As a long, eccentrically loaded column, the femur bows very slightly when subjected to the weight of the body. Consequently, stress along the bone is dissipated through compression along its posterior shaft and through tension along its anterior shaft. Ultimately this bowing allows the femur to bear a greater load than if the femur were perfectly straight.

Anteriorly, the *intertrochanteric line* marks the distal attachment of the capsular ligaments (see Figure 12-4). The *greater trochanter* extends laterally and posteriorly from the junction of the femoral neck and shaft (see Figure 12-5, *B*). This promi-

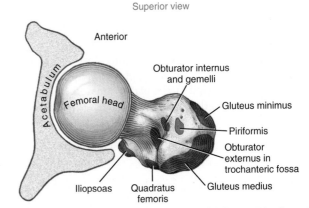

Superior view

Anterior
Obturator internus and gemelli
Gluteus minimus
Femoral head
Piriformis
Acetabulum
Obturator externus in trochanteric fossa
Iliopsoas
Quadratus femoris
Gluteus medius

FIGURE 12-6. The superior aspect of the right femur. Distal attachments of muscles are shown in gray.

nent and easily palpable structure serves as the distal attachment for many muscles. On the medial surface of the greater trochanter is a small pit called the *trochanteric fossa* (see Figures 12-5, *A* and 12-6). This fossa marks the distal attachment of the obturator externus muscle.

Posteriorly, the femoral neck joins the femoral shaft at the raised *intertrochanteric crest* (see Figure 12-5, *B*). The *quadrate tubercle,* the distal attachment of the quadratus femoris muscle, is a slightly raised area on the crest just inferior to the trochanteric fossa. The *lesser trochanter* projects sharply from the inferior end of the crest in a posterior-medial direction. The lesser trochanter serves as the distal attachment for the iliopsoas muscle, an important hip flexor and vertical stabilizer of the lumbar spine.

The middle third of the posterior side of the femoral shaft is clearly marked by a vertical ridge called the *linea aspera* (Latin words *linea,* line + *aspera,* rough). This raised line serves as an attachment site for the vasti muscles of the quadriceps group, many of the adductor muscles, and the intermuscular fascia of the thigh. Proximally, the linea aspera splits into the *pectineal (spiral) line* medially and the *gluteal tuberosity* laterally (see Figure 12-5, *B*). At the distal end of the femur, the linea aspera divides into the *lateral* and *medial supracondylar lines.* The *adductor tubercle* is located at the extreme distal end of the medial supracondylar line.

SHAPE OF THE PROXIMAL FEMUR

The ultimate shape and configuration of the developing proximal femur are determined by several factors, including differential growth of the bone's ossification centers, the force of muscle activation and weight bearing, and circulation.[171] Abnormal growth and development resulting in a misshaped proximal femur is referred to generically as femoral *dysplasia* (from the Greek *dys,* ill or bad, + *plasia,* growth). Trauma or other acquired factors can also affect the shape of the proximal femur. The shape and configuration of the proximal femur have important implications on the congruity and stability of the joint, as well as the stress placed on the joint structures. This topic will be revisited throughout this chapter.

Two specific angulations of the proximal femur help define its shape: the angle of inclination and the torsional angle.

Angle of Inclination

The *angle of inclination* of the proximal femur describes the angle within the frontal plane between the femoral neck and the medial side of the femoral shaft (Figure 12-7). At birth this angle measures about 140 to 150 degrees. Primarily because of the loading across the femoral neck during walking, this angle usually reduces to its normal adulthood value of about 125 degrees.[16,132] As depicted by the pair of red dots in Figure 12-7, this angle optimizes the alignment of the joint surfaces.

A change in the normal angle of inclination is referred to as either *coxa vara* or *coxa valga. Coxa vara* (Latin *coxa,* hip, + *vara,* to bend inward) describes an angle of inclination markedly *less than* 125 degrees; *coxa valga* (Latin *valga,* to bend outward) describes an angle of inclination markedly *greater than* 125 degrees (see Figure 12-7, *B* and *C*). These abnormal angles can significantly alter the articulation between the femoral head and the acetabulum, thereby affecting hip biomechanics. Severe malalignment may lead to dislocation or stress-induced degeneration of the joint.

Femoral Torsion

Femoral torsion describes the relative rotation (twist) between the bone's shaft and neck. Normally, as viewed from above, the femoral neck projects about 15 degrees anterior to a medial-lateral axis through the femoral condyles.[43] This degree of torsion is called *normal anteversion* (Figure 12-8, *A*). In conjunction with the normal angle of inclination, an approximate 15-degree angle of anteversion affords optimal alignment and joint congruence (see alignment of red dots in Figure 12-8, *A*).

Femoral torsion that is markedly different from 15 degrees is considered abnormal. Torsion significantly greater than 15 degrees is called *excessive anteversion* (see Figure 12-8, *B*). In contrast, torsion significantly less than 15 degrees (i.e., approaching 0 degrees) is called *retroversion* (see Figure 12-8, *C*).

Typically a healthy infant is born with about 40 degrees of femoral anteversion.[43] With continued bone growth, increased weight bearing, and muscle activity, this angle usually decreases to about 15 degrees by 16 years of age. Excessive anteversion that persists into adulthood can increase the likelihood of hip dislocation, articular incongruence, increased joint contact force, and increased wear on the articular cartilage.[57] These factors may lead to secondary osteoarthritis of the hip.[147]

Excessive anteversion in children may be associated with an abnormal gait pattern called "in-toeing." In-toeing is a walking pattern with exaggerated posturing of hip internal rotation. The amount of in-toeing is generally related to the amount of femoral anteversion. This gait pattern apparently is a compensatory mechanism used to guide the excessively anteverted femoral head more directly into the acetabulum (Figure 12-9). In addition, Arnold and colleagues have shown that the exaggerated internally rotated position during walking serves to increase the moment arm of the important hip abductor muscles—leverage that is substantially reduced with excessive femoral anteversion.[9] Regardless of the reason for the internal rotated position, children may,

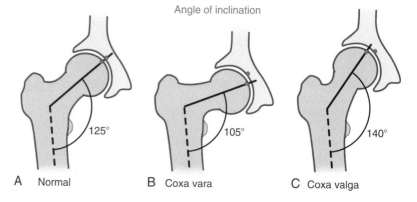

FIGURE 12-7. The proximal femur is shown: **A,** normal angle of inclination; **B,** coxa vara; and **C,** coxa valga. The pair of red dots in each figure indicates the different alignments of the hip joint surfaces. Optimal alignment is shown in **A.**

Angle of inclination

A Normal   125°

B Coxa vara   105°

C Coxa valga   140°

over time, develop shortening of the internal rotator muscles and various ligaments, thereby reducing external rotation range of motion. Fortunately, most children with in-toeing eventually walk normally.[163] The gait pattern typically improves with time because of a natural normalization of the anteversion or a combined structural compensation in other parts of the lower extremity, most commonly the tibia.[60] There is no evidence that nonoperative treatment can reduce excessive femoral anteversion.

Excessive femoral anteversion of 25 to 45 degrees is common in persons with cerebral palsy, and even anteversion as high as 60 to 80 degrees has been reported.[8,16] In-toeing typically persists in children with cerebral palsy who are ambulatory and usually does not resolve.[149]

SPECIAL FOCUS 12-1

Natural Anteversion of the Femur: a Reflection of the Prenatal Development of the Lower Limb

During prenatal development, the upper and lower extremities both undergo significant axial rotation. By about 54 days after conception, the lower limbs have rotated *internally* (medially) about 90 degrees.[115] This rotation turns the kneecap region to its final anterior position. In essence, the lower limbs have become permanently "pronated." This helps to explain why the "extensor" muscles—such as the quadriceps and tibialis anterior—face anteriorly, and the "flexor" muscles—such as the hamstrings and gastrocnemius—face posteriorly after birth. The torsion angle between the shaft and the neck of the femur at birth partially reflects the degree of this medial rotation.

The functional consequence of the medial rotation of the lower limbs is that the plantar surfaces of the feet assume a plantigrade position suitable for walking. The fixed pronated position is evidenced by the medial position of the great toe of the lower limb, similar to the thumb in the fully pronated forearm. Additional anatomic features that may reflect this developmental medial rotation include the spiraled path of the lower extremity dermatomes (see Appendix IV, Part C), the twisted or spiraled ligaments of the hip (described ahead), and the oblique course of the sartorius muscle.

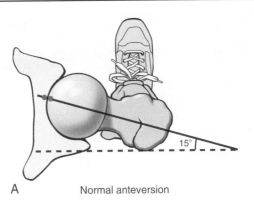

A   Normal anteversion

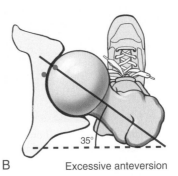

B   Excessive anteversion

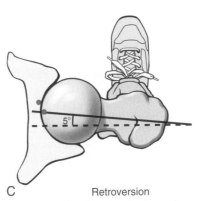

C   Retroversion

FIGURE 12-8. The angle of torsion is shown between the neck and shaft of the femur: **A,** normal anteversion; **B,** excessive anteversion; and **C,** retroversion. The pair of red dots in each figure indicates the different alignments of the hip joint surfaces. Optimal alignment is shown in **A.**

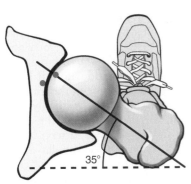

A   Excessive anteversion

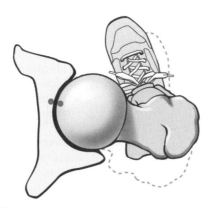

B   Excessive anteversion with "in-toeing"

FIGURE 12-9. Two situations show the same individual with excessive anteversion of the proximal femur. **A,** Offset red dots indicate malalignment of the hip while a subject stands in the anatomic position. **B,** As evidenced by the alignment of the red dots, standing with the hip internally rotated ("in-toeing") improves the joint congruity.

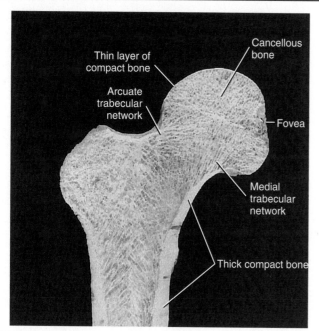

FIGURE 12-10. A frontal plane cross-section showing the internal architecture of the proximal femur. Note the thicker areas of compact bone around the shaft, and the cancellous bone occupying most of the medullary (internal) region. Two trabecular networks within the cancellous bone are also indicated. (From Neumann DA: *An arthritis home study course. The synovial joint: anatomy, function, and dysfunction,* LaCrosse, Wisc, 1998, Orthopedic Section of the American Physical Therapy Association.)

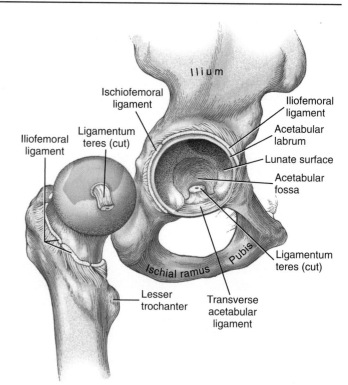

FIGURE 12-11. The right hip joint is opened to expose its internal components. The regions of thickest cartilage are highlighted (in blue) on the articular surfaces of the femoral head and acetabulum.

INTERNAL STRUCTURE OF THE PROXIMAL FEMUR

Compact and Cancellous Bone

Walking produces tension, compression, bending, shear, and torsion on the proximal femur. Many of these forces are large, exceeding one's body weight. Throughout a lifetime, the proximal femur typically resists and absorbs these repetitive forces without incurring injury. This is accomplished by two strikingly different compositions of bone. *Compact bone* is very dense and unyielding, with an ability to withstand large loads. This type of bone is particularly thick in the cortex, or outer shell, of the lower femoral neck and entire shaft (Figure 12-10). These regions are subjected to large shear and torsion forces. *Cancellous bone,* in contrast, is relatively porous, consisting of a spongy, three-dimensional trabecular lattice, as shown in Figure 12-10. The relative elasticity of cancellous bone is ideal for repeatedly absorbing external forces. Cancellous bone tends to concentrate along lines of stress, forming *trabecular networks.* A *medial trabecular* and an *arcuate trabecular network* are visible within the femur shown in Figure 12-10. The overall pattern of the trabecular network changes when the proximal femur is subjected to abnormal forces over an extended time.

ARTHROLOGY

Functional Anatomy of the Hip Joint

The hip is the classic ball-and-socket joint of the body, secured within the acetabulum by an extensive set of connective tissues and muscles. Thick layers of articular cartilage, muscle,

and cancellous bone in the proximal femur help dampen the large forces that routinely cross the hip. Failure of any of these protective mechanisms because of disease, congenital or developmental malalignment or malformation, or trauma often leads to a deterioration of the joint structure.

FEMORAL HEAD

The femoral head is located just inferior to the middle one third of the inguinal ligament. On average, the centers of the two adult femoral heads are 17.5 cm (6.9 inches) apart from each other.[127] The head of the femur forms about two thirds of a nearly perfect sphere (Figure 12-11). Located slightly posterior to the center of the head is a prominent pit, or *fovea* (see Figure 12-5, *A*). The entire surface of the femoral head is covered by articular cartilage, except for the region of the fovea. The cartilage is thickest (about 3.5 mm) in a broad region above and slightly anterior to the fovea (see highlighted region in Figure 12-11).[86]

The *ligamentum teres* (also known as the ligament to the head of the femur) is a tubular sheath of synovial-lined connective tissue that runs between the transverse acetabular ligament and the fovea of the femoral head (see Figure 12-11). Although the ligament is stretched during flexion and adduction, it likely contributes only a small amount of stability to the articulation.[160] Interestingly, the ligament functions primarily as a protective conduit, or sheath, for the passage of the small acetabular artery (a branch from the obturator artery) to the femoral head. The small and inconstant acetabular artery provides only a minor source of blood to the femur.[28,160] The primary blood supply to the head and neck of the femur is through the medial and lateral circumflex arteries, which pierce the capsule of the joint adjacent to the femoral neck.

ACETABULUM

The acetabulum (from Latin, meaning "vinegar cup") is a deep, hemispheric cuplike socket that accepts the femoral head. About 60 to 70 degrees of the rim of the acetabulum are incomplete near its inferior pole, creating the *acetabular notch* (see Figure 12-2).

The femoral head contacts the acetabulum only along its horseshoe-shaped *lunate surface* (see Figure 12-11). This surface is covered with articular cartilage, thickest along the superior-anterior region of its dome.[38,86] The region of thickest cartilage (about 3.5 mm) corresponds to approximately the same region of highest joint force during walking.[31] During walking, hip forces fluctuate from 13% of body weight during mid-swing phase to over 300% of body weight during the mid-stance phase. During the stance phase—when forces are the greatest—the lunate surface flattens slightly as the acetabular notch widens slightly, thereby increasing contact area as a means to reduce peak pressure (Figure 12-12).[38,101] This natural dampening mechanism represents yet another design that strives to keep the stress on the subchondral bone within physiologic tolerable levels.

The *acetabular fossa* is a depression located deep within the floor of the acetabulum. Because the fossa does not normally contact the femoral head, it is devoid of cartilage. Instead, the fossa contains the teres ligament, fat, synovial membrane, and blood vessels.

Anatomic Features of the Hip Joint

Femoral Head
- Fovea
- Ligamentum teres

Acetabulum
- Acetabular notch
- Lunate surface
- Acetabular fossa
- Labrum
- Transverse acetabular ligament

ACETABULAR LABRUM

The *acetabular labrum* is a flexible ring of primary fibrocartilage that surrounds the outer circumference (rim) of the acetabulum (see Figure 12-11).[142] Adjacent to the acetabular notch, the labrum widens as it is transformed into the *transverse acetabular ligament*.[160]

The acetabular labrum is nearly triangular in cross-section, with its apex projecting outward about 5 mm toward the femoral head.[164] The base of the labrum attaches along the internal and external surfaces of the acetabulum rim. The part of the labrum that attaches to the internal surface gradually fuses with the articular cartilage within the acetabulum.

The acetabular labrum provides significant stability to the hip by "gripping" the femoral head and by deepening the volume of the socket by approximately 30%.[164] The seal formed around the joint by the labrum helps maintain a negative intra-articular pressure, thereby creating a modest suction that resists distraction of the joint surfaces. The circumferential seal also holds the synovial fluid within the joint; therefore the labrum indirectly enhances the lubrication and load dissipation functions of the articular cartilage.[44] The labrum directly protects the articular cartilage by reduc-

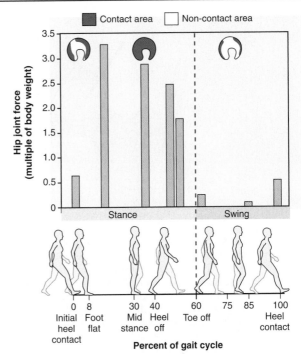

FIGURE 12-12. Graph shows a computer model's estimate of the hip joint compression force as a multiple of body weight during the gait cycle. The stance phase is between 0% and 60% of the gait cycle, and the swing phase is between 60% and 100% of the gait cycle (vertical stippled line separates these major divisions of the gait cycle). The images above the graph indicate the approximate area of acetabular contact at three selected magnitudes of hip joint force, estimated by data published in the literature.[38] The area of joint contact increases from about 20% of the lunate surface during the swing phase to about 98% during mid stance phase.

ing contact stress (force/area) by increasing the surface area of the acetabulum.[164]

Consisting primarily of fibrocartilage, the labrum is poorly vascularized, receiving only modest blood supply to its outer one third.[109,142] For this reason, a torn labrum has a very limited ability to heal. In contrast to its poor vascularization, the labrum is well supplied by afferent nerves capable of providing proprioceptive feedback and, when the labrum is acutely injured, the sensation of pain.[82]

ACETABULAR ALIGNMENT

In the anatomic position the acetabulum typically projects laterally from the pelvis with a varying amount of inferior and anterior tilt. Congenital or developmental conditions may cause an abnormally shaped acetabulum. A malshaped, *dysplastic acetabulum* that does not adequately cover the femoral head may lead to chronic dislocation and increased stress, often leading to degeneration or osteoarthritis. Two measurements are commonly used to describe the extent to which the acetabulum naturally covers and helps secure the femoral head: the center-edge angle and the acetabular anteversion angle.

Center-Edge Angle

The *center-edge angle* is highly variable but on average measures about 35 degrees in radiographs from adults (Figure 12-13, *A*).[4,50] As described in the legend of Figure 12-13, a significantly lower central-edge angle reduces the acetabular coverage of

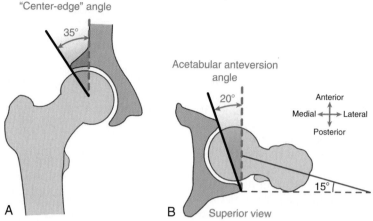

FIGURE 12-13. A, The *center-edge angle* measures the fixed orientation of the acetabulum within the frontal plane, relative to the pelvis. This measurement defines the extent to which the acetabulum covers the *top* of the femoral head. The center-edge angle is measured as the intersection of a vertical, fixed *reference line (stippled)* with the *acetabular reference line (bold solid line)* that connects the upper lateral edge of the acetabulum with the center of the femoral head. A more vertical acetabular reference line results in a smaller center-edge angle, providing *less* superior coverage of the femoral head. **B,** The *acetabular anteversion angle* measures the fixed orientation of the acetabulum within the horizontal plane, relative to the pelvis. This measurement indicates the extent to which the acetabulum covers the *front* of the femoral head. The angle is formed by the intersection of a fixed *anterior-posterior reference line (stippled)* with an *acetabular reference line (bold solid line)* that connects the anterior and posterior rim of the acetabulum. A larger acetabular anteversion angle creates *less* acetabular containment of the anterior side of the femoral head. (A normal femoral anteversion of 15 degrees is also shown.)

the femoral head. This reduced coverage increases the risk of dislocation and, equally important, reduces the contact area within the joint.[108] A central-edge angle of only 15 degrees, for example, reduces normal contact area by as much as 35%.[50] During the single-limb–support phase of walking, for instance, this reduced surface area would theoretically *increase* joint pressure (force/area) by about 50%. Over many years of walking, this scenario may lead to premature hip osteoarthritis, often starting with degeneration of the acetabular labrum.[26,94,111]

Acetabular Anteversion Angle

The *acetabular anteversion angle* measures the extent to which the acetabulum projects *anteriorly* within the horizontal plane, relative to the pelvis. Such a perspective can be measured through computed tomography. Observed from above, the acetabular anteversion angle is normally about 20 degrees (Figure 12-13, *B*).[4,148] Even when normal, this orientation exposes part of the anterior side of the femoral head. The thick anterior capsular ligament of the hip and the iliopsoas tendon naturally cover and support this vulnerable side of the joint. A hip demonstrating *excessive acetabular anteversion* is more exposed anteriorly: when anteversion is severe, the hip is more prone to anterior dislocation and associated lesions of the anterior labrum, especially at the extremes of external rotation. The likelihood of these associated pathologies increases when acetabular anteversion is combined with excessive femoral anteversion.[95]

An acetabulum that projects directly laterally, or even slightly posterior-laterally, within the horizontal plane is described as being abnormally *retroverted*.

CAPSULE AND LIGAMENTS OF THE HIP

A *synovial membrane* lines the internal surface of the hip joint capsule. The iliofemoral, pubofemoral, and ischiofemoral

TABLE 12-1. **Connective Tissues and Selected Muscles That Become Taut at the End-Ranges of Passive Hip Motion**	
End-Range Position	**Taut Tissue**
Hip flexion (knee extended)	Hamstrings
Hip flexion (knee flexed)	Inferior and posterior capsule; gluteus maximus
Hip extension (knee extended)	Primarily iliofemoral ligament, some fibers of the pubofemoral and ischiofemoral ligaments; psoas major
Hip extension (knee flexed)	Rectus femoris
Abduction	Pubofemoral ligament; adductor muscles
Adduction	Superior fibers of ischiofemoral ligament; iliotibial band; and abductor muscles such as the tensor fasciae latae and gluteus medius
Internal rotation	Ischiofemoral ligament; external rotator muscles, such as the piriformis or gluteus maximus
External rotation	Iliofemoral and pubofemoral ligaments; internal rotator muscles, such as the tensor fasciae latae or gluteus minimus

ligaments reinforce the external surface of the capsule (Figures 12-14 and 12-15). Passive tension in stretched ligaments, the adjacent capsule, and the surrounding muscles help define the end-range of movements of the hip (Table 12-1).[47] Increasing the flexibility in various parts of the capsule is an impor-

Anterior view

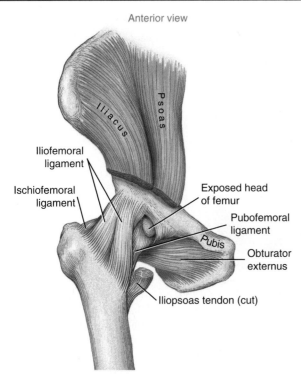

FIGURE 12-14. The anterior capsule and ligaments of the right hip. The iliopsoas is cut to expose the anterior side of the joint. Note that part of the femoral head protrudes just medial to the iliofemoral ligament. This region may be covered by a bursa.

Posterior view

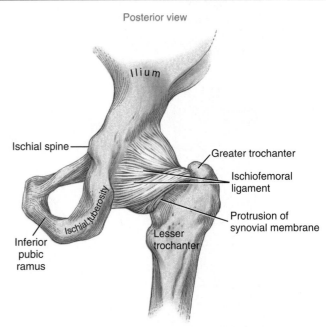

FIGURE 12-15. The posterior capsule and ligaments of the right hip.

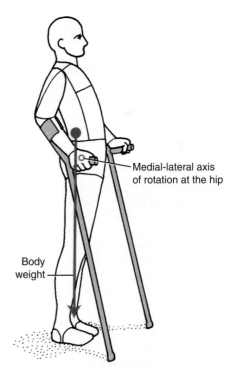

FIGURE 12-16. A person with paraplegia is shown standing with the aid of braces at the knees and ankles. Leaning the pelvis and trunk posteriorly orients the body weight vector *(red arrow)* posterior to the hip joints *(small green circle)*, thereby stretching the iliofemoral ligaments. This stretch provides a passive flexion torque at the hip, which helps to balance the extension torque generated by gravity. Once counterbalanced, these opposing torques can stabilize the pelvis and trunk, relative to the femur, during standing. (Modified from Somers MF: *Spinal cord injury: functional rehabilitation*, Norwalk, 1992, Appleton & Lange.)

tant component of manual physical therapy for restricted motion of the hip.[66,103]

The *iliofemoral ligament* (or Y-ligament) is a thick and strong sheet of connective tissue, resembling an inverted Y. Proximally, the iliofemoral ligament attaches near the anterior-inferior iliac spine and along the adjacent margin of the acetabulum. Fibers form distinct medial and lateral fasciculi, each attaching to either end of the intertrochanteric line of the femur (see Figure 12-14). Full hip extension stretches the iliofemoral ligament and anterior capsule. Full external rotation also elongates fibers of the iliofemoral ligament, especially those within the lateral fasciculus.[47,106]

The iliofemoral ligament is the strongest and stiffest ligament of the hip.[61,162] The mean maximal force required to disrupt either fasciculus is approximately 330 N (75 lb).[61] When a person stands with the hip fully extended, the anterior surface of the femoral head presses firmly against the iliofemoral ligament and superimposed iliopsoas muscle.[181] From a position of standing, passive tension in these structures forms an important stabilizing force that *resists further hip extension*. Persons with paraplegia often rely on the passive tension in an elongated and taut iliofemoral ligament to assist with standing (Figure 12-16).

Although thinner and more circular than the fibers of the iliofemoral ligament, the pubofemoral and ischiofemoral ligaments blend with and strengthen adjacent aspects of the capsule. The *pubofemoral ligament* attaches along the anterior and inferior rim of the acetabulum and adjacent parts of the superior pubic ramus and obturator membrane (see Figure 12-14). The fibers blend with the medial fasciculus of the

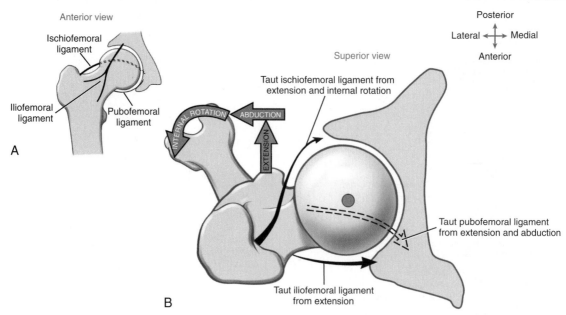

FIGURE 12-17. A, The hip is shown in a neutral position, with all three capsular ligaments identified. **B,** Superior view of the hip in its close-packed position (i.e., fully extended with slight abduction and internal rotation). This position elongates at least some component of all three capsular ligaments.

iliofemoral ligament, becoming taut in hip abduction and extension and, to a lesser degree, external rotation.[106]

The *ischiofemoral ligament* attaches from the posterior and inferior aspects of the acetabulum, primarily from the adjacent ischium (see Figure 12-15). Fibers from this ligament join circular fibers located deeper within the posterior and inferior capsule. Other more superficial fibers spiral superiorly and laterally across the posterior neck of the femur to attach near the apex of the greater trochanter (see Figure 12-14). These superficial fibers become taut in full internal rotation and extension[106]; other more superior fibers become taut in full adduction.

Close-Packed Position of the Hip

Full extension of the hip (i.e., about 20 degrees beyond the neutral position) in conjunction with slight internal rotation and slight abduction twists or "spirals" most of the fibers within the capsular ligaments to their most taut position (Figure 12-17). This position is useful therapeutically during attempts to stretch the entirety of the hip's capsular ligaments. Because the position of full extension, slight internal rotation and abduction elongates most of the capsule, it is considered the *close-packed position* at the hip.[160] The passive tension generated especially by full extension lends stability to the joint and reduces passive accessory movement or "joint play." The hip is one of a very few joints in the body in which the close-packed position is *not* also associated with the position of maximal joint congruency. The hip joint surfaces fit most congruently in about 90 degrees of flexion with moderate abduction and external rotation. In this position, most of the capsule and associated ligaments have "unraveled" to a more slackened state, adding only little passive tension to the joint.

Osteokinematics

This section describes the range of motion allowed by the adult hip, including the factors that permit and restrict this motion. Reduced hip motion may be an early indicator of disease or trauma, either at the hip or elsewhere in the body.[41] Limited hip motion can impose significant functional limitations in activities such as walking, standing upright comfortably, or picking up objects off the floor.

Two terms are used to describe the kinematics at the hip. *Femoral-on-pelvic hip osteokinematics* describes the rotation of the femur about a relatively fixed pelvis. *Pelvic-on-femoral hip osteokinematics*, in contrast, describes the rotation of the pelvis, and often the superimposed trunk, over relatively fixed femurs. Regardless of whether the femur or the pelvis is the moving segment, the osteokinematics are described from the anatomic position. The names of the movements are as follows: *flexion* and *extension* in the sagittal plane, *abduction* and *adduction* in the frontal plane, and *internal* and *external rotation* in the horizontal plane (Figure 12-19).

Reporting the range of motion at the hip uses the anatomic position as the 0-degree or neutral reference point. Within the sagittal plane, for example, femoral-on-pelvic (hip) flexion occurs as the femur rotates anteriorly beyond the 0-degree reference position. Extension, the reverse movement, occurs as the femur rotates posteriorly toward and beyond the 0-degree reference position. The term hyperextension is *not* used to describe normal range of motion at the hip.

As depicted in Figure 12-19, each plane of motion is associated with a unique *axis of rotation*. The axis of rotation for internal and external rotation is often referred to as a "longitudinal" or vertical axis. (The vertical description assumes the subject is standing with the hip in the anatomic position.) This longitudinal axis of rotation extends as a straight line between the center of the femoral head and the center of the knee joint. Because of the angle of inclination of the proximal femur and the anterior bowing of the femoral shaft, most of the longitudinal axis of rotation lies *outside* the femur itself (see Figure 12-19, *A* and *B*). The extramedullary axis has implications on some of the actions of hip muscles, a point discussed later in this chapter.

SPECIAL FOCUS 12-2

Intracapsular Pressure within the Hip

As described earlier, the intracapsular pressure within the healthy hip is normally less than atmospheric pressure. This relatively low pressure creates a partial suction that provides some stability to the hip.

Wingstrand and colleagues studied the effect of joint position and capsular swelling on the intracapsular pressure within cadaveric hips.[175] Except in the extremes of motion, pressures remained relatively low throughout most of flexion and extension. When fluid was injected into the joint to simulate capsular swelling, pressures rose dramatically throughout a greater portion of the range of motion (Figure 12-18). Regardless of the amount of injected fluid, however, pressures always remained lowest in the middle of the range of motion. These data help to explain why persons with capsulitis and swelling within the hip tend to feel most comfortable holding the hip in partial flexion. Reduced intracapsular pressure decreases distension of the inflamed capsule. Unfortunately, over time, the flexed position may lead to contracture caused by the adaptive shortening of the hip flexor muscles and capsular ligaments.

Persons with an inflamed synovium, capsule, or bursa of the hip are susceptible to flexion contracture. It is important to reduce the inflammation through medicine and physical therapy so that activities that favor the extended position can be tolerated. When tolerated, exercises should be devised that strengthen hip extensor muscles while also stretching the hip flexor muscles and anterior capsular structures.

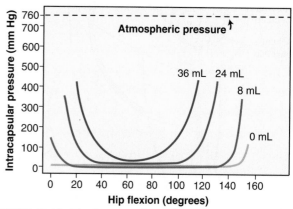

FIGURE 12-18. The intracapsular pressure in the hip joints of cadavers as a function of hip flexion angle. The four curved lines indicate the pressure-angle relationships after the injection of different volumes of fluid into the capsule of the hip.[175]

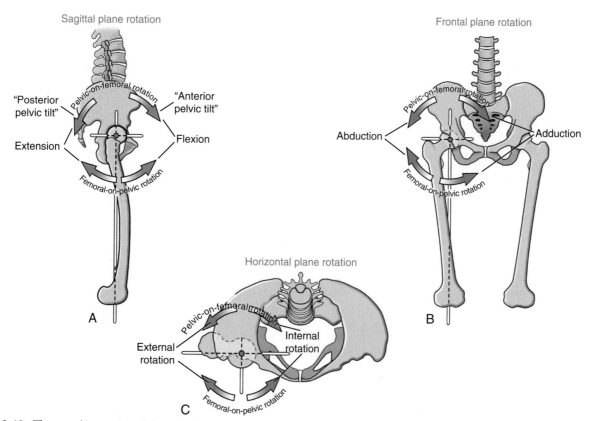

FIGURE 12-19. The osteokinematics of the right hip joint. Femoral-on-pelvic and pelvic-on-femoral rotations occur in three planes. The axis of rotation for each plane of movement is shown as a colored dot, located at the center of the femoral head. **A,** Side view shows *sagittal plane rotations* around a medial-lateral axis of rotation. **B,** Front view shows *frontal plane rotations* around an anterior-posterior axis of rotation. **C,** Top view shows *horizontal plane rotations* around a longitudinal, or vertical, axis of rotation.

Femoral-on-pelvic hip rotation

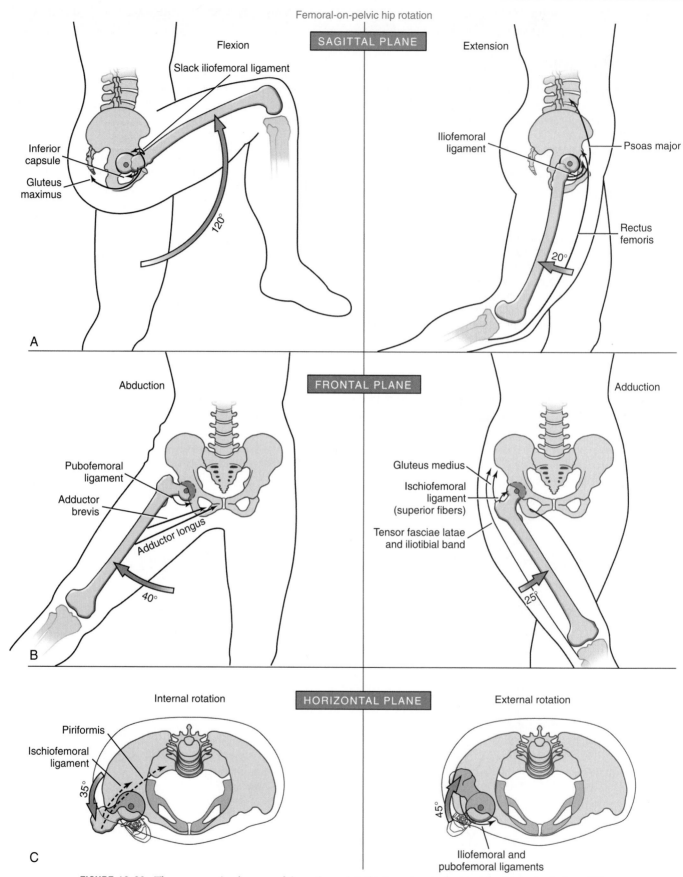

FIGURE 12-20. The near maximal range of *femoral-on-pelvic* (hip) motion is depicted in the sagittal plane **(A),** frontal plane **(B),** and horizontal plane **(C).** Tissues that are elongated or pulled taut are indicated by straight black or dashed black arrows. Slackened tissue is indicated by a wavy black arrow.

Unless otherwise specified, the following discussions include *passive* ranges of motion. The connective tissues and selected muscles that limit motion are also described and are summarized in Table 12-1. The muscles used to produce and control hip motion are discussed later in this chapter. Although femoral-on-pelvic and pelvic-on-femoral movements often occur simultaneously, they are presented here separately.

FEMORAL-ON-PELVIC OSTEOKINEMATICS

Rotation of the Femur in the Sagittal Plane

On average, with the knee flexed, the hip *flexes* to about 120 degrees (Figure 12-20, *A*).[41,150] Tasks such as comfortably squatting or tying a shoelace typically require this amount of hip flexion.[77] Full hip flexion slackens the three primary capsular ligaments but stretches the inferior capsule and muscles such as the gluteus maximus. With the knee fully extended, hip flexion is typically limited to 70 to 80 degrees by increased tension in the hamstring muscles. Considerable variability can be expected in this movement because of high inter-subject variability in hamstring muscle flexibility.

The hip normally *extends* about 20 degrees beyond the neutral position.[150] Full hip extension increases the passive tension throughout the capsular ligaments—especially the ilio-femoral ligament and the hip flexor muscles. When the knee is fully flexed during hip extension, passive tension in the stretched rectus femoris, which crosses both the hip and the knee, reduces hip extension to about the neutral position.

Rotation of the Femur in the Frontal Plane

The hip *abducts* on average about 40 degrees, limited primarily by the pubofemoral ligament and the adductor muscles (see Figure 12-20, *B*).[150] The hip *adducts* about 25 degrees beyond the neutral position.[17] In addition to interference with the contralateral limb, passive tension in stretched hip abductor muscles, iliotibial band, and superior fibers of the ischiofemoral ligament limits full adduction.

Rotation of the Femur in the Horizontal Plane

The magnitude of internal and external rotation of the hip is particularly variable among subjects. On average, the hip *internally rotates* about 35 degrees from the neutral position (see Figure 12-20, *C*).[150,156] With the hip in extension, maximal internal rotation elongates the external rotator muscles, such as the piriformis, and parts of the ischiofemoral ligament.

The extended hip *externally rotates* on average about 45 degrees. Excessive tension in the lateral fasciculus of the iliofemoral ligament can limit full external rotation. In addition, external rotation can be limited by excessive tension in any internal rotator muscle.

PELVIC-ON-FEMORAL OSTEOKINEMATICS

Lumbopelvic Rhythm

The caudal end of the axial skeleton is firmly attached to the pelvis by way of the sacroiliac joints. As a consequence, rotation of the pelvis over the femoral heads typically changes the configuration of the lumbar spine. This important kinematic relationship is known as *lumbopelvic rhythm*, introduced in Chapter 9. This concept is revisited in this chapter with a focus on the kinesiology at the hip.

Figure 12-21 shows two contrasting types of lumbopelvic rhythms frequently used during pelvic-on-femoral (hip) flexion. Although the kinematics depicted are limited to the sagittal plane, the concepts can also be applied to pelvic rotations in frontal and horizontal planes. Figure 12-21, *A* shows an example of an *ipsidirectional lumbopelvic rhythm,* in which the pelvis and lumbar spine rotate in the *same* direction.[90] The effect of this movement is to maximize the angular displacement of the *entire* trunk relative to the lower extremities—an effective strategy for increasing reach of the upper extremities. The kinematics of the ipsidirectional lumbopelvic rhythm are discussed in detail in Chapter 9. In contrast, during *contradirectional lumbopelvic rhythm,* the pelvis rotates in one direction while the lumbar spine simultaneously rotates in the *opposite* direction (see Figure 12-21, *B*). The important consequence of this movement is that the supralumbar trunk (i.e., that part of the body located above the first lumbar vertebra) can remain nearly stationary as the pelvis rotates over the femurs. This type of rhythm is used during walking, for example, when the position of the supralumbar trunk—including the head and eyes—needs to be held relatively fixed in space, independent of the rotation of the pelvis. In this manner the lumbar spine functions as a mechanical "decoupler," allowing the pelvis and the supralumbar trunk to move independently.[152] A person with a fused lumbar spine, therefore, is

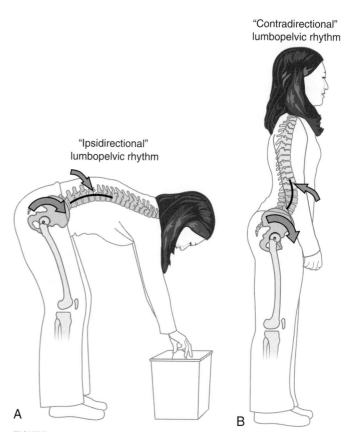

FIGURE 12-21. Two contrasting types of lumbopelvic rhythms used to rotate the pelvis over fixed femurs. **A,** An "ipsidirectional" rhythm describes a movement in which the lumbar spine and pelvis rotate in the *same* direction, thus amplifying overall trunk motion. **B,** A "contradirectional" rhythm describes a movement in which the lumbar spine and pelvis rotate in *opposite* directions. See text for further explanation.

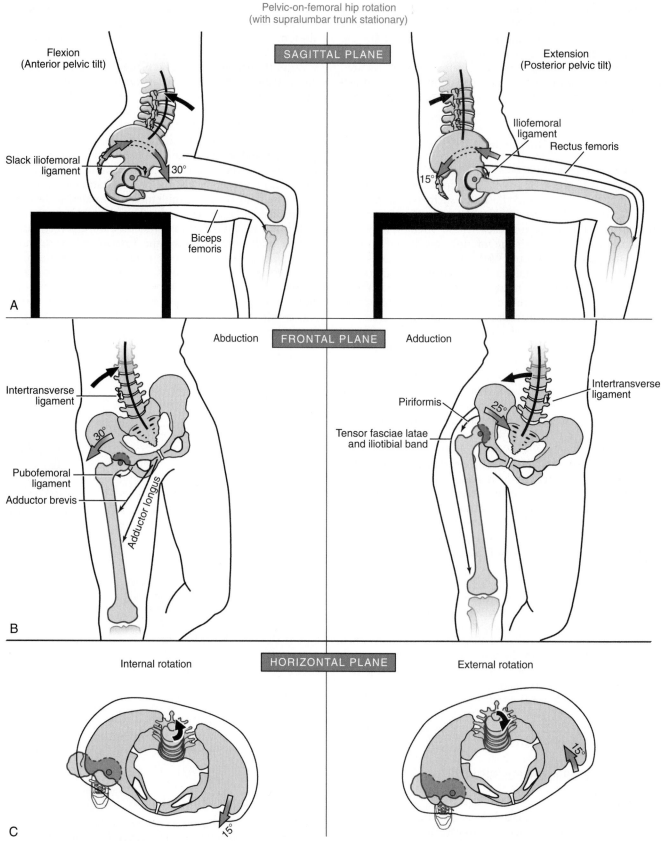

FIGURE 12-22. The near-maximal range of *pelvic-on-femoral* (hip) motion is shown in the sagittal plane **(A)**, frontal plane **(B)**, and horizontal plane **(C)**. The motion assumes that the supralumbar trunk remains nearly stationary during the hip motion (i.e., kinematics based on a *contradirectional* lumbopelvic rhythm). The large colored and black arrows depict pelvic rotation and the associated "offsetting" lumbar motion (see text for further explanation). Tissues that are elongated or pulled taut are indicated by thin, straight black arrows; tissues slackened are indicated by thin wavy black arrows. The range of motions depicted in each figure has been estimated by observing photographs of healthy young adults.

unable to rotate the pelvis about the hips without a similar rotation of parts of the supralumbar trunk. This abnormal situation is readily apparent when the individual walks.

Figure 12-22 shows pelvic-on-femoral osteokinematics at the hip, organized by plane of motion. These kinematics are all based on the *contradirectional* lumbopelvic rhythm. In many cases the amount of pelvic-on-femoral rotation is restricted by natural limitations of movement within the lumbar spine.

Pelvic Rotation in the Sagittal Plane: Anterior and Posterior Pelvic Tilting

Hip flexion can occur through an *anterior pelvic tilt* (see Figure 12-22, *A*). As defined in Chapter 9, a "pelvic tilt" is a short-arc, sagittal plane rotation of the pelvis relative to stationary femurs. The direction of the tilt—either anterior or posterior—is based on the direction of rotation of a point on the iliac crest. The anterior tilt of the pelvis occurs about a medial-lateral axis of rotation through both femoral heads. The associated increased lumbar lordosis offsets most of the tendency of the supralumbar trunk to follow the forward rotation of the pelvis. While sitting with 90 degrees of hip flexion, the normal adult can perform about 30 degrees of additional pelvic-on-femoral hip flexion before being restricted by a completely extended lumbar spine. Full anterior tilt of the pelvis slackens most of the ligaments of the hip, most notably the iliofemoral ligament. Marked tightness in any hip extensor muscle—such as the hamstrings—could theoretically limit the extremes of an anterior pelvic tilt. As depicted in Figure 12-22, *A*, however, because the knees are flexed, the partially slackened hamstring muscles would not normally produce any noticeable resistance to an anterior pelvic rotation. During *standing* (and with knees fully extended), however, the more elongated hamstrings are more likely to resist an anterior pelvic tilt, but the amount of resistance is usually insignificant unless the muscle is physiologically impaired and generating extreme resistance to elongation.[97]

As depicted in Figure 12-22, *A*, the hips can be *extended* about 10 to 20 degrees from the 90-degree sitting posture via a *posterior tilt* of the pelvis. During sitting, this short-arc pelvic rotation would increase the length (and therefore tension) only minimally in the iliofemoral ligament and rectus femoris muscle. As depicted in the figure, the lumbar spine flexes, or flattens, as the pelvis posteriorly tilts.

Pelvic Rotation in the Frontal Plane

Pelvic-on-femoral rotation in the frontal and horizontal planes is best described assuming a person is standing on one limb. The weight-bearing extremity is referred to as the *support hip*.

Abduction of the support hip occurs by raising or "hiking" the iliac crest on the side of the nonsupport hip (see Figure 12-22, *B*). Assuming that the supralumbar trunk remains nearly stationary, the lumbar spine must bend in the direction opposite the rotating pelvis. A slight lateral convexity occurs within the lumbar region toward the side of the abducting hip.

Pelvic-on-femoral hip abduction is restricted to about 30 degrees, primarily because of the natural limits of lateral bending in the lumbar spine. Marked tightness in hip adductor muscles or the pubofemoral ligament can limit pelvic-on-femoral hip abduction. In the event of a marked adductor contracture, the iliac crest on the side of the nonsupport hip remains *lower* than the iliac crest of the support hip, which may interfering with walking.

Adduction of the support hip occurs by a *lowering* of the iliac crest on the side of the nonsupport hip. This motion causes a slight lateral concavity within the lumbar region on the side of the adducted hip. A hypomobile lumbar spine and/or reduced extensibility in the iliotibial band or hip abductor muscles, such as the gluteus medius, piriformis, or tensor fasciae latae, may restrict the extremes of this motion.

Pelvic Rotation in the Horizontal Plane

Pelvic-on-femoral rotation occurs in the horizontal plane about a longitudinal axis of rotation (see green circle at femoral head in Figure 12-22, *C*). *Internal rotation* of the support hip occurs as the iliac crest on the side of the nonsupport hip rotates *forward* in the horizontal plane. During *external rotation*, in contrast, the iliac crest on the side of the nonsupport hip rotates *backward* in the horizontal plane. If the pelvis is rotating beneath a relatively stationary trunk, the lumbar spine must rotate (or twist) in the opposite direction as the rotating pelvis. The small amount of axial rotation normally permitted in the lumbar spine significantly limits the full expression of horizontal plane rotation of the support hip. The full potential of pelvic-on-femoral rotation requires that the lumbar spine *and* trunk follow the rotation of the pelvis—a movement strategy more consistent with an ipsidirectional lumbopelvic rhythm.

Arthrokinematics

During hip motion, the nearly spherical femoral head normally remains snugly seated within the confines of the acetabulum. The steep walls of the acetabulum, in conjunction with the tightly fitting acetabular labrum, limit significant translation between the joint surfaces. Hip arthrokinematics are based on the traditional convex-on-concave or concave-on-convex principles (see Chapter 1).

Figure 12-23 shows a highly mechanical illustration of a hip opened to enable visualization of the paths of articular motion. *Abduction* and *adduction* occur across the longitudinal diameter of the joint surfaces. With the hip extended, *internal* and *external* *rotation* occur across the transverse diameter of the joint surfaces. *Flexion* and *extension* occur as a spin between the femoral head and the lunate surfaces of the acetabulum. The axis of rotation for this spin passes through the femoral head.

MUSCLE AND JOINT INTERACTION

Innervation of the Muscles and Joint

INNERVATION OF MUSCLES

The lumbar plexus and the sacral plexus arise from the ventral rami of spinal nerve roots T^{12} through S^4. Nerves from the lumbar plexus innervate the muscles of the anterior and medial thigh, including the quadriceps femoris. Nerves from the sacral plexus innervate the muscles of the posterior and lateral hip, posterior thigh, and entire lower leg.

Lumbar Plexus

The lumbar plexus is formed from the ventral rami of spinal nerve roots T^{12}-L^4. This plexus gives rise to the femoral and obturator nerves (Figure 12-24, *A*). The *femoral nerve*, the largest branch of the lumbar plexus, is formed by L^2-L^4 nerve roots. *Motor branches* innervate most hip flexors and all knee extensors. Within the pelvis, proximal to the inguinal liga-

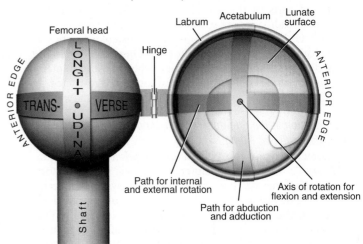

Articular paths of hip motion

FIGURE 12-23. A mechanical drawing of the right hip. The joint surfaces are exposed by swinging the femur open like a door on a hinge. The articular paths of hip frontal and horizontal plane motion occur along the longitudinal *(purple)* and transverse *(blue)* diameters, respectively. Consider these paths of motion for both femoral-on-pelvic and pelvic-on-femoral motions.

ment, the femoral nerve innervates the psoas major and iliacus. Distal to the inguinal ligament, the femoral nerve innervates the sartorius, part of the pectineus, and the quadriceps muscle group. The femoral nerve has an extensive *sensory distribution* covering much of the skin of the anterior-medial aspect of the thigh. The sensory branches of the femoral nerve innervate the skin of the anterior-medial aspect of the lower leg, via the saphenous cutaneous nerve.

Motor Innervation of the Lower Extremity Originating from the Lumbar Plexus

- Femoral nerve (L^2-L^4)   • Obturator nerve (L^2-L^4)

Like the femoral nerve, the *obturator nerve* is formed from L^2-L^4 nerve roots. *Motor branches* innervate the hip adductor muscles. The obturator nerve divides into anterior and posterior branches as it passes through the obturator foramen. The posterior branch innervates the obturator externus and anterior head of the adductor magnus. The anterior branch innervates part of the pectineus, the adductor brevis, the adductor longus, and the gracilis. The obturator nerve has a *sensory distribution* to the skin of the medial thigh.

Sacral Plexus
The sacral plexus, located on the posterior wall of the pelvis, is formed from the ventral rami of L^4-S^4 spinal nerve roots. Most nerves from the sacral plexus exit the pelvis via the greater sciatic foramen to innervate the posterior hip muscles (see Figure 12-24, *B*).

Motor Innervation of the Lower Extremity Originating from the Sacral Plexus

- Nerve to the piriformis (S^1-S^2)
- Nerve to the obturator internus and gemellus superior (L^5-S^2)
- Nerve to the quadratus femoris and gemellus inferior (L^4-S^1)
- Superior gluteal nerve (L^4-S^1)
- Inferior gluteal nerve (L^5-S^2)
- Sciatic nerve (L^4-S^3), including tibial and common fibular (peroneal) portions

---

Three small nerves innervate five of the six "short external rotators" of the hip. The nerves are named simply by the muscles that they innervate. The *nerve to the piriformis* (S^1-S^2) innervates the piriformis. External to the pelvis, the *nerve to the obturator internus* and *gemellus superior* (L^5-S^2) and the *nerve to the quadratus femoris* and *gemellus inferior* (L^4-S^1) travel to and innervate their respective muscles.

The *superior* and *inferior gluteal nerves* are named according to their position relative to the piriformis muscle as they exit the greater sciatic notch. The *superior gluteal nerve* (L^4-S^1) innervates the gluteus medius, gluteus minimus, and tensor fasciae latae. The *inferior gluteal nerve* (L^5-S^2) provides the sole innervation to the gluteus maximus.

The *sciatic nerve*, the widest and longest nerve in the body, is formed from L^4-S^3 nerve roots. This nerve exits the pelvis through the greater sciatic foramen, usually inferior to the piriformis. The sciatic nerve consists of two nerves: the tibial and the common fibular (peroneal), both enveloped in one connective tissue sheath. In the posterior thigh, the *tibial portion* of the sciatic nerve innervates all the biarticular muscles within the hamstring group and the posterior head of the adductor magnus. The *common fibular portion* of the sciatic nerve innervates the short head of the biceps femoris.

The sciatic nerve branches into separate tibial and common fibular components usually just proximal to the knee. It is not uncommon, however, that the division occurs more proximally near the pelvis. A division proximal to the greater sciatic foramen usually results in the common fibular nerve piercing the piriformis as the nerve exits the pelvis.

As a reference, the primary spinal nerve roots that supply the muscles of the lower extremity are listed in Appendix IV, Part A. In addition, Appendix IV, Parts B and C include additional reference items to help guide the clinical assessment of the functional status of the L^2-S^3 nerve roots.

SENSORY INNERVATION OF THE HIP

As a general rule, the hip capsule, ligaments, and parts of the labrum receive sensory innervation through the same nerve roots that supply the overlying muscles. The anterior part of the capsule of the hip receives sensory fibers from the femoral nerve. The posterior capsule receives sensory fibers from all nerve roots originating from the sacral plexus.[74,160] The con-

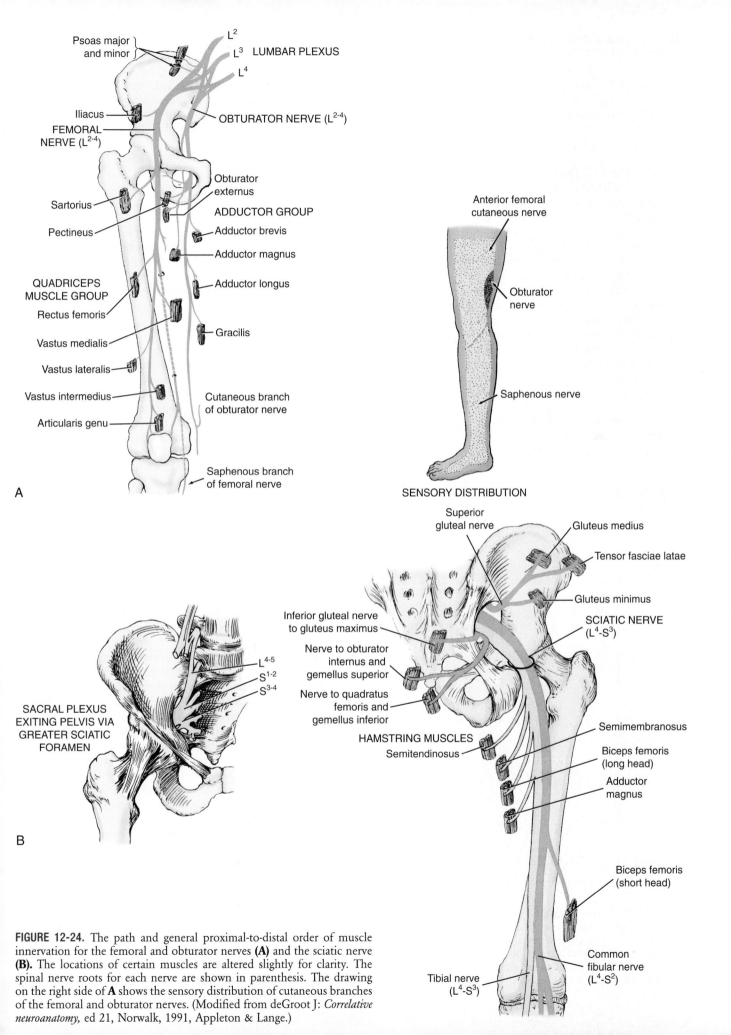

FIGURE 12-24. The path and general proximal-to-distal order of muscle innervation for the femoral and obturator nerves **(A)** and the sciatic nerve **(B).** The locations of certain muscles are altered slightly for clarity. The spinal nerve roots for each nerve are shown in parenthesis. The drawing on the right side of **A** shows the sensory distribution of cutaneous branches of the femoral and obturator nerves. (Modified from deGroot J: *Correlative neuroanatomy,* ed 21, Norwalk, 1991, Appleton & Lange.)

nective tissues of the medial aspects of the hip and knee joints receive sensory fibers from the obturator nerve; this may explain why inflammation of the hip may be perceived as pain in the medial knee region.

Muscular Function at the Hip

Throughout this chapter, the line of force of several muscles is illustrated relative to the axes of rotation at the hip. Figure 12-25, for example, shows a sagittal plane representation of the significant flexor and extensor muscles of the hip.[35,36] Although Figure 12-25 provides useful insight into the potential function of several muscles of the hip, two limitations must be considered. First, the line of force of each muscle does *not* represent a force vector, but the overall *direction* of the muscle's force within the sagittal plane. The figure therefore does not provide the information needed to compare the "strength"—or torque—potential between the muscles. This comparison requires additional information, such as the muscle's three-dimensional orientation to the hip and its cross-sectional area. Second, the lines of force and subsequent lengths of the moment arms depicted in Figure 12-25 apply only when the hip is in the anatomic position. Once the hip moves out of this position, the potential action and torque potential of each muscle change.[15] This partially explains why the maximal-effort internal torque of a muscle group varies throughout the range of motion.

Throughout this chapter, a muscle's action is considered as either primary or secondary (Table 12-2). The designation of muscle action is based on data such as moment arm length, muscle size and overall fiber direction, and, when available,

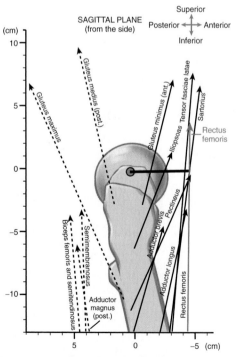

FIGURE 12-25. A view from the side that depicts the sagittal plane line of force of several muscles that cross the hip. The axis of rotation is directed in the medial-lateral direction through the femoral head. The flexors are indicated by solid lines and the extensors by dashed lines. The internal moment arm, used by the rectus femoris, is represented by the thick black line.

reports from electromyography (EMG)-based and anatomic studies. Unless otherwise specified, muscle actions are based on a concentric contraction, originating from the anatomic position. A muscle with a relatively insignificant action, or an action that is more substantial in a hip position other than the anatomic position, is not included in Table 12-2. Consult Appendix IV, Part D for a listing of detailed attachments and innervation of all muscles of the hip.

HIP FLEXOR MUSCLES

The primary hip flexors are the iliopsoas, sartorius, tensor fasciae latae, rectus femoris, adductor longus, and pectineus (Figure 12-26).[36] Figure 12-25 shows the excellent flexion leverage of many of these muscles. Secondary hip flexors are the adductor brevis, gracilis, and anterior fibers of the gluteus minimus.

Anatomy and Individual Action

The *iliopsoas* is large and long, spanning the area between the last thoracic vertebra and the proximal femur (see Figure 12-26). Anatomically, the iliopsoas consists of two muscles: the iliacus and the psoas major. The *iliacus* attaches on the iliac fossa and extreme lateral edge of sacrum, just over the sacroiliac joint. The *psoas major* attaches along the transverse processes of the last thoracic and all lumbar vertebrae, including the intervertebral discs.[53] The fibers of the iliacus and the psoas major usually fuse just anterior to the femoral head (see Figure 12-26, left hip). A tendon forms that anchors the muscle to the femur, on the lesser trochanter. En route to its distal insertion, the broad tendon of the iliopsoas is deflected posteriorly about 35 to 45 degrees, immediately after it crosses the superior pubic ramus. With the hip in full extension, this deflection raises the tendon's angle-of-insertion to the femur, thereby increasing the muscle's leverage for hip flexion.

The iliopsoas is a potent hip flexor from both a femoral-on-pelvic and pelvic-on-femoral perspective. From the anatomic position, the iliopsoas is not an effective rotator, although with the hip abducted the iliopsoas assists with external rotation.[157]

The iliopsoas muscle produces force that crosses the lumbar and lumbosacral regions as well as the hip.[5,78,154] Because of its strong anterior tilting action on the pelvis, the iliopsoas can accentuate the lumbar lordosis if the pelvis is not well stabilized by an abdominal muscle such as the rectus abdominis. The psoas major provides excellent vertical stability to the lumbar spine, especially in near full hip extension, where the passive tension in the muscle is greatest (see Chapter 10).[181]

The *psoas minor* lies anterior to the muscle belly of the psoas major, although it may be absent in about 40% of people.[160] This slender muscle attaches proximally between the twelfth thoracic and first lumbar vertebra and distally to the pelvis near the pectineal line. The psoas minor has no ability to flex the hip; isolated biteral contraction of the psoas minor may have the ability to posteriorly tilt the pelvis.

The *sartorius*, the longest muscle in the body, originates at the anterior-superior iliac spine (see Figure 12-26). This thin, fusiform muscle courses distally and medially across the thigh to attach on the medial surface of the proximal tibia (see Figure 13-7). The name *sartorius* is based on the Latin root *sartor*, referring to a tailor's position of cross-legged sitting. This name describes the muscle's combined action of hip flexion, external rotation, and abduction.

TABLE 12-2. Muscles of the Hip, Organized According to Primary or Secondary Actions*

	Flexors	Adductors	Internal Rotators	Extensors	Abductors	External Rotators
Primary	Iliopsoas Sartorius Tensor fasciae latae Rectus femoris Adductor longus Pectineus	Pectineus Adductor longus Gracilis Adductor brevis Adductor magnus	Not applicable	Gluteus maximus Biceps femoris (long head) Semitendinosus Semimembranosus Adductor magnus (posterior head)	Gluteus medius Gluteus minimus Tensor fasciae latae	Gluteus maximus Piriformis Obturator internus Gemellus superior Gemellus inferior Quadratus femoris
Secondary	Adductor brevis Gracilis Gluteus minimus (anterior fibers)	Biceps femoris (long head) Gluteus maximus (lower fibers) Quadratus femoris	Gluteus minimus (anterior fibers) Gluteus medius (anterior fibers) Tensor fasciae latae Adductor longus Adductor brevis Pectineus	Gluteus medius (posterior fibers) Adductor magnus (anterior head)	Piriformis Sartorius	Gluteus medius (posterior fibers) Gluteus minimus (posterior fibers) Obturator externus Sartorius Biceps femoris (long head)

*Each action assumes a muscle contraction that originates from the anatomic position. Several of these muscles may have a different action when they contract from a position other than the anatomic position.

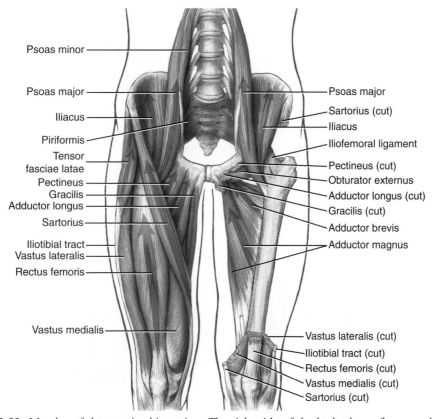

FIGURE 12-26. Muscles of the anterior hip region. The right side of the body shows flexors and adductor muscles. Many muscles on the left side are cut to expose the adductor brevis and adductor magnus.

The *tensor fasciae latae* attaches to the ilium just lateral to the sartorius (see Figure 12-26). This relatively short muscle attaches distally to the proximal part of the iliotibial band. The band extends distally across the knee to attach to the lateral tubercle of the tibia.

The iliotibial band is a component of a more extensive connective tissue known as the *fascia lata of the thigh*.[160] Laterally, the fascia lata is thickened by attachments from the tensor fasciae latae and the gluteus maximus. At multiple locations the fascia lata turns inward between muscles,

forming distinct fascial sheets known as *intermuscular septa*. These septa partition each of the main muscle groups of the thigh according to innervation. The intermuscular septa of the thigh ultimately attach to the linea aspera on the posterior surface of the femur, along with attachments of most of the adductor muscles and several of the vasti muscles (components of the quadriceps).

From the anatomic position, the tensor fasciae latae is a primary flexor and abductor of the hip. The muscle is also a secondary internal rotator.[136] As indicated by its name, the tensor fasciae latae increases tension throughout the fascia lata. Tension passed inferiorly through the iliotibial band may help stabilize the extended knee. Repetitive tension within the iliotibial band may cause inflammation at its insertion site near the lateral tubercle of the tibia. Stretching a tightened iliotibial band with the knee extended often incorporates various combinations of hip adduction and extension.[48]

The proximal part of the *rectus femoris* emerges between the limbs of an inverted V formed by the sartorius and tensor fasciae latae (see Figure 12-26). This large bipennate-shaped muscle has its proximal attachment on the anterior-inferior iliac spine and along the superior rim of the acetabulum and in the joint capsule.[160] Along with the other members of the quadriceps, the rectus femoris attaches to the tibia via the patellar tendon. The rectus femoris is responsible for about one third of the total isometric, flexion torque at the hip.[105] In addition, the rectus femoris is a primary knee extensor. The combined two-joint actions of this important muscle are considered in Chapter 13. The anatomy and function of the pectineus and adductor longus are described in the section on the adductors of the hip.

Overall Function

Pelvic-on-Femoral Hip Flexion: Anterior Pelvic Tilt

The anterior pelvic tilt is performed by a force-couple between the hip flexors and low-back extensor muscles (Figure 12-27). With fixed femurs, contraction of the hip flexors rotates the pelvis about the medial-lateral axis through both hips. Although Figure 12-27 illustrates the iliopsoas and sartorius, *any muscle capable of femoral-on-pelvic flexion is equally capable of tilting the pelvis anteriorly.* Clinically, an important aspect of the anterior tilt is related to the increase in lordosis at the lumbar spine. Greater lordosis increases the compressive loads on the lumbar apophyseal joints and increases anterior shear force at the lumbosacral junction.

A lumbopelvic posture with normal lumbar lordosis optimizes the alignment of the entire spine (see Chapter 9). Some persons, however, have difficulty maintaining lumbar lordosis and therefore have a relatively flat (i.e., slightly flexed) lumbar spine. This abnormal posture may be caused by a combination of factors, including habit, pain avoidance, compensation from another poorly aligned region of the body, increased stiffness in connective tissue around the lumbar spine, and, in extreme cases, tension emanating from hip extensor muscles. The quantitative relationship between tightness in the hamstring muscles and the posture of the pelvis-and-lumbar region during standing remains controversial.[97]

Femoral-on-Pelvic Hip Flexion

Femoral-on-pelvic hip flexion often occurs simultaneously with knee flexion as a means to shorten the functional length of the lower extremity during the swing phase of walking or running. The action of moderate- to high-power hip flexion requires coactivation of the hip flexor and abdominal muscles. This intermuscular cooperation is apparent when the leg is lifted while the knee is held in extension (i.e., a "straight-leg-raise" movement). This action requires that the rectus abdominis (a representative "abdominal" muscle) generate a potent *posterior* pelvic tilt effort that is strong enough to neutralize the strong *anterior* pelvic tilt potential of the hip flexor muscles (Figure 12-28, *A*).[65] The degree to which the abdominal muscles actually neutralize the anterior pelvic tilt depends on the demands of the activity and the relative forces produced by the contributing muscle groups.[34] Without sufficient stabilization from the abdominal muscles, however, contraction of the hip flexor muscles is inefficiently spent tilting the pelvis anteriorly (see Figure 12-28, *B*). As stated, the excessive anterior tilt of the pelvis accentuates the lumbar lordosis.

The pathomechanics depicted in Figure 12-28, *B* are most severe in situations in which the abdominal muscles are markedly weakened but the hip flexors remain relatively strong. With the exception of pathology such as poliomyelitis or muscular dystrophy, this pattern of weakness is relatively rare. More commonly, the abdominal muscles are only moderately weak, secondary to disuse or abdominal surgery. In this case, persons may develop low-back pain because of the increased compression on the apophyseal joints of the chronically, fully extended lumbar vertebrae.

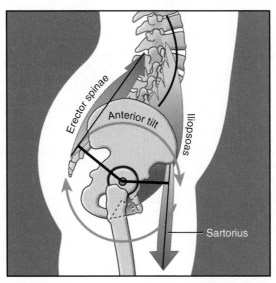

FIGURE 12-27. The force couple is shown between two representative hip flexor muscles and the erector spinae to anteriorly tilt the pelvis. The moment arms for the erector spinae and sartorius are indicated by the dark black lines. Note the increased lordosis at the lumbar spine.

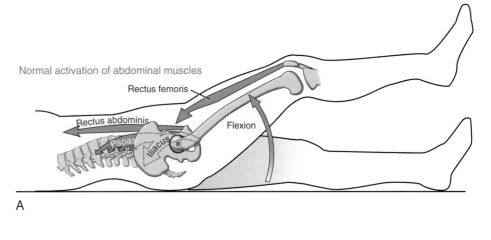

Normal activation of abdominal muscles

A

Reduced activation of abdominal muscles

B

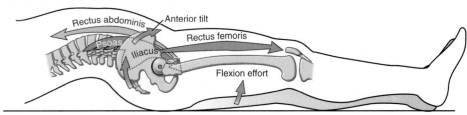

FIGURE 12-28. The stabilizing role of the abdominal muscles is shown during a unilateral straight-leg-raise. **A,** With normal activation of the abdominal muscles (such as the rectus abdominis), the pelvis is stabilized and prevented from anterior tilting by the inferior pull of the hip flexor muscles. **B,** With reduced activation of the rectus abdominis, contraction of the hip flexor muscles causes a marked anterior tilt of the pelvis. Note the increase in lumbar lordosis that accompanies the anterior tilt of the pelvis. The reduced activation in the abdominal muscle is indicated by the lighter red.

HIP ADDUCTOR MUSCLES

The primary adductors of the hip are the pectineus, adductor longus, gracilis, adductor brevis, and adductor magnus (see Figure 12-26). Secondary adductors are the biceps femoris (long head), the gluteus maximus, especially the lower fibers, and the quadratus femoris. The line of force of many of these muscles is shown in Figure 12-29.

Functional Anatomy

The adductor muscle group occupies the medial quadrant of the thigh. Topographically, the adductor muscles are organized into three layers (Figure 12-31). The pectineus, adductor longus, and gracilis occupy the *superficial layer.* Proximally, these muscles attach along the superior and inferior pubic ramus and adjacent body of the pubis. Distally, the pectineus and the adductor longus attach to the posterior surface of the femur—near and along varying regions of the linea aspera. The long and slender gracilis attaches distally to the medial side of the proximal tibia (see Figure 13-7). The *middle layer* of the adductor group is occupied by the triangular-shaped *adductor brevis.* The adductor brevis attaches to the pelvis on the inferior pubic ramus and to the femur along the proximal one third of the linea aspera.

The *deep layer* of the adductor group is occupied by the massive, triangular *adductor magnus* (see Figure 12-26, left side, and Figure 12-37, right side). This large muscle attaches primarily from the ischial ramus and part of the ischial tuberosity. From its proximal attachment the adductor magnus forms anterior and posterior heads.

The *anterior head of the adductor magnus* has two sets of fibers: horizontal and oblique. The relatively small (and often poorly defined) set of horizontally directed fibers crosses from the inferior pubic ramus to the extreme proximal end

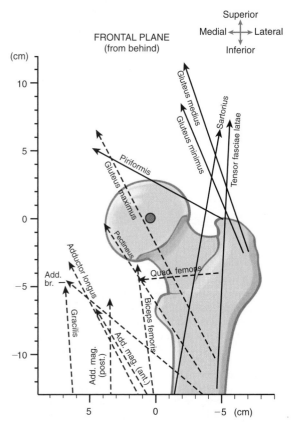

FIGURE 12-29. A posterior view depicts the frontal plane line of force of several muscles that cross the right hip. The axis of rotation is directed in the anterior-posterior direction through the femoral head. The abductors are indicated by solid lines and the adductors by dashed lines. (The actual scale of the image is indicated on the vertical and horizontal axes of the graph.)

SPECIAL FOCUS 12-3

The Functional Importance of the Fully Extendable Hip

Hips that remain flexed for a prolonged time often develop flexion contracture. This situation may be associated with spasticity of the hip flexors, gross weakness of the hip extensors, a painful or inflamed hip joint capsule, a chronically subluxed hip, or confinement to the seated position. Over time, adaptive shortening occurs in the flexor muscles and capsular ligaments, thereby limiting full hip extension.

One consequence of a hip flexion contracture is a disruption in the normal biomechanics of standing. Normally, upright walking in humans is relatively efficient from a metabolic perspective.[22] Upright standing in healthy persons can usually be maintained with relatively little muscular activation across the hips. The extended hip can be passively stabilized through an interaction of two opposing torques: body weight and passive tension from stretched capsular ligaments, especially the iliofemoral ligament (Figure 12-30, *A*). As illustrated, standing with the hips near full extension typically directs the force of body weight slightly *posterior* to the medial-lateral axis of rotation at the hip (small green circle). The force of body weight, therefore, is converted to a very small, but nevertheless useful, hip extension torque. The hip is prevented from further extension by a passive flexion torque created by the stretched capsular ligaments, such as the iliofemoral ligament. The pair of red dots placed in Figure 12-30, *A*, indicates the approximate location of the relatively thicker regions of articular cartilage covering the femoral head and acetabulum. The normal upright posture tends to align the hip such that the thicker regions of articular cartilage overlap, producing maximal protection of the underlying subchondral bone.

The static equilibrium formed between the forces of gravity and stretched connective tissues minimizes the need for metabolically "expensive" muscle activation during quiet standing. Of course, the muscles of the hip can contract strongly to provide greater stability when needed, especially when the body is subjected to potentially destabilizing external forces.

With a hip flexion contracture, the hip remains partially flexed while the person attempts to stand upright. This posture redirects the force of body weight *anterior* to the hip, creating a hip flexion torque (see Figure 12-30, *B*). Whereas gravity normally extends the hip during standing, *gravity now acts as a hip flexor*. In order to prevent collapse into full hip and knee flexion, active forces are required from hip extensor muscles. In turn, the metabolic cost of standing increases and in some persons, over time, increases the desire to sit. Often, prolonged sitting perpetuates the circumstances that initiated the flexion contracture.

Standing with a hip flexion contracture interferes with the joint's ability to optimally dissipate compression loads across the hip. Hip joint forces increase in response to the greater muscular demand to support the flexed posture. Furthermore, as indicated by the pair of red dots in Figure 12-30, *B*, standing with partially flexed hips realigns the joint surfaces such that the regions of thicker articular cartilage *no longer* optimally overlap. This arrangement theoretically increases the stress across the hip, which over time may increase the wear on the joint surfaces.

Therapeutic goals for most impairments of the hip should include, when appropriate, maximizing hip extension. In general, this is achieved through strengthening the hip extensor muscles and stretching the hip flexors muscles and the capsular ligaments—most important, the iliofemoral ligament. Activation of the abdominal muscles through posterior tilting of the pelvis may also encourage extension of the hip joint. The capsular ligaments of the hip may be further stretched when extension is combined with slight abduction and internal rotation—the close-packed position of the hip.

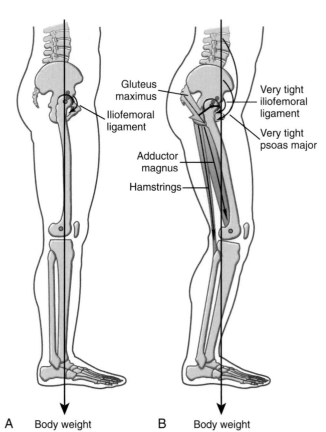

FIGURE 12-30. The effect of a hip flexion contracture on the biomechanics of standing. **A,** Ideal standing posture. **B,** Attempts at standing upright with a hip flexion contracture. Hip extensor muscles are shown active (in red) to varying magnitudes to prevent further hip flexion. The moment arms used by the muscles and body weight are indicated as short black lines originating at the hip's axis of rotation. In **A** and **B,** the green dot at the center of the femoral head represents the axis of rotation. The pair of red circles denotes the overlap of the relatively thicker areas of articular cartilage. (See text for further description.) (From Neumann DA: An arthritis home study course. The synovial joint: anatomy, function, and dysfunction. LaCrosse, Wisc, 1998, Orthopaedic Section of the American Physical Therapy Association.)

Adductor muscle group

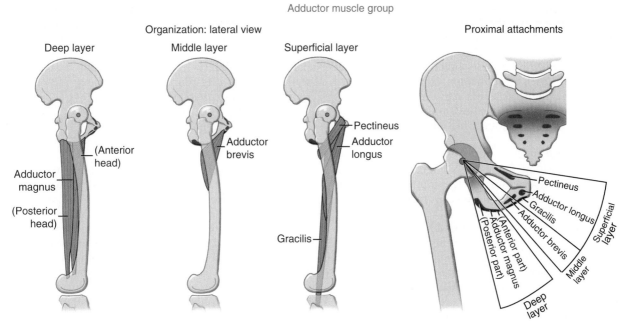

FIGURE 12-31. The anatomic organization and proximal attachments of the adductor muscle group.

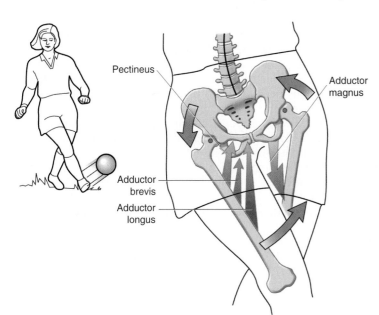

FIGURE 12-32. The bilateral cooperative action of selected adductor muscles while a soccer ball is kicked. The left adductor magnus is shown actively producing *pelvic-on-femoral adduction*. Several right adductor muscles are shown actively producing *femoral-on-pelvic adduction torque*, needed to accelerate the ball.

of the linea aspera, often called the *adductor minimus*. The larger obliquely directed fibers run from the ischial ramus to nearly the entire length of the linea aspera, as far distally as the medial supracondylar line. Both parts of the anterior head are innervated by the obturator nerve, which is typical of the adductor muscles.

The *posterior head of the adductor magnus* consists of a thick mass of the fibers arising from the region of the pelvis adjacent to the ischial tuberosity. From this posterior attachment the fibers run vertically and attach as a tendon on the adductor tubercle on the medial side of the distal femur. The posterior head of the adductor magnus is innervated by the tibial branch of the sciatic nerve, as are most hamstring muscles. Because of a location, innervation, and action similar to those of the hamstring muscles, the posterior head is often referred to as the *extensor head* of the adductor magnus.

Overall Function

The line of force of the adductors approaches the hip from many different orientations. Functionally, therefore, the adductor muscles produce torques in all three planes at the hip.[36,119] The following section considers the primary actions of the adductors in the frontal and sagittal planes. The action of these muscles as secondary internal rotators is discussed later in this chapter.

Frontal Plane Function

The most obvious function of the adductor muscles is production of adduction torque. The torque controls the kinematics of both femoral-on-pelvic and pelvic-on-femoral hip adduction. Figure 12-32 shows an example of selected adductor muscles contracting bilaterally to control both forms of motion. On the right side, several adductors are shown accelerating the femur toward the ball. Adding to the forcefulness of this action is the downward rotation or lowering of the right iliac crest–a motion occurring by pelvic-on-femoral adduction of the left hip. Although only the adductor magnus is shown on the left side, other adductor muscles assist in this action. Such an adduction action of the planted left hip likely also requires eccentric activation of the left hip *abductors* (such as the gluteus medius), which are well suited to decelerate the pelvic-on-femoral hip adduction.

Sagittal Plane Function

Regardless of hip position, the posterior fibers of the adductor magnus are powerful extensors of the hip, similar to the hamstring muscles. Of interest, however, is that within an arc of about 40 to 70 degrees of hip flexion, the line of force of most of the other adductor muscles runs *directly through or close to* the medial-lateral axis of rotation of the hip. At this point, the adductor muscles lose their potential to produce any torque in the sagittal plane.[67] When *outside* the 40- to 70-degree flexed position, however, the individual adductor muscles regain leverage as significant flexors *or* extensors of the hip.[36,67] Consider, for example, the adductor longus as a representative adductor muscle during a fast sprint (Figure 12-33, *A*). From a position of about 100 degrees of hip flexion, the line of force of the adductor longus is well *posterior* to the medial-lateral axis of the joint. At this position the adductor longus has an extensor moment arm and is capable of generating an extension torque–similar to the posterior head of the adductor magnus. From a hip position of near extension, however, the line of force of the adductor longus is well *anterior* to the medial-lateral axis of rotation (see Figure 12-33, *B*). The adductor longus now has a flexor moment arm and generates a flexion torque similar to that of the rectus femoris, for example. The adductor muscles therefore provide a useful source of flexion *and* extension torque at the hip. The bidirectional torques are useful during high-power, cyclic motions such as sprinting, cycling, running up a steep hill, and descending and rising from a deep squat. When the hip is near full flexion, the adductors are most mechanically prepared to augment the extensors. In contrast, when the hip is near full extension, they are most mechanically prepared to augment the flexors. This utilitarian function of the adductors may partially explain their relatively high susceptibility to strain injury during running and jumping, especially while quickly changing directions.

HIP INTERNAL ROTATOR MUSCLES

Overall Function

An "ideal" primary internal rotator muscle of the hip would theoretically be oriented in the horizontal plane during standing, at some linear distance from the longitudinal or vertical axis of rotation at the hip. From the anatomic position, however, there are *no* primary internal rotators because no muscle is oriented even close to the horizontal plane. Several secondary internal rotators exist, however, including the anterior fibers of the gluteus minimus and the gluteus medius, tensor fasciae latae, adductor longus, adductor brevis, and pectineus. The horizontal line of force of many of these muscles is depicted in Figure 12-34.[36,91,104] The anatomy of each of the internal rotators is described in other sections (see Figures 12-26 and 12-41).

With the hip approaching 90 degrees of flexion, the internal rotation torque potential of the internal rotator muscles dramatically increases.[33,36,104] This becomes clear with the help of a skeleton model and piece of string to mimic the line of force of muscles, such as the anterior fibers of the gluteus minimus or gluteus medius. Flexing the hip close to 90 degrees reorients the line of force of these muscles from nearly parallel to nearly *perpendicular* to the longitudinal axis of rotation at the hip. This occurs because the longitudinal axis of rotation remains parallel with the shaft of the repositioned femur. Delp and co-workers have reported that the internal rotation moment arm of the anterior part of the gluteus medius, for example, increases eightfold between 0 and 90 degrees of flexion.[33] Even some *external* rotator muscles (such as the piriformis, anterior fibers

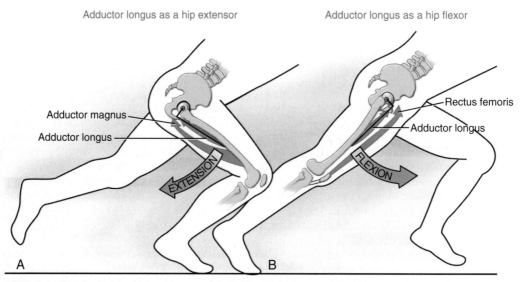

FIGURE 12-33. The dual sagittal plane action of the adductor longus muscle is demonstrated during sprinting. **A,** With the hip flexed, the adductor longus is in position to extend the hip, along with the adductor magnus. **B,** With hip extended, the adductor longus is in position to flex the hip, along with the rectus femoris. These contrasting actions are based on the change in line of force of the adductor longus, relative to the medial-lateral axis of rotation at the hip.

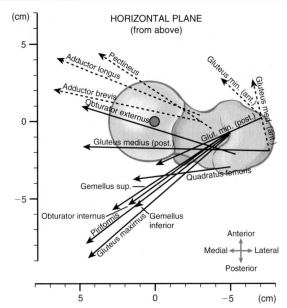

FIGURE 12-34. A superior view depicts the horizontal plane line of force of several muscles that cross the hip. The longitudinal axis of rotation is in the superior-inferior direction through the femoral head. For clarity, the tensor fasciae latae and sartorius muscles are not shown. The external rotators are indicated by solid lines and the internal rotators by dashed lines. (The actual scale of the image is indicated on the vertical and horizontal axes of the graph.)

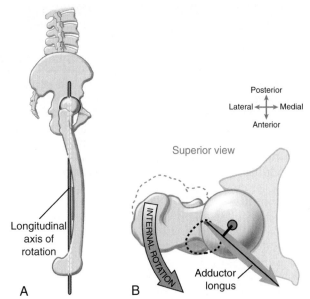

FIGURE 12-35. The adductor muscles as secondary internal rotators of the hip. **A,** Because of the anterior bowing of the femoral shaft, a large segment of the linea aspera *(short red line)* runs *anterior* to the longitudinal axis of rotation *(blue rod)*. **B,** A superior view of the right hip shows the horizontal line of force of the adductor longus. The muscle causes an internal rotation torque by producing a force that passes anterior to the axis of rotation *(small blue circle at femoral head)*. The moment arm used by the adductor longus is indicated by the thick dark line. The oval set of dashed black lines represents the outline of the midshaft of the femur at the region of the distal attachment of the adductor longus.

of the gluteus maximus, and posterior fibers of the gluteus minimus) *switch* actions and become internal rotators beyond about 90 degrees of flexion.[33] These changes in muscle action help explain why maximal-effort internal rotation torque in healthy persons has been shown to be about 50% greater with the hip flexed rather than extended.[99]

The kinesiologic phenomenon just described also helps explain the excessively internally rotated and flexed ("crouched") gait pattern often observed in persons with cerebral palsy.[62,166] With poor active control of hip extension (especially combined with contracture of the hip flexor muscles), the flexed posture of the hip exaggerates the internal rotation torque potential of many muscles of the hip.[6,7,33] This gait pattern may be better controlled by enhanced activation of the gluteus maximus, a potent extensor and external rotator.[6]

Biomechanics of the Adductor Muscles as Internal Rotators of the Hip

In general, most of the adductor muscles are capable of producing a modest internal rotation torque at the hip when the body is in or near the anatomic position.[36,91,104] This action, however, may be difficult to reconcile considering that most adductors attach to the *posterior* side of the femur along the linea aspera. With normal anatomy of the hip, a shortening of these muscles would appear to rotate the femur *externally* instead of internally. What must be considered, however, is the effect that the natural anterior bowing of the femoral shaft has on the line of force of the muscles. Bowing places much of the linea aspera *anterior* to the longitudinal axis of rotation at the hip (Figure 12-35, *A*). As depicted in Figure 12-35, *B,* the horizontal force component of an adductor muscle, such as the adductor longus, lies *anterior* to the axis of rotation. Force from this muscle therefore acts with a moment arm to produce internal rotation.

HIP EXTENSOR MUSCLES

Anatomy and Individual Action

The primary hip extensors are the gluteus maximus, the hamstrings (i.e., the long head of the biceps femoris, the semitendinosus, and the semimembranosus), and the posterior head of the adductor magnus (Figure 12-37).[36] The posterior fibers of the gluteus medius and anterior fibers of the adductor magnus are secondary extensors. With the hip flexed to at least about 70 degrees and beyond, most adductors muscles (with the possible exception of the pectineus) are capable of assisting with hip extension.

The *gluteus maximus* has numerous proximal attachments from the posterior side of the ilium, sacrum, coccyx, sacrotuberous and posterior sacroiliac ligaments, and adjacent fascia. The muscle attaches into the iliotibial band of the fascia lata (along with the tensor fasciae latae), and the gluteal tuberosity on the femur. The gluteus maximus is a primary extensor and external rotator of the hip.

The *hamstring muscles* have their proximal attachment on the posterior side of the ischial tuberosity and attach distally to the tibia and fibula. Based on these attachments, the hamstrings extend the hip *and* flex the knee. The anatomy and function of the posterior head of the *adductor magnus* is described under the section on adductors of the hip.

Figure 12-25 depicts the line of force of the primary hip extensors. In the extended position the posterior head of the adductor magnus has the greatest moment arm for extension. The adductor magnus and the gluteus maximus have the greatest cross-sectional areas of all the extensors.[176]

SPECIAL FOCUS 12-4

Function of the Internal Rotator Muscles during Walking

From a pelvic-on-femoral perspective, the internal rotators perform a subtle but useful function during walking. During the stance phase of gait, the internal rotators rotate the pelvis in the horizontal plane over a relatively fixed femur.[73] These pelvic-on-femoral kinematics are illustrated for the first 30% of the gait cycle in Figure 12-36. The pelvic rotation about the right hip is shown by the forward rotation of the *left* iliac crest (seen from above). The right internal rotator muscles therefore can provide some of the drive to the contralateral (left) swinging limb, especially useful during rapid walking. As described later in this chapter, the tensor fasciae latae and the gluteus minimus and gluteus medius are also functioning as hip abductors during this part of the gait cycle. Activation of these muscles is necessary to stabilize the pelvis in the frontal plane during this part of the gait cycle.

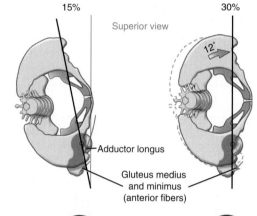

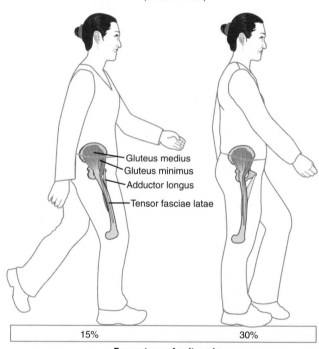

FIGURE 12-36. The activation pattern of several internal rotator muscles of the right hip is depicted during the first 30% of the gait cycle. (Brighter red indicates greater muscle activation.) Specifically, the tensor fasciae latae, anterior fibers of the gluteus minimus and gluteus medius, and adductor longus are shown rotating the pelvis in the horizontal plane over a relatively fixed right femur. (Compare the bottom and top views.)

Overall Function

Pelvic-on-Femoral Hip Extension

The following sections describe two different situations in which the hip extensor muscles control pelvic-on-femoral extension.

Hip Extensors Performing a Posterior Pelvic Tilt. With the supra-lumbar trunk held relatively stationary, the hip extensor and abdominal muscles act as a force-couple to posteriorly tilt the pelvis (Figure 12-38). The posterior tilt extends the hip joints slightly and reduces the lumbar lordosis.

The muscular mechanics involved with posterior tilting of the pelvis are generally similar to those described for the anterior tilting of the pelvis (compare Figures 12-27 and 12-38). In both tilting actions, a force-couple exists between the hip and trunk muscles. Consequently the pelvis rotates through a relatively short arc, using the femoral heads as a pivot point.

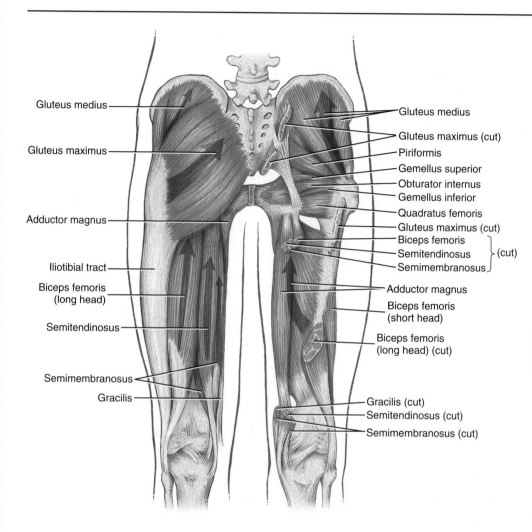

Gluteus medius

Gluteus maximus

Adductor magnus

Iliotibial tract

Biceps femoris
(long head)

Semitendinosus

Semimembranosus

Gracilis

Gluteus medius

Gluteus maximus (cut)

Piriformis

Gemellus superior

Obturator internus

Gemellus inferior

Quadratus femoris

Gluteus maximus (cut)

Biceps femoris
Semitendinosus   } (cut)
Semimembranosus

Adductor magnus

Biceps femoris
(short head)

Biceps femoris
(long head) (cut)

Gracilis (cut)
Semitendinosus (cut)
Semimembranosus (cut)

FIGURE   12-37. The posterior muscles of the hip. The left side highlights the gluteus maximus and hamstring muscles (long head of the biceps femoris, semitendinosus, and semimembranosus). The right side shows the hamstring muscles cut to expose the adductor magnus and short head of the biceps femoris. The right side shows the gluteus medius and five of the six short external rotators (i.e., piriformis, gemellus superior and inferior, obturator internus, and quadratus femoris).

During standing, a combination of tension in the hip's capsular ligaments and hip flexor muscles normally determines the end-range of the posterior pelvic movement. Interestingly, unlike the end-range of an anterior pelvic tilt, the lumbar spine does not normally restrict the end-range of the posterior pelvic tilt.

Hip Extensors Controlling a Forward Lean of the Body. Leaning forward while standing is a very common activity. Consider, for example, the forward lean used to brush your teeth over a sink. The muscular support at the hip for this near static posture is primarily the responsibility of the hamstring muscles. Consider two phases of a forward lean shown in Figure 12-39. During a slight forward lean (see Figure 12-39, *A*), body weight is displaced just anterior to the medial-lateral axis of rotation at the hips. This slightly flexed posture is restrained by minimal activation from the gluteus maximus and hamstring muscles. A more significant forward lean, however, displaces body weight farther in front of the hips (see Figure 12-39, *B*). Supporting this markedly flexed posture requires greater muscle activation from the hamstring muscles. The gluteus maximus, however, remains relatively inactive in this position—a point verifiable by palpation and inferred from electromyographic data.[45] The apparent increased responsibility of the hamstrings (in contrast to the gluteus maximus) can be explained biomechanically and physiologically. Forward leaning *increases* the hip extension moment arm of the hamstring muscles while it *decreases* the hip extensor

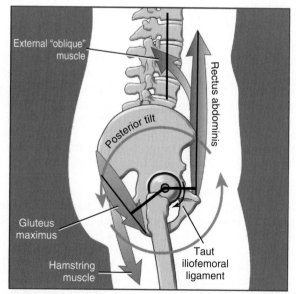

External "oblique" muscle

Rectus abdominis

Posterior tilt

Gluteus maximus

Taut iliofemoral ligament

Hamstring muscle

FIGURE 12-38. The force couple between representative hip extensors (gluteus maximus and hamstrings) and abdominal muscles (rectus abdominis and obliquus externus abdominis) used to posteriorly tilt the pelvis. The moment arms for each muscle group are indicated by the dark black line. Note the decreased lordosis at the lumbar spine. The extension at the hip stretches the iliofemoral ligament.

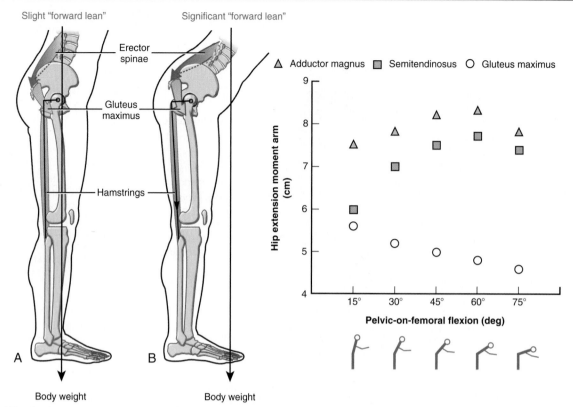

FIGURE 12-39. The hip extensor muscles are shown controlling a forward lean of the pelvis over the thighs. **A,** Slight forward lean of the upper body displaces the body weight force slightly anterior to the medial-lateral axis of rotation at the hip. **B,** A more significant forward lean displaces the body weight force even farther anteriorly. The greater flexion of the hips rotates the ischial tuberosities posteriorly, thereby increasing the hip extension moment arm of the hamstrings. The taut line (with arrow head within the stretched hamstring muscles) indicates the increased passive tension. In both **A** and **B,** the relative demands placed on the muscles are shown by relative shades of red. At right is a graph showing the length of hip extension moment arms of selected hip extensors as a function of forward lean.[145]

moment arm of the gluteus maximus.[145] (Compare the 15-degree and 30-degree points in the graph in Figure 12-39.) Leaning forward, therefore, mechanically optimizes the extension torque potential of the hamstrings.[67] A significant forward lean also elongates the hamstring muscles across both the hip and the knee joints. The resulting increased passive tension in these elongated biarticular muscles helps support the partially flexed position of the hips. For these reasons the hamstrings appear uniquely equipped to support the hip during a forward lean. Apparently the nervous system holds the gluteus maximus partially in reserve for more powerful hip extension activities, such as rapidly climbing a flight of stairs.

Femoral-on-Pelvic Hip Extension

As a group, the hip extensor muscles are frequently required to produce large and powerful femoral-on-pelvic hip extension torque to accelerate the body forward and upward. Consider, for example, the demands placed on the right hip extensors while one climbs a steep hill (Figure 12-40). The flexed position of the right hip while the climber is carrying a heavy pack imposes a large external (flexion) torque at the hip. The flexed position, however, favors greater extension torque generation from the hip extensor muscles. Furthermore, with the hip markedly flexed, many of the adductor muscles can produce an extension torque, thereby assisting the primary hip extensors. Activation of the low-back extensor muscles helps support the flexed trunk, as well as stabilizing the pelvis for the strongly activated hip extensor muscles.

HIP ABDUCTOR MUSCLES

Anatomy and Individual Action

The primary hip abductor muscles are the gluteus medius, gluteus minimus, and tensor fasciae latae.[23] The piriformis and sartorius are considered secondary hip abductors.

The *gluteus medius* attaches on the external surface of the ilium above the anterior gluteal line. The muscle attaches distally on the lateral aspect of the greater trochanter (see Figure 12-37). The distal attachment provides the gluteus medius with the greatest abductor moment arm of all the abductor muscles (see Figure 12-29). The gluteus medius is also the largest of the hip abductor muscles, occupying about 60% of the total abductor cross-sectional area.[23] The broad and fan-shaped gluteus medius has been considered as having three functional sets of fibers: anterior, middle, and posterior.[23,159] All fibers contribute to abduction of the hip; however, from the anatomic position the anterior fibers also produce internal rotation, and the posterior fibers also produce extension and external rotation. These actions may change considerably when muscle activation is initiated from outside the anatomic position.[8]

The *gluteus minimus* lies deep and slightly anterior to the gluteus medius. This muscle attaches proximally on the ilium—between the anterior and inferior gluteal lines—and distally on the anterior-lateral aspect of the greater trochanter (Figure 12-41). The muscle also attaches into the superior capsule of the joint.[169] These attachments may retract this part of the capsule away from the joint during motion—a mechanism that may prevent capsular impingement.

All the fibers of the gluteus minimus contribute to abduction; the more anterior fibers also contribute to internal rotation and flexion.[23,85] The gluteus minimus is smaller than the gluteus medius, occupying about 20% of the total abductor cross-sectional area.[23]

The *tensor fasciae latae* is the smallest of the three primary hip abductors, occupying about 11% of the total abductor cross-sectional area.[23] The anatomy of the tensor fasciae latae is discussed elsewhere in this text.

It is interesting to note that all the hip abductor muscles have an action as either internal or external rotators of the hip. The production of a *pure* frontal plane abduction torque therefore requires that the abductors completely neutralize one another's horizontal plane torque potential.

Hip Abductor Mechanism: Control of Frontal Plane Stability of the Pelvis during Walking

The abduction torque produced by the hip abductor muscles is essential to the control of the frontal plane pelvic-on-femoral kinematics during walking. During most of the stance phase, the hip abductors stabilize the pelvis over the relatively fixed femur (see Figure 12-36).[71,72] During the stance phase, therefore, the hip abductor muscles have a role in controlling the pelvis in the frontal plane and, as discussed earlier, the horizontal plane.

The abduction torque produced by the hip abductor muscles is particularly important during the single-limb–support phase of gait. During this phase the opposite leg is off the ground and swinging forward. Without adequate

abduction torque on the stance limb, the pelvis and trunk may drop uncontrollably toward the side of the swinging limb. The activation of the hip abductor muscle can be easily appreciated by palpating the gluteus medius just superior to the greater trochanter. The right muscle, for example, becomes firm as the left leg lifts off the ground.

The frontal plane stabilizing function of hip abductor muscles is a very important component of walking. Furthermore, the force produced by the abductors during stance accounts for most of the compressive forces generated between the acetabulum and femoral head.

Hip Abductor Mechanism: Role in the Production of Compression Force at the Hip

Figure 12-42 shows the major factors involved with maintaining frontal plane stability of the right hip during single-limb-support, similar to that required during the mid-stance phase of walking. The forces created by active hip abductors and body weight create opposing torques that control the position and stability of the pelvis (within the frontal plane) over the femoral head. During single-limb support, the pelvis is comparable to a seesaw, with its fulcrum represented by the femoral head. When the seesaw is balanced, the counterclockwise (internal) torque produced by the right hip abductor force (HAF) equals the clockwise (external) torque caused by body weight (BW). Balance of opposing torques is called *static rotary equilibrium*.

During single-limb support, the hip abductor muscles—in particular the gluteus medius—produce most of the compression force across the hip.[31] This important point is demonstrated by the model in Figure 12-42.[121,123] Note that the

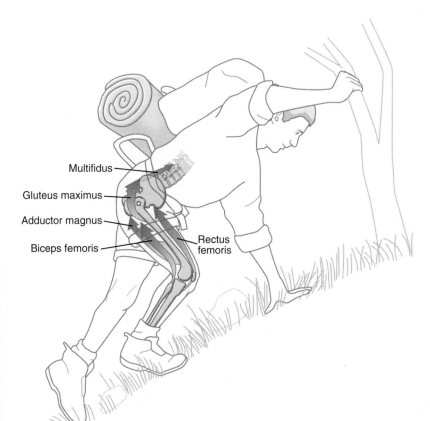

Multifidus
Gluteus maximus
Adductor magnus
Biceps femoris
Rectus femoris

FIGURE 12-40. Relatively high demands are placed on hip extensor muscles while one climbs a mountain supporting an external load. Activation is also required in low-back extensor muscles (such as, for example, the lower multifidus) to stabilize the position of the pelvis.

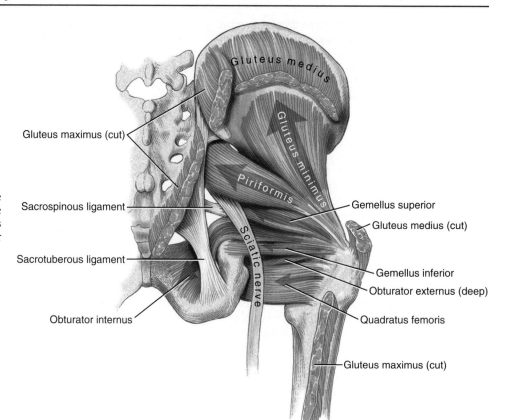

FIGURE 12-41. Deep muscles of the posterior and lateral hip region. The gluteus medius and the gluteus maximus are cut to expose deeper muscles.

Gluteus medius

Gluteus minimus

Gluteus maximus (cut)

Piriformis

Sacrospinous ligament

Sciatic nerve

Gemellus superior

Gluteus medius (cut)

Sacrotuberous ligament

Gemellus inferior

Obturator externus (deep)

Obturator internus

Quadratus femoris

Gluteus maximus (cut)

internal moment arm (D) used by the hip abductor muscles is about half the length of the external moment arm (D₁) used by body weight.[127] Given this length disparity, the hip abductor muscles must produce a force *twice* that of body weight in order to achieve stability during single-limb support. On every step, therefore, the acetabulum is pulled against the femoral head by the combined forces produced by the hip abductor muscles *and* the pull of body weight. To achieve static linear equilibrium, this downward force is counteracted by a joint reaction force (JRF) of equal magnitude but oriented in nearly the opposite direction (see Figure 12-42). The joint reaction force is directed 10 to 15 degrees off vertical–an angle that is strongly influenced by the orientation of the hip abductor muscle force vector.[72]

The sample data supplied in Figure 12-42 show how to estimate the approximate magnitude of the hip abductor force and hip joint reaction force. (For simplicity, it is assumed that all forces act vertically, as shown in the seesaw model.) As shown in the calculations, an upward-directed joint reaction force (JRF) of 1873.8 N (421.3 lb) occurs when a person weighing 760.6 N (171 lb) is in single-limb support over the right limb. This reaction force is about 2.5 times body weight, *66% of which comes from the hip abductor muscles.* During walking, the joint reaction force is even greater because of the acceleration of the pelvis over the femoral head. Data based on computer modeling or direct measurements from strain gauges implanted into a hip prosthesis show that joint compression forces reach three times body weight during walking.[71,161] These forces can increase to at least 5 or 6 times body weight while running or ascending and descending stairs or ramps.[12,153] Even ordinary daily functional activities can generate surprisingly large hip joint forces.[64] In general, these

forces serve important physiologic functions, such as stabilizing the femoral head within the acetabulum, assisting in the nutrition of the articular cartilage, and providing the stimulus for normal development and shape of joint structure in the growing child. The articular cartilage and trabecular bone normally protect the joint by safely dispersing large forces. A hip with arthritis, however, may no longer be able to provide this protection.

Maximal Abduction Torque Varies According to Hip Joint Angle

The unique relationship between a muscle group's internal torque and joint angle provides insight into the functional demands naturally placed on the muscles. The shape of the plot depicted in Figure 12-43, for example, clearly shows that the abductor muscles produce their peak torque (greatest strength) when elongated.[127] The maximal torque is produced when the hip is slightly adducted or in a neutral (0-degree) hip position. This frontal plane hip angle naturally occurs when the body is in or close to the single-limb support phase of walking: precisely when these muscles are needed to provide frontal plane stability to the hip. In essence, the abductor muscles have their greatest torque reserve at muscle lengths that correspond to their greatest functional demands.

The adducted position of the hip also increases the passive tension in the naturally stiff iliotibial band. This passive tension, although likely relatively small, can nevertheless augment the abduction torque required during the single-limb support phase of walking.[128]

In contrast, hip abduction torque potential is *least* at the near–fully shortened muscle length that corresponds to 40 degrees of abduction (see Figure 12-43). Ironically, the near–maximally abducted hip is in the position traditionally

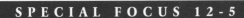

SPECIAL FOCUS 12-5

Greater Trochanteric Pain Syndrome

Excessive or repetitive activation of the gluteus medius and minimus can cause point tenderness adjacent to the greater trochanter—the primary distal attachment of these muscles. This painful response suggests injury or inflammation within the hip abductor mechanism. Pain associated with activation of the hip abductor mechanism can be disabling considering the frequent and relatively large demands placed on these muscles during the single-limb–support phase of the gait cycle.

It was traditionally believed that the source of greater trochanteric pain was inflamed *bursa* associated with the distal attachment of the gluteus medius and minimus.[144] This "trochanteric bursitis" may be caused by excessive and repetitive tension in the hip abductor mechanism, or frictional stress created by the overlying iliotibial band. More recent magnetic resonance imaging and

other clinical observations suggest that tears or degenerative changes in the distal tendons of the gluteal medius and minimus—at the site of their distal attachment—may also cause pain in the region of the greater trochanter and associated weakness of the hip abductor muscles.[180]

Because pain near the greater trochanter may involve either the bursa or tendons of the hip abductor muscles, some clinicians have suggested the more general term *greater trochanteric pain syndrome* to describe the condition. Continued advances in musculoskeletal imaging may improve the ability to make a more specific diagnosis. This is useful because continued pain in the area of the greater trochanter may be "referred" pain originating from hip osteoarthritis or pathology involving the low-back region.

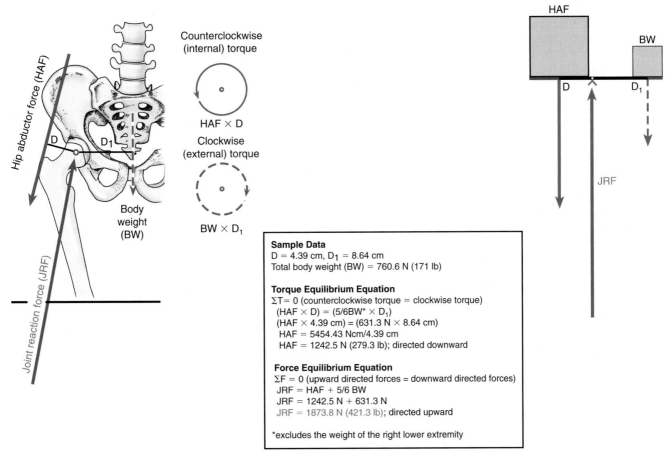

Sample Data
D = 4.39 cm, D_1 = 8.64 cm
Total body weight (BW) = 760.6 N (171 lb)

Torque Equilibrium Equation
ΣT = 0 (counterclockwise torque = clockwise torque)
(HAF × D) = (5/6BW* × D_1)
(HAF × 4.39 cm) = (631.3 N × 8.64 cm)
HAF = 5454.43 Ncm/4.39 cm
HAF = 1242.5 N (279.3 lb); directed downward

Force Equilibrium Equation
ΣF = 0 (upward directed forces = downward directed forces)
JRF = HAF + 5/6 BW
JRF = 1242.5 N + 631.3 N
JRF = 1873.8 N (421.3 lb); directed upward

*excludes the weight of the right lower extremity

FIGURE 12-42. A frontal plane diagram shows the function of the right hip abductor muscles during single-limb support on the right hip. The illustration on the left assumes that the pelvis and trunk are in static (linear and rotary) equilibrium about the right hip. The *counterclockwise torque (solid circle)* is the product of the right hip abductor force *(HAF)* times internal moment arm *(D)*; the *clockwise torque (dashed circle)* is the product of body weight *(BW)* times external moment arm *(D₁)*. Because the system is assumed to be in equilibrium, the torques in the frontal plane are equal in magnitude and opposite in direction: HAF × D = BW × D₁. The seesaw model *(right)* simplifies the major kinetic events during single-limb support. A joint reaction force *(JRF)* is directed through the fulcrum of the seesaw (hip joint). The sample data in the box are used in the torque and force equilibrium equations. These equations allow an estimate of the approximate magnitude of the hip abductor force and joint reaction force needed during single-limb support. (To simplify the mathematics, the calculations assume that all forces are acting in a vertical direction. This assumption introduces modest error in the results. Again, for simplicity, all moment arm directions are assigned positive values.) (From Neumann DA: Biomechanical analysis of selected principles of hip joint protection, *Arthritis Care Res* 2:146, 1989. Reprinted with permission from *Arthritis Care and Research*, American College of Rheumatology.)

SPECIAL FOCUS 12-6

Hip Abductor Muscle Weakness

Several medical conditions are associated with weakness of the hip abductor muscles. These conditions include muscular dystrophy, Guillain-Barré syndrome, spinal cord injury, greater trochanteric pain syndrome, hip osteoarthritis or rheumatoid arthritis, poliomyelitis, and undefined hip pain or weakness. The abductors may also be weakened after hip surgery, especially when the muscles have been incised to expose the joint. Persons with a painful or unstable hip often experience "disuse" weakness and atrophy in the abductor muscles—a consequence of purposely avoiding their strong muscular activation as a way to minimize the associated compression force across the joint.

The classic indicator of hip abductor weakness is the positive *Trendelenburg sign*.[54] The patient is asked to stand in single-limb support over the weak hip. A positive sign occurs if the pelvis drops to the side of the unsupported limb; in other words, the weak hip "falls" into pelvic-on-femoral adduction (see Figure 12-22, *B*). The clinician needs to be cautious in interpreting and documenting the results of this test. The patient with a weak right hip abductor muscle, for example, may indeed drop the pelvis to the left when asked to stand only on the right limb. The weakness may be masked, however, by a compensatory lean of the *trunk* to the right, especially if the weakness is marked. Leaning the trunk *to the side of the weakness* reduces the external torque demand on the abductor muscles by reducing the length of the external moment arm (see Figure 12-42, D_1). When observed while a person is walking, this compensatory lean to the side of weakness is referred to as a "gluteus medius limp" or "compensated Trendelenburg gait." Using a cane in the hand opposite the weakened hip abductors often corrects this abnormal gait pattern.

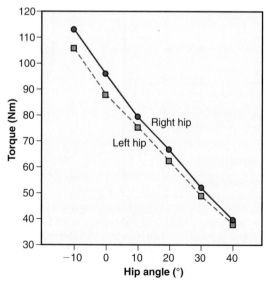

FIGURE 12-43. This plot shows the effect of frontal plane range of hip motion on the maximal-effort, isometric hip abduction torque in 30 healthy persons.[127] The −10-degree hip angle represents the adducted position at which the muscles are at their longest. Data are shown for both right and left sides.

suggested for manually testing the strength of the hip abductors.[80]

HIP EXTERNAL ROTATOR MUSCLES

The primary external rotator muscles of the hip are the gluteus maximus and five of the six "short external rotators." In the anatomic position, muscles considered as secondary external rotators are the posterior fibers of the gluteus medius and minimus, obturator externus, sartorius, and long head of the biceps femoris. The obturator externus is considered a secondary rotator because in the anatomic position its line of force lies only a few millimeters posterior to the longitudinal axis of rotation (see Figure 12-34).

The attachments of the gluteus maximus and sartorius were previously described under the topic of hip extensors and hip flexors, respectively.

Functional Anatomy of the "Short External Rotators"

The six "short external rotators" of the hip are the piriformis, obturator internus, gemellus superior, gemellus inferior, quadratus femoris, and obturator externus (see Figures 12-14, 12-37, and 12-41). The line of force of these muscles is oriented primarily in the horizontal plane. This orientation is optimal for the production of external rotation torque, as most of the force component of each muscle has a perpendicular intersection with the vertical axis of rotation. In a manner similar to the infraspinatus and teres minor at the shoulder, the short external rotators also provide stability to the posterior side of the joint.

The *piriformis* attaches proximally on the anterior surface of the sacrum, among the ventral sacral foramina (see Figure 12-26). Exiting the pelvis posteriorly through the greater sciatic foramen, the piriformis attaches to the superior aspect of the greater trochanter (see Figure 12-41).

In addition to the action of external rotation, the piriformis is a secondary hip abductor. Both actions are apparent in the muscle's line of force relative to the axis of rotation at the hip (see Figures 12-29 and 12-34).

The sciatic nerve usually exits the pelvis inferior to the piriformis. As described earlier in this chapter, the sciatic nerve may pass *through* the belly of the piriformis. A shortened or "tight" piriformis may compress and irritate the sciatic nerve, a condition known as "piriformis syndrome."

The *obturator internus* muscle arises from the internal side of the obturator membrane and from the adjacent ilium (see Figure 12-41). From this origin, the fibers converge to a central tendon after exiting the pelvis through lesser sciatic foramen. This notch, which is lined with hyaline cartilage, functions as a pulley by deflecting the tendon of the obturator internus by about 130 degrees on its approach to the trochanteric fossa of the femur (Figure 12-44, *A*).[160] With the femur firmly fixed during standing, strong contraction of this muscle rotates the pelvis (and superimposed trunk) relative to the femoral head (see Figure 12-44, *B*). In addition to rotating the pelvis, the force produced by the obturator internus compresses the surfaces of the joint, thereby providing an element of dynamic stability to the hip.

The *gemellus superior* and *inferior* (from the Latin root *geminus*, meaning twins) are two, small, nearly identically sized muscles with proximal attachments on either side of the lesser sciatic notch (see Figure 12-41). Each muscle blends in

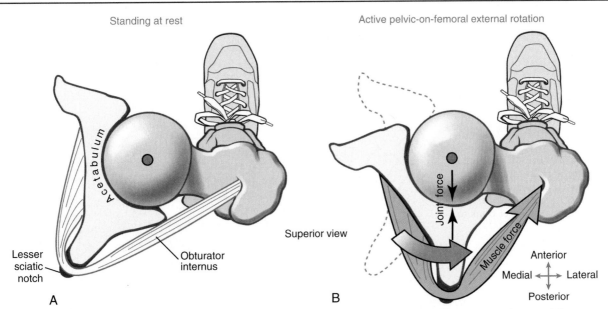

Standing at rest

Active pelvic-on-femoral external rotation

Acetabulum

Lesser
sciatic
notch

Obturator
internus

Joint force

Muscle force

Superior view

Anterior

Medial ↔ Lateral

Posterior

A

B

FIGURE 12-44. Superior view depicts the orientation and action of the obturator internus muscle. **A,** While one stands at rest, the obturator internus muscle makes a 130-degree deflection as it courses through the pulley formed by the lesser sciatic notch. **B,** With the femur fixed during standing, contraction of this muscle causes pelvic-on-femoral (hip) external rotation. (The external rotation of the hip is apparent by the reduced distance between the posterior side of the greater trochanter and the lateral side of the pelvis.) Note the compression force generated into the joint as the result of the muscle contraction.

with the central tendon of the obturator internus for a common attachment to the femur. Immediately below the gemellus inferior is the *quadratus femoris* muscle. This flat muscle arises from the external side of the ischial tuberosity and inserts on the posterior side of the proximal femur.

The *obturator externus* muscle arises from the external side of the obturator membrane and adjacent ilium (see Figure 12-14). The belly of this muscle is visible from the anterior side of the pelvis after removal of the adductor longus and pectineus muscles (see Figure 12-26, left side). The muscle attaches posteriorly on the femur at the trochanteric fossa (see Figure 12-6). (Based on its location and innervation, the obturator externus is more anatomically associated with the *adductor group* of muscles, rather than the other five short external rotators. The obturator externus is innervated by nerve roots that originate from the lumbar plexus [via the obturator nerve], as are most of the other adductor muscles. The other small external rotators, in contrast, are innervated through the sacral plexus, with nerve roots as low as S^2.)

Overall Function

The functional potential of the external rotators is most evident during pelvic-on-femoral rotation. Consider, for example, the external rotator muscles contracting to rotate the pelvis over the femur (Figure 12-45). With the right lower extremity firmly in contact with the ground, contraction of the right external rotators accelerates the anterior side of the pelvis and attached trunk to the left—*contralateral* to the fixed femur. This action of planting a foot and "cutting" to the opposite side is the natural way to abruptly change direction while running. As indicated in Figure 12-45, activation of the right gluteus maximus, for instance, is very capable of imparting both the extension and external rotation thrust to the hip

during this action. If needed, the external rotation torque can be decelerated by eccentric action of internal rotator muscles. Extremely rapid eccentric activation of the adductor longus or brevis, for example, may be used to decelerate the contralateral-directed pelvic rotation—an action that may cause "strain" injury to these muscles. The mechanism of injury may partially explain the relatively high incidence of adductor muscle strain during many sporting activities that involve rapid rotation of the pelvis and trunk while running.

MAXIMAL TORQUE PRODUCED BY THE HIP MUSCLES

Normative data on the maximal-effort torque production of the hip muscles can serve as useful information in assessment of progress and setting of goals for persons involved in rehabilitation and training programs. Figure 12-46 depicts the average, maximal internal torque produced by a sample of healthy males.[21] It is interesting to observe the ranking of the peak torques across the three planes of motion. The greatest torque is produced within the sagittal plane, with extension torque slightly exceeding flexion torque. The predominant strength of the hip extensors compared with all other muscle groups is not surprising: these muscles must lift or propel the body upward (and often forward) against gravity or control the descent of the body. The relatively high strength of the hip flexor muscles reflects the need to rapidly accelerate the lower limb during running, in addition to controlling the entire trunk and pelvis relative to fixed lower extremities. Consider in the latter case the physically powerful iliopsoas, for example—a muscle that likely accounts for a significant proportion of the flexion torque potential at the hip.

The internal and external rotator muscles produce the least magnitude of torque of all muscle groups of the hip.

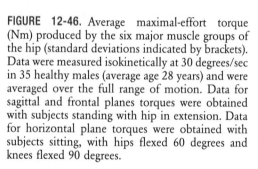

FIGURE 12-45. Action of the right external rotator muscles during pelvic-on-femoral external rotation of the right hip. Back extensor muscles are also shown rotating the lower trunk to the left.

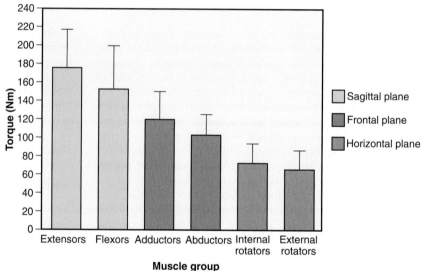

FIGURE 12-46. Average maximal-effort torque (Nm) produced by the six major muscle groups of the hip (standard deviations indicated by brackets). Data were measured isokinetically at 30 degrees/sec in 35 healthy males (average age 28 years) and were averaged over the full range of motion. Data for sagittal and frontal planes torques were obtained with subjects standing with hip in extension. Data for horizontal plane torques were obtained with subjects sitting, with hips flexed 60 degrees and knees flexed 90 degrees.

Such a ranking reflects the fact that in the upright position these muscles produce a rotary torque between the femur and pelvis in a plane that does *not* typically oppose the force of gravity.

EXAMPLES OF HIP DISEASE: RATIONALE FOR SELECTED THERAPEUTIC AND SURGICAL INTERVENTIONS

Two of the most common causes of hip impairment are fracture of the proximal femur and osteoarthritis. This section describes each of these conditions, followed by a discussion of clinical biomechanics associated with selected therapeutic and surgical interventions.

Fracture of the Hip

Fracture of the hip (i.e., proximal femur) is a major health and economic problem in the United States.[167,170] About 95% of all fractures of the hip are the result of falls.[137] The incidence of hip fracture increases with advanced age, and hip fracture is the second leading cause of hospitalization in the elderly.[174] Two primary factors often associated with the higher incidence of hip fracture in the elderly are age-related osteoporosis and the higher incidence of falling.[30,170]

The number of hip fractures in the United States is expected to triple by the year 2050 because of the rapidly increasing number of persons aged 85 years and older.[170] Large increases in the number of hip fractures are also anticipated over the next several decades worldwide.[51]

Mortality is surprisingly high after hip fracture: studies report 12% to 25% of persons die within 1 year of fracturing a hip.[68,134,170] Much of this mortality is associated with an underlying medical condition rather than the actual trauma of the fracture.[140] Although nearly 80% of persons over 65 years of age who sustain hip fractures are women, the mortality rate in men is almost twice as high after a hip fracture.[79,170]

Hip fracture can result in significant loss of function.[135] Research indicates that only about 40% of persons are able to independently perform their basic functional activities 6 to 12 months after hip fracture.[37,68,179] About half these persons also continue to require an assistive device to aid their walking.

Osteoarthritis of the Hip

Hip osteoarthritis is a disease manifested primarily by deterioration of the joint's articular cartilage, loss of joint space, sclerosis of subchondral bone, and the presence of osteophytes.[3] Without an adequate dampening mechanism to dissipate joint forces, the hip can experience marked degeneration and change in shape. The American College of Rheumatology recommends the following criteria for diagnosing hip osteoarthritis without the use of radiography: hip pain, less than 115 degrees of hip flexion, and less than 15 degrees of internal rotation.[2] The reduced range of motion may be caused by restrictions in soft tissue (such as posterior and inferior capsule or parts of the ischiofemoral ligament) and, in more severe cases, articular malalignment and osteophyte formation. Additional symptoms may include atrophy and weakness of hip muscles, morning stiffness, crepitus, inflammation of soft tissues, and abnormal gait pattern (such as a compensated Trendelenburg gait) or altered step length.[103]

Hip osteoarthritis can cause major disability and occurs in 10% to 20% of persons in the aging population.[39,131] Impairments associated with hip osteoarthritis can cause significant loss in function, such as difficulty climbing stairs, bathing, dressing the lower extremities, and rising from a low chair.

Hip osteoarthritis may be classified as either a primary or secondary disease. *Primary* or idiopathic *hip osteoarthritis* is an arthritic condition without a known cause. *Secondary hip osteoarthritis*, in contrast, is an arthritic condition resulting from a known mechanical disruption of the joint. This may occur from trauma or overuse; structural failure, such as a slipped capital femoral epiphysis; anatomic asymmetry or dysplasia, such as excessive acetabular anteversion or a malshaped proximal femur, leg length discrepancy, or avascular necrosis of the femoral head (i.e., Legg-Calvé-Perthes disease); or repeated dislocation and instability.

The exact cause of primary hip osteoarthritis remains unclear. Although the frequency of osteoarthritis at any joint increases with age, the disease is not triggered solely *by* the aging process.[102] If this were true, then *all* elderly persons would eventually develop this disease. The causes of osteoarthritis are complicated and not exclusively based on a simple wear-and-tear phenomenon. Although physical stress may increase the rate and amount of wear at the hip, this does not always lead to osteoarthritis.[98,143,147] Other mechanisms that may be related to osteoarthritis are metabolism of the ground matrix of the cartilage, genetics, immune system factors, neuromuscular disorders, and biochemical factors.[63,102]

Therapeutic Intervention for a Painful or Mechanically Unstable Hip

USING A CANE AND PROPER METHODS FOR CARRYING EXTERNAL LOADS

Severe fracture or osteoarthritis of the hip can lead to chronic pain and mechanical instability. These potentially disabling impairments can also occur in a hip that is either acutely inflamed, brittle because of severe osteoporosis, or markedly dysplastic. Conservative treatment for such conditions may include instructions in assisted gait and functional activities,[84,122,123] modalities for relieving pain, and, when appropriate, graded aerobic conditioning and exercise.[151] In addition, clinicians frequently provide advice on how to limit the magnitude of potentially large forces that may exacerbate or further complicate the underlying pathology.[123] Such advice on hip "joint protection" may include reducing body weight; walking with reduced speed, cadence, and stride length; using an assistance device such as a cane; and methods of carrying loads.[13,120,121,161]

One of the most practical and effective methods of reducing compression forces on the hip during walking is to use a cane held in the hand *opposite* the affected hip.[1] Use of the cane in this fashion reduces joint reaction forces caused by activation of the hip abductor muscles.[120] Figure 12-47 shows that applying a cane force (CF) by the left hand results in a joint reaction force at the right hip of 1195.4 N (268.8 lb).[120] This correlates with a 36% reduction in joint reaction force compared with that produced when a cane is not used (see Figure 12-42 for comparison). In essence, the force applied to the cane (held in the left hand) produces a torque about the right hip that is in the *same rotary direction* as that produced by the overlying hip abductor muscles. Pushing on the cane, therefore, can substitute for part of the force that is naturally required by the hip abductor muscles: reduced demands placed on the hip abductor muscles during single-limb support equates to reduced compression force on the hip joint.[112]

Methods of carrying external loads significantly influence the demands placed on the hip abductor muscles and therefore on the underlying hip joint. Persons with painful, unstable, or surgically replaced hips are to be cautioned about the consequences of carrying relatively large hand-held loads *opposite*, or contralateral to, the affected hip.[13,121,124,126] As shown in Figure 12-48, the contralateral load has a very large external moment arm (D_2), creating a substantial clockwise torque about the right hip.[121] For frontal plane stability, the right hip abductors must create a counterclockwise torque large enough to balance the clockwise torques caused by the external load ($CL \times D_2$) *and* body weight ($BW \times D_1$). As a result of the relatively small moment arm available to the hip abductor muscles (D), the hip abductor force during single-limb support is very large. As shown by the calculations in Figure 12-48, carrying a contralaterally held load of 15% of body weight (114.1 N or 25.7 lb) produces a joint reaction force of 2897.6 N (651.1 lb). A healthy hip can usually toler-

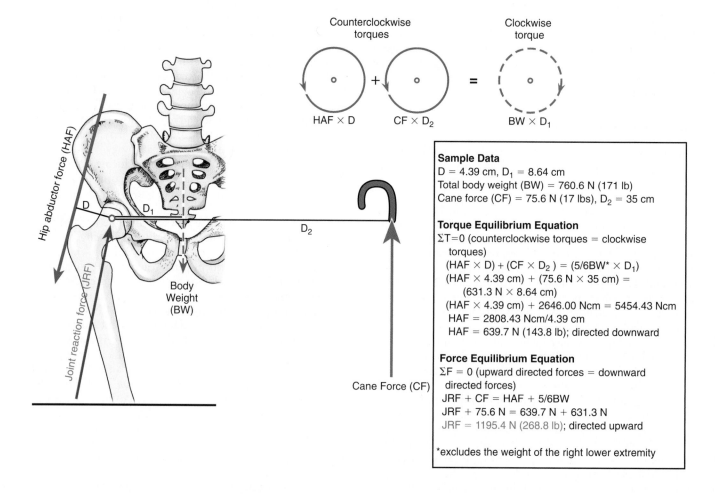

Counterclockwise torques

Clockwise torque

$HAF \times D$ $CF \times D_2$ $BW \times D_1$

Hip abductor force (HAF)

Joint reaction force (JRF)

D D_1

D_2

Body Weight (BW)

Cane Force (CF)

Sample Data
$D = 4.39$ cm, $D_1 = 8.64$ cm
Total body weight (BW) = 760.6 N (171 lb)
Cane force (CF) = 75.6 N (17 lbs), $D_2 = 35$ cm

Torque Equilibrium Equation
$\Sigma T = 0$ (counterclockwise torques = clockwise torques)
$(HAF \times D) + (CF \times D_2) = (5/6BW^* \times D_1)$
$(HAF \times 4.39$ cm$) + (75.6$ N $\times 35$ cm$) =$
$\quad (631.3$ N $\times 8.64$ cm$)$
$(HAF \times 4.39$ cm$) + 2646.00$ Ncm $= 5454.43$ Ncm
$HAF = 2808.43$ Ncm/4.39 cm
$HAF = 639.7$ N (143.8 lb); directed downward

Force Equilibrium Equation
$\Sigma F = 0$ (upward directed forces = downward directed forces)
$JRF + CF = HAF + 5/6BW$
$JRF + 75.6$ N $= 639.7$ N $+ 631.3$ N
$JRF = 1195.4$ N (268.8 lb); directed upward

*excludes the weight of the right lower extremity

FIGURE 12-47. A frontal plane diagram shows how a cane force *(CF)* applied by the left hand produces a frontal plane torque about the right hip in single-limb support. The pelvis and trunk are assumed to be in static (linear and rotary) equilibrium about the right hip. The cane-produced torque minimizes the torque and force demands on the right hip abductor muscles. Note that the *clockwise torque (dashed circle)* resulting from body weight *(BW × D₁)* is balanced by the *counterclockwise torques (solid circles)* resulting from the hip abductor force *(HAF × D) and* the cane force *(CF × D₂)*. The data shown in the box are used in the torque and force equilibrium equations to estimate the approximate magnitude of hip abductor force and joint reaction force *(JRF)*. The moment arm used by cane force is represented by D_2. (See Figure 12-42 for additional abbreviations and background.) (To simplify the mathematics, the calculations assume that all forces are acting in a vertical direction. This assumption introduces modest error in the results. All moment arm directions are assigned positive values.) (From Neumann DA: Hip abductor muscle activity as subjects with hip prosthesis walk with different methods of using a cane, *Phys Ther* 78:490, 1998. With permission of the American Physical Therapy Association.)

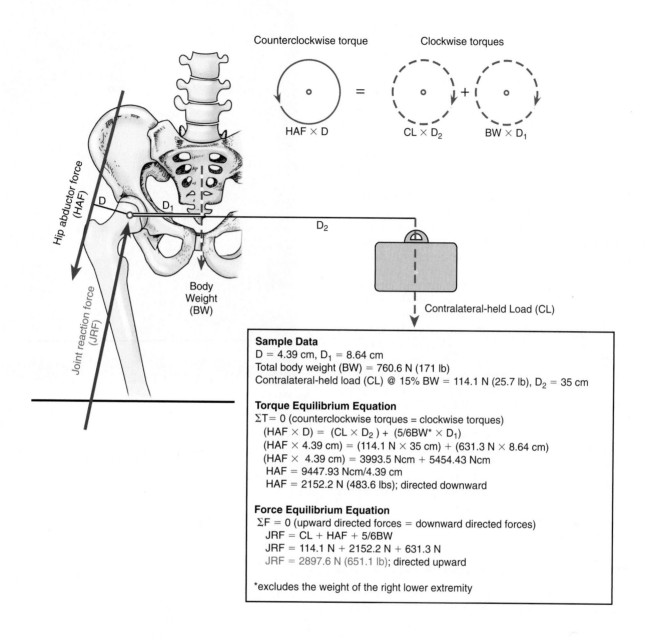

Counterclockwise torque
HAF × D

Clockwise torques
CL × D₂ + BW × D₁

Hip abductor force (HAF)

Joint reaction force (JRF)

D

D₁

D₂

Body Weight (BW)

Contralateral-held Load (CL)

Sample Data
D = 4.39 cm, D₁ = 8.64 cm
Total body weight (BW) = 760.6 N (171 lb)
Contralateral-held load (CL) @ 15% BW = 114.1 N (25.7 lb), D₂ = 35 cm

Torque Equilibrium Equation
ΣT = 0 (counterclockwise torques = clockwise torques)
  (HAF × D) = (CL × D₂) + (5/6BW* × D₁)
  (HAF × 4.39 cm) = (114.1 N × 35 cm) + (631.3 N × 8.64 cm)
  (HAF × 4.39 cm) = 3993.5 Ncm + 5454.43 Ncm
  HAF = 9447.93 Ncm/4.39 cm
  HAF = 2152.2 N (483.6 lbs); directed downward

Force Equilibrium Equation
ΣF = 0 (upward directed forces = downward directed forces)
  JRF = CL + HAF + 5/6BW
  JRF = 114.1 N + 2152.2 N + 631.3 N
  JRF = 2897.6 N (651.1 lb); directed upward

*excludes the weight of the right lower extremity

FIGURE 12-48. A frontal plane diagram shows how a load held in the left hand significantly increases the right hip abductor force *(HAF)* during single-limb support. Two clockwise torques *(dashed circles)* are produced about the right hip because of the contralateral-held load *(CL × D₂) and* body weight *(BW × D₁)*. For equilibrium about the right hip, the clockwise torques must be balanced by a counterclockwise torque *(solid circle)* produced by the hip abductor force *(HAF × D)*. The data shown in the box are used in the torque and force equilibrium equations to estimate the approximate magnitude of hip abductor force and joint reaction force *(JRF)*. D₂ designates the moment arm used by the contralateral-held load *(CL)*. Refer to Figure 12-42 for background and other abbreviations. (To simplify the mathematics, the calculations assume that all force vectors are acting in a vertical direction. This assumption introduces modest error in the results. All moment arm directions are assigned positive values.) (From Neumann DA: Hip abductor muscle activity in persons with a hip prosthesis while carrying loads in one hand, *Phys Ther* 76:1320, 1996. With permission of the American Physical Therapy Association.)

ate this amount of force without difficulty. Caution must be exercised, however, if structural stability of the hip is compromised.

As a general principle, persons with an unstable or painful hip should be advised to avoid or limit the carrying of any external loads. For most ambulatory persons, however, this advice is impractical. More practically, when loads *must* be carried, they should be as light as possible, carried in a backpack or by hand ipsilateral to the affected hip, or divided in half and carried bilaterally.[13,124,125] Research has shown that a strategy of *combining* the use of a contralaterally held cane with an ipsilaterally held load (equal to or less than 15% of body weight) reduces the demands on the hip abductor muscles to a greater degree than either method implemented separately.[122]

The previous discussion focuses on methods that reduce the force demands on the hip abductor muscles as a means to reduce the force on a painful or an unstable hip. The same methods also apply to protecting an unstable hip associated with an arthroplasty (joint replacement). Although these methods may have their desired effect, the reduced functional demand placed on the hip may also perpetuate prolonged weakness in the hip abductor muscles, which in turn leads to deviations in gait.[141] A study on a group of persons with hip osteoarthritis awaiting arthroplastic surgery reported a 31% average loss in hip abduction torque compared with aged-match controls.[10] This loss in strength exceeded that of the hip flexors, extensors, and adductor muscles. Clinicians must meet the dual challenge of protecting a vulnerable hip from excessive and potentially damaging forces from the abductor muscles while simultaneously increasing the functional strength and endurance of these muscles. This requires knowledge of the normal and abnormal frontal plane mechanics of the hip, the pathology specific to the patient's condition, and the symptoms that suggest the hip is being subjected to potentially damaging forces. These signs and symptoms include excessive pain, marked gait deviation, generalized hip instability, and abnormal positioning of the lower limb.

Surgical Intervention after Fracture or Osteoarthritis

Surgery is often indicated to repair a fractured hip. The type of surgical repair depends on the patient's age and activity level, plus the location and severity of the fracture.

A *hip arthroplasty* is often performed when a person with hip disease, most often osteoarthritis, has constant pain that significantly limits function and quality of life. This operation replaces the diseased or degenerated acetabulum and/or femoral head with biologically inert materials. The arthroplasty may totally replace or resurface the femoral head.[133] A prosthetic hip may be secured by cement, or through biologic fixation provided by bone growth into the surface of the implanted components. Although the total hip arthroplasty is typically a successful procedure,[114] premature loosening or dislocation of the femoral and/or acetabular component can be a postoperative problem.[18,83,92,116] Large torsional loads between the prosthetic implant and the bony interface may contribute to the loss of fixation. Until sufficient long-term data emerge from clinical trials, debate regarding the most durable materials and effective methods of fixation and implantation continues.[29,58,70,113]

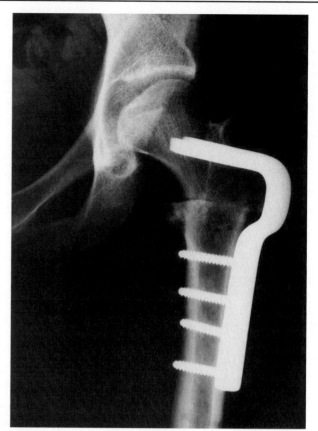

FIGURE 12-49. A varus osteotomy was performed on a hip with avascular necrosis of the femoral head. The removed wedge of bone is apparent at the extreme proximal femoral shaft. The increased varus position in this particular patient improved the congruency of the weight-bearing surface of the hip. The osteotomy site was stabilized with a blade plate. (Courtesy Michael Anderson, MD, Blount Orthopedic Clinic, Milwaukee, Wisconsin.)

BIOMECHANICAL CONSEQUENCES OF COXA VARA AND COXA VALGA

As previously described in this chapter, the average angle of inclination of the femoral neck is approximately 125 degrees (see Figure 12-7, *A*). The angle may be changed as a result of a surgical repair of a fractured hip or the specific design of a prosthetic hip. In addition, a surgical operation known as a *coxa vara* (or *valga*) *osteotomy* intentionally alters a preexisting angle of inclination. This operation involves cutting a wedge of bone from the proximal femur, thereby changing the orientation of the femoral head to the acetabulum. A goal of this operation is often to improve the congruency of the weight-bearing surfaces of the hip (Figure 12-49).

Regardless of the type of and rationale for the hip surgery, changing the angle of inclination of the proximal femur alters the biomechanics of the joint. These alterations can have positive or negative biomechanical effects. Figure 12-50, *A* shows two potentially positive biomechanical effects of *coxa vara*. The varus position increases the moment arm of the hip abductor force (indicated by D'). The greater leverage increases the abduction torque produced per unit of hip abductor muscle force. This situation may benefit persons with hip abductor weakness. Also, increasing the leverage of the abductor muscles may allow a given level of abduction torque

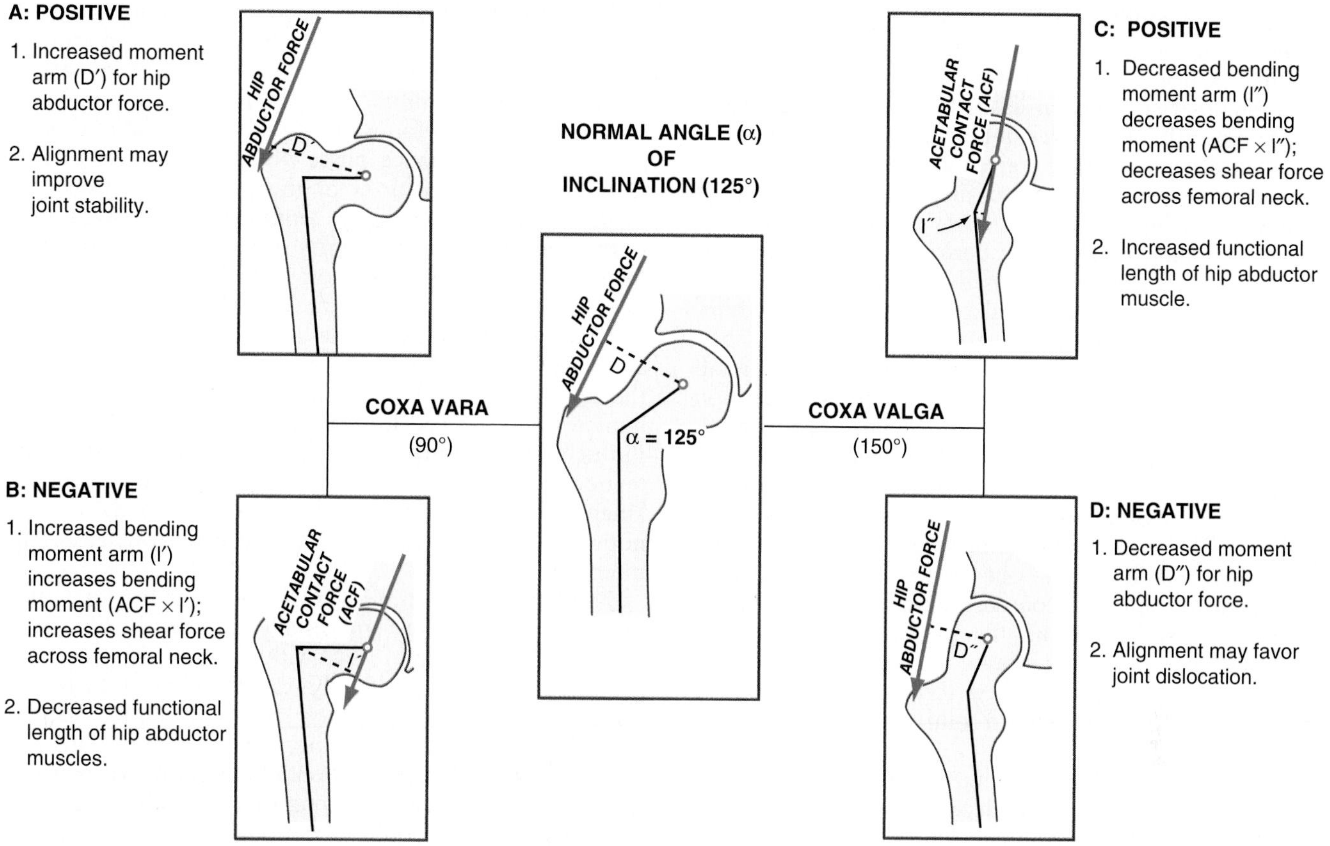

A: POSITIVE

1. Increased moment arm (D') for hip abductor force.

2. Alignment may improve joint stability.

NORMAL ANGLE (α) OF INCLINATION (125°)

COXA VARA
(90°)

α = 125°

COXA VALGA
(150°)

C: POSITIVE

1. Decreased bending moment arm (I") decreases bending moment (ACF × I"); decreases shear force across femoral neck.

2. Increased functional length of hip abductor muscle.

B: NEGATIVE

1. Increased bending moment arm (I') increases bending moment (ACF × I'); increases shear force across femoral neck.

2. Decreased functional length of hip abductor muscles.

D: NEGATIVE

1. Decreased moment arm (D") for hip abductor force.

2. Alignment may favor joint dislocation.

FIGURE 12-50. The negative and positive biomechanical effects of coxa vara and coxa valga are contrasted. As a reference, a hip with a normal angle of inclination (α = 125 degrees) is shown in the center of the display. D is the internal moment arm used by hip abductor force; I is the bending moment arm across the femoral neck.

required during the stance phase of walking to be generated by less muscle force. Reducing the magnitude of muscular-based joint forces can help protect an arthritic or unstable prosthetic hip from excessive wear during walking. A varus osteotomy may in some patients improve the stability of the joint by aligning the femoral head more directly into the acetabulum.

A potentially negative effect of coxa vara is an increased bending moment (or torque) generated across the femoral neck (see Figure 12-50, *B*). The bending moment arm (dashed line indicated by I') increases as the angle of inclination approaches 90 degrees. Increasing the bending moment raises the tension across the superior aspect of the femoral neck. This situation may cause a fracture of the femoral neck or a structural failure of a prosthesis. Marked coxa vara increases the vertical shear between the femoral head and the adjacent epiphysis. In children this situation may lead to a condition known as a *slipped capital femoral epiphysis*.[100] Coxa vara may decrease the functional length of the hip abductor muscles, thereby reducing the force-generating capability of these muscles and increasing the likelihood of a "gluteus medius limp." The loss in muscle force may offset the increased abduction torque potential gained by the increased hip abductor moment arm.

Coxa valga may result from a surgical intervention or from pathology such as hip dysplasia. A potentially positive effect of the valgus position is a decrease in bending moment arm across the femoral neck (see I" in Figure 12-50, *C*). This situation also decreases the vertical shear across the femoral neck. The valgus position, however, may increase the functional length of the hip abductor muscles, thus improving their force-generating ability. In contrast, a potentially negative effect of coxa valga is the decreased moment arm available to the hip abductor force (indicated by D" in Figure 12-50, *D*). In extreme coxa valga, the femoral head may be positioned more lateral to the acetabulum, possibly favoring dislocation.

SYNOPSIS

The hip joints function as basilar joints for both the axial skeleton and the lower extremities. As such, the hips form the central pivot point for common movements of the body as a whole, especially those involving flexion and extension. Consider, for instance, lifting the leg to ascend a steep stair, or bending down at the waist to pick up an object from the floor. Both motions demand a significant amount of movement and production of muscular force between the proximal femurs and the pelvis. Weakness, instability, or pain in the hips therefore typically causes marked difficulty in performing a wide range of activities—from getting in and out of a chair to engaging in even moderate aerobic exercise.

The osteology and arthrology of the healthy hip joint are designed more for ensuring stability than for providing excessive mobility, a condition essentially the opposite of that for the glenohumeral joint—the analogous joint of the upper extremity. A deep-seated and well-contained femoral head, surrounded by thick capsular ligaments and muscles, ensures stability especially in the weight-bearing phase of walking—a phase that occupies 60% of a given gait cycle.

A surprisingly small amount of muscle activity is required to stabilize the hips while one stands in an upright relaxed posture, assuming that one or both of the hips are fully extended. Such a posture orients the body's line of gravity just posterior to the medial-lateral axis of rotation at the hips. The force of gravity therefore acts to maintain the hips passively extended. Being pulled relatively taut in near or full hip extension, the ligaments of the hip create useful tension that adds further to the stability of the extended hips. Indeed, muscle forces are periodically required to augment or readjust the stability of the hips while one stands at ease; however, this active mechanism is normally used as a reserve or secondary source. This is not the case, however, with a hip flexion contracture; stability while one stands in partial flexion demands significant and constant activation from the hip extensor muscles. Such a condition not only is metabolically "expensive" but places unnecessarily large muscular-based forces across the hip joints. These forces, acting over time, may be harmful in a malaligned joint that cannot properly dissipate stress.

The full extent to which the hip joints contribute to full body movement requires an understanding of both femoral-on-pelvic and pelvic-on-femoral kinematics. Femoral-on-pelvic movements are often associated with a change in location of the body as a whole relative to the surroundings, such as while walking. Pelvic-on-femoral movements, on the other hand, are often performed to change the position of the pelvis—and often the entire superimposed trunk—relative to fixed lower extremities. Pelvic-on-femoral movements are expressed in many forms, from subtle oscillations of the pelvis during the stance phase of each gait cycle to more obvious large-arc rotations of the pelvis (and trunk) as a figure skater spins on the ice while bending forward at the waist. Adding to the complexity of pelvic-on-femoral movements is the strong association with the kinematics of the lumbar spine. Clinical evaluation of the causes of reduced or abnormal motions at the hip must therefore include an evaluation of the flexibility and prevailing posture of the lumbar region. Limitations of movement at *either* the lumbar spine or the hips alter the kinematic sequencing throughout the trunk and proximal end of the lower kinematic chain. Being able to localize the source of abnormal kinematics within this broad area of the body certainly improves the likelihood of successful clinical diagnosis and intervention.

Nearly one third of muscles that cross the hip joint attach proximally to the pelvis and distally to either the tibia or the fibula. An imbalance of force within any of these muscles—generated actively or passively—can therefore influence the posture and range of motion across multiple segments, including the lumbar spine, hip, and knee. Clinicians regularly evaluate and treat functional limitations that may arise from impairments in and among these and other synergistic muscles. Treatment requires a thorough understanding of the muscular interactions that exist across a very mechanically interrelated region of the body.

ADDITIONAL CLINICAL CONNECTIONS

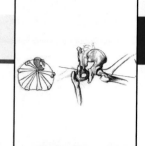

CLINICAL CONNECTION 12-1
Justifying a Standard Method of Stretching the Piriformis Muscle

Restrictions in the extensibility of the piriformis muscle may limit hip internal rotation, compress the underlying sciatic nerve, or produce abnormal stress on the sacroiliac joint. Some clinicians believe that an inflamed and tight piriformis may also create a painful "trigger" point deep in the buttock region, in the area of the posterior-superior iliac spine. This poorly defined condition is often referred to as "piriformis syndrome." The degree to which this condition actually exists has been questioned for many years.[19]

Treatment for piriformis syndrome often involves stretching of the tightened muscle. A common strategy for stretching the piriformis combines full flexion and *external rotation* of the hip, typically performed with the knee flexed to reduce tension from the biarticular hamstring muscles. The amount of piriformis elongation caused by this stretching technique is uncertain, although the position of cross-legged sitting has been shown to increase the length of the piriformis by 21% as compared with the muscle's

length when the subject stands in the anatomic position.[158] At first thought, the external rotation component of the standard piriformis stretch position appears counterintuitive, based on the muscle's action as a primary *external* rotator of the hip. Further kinesiologic consideration, however, can justify this method of stretch. As described earlier in this chapter, with the hip flexed the piriformis switches its action from an external rotator (in hip extension) to an internal rotator.[33] This can be visualized nicely with a skeleton model and piece of flexible cord that mimics the muscle's line of force (Figure 12-51, *A*). Flexing the hip beyond 90 degrees, therefore, allows external rotation of the hip to cause *further elongation* of the piriformis (Figure 12-51, *B*).

In closing, even though the piriformis switches its rotary action in flexion, the principle used to stretch this muscle is not violated: stretching a muscle requires that the muscle be placed in a position *opposite* to its primary actions.

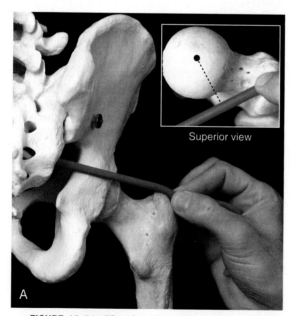
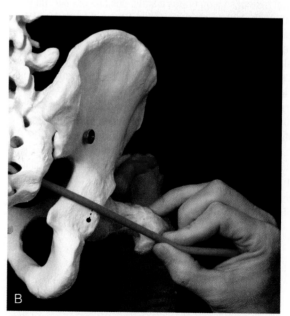

FIGURE 12-51. The changing action of the piriformis is shown with hip flexion. **A,** With the hip extended, the piriformis *(red cord)* has a line of force to externally rotate the hip. As shown from a superior view in the inset, the muscle's line of pull is posterior to the vertical axis of rotation. The muscle's moment arm for this action is shown as a dashed line. **B,** With the hip flexed, the line of force of the piriformis shifts its position to the opposite side of the longitudinal axis of rotation. Although acting with a relatively small moment arm, the muscle is now an internal rotator of the hip.

ADDITIONAL CLINICAL CONNECTIONS

CLINICAL CONNECTION 12-2
Augmenting the Therapeutic Stretch of Selected Biarticular Muscles of the Hip

Clinicians frequently employ methods of stretching muscles to treat or prevent musculoskeletal disorders.[76] Biarticular muscles of the hip receive specific attention from physical therapists and athletic trainers, especially the hamstrings and rectus femoris. Reduced flexibility within these muscles can alter the posture and range of motion across multiple segments; including the lumbar spine, hip, and knee.[25,80] Especially significant, the increased stiffness in these muscles has been associated with impairments in these regions.[42,52] Some evidence supports the premise that stretching of muscles can prevent injury. It has been shown, for example, that incorporating a regular hamstring stretching program can reduce the incidence of injury in military basic trainees.[56]

Because the aforementioned muscles cross so many joints, different combinations of active movements and static positions can be used to perform the stretch. Methods used for a person to augment a self-stretch of some of these biarticular muscles are the topics of this discussion.

As the first of two examples, consider methods used by persons to stretch their *hamstring* muscles. One of the more traditional methods incorporates a static position of near full knee extension with varying amounts of hip flexion (Figure 12-52, *A*). As depicted in this figure, the increased muscular tension in the stretched hamstrings pulls the ischial tuberosity forward, thereby increasing the posterior tilt of the pelvis and reducing the lordosis in the subject's lumbar spine. This posterior pelvic tilt would theoretically reduce the effectiveness of the stretch on the hamstring muscles. As a way to augment the extent of this stretch, the subject can be instructed to *actively contract* muscles that are antagonists to the tightened hamstring group, such as the rectus femoris and multifidus (see Figure 12-52, *B*). These muscles are considered antagonists to the hamstrings because of their ability to perform *pelvic-on-femoral (hip) flexion* by rotating the pelvis anteriorly relative to the fixed femurs. Active contraction of this pair of muscles elongates the right hamstrings, which, as noted in Figure 12-52, *B*, is evidenced by the increased lumbar lordosis.

By contracting the quadriceps, the rectus femoris can flex the hip (via a pelvic-on-femoral perspective) while also stabilizing the knee in extension. This stabilizing action of the quadriceps can resist a possible knee flexion response created by the taut hamstrings, which may reduce the effectiveness of the stretch.

Consider a second example involving a similar strategy for augmenting the self-stretch of the *rectus femoris* muscle. Figure 12-53, *A* shows a woman positioned to stretch her rectus femoris muscle by maintaining the combined position of hip extension and knee flexion. The increased passive tension in the stretched biarticular rectus femoris rotates the pelvis anteriorly, thus increasing the anterior pelvic tilt and lumbar lordosis. As depicted in Figure 12-53, *B*, active contraction of the subject's abdominal muscles and gluteus maximus (among other hip extensors) can be used to stretch all hip flexor muscles, including the rectus femoris. Both of these activated muscles are antagonists to the rectus femoris because of their ability to perform *pelvic-on-femoral (hip) extension* by rotating the pelvis posteriorly relative to the fixed femurs. This posterior pelvic tilt would also assist in stretching much of the capsule of the hip, especially regions near the iliofemoral ligament.

The two aforementioned examples demonstrate methods of stretching polyarticular muscles of the hip. In each case the standard stretching procedure was augmented by a volitional contraction of a muscle group considered antagonistic to the tight muscle. This therapeutic approach requires a sound understanding of how multiple muscles can affect the hip, either directly or indirectly. Whether activation of these antagonist muscles in the manner described produces greater and prolonged flexibility in tightened biarticular hip muscle as compared with a standard passive stretch is an interesting area of research.[177] Through "reciprocal inhibition," perhaps a strong contraction of an antagonist muscle can inhibit the resistance in the tightened muscle. A more certain benefit of this therapeutic approach is that the patient or client is more actively involved in the treatment, which may enhance his or her ability to learn and thereby better control the biomechanics of this region of the body.

Additional Clinical Connections

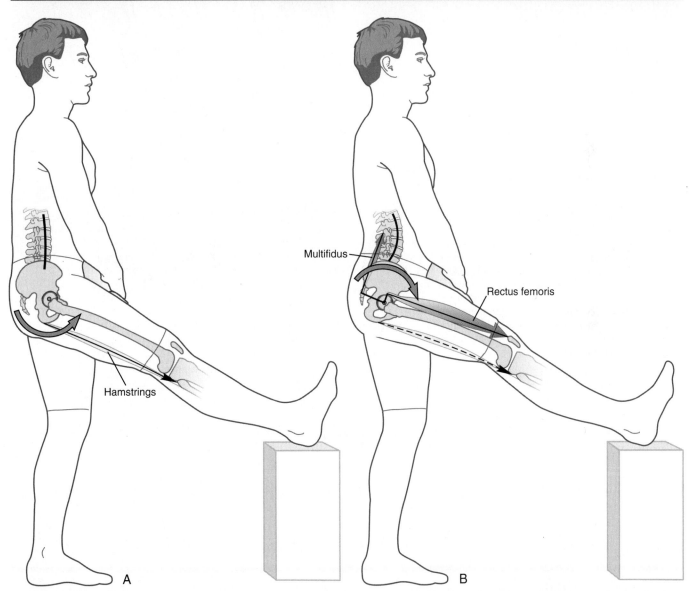

Multifidus

Rectus femoris

Hamstrings

A   B

FIGURE 12-52. Method for augmenting the stretch of the biarticular hamstring muscles. **A,** The traditional starting position for stretching hamstring muscles combines hip flexion and knee extension. The green counterclockwise arrow depicts the passive, posterior pelvic tilt caused by the tension in the stretched hamstrings. **B,** Active contraction of the multifidus and rectus femoris creates an anterior tilt of the pelvis *(green clockwise arrow),* increasing the elongation and subsequent stretch within the hamstring muscles *(dashed arrow).* The moment arms of the activated muscles are shown as black lines, originating at the axis of rotation of the hip (small green circle at the femoral head).

Continued

ADDITIONAL CLINICAL CONNECTIONS

CLINICAL CONNECTION 12-2
Augmenting the Therapeutic Stretch of Selected Biarticular Muscles of the Hip—cont'd

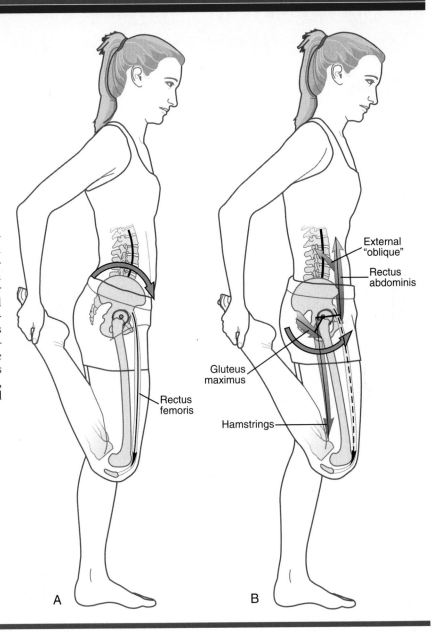

FIGURE 12-53. Method for augmenting the self-stretch of the rectus femoris muscle. **A,** A position typically used to stretch the rectus femoris combines hip extension with knee flexion. The green clockwise arrow depicts the passive, anterior pelvic tilt caused by the tension in the stretched rectus femoris. **B,** Active contraction of representative hip extensors and abdominal muscles causes a posterior tilt of the pelvis *(green counterclockwise arrow),* increasing the stretch within the rectus femoris *(dashed arrow).* The moment arms of the activated muscles are shown as black lines, originating at the axis of rotation of the hip (small green circle at the femoral head).

External "oblique"

Rectus abdominis

Gluteus maximus

Hamstrings

Rectus femoris

A   B

ADDITIONAL CLINICAL CONNECTIONS

CLINICAL CONNECTION 12-3
Injury or Degeneration of the Acetabular Labrum

Essentially any movement between the trunk and pelvis and the femur will produce some compressive, tensile, or shearing force against the acetabular labrum. The labrum therefore is particularly vulnerable to mechanical-based pathology. Clinical awareness of this pathology has increased in recent years as a result of the technical advances in arthroscopic surgery and imaging techniques such as magnetic resonance arthrography (Figure 12-54).[46]

The mechanism of injuring the acetabular labrum varies considerably, and injury can occur across all age groups. In the aged hip, degeneration of the labrum is a very common finding and often is asymptomatic.[93] This suggests that labral degeneration may be associated with natural wear of the hip. A less frequent but more isolated injury of the labrum occurs in young or middle-aged, active persons, often after repetitive or extreme motions of the hip.[96,107,109] This type of injury typically involves a tear along the anterior quadrant of the acetabulum—at the junction of the articular cartilage and labrum. Mechanical symptoms most often include a clicking, "catching," or buckling sensation.[109] Pain is typically reported over the region of the anterior groin. Suspicion of a labral injury increases when these symptoms are associated with activities such as soccer, golf, karate, long-distance running, ballet, or baseball.[118]

Other mechanisms of labral injury include significant trauma, such as that associated with a hip dislocation, falling, or a motor vehicle accident. Often, however, the onset of painful symptoms from a torn labrum is insidious and not related to a specific event. Unfortunately, labral tears may be difficult to diagnose and, unless observed arthroscopically, may evade detection for many years.[20] Arthroscopic treatment of isolated labral tears usually involves debridement of the torn region.[110]

A torn or otherwise degenerated labrum theoretically results in decreased joint stability, greater joint stress, and reduced articular congruence—factors often associated with the development or exacerbation of hip degeneration.[109,111] This assertion is strengthened by data published on the arthroscopic observation of 456 patients suspected of labral tears, with a mean age of 38 years. McCarthy and colleagues found that, overall, 73% of the patients with lesions of their labrum also had chondral (cartilage) lesions within the acetabulum; most of which were located anteriorly, in the same region as the labral tear.[111] Furthermore, chondral lesions were found in only 6% of the patients who did *not* have a labral tear. The presence of degenerative lesions involving both the labrum and articular cartilage strongly suggests an environment of damaging mechanical stress. Individuals at risk for developing these intra-arthritic lesions often have a history of acute trauma, repetitive microtrauma, or structural malformations (dysplasia) of the acetabulum or proximal femur.[139] Whether the dysplasia is mild or severe, structural malformations that affect the joint alter the fit and clearance between the femoral head and acetabulum, ultimately increasing stress on intra-articular structures, especially the acetabular labrum.[11,27] Examples of these structural malformations are described in the following paragraphs.

The normal skeletal configuration of the hip usually minimizes excessive contact between the proximal end of the femur and the rim of the acetabulum. Relatively slight deviations in the bones' morphology, however, can compromise the dynamic clearance between these two regions. Cyclic and continued abutment of the proximal femur against the acetabular rim (or vice versa) can damage the relatively delicate acetabular labrum—a condition often described as *femoral-acetabular impingement.*[27,178] This usually painful condition tends to occur more frequently in active young or middle-aged persons, especially those who regularly engage in full hip flexion activities.[14] Research strongly suggests that labral damage from this impairment may be an early sign of a more progressive degenerative process, often culminating in hip osteoarthritis.[11,93,139]

The bony anomalies that predispose to femoral-acetabular impingement may have occurred secondary to trauma but more

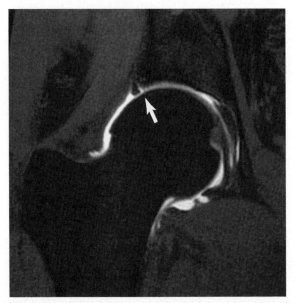

FIGURE 12-54. Frontal plane (T1 fat-saturated) magnetic resonance (MR) arthrogram showing a torn acetabular labrum *(arrow)*. The MR arthrogram involves an intra-articular injection of gadolinium contrast. The labral tear was confirmed and excised during arthroscopic surgery. (Courtesy of Michael O'Brien MD, Musculoskeletal Radiology Fellow, University of Wisconsin.)

Continued

ADDITIONAL CLINICAL CONNECTIONS

CLINICAL CONNECTION 12-3
Injury or Degeneration of the Acetabular Labrum—cont'd

often are related to a relatively mild and previously undetected hip dysplasia.[94,173] The most common anomaly involving the proximal femur is an enlarged and slightly distorted femoral head, coupled with a *reduced "femoral head-neck offset."*[75,130] (Here, *offset* refers to the normal constriction or tapering of the femoral head at its junction with the femoral neck.) Without this normal offset, a thicker, nonspherical femoral head compresses against the acetabular labrum during extreme flexion. This mechanism has been referred to as *cam impingement.*[11]

Acetabular dysplasia may also contribute to femoral-acetabular impingement. An acetabulum that is unusually deep *(acetabular profunda),* or excessively *retroverted* may abnormally surround and embrace the head and part of the neck of the femur.[81,155,173] Extreme flexion in this case can cause the anterior side of the femoral head and neck to abut against the anterior acetabular rim and labrum. This potentially damaging situation is often referred to as *pincer impingement,* reflecting the manner of the abnormal contact between the acetabular labrum and the proximal femur.[11]

Both cam and pincer impingement are usually more pronounced when excessive hip flexion is combined with internal rotation and adduction.[107] Over many cycles of compression, the mechanically fatigued labrum may become torn and fragmented and may partially ossify.[27] Labral pathology secondary to femoral-acetabular impingement occurs most often in the anterior-superior quadrant of the acetabulum and is frequently associated with fragmentation of the adjacent articular cartilage.[94] The damaged labrum may further reduce the stability and congruity of the articulation—factors that often predispose the hip to osteoarthritis.[49,165]

Conservative treatment of femoral-acetabular impingement may involve using nonsteroidal anti-inflammatory drugs and modifying the activities that create the impingement. This may include reducing extreme hip flexion movements or minimizing activities that cause excessive compression forces on the anterior side of the joint.[40,95] Surgical intervention often involves debridement of the fragmented labrum, as well as procedures to realign the malformed bones.[88,155]

ADDITIONAL CLINICAL CONNECTIONS

CLINICAL CONNECTION 12-4
Developmental Dysplasia of the Hip: Often an Evolving Pathology

Developmental dysplasia of the hip (DDH) is one of the most common orthopedic disorders to affect the hip, often manifesting at birth or within the first few years of life. The condition involves a continuum of disorders associated primarily with the abnormal structural development and growth (i.e., *dysplasia*) of the bones that constitute the hip. Because the hip naturally continues to develop after birth and throughout childhood, a specific diagnosis and prognosis of DDH is not always made in the newborn child. The presence of a dislocated or subluxed hip in the neonate is a classic sign of DDH.

Most symptoms associated with mild DDH in an otherwise healthy child spontaneously resolve without treatment.[171] Unfortunately, it is not always possible to predict at an early age which child's symptoms will resolve and which will not. Those whose symptoms continue or worsen often present an evolving clinical picture that can persist until late adolescence. Although relatively rare, these symptoms may lead to permanent physical impairments in the younger adult if not properly treated. Ideally, DDH is diagnosed at birth by physical examination and, when appropriate, imaging techniques such as ultrasonography.[138] In very mild or subclinical cases, however, a diagnosis is often not made or is made later when the patient is an adolescent or adult—typically because of symptoms related to the premature development of hip osteoarthritis.

The underlying and constant feature of DDH is an abnormally formed, poorly articulated hip joint. Although most attention is given to the abnormally developed acetabulum (and subsequent short and shallow acetabular "roof" over the femoral head), the femur is frequently malformed, exhibiting a slightly flattened head, excessive anteversion, or coxa varus or valgus.

Although the cause of DDH is not completely understood, genetic predisposition and the local forces affecting the developing hip are likely important factors.[171] Furthermore, the natural course of fetal development of the human hip may indirectly predispose to this condition. In the 12-week-old fetus the developing femoral head is completely covered and secured within the developing acetabulum. The percentage of coverage, however, naturally *diminishes* until birth and then gradually begins to increase with normal postnatal development.[146] In the perinatal period, therefore, the hip is potentially unstable, consisting of a shallow and relatively flat acetabulum and a partially exposed femoral head—both of which are composed chiefly of soft cartilage. Subsequent normal growth and development of the hip are strongly influenced by the contact forces made by a well-centered femoral head. Such contact helps mold the concavity of the pliable acetabulum to the spherical shape of the femoral head and vice versa, eventually facilitating the formation of a normal and stable joint. The hip that forms abnormally is typically unstable and prone to recurrent dislocation and chronic subluxation, situations that interfere with the natural molding process of the joint.

Abnormally applied forces to the hip at the very plastic and vulnerable perinatal phase of development can directly affect the ultimate morphology of the joint. The sources of some of these potentially deforming forces are further described in the following paragraphs.

EXCESSIVE JOINT LAXITY: Excessive laxity in the capsule and ligaments of the hip can lead to increased shear force between the joint surfaces. In cases of severe laxity the unstable hip demonstrates increased translation and joint "play," often resulting in a greater risk of dislocation and subluxation. An abnormally aligned or dislocated hip lacks the normal kinetic stimulus to guide its growth and development.[171]

Increased laxity in the child's connective tissues is often associated with genetic predisposition. The increased laxity may also be caused by an exaggerated response to the maternal hormone relaxin, normally intended to induce pelvic laxity in the mother during childbirth. Females are more responsive to the effects of relaxin, which may partially explain the higher incidence of DDH in female infants.[59]

ABNORMAL INTRAUTERINE POSITIONING: Abnormal positioning of the fetus within the uterus may place abnormal forces on the developing hip. This relationship is suggested by the fact that DDH occurs with increased frequency in children born by breech delivery, especially when both knees are extended.[59] Furthermore, children with DDH have a slightly higher incidence of other structural abnormalities thought to be associated with abnormal prenatal positioning, such as torticollis[69] (see Chapter 10) or foot deformities (such as metatarsus adductus or forefoot varus [see Chapter 14]).

POSTNATAL POSITIONING: Postnatal positioning may also have some influence on the structural development of the infant's hip. Some evidence of this relationship exists in cultures in which infants are traditionally swaddled in a manner that maintains the hips in full extension.[24] Such a chronically extended position in the young infant may create abnormal stress on hips that are normally flexed in the "fetal position." Cultures in which infants are routinely swaddled with hips *flexed and abducted* have shown a reduced frequency of DDH.

ABNORMAL NEUROMUSCULAR DEVELOPMENT:
Children with pathology involving the neuromuscular system have a higher than normal incidence of DDH. This association exists, for example, in children with cerebral palsy and may be explained by abnormal muscle tone, retained primitive reflexes, and lack of normal weight-bearing activities.[16] Figure 12-55 shows significant hip dysplasia in an adolescent female with severe cerebral palsy.

Continued

ADDITIONAL CLINICAL CONNECTIONS

CLINICAL CONNECTION 12-4
Developmental Dysplasia of the Hip: Often an Evolving Pathology—cont'd

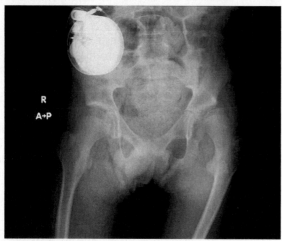

FIGURE 12-55. Pelvic radiograph of a dysplastic and subluxed left hip of an adolescent girl with severe cerebral palsy. The subject is nonambulatory. (Courtesy Jeffrey P. Schwab, MD, Department of Orthopaedic Surgery, Medical College of Wisconsin.)

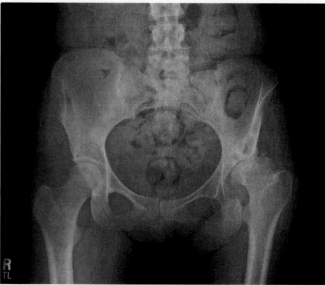

FIGURE 12-56. Pelvic radiograph showing degenerative arthritis of the left hip in a 38-year-old woman, secondary to the residual effects of hip dysplasia as an infant. Note the laterally displaced and flattened femoral head, and inadequate coverage provided by the acetabulum. The patient's left leg is also approximately 3.8 cm shorter than the right. The patient went on to have left total hip arthroplasty. The right hip is normal and asymptomatic. (Courtesy Michael O'Brien MD, Musculoskeletal Radiology Fellow, University of Wisconsin.)

Persisting or severe cases of untreated DDH can create significant functional problems in the maturing child, especially related to walking. If the hip joint is unstable, the femoral head may "drift" superiorly and posterior-laterally from the acetabulum. The dislocated or subluxed joint typically creates an unstable fulcrum for the actions of muscles, especially the hip abductor group. Pelvic stability is lost during the mid-stance phase of walking, causing the characteristic compensated Trendelenburg gait pattern.

The specific treatment for DDH depends on the age of the patient, his or her functional limitations, and the natural progression of the disease. In the very young child, splinting the hip in flexion and abduction using a Pavlik harness is often performed in an attempt to "seat" the femoral head more directly into the acetabulum.[117,172] Over time, this position may stimulate the for-

mation of a more normal formed acetabulum. Surgical realignment of the pelvis and/or the proximal femur may be required to improve stability and increase the surface area for weight bearing.[87] An underlying goal of both surgical and nonsurgical treatment is to restore a stable articulation and facilitate optimum growth and development of the joint. Residual bony abnormalities associated with untreated or undetected DDH are a leading cause of premature hip osteoarthritis later in life[55,171,172] (Figure 12-56), often necessitating a total hip replacement.[32,129]

REFERENCES

1. Ajemian S, Thon D, Clare P, et al: Cane-assisted gait biomechanics and electromyography after total hip arthroplasty, *Arch Phys Med Rehabil* 85:1966-1971, 2004.
2. Altman R, Alarcón G, Appelrouth D, et al: The American College of Rheumatology criteria for the classification and reporting of osteoarthritis of the hip, *Arthritis Rheum* 34:505-514, 1991.
3. Altman RD, Bloch DA, Dougados M, et al: Measurement of structural progression in osteoarthritis of the hip: the Barcelona consensus group, *Osteoarthritis Cartilage* 12:515-524, 2004.
4. Anda S, Svenningsen S, Dale LG, Benum P: The acetabular sector angle of the adult hip determined by computed tomography, *Acta Radiol Diagn (Stockh)* 27:443-447, 1986.
5. Andersson E, Oddsson L, Grundström H, Thorstensson A: The role of the psoas and iliacus muscles for stability and movement of the lumbar spine, pelvis and hip, *Scand J Med Sci Sports* 5:10-16, 1995.
6. Arnold AS, Anderson FC, Pandy MG, Delp SL: Muscular contributions to hip and knee extension during the single limb stance phase of normal gait: a framework for investigating the causes of crouch gait, *J Biomech* 38:2181-2189, 2005.
7. Arnold AS, Asakawa DJ, Delp SL: Do the hamstrings and adductors contribute to excessive internal rotation of the hip in persons with cerebral palsy? *Gait Posture* 11:181-190, 2000.
8. Arnold AS, Delp SL: Rotational moment arms of the medial hamstrings and adductors vary with femoral geometry and limb position: implications for the treatment of internally rotated gait, *J Biomech* 34:437-447, 2001.
9. Arnold AS, Komattu AV, Delp SL: Internal rotation gait: a compensatory mechanism to restore abduction capacity decreased by bone deformity, *Dev Med Child Neurol* 39:40-44, 1997.
10. Arokoski MH, Arokoski JP, Haara M, et al: Hip muscle strength and muscle cross sectional area in men with and without hip osteoarthritis, *J Rheumatol* 29:2187-2195, 2002.
11. Beck M, Kalhor M, Leunig M, Ganz R: Hip morphology influences the pattern of damage to the acetabular cartilage: femoroacetabular impingement as a cause of early osteoarthritis of the hip, *J Bone Joint Surg Br* 87:1012-1018, 2005.
12. Bergmann G, Graichen F, Rohlmann A: Hip joint loading during walking and running, measured in two patients, *J Biomech* 26:969-990, 1993.
13. Bergmann G, Graichen F, Rohlmann A, Linke H: Hip joint forces during load carrying, *Clin Orthop Relat Res* 335:190-201, 1997.
14. Bizzini M, Notzli HP, Maffiuletti NA: Femoroacetabular impingement in professional ice hockey players: a case series of 5 athletes after open surgical decompression of the hip, *Am J Sports Med* 35:1955-1959, 2007.
15. Blemker SS, Delp SL: Three-dimensional representation of complex muscle architectures and geometries, *Ann Biomed Eng* 33:661-673, 2005.
16. Bobroff ED, Chambers HG, Sartoris DJ, et al: Femoral anteversion and neck-shaft angle in children with cerebral palsy, *Clin Orthop Relat Res* 364:194-204, 1999.
17. Boone DC, Azen SP: Normal range of motion of joints in male subjects, *J Bone Joint Surg Am* 61:756-759, 1979.
18. Bordini B, Stea S, De CM, et al: Factors affecting aseptic loosening of 4750 total hip arthroplasties: multivariate survival analysis, *BMC Musculoskelet Disord* 8:69, 2007.
19. Broadhurst NA, Simmons DN, Bond MJ: Piriformis syndrome: correlation of muscle morphology with symptoms and signs, *Arch Phys Med Rehabil* 85:2036-2039, 2004.
20. Burnett RS, la Rocca GJ, Prather H, et al: Clinical presentation of patients with tears of the acetabular labrum, *J Bone Joint Surg Am* 88:1448-1457, 2006.
21. Cahalan TD, Johnson ME, Liu S, Chao EY: Quantitative measurements of hip strength in different age groups, *Clin Orthop Relat Res* 246:136-145, 1989.
22. Carey TS, Crompton RH: The metabolic costs of "bent-hip, bent-knee" walking in humans, *J Hum Evol* 48:25-44, 2005.
23. Clark JM, Haynor DR: Anatomy of the abductor muscles of the hip as studied by computed tomography, *J Bone Joint Surg Am* 69:1021-1031, 1987.
24. Coleman SS: Congenital dysplasia of the hip in the Navajo infant, *Clin Orthop Relat Res* 56:179-193, 1968.
25. Congdon R, Bohannon R, Tiberio D: Intrinsic and imposed hamstring length influence posterior pelvic rotation during hip flexion, *Clin Biomech (Bristol, Avon)* 20:947-951, 2005.
26. Cooperman DR, Wallensten R, Stulberg SD: Acetabular dysplasia in the adult, *Clin Orthop Relat Res* 175:79-85, 1983.
27. Crawford JR, Villar RN: Current concepts in the management of femoroacetabular impingement, *J Bone Joint Surg Br* 87:1459-1462, 2005.
28. Crock HV: An atlas of the arterial supply of the head and neck of the femur in man, *Clin Orthop Relat Res* 152:17-27, 1980.
29. Cuckler JM: The rationale for metal-on-metal total hip arthroplasty, *Clin Orthop Relat Res* 441:132-136, 2005.
30. Cummings SR, Nevitt MC: A hypothesis: the causes of hip fractures, *J Gerontol* 44:M107-M111, 1989.
31. Dalstra M, Huiskes R: Load transfer across the pelvic bone, *J Biomech* 28:715-724, 1995.
32. de Jong PT, Haverkamp D, van der Vis HM, Marti RK, et al: Total hip replacement with a superolateral bone graft for osteoarthritis secondary to dysplasia: a long-term follow-up, *J Bone Joint Surg Br* 88:173-178, 2006.
33. Delp SL, Hess WE, Hungerford DS, Jones LC: Variation of rotation moment arms with hip flexion, *J Biomech* 32:493-501, 1999.
34. Dewberry MJ, Bohannon RW, Tiberio D, et al: Pelvic and femoral contributions to bilateral hip flexion by subjects suspended from a bar, *Clin Biomech (Bristol, Avon)* 18:494-499, 2003.
35. Dostal WF, Andrews JG: A three-dimensional biomechanical model of hip musculature, *J Biomech* 14:803-812, 1981.
36. Dostal WF, Soderberg GL, Andrews JG: Actions of hip muscles, *Phys Ther* 66:351-361, 1986.
37. Eastwood EA, Magaziner J, Wang J, et al: Patients with hip fracture: subgroups and their outcomes, *J Am Geriatr Soc* 50:1240-1249, 2002.
38. Eckstein F, von Eisenhart-Rothe R, Landgraf J, et al: Quantitative analysis of incongruity, contact areas and cartilage thickness in the human hip joint, *Acta Anat (Basel)* 158:192-204, 1997.
39. Elders MJ: The increasing impact of arthritis on public health, *J Rheumatol Suppl* 60:6-8, 2000.
40. Enseki KR, Martin RL, Draovitch P, et al: The hip joint: arthroscopic procedures and postoperative rehabilitation, *J Orthop Sports Phys Ther* 36:516-525, 2006.
41. Escalante A, Lichtenstein MJ, Dhanda R, et al: Determinants of hip and knee flexion range: results from the San Antonio Longitudinal Study of Aging, *Arthritis Care Res* 12:8-18, 1999.
42. Esola MA, McClure PW, Fitzgerald GK, Siegler S: Analysis of lumbar spine and hip motion during forward bending in subjects with and without a history of low back pain, *Spine* 21:71-78, 1996.
43. Fabry G, MacEwen GD, Shands AR Jr: Torsion of the femur. A follow-up study in normal and abnormal conditions, *J Bone Joint Surg Am* 55:1726-1738, 1973.
44. Ferguson SJ, Bryant JT, Ganz R: An in vitro investigation of the acetabular labrum seal in hip joint mechanics, *J Biomech* 36:171-178, 2003.
45. Fischer FJ, Houtz SJ: Evaluation of the function of the gluteus maximus muscle. An electromyographic study, *Am J Phys Med* 47:182-191, 1968.
46. Freedman BA, Potter BK, Dinauer PA, et al: Prognostic value of magnetic resonance arthrography for Czerny stage II and III acetabular labral tears, *Arthroscopy* 22:742-747, 2006.
47. Fuss FK, Bacher A: New aspects of the morphology and function of the human hip joint ligaments, *Am J Anat* 192:1-13, 1991.
48. Gajdosik RL, Sandler MM, Marr HL: Influence of knee positions and gender on the Ober test for length of the iliotibial band, *Clin Biomech (Bristol, Avon)* 18:77-79, 2003.
49. Ganz R, Leunig M, Leunig-Ganz K, Harris WH: The etiology of osteoarthritis of the hip: an integrated mechanical concept, *Clin Orthop Relat Res* 466:264-272, 2008.
50. Genda E, Iwasaki N, Li G, et al: Normal hip joint contact pressure distribution in single-leg standing—effect of gender and anatomic parameters, *J Biomech* 34:895-905, 2001.
51. Gullberg B, Johnell O, Kanis JA: World-wide projections for hip fracture, *Osteoporos Int* 7:407-413, 1997.
52. Halbertsma JP, Göeken LN, Hof AL, et al: Extensibility and stiffness of the hamstrings in patients with nonspecific low back pain, *Arch Phys Med Rehabil* 82:232-238, 2001.
53. Hansen L, de Zee M, Rasmussen J, et al: Anatomy and biomechanics of the back muscles in the lumbar spine with reference to biomechanical modeling, *Spine* 31:1888-1899, 2006.
54. Hardcastle P, Nade S: The significance of the Trendelenburg test, *J Bone Joint Surg Br* 67:741-746, 1985.
55. Harris WH: Etiology of osteoarthritis of the hip, *Clin Orthop Relat Res* 213:20-33, 1986.

56. Hartig DE, Henderson JM: Increasing hamstring flexibility decreases lower extremity overuse injuries in military basic trainees, *Am J Sports Med* 27:173-176, 1999.

57. Heller MO, Bergmann G, Deuretzbacher G, et al: Influence of femoral anteversion on proximal femoral loading: measurement and simulation in four patients, *Clin Biomech (Bristol, Avon)* 16:644-649, 2001.

58. Helm CS, Greenwald AS: The rationale and performance of modularity in total hip arthroplasty, *Orthopedics* 28:S1113-S1115, 2005.

59. Herring JA: *Tachdjian's pediatric orthopaedics*, Vol 1, Philadelphia, 2002, Saunders.

60. Herring JA: *Tachdjian's pediatric orthopaedics*, Vol 3, Philadelphia, 2002, Saunders.

61. Hewitt JD, Glisson RR, Guilak F, Vail TP: The mechanical properties of the human hip capsule ligaments, *J Arthroplasty* 17:82-89, 2002.

62. Hicks JL, Schwartz MH, Arnold AS, Delp SL: Crouched postures reduce the capacity of muscles to extend the hip and knee during the single-limb stance phase of gait, *J Biomech* 41:960-967, 2008.

63. Hoaglund FT, Steinbach LS: Primary osteoarthritis of the hip: etiology and epidemiology, *J Am Acad Orthop Surg* 9:320-327, 2001.

64. Hodge WA, Carlson KL, Fijan RS, et al: Contact pressures from an instrumented hip endoprosthesis, *J Bone Joint Surg Am* 71:1378-1386, 1989.

65. Hodges PW, Richardson CA: Contraction of the abdominal muscles associated with movement of the lower limb, *Phys Ther* 77:132-142, 1997.

66. Hoeksma HL, Dekker J, Ronday HK, et al: Comparison of manual therapy and exercise therapy in osteoarthritis of the hip: a randomized clinical trial, *Arthritis Rheum* 51:722-729, 2004.

67. Hoy MG, Zajac FE, Gordon ME: A musculoskeletal model of the human lower extremity: the effect of muscle, tendon, and moment arm on the moment-angle relationship of musculotendon actuators at the hip, knee, and ankle, *J Biomech* 23:157-169, 1990.

68. Huddleston JM, Whitford KJ: Medical care of elderly patients with hip fractures, *Mayo Clin Proc* 76:295-298, 2001.

69. Hummer CD, MacEwen GD: The coexistence of torticollis and congenital dysplasia of the hip, *J Bone Joint Surg Am* 54:1255-1256, 1972.

70. Huo MH, Parvizi J, Bal BS, et al: What's new in total hip arthroplasty, *J Bone Joint Surg Am* 90:2043-2055, 2008.

71. Hurwitz DE, Foucher KC, Andriacchi TP: A new parametric approach for modeling hip forces during gait, *J Biomech* 36:113-119, 2003.

72. Inman VT: Functional aspects of the abductor muscles of the hip, *J Bone Joint Surg Am* 29:607-619, 1947.

73. Inman VT, Ralston HJ, Todd F: *Human walking*, Baltimore, 1981, Williams & Wilkins.

74. Inman VT, Saunders JB: Referred pain from skeletal structures, *J Nerv Ment Dis* 99:660-667, 1944.

75. Ito K, Minka MA 2nd, Leunig M, et al: Femoroacetabular impingement and the cam-effect. A MRI-based quantitative anatomical study of the femoral head-neck offset, *J Bone Joint Surg Br* 83:171-176, 2001.

76. Jette AM, Delitto A: Physical therapy treatment choices for musculoskeletal impairments, *Phys Ther* 77:145-154, 1997.

77. Johnston RC, Smidt GL: Hip motion measurements for selected activities of daily living, *Clin Orthop Relat Res* 72:205-215, 1970.

78. Keagy RD, Brumlik J, Bergan JL: Direct electromyography of the psoas major muscle in man, *J Bone Joint Surg Am* 48:1377-1382, 1966.

79. Kelsey JL: The epidemiology of diseases of the hip: a review of the literature, *Int J Epidemiol* 6:269-280, 1977.

80. Kendall FP, McCreary AK, Provance PG: *Muscles: testing and function*, ed 4, Baltimore, 1993, Williams & Wilkins.

81. Kim WY, Hutchinson CE, Andrew JG, Allen PD: The relationship between acetabular retroversion and osteoarthritis of the hip, *J Bone Joint Surg Br* 88:727-729, 2006.

82. Kim YT, Azuma H: The nerve endings of the acetabular labrum, *Clin Orthop Relat Res* 320:176-181, 1995.

83. Kinov P, Leithner A, Radl R, et al: Role of free radicals in aseptic loosening of hip arthroplasty, *J Orthop Res* 24:55-62, 2006.

84. Krebs DE, Elbaum L, Riley PO, et al: Exercise and gait effects on in vivo hip contact pressures, *Phys Ther* 71:301-309, 1991.

85. Kumagai M, Shiba N, Higuchi F, et al: Functional evaluation of hip abductor muscles with use of magnetic resonance imaging, *J Orthop Res* 15:888-893, 1997.

86. Kurrat HJ, Oberlander W: The thickness of the cartilage in the hip joint, *J Anat* 126:145-155, 1978.

87. Lalonde FD, Frick SL, Wenger DR: Surgical correction of residual hip dysplasia in two pediatric age-groups, *J Bone Joint Surg Am* 84:1148-1156, 2002.

88. Lavigne M, Parvizi J, Beck M, et al: Anterior femoroacetabular impingement: part I. Techniques of joint preserving surgery, *Clin Orthop Relat Res* 418:61-66, 2004.

89. Leadbetter RE, Mawer D, Lindow SW: Symphysis pubis dysfunction: a review of the literature, *J Matern Fetal Neonatal Med* 16:349-354, 2004.

90. Lee RY, Wong TK: Relationship between the movements of the lumbar spine and hip, *Hum Mov Sci* 21:481-494, 2002.

91. Lengsfeld M, Pressel T, Stammberger U: Lengths and lever arms of hip joint muscles: geometrical analyses using a human multibody model, *Gait Posture* 6:18-26, 1997.

92. Lennon AB, Britton JR, MacNiocaill RF, et al: Predicting revision risk for aseptic loosening of femoral components in total hip arthroplasty in individual patients—a finite element study, *J Orthop Res* 25:779-788, 2007.

93. Leunig M, Beck M, Woo A, et al: Acetabular rim degeneration: a constant finding in the aged hip, *Clin Orthop Relat Res* 413:201-207, 2003.

94. Leunig M, Podeszwa D, Beck M, et al: Magnetic resonance arthrography of labral disorders in hips with dysplasia and impingement, *Clin Orthop Relat Res* 418:74-80, 2004.

95. Lewis CL, Sahrmann SA: Acetabular labral tears, *Phys Ther* 86:110-121, 2006.

96. Lewis CL, Sahrmann SA, Moran DW: Anterior hip joint force increases with hip extension, decreased gluteal force, or decreased iliopsoas force, *J Biomech* 40:3725-3731, 2007.

97. Li Y, McClure PW, Pratt N: The effect of hamstring muscle stretching on standing posture and on lumbar and hip motions during forward bending, *Phys Ther* 76:836-845, 1996.

98. Lievense AM, Bierma-Zeinstra SM, Verhagen AP, et al: Influence of sporting activities on the development of osteoarthritis of the hip: a systematic review, *Arthritis Rheum* 49:228-236, 2003.

99. Lindsay DM, Maitland ME, Lowe RC: Comparison of isokinetic internal and external hip rotation torques using different testing positions, *J Orthop Sports Phys Ther* 16:43-50, 1992.

100. Loder RT, Aronsson DD, Dobbs MB, et al: Slipped capital femoral epiphysis, *Instr Course Lect* 50:555-570, 2001.

101. Löhe F, Eckstein F, Sauer T, Putz R: Structure, strain and function of the transverse acetabular ligament, *Acta Anat (Basel)* 157:315-323, 1996.

102. Lohmander LS: Articular cartilage and osteoarthrosis. The role of molecular markers to monitor breakdown, repair and disease, *J Anat* 184:477-492, 1994.

103. MacDonald CW, Whitman JM, Cleland JA, et al: Clinical outcomes following manual physical therapy and exercise for hip osteoarthritis: a case series, *J Orthop Sports Phys Ther* 36:588-599, 2006.

104. Mansour JM, Pereira JM: Quantitative functional anatomy of the lower limb with application to human gait, *J Biomech* 20:51-58, 1987.

105. Markhede G, Stener B: Function after removal of various hip and thigh muscles for extirpation of tumors, *Acta Orthop Scand* 52:373-395, 1981.

106. Martin HD, Savage A, Braly BA, et al: The function of the hip capsular ligaments: a quantitative report, *Arthroscopy* 24:188-195, 2008.

107. Martin RL, Enseki KR, Draovitch P, et al: Acetabular labral tears of the hip: examination and diagnostic challenges, *J Orthop Sports Phys Ther* 36:503-515, 2006.

108. Mavcic B, Pompe B, Antolic V, et al: Mathematical estimation of stress distribution in normal and dysplastic human hips, *J Orthop Res* 20:1025-1030, 2002.

109. McCarthy J, Noble P, Aluisio FV, et al: Anatomy, pathologic features, and treatment of acetabular labral tears, *Clin Orthop Relat Res* 406:38-47, 2003.

110. McCarthy JC: The diagnosis and treatment of labral and chondral injuries, *Instr Course Lect* 53:573-577, 2004.

111. McCarthy JC, Noble PC, Schuck MR, et al: The Otto E. Aufranc Award: the role of labral lesions to development of early degenerative hip disease, *Clin Orthop Relat Res* 393:25-37, 2001.

112. McGibbon CA, Krebs DE, Mann RW: In vivo hip pressures during cane and load-carrying gait, *Arthritis Care Res* 10:300-307, 1997.

113. Mehmood S, Jinnah RH, Pandit H: Review on ceramic-on-ceramic total hip arthroplasty, *J Surg Orthop Adv* 17:45-50, 2008.

114. Montin L, Leino-Kilpi H, Suominen T, Lepistö J: A systematic review of empirical studies between 1966 and 2005 of patient outcomes of total hip arthroplasty and related factors, *J Clin Nurs* 17:40-45, 2008.

115. Moore KL, Persaud TVN: *The developing human: clinically oriented embryology*, ed 7, St Louis, 2003, Elsevier.

116. Münger P, Röder C, Ackermann-Liebrich U, Busato A: Patient-related risk factors leading to aseptic stem loosening in total hip arthroplasty: a case-control study of 5,035 patients, *Acta Orthop* 77:567-574, 2006.

117. Nakamura J, Kamegaya M, Saisu T, et al: Treatment for developmental dysplasia of the hip using the Pavlik harness: long-term results, *J Bone Joint Surg Br* 89:230-235, 2007.

118. Narvani AA, Tsiridis E, Tai CC, Thomas P: Acetabular labrum and its tears, *Br J Sports Med* 37:207-211, 2003.

119. Nemeth G, Ohlsen H: Moment arms of the hip abductor and adductor muscles measured in vivo by computed tomography, *Clin Biomech (Bristol, Avon)* 4:133-136, 1989.

120. Neumann DA: Hip abductor muscle activity as subjects with hip prostheses walk with different methods of using a cane, *Phys Ther* 78:490-501, 1998.

121. Neumann DA: Hip abductor muscle activity in persons with a hip prosthesis while carrying loads in one hand, *Phys Ther* 76:1320-1330, 1996.

122. Neumann DA: An electromyographic study of the hip abductor muscles as subjects with a hip prosthesis walked with different methods of using a cane and carrying a load, *Phys Ther* 79:1163-1173, 1999.

123. Neumann DA: Biomechanical analysis of selected principles of hip joint protection, *Arthritis Care Res* 2:146-155, 1989.

124. Neumann DA, Cook TM: Effect of load and carrying position on the electromyographic activity of the gluteus medius muscle during walking, *Phys Ther* 65:305-311, 1985.

125. Neumann DA, Cook TM, Sholty RL, Sobush DC: An electromyographic analysis of hip abductor muscle activity when subjects are carrying loads in one or both hands, *Phys Ther* 72:207-217, 1992.

126. Neumann DA, Hase AD: An electromyographic analysis of the hip abductors during load carriage: implications for hip joint protection, *J Orthop Sports Phys Ther* 19:296-304, 1994.

127. Neumann DA, Soderberg GL, Cook TM: Comparison of maximal isometric hip abductor muscle torques between hip sides, *Phys Ther* 68:496-502, 1988.

128. Neumann DA, Soderberg GL, Cook TM: Electromyographic analysis of hip abductor musculature in healthy right-handed persons, *Phys Ther* 69:431-440, 1989.

129. Noble PC, Kamaric E, Sugano N, et al: Three-dimensional shape of the dysplastic femur: implications for THR, *Clin Orthop Relat Res* 417:27-40, 2003.

130. Notzli HP, Wyss TF, Stoecklin CH, et al: The contour of the femoral head-neck junction as a predictor for the risk of anterior impingement, *J Bone Joint Surg Br* 84:556-560, 2002.

131. Odding E, Valkenburg HA, Stam HJ, Hofman A: Determinants of locomotor disability in people aged 55 years and over: the Rotterdam Study, *Eur J Epidemiol* 17:1033-1041, 2001.

132. Oguz O: Measurement and relationship of the inclination angle, Alsberg angle and the angle between the anatomical and mechanical axes of the femur in males, *Surg Radiol Anat* 18:29-31, 1996.

133. Ong KL, Kurtz SM, Manley MT, et al: Biomechanics of the Birmingham hip resurfacing arthroplasty, *J Bone Joint Surg Br* 88:1110-1115, 2006.

134. Paksima N, Koval KJ, Aharanoff G, et al: Predictors of mortality after hip fracture: a 10-year prospective study, *Bull NYU Hosp Jt Dis* 66:111-117, 2008.

135. Palombaro KM, Craik RL, Mangione KK, Tomlinson JD: Determining meaningful changes in gait speed after hip fracture, *Phys Ther* 86:809-816, 2006.

136. Pare EB, Stern JT, Jr, Schwartz JM: Functional differentiation within the tensor fasciae latae. A telemetered electromyographic analysis of its locomotor roles, *J Bone Joint Surg Am* 63:1457-1471, 1981.

137. Parkkari J, Kannus P, Palvanen M, et al: Majority of hip fractures occur as a result of a fall and impact on the greater trochanter of the femur: a prospective controlled hip fracture study with 206 consecutive patients, *Calcif Tissue Int* 65:183-187, 1999.

138. Paton RW, Hinduja K, Thomas CD: The significance of at-risk factors in ultrasound surveillance of developmental dysplasia of the hip. A ten-year prospective study, *J Bone Joint Surg Br* 87:1264-1266, 2005.

139. Peelle MW, la Rocca GJ, Maloney WJ, et al: Acetabular and femoral radiographic abnormalities associated with labral tears, *Clin Orthop Relat Res* 441:327-333, 2005.

140. Penrod JD, Litke A, Hawkes WG, et al: The association of race, gender, and comorbidity with mortality and function after hip fracture, *J Gerontol A Biol Sci Med Sci* 63:867-872, 2008.

141. Perron M, Malouin F, Moffet H, McFadyen BJ: Three-dimensional gait analysis in women with a total hip arthroplasty, *Clin Biomech (Bristol, Avon)* 15:504-515, 2000.

142. Petersen W, Petersen F, Tillmann B: Structure and vascularization of the acetabular labrum with regard to the pathogenesis and healing of labral lesions, *Arch Orthop Trauma Surg* 123:283-288, 2003.

143. Peyron JG: Osteoarthritis. The epidemiologic viewpoint, *Clin Orthop Relat Res* 213:13-19, 1986.

144. Pfirrmann CW, Chung CB, Theumann NH, et al: Greater trochanter of the hip: attachment of the abductor mechanism and a complex of three bursae—MR imaging and MR bursography in cadavers and MR imaging in asymptomatic volunteers, *Radiology* 221:469-477, 2001.

145. Pohtilla JF: Kinesiology of hip extension at selected angles of pelvifemoral extension, *Arch Phys Med Rehabil* 50:241-250, 1969.

146. Ralis Z, McKibbin B: Changes in shape of the human hip joint during its development and their relation to its stability, *J Bone Joint Surg Br* 55:780-785, 1973.

147. Recnik G, Kralj-Iglic V, Iglic A, et al: Higher peak contact hip stress predetermines the side of hip involved in idiopathic osteoarthritis, *Clin Biomech (Bristol, Avon)* 22:1119-1124, 2007.

148. Reikeras O, Bjerkreim I, Kolbenstvedt A: Anteversion of the acetabulum and femoral neck in normals and in patients with osteoarthritis of the hip, *Acta Orthop Scand* 54:18-23, 1983.

149. Rethlefsen SA, Healy BS, Wren TA, et al: Causes of intoeing gait in children with cerebral palsy, *J Bone Joint Surg Am* 88:2175-2180, 2006.

150. Roach KE, Miles TP: Normal hip and knee active range of motion: the relationship to age, *Phys Ther* 71:656-665, 1991.

151. Roddy E, Zhang W, Doherty M, et al: Evidence-based recommendations for the role of exercise in the management of osteoarthritis of the hip or knee—the MOVE consensus, *Rheumatology (Oxford)* 44:67-73, 2005.

152. Rozumalski A, Schwartz MH, Wervey R, et al: The in vivo three-dimensional motion of the human lumbar spine during gait, *Gait Posture* 28:378-384, 2008.

153. Rydell N: Biomechanics of the hip-joint, *Clin Orthop Relat Res* 92:6-15, 1973.

154. Santaguida PL, McGill SM: The psoas major muscle: a three-dimensional geometric study, *J Biomech* 28:339-345, 1995.

155. Siebenrock KA, Schoeniger R, Ganz R: Anterior femoro-acetabular impingement due to acetabular retroversion. Treatment with periacetabular osteotomy, *J Bone Joint Surg Am* 85-A:278-286, 2003.

156. Simoneau GG, Hoenig KJ, Lepley JE, Papanek PE: Influence of hip position and gender on active hip internal and external rotation, *J Orthop Sports Phys Ther* 28:158-164, 1998.

157. Skyrme AD, Cahill DJ, Marsh HP, Ellis H: Psoas major and its controversial rotational action, *Clin Anat* 12:264-265, 1999.

158. Snijders CJ, Hermans PF, Kleinrensink GJ: Functional aspects of cross-legged sitting with special attention to piriformis muscles and sacroiliac joints, *Clin Biomech (Bristol, Avon)* 21:116-121, 2006.

159. Soderberg GL, Dostal WF: Electromyographic study of three parts of the gluteus medius muscle during functional activities, *Phys Ther* 58:691-696, 1978.

160. Standring S: *Gray's anatomy: the anatomical basis of clinical practice*, ed 40, St Louis, 2009, Elsevier.

161. Stansfield BW, Nicol AC: Hip joint contact forces in normal subjects and subjects with total hip prostheses: walking and stair and ramp negotiation, *Clin Biomech (Bristol, Avon)* 17:130-139, 2002.

162. Stewart K, Edmonds-Wilson R, Brand R, Brown TD: Spatial distribution of hip capsule structural and material properties, *J Biomech* 35:1491-1498, 2002.

163. Svenningsen S, Apalset K, Terjesen T, Anda S: Regression of femoral anteversion. A prospective study of intoeing children, *Acta Orthop Scand* 60:170-173, 1989.

164. Tan V, Seldes RM, Katz MA, et al: Contribution of acetabular labrum to articulating surface area and femoral head coverage in adult hip joints: an anatomic study in cadavera, *Am J Orthop* 30:809-812, 2001.

165. Tanzer M, Noiseux N: Osseous abnormalities and early osteoarthritis: the role of hip impingement, *Clin Orthop Relat Res* 429:170-177, 2004.

166. Thelen DD, Riewald SA, Asakawa DS, et al: Abnormal coupling of knee and hip moments during maximal exertions in persons with cerebral palsy, *Muscle Nerve* 27:486-493, 2003.

167. Toussaint EM, Kohia M: A critical review of literature regarding the effectiveness of physical therapy management of hip fracture in elderly persons, *J Gerontol A Biol Sci Med Sci* 60:1285-1291, 2005.

168. Walheim GG, Selvik G: Mobility of the pubic symphysis. In vivo measurements with an electromechanic method and a roentgen stereophotogrammetric method, *Clin Orthop Relat Res* 191:129-135, 1984.

169. Walters J, Solomons M, Davies J: Gluteus minimus: observations on its insertion, *J Anat* 198:239-242, 2001.

170. Wehren LE, Magaziner J: Hip fracture: risk factors and outcomes, *Current Osteoporosis Reports* 1:78-85, 2003.

171. Weinstein SL, Mubarak SJ, Wenger DR: Developmental hip dysplasia and dislocation: Part I, *Instr Course Lect* 53:523-530, 2004.

172. Weinstein SL, Mubarak SJ, Wenger DR: Developmental hip dysplasia and dislocation: Part II, *Instr Course Lect* 53:531-542, 2004.

173. Wenger DE, Kendell KR, Miner MR, Trousdale RT: Acetabular labral tears rarely occur in the absence of bony abnormalities, *Clin Orthop Relat Res* 426:145-150, 2004.

174. Wilkins K: Health care consequences of falls for seniors, *Health Rep* 10:47-55, 1999.

175. Wingstrand H, Wingstrand A, Krantz P: Intracapsular and atmospheric pressure in the dynamics and stability of the hip. A biomechanical study, *Acta Orthop Scand* 61:231-235, 1990.

176. Winter DA: *Biomechanics and motor control of human movement*, New Jersey, 2005, John Wiley & Sons.

177. Winters MV, Blake CG, Trost JS, et al: Passive versus active stretching of hip flexor muscles in subjects with limited hip extension: a randomized clinical trial, *Phys Ther* 84:800-807, 2004.

178. Wisniewski SJ, Grogg B: Femoroacetabular impingement: an overlooked cause of hip pain, *Am J Phys Med Rehabil* 85:546-549, 2006.

179. Wolinsky FD, Fitzgerald JF, Stump TE: The effect of hip fracture on mortality, hospitalization, and functional status: a prospective study, *Am J Public Health* 87:398-403, 1997.

180. Woodley SJ, Nicholson HD, Livingstone V, et al: Lateral hip pain: findings from magnetic resonance imaging and clinical examination, *J Orthop Sports Phys Ther* 38:313-328, 2008.

181. Yoshio M, Murakami G, Sato T, et al: The function of the psoas major muscle: passive kinetics and morphological studies using donated cadavers, *J Orthop Sci* 7:199-207, 2002.

STUDY QUESTIONS

1 What structures convert the greater sciatic notch to a foramen? List three structures (nerves or muscles) that pass through this foramen.

2 A patient has excessive anteversion of the femur *and* acetabulum. Which extreme hip motion (in the horizontal plane) would most likely be associated with a spontaneous anterior dislocation?

3 What characteristics define the close-packed position of the hip? How do these characteristics differ from those of most other synovial joints of the body?

4 Explain why a patient with an inflamed capsule of the hip joint may be susceptible to a hip flexion contracture.

5 Describe how the ischiofemoral ligament becomes taut in full internal rotation and extension of the hip. Include both femoral-on-pelvic and pelvic-on-femoral perspectives in your description.

6 While standing, a person performs a full *posterior* pelvic tilt while keeping the trunk essentially stationary. Describe how this movement could indirectly alter the tension in the anterior longitudinal ligament and the ligamentum flavum in the lumbar region.

7 Using a ruler and Figure 12-29 as a reference, which muscle appears to have the greatest moment arm for hip abduction?

8 Based on Figure 12-34, which muscle has (a) the *least* leverage and (b) the *greatest* leverage for producing internal rotation torque?

9 A patient sustained a severe fracture of the femoral head and the acetabulum, with marked reduction in contact area between the articular surfaces of the joint. As part of the reconstructive surgery, the surgeon decides to slightly increase the internal moment arm of the hip abductor muscles. What is the likely rationale for this procedure?

10 Explain how a reduced *center-edge angle* of the acetabulum could favor a dislocation of the hip.

11 Contrast the arthrokinematics of (femoral-on-pelvic) hip flexion and extension with those of internal and external rotation.

12 As indicated in Figure 12-12, during the *swing phase* of walking the hip experiences (compression) forces of about 10% to 20% of body weight. What causes this force?

13 Figure 12-22, *A* shows a seated person performing a 30-degree anterior pelvic tilt. What structure(s) is (are) most likely responsible for determining the end-range of this motion?

14 A person sustained an injury of the cauda equina resulting in reduced function of spinal nerve roots L^3 and below. What pattern of muscular tightness may develop without adequate physical therapy intervention? (Consult Appendix IV, Part A, for assistance in responding to this question.)

15 Justify how bilateral tightness in the adductor longus and brevis could contribute to excessive lumbar lordosis during standing.

Answers to the study questions can be found on the Evolve website.

Knee

DONALD A. NEUMANN, PT, PhD, FAPTA

The knee consists of the lateral and medial compartments of the tibiofemoral joint and the patellofemoral joint (Figure 13-1). Motion at the knee occurs in two planes, allowing flexion and extension, and internal and external rotation. Functionally, however, these movements rarely occur independent of movement at other joints within the lower limb. Consider, for example, the interaction among the hip, knee, and ankle during running, climbing, or standing from a seated position. The strong functional association within the joints of the lower limb is reflected by the fact that about two thirds of the muscles that cross the knee also cross either the hip or the ankle.

The knee has important biomechanical functions, many of which are expressed during walking and running. During the swing phase of walking, the knee flexes to shorten the functional length of the lower limb; otherwise, the foot would not easily clear the ground. During the stance phase, the knee remains slightly flexed, allowing shock absorption, conservation of energy, and transmission of forces through the lower limb. Running requires that the knee move through a greater range of motion than walking, especially in the sagittal plane. In addition, rapidly changing direction during walking or running demands adequate internal and external rotation of the knee.

Stability of the knee is based primarily on its soft-tissue constraints rather than on its bony configuration. The massive femoral condyles articulate with the nearly flat proximal articular surfaces of the tibia, held in place by extensive ligaments, joint capsule and menisci, and large muscles. With the foot firmly in contact with the ground, these soft tissues are often subjected to large forces, from both muscles and external sources. Injuries to ligaments, menisci, and articular cartilage are unfortunately common consequences of the large functional demands placed on the knee. Knowledge of the anatomy and kinesiology of the knee is an essential prerequisite to the understanding of most mechanisms of injury and effective therapeutic intervention.

OSTEOLOGY

Distal Femur

At the distal end of the femur are the large *lateral* and *medial condyles* (from the Greek *kondylos*, knuckle) (Figure 13-2). *Lateral* and *medial epicondyles* project from each condyle, providing elevated attachment sites for the collateral ligaments. A large *intercondylar notch* separates the lateral and medial condyles, forming a passageway for the cruciate ligaments. A

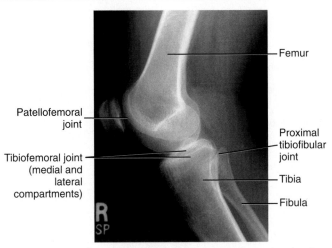

FIGURE 13-1. Radiograph showing the bones and associated articulations of the knee.

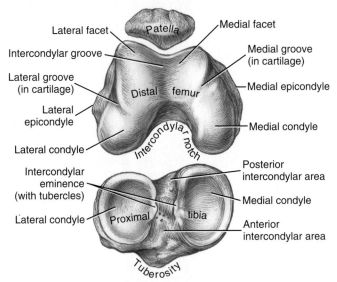

FIGURE 13-2. Osteology of the right patella, articular surfaces of the distal femur, and proximal tibia.

> **Osteologic Features of the Distal Femur**
> - Lateral and medial condyles
> - Lateral and medial epicondyles
> - Intercondylar notch
> - Intercondylar (trochlear) groove
> - Lateral and medial facets (for the patella)
> - Lateral and medial grooves (etched in the cartilage of the femoral condyles)
> - Popliteal surface

The articular capsule of the knee extends across all sides of the tibiofemoral joint and the patellofemoral joint (see dotted lines in Figure 13-3). Posteriorly, the capsule attaches just proximal to the femoral condyles, immediately distal to the *popliteal surface* of the femur.

Proximal Tibia and Fibula

Although the fibula has no direct function at the knee, the slender bone splints the lateral side of the tibia and helps maintain its alignment. The *head* of the fibula serves as an attachment for the biceps femoris and the lateral collateral ligament. The fibula is attached to the lateral side of the tibia by proximal and distal tibiofibular joints (see Figure 13-3). The structure and function of these joints are discussed in Chapter 14.

> **Osteologic Features of the Proximal Tibia and Fibula**
> *Proximal Fibula*
> - Head
>
> *Proximal Tibia*
> - Medial and lateral condyles
> - Intercondylar eminence (with tubercles)
> - Anterior intercondylar area
> - Posterior intercondylar area
> - Tibial tuberosity
> - Soleal line

The primary function of the tibia is to transfer weight across the knee and to the ankle. The proximal end of the tibia flares into *medial* and *lateral condyles,* which form articular surfaces with the distal femur (see Figure 13-3). The superior surfaces of the condyles form a broad region, often referred to as the *tibial plateau.* The plateau supports two smooth articular surfaces that accept the large femoral condyles, forming medial and lateral compartments of the tibiofemoral joint. The larger, medial articular surface is slightly concave, whereas the lateral articular surface is flat to slightly convex. The articular surfaces are separated down the midline by an *intercondylar eminence,* formed by irregularly shaped medial and lateral tubercles (see Figure 13-2). Shallow anterior and posterior *intercondylar areas* flank both ends of the eminence. The cruciate ligaments and menisci attach along the intercondylar region of the tibia.

The prominent *tibial tuberosity* is located on the anterior surface of the proximal shaft of the tibia (see Figure 13-3, *A*). The tibial tuberosity serves as the distal attachment for the quadriceps femoris muscle, via the patellar tendon. On

narrower than average notch may increase the likelihood of injury to the anterior cruciate ligament.[267]

The femoral condyles fuse anteriorly to form the *intercondylar (trochlear) groove* (see Figure 13-2). This groove articulates with the posterior side of the patella, forming the patellofemoral joint. The intercondylar groove is concave from side to side and slightly convex from front to back. The sloping sides of the intercondylar groove form *lateral* and *medial facets.* The more pronounced lateral facet extends more proximally and anteriorly than the medial facet. The steeper slope of the lateral facet helps to stabilize the patella within the groove during knee movement.

Lateral and *medial grooves* are etched faintly in the cartilage that covers much of the articular surface of the femoral condyles (see Figure 13-2). When the knee is fully extended, the anterior edge of the tibia is aligned with these grooves. The position of the grooves highlights the asymmetry in the shape of the medial and lateral articular surfaces of the distal femur. As explained later in this chapter, the asymmetry in the shape of the condyles affects the sagittal plane kinematics.

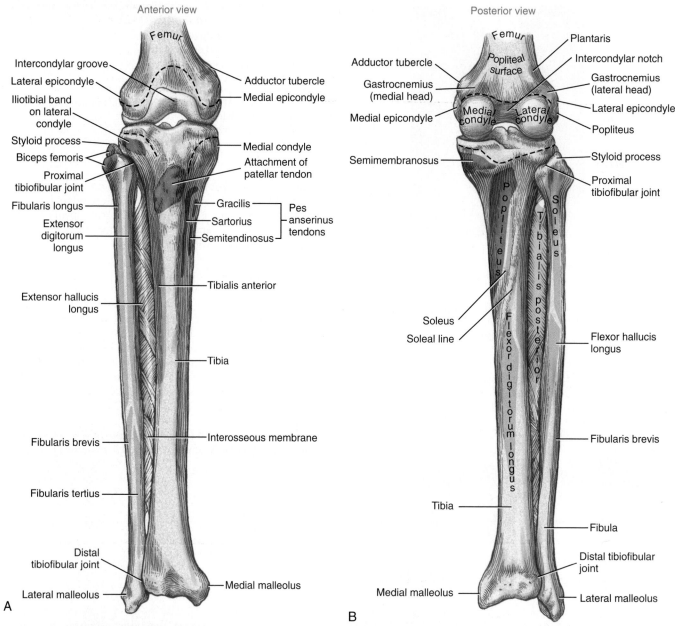

FIGURE 13-3. Right distal femur, tibia, and fibula. **A,** Anterior view. **B,** Posterior view. Proximal attachments of muscles are shown in red, distal attachments in gray. The dashed lines show the attachment of the joint capsule of the knee.

the posterior side of the proximal tibia is a roughened *soleal line,* coursing diagonally in a distal-to-medial direction (see Figure 13-3, *B*).

Patella

The patella (from the Latin, "small plate") is a nearly triangular bone embedded within the quadriceps tendon. It is the largest sesamoid bone in the body. The patella has a curved *base* superiorly and a pointed *apex* inferiorly (Figures 13-4 and 13-5). The thick patellar tendon attaches to and between the apex of the patella and the tibial tuberosity. In a relaxed standing position, the apex of the patella lies just proximal to the knee joint line. The subcutaneous *anterior surface* of the patella is convex in all directions.

The *posterior articular surface* of the patella is covered with articular cartilage up to 4 to 5 mm thick (see Figure 13-5).[65] Part of this surface articulates with the intercondylar groove of the femur, forming the patellofemoral joint. The thick cartilage helps to disperse the large compression forces that cross the joint. A rounded *vertical ridge* runs longitudinally

---

Osteologic Features of the Patella

- Base
- Apex
- Anterior surface
- Posterior articular surface
- Vertical ridge
- Lateral, medial, and "odd" facets

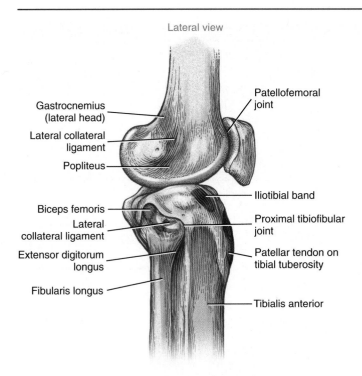

FIGURE 13-4. Lateral view of the right knee. Note the curved articular surface of the lateral femoral condyle. Proximal attachments of muscles and ligaments are shown in red, distal attachments in gray.

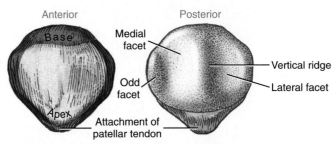

FIGURE 13-5. Anterior and posterior surfaces of the right patella. The attachment of the tendon of the quadriceps muscle is indicated in gray; the proximal attachment of the patellar tendon is indicated in red. Note the smooth articular cartilage covering the posterior articular surface of the patella.

from top to bottom across the posterior surface of the patella. On either side of this ridge is a lateral or a medial facet. The larger and slightly concave *lateral facet* matches the general contour of the lateral facet on the intercondylar groove of the femur (see Figure 13-2). The *medial facet* shows significant anatomic variation. A third *"odd" facet* exists along the extreme medial border of the medial facet.

ARTHROLOGY

General Anatomic and Alignment Considerations

The shaft of the femur angles slightly medially as it descends toward the knee. This oblique orientation is a result of the natural 125-degree angle of inclination of the proximal femur (Figure 13-6, *A*). Because the articular surface of the proximal tibia is oriented nearly horizontally, the knee forms an angle

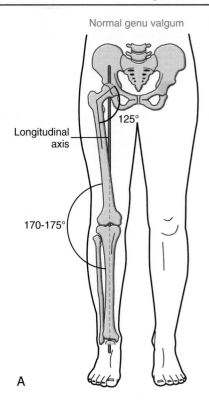

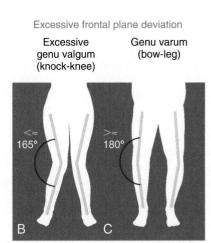

FIGURE 13-6. Frontal plane deviations of the knee. **A,** Normal genu valgum. The normal 125-degree angle of inclination of the proximal femur and the longitudinal axis of rotation throughout the entire lower extremity are also shown. **B** and **C** illustrate excessive frontal plane deviations.

on its lateral side of about 170 to 175 degrees. This normal alignment of the knee within the frontal plane is referred to as *genu valgum.*

Variation in normal frontal plane alignment at the knee is not uncommon. A lateral angle less than 170 degrees is called *excessive genu valgum,* or "knock-knee" (see Figure 13-6, *B*). In contrast, a lateral angle that exceeds about 180 degrees is called *genu varum,* or "bow-leg" (Figure 13-6, *C*).

The longitudinal or vertical axis of rotation at the hip is defined in Chapter 12 as a line connecting the femoral head with the center of the knee joint. As depicted in Figure 13-6, *A,* this longitudinal axis can be extended inferiorly through the knee to the ankle and foot. The axis mechanically links

TABLE 13-1. Ligaments, Fascia, and Muscles That Reinforce the Capsule of the Knee

Region of the Capsule	Connective Tissue Reinforcement	Muscular-Tendinous Reinforcement
Anterior	Patellar tendon Patellar retinacular fibers	Quadriceps
Lateral	Lateral collateral ligament Lateral patellar retinacular fibers Iliotibial band	Biceps femoris Tendon of the popliteus Lateral head of the gastrocnemius
Posterior	Oblique popliteal ligament Arcuate popliteal ligament	Popliteus Gastrocnemius Hamstrings, especially the tendon of the semimembranosus
Posterior-lateral	Arcuate popliteal ligament Lateral collateral ligament	Tendon of the popliteus
Medial	Medial patellar retinacular fibers* Medial collateral ligament Thickened fibers posterior-medially†	Expansions from the tendon of the semimembranosus Tendons of the sartorius, gracilis, and semitendinosus

*Often referred to as the medial patellofemoral ligament.
†Often referred to as the *posterior-medial capsule* or the *posterior oblique ligament.*

the horizontal plane movements of the major joints of the entire lower limb. Horizontal plane rotations that occur in the hip, for example, affect the posture of the joints throughout the lower limb as far distal as those in the foot, and vice versa.

Capsule and Reinforcing Ligaments

The fibrous capsule of the knee encloses the medial and lateral compartments of the tibiofemoral joint and the patellofemoral joint. The proximal and distal attachments of the capsule to bone are indicated by the dotted lines in Figure 13-3, *A* and *B*. The capsule of the knee receives significant reinforcement from muscles, ligaments, and fascia. Five reinforced regions of the capsule are described next and are summarized in Table 13-1.

The *anterior capsule* of the knee attaches to the margins of the patella and the patellar tendon, being reinforced by the quadriceps muscle and *medial* and *lateral patellar retinacular fibers* (Figure 13-7). The retinacular fibers are extensions of the connective tissue covering the vastus lateralis, vastus medialis, and iliotibial band. The extensive set of netlike fibers has connection to and among the femur, tibia, patella, quadriceps and patellar tendon, collateral ligaments, and menisci.

The *lateral capsule* of the knee is reinforced by the lateral (fibular) collateral ligament, lateral patellar retinacular fibers, and iliotibial band (Figure 13-8).[232] Muscular stability is provided by the biceps femoris, the tendon of the popliteus, and the lateral head of the gastrocnemius.

The *posterior capsule* is reinforced by the oblique popliteal ligament and the arcuate popliteal ligament (Figure 13-9). The *oblique popliteal ligament* originates medially from the posterior-medial capsule and the semimembranosus tendon. Laterally and superiorly, the fibers blend with the capsule adjacent to the lateral femoral condyle. This ligament is pulled taut in full knee extension, a position that naturally includes slight external rotation of the tibia relative to the femur. The *arcuate popliteal ligament* originates from the fibular head and then divides into two limbs. The larger and more prominent limb arches (hence the term "arcuate") across the tendon of the popliteus muscle to attach to the posterior intercondylar area of the tibia. An inconsistent and smaller limb attaches to the

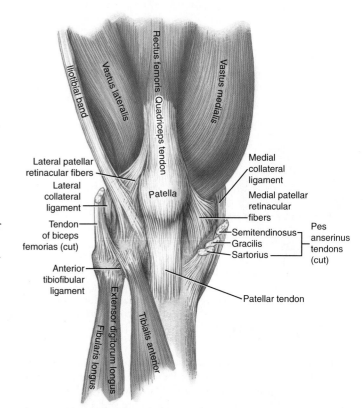

FIGURE 13-7. Anterior view of the right knee, highlighting many muscles and connective tissues. The pes anserinus tendons are cut to expose the medial collateral ligament and the medial patellar retinaculum.

posterior side of the lateral femoral condyle, and often to a sesamoid bone (or *fabella*, meaning "little bean") embedded within the lateral head of the gastrocnemius. The posterior capsule is further reinforced by the popliteus, gastrocnemius, and hamstring muscles, especially by the fibrous extensions of the semimembranosus tendon. Unlike the elbow, the knee has no bony block against hyperextension. The muscles and posterior capsule limit hyperextension.

Lateral view

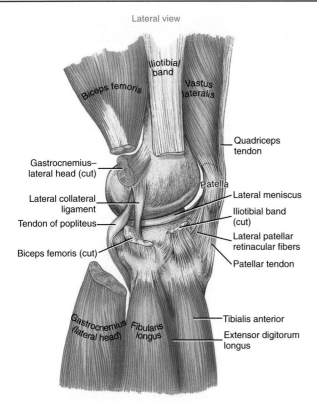

FIGURE 13-8. Lateral view of the right knee shows many muscles and connective tissues. The iliotibial band, lateral head of the gastrocnemius, and biceps femoris are cut to better expose the lateral collateral ligament, popliteus tendon, and lateral meniscus.

Posterior view

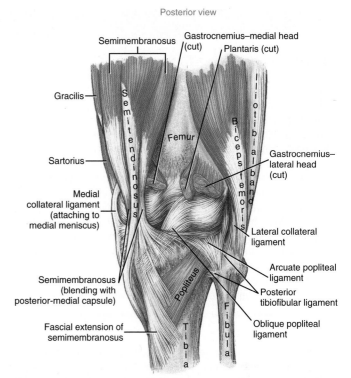

FIGURE 13-9. Posterior view of the right knee that emphasizes the major parts of the posterior capsule: the oblique popliteal and arcuate popliteal ligaments. The lateral and medial heads of the gastrocnemius and plantaris muscles are cut to expose the posterior capsule. Note the popliteus muscle deep in the popliteal fossa, lying partially covered by the fascial extension of the semimembranosus.

The *posterior-lateral capsule* of the knee is reinforced by the arcuate popliteal ligament, lateral collateral ligament, and popliteus muscle and tendon. This set of tissues is often referred to as the *arcuate complex.*

The *medial capsule* of the knee extends in varying thickness from the patellar tendon to the posterior capsule.[226,258] Its anterior one third consists of a thin layer of fascia reinforced by the medial patellar retinacular fibers (Figure 13-10). The middle one third of the capsule is reinforced by a continuation of the medial patellar retinacular fibers and, more substantially, by the superficial and deep fibers of the medial collateral ligament (the deep fibers are not exposed in Figure 13-10). The posterior one third of the capsule is relatively thick, originating near the adductor tubercle and blending with tendinous expansions of the semimembranosis and to the adjacent posterior capsule.[226] The posterior one third of the medial capsule is relatively well defined and is frequently described as a discrete structure, often under the name of the *posterior-medial capsule* or, less frequently, the *posterior oblique ligament.*[203,226] The posterior-medial capsule is reinforced by the flat conjoined tendons of the sartorius, gracilis, and semitendinosus—collectively referred to as the *pes anserinus* (from the Latin, "goose's foot") *tendons.* The posterior two thirds of the medial capsule and its associated structures provide an important source of stabilization to the knee.[225]

Synovial Membrane, Bursae, and Fat Pads

The internal surface of the capsule of the knee is lined with a synovial membrane. The anatomic organization of this

Medial view

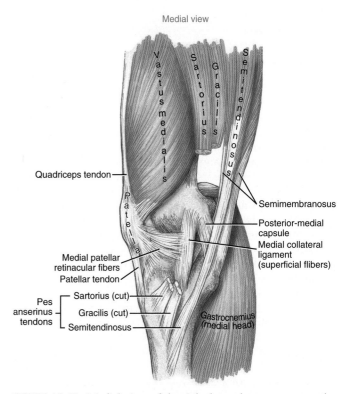

FIGURE 13-10. Medial view of the right knee shows many muscles and connective tissues. The tendons of the sartorius and gracilis are cut to better expose the superficial part of the medial collateral ligament and the posterior-medial capsule.

Development of Knee Plicae

During embryonic development, the knee experiences significant physical transformation. Mesenchymal tissues thicken and then reabsorb, forming primitive joint compartments, ligaments, and menisci. Incomplete resorption of mesenchymal tissue during development forms tissues known as *plicae*.[46,258] Plicae, or synovial pleats, appear as folds in the synovial membranes. Plicae may be very small and unrecognizable, or so large that they nearly separate the knee into medial and lateral joint compartments. The literature reports a wide range in the presence of plicae within the knee, ranging from 20% and 70%.[46,199] Plicae may serve to reinforce the synovial membrane of the knee, although this is only speculation. Other synovial joints of the body besides the knee may have plicae.

The three most commonly described plicae in the knee are the (1) superior or suprapatellar plica, (2) inferior plica, first called the ligamentum mucosum by Vesalius in the sixteenth century,[46] and (3) medial plica. The most prominent *medial plica* is known by about 20 names, including *alar ligament, synovialis patellaris,* and *intra-articular medial band.* Plicae that are unusually large, or are thickened owing to irritation or trauma, can cause knee pain. Because this pathology occurs most often in the medial plica, pain is often reported in the anterior-medial region of the knee. If particularly large, some medial plicae are visible or palpable under the skin.[245] Observations during arthroscopy suggest that an enlarged medial plica can cause abrasion of the facing articular cartilage of the medial femoral condyle.[149] Inflammation and pain of the medial plica may be easily confused with patellar tendonitis, a torn medial meniscus, or patellofemoral joint pain. Treatment includes rest, anti-inflammatory medication, physical therapy, and, in some cases, arthroscopic resection.

TABLE 13-2. Examples of Bursae at Various Inter-tissue Junctions

Inter-tissue Junction	Examples
Ligament and tendon	Bursa between the lateral collateral ligament and tendon of the biceps femoris Bursa between the medial collateral ligament and tendons of the pes anserinus (i.e., gracilis, semitendinosus, and sartorius)
Muscle and capsule	Unnamed bursa between the medial head of the gastrocnemius and the medial side of the capsule
Bone and skin	*Subcutaneous prepatellar bursa* between the inferior border of the patella and the skin
Tendon and bone	*Semimembranosus bursa* between the tendon of the semimembranosus and the medial condyle of the tibia
Bone and muscle	*Suprapatellar bursa* between the femur and the quadriceps femoris (largest of the knee)
Bone and ligament	*Deep infrapatellar bursa* between the tibia and patellar tendon

membrane is complicated, in part, by the knee's convoluted embryonic development.[258]

The knee has as many as 14 bursae, which form at inter-tissue junctions that encounter high friction during movement.[258] These inter-tissue junctions involve tendon, ligament, skin, bone, capsule, and muscle (Table 13-2). Although some bursae are simply extensions of the synovial membrane, others are formed external to the capsule. Activities that involve excessive and repetitive forces at these inter-tissue junctions potentially lead to bursitis, an inflammation of the bursa.

Fat pads are often associated with bursae around the knee. Fat and synovial fluid reduce friction between moving parts. At the knee, the most extensive fat pads are associated with the suprapatellar and deep infrapatellar bursae.

Tibiofemoral Joint

The tibiofemoral joint consists of the articulations between the large, convex femoral condyles and the nearly flat and smaller tibial condyles (see Figure 13-4). The large articular surface area of the femoral condyles permits extensive knee motion in the sagittal plane for activities such as running, squatting, and climbing. Joint stability is provided not by a tight bony fit, but by forces and physical containment provided by muscles, ligaments, capsule, menisci, and body weight.

MENISCI

Anatomic Considerations

The medial and lateral menisci are crescent-shaped, fibrocartilaginous structures located within the knee joint (Figure 13-11). The menisci transform the articular surfaces of the tibia into shallow seats for the larger convex femoral condyles. This transformation is most important laterally because of the flat to slightly convex shape of the tibia's lateral articular surface.

The menisci are anchored to the intercondylar region of the tibia by their free ends, known as *anterior* and *posterior horns*. The external edge of each meniscus is attached to the tibia and the adjacent capsule by *coronary* (or *meniscotibial*) *ligaments* (see Figure 13-11, *A*). The coronary ligaments are relatively loose, thereby allowing the menisci, especially the lateral meniscus, to pivot freely during movement.[232] A slender *transverse ligament* connects the two menisci anteriorly.

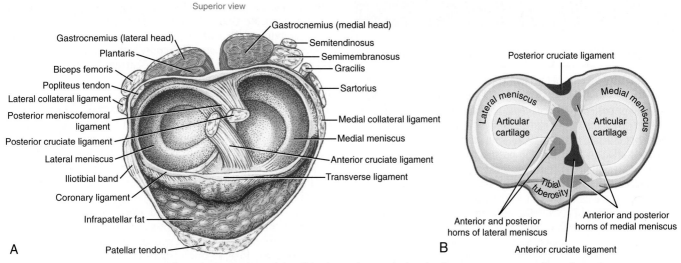

FIGURE 13-11. **A,** The superior surface of the tibia shows the menisci and other cut structures: collateral, cruciate, and posterior meniscofemoral ligaments, as well as muscles and tendons. (This specimen does not have an anterior meniscofemoral ligament.) **B,** The superior view of the right tibia marks the attachment points of the menisci and cruciate ligaments within the intercondylar region.

Several muscles have secondary attachments into the menisci. The quadriceps and semimembranosus attach to both menisci,[124] whereas the popliteus attaches to the lateral meniscus.[54,232] Through these attachments, the muscles help stabilize the position of the menisci.

Blood supply to the menisci is greatest near the peripheral (external) border. Blood comes from capillaries located within the adjacent synovial membrane and capsule.[258] The internal border of the menisci, in contrast, is essentially avascular.

The two menisci have different shapes and methods of attaching to the tibia. The medial meniscus has an oval shape, with its external border attaching to the deep surface of the medial collateral ligament and adjacent capsule; the lateral meniscus has more of a circular shape, with its external border attaching only to the lateral capsule. The tendon of the popliteus passes between the lateral collateral ligament and the external border of the lateral meniscus (Figure 13-12).

Functional Considerations

The primary function of the menisci is to reduce the compressive stress* across the tibiofemoral joint.[123,137] Other functions of the menisci include stabilizing the joint during motion, lubricating the articular cartilage, providing proprioception,[284] and helping to guide the knee's arthrokinematics.

Compression forces at the knee joint routinely reach 2.5 to 3 times body weight while one is walking, and over 4 times body weight while one ascends stairs.[176,283] By nearly tripling the area of joint contact, the menisci significantly reduce pressure (i.e., force per unit area) on the articular cartilage. This method of attenuating peak pressure is essential to the health and protection of the knee joint.[51] A complete lateral meniscectomy has been shown to increase peak contact pressures at the knee by 230%, which increases the risk of development of

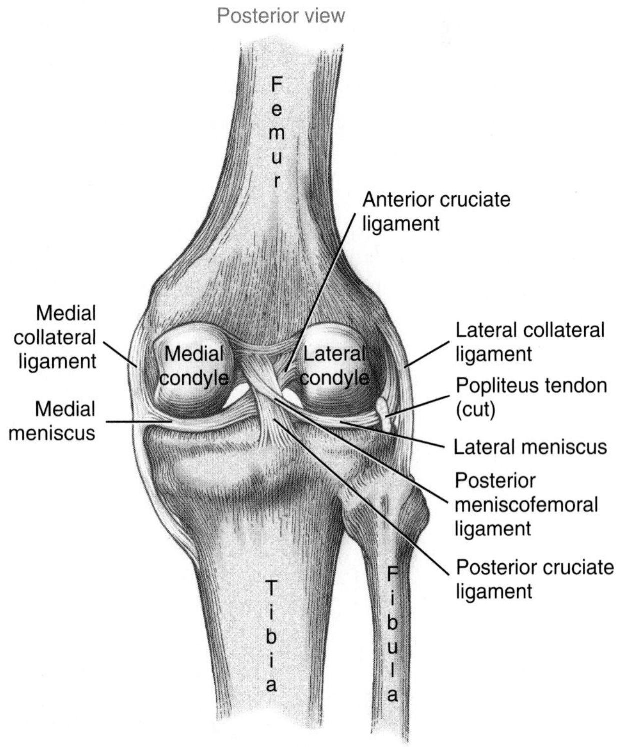

FIGURE 13-12. Posterior view of the deep structures of the right knee after all muscles and the posterior capsule have been removed. Observe the menisci, collateral ligaments, and cruciate ligaments. Note the popliteus tendon, which courses between the lateral meniscus and lateral collateral ligament.

stress-related arthritis.[52,163,192] Even a tear or a partial meniscectomy significantly increases local stress, which is strongly believed to cause excessive wear on the articular cartilage.[137] When possible, surgically repairing a meniscus instead of removing the damaged regions is clearly the treatment of

*Throughout this chapter the terms *stress* and *pressure* are used interchangeably; both are similarly defined as a force (or tension) divided by area.

A Closer Look at the Meniscofemoral Ligaments

The posterior horn of the lateral meniscus is usually attached to the lateral aspect of the medial condyle of the femur by anterior or posterior *meniscofemoral ligaments*.[77,78] The meniscofemoral ligaments are named for their position relative to the posterior cruciate ligament (PCL), with which they share similar femoral attachments. Only the posterior meniscofemoral ligament is present in the specimen illustrated in Figure 13-11, *A*.

Cadaveric studies reveal that at least one of the meniscofemoral ligaments is present in 92% of knees, and both are present in 32% of knees.[76] The posterior meniscofemoral ligament is usually the more substantial of the two structures. After arising from the posterior horn of the lateral meniscus, the posterior meniscofemoral ligament attaches to the femur just posterior and slightly medial to the PCL (see Figure 13-12). The meniscofemoral ligaments sometimes serve as the only bony attachment of the posterior horn of the lateral meniscus.[258] The exact function of the meniscofemoral ligaments is not certain. The ligaments may help stabilize the posterior horn of the lateral meniscus during movement. In addition, these ligaments may provide secondary (and likely minor) sagittal plane dynamic stability to the knee, an assumption based on research showing that the anterior ligament becomes more taut in flexion and the posterior ligament more taut in extension.[175]

tension (known as *hoop stress*) throughout each meniscus. Studies indicate that a torn medial meniscus, most notably with an avulsion tear of its posterior horn, loses its ability to optimally resist hoop stress, thereby reducing the capacity for protecting the underlying articular cartilage and bone.[161]

Common Mechanisms of Injury

Tears of the meniscus are the most common injury of the knee, occurring relatively frequently in both the athletic and the general population.[145,187] According to research cited by Lohmander and colleagues, 50% of all acute injuries of the anterior cruciate ligaments are associated with a concurrent injury to a meniscus.[145] In general, meniscal tears are often associated with a forceful, axial rotation of the femoral condyles over a partially flexed and weight-bearing knee. The axial torsion within the compressed knee can pinch and dislodge the meniscus. A dislodged or folded flap of meniscus (often referred to as a "bucket-handle tear") can mechanically block knee movement.

The medial meniscus is injured twice as frequently as the lateral meniscus.[29] The mechanism of injury for a medial meniscus tear often involves axial rotation, and also may involve an external force applied to the lateral aspect of the knee. This force—typically described as a "valgus force"—can cause an excessive valgus position of the knee and subsequent large stress on the medial collateral ligament and posterior-medial capsule. Because of the anatomic connections between the medial meniscus and these connective tissues, a significant valgus force delivered to the knee can indirectly strain and thereby injure the medial meniscus.

This risk of developing tears in the meniscus of the knee increases if the knee is malaligned or has a history of ligamentous instability, most notably in the anterior cruciate.[145,163]

choice.[163,216] In certain cases, after a complete meniscectomy a meniscal allograft transplantation may be indicated, with goals of limiting the degeneration of the articular cartilage.[35,229]

At every step, the menisci deform peripherally as they are compressed.[123,248] This mechanism allows part of the compression force at the knee to be absorbed as a circumferential

OSTEOKINEMATICS AT THE TIBIOFEMORAL JOINT

The tibiofemoral joint possesses two degrees of freedom: flexion and extension in the sagittal plane and, provided the

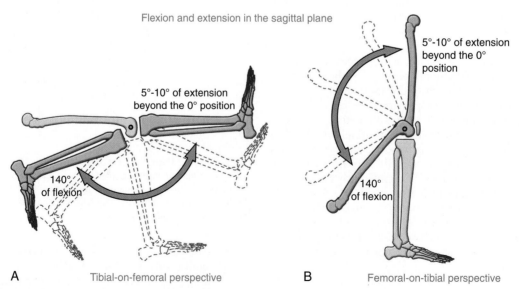

Flexion and extension in the sagittal plane

FIGURE 13-13. Sagittal plane motion at the knee. **A,** Tibial-on-femoral perspective (femur is stationary). **B,** Femoral-on-tibial perspective (tibia is stationary).

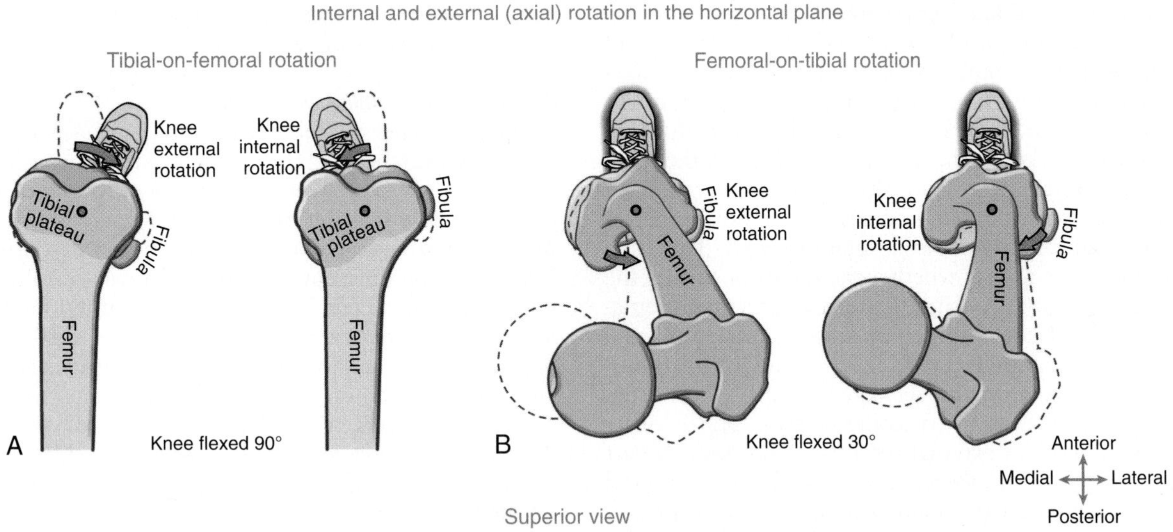

Internal and external (axial) rotation in the horizontal plane

Tibial-on-femoral rotation

Knee external rotation

Knee internal rotation

Tibial plateau

Tibial plateau

Fibula

Fibula

Femur

Femur

A   Knee flexed 90°

Femoral-on-tibial rotation

Fibula

Knee external rotation

Femur

Knee internal rotation

Fibula

Femur

B   Knee flexed 30°

Anterior

Medial ←→ Lateral

Posterior

Superior view

FIGURE 13-14. Internal and external (axial) rotation of the right knee. **A,** Tibial-on-femoral (knee) rotation. In this case the direction of the knee rotation (internal or external) is the same as the motion of the tibia; the femur is stationary. **B,** Femoral-on-tibial rotation. In this case the tibia is stationary and the femur is rotating. The direction of the knee rotation (external or internal) is the opposite of the motion of the moving femur: *external rotation* of the knee occurs by internal rotation of the femur; *internal rotation* of the knee occurs by external rotation of the femur.

knee is at least slightly flexed, internal and external rotation. These motions are shown for *tibial-on-femoral* and *femoral-on-tibial* situations in Figures 13-13 and 13-14. Frontal plane motion at the knee occurs passively only, limited to about 6 to 7 degrees.[159]

Flexion and Extension

Flexion and extension at the knee occur about a medial-lateral axis of rotation. Range of motion varies with age and gender, but in general the healthy knee moves from 130 to 150 degrees of flexion to about 5 to 10 degrees beyond the 0-degree (straight) position.[83,224]

The medial-lateral axis of rotation for flexion and extension is not fixed, but migrates within the femoral condyles.[251] The curved path of the axis is known as an "evolute" (Figure 13-15). The path of the axis is influenced by the eccentric curvature of the femoral condyles.[97,251]

The migrating axis of rotation has biomechanical and clinical implications. First, the migrating axis alters the length of the internal moment arm of the flexor and extensor muscles of the knee. This fact explains, in part, why maximal-effort internal torque varies across the range of motion. Second, many external devices that attach to the knee, such as a goniometer, an isokinetic testing device, or a hinged knee orthosis, rotate about a *fixed* axis of rotation. During knee motion, therefore, the external devices may rotate in a slightly dissimilar arc than the leg. As a consequence, a hinged orthosis, for example, may act as a piston relative to the leg, causing rubbing against and abrasion to the skin. To minimize this consequence, care must be taken to align the fixed axis of the external device as close as possible to the "average" axis of rotation of the knee, which is close to the lateral epicondyle of the femur.

Internal and External (Axial) Rotation

Internal and external rotation of the knee occurs about a vertical or longitudinal axis of rotation. This motion is also called "axial" rotation. In general, the freedom of axial rota-

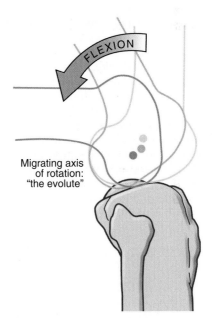

FLEXION

Migrating axis of rotation: "the evolute"

FIGURE 13-15. The flexing knee generates a migrating medial-lateral axis of rotation (shown as three small circles). This migration is described as "the evolute."

tion increases with greater knee flexion. A knee flexed to 90 degrees can perform about 40 to 45 degrees of total axial rotation.[178,190] External rotation range of motion generally exceeds internal rotation by a ratio of nearly 2:1.[178] Once the knee is in full extension, however, axial rotation is maximally restricted. Rotation of the knee is significantly blocked by passive tension in the stretched ligaments, parts of the capsule, and increased bony congruity within the joint.

As depicted in Figure 13-14, axial rotation of the knee occurs by either tibial-on-femoral or femoral-on-tibial rotation. (Although not depicted, axial rotation can also occur as a result of both rotational perspectives occuring simultaneously.) Axial rotation of the knee provides an important functional element of mobility to the lower extremity as a whole. The terminology used to describe axial rotation of the knee is important to understand. As a rule, the naming of axial rotation of the knee is based on the position of the tibial tuberosity relative to the anterior distal femur. External rotation of the knee, for example, occurs when the tibial tuberosity is located lateral to the distal anterior femur. This rule, however, does *not* stipulate whether the femur or tibia is the moving bone; it only stipulates the relative articular orientation of the rotated knee. To demonstrate, compare external rotation of the knee in Figures 13-14, *A* and *B.* Tibial-on-femoral external rotation of the knee occurs as the tibia rotates *externally* relative to a stationary femur. On the other hand, femoral-on-tibial external rotation of the knee occurs as the femur rotates *internally* relative to a stationary tibia (and foot). Both examples fit the definition of external rotation of the knee because both motions end up with a similar articular orientation: the tibial tuberosity is located lateral to the anterior distal femur. The distinction between *bony* rotation (tibial or femoral) and *knee joint* rotation must always be clear to avoid misinterpretation. This point is particularly important in describing femoral-on-tibial osteokinematics.

ARTHROKINEMATICS AT THE TIBIOFEMORAL JOINT

Extension of the Knee

Figure 13-16 depicts the arthrokinematics of the last 90 degrees of active knee extension. During *tibial-on-femoral extension,* the articular surface of the tibia rolls and slides anteriorly on the femoral condyles (see Figure 13-16, *A*). The menisci are shown pulled anteriorly by the contracting quadriceps muscle.

During *femoral-on-tibial extension,* as in standing up from a deep squat position, the femoral condyles simultaneously roll anteriorly and slide posteriorly on the articular surface of the tibia (see Figure 13-16, *B*). These "offsetting" arthrokinematics limit the magnitude of anterior translation of the femur on the tibia. The quadriceps muscle directs the roll of the femoral condyles and stabilizes the menisci against the horizontal shear caused by the sliding femur.

"Screw-Home" Rotation of the Knee

Locking the knee in full extension requires about 10 degrees of external rotation.[109] The rotary locking action has historically been referred to as the *"screw-home"* rotation, based on the observable twisting of the knee during the last 30 or so degrees of extension. The external rotation described here is fundamentally different from the axial rotation illustrated in Figure 13-14. Screw-home (external) rotation has been described as a *conjunct rotation,* emphasizing the fact that it is mechanically linked (or coupled) to the flexion and extension kinematics and cannot be performed independently.[200,258] The combined external rotation and knee extension maximizes the overall contact area of the adult knee: 375 mm^2 in the medial tibiofemoral joint and about 275 mm^2 in the lateral tibiofemoral joint.[200] This final position of extension increases joint congruence and favors stability.

To observe the screw-home rotation at the knee, have a partner sit with the knee flexed to about 90 degrees. Draw a line on the skin between the tibial tuberosity and the apex of the patella. After the partner completes full tibial-on-femoral extension, redraw this line between the same landmarks and note the change in position of the externally rotated tibia. A similar but less obvious locking mechanism also functions during femoral-on-tibial extension (compare Figure 13-16, *A* with *B*). When one rises up from a squat position, for example, the knee locks into extension as the femur internally rotates relative to the fixed tibia. Regardless of whether the thigh or leg is the moving segment, both knee extension movements depicted in Figure 13-16, *A* and *B* show a knee *joint* that is relatively *externally* rotated when fully extended.

The screw-home rotation mechanics are driven by at least three factors: the shape of the medial femoral condyle, the passive tension in the anterior cruciate ligament, and the slight lateral pull of the quadriceps muscle (Figure 13-17). The most important (or at least obvious) factor is the shape of the medial femoral condyle. As depicted in Figure 13-17, *B,* the

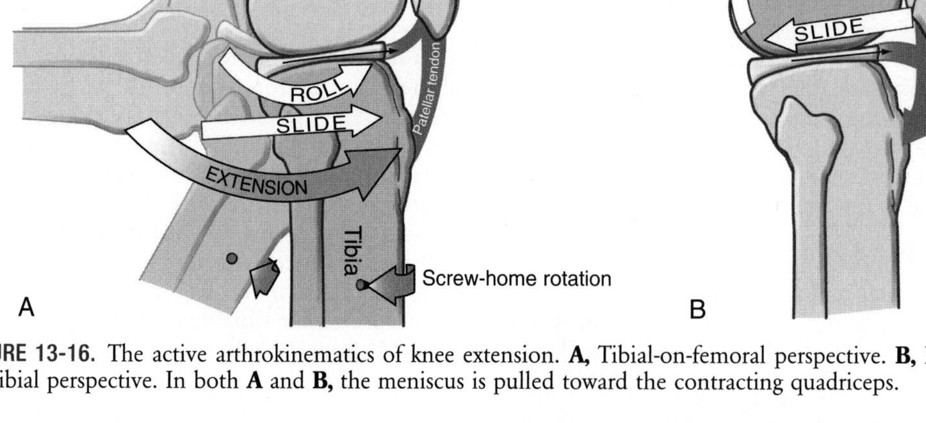

Tibial-on-femoral extension

Femoral-on-tibial extension

A   **B**

FIGURE 13-16. The active arthrokinematics of knee extension. **A,** Tibial-on-femoral perspective. **B,** Femoral-on-tibial perspective. In both **A** and **B,** the meniscus is pulled toward the contracting quadriceps.

articular surface of the medial femoral condyle curves about 30 degrees laterally, as it approaches the intercondylar groove. Because the articular surface of the medial condyle extends farther anteriorly than the lateral condyle, the tibia is obliged to "follow" the laterally curved path into full tibial-on-femoral extension. During femoral-on-tibial extension, the femur follows a medially curved path on the tibia. In either case, the result is external rotation of the knee at full extension.

Flexion of the Knee

The arthrokinematics of knee flexion occur by a reverse fashion as that depicted in Figure 13-16. For a knee that is fully extended to be unlocked, the joint must first internally rotate slightly.[200,206,225] This action is driven primarily by the popliteus muscle. The muscle can rotate the femur externally to initiate femoral-on-tibial flexion or can rotate the tibia internally to initiate tibial-on-femoral flexion.

Internal and External (Axial) Rotation of the Knee

As described earlier, the knee must be flexed to maximize independent axial rotation between the tibia and femur. Once the knee is flexed, the arthrokinematics of internal and external rotation involve primarily a *spin* between the menisci and the articular surfaces of the tibia and femur. Axial rotation of the femur over the tibia causes the menisci to deform slightly, as they are compressed between the spinning femoral condyles. The menisci are stabilized by connections from active musculature such as the popliteus and semimembranosus.

MEDIAL AND LATERAL COLLATERAL LIGAMENTS

Anatomic Considerations

The *medial (tibial) collateral ligament* (MCL) is a flat, broad structure that crosses the medial side of the joint.[258] Although different terminology exists, this chapter describes the MCL as having superficial and deep parts.[225,226] The larger *superficial part* consists of a relatively well-defined set of parallel running fibers about 10 cm in length (see Figure 13-10).[226] After arising from the medial epicondyle of the femur, the superficial fibers course distally to blend with medial patellar retinacular fibers before attaching to the medial-proximal aspect of the tibia. The fibers attach just posterior to the distal attachments of the closely aligned tendons of the sartorius and the gracilis.

The *deep part* of the MCL consists of a shorter and more oblique set of fibers, lying immediately deep and slightly posterior and distal to the proximal attachment of the superficial fibers. Although not visible on Figure 13-10, the deep fibers attach distally to the posterior-medial joint capsule, medial meniscus, and tendon of the semimembranosus muscle.[226,258]

The *lateral (fibular) collateral ligament* consists of a round, strong cord that runs nearly vertically between the lateral epicondyle of the femur and the head of the fibula (see Figure 13-8).[135,232] Distally, the lateral collateral ligament blends with the tendon of the biceps femoris muscle. Unlike its medial counterpart, the MCL, the lateral collateral ligament does not attach to the adjacent lateral meniscus (see Figure 13-12). As described later in this chapter, the tendon of the popliteus courses *between* these two structures.

Functional Considerations

The primary function of the collateral ligaments is to limit excessive knee motion within the frontal plane. With the knee

extended, the superficial part of the MCL provides the primary resistance against a valgus (abduction) force.[74,225] The lateral collateral ligament, in comparison, provides the primary resistance against a varus (adduction) force.[95,237] Table 13-3 lists several other tissues that provide restraint against valgus and varus applied forces to the knee.

A secondary function of the collateral ligaments is to produce a generalized stabilizing tension at the knee throughout the sagittal plane range of motion. Although some of the fibers that constitute the collateral ligaments are taut throughout the full range of knee flexion and extension, most are

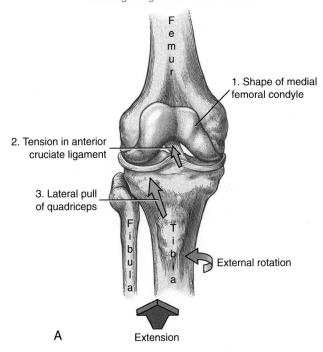

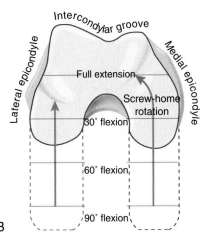

FIGURE 13-17. The "screw-home" locking mechanism of the knee. **A,** During terminal tibial-on-femoral extension, three factors contribute to the locking mechanism of the knee. Each factor contributes bias to external rotation of the tibia, relative to the femur. **B,** The two arrows depict the path of the tibia across the femoral condyles during the last 90 degrees of extension. Note that the curved medial femoral condyle helps to direct the tibia to its externally rotated and locked position.

TABLE 13-3. Tissues That Provide Primary and Secondary Restraint to the Knee in the Frontal Plane*

	Valgus Force	Varus Force
Primary restraint	Medial collateral ligament, especially the superficial fibers	Lateral collateral ligament
Secondary restraint	Posterior-medial capsule (includes semimembranosus tendon) Anterior and posterior cruciate ligaments Joint contact laterally Compression of the lateral meniscus Medial retinacular fibers Pes anserinus (i.e., tendons of the sartorius, gracilis, and semitendinosus) Gastrocnemius (medial head)	Arcuate complex (includes lateral collateral ligament, posterior-lateral capsule, popliteus tendon, and arcuate popliteal ligament) Iliotibial band Biceps femoris tendon Joint contact medially Compression of the medial meniscus Anterior and posterior cruciate ligaments Gastrocnemius (lateral head)

*Assume a fully extended knee.

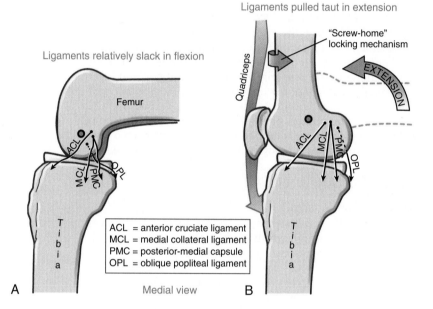

FIGURE 13-18. Medial view of the knee shows the relative elongation of some fibers of the medial collateral ligament, oblique popliteal ligament, posterior capsule, and components of the anterior cruciate ligament *(ACL)* during active femoral-on-tibial extension. **A,** In knee flexion the structures are shown in a relatively slackened (or least taut) state. **B,** The structures are pulled relatively taut as the knee actively extends by contraction of the quadriceps. Note the "screw-home" rotation of the knee during end-range extension. The combined external rotation and extension on the knee specifically elongate the posterior-medial capsule and oblique popliteal ligament (within the posterior capsule).

positioned slightly posterior to the medial-lateral axis of rotation of the knee and therefore are pulled relatively taut in full extension.[197,225,268] Other structures that become more taut in full extension are the posterior-medial capsule, the oblique popliteal ligament (representative of the posterior capsule), the knee flexor muscles, and the components of the anterior cruciate ligament.[197,203,225] Figure 13-18 demonstrates these tissues as being relatively slack in flexion *(A)* and more taut as the knee assumes the locked position of full femoral-on-tibial extension *(B)*. Full extension—which includes the kinematics of the screw-home rotation—elongates the collateral ligaments roughly 20% beyond their length at full flexion.[270] Although a valuable stabilizer in full extension, a taut MCL and posterior-medial capsule are especially vulnerable to injury from a valgus (i.e., an abduction) load delivered over a planted foot. Because the deeper fibers of the MCL are shorter than the superficial, the deeper fibers experience a greater percentage of stretch when subjected to similar valgus (abduction) strain.[225] Primarily for this reason, the deeper fibers of the MCL are more frequently injured than the superficial fibers during an excessive valgus-related trauma, such as what typically occurs in the "clip" injury in American football.[250]

The collateral ligaments and adjacent capsule also provide resistance to the extremes of internal and external rotation.[232,270] Most notable in this regard are the elongation and subsequent increased passive tension in the superficial fibers of the MCL at the extremes of external rotation of the knee.[74,225] Planting the right foot securely on the ground and vigorously rotating the superimposed femur (and body) to the left, for example, may damage the superficial fibers of the right MCL. This potential for injury increases if the externally rotating knee (i.e., internally rotating femur) is simultaneously experiencing a substantial valgus load.

Table 13-4 provides a summary of the functions and common mechanisms of injury for the major ligaments of the knee, including the posterior-medial and posterior capsule.

ANTERIOR AND POSTERIOR CRUCIATE LIGAMENTS

General Considerations

Cruciate, meaning cross-shaped, describes the spatial relation of the anterior and posterior cruciate ligaments as they cross within the intercondylar notch of the femur (Figure 13-19). The cruciate ligaments are intracapsular and covered by an extensive synovial lining. The ligaments are supplied with

TABLE 13-4. Function of Ligaments at the Knee and Common Mechanisms of Injury

Structure	Function	Common Mechanisms of Injury
Medial collateral ligament (and posterior-medial capsule)	1. Resists valgus (abduction) 2. Resists knee extension 3. Resists extremes of axial rotation (especially knee external rotation)	1. Valgus-producing force with foot planted (e.g., "clip" in football) 2. Severe hyperextension of the knee
Lateral collateral ligament	1. Resists varus (adduction) 2. Resists knee extension 3. Resists extremes of axial rotation	1. Varus-producing force with foot planted 2. Severe hyperextension of the knee
Posterior capsule	1. Resists knee extension 2. Oblique popliteal ligament resists knee external rotation 3. Posterior-lateral capsule resists varus	1. Hyperextension or combined hyperextension with external rotation of the knee
Anterior cruciate ligament	1. Most fibers resist extension (either excessive anterior translation of the tibia, posterior translation of the femur, or a combination thereof) 2. Resists extremes of varus, valgus, and axial rotation	1. Large valgus-producing force with the foot firmly planted 2. Large axial rotation torque applied to the knee (in either rotation direction), with the foot firmly planted 3. Any combination of the above, especially involving strong quadriceps contraction with the knee in full or near-full extension 4. Severe hyperextension of the knee
Posterior cruciate ligament	1. Most fibers resist knee flexion (either excessive posterior translation of the tibia or anterior translation of the femur, or a combination thereof) 2. Resists extremes of varus, valgus, and axial rotation	1. Falling on a fully flexed knee (with ankle fully plantar flexed) such that the proximal tibia first strikes the ground 2. Any event that causes a forceful posterior translation of the tibia (i.e., "dashboard" injury) or anterior translation of the femur, especially while the knee is flexed 3. Large axial rotation or valgus-varus applied torque to the knee with the foot firmly planted, especially while the knee is flexed 4. Severe hyperextension of the knee causing a large gapping of the posterior side of the joint

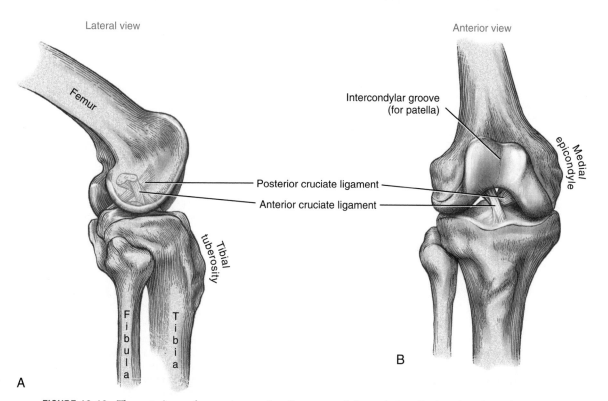

FIGURE 13-19. The anterior and posterior cruciate ligaments. **A,** Lateral view. **B,** Anterior view. The two fiber bundles within the anterior cruciate ligament are evident in **A.**

blood from small vessels located in the synovial membrane and nearby tissues.

The cruciate ligaments are named according to their attachment to the tibia (see Figure 13-11). Both ligaments are thick and strong, reflecting their important role in providing multiplanar stability to the knee. Acting together, the anterior and posterior cruciate ligaments resist the extremes of *all* knee movements (review Table 13-4).* Most important, however, the cruciate ligaments provide most of the resistance to anterior-posterior shear forces created between the tibia and femur. These forces reflect the natural sagittal plane kinematics associated with walking, running, squatting, and jumping.

In addition to stabilizing the knee, tension in the anterior and posterior cruciate ligaments helps guide the knee's arthrokinematics. Furthermore, because the cruciates contain mechanoreceptors, they indirectly provide the nervous systems with proprioceptive feedback.[234,236] In addition to helping control movement, these sensory receptors may also play a protective role by reflexively limiting muscle activation that could create large and potentially damaging strain on the anterior cruciate ligament.[253,266]

> **General Functions of the Anterior and Posterior Cruciate Ligaments**
> * Provide multiple plane stability to the knee, most notably in the sagittal plane
> * Guide the natural arthrokinematics, especially those related to the restraint of sliding motions between the tibia and femur
> * Contribute to proprioception of the knee

ANTERIOR CRUCIATE LIGAMENT

Anatomy and Function

The anterior cruciate ligament (ACL) attaches along an impression on the anterior intercondylar area of the tibial plateau. From this attachment, the ligament runs obliquely in a posterior, superior, and lateral direction to attach on the medial side of the lateral femoral condyle (see Figure 13-19). The collagen fibers within the ACL twist on one another, forming two often indistinct spiraling bundles.[14] The bundles are often referred to as *anterior-medial* and *posterior-lateral*, named according to their relative attachments to the tibia.[48,49,56]

The tension and orientation of the ACL change as the knee flexes and extends.[48,114,181] Although some fibers of the ACL remain relatively taut throughout the full range of sagittal plane motion, most fibers, especially those within the posterior-lateral bundle, become *increasingly taut as the knee approaches and reaches full extension.*[13,32,114,166] In addition to most fibers of the ACL, the posterior capsule, parts of the collateral ligaments, and all knee flexor muscles also become relatively taut in extension, which helps stabilize the knee, especially during weight-bearing activities (review Figure 13-18, *B*).

During the last approximately 50 to 60 degrees of complete knee extension, the active force generated by the contracting quadriceps pulls the tibia anteriorly, thereby powering the anterior slide arthrokinematics (Figure 13-20, *A*).[14,142,143,157,160] The resulting tension in the stretched fibers of the ACL helps limit the extent of this anterior slide. Clinically, it is useful

---

*References 14, 37, 59, 90, 196, 246.

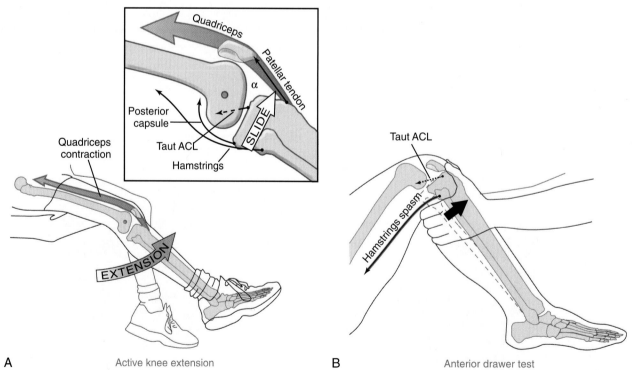

A   Active knee extension

B   Anterior drawer test

FIGURE 13-20. The interaction between muscle contraction and tension changes in the anterior cruciate ligaments. **A,** Contraction of the quadriceps muscle extends the knee and slides the tibia anterior relative to the femur. Knee extension also elongates most of the anterior cruciate ligament *(ACL)*, posterior capsule, hamstring muscles, collateral ligaments and adjacent capsule (the last two structures not depicted). Note that the quadriceps and ACL have an antagonistic relationship throughout most of the terminal range of extension. (The angle-of-insertion between the patellar tendon and the tibia is indicated by α). **B,** The anterior drawer test evaluates the integrity of the ACL. Note that spasm in the hamstring muscles places a posterior force on the tibia, which can limit the tension on the ACL.

to appreciate the general similarity between the anterior force placed on the ACL by quadriceps contraction and the anterior-directed pull applied to the tibia as a clinician performs an *anterior drawer* test (see Figure 13-20, *B*). This test is one of several used by clinicians to assess the relative amount of laxity in a knee with a suspected injured ACL. The basic component of this test involves pulling the proximal end of the tibia (leg) forward with the knee flexed to about 90 degrees. In the normal knee the ACL provides about 85% of the total passive resistance to the anterior translation of the tibia.[26] An anterior translation of 8 mm (⅓ inch) greater than the contralateral knee suggests a possible tear of the ACL. As illustrated in Figure 13-20, *B*, protective spasm in the hamstring muscles may limit anterior translation of the tibia, thereby masking a torn ACL.

Clinically, the quadriceps muscle is often referred to as an "ACL antagonist." This naming reflects the fact that the contraction force from the quadriceps at relatively low flexion angles stretches (or antagonizes) most fibers of the ACL.[108,166,194,241] Studies have reported a 4.4% strain on the ACL after a maximal-effort, isometric activation of the quadriceps at 15 degrees of flexion.[12] This level of strain would increase as a result of a forceful contraction of the quadriceps that abruptly brings the tibia into full knee extension. The ability of the quadriceps to strain the ACL is greatest at full extension because this position maximizes the angle-of-insertion of the patellar tendon relative to the tibia (see α in Figure 13-20, *A*).[168] The greater this angle-of-insertion, the greater the proportion of quadriceps force is available to slide the tibia *anteriorly* relative to the femur. The angle-of-insertion is progressively reduced with greater knee flexion, thereby reducing the muscle's ability to slide the tibia anteriorly and stretch the ACL.[13,16,120,157,167] Understanding factors that naturally strain the ACL becomes important when considering mechanisms that cause ACL injury or ways to protect an ACL graft early after surgery.[45] These issues will be revisited later in this chapter.

Common Mechanisms of Injury

The oblique manner by which the ACL courses through the knee allows for at least a part of its structure to resist the extremes of essentially all movements of the knee.[14,59] Although this spatial orientation is ideal for providing a wide range of stability, it also renders the ligament vulnerable to injury from many combinations of extreme movements. One variable that is common to essentially all ACL injuries is the presence of a high-velocity stretch to a ligament that is already under tension; the ligament ruptures when the tensile stress exceeds its physiologic strength.[14] Biomechanical factors associated with the amount of tension in the ACL at any given instant are interrelated and complex. These factors include the direction and magnitude of the ground reaction force; the amount, control, and precise sequencing of protective muscular forces; the integrity and strength of the surrounding tissues; and the alignment and position of the knee.[92]

The ACL is the most frequently totally ruptured ligament of the knee. Approximately half of all ACL injuries occur in persons between 15 and 25 years of age, often during high-velocity sporting activities such as American football, downhill skiing, lacrosse, basketball, and soccer.[99] Most ACL tears involve a transient subluxation of the knee, causing secondary trauma to other tissues, including bone, articular cartilage, menisci, or the MCL.[152,188,256]

Injury to the ACL can lead to marked instability of the knee and potentially stressful kinematics.[269] An ACL-deficient knee is also more vulnerable to injury or deterioration of other structures.[185,268] Furthermore, because the ligament does not spontaneously heal on its own, surgical reconstruction is often recommended, requiring an autograft (using the person's own patellar tendon or hamstring-adductor tendon) or an allograft.[9,14,207] Although these reconstructions are reasonably successful at restoring basic stability and function to the knee, the natural kinematics and in some cases the preinjury muscle strength are not fully restored.[14,136,262,274] Even after surgical reconstruction, persons who have had an ACL rupture are at an elevated risk for developing stress-related osteoarthritis of the knee at some point in their lives.[145,183]

Approximately 70% of ACL sporting-related injuries occur through noncontact, or at least minimal contact, situations.[128,171] Many noncontact injuries occur while landing from a jump, or while quickly and forcefully decelerating, cutting, or pivoting over a single planted lower limb.[67] The mechanisms causing the injury are often unpredictable and occur very rapidly; therefore the precise position and prevailing direction of the forces applied to the knee at the time of injury are not always certain. Much of what is known about the mechanisms associated with noncontact ACL injury are from reports from the injured players; careful video analysis of the injury; and simulated injury and stress-strain relationships using ligaments of cadavers, implanted strain gauges in the ACL in live persons and cadavers, and computer-based biomechanical models.* As stated earlier, one movement situation that is frequently associated with a noncontact injury of the ACL involves landing from a jump.[246,278] Self-reports, video analysis, and other study methods frequently confirm at least three factors associated with this potentially harmful event: (1) strong activation of the quadriceps muscle over a slightly flexed or fully extended knee, (2) a marked "valgus collapse" of the knee, and (3) excessive external rotation of the knee (i.e., the femur excessively rotated *internally* at the hip relative to a fixed tibia).** All three of these elements are present in Figure 13-21. Research has indeed confirmed that the kinetic and kinematic situations described relative to Figure 13-21 can, when combined or extreme, overload the tensile strength of the ACL.† Although not depicted in Figure 13-21, excessive *internal* rotation of the knee (when combined with extension and extreme valgus) has also been shown to be a predisposing factor to ACL injury.‡[59,160,246]

Another common mechanism for injuring the ACL involves excessive hyperextension of the knee while the foot is firmly planted on the ground.[19] Normal extension kinematics would, in theory, involve an excessive posterior slide of the femur relative to the tibia (review Figure 13-16, *B*). During hyperextension, however, the posterior femoral slide relative to the fixed tibia may overstretch and rupture the ACL. A large concurrent activation of the quadriceps muscle may pull the tibia forward relative to the posterior sliding femur, thereby adding to the likelihood of injury.[45] Often, hyperextension-related ACL injuries are associated with large axial rotation or valgus-producing forces, thereby further

---

*References 16, 34, 58, 160, 243, 247, 278.

**References 45, 91, 128, 160, 164, 246.

†References 45, 63, 91, 92, 128, 246, 278.

‡As defined earlier in Figure 13-14, from a femoral-on-tibial (weight-bearing) perspective, knee internal rotation occurs by the femur rotating externally relative to a fixed tibia.

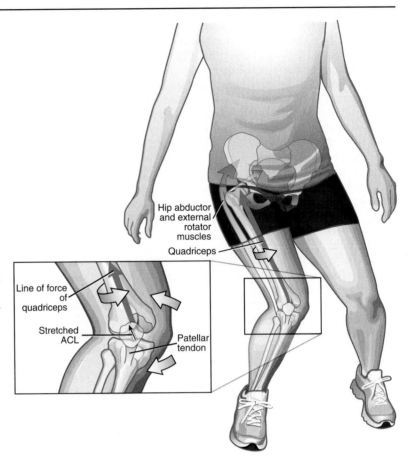

FIGURE 13-21. An image of a young healthy woman immediately after landing from a jump. Note the combined and excessive valgus and external rotated position of the right knee (via internal femoral rotation over a fixed tibia). Note that in a weight-bearing position, the positions of the right hip and foot strongly influence the positions of the femur and tibia, respectively. In particular, the right hip is adducted and internally rotated, which strongly contributes to the exaggerated valgus and externally rotated position of the knee. Reduced activation of hip abductors and external rotator muscles could contribute to this position of the hip. The inset on the left shows the increased tension in the ACL and the line of force of the quadriceps muscle. Note the relative lateral displacement of the patella relative to the intercondylar groove of the femur. (Purple arrows depict excessive valgus alignment; blue arrows depict the excessive internal rotation of the femur.)

increasing the tension on the ACL.[160,246] In addition to injuring the ACL, marked hyperextension frequently causes injury to the posterior capsule and MCL. Table 13-4 summarizes many of the common mechanisms of injury that may be associated with the ACL.

POSTERIOR CRUCIATE LIGAMENT

Anatomy and Function

Slightly thicker than the ACL, the posterior cruciate ligament (PCL) attaches from the posterior intercondylar area of the tibia to the lateral side of the medial femoral condyle (see Figures 13-11, 13-12, and 13-19). The specific anatomy of the PCL is usually described as having two primary bundles: a larger *anterior set* (anterior-lateral), forming the bulk of the ligament, and a smaller *posterior set* (posterior-medial).[2,158,196] Some authors have proposed four distinct fiber bundles within the PCL.[37,158]

As the knee flexes, the PCL undergoes a complex twisting and changing in its length and orientation.[43,196] The precise mechanical effect of this dynamic deformation is not completely understood. Because of the relative low incidence of PCL injury, research regarding its specific function has lagged behind that of the ACL. What is known, however, is that some fibers within the PCL remain taut throughout most of flexion and extension, although the majority of the ligament *becomes increasingly taut with greater flexion*.[131,196,217] Between full extension and approximately 30 to 40 degrees of flexion, most of the PCL is relatively slackened; tension peaks between 90 and 120 degrees of flexion.[37,141,196] In vivo analysis through magnetic resonance imaging (MRI) shows that, on average, the bulk of the PCL elongates approximately 30% of its

length between full extension and 90 degrees of flexion; this correlates to an approximate 3% increase in length per 10 degrees of flexion.[196] This relative sharp increase in tension explains, in part, why many PCL injuries involve significant knee flexion. In addition to becoming taut in flexion, the PCL provides a secondary restraint to varus-and-valgus loads, as well as excessive axial rotation.[37]

While a person actively flexes the knee against gravity, such as when lying prone, the knee flexor muscles (such as the hamstrings) actively slide the tibia (along with the fibula) posteriorly relative to the femur. The extent of the posterior slide arthrokinematics is limited, in part, by passive tension in the PCL (Figure 13-22, *A*).[141] For this reason, the hamstrings are often referred to as a "PCL antagonist," especially at flexion angles closer to a 90-degree position, which aligns the hamstrings nearly perpendicular to the long axis of the tibia. Adding a forceful contraction of the quadriceps to an existing hamstring contraction reduces the strain on the PCL.[69,96]

One of the most commonly performed tests to evaluate the integrity of the PCL is the *"posterior drawer" test*. This test involves pushing the proximal end of the tibia (leg) posteriorly with the knee flexed to about 90 degrees (see Figure 13-22, *B*). In this position the PCL provides about 95% of the total passive resistance to the posterior translation of the tibia.[6] With the knee held between 0 and about 30 degrees flexion, the PCL provides only negligible passive resistance to posterior translation of the tibia; most of the resistance is furnished by the posterior capsule and the majority of the fibers within the collateral ligaments—tissues that are naturally stretched in near extension.[37]

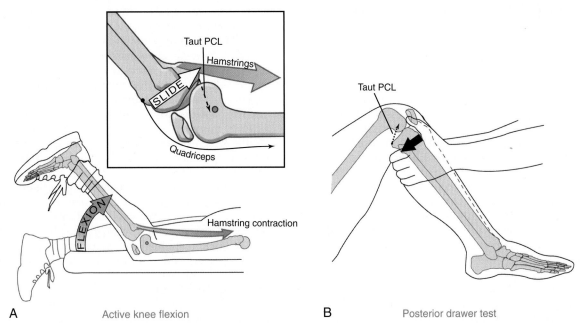

FIGURE 13-22. A, Contraction of the hamstring muscles flexes the knee and slides the tibia posterior relative to the femur. Knee flexion elongates the quadriceps muscle and most of the fibers within the posterior cruciate ligament (PCL). **B,** The posterior drawer test evaluates the integrity of the PCL. Tissues pulled taut are indicated by thin black arrows.

Another function of the PCL is to limit the extent of anterior translation of the *femur* relative to the fixed lower leg. Activities such as rapid descent into a deep squat can create a potential anterior translation of the femur relative to the tibia. The femur is prevented from sliding off the anterior edge of the tibia by tension in the PCL as well as the surrounding capsule and compression forces within the tibiofemoral joint caused by gravity and muscular coactivation. As apparent in Figure 13-8, the stout tendon of the popliteus, by crossing obliquely across the posterior-lateral side of the knee, can resist anterior translation of the femur relative to the tibia (or posterior translation of the tibia relative to the femur).[232] The importance of the restraining function of the popliteus is more evident in persons with a PCL-deficient knee.[232]

Common Mechanisms of Injury

Most PCL injuries are associated with high-energy trauma, such as being in an automobile accident or playing contact sports like American football.[198,235] It is generally reported that isolated sports-related PCL injuries are rare.[156] The cited percentage of sports-related injuries involving isolated PCL tears is generally within the 2% to 10% range.[33,156,204] Approximately half of all PCL injuries also involve other knee structures, including the meniscus, ACL, and posterior-lateral capsule.[235]

Several mechanisms have been described for injury to the PCL.[110,204,235] One relatively frequent mechanism involves *falling over a fully flexed knee* (with the ankle plantar flexed) such that the proximal tibia first strikes the ground.[156,235] One of the most common high-energy injuries to the PCL is the *"dashboard" injury,* in which the knee of a passenger in an automobile strikes the dashboard subsequent to a front-end collision, driving the tibia posteriorly relative to the femur. Other mechanisms of injury are listed in Table 13-4.

Often after a PCL injury the proximal tibia sags posteriorly relative to the femur when the lower leg is subjected to the pull of gravity. This observation, in conjunction with a positive posterior drawer sign, suggests a ruptured PCL. Often, isolated PCL injuries can be managed conservatively without tendon graft reconstructive surgery. Surgery is often recommended, however, if marked posterior instability or subluxation is evident and (as frequently is the case) the PCL is injured along with other ligaments. Data on long-term function of the knee after PCL injury are lacking. Most studies suggest that the PCL-deficient knee is more likely to develop posttraumatic knee osteoarthritis.[22,223,240] Whether PCL reconstruction following injury prevents the knee from significant instability and degeneration later in life is a controversial topic.[156]

Patellofemoral Joint

The patellofemoral joint is the interface between the articular side of the patella and the intercondylar (trochlear) groove of the femur. Local stabilizers of this joint include forces produced by the quadriceps muscle, the fit of the joint surfaces, and passive restraint from the surrounding retinacular fibers and capsule. Abnormal kinematics and possible instability of the patellofemoral joint are all too common and often are implicated with chronic anterior knee pain and even joint degeneration. These pathomechanics are addressed later in this chapter. As a background to this topic, the following sections describe the normal kinematics at the patellofemoral joint.

As the knee flexes and extends, a sliding motion occurs between the articular surfaces of the patella and the intercondylar groove of the femur. During *tibial-on-femoral movements,* the patella slides relative to the fixed intercondylar groove of the femur. Because of the bony attachment of the patellar tendon to the tibial tuberosity, the patella follows the direction of the tibia during knee flexion. During *femoral-on-tibial movements (*such as during descent into a squat position), the intercondylar groove of the femur slides relative to the fixed patella. The patella is held in place primarily by its connection to the tibia via the patellar tendon.

PATELLOFEMORAL JOINT KINEMATICS

Path and Area of Patellar Contact on the Femur

Data from in vivo and in vitro studies have provided detailed descriptions of the kinematics and contact areas within the patellofemoral joint during flexion and extension.* Most in vivo measurements are made using MRI scanners or fluoroscopy or by inserting metallic pins into bone. Data primarily from the work of Goodfellow and Hungerford were used to help construct the model illustrated in Figure 13-23.[70] At 135 degrees of flexion, the patella contacts the femur primarily near its superior pole (see Figure 13-23, *A*). At this near fully flexed position, the patella rests below the intercondylar groove, bridging the intercondylar notch of the femur (see Figure 13-23, *D*). In this position, the lateral edge of the lateral facet and the "odd" facet of the patella share articular contact with the femur (see Figure 13-23, *E*). As the knee extends toward 90 degrees of flexion, the primary contact region on the patella starts to migrate toward its inferior pole (see Figure 13-23, *B*).[220,231] Between 90 and 60 degrees of flexion, the

_____

*References 4, 10, 126, 133, 134, 186, 189.

patella is usually engaged within the intercondylar groove of the femur. Within this arc of motion, the contact area between the patella and femur is therefore greatest (see Figure 13-23, *D* and *E*).[41,102] Even at its maximum, however, the contact area is only about one third of the total surface area of the posterior side of the patella. Joint pressure (i.e., compression force per unit area), therefore, can rise to very large levels within the patellofemoral joint, given strong activation of the quadriceps muscle.

As the knee extends through the last 20 to 30 degrees of flexion, the primary contact point on the patella migrates to its inferior pole (see Figure 13-23, *C*). Within this arc the patella loses much of its mechanical engagement with the intercondylar groove. Once in full extension, the patella rests completely proximal to the groove and against the suprapatellar fat pad. In this position, with the quadriceps relaxed, the patella can be moved freely relative to the femur. The overall reduced fit of the patella within the intercondylar groove in the first 20 or 30 degrees of flexion explains, in part, why most chronic lateral dislocations of the patella occur near this position.[1] The reason why the patella typically dislocates *laterally* is based primarily on the overall lateral line of force of the quadriceps muscle relative to the long axis of the patellar tendon—a topic that is covered in the upcoming sections that describe the structure and function of the quadriceps muscles.

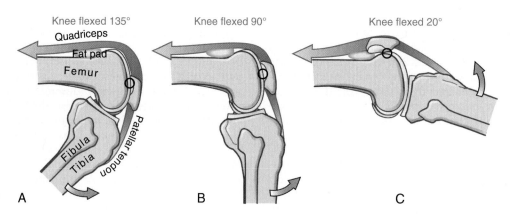

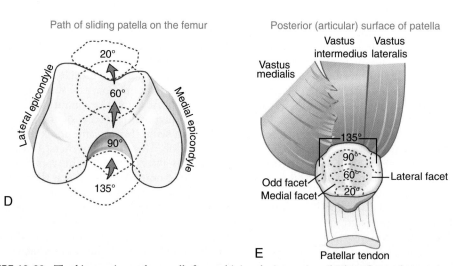

FIGURE 13-23. The kinematics at the patellofemoral joint during active tibial-on-femoral extension. The circle depicted in **A** to **C** indicates the point of maximal contact between the patella and the femur. As the knee extends, the contact point on the patella migrates from its superior pole to its inferior pole. Note the suprapatellar fat pad deep to the quadriceps. **D** and **E** show the path and contact areas of the patella on the intercondylar groove of the femur. The values 135, 90, 60, and 20 degrees indicate flexed positions of the knee.

Accessory Patellar Kinematics

Relatively recent technologic advances in magnetic resonance imaging (MRI) and dual orthogonal fluoroscopy have provided researchers the ability to measure in vivo patellofemoral joint kinematics in far greater detail than the relative global patellar movements depicted in Figure 13-23.[151,186] These more detailed *accessory patellar kinematics* include patellar *tilt* (near horizontal plane rotation about a near vertical axis), *spin** (frontal plane rotation about an anterior-posterior axis) and lateral-medial *shift* (translation).[151,186,220] These relatively slight and often overlooked accessory patellar kinematics accompany all patellofemoral movements. Several factors cause accessory patellar kinematics. Consider, for example, active tibial-on-femoral knee flexion, starting from full extension. The moving tibia pulls the patellar tendon and patella distally relative to the femur, causing the patella to undulate slightly in accord with the irregular contours of the patellofemoral joint. In addition, accessory patellar kinematics are caused by concurrent axial rotation of the tibia (related to the unlocking of the knee), as well as the fluctuating passive tension in the patellofemoral retinacular fibers and stretched quadriceps.

The amount and direction of the accessory patellar kinematics vary considerably among persons, types of movement (tibia fixed versus femur fixed), types of muscle activation or coactivation (eccentric, isometric, etc), and the magnitude of the external load placed on the muscles.[116,134,150] The reported high variability also reflects the different and poorly standardized methodology used to measure these elusive kinematics. It is difficult, therefore, to make meaningful comparisons of accessory kinematics across research studies or loading conditions. Although tempting, it is equally difficult to offer a biomechanical reason for the extent and direction of many of the reported patellar kinematics.

Perhaps the most consistently described accessory patellar kinematics during flexion and extension of the knee are medial or lateral *shifts* of the patella within the intercondylar groove.[1,150,186,276] Using MRI, Nha and colleagues studied a weight-bearing lunging motion through 90 degrees of knee flexion in eight healthy subjects.[186] With full extension as a starting point, the data showed that, on average, the patella first shifted *medially* 2.8 mm by 30 degrees of flexion, then back *laterally* 2 mm by 90 degrees of flexion. Net patellar shift was negligible throughout the reported range of flexion. In another study using comparable weight-bearing movements, MacIntyre and co-workers compared patellar kinematics in healthy subjects to those with chronic anterior knee pain.[150,151] The trends in the patellar kinematic data were similar in the two groups except for the symptomatic (painful) group showed a statistically greater *lateral* shift of the patella compared with the control group, most notably at about 20 degrees of flexion. As described later in this chapter, excessive lateral shift of the patella during knee movement is often associated with patellofemoral joint instability and pain.

In summary, accessory patellar kinematics normally accompany all knee motions. Although not well understood or predictable, there is likely an optimal amount and pattern of patellar accessory kinematics that help minimize the stress within the patellofemoral joint. Much more clinical and basic research is needed to better define and recognize the pattern of accessory patellar kinematics, both in normal subjects and in those with suspected degeneration or instability of the patellofemoral joint. A better understanding of this topic would provide a clearer picture of the underlying pathology associated with patellofemoral joint pain and degeneration, as well as assisting with its treatment.

*Also referred to as rotation.

MUSCLE AND JOINT INTERACTION

Innervation of the Muscles

The quadriceps femoris is innervated by the *femoral nerve* (see Figure 12-24, *A*). Like the triceps at the elbow, the knee's sole extensor group is innervated by just one peripheral nerve. A complete femoral nerve lesion, therefore, can cause total paralysis of the knee extensors. The flexors and rotators of the knee are innervated by several nerves from both the lumbar and sacral plexus, but primarily by the *tibial portion of the sciatic nerve* (see Figure 12-24, *B*). Table 13-5 lists the motor innervation of all muscles that cross the knee.

As an additional reference, the primary spinal nerve roots that supply the muscles of the lower extremity are listed in Appendix IV, Part A. In addition, Appendix IV, Parts B and C include additional reference items to help guide the clinical assessment of the functional status of the L^2-S^3 spinal nerve roots.

Sensory Innervation of the Knee Joint

Sensory innervation of the knee and associated ligaments is supplied primarily from L^3 through L^5 spinal nerve roots, which travel to the spinal cord primarily in the posterior tibial, obturator, and femoral nerves.[106,119] The *posterior tibial nerve* (a branch of the tibial portion of the sciatic) is the largest afferent supply to the knee joint. It supplies sensation to the posterior capsule and associated ligaments and most of the internal structures of the knee as far anterior as the infrapatellar fat pad. Afferent fibers within the *obturator* nerve carry sensation from the skin over the medial aspect of the knee and parts of the posterior and posterior-medial capsule. Afferent fibers from the *femoral* nerve supply most of the anterior-medial and anterior-lateral capsule.

Muscular Function at the Knee

Muscles of the knee are described as two groups: the *knee extensors* (i.e., quadriceps femoris) and the *knee flexor-rotators*. The anatomy of many of these muscles is presented in Chapter 12. Consult Appendix IV, Part D for a summary of the attachments and nerve supply to the muscles of the knee.

EXTENSORS OF THE KNEE: QUADRICEPS FEMORIS MUSCLE

Anatomic Considerations

The *quadriceps femoris* is a large and powerful extensor muscle, consisting of the rectus femoris, vastus lateralis, vastus media-

TABLE 13-5. Actions and Innervation of Muscles that Cross the Knee*

Muscle	Action	Innervation	Plexus
Sartorius	Hip flexion, external rotation, and abduction **Knee flexion and internal rotation**	Femoral nerve	Lumbar
Gracilis	Hip flexion and adduction **Knee flexion and internal rotation**	Obturator nerve	Lumbar

Quadriceps femoris
  Rectus femoris
  Vastus group
	
	Knee extension and hip flexion
	Knee extension
		Femoral nerve	Lumbar

Popliteus	**Knee flexion and internal rotation**	Tibial nerve	Sacral
Semimembranosus	Hip extension **Knee flexion and internal rotation**	Sciatic nerve (tibial portion)	Sacral
Semitendinosus	Hip extension **Knee flexion and internal rotation**	Sciatic nerve (tibial portion)	Sacral
Biceps femoris (short head)	**Knee flexion and external rotation**	Sciatic nerve (common fibular portion)	Sacral
Biceps femoris (long head)	Hip extension **Knee flexion and external rotation**	Sciatic nerve (tibial portion)	Sacral
Gastrocnemius	**Knee flexion** Ankle plantar flexion	Tibial nerve	Sacral
Plantaris	**Knee flexion** Ankle plantar flexion	Tibial nerve	Sacral

*The actions involving the knee are shown in **bold.** Muscles are listed in descending order of nerve root innervations.

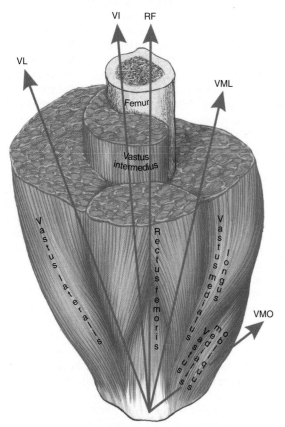

FIGURE 13-24. A cross-section through the right quadriceps muscle. The arrows depict the approximate line of force of each part of the quadriceps: vastus lateralis *(VL)*, vastus intermedius *(VI)*, rectus femoris *(RF)*, vastus medialis longus *(VML)*, and vastus medialis obliquus *(VMO)*. Much of the vastus medialis and vastus lateralis muscles originate on the posterior side of the femur, at the linea aspera.

lis, and deeper vastus intermedius (see Figures 13-7 and 13-24). The large vastus group of muscles produces about 80% of the total extension torque at the knee, and the rectus femoris produces about 20%.[101] Contraction of the vastus muscles extends the knee only. Contraction of the rectus femoris, however, causes hip flexion and knee extension.

All heads of the quadriceps unite to form a strong *quadriceps tendon* that attaches to the base and sides of the patella. The *patellar tendon* connects the apex of the patella to the tibial tuberosity. The vastus lateralis and vastus medialis muscles attach into the capsule and menisci via patellar retinacular fibers (see Figure 13-7). Together, the quadriceps muscle and tendon, patella, and patellar tendon are referred to as the *knee extensor mechanism.*

The *rectus femoris* attaches to the pelvis near the anterior-inferior iliac spine. The vastus muscles, however, attach to an extensive part of the femur, particularly the anterior-lateral shaft and the linea aspera (Figure 12-5). Although the *vastus lateralis* has the largest cross-sectional area of the quadriceps muscles, the vastus medialis extends farther distally toward the knee.[277]

The *vastus medialis* consists of fibers that form two distinct fiber directions. The more distal oblique fibers (the vastus medialis "obliquus") approach the patella at 50 to 55 degrees medial to the quadriceps tendon (see Figure 13-24). The remaining more longitudinal fibers (the vastus medialis "longus") approach the patella at 15 to 18 degrees medial to the quadriceps tendon.[144] The oblique fibers of the vastus medialis extend further distally than other muscular components of the quadriceps. Although the oblique fibers account for only 30% of the cross-sectional area of the entire vastus medialis muscle,[218] the oblique pull on the patella has important implications for the stabilization and orientation of the patella as it slides (tracks) through the intercondylar groove of the femur.

The deepest quadriceps muscle, the *vastus intermedius,* is located under the rectus femoris. Deep to the vastus intermedius is the poorly defined *articularis genu.* This muscle contains a few slips of fibers that attach proximally to the anterior side of the distal femur, and then distally into the anterior capsule. This muscle pulls the capsule and synovial membrane proximally during active knee extension.[258] The articularis genu is analogous to the poorly defined *articularis cubiti* at the elbow.

Functional Considerations

In general, the knee extensor muscles produce a torque about two thirds greater than that produced by the knee flexor muscles.[28,71] Through their isometric, eccentric, and concentric activations, this extensor torque is used to perform multiple functions at the knee. Through *isometric activation,* the quadriceps stabilizes and helps to protect the knee; through *eccentric activation,* the quadriceps controls the rate of descent of the body's center of mass, such as during sitting or squatting. Eccentric activation of these muscles also provides shock absorption to the knee. At the heel contact phase of walking, the knee flexes slightly in response to the ground reaction force. Eccentrically active quadriceps controls the extent of the knee flexion. Acting as a spring, the muscle helps dampen the impact of loading on the joint. This protection is especially useful during high-impact loading, such as during landing from a jump, the initial foot contact phase of running, or descending from a high step. A person whose knee is braced or fused in extension lacks this natural shock absorption mechanism.

In the previous examples, eccentric activation of the quadriceps is employed to decelerate knee flexion. *Concentric contraction* of this muscle, in contrast, accelerates the tibia or femur toward knee extension. This action is often used to raise the body's center of mass, such as during running uphill, jumping, or standing from a seated position.

Quadriceps Action at the Knee: Understanding the Biomechanical Interactions between External and Internal Torques

In many upright activities, an *external* (flexor) torque is acting on the knee. This external torque is equal to the external load being moved or supported, multiplied by its external moment arm. The external flexor torque must often be met or exceeded by an opposing *internal* (extensor) torque, which is the product of quadriceps force multiplied by its internal moment arm. An understanding of how these opposing torques are produced and functionally interact is the focus of this section. This topic is an important component of many aspects of strengthening the quadriceps as part of a rehabilitation program.[279]

External Torque Demands Placed against the Quadriceps: Contrasting "Tibial-on-Femoral" with "Femoral-on-Tibial" Methods of Knee Extension

Many strengthening exercises designed to challenge the quadriceps muscle rely on resistive, external torques generated by gravity acting on the body. The magnitude of the external torque is highly dependent on the specific manner in which the knee is being extended. These differences are illustrated in Figure 13-25. During *tibial-on-femoral* knee extension, the external moment arm of the weight of the lower leg *increases* from 90 to 0 degrees of knee flexion (see Figure 13-25, *A* to *C*). In contrast, during *femoral-on-tibial* knee extension (as in rising from a squat position), the external moment arm of the

upper body weight *decreases* from 90 to 0 degrees of knee flexion (see Figure 13-25, *D* to *F*). The graph included in Figure 13-25 contrasts the external torque–knee angle relationships for the two methods of extending the knee between 90 degrees of flexion and full extension.

Information contained in the graph in Figure 13-25 is useful for designing quadriceps strengthening exercises. By necessity, exercises that significantly challenge the quadriceps also stress the knee joint and its associated periarticular connective tissues. Clinically, this stress may be considered potentially damaging or therapeutic, depending on the medical history of the person performing the exercise. A person with marked patellofemoral joint pain or painful knee arthritis, for example, is typically advised against producing large muscular-based stresses on the knee. A completely healthy person or a high-level athlete in the later phases of postsurgical ACL rehabilitation, in contrast, may actually benefit from such judiciously applied muscular stresses to the knee.

External torques applied to the knee by a constant load vary in a predictable fashion, based on knee angle and orientation of the limb segments. As depicted by the red shading in the graph in Figure 13-25, external torques are relatively large from 90 to 45 degrees of flexion via femoral-on-tibial extension, and from 45 to 0 degrees of flexion via tibial-on-femoral extension. Reducing these external torques can be accomplished by several strategies. An external load, for example, can be applied at the ankle during tibial-on-femoral knee extension between 90 and 45 degrees of flexion. This activity can be followed by an exercise that involves rising from a partial squat position, a motion that incorporates femoral-on-tibial extension between 45 and 0 degrees of flexion. Combining both exercises in the manner described provides only moderate to minimal external torques against the quadriceps, throughout a continuous range of motion.

Internal Torque–Joint Angle Relationship of the Quadriceps Muscle

Maximal knee extension (internal) torque typically occurs between 45 and 70 degrees of knee flexion, with less torque produced at the near extremes of flexion and extension.[129,130,205,219,251] The specific shape of this torque-angle curve varies, however, based on the type and speed of activation and position of the hip.[130,205] A representative maximal-effort torque versus joint angle curve obtained from healthy male subjects is displayed in Figure 13-26. In this study, subjects produced maximal-effort (isometric) knee extension torque with hips held fixed in extension.[251] As depicted by the red line in Figure 13-26, maximal-effort knee extension torque remains at least 90% of maximum between 80 and 30 degrees of flexion. This high-torque potential of the quadriceps within this arc of motion is used during many functional activities that incorporate femoral-on-tibial kinematics, such as ascending a high step, rising from a chair, or holding a partial squat position while participating in sports, such as basketball or speed skating. Note the rapid decline in internal torque potential as the knee angle approaches full extension. Most studies report a 50% to 70% reduction in maximal internal torque as the knee approaches full extension.[130,205,251] Of interest, the *external torque* applied against the knee during femoral-on-tibial extension also declines rapidly during this same range of motion (see Figure 13-25, graph). There appears to be a general biomechanical match in the internal torque potential of the quadriceps and the external torques applied

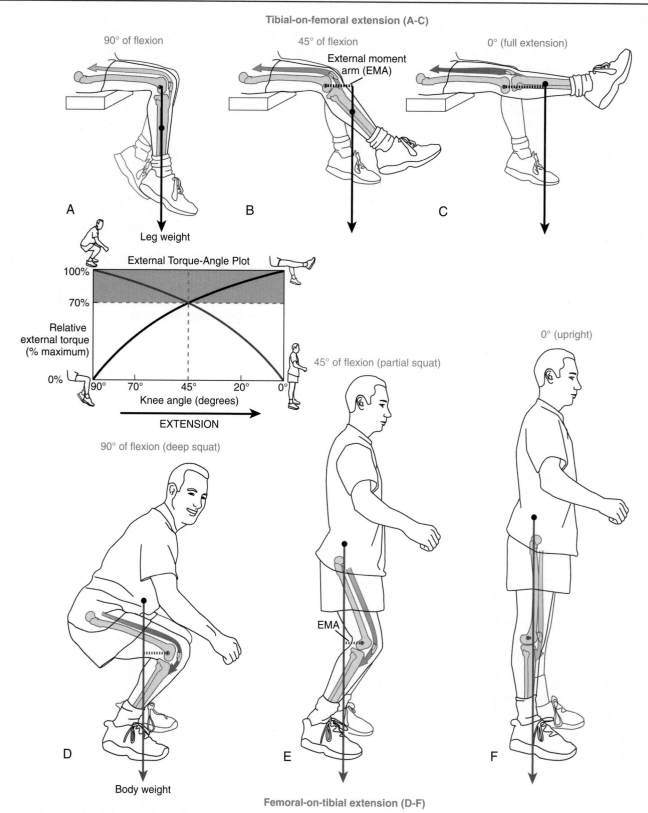

Tibial-on-femoral extension (A-C)

90° of flexion

45° of flexion

External moment arm (EMA)

0° (full extension)

A

Leg weight

B

C

External Torque-Angle Plot

100%

70%

Relative external torque (% maximum)

0%

90°   70°   45°   20°   0°

Knee angle (degrees)

EXTENSION

90° of flexion (deep squat)

45° of flexion (partial squat)

0° (upright)

EMA

D

Body weight

E

F

Femoral-on-tibial extension (D-F)

FIGURE 13-25. The external (flexion) torques are shown imposed on the knee between flexion (90 degrees) and full extension (0 degrees). *Tibial-on-femoral* extension is shown in **A** to **C**, and *femoral-on-tibial* extension is shown in **D** to **F**. The external torques are equal to the product of body or leg weight times the external moment arm *(EMA)*. The increasing red color of the quadriceps muscle denotes the increasing demand on the muscle and underlying joint, in response to the increasing external torque. The graph shows the relationship between the external torque—normalized to a maximum (100%) torque for each method of extending the knee—for selected knee joint angles. (Tibial-on-femoral extension is shown in black; femoral-on-tibial extension is shown in gray.) External torques above 70% for each method of extension are shaded in red.

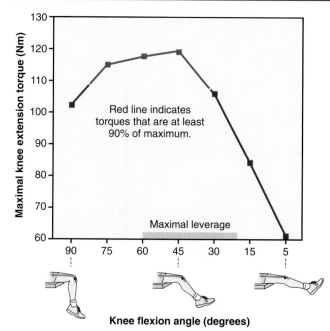

FIGURE 13-26. A plot showing the maximal-effort knee extensor torques produced between about 90 and 5 degrees of flexion. The internal moment arm (leverage) used by the quadriceps is greatest between about 60 and 20 degrees of knee flexion. Knee extensor torques are produced isometrically by maximal effort, with the hip held in extension. Data from 26 healthy males, average age 28 years old. (Data from Smidt GL: Biomechanical analysis of knee flexion and extension, *J Biomech* 6:79-92, 1973.)

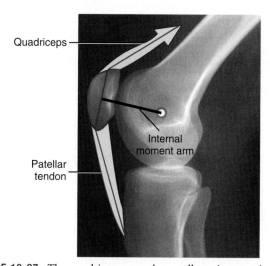

FIGURE 13-27. The quadriceps uses the patella to increase its internal moment arm (thick black line). The axis of rotation is shown as the open circle near the lateral epicondyle of the femur.

against the quadriceps during the last approximately 45 to 70 degrees of complete femoral-on-tibial knee extension. This match accounts, in part, for the popularity of "closed-kinematic chain" exercises that focus on applying resistance to the quadriceps while the upright person moves the body through this arc of femoral-on-tibial knee extension.[279]

Functional Role of the Patella. The patella acts as a "spacer" between the femur and quadriceps muscle, which increases the *internal moment arm* of the knee extensor mechanism (Figure

---

SPECIAL FOCUS 13-4

Quadriceps Weakness: Pathomechanics of "Extensor Lag"

Persons with significant weakness in the quadriceps often show considerable difficulty completing the full range of tibial-on-femoral extension of the knee, commonly displayed while sitting. This difficulty persists even when the external load is limited to just the weight of the lower leg. Although the knee can be fully extended passively, efforts at active extension typically fail to produce the last 15 to 20 degrees of extension. Clinically, this characteristic demonstration of quadriceps weakness is referred to as an "extensor lag."

Extensor lag at the knee is often a persistent and perplexing problem during rehabilitation of the postsurgical or posttraumatized knee. The mechanics that create this condition during the seated position are as follows. As the knee approaches terminal extension, the maximal internal torque potential of the quadriceps is *least* while the opposing external (flexor) torque is *greatest* (compare graphs in Figures 13-25 and 13-26). This natural disparity is not observed in persons with normal quadriceps strength. With significant muscle weakness, however, the disparity often results in extensor lag.

Swelling or effusion of the knee increases the likelihood of an extensor lag. Swelling increases intra-articular pressure, which can physically impede full knee extension.[280] Increased intra-articular pressure can also reflexively inhibit the neural activation of the quadriceps muscle.[42,165,193] Methods that reduce swelling of the knee, therefore, can have an important role in a therapeutic exercise program of the knee. Passive resistance from hamstring muscles that are stretched across a flexed hip in a seated position can also play a role in limiting full extension.

13-27). By definition, the knee extensor internal moment arm is the perpendicular distance between the medial-lateral axis of rotation and the line of force of the muscle. Because torque is the product of force and its moment arm, the presence of the patella augments the extension torque at the knee.

Researchers have shown that the knee extensor internal moment arm changes considerably across the full arc of knee flexion and extension.[127,251,257] Although the data published on this topic differ considerably based on methodology and natural variability, most studies report that the knee extensor moment arm is greatest between about 20 and 60 degrees of knee flexion (see bar on horizontal axis in graph of Figure 13-26).[24,127,251] This range of relatively high leverage partially explains why knee extension torques are typically highest across a significant part of this same range of motion. Maximal-effort knee extension torque typically falls off dramatically in the last 30 degrees of extension, likely because of a combination of reduced extension leverage and shortened muscle length.

At least three factors affect the length of the knee extension moment arm across the sagittal plane range of motion. These include (1) the shape and position of the patella, (2) the shape of the distal femur (including the depth of the intercondylar groove), and (3) the migrating medial-lateral axis of rotation

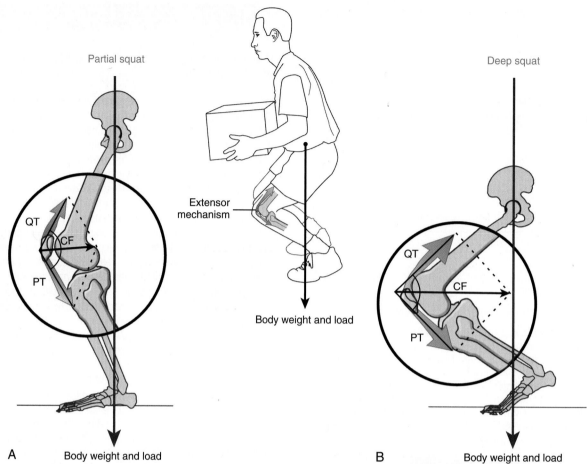

FIGURE 13-28. The relationship between quadriceps activation, depth of a squat position, and the compression force within the patellofemoral joint is shown. **A,** Maintaining a partial squat requires that the quadriceps transmit a force through the quadriceps tendon *(QT)* and the patellar tendon *(PT)*. The vector addition of QT and PT provides an estimation of the patellofemoral joint compression force *(CF)*. **B,** A deeper squat requires greater force from the quadriceps owing to the greater external (flexion) torque on the knee. Furthermore, the greater knee flexion **(B)** decreases the angle between QT and PT and consequently produces a greater joint force between the patella and femur.

at the knee (referred to as the *evolute* earlier in this chapter). Exactly how the changing length of the internal moment arm influences the shape of the extensor torque–joint angle curve, such as that depicted in Figure 13-26 is uncertain. It is technically difficult to isolate the effects of leverage from those of changing muscle length: both factors simultaneously change throughout the range of motion, and both directly or indirectly affect knee extension torque.

PATELLOFEMORAL JOINT KINETICS

The patellofemoral joint is routinely exposed to high magnitudes of compression force. A sampling of these forces include 1.3 times body weight during walking on level surfaces, 2.6 times body weight during performance of a straight leg raise, 3.3 times body weight during climbing of stairs, and up to 7.8 times body weight during performance of deep knee bends.[55,139,221,242] Although these compression forces originate primarily from active forces produced from the overlying quadriceps, their magnitude is strongly influenced by the amount of knee flexion at the time of muscle activation. To illustrate this important interaction, consider the compression force on the patellofemoral joint in a partial squat position (Figure 13-28, *A*). Forces within the extensor mechanism are transmitted proximally and distally through the quadriceps tendon (QT) and patellar tendon (PT), much like a cable crossing a pulley. The resultant, or combined, effect of these forces is directed toward the intercondylar groove of the femur as a joint compression force (CF). Increasing knee flexion by descending into a deeper squat significantly raises the force demands throughout the extensor mechanism, and ultimately on the patellofemoral joint (see Figure 13-28, *B*). The increased knee flexion associated with the deeper squat also reduces the angle formed by the intersection of force vectors QT and PT. As shown by vector addition, reducing the angle of these force *increases* the magnitude of the CF directed between the patella and the femur. In theory, if the QT and PT vectors were collinear and oriented in opposite directions, the muscular-based compression force on the patellofemoral joint would be zero.

Two Interrelated Factors Associated with Joint Compression Force on the Patellofemoral Joint

1. Force within the quadriceps muscle
2. Knee flexion angle

Both the compression force and area of articular contact on the patellofemoral joint increase with knee flexion, reaching a maximum between 60 and 90 degrees of knee flexion.[102,148,167,231] As described earlier, the compression force can rise to very high levels during descent into a squat position. Because increased flexion is associated with a greater relative increase in compression force than relative increase in articular contact area, the *stress* (force/area) is also greatest in the patellofemoral joint in the position of 60 to 90 degrees of knee flexion. Without the relatively large contact area to disperse the large compression force produced by the quadriceps, the stress within the joint would rise to intolerable physiologic levels.[11,55,148] Having the area of joint contact greatest at positions that are generally associated with the largest muscular-based compression force naturally protects the joint against stress-induced cartilage degeneration. This mechanism allows most healthy and normally aligned patellofemoral joints to tolerate large compression forces over a lifetime, often with little or no appreciable discomfort or degeneration of the articular cartilage or subchondral bone. As will be explained, for many persons, however, the natural high force environment within the patellofemoral joint is a contributing factor to the development of *patellofemoral pain syndrome.*

FACTORS AFFECTING THE TRACKING OF THE PATELLA ACROSS THE PATELLOFEMORAL JOINT

The large compression forces that naturally occur at the patellofemoral joint are typically well tolerated, provided that the forces are evenly dispersed across the largest possible area of articular surface. A joint with less than optimal congruity, or one with subtle structural anomalies, will likely experience abnormal "tracking" of the patella. As a consequence, the patellofemoral joint is exposed to higher joint contact stress, thereby increasing its risk for developing degenerative lesions and pain.[53,132,220] Such a scenario may ultimately lead to patellofemoral pain syndrome or potentially trigger osteoarthritis.

Role of the Quadriceps Muscle in Patellar Tracking

Among the most important influences on patellofemoral joint biomechanics are the magnitude and direction of force produced by the overlying quadriceps muscle. As the knee is extending, the contracting quadriceps pulls the patella not only superiorly within the intercondylar groove, but also slightly laterally and posteriorly. The slight but omnipresent *lateral* line of force exerted by the quadriceps results, in part, from the larger cross-sectional area and force potential of the vastus lateralis. Because of the purported association between patellofemoral joint pain and excessive lateral tracking (and subluxation) of the patella, assessing the overall lateral line of pull of the quadriceps relative to the patella is a meaningful clinical measure. Such a measure is referred to as the *quadriceps angle,* or more commonly the *Q-angle* (Figure 13-29, *A*).[62,195] The Q-angle is formed between (1) a line representing the resultant line of force of the quadriceps, made by connecting a point near the anterior-superior iliac spine to the midpoint of the patella, and (2) a line representing the long axis of the patellar tendon, made by connecting a point on the tibial tuberosity with the midpoint of the patella. Q-angles average about 13 to 15 degrees (± 4.5 degrees) when measured across a healthy adult population.[195] The Q-angle assessment has been criticized for its low association with pathology at the patellofemoral joint, poorly standardized measurement pro-

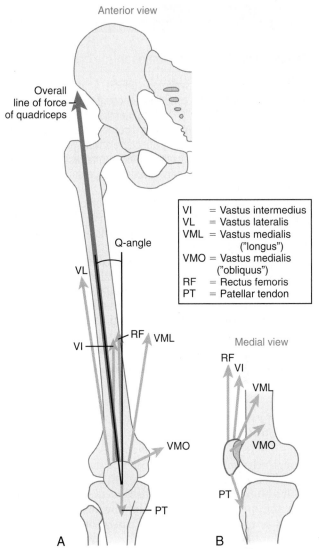

Anterior view

Overall line of force of quadriceps

Q-angle

VL

VI

RF   VML

VMO

PT

A

VI	= Vastus intermedius
VL	= Vastus lateralis
VML	= Vastus medialis ("longus")
VMO	= Vastus medialis ("obliquus")
RF	= Rectus femoris
PT	= Patellar tendon

Medial view

RF
VI

VML

VMO

PT

B

FIGURE 13-29. **A,** The overall line of force of the quadriceps is shown as well as the separate line of force of each of the muscular components of the quadriceps. The vastus medialis is divided into its two predominant fiber groups: the obliquus and the longus. The net lateral pull exerted on the patella by the quadriceps is indicated by the Q-angle. The larger the Q-angle, the greater the lateral muscle pull on the patella (see text for further details.). **B,** The line of force of several of the muscular components is observed from a medial view, emphasizing the posterior pull of the oblique fibers of the vastus medialis.

tocol,[87,211] and inability to measure dynamic alignment. Nevertheless, the Q-angle remains the most popular and simple clinical index for assessing the relative lateral pull of the quadriceps on the patella.[62,102,195] Factors that naturally offset or limit the lateral pull of the patella are described in the next section. If these factors fail to operate in a coordinated fashion, the patella may track (shift and tilt) more laterally within the intercondylar groove—kinematics that reduce contact area, increase patellofemoral joint stress,[64,82] and increase the likelihood of chronic lateral dislocation of the patella.[1,220,231]

Activation of the quadriceps as a whole also pulls and compresses the patella *posteriorly,* thereby stabilizing its path of movement relative to the distal femur. This stabilization effect increases with greater knee flexion (review Figure 13-28). Even in full knee extension, however, some fibers of the quadriceps are aligned to produce a posterior compression

Patellofemoral Pain Syndrome: an All Too Common Condition Affecting the Knee

*P*atellofemoral pain syndrome (PFPS) is one of the most common orthopedic conditions encountered in sports medicine outpatient settings.[263,264] This potentially disabling condition accounts for about 30% of all knee disorders in women and 20% in men.[44] PFPS most frequently affects relatively young and active persons and is often associated with overuse activities.[113] Less frequently, however, PFPS affects sedentary persons or those with no history of overuse or trauma.

Persons with PFPS typically experience diffuse peripatellar or retropatellar pain with an insidious onset. Pain is aggravated by squatting or climbing stairs, or sitting with knees flexed for a prolonged period of time. Cases of PFPS may be mild, involving only a generalized aching about the anterior knee, or they may be severe and may involve recurrent lateral dislocation or subluxation of the patella from the intercondylar groove of the femur. Pain or fear of repeated spontaneous dislocations may be severe enough to significantly limit functional or sporting activities.

The exact pathogenesis of PFPS is unknown and may involve neurologic, genetic, neuromuscular, or biomechanical factors acting either in isolation or in some combination.[1,23,66,186,260] This chapter focuses primarily on the biomechanical causes of PFPS, with an underlying assumption that the condition results primarily from stress intolerance of the articular cartilage and innervated subchondral bone.[4,55,148,151] Excessive stress typically results from abnormal movement (tracking) and alignment of the patella within the intercondylar groove.[169] Complicating these pathomechanics is the strong relationship between the kinematics and kinetics of the patellofemoral joint with those of other joints of the lower extremity, especially in a weight-bearing situation.[255] Furthermore, knowing whether the pathomechanics are the primary cause *or* consequence of increased stress and associated discomfort within the patellofemoral joint is not always certain. The lack of understanding of the exact cause and underlying pathology of PFPS can make this condition one of the most difficult treatment challenges in physical and sports medicine.[62,146,273] The biomechanical rationale behind many of the traditional treatment approaches to PFPS will become clear as this chapter progresses.

---

through the patellofemoral joint. This is particularly apparent by observing a side-view diagram of the line of force of the oblique fibers of the vastus medialis (see Figure 13-29, *B*). Although relatively small, this posterior stabilizing effect on the patella is especially useful in the last 20 degrees of extension, at a point when (1) the patella is no longer fully engaged within the intercondylar groove of the femur and (2) the resultant joint compression (stabilizing) force produced by the quadriceps as a whole is least.[1]

Factors that Naturally Oppose the Lateral Pull of the Quadriceps on the Patella

Several factors throughout the lower extremity oppose and thereby limit the lateral bias in pull of the quadriceps relative to the patellofemoral joint. These factors are important to optimal tracking. In this context, *optimal tracking* is defined as movement between the patella and femur across the greatest possible area of articular surface with the least possible stress. Understanding the factors that favor optimal tracking provides insight into most pathomechanics and many treatments for pain and other dysfunctions of the patellofemoral joint. Both local and global factors will be described. *Local factors* are those that act directly on the patellofemoral joint. *Global factors*, on the other hand, are those related to the alignment of the bones and joints of the lower limb. Although these factors are described as separate entities, in reality, their effectiveness in optimizing patellar tracking is based on the sum of their combined influences.

Local Factors

As previously introduced, the overall line of force of the quadriceps is indicated by the Q-angle (see Figure 13-29, *A*). Biomechanically, this net lateral pull of the quadriceps produces a lateral "bowstringing" force on the patella (Figure 13-30). As

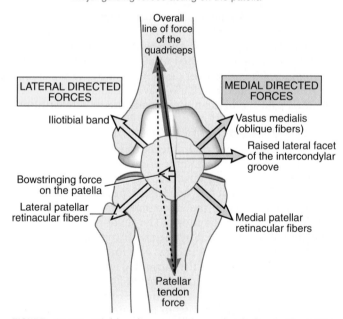

FIGURE 13-30. Highly diagrammatic and idealized illustration showing the interaction of locally produced forces acting on the patella as it moves through the intercondylar groove of the femur. Each force has a tendency to pull (or push in the case of the raised lateral facet of the intercondylar groove of the femur) the patella generally laterally *or* medially. Ideally, the opposing forces counteract one another so that the patella tracks optimally during flexion and extension of the knee. Note that the magnitude of the lateral bowstringing force is determined by the parallelogram method of vector addition (see Chapter 4). In theory, if the line of force of the quadriceps is collinear with the patellar tendon force, the lateral bowstringing force would be zero. Vectors are not drawn to scale.

apparent by the vector addition in Figure 13-30, a larger Q-angle creates a larger lateral bowstringing force.[102,220] A large lateral bowstringing force has the tendency to pull the patella laterally over a region of reduced contact area, thereby increasing the stress on its articular surfaces and potentially increasing the likelihood of dislocation.[115]

As indicated in Figure 13-30, excessive tension in the iliotibial band or lateral patellar retinacular fibers can add to the natural lateral pull on the patella. Although the procedure is controversial, some surgeons perform a partial release of the lateral retinacular fibers in efforts to reduce excessive lateral tracking of the patella.[55]

Structures that oppose the lateral bowstringing force on the patella are shown on the right side of Figure 13-30. The *lateral facet of the intercondylar groove* is normally steeper than the medial facet (compare facets in Figure 13-23, *D*). This steeper slope naturally blocks, or at least resists, an approaching patella and thereby limits its excessive lateral shift.[209] For a patella to laterally dislocate, it must traverse completely up and over this relatively steep slope. Researchers who experimentally flattened the lateral facet of the intercondylar groove on cadaver specimens report an average 55% loss in medial patellar stability across the tested knee range of motion; in other words, the patella could be shifted laterally with 55% *less* force than before the facet was flattened.[238] The normally steep slope of the lateral facet of the intercondylar groove provides the single most important source of local resistance to excessive lateral translation of the patella. A dysplastic (or "shallow") intercondylar groove may occur in otherwise healthy persons and is one of several recognized risk factors for excessive lateral tracking or chronic dislocation of the patella.[153]

The *oblique fibers of the vastus medialis* (frequently abbreviated as VMO) appear uniquely oriented to help balance the lateral pull exerted on the patella by the quadriceps muscle as a whole (review Figure 13-24). Selectively cutting fibers of the VMO in cadaver specimens produces an average 27% loss in medial patellar stability across the tested knee range of motion.[4] This finding may be difficult to apply to clinical settings because it is extremely rare for a person to have isolated paralysis of the VMO. For decades, however, anecdotal evidence has suggested a preferential *atrophy* in the VMO in persons with chronic patellofemoral pain or history of chronic subluxation or dislocation, apparently from disuse or neurogenic inhibition.[5] It is not certain, however, if the observed atrophy of the VMO is any more extreme than the atrophy often observed across the entire quadriceps muscle. Nevertheless, the suspicion of preferential atrophy or inhibition of the VMO has led to the development of multiple conservative treatments designed to selectively recruit, strengthen, or otherwise augment the action of this relatively small portion of the quadriceps. Although the biomechanical rationale for this approach is sound,[50] the ability to selectively recruit and functionally strengthen one component of the quadriceps remains a controversial topic.*

Finally, the *medial patellar retinacular fibers* are oriented in medial-distal and medial directions (see Figure 13-7). The clinical and research literature often refers to these fibers as the *medial patellofemoral ligament*, which includes a broad but thin set of fibers interconnecting the medial patella, femur,

---

tibia, medial meniscus, and undersurface of the VMO.[3,17] This ligament is well known medically because it is usually ruptured after a complete lateral dislocation of the patella. Selectively cutting the medial patellofemoral ligament in cadaver specimens produces an average 27% loss in medial patellar stability across the tested knee range of motion.[238] It is noteworthy that the loss in medial patellar stability increases sharply to 50% when the knee is in full extension.

The medial patellofemoral ligament is drawn most taut in the last 20 degrees of extension.[3] Bicos and colleagues suggest that the ligament is pulled taut in extension with the aid of the activated VMO, to which the ligament partially attaches.[17] These combined active and passive actions provide a useful source of medial stability to the patella at a point in the knee's range of motion at which the patella is least stable because, in part, it is relatively disengaged from the bony "grip" of the intercondylar groove of the femur.

Global Factors

The magnitude of the lateral bowstringing force applied to the patella is strongly influenced by the frontal and horizontal plane alignment of the bones associated with the knee extensor mechanism. As a general principle, *factors that resist excessive valgus or the extremes of axial rotation of the tibiofemoral joint favor optimal tracking of the patellofemoral joint.* These factors are referred to as "global" in the sense that they are associated with joints distant to the patellofemoral joint, as far removed as the hip and the subtalar joint of the foot.

Excessive genu valgum can increase the Q-angle and thereby increase the lateral bowstringing force on the patella (compare Figure 13-31, *A* and *B*).[173,211] If persistent, the lateral force on the patella can alter its alignment and thereby increase the stress at the patellofemoral joint. Increased valgus of the knee can occur from laxity of or injury to the MCL of the knee, but also indirectly from a chronic posture of the hip that involves increased *adduction* of the femur in an upright position.[211] Weakness of the hip abductor muscles, tightness of the hip adductor muscles, or a condition of *coxa vara* (see Chapter 12) can allow the femur to slant excessively medially toward the midline during standing, thereby placing excessive tension on the medial structures of the knee—often a precursor to excessive valgus of the knee.[107,162,255] Furthermore, excessive pronation (eversion) of the subtalar joint can, in some cases, create an excessive valgus load and posturing at the knee in a weight-bearing position. This issue is described in greater detail in Chapter 14.

As depicted in the drawing of the woman's knee in Figure 13-31, *B*, excessive *external rotation of the knee* often occurs in conjunction with an excessive valgus load. External rotation of the knee places the tibial tuberosity and attached patellar tendon in a more lateral position relative to the distal femur.[211] As shown by comparing Figure 13-31, *A* and *B*, excessive external rotation of the knee can also increase the Q-angle and thereby amplify the lateral bowstringing force on the patella.[139,211] As indicated by the pair of blue arrows in Figure 13-31, external rotation of the knee can occur as a combination of femoral-on-tibial and tibial-on-femoral perspectives. Often, however, excessive external rotation of the knee is expressed in a weight-bearing position, as the *femur is internally rotated* relative to a fixed or nearly fixed lower leg. Persistent internal rotation posturing of the femur during weight-bearing activities may occur from reduced strength or neuromuscular

---

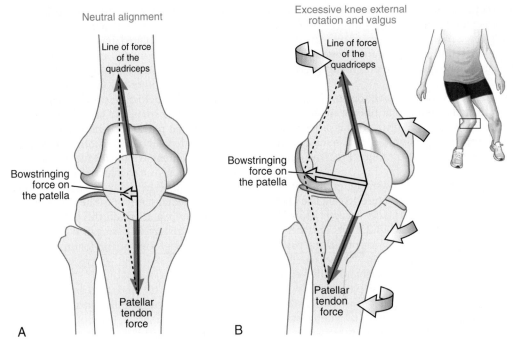

FIGURE 13-31. A, Neutral alignment of knee, showing the characteristic lateral bowstringing force acting on the patella. **B,** Excessive knee valgus and knee external rotation can increase the Q-angle and thereby increase the lateral bowstringing force on the patella. Blue arrows indicate bone movement that can increase knee external rotation, and purple arrows indicate an increased valgus load placed on the knee. Note that the increased external rotation of the knee can occur as a combination of excessive internal rotation of the femur and external rotation of the tibia.

control of the external rotator muscles of the hip,[162,211,255] tightness of the hip internal rotator muscles, or as a compensation for excessive femoral anteversion (see Chapter 12)[138] or excessive tibial (external) torsion. When weakness or poor control of the hip muscles is present, the posture of excessive hip internal rotation is often combined with varying amounts of hip adduction.[107] Although this postural weakness can be subtle, it is often observed when a person is asked to slowly descend a step or assume a partial single-leg squat position. During this maneuver, the distal femur may be observed to "roll" inward slightly, despite conscious effort to resist this motion by activation of hip muscles.

Postural weakness of the hip external rotators and abductors is surprisingly common in otherwise normal and healthy females[21,154,227] and is believed by many who study this phenomenon to be an important global factor that may increase the risk of developing patellofemoral joint pain and recurrent dislocation.[98,107,125,275] Powers and colleagues used kinematic MRI to evaluate the patellofemoral kinematics in a group of young females with a history of patellofemoral joint pain.[215] One component of the study instructed subjects to actively rise from a partial one-legged squat position, from 45 degrees of flexion to full knee extension. On average, the femurs of the extending hips rotated internally rather sharply throughout the last 20 degrees of full knee extension. On close individual analysis, images showed that the intercondylar groove of the femur rotated *medially under the patella* which was held fixed by the strong contraction of the quadriceps. Such *femoral-on-patellar* kinematics aligned the extensor mechanism and embedded patella more laterally and closer to the raised lateral facet of the intercondylar groove of the femur. This precarious alignment places the patella closer to a point of lateral subluxation or dislocation. These observations suggest

that the pathomechanics of lateral patellofemoral dislocation can result from the femur dislocating medially under the patella, as well as the patella dislocating laterally over the femur, as is generally described.

Excessive *internal rotation of the knee* has also been suggested as a predisposing factor to patellofemoral joint pain.[211] Although excessive internal rotation of the knee would theoretically *decrease* the Q-angle and associated lateral bowstringing force on the patella, it has been theorized that this posture could adversely alter the kinematics at the patellofemoral joint.[139,231] Clinically, this issue is most often associated with the pathomechanics of excessive *pronation* of the subtalar joint in the early and mid-stance phase of walking.[212] As will be described in Chapter 14, excessive pronation of the foot during this part of the gait cycle is usually mechanically coupled with excessive internal rotation of the leg.[222] For this reason, the use of foot orthotics may be an appropriate treatment strategy for someone with patellofemoral pain syndrome.[75,112]

Evidence consistently suggests that females experience a greater incidence of abnormal kinematics and related pathology at the patellofemoral joint than males.[57,263] Data collected at a large sports medicine clinic, for instance, showed that recurrent lateral dislocation of the patella accounted for 58.4% of all joint dislocations in women, compared with only 14% in men.[44] It has been speculated that the gender bias in chronic patellar dislocation may in some persons be biomechanically associated with the 3 to 4 degrees of greater Q-angle often measured in females.[100] A greater Q-angle may reflect a greater pelvic width–to–femoral length ratio in females.[195] Whether the apparent greater Q-angle in females (and assumed greater lateral bowstringing force on the patella) alters patellar tracking and stress to a point of actually *causing* an increased incidence in dislocation and pain is difficult to prove, although this is an important and logical point to consider.[84]

Summary

Table 13-6 provides a list of potential indirect and direct causes of excessive lateral tracking of the patella. Although many of the causes listed in Table 13-6 are described as separate entities, in reality many occur in combinations. Clinical evaluation of persons with patellofemoral joint pathology must therefore consider several potential interrelated factors that can contrib-

ute to the problem. Much more clinical research is needed in this area to improve the conservative and surgical treatment of patellofemoral joint pain and chronic dislocation.

KNEE FLEXOR-ROTATOR MUSCLES

With the exception of the gastrocnemius, all muscles that cross posterior to the knee have the ability to flex and to internally or externally rotate the knee.[25] The so-called *flexor-rotator group* of the knee includes the hamstrings, sartorius,

TABLE 13-6. Potential Indirect and Direct Causes of Excessive Lateral Tracking of the Patella	
Structural or Functional Causes	**Specific Examples**
Bony dysplasia	Dysplastic lateral facet of the intercondylar groove of the femur ("shallow" groove) Dysplastic or "high" patella (patella alta)
Excessive laxity in periarticular connective tissue	Laxity of the medial patellar retinacular fibers (medial patellofemoral ligament) Laxity or attrition of the medial collateral ligament of the knee Laxity and reduced height of the medial longitudinal arch of the foot (related to overpronation of the subtalar joint)
Excessive stiffness or tightness in periarticular connective tissue and muscle	Increased tightness in the lateral patellar retinacular fibers or iliotibial band Increased tightness of the internal rotator or adductor muscles of the hip
Extremes of bony or joint alignment	Coxa varus Excessive anteversion of the femur External tibial torsion Large Q-angle Excessive genu valgum
Muscle weakness	Weakness or poor control of • hip external rotator and abductor muscles • the vastus medialis (oblique fibers) • the tibialis posterior muscle (related to overpronation of the foot)

SPECIAL FOCUS 13-6

Traditional Treatment Principles for Abnormal Tracking and Chronic Dislocation of the Patellofemoral Joint

Much of the conservative orthopedic treatment and physical therapy for abnormal tracking of the patella and chronic lateral dislocation focus on addressing many of the underlying pathomechanics described in this chapter.[146,162,213,259] Unfortunately, there is no universally accepted gold standard approach to treatment.[40] Generally, however, attempts are made to alter, as much as possible, the alignment of the tibiofemoral and patellofemoral joints as a way to reduce the magnitude of the lateral bowstringing force on the patella. This may involve exercises aimed at strengthening or challenging the control over the hip abductor and external rotator muscles, quadriceps (particularly oblique fibers of the vastus medialis), and other muscles that normally support the medial longitudinal arch of the foot.[85,146] In addition, physical therapy may also include stretching tight periarticular connective tissues of the hip and knee, mobilizing the patella, using a patellar brace or using a foot orthosis to reduce excessive pronation of the foot.* Patellar taping has also been used in attempts to more optimally guide the patella's tracking, alter the

muscle activation pattern of the oblique fibers of the vastus medialis, or provide increased biofeedback from the region.[39,93,140,146,230] The effectiveness of much of the conservative treatment for excessive lateral tracking and chronic dislocation of the patella is controversial.[18,146,210] Perhaps the most universally accepted treatment relies on providing advice on ways to modify physical activities that create unnecessarily large stress on the patellofemoral joint.

Surgery is often performed to lessen the effect of exaggerated lateral forces on the patella. Examples include lateral retinacular release, trochleaplasty, repair of a torn or lax medial patellofemoral ligament, realignment of the extensor mechanism, in particular the oblique fibers of the vastus medialis, and a medial transfer or elevation of the tibial tuberosity.[55,189,220,233,252] Several of these procedures may be combined. In extreme cases of excessive femoral anteversion, de-rotation osteotomies may be considered to reduce the internal rotation posturing of the hip. As with the many conservative approaches to treatment of impairments of the patellofemoral joint, there are also many surgical approaches to this problem—many of which remain controversial. The myriad treatment approaches reflect, in part, the lack of understanding of the potentially complex pathogenesis of the problem.

---

*References 55, 85, 86, 112, 146, 214.

gracilis, and popliteus. Unlike the knee extensor group, which is innervated by the femoral nerve, the flexor-rotator muscles have three sources of innervation: femoral, obturator, and sciatic.

Functional Anatomy

The *hamstring muscles* (i.e., semimembranosus, semitendinosus, and long head of the biceps femoris) have their proximal attachment on the ischial tuberosity. The short head of the biceps has its proximal attachment on the lateral lip of the linea aspera of the femur. Distally, the hamstrings cross the knee joint and attach to the tibia and fibula (see Figures 13-9 to 13-10).

The *semimembranosus* attaches distally to the posterior side of the medial condyle of the tibia. Additional distal attachments of this muscle include the MCL, both menisci, the oblique popliteal ligament, and the popliteus muscle. For most of its course, the sinewy *semitendinosus* tendon lies posterior to the semimembranosus muscle. Just proximal to the knee, however, the tendon of the semitendinosus courses anteriorly toward its distal attachment on the anterior-medial aspect of tibia. Both heads of the *biceps femoris* attach primarily to the head of the fibula, with lesser insertions to the lateral collateral ligament, lateral capsule of the knee, and lateral tubercle of the tibia.[232,258]

All hamstring muscles, except the short head of the biceps femoris, cross the hip and knee. As described in Chapter 12, the three biarticular hamstrings are very effective hip extensors, especially in the control of the position of the pelvis and trunk over the femur.

In addition to flexing the knee, the medial hamstrings (i.e., semimembranosus and semitendinosus) internally rotate the knee. The biceps femoris flexes and externally rotates the knee. Active axial rotation in either direction is freest with the knee partially flexed. This axial rotation action of the hamstrings can be appreciated by palpating the tendons of semitendinosus and biceps femoris behind the knee as the leg is actively internally and externally rotated repeatedly. This is performed while the subject sits with the knee flexed 70 to 90 degrees. As the knee is gradually extended, the pivot point of the rotating lower leg shifts from the knee to the hip. At full extension, active rotation at the knee is restricted because the knee is mechanically locked and most ligaments are pulled taut. Furthermore, the moment arm of the hamstrings for internal and external rotation of the knee is reduced significantly in full extension.[25]

The *sartorius* and *gracilis* have their proximal attachments on different parts of the pelvis (see Chapter 12). At the hip, both muscles are hip flexors, but they have opposite actions in the frontal and horizontal planes. Distally, the tendons of the sartorius and gracilis travel side by side across the medial side of the knee to attach to the proximal shaft of the tibia, near the semitendinosus (see Figure 13-10). The three juxtaposed tendons of the sartorius, gracilis, and semitendinosus attach to the tibia using a common, broad sheet of connective tissue known as the *pes anserinus*. As a group the "pes muscles" are effective internal rotators of the knee. Connective tissues hold the tendons of the pes group just *posterior* to the medial-lateral axis of rotation of the knee. The three pes muscles therefore flex and internally rotate the knee.

The pes anserinus group adds significant dynamic stability to the medial side of the knee.[174] Along with the MCL and

posterior-medial capsule, active tension in the pes muscles resists knee *external* rotation and valgus loads applied to the knee.

The *popliteus* is a triangular muscle located deep to the gastrocnemius within the popliteal fossa (see Figure 13-9). By a strong intracapsular tendon, the popliteus attaches proximally to the lateral condyle of the femur, between the lateral collateral ligament and the lateral meniscus (see Figures 13-8 and 13-11). The popliteus is the only muscle of the knee that attaches *within* the capsule of the knee joint. More distally, the popliteus has an extensive attachment to the posterior side of the tibia. Fibers from the popliteus attach to the lateral meniscus and blend with the arcuate popliteal ligament.

The anatomy and action of the gastrocnemius and plantaris are considered in Chapter 14.

Group Action of Flexor-Rotator Muscles

Many of the overall functions of the flexor-rotator muscles of the knee are expressed during walking and running activities. Examples of these functions are considered separately for tibial-on-femoral and femoral-on-tibial movements of the knee.

SPECIAL FOCUS 13-7

Popliteus Muscle: the "Key to the Knee," and More

The popliteus is an important internal rotator and flexor of the knee joint. As the extended and locked knee prepares to flex, the popliteus provides an important *internal rotation* torque that helps mechanically *unlock* the knee.[3] (Recall that the knee is mechanically locked by a combination of extension and external rotation of the knee.) Unlocking the knee to flex into a squat position, for example, requires that the *femur externally rotate* slightly over a relatively fixed tibia. The ability of the popliteus to externally rotate the femur (and hence internally rotate the knee) is apparent by observing the muscle's oblique line of force as it crosses behind the knee (see Figure 13-9).

The popliteus muscle's oblique line of pull furnishes it with the most favorable leverage of all knee flexor muscles to produce a horizontal plane rotation torque on an extended knee. The line of force of the other knee flexor muscles is nearly vertical when the knee is extended, which greatly minimizes their axial rotation torque potential. Because of the popliteus muscle's enhanced leverage to initiate internal rotation of the locked knee, it has been referred to as the "key to the knee."

Another important function of the popliteus is to help dynamically stabilize both the lateral and the medial sides of the knee. The strong intracapsular tendon of the popliteus provides a significant resistance to a *varus* load applied to the knee. The muscle also stabilizes the medial side of the knee by decelerating and limiting excessive *external rotation of the knee*. This action, performed through eccentric activation, reduces the stress placed on the medial collateral ligament, posterior-medial capsule, and anterior cruciate ligament.

Control of Tibial-on-Femoral Osteokinematics

An important action of the flexor-rotator muscles is to accelerate or decelerate the lower leg during the swing phase of walking or running. Typically, these muscles produce relatively low-to-moderate forces but at relatively high shortening or lengthening velocities. One of the more important functions of the hamstring muscles, for example, is to decelerate the advancing lower leg at the late swing phase of walking. Through eccentric action, the muscles help dampen the impact of full knee extension. Consider also sprinting or rapidly walking. These same muscles rapidly contract to accelerate knee flexion in order to shorten the functional length of the lower limb during the swing phase.

Control of Femoral-on-Tibial Osteokinematics

The muscular demand needed to control femoral-on-tibial motions is generally larger and more complex than that needed to control most ordinary tibial-on-femoral knee motions. A muscle such as the sartorius, for example, may have to simultaneously control up to five degrees of freedom (i.e., two at the knee and three at the hip). Consider the action of several knee flexor-rotator muscles while one runs to catch a ball (Figure 13-32, *A*). While the right foot is firmly fixed to the ground, the right femur, pelvis, trunk, neck, head, and eyes all rotate to the left. Note the diagonal flow of activated muscles between the right fibula and left side of the neck. The muscle action epitomizes intermuscular synergy. In this case the short head of the biceps femoris anchors the bottom of the diagonal kinetic chain to the fibula. The fibula, in turn, is anchored to the tibia via the interosseous membrane and other muscles.

Stability and control at the knee require interaction of forces produced by surrounding muscles and ligaments. Interaction is especially important for control of high-velocity movements in the horizontal and frontal planes. To illustrate, refer to Figure 13-32, *B*. With the right foot planted, the short head of the biceps femoris accelerates the femur internally. By way of eccentric activation, the pes anserinus muscles help decelerate the internal rotation of the femur over the tibia. The pes anserinus group may be regarded as a "dynamic medial collateral ligament" by resisting not only the external rotation of the knee but also any valgus loads. The pes group of muscles may help compensate for a weak or lax MCL or posterior-medial capsule. Although not depicted in Figure 13-32, *B*, eccentric activation of the popliteus can assist the pes group with decelerating external rotation of the knee.[135,232]

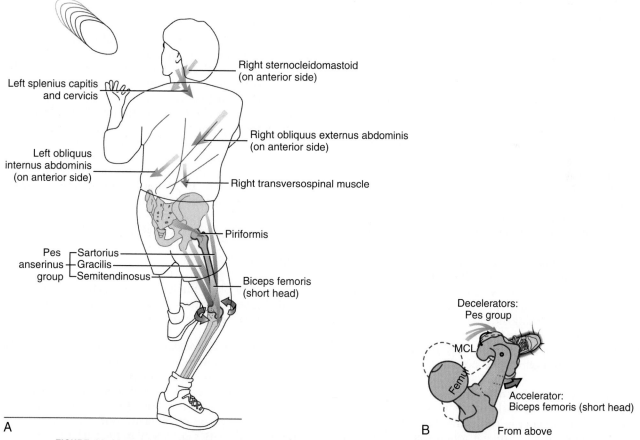

FIGURE 13-32. A, Several muscles are shown controlling the rotation of the head, neck, trunk, pelvis, and femur toward the approaching ball. Because the right foot is fixed to the ground, the right knee functions as an important pivot point. **B,** Control of axial rotation of the right knee is illustrated from above. The short head of the biceps femoris contracts to accelerate the femur internally (i.e., the knee joint moves into external rotation). Active force from the pes anserinus muscles in conjunction with a passive force from the stretched medial collateral ligament (MCL) and oblique popliteal ligament (not shown) helps to decelerate, or limit, the external rotation at the knee.

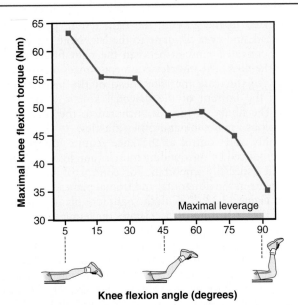

FIGURE 13-33. A plot showing the maximal-effort knee flexor torques produced between 5 degrees and about 90 degrees of flexion. The internal moment arm (leverage) used by the knee flexors (hamstrings) is greatest between about 50 and 90 degrees of knee flexion. Knee flexor torques are produced isometrically by maximal effort, with the hip held in extension. Data from 26 healthy males, average age 28 years old. (Data from Smidt GL: Biomechanical analysis of knee flexion and extension, *J Biomech* 6:79-92, 1973.)

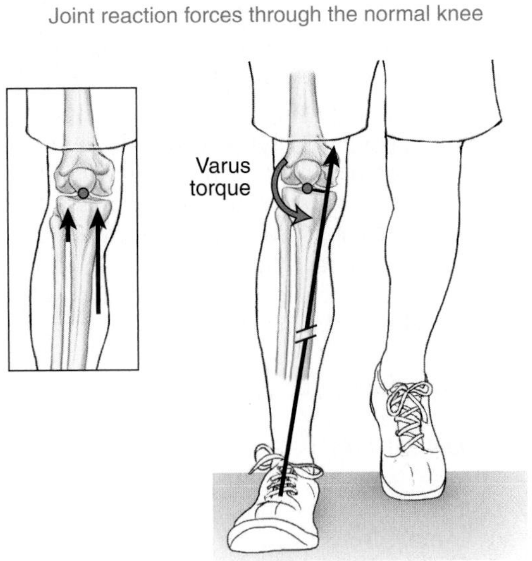

Maximal Torque Production of the Knee Flexor-Rotator Muscles

Maximal-effort knee flexion torque is generally greatest with the knee in the last 20 degrees of full extension and then declines steadily as the knee is progressively flexed.[130,251] A representative plot of published torque data from healthy males is shown in Figure 13-33.[251] Subjects produced maximal-effort isometric knee flexion torque with hips held in extension. Although a wide range of values have been reported, in general the hamstrings have their greatest flexor moment arm (leverage) at 50 to 90 degrees of knee flexion (see bar on horizontal axis in graph of Figure 13-33).[24,118,147,191,251] The torque-angle data depicted in Figure 13-33 clearly indicate that the hamstrings (and presumably other knee flexors) generate their greatest torque at knee angles that coincide with relative elongated muscle length, rather than high leverage. (As noted in Figure 13-26, this is in slight contrast to the quadriceps, where maximal-effort knee extensor torque partially overlaps the point in the range of motion where leverage is greatest.) Flexing the hip to elongate the hamstrings promotes even greater knee flexion torque.[20] The length-tension relationship appears to be a very influential factor in determining the flexion torque potential of the hamstring muscles.[118]

Few data are available on the maximal torque potential of the internal and external rotator muscles of the knee. When tested isokinetically with the knee flexed to 90 degrees, the internal and external rotators at the knee have been shown to produce nearly equal peak torques.[8] At first thought, these results may be surprising considering the far greater number of internal rotator muscles compared with just one external rotator muscle at the knee (i.e., the biceps femoris). The apparent conflict can be partially reconciled by the fact that, with the knee flexed to 90 degrees, the

Joint reaction forces through the normal knee

FIGURE 13-34. The ground reaction force (long straight arrow originating from the ground) passes medial to the knee joint, creating a varus torque at the knee with every step. The moment arm available to the ground reaction force is shown, extending between the anterior-posterior axis *(small purple circle)* and the ground reaction force. As depicted by the pair of arrows in the inset to the left, greater compression force is generated over the medial articular surface of the joint.

biceps femoris muscle has a threefold greater axial rotation moment arm than the average of all the internal rotators.[25] The laterally displaced distal attachment of the biceps femoris to the head of the fibula apparently augments this muscle's rotational leverage.

The average axial rotation leverage for virtually all rotators of the knee is greatest between 70 and 90 degrees of knee flexion, where the muscles' line of force is nearly perpendicular to the longitudinal (vertical) axis of rotation through the tibia.[25] The only exception to this design is the popliteus muscle, which has its greatest moment arm to internally rotate the knee at about 40 degrees of flexion.

Abnormal Alignment of the Knee

FRONTAL PLANE

In the frontal plane the knee is normally aligned in about 5 to 10 degrees of valgus. Deviation from this alignment is referred to as excessive genu valgum or genu varum.

Genu Varum with Unicompartmental Osteoarthritis of the Knee

During walking at normal speeds across level terrain, the joint reaction force at the knee reaches about 2.5 to 3 times body weight.[243,283] This force is created by the combined effect of muscle activation and the ground reaction force. During the loading (early) phase of the gait cycle, the ground reaction force normally passes just lateral to the heel, then upward and *medial* to the knee as it continues toward the center of gravity of the body as a whole.[104] As depicted in Figure 13-34, by passing medial to an anterior-posterior axis at the knee, the ground reaction force produces a *varus torque* at the knee with every step.[61,94] As a result, joint reaction force at the knee during walking is normally several times greater on the *medial*

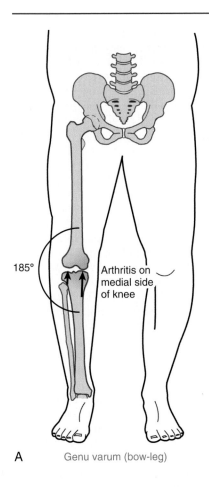

A   Genu varum (bow-leg)

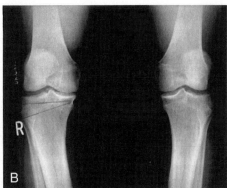

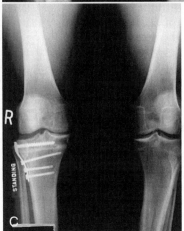

FIGURE 13-35. Bilateral genu varum with osteoarthritis in the medial compartment of the right knee. **A,** The varus deformity of the right knee is shown with greater joint reaction force on the medial compartment. **B,** An anterior x-ray view with subject (a 43-year-old man) standing, showing bilateral genu varum and medial joint osteoarthritis. Both knees have a loss of medial joint space and hypertrophic bone around the medial compartment. To correct the deformity on the right *(R)* knee, a wedge of bone will be surgically removed by a procedure known as a *high tibial osteotomy.* **C,** The x-ray film shows the right knee after the removal of the wedge of bone. Note the change in joint alignment compared with the same knee in **B.** (Courtesy Joseph Davies, MD, Aurora Advanced Orthopedics, Milwaukee.)

joint compartment than on the lateral joint compartment (see inset in Figure 13-34).[244] Throughout one's lifetime, this repetitive varus loading is partially absorbed by tension in lateral structures at the knee, such as the lateral collateral ligament and iliotibial band.

Most persons tolerate the asymmetrical dynamic loading of the knee with little or no difficulty. In some persons, however, the asymmetry may lead to excessive wear of the articular cartilage, ultimately leading to (medial) unicompartmental osteoarthritis.[47,239] A 20% increase in peak varus torque at the knee during walking has been shown to be associated with a sixfold increase in the risk of developing medial compartment knee osteoarthritis.[172] Thinning of the articular cartilage and meniscus on the medial side can tilt the knee into genu varum, or a bow-legged deformity (Figure 13-35, *A*). A vicious circle may develop: the varus deformity increases medial joint compartment loading, resulting in greater loss of medial joint space, causing greater varus deformity, and so on. Figure 13-35, *B* is an anterior view x-ray film showing bilateral genu varum. Both knees show signs of medial joint osteoarthritis (i.e., loss of medial joint space and hypertrophic reactive bone around the medial compartment). Management of severe genu varum often involves surgery, such as a high tibial (wedge) osteotomy. The goal of this surgery is to correct the varus deformity and reduce the stress over the medial joint compartment (Figure 13-35, *C*). In addition to surgery, foot orthoses, valgus knee bracing, reduced walking velocity, and the use of a cane held in the contralateral hand have all been shown to reduce stress on

the medial side of the knee.[180,244] A laterally wedged insole worn within the shoe typically produces a *valgus* torque on the knee during the stance phase. This, in turn, reduces the net varus torque at every step, which reduces the compression load on the medial joint compartment of the knee.[94,122,244] This relatively simple orthotic approach has been shown to reduce pain and improve function in persons with medial compartment osteoarthritis.[38,94]

Excessive Genu Valgum

Several factors can lead to excessive genu valgum, or knock-knee (Figure 13-36). These include previous injury, genetic predisposition, high body mass index, and laxity of ligaments. Genu valgum may also result from or be exacerbated by abnormal alignment or muscle weakness at either end of the lower extremity. As indicated in Figure 13-36, coxa vara (i.e., a femoral neck-shaft angle less than 125 degrees) or weakened hip muscles (such as the gluteus medius) can, at least in theory, increase the valgus load on the knee. In some cases excessive foot pronation may increase the valgus load on the knee by allowing the distal end of the tibia to slant ("abduct") farther away from the midline of the body. Over time, the tensional stress placed on the MCL and adjacent capsule may weaken the tissue. As described earlier in this chapter, excessive valgus of the knee may negatively affect patellofemoral joint tracking and create additional stress on the ACL.

Standing with a valgus deformity of approximately 10 degrees greater than normal directs most of the joint compression force to the lateral joint compartment.[111] This increased

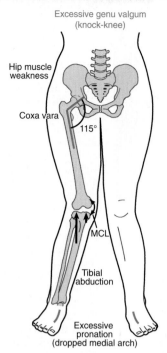

Excessive genu valgum
(knock-knee)

Hip muscle
weakness

Coxa vara

115°

MCL

Tibial
abduction

Excessive
pronation
(dropped medial arch)

FIGURE 13-36. Excessive genu valgum of the right knee. In this example the valgus deformity is assumed to be the result of abnormal alignment or muscle weakness at either the proximal or distal end of the lower limb. The pair of vertical arrows representing force vectors at the knee indicates the greater compression force on the lateral compartment. See text for more details.

regional stress may lead to lateral unicompartmental osteoarthritis.[47,239] Knee replacement surgery may be indicated to correct a valgus deformity, especially if it is progressive, is painful, or causes loss of function. Figure 13-37, *A* and *B* show severe bilateral osteoarthritis of the knee, with severe genu valgum on the right and genu varum on the left. This "wind-swept" deformity was corrected surgically with bilateral knee replacements (see Figure 13-37, *C*).

SAGITTAL PLANE

Genu Recurvatum

Full extension with slight external rotation is the knee's close-packed, most stable position. The knee may be extended beyond neutral an additional 5 to 10 degrees, although this is highly variable among persons. Standing with the knee in full extension usually directs the line of gravity from body weight slightly *anterior* to the medial-lateral axis of rotation at the knee. Gravity, therefore, produces a slight knee extension torque that can naturally assist with locking of the knee, allowing the quadriceps to relax intermittently during standing. Normally this gravity-assisted extension torque is resisted primarily by passive tension in the stretched posterior capsule and stretched flexor muscles of the knee, including the gastrocnemius.

Hyperextension beyond 10 degrees of neutral is frequently called *genu recurvatum* (from the Latin *genu*, knee, + *recurvare*, to bend backward). Mild cases of recurvatum may occur in otherwise healthy persons, often because of generalized laxity of the posterior structures of the knee. The primary cause of more severe genu recurvatum is a chronic, overpowering (net) knee extensor torque that eventually overstretches the posterior structures of the knee. The overpowering knee extension torque may stem from poor postural control or from neuromuscular disease that causes spasticity of the quadriceps muscles and/or paralysis of the knee flexors.

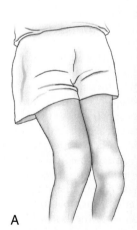
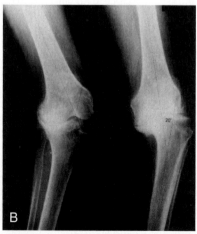
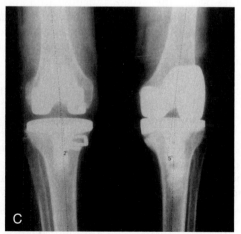

A   B   C

FIGURE 13-37. Bilateral frontal plane malalignment in the knees of an 83-year-old woman. **A,** The classic "wind-swept" deformity, with excessive genu valgum on the right and genu varum on the left. **B** and **C** are the x-ray films of the patient in **A,** before and after bilateral knee replacement. Note in **B,** the hypertrophic bone formation in areas of increased stress. With excessive genu valgum, the stress is greater on the lateral compartment; with genu varum, the stress is greater on the medial compartment. (Courtesy Joseph Davies, MD, Aurora Advanced Orthopedics, Milwaukee.)

Case Report: Pathomechanics and Treatment of Severe Genu Recurvatum

Figure 13-38, *A* shows a case of severe genu recurvatum of the left knee caused by a flaccid muscle paralysis from polio, contracted 30 years earlier. The deformity progressed slowly over the previous 20 years as the individual continued to walk without a knee brace. She has partial paralysis of the left quadriceps and hip flexors but complete paralysis of the left knee flexors. Her completely paralyzed left ankle joint was surgically fused in about 25 degrees of plantar flexion.

Several interrelated factors are responsible for the development of the severe deformity depicted in Figure 13-38, *A*. Because of the fixed plantar flexion position of the ankle, the tibia must be tilted posteriorly so that the bottom of the foot makes full contact with the ground. This surgery had been designed 30 years earlier as a way to provide the knee with greater stability in extension. Over the years, however, the posterior tilted position of the tibia led to an overstretching of the posterior structures of the knee, which ultimately led to the hyperextension deformity. Of particular importance is the fact that total paralysis of the knee's flexor muscles provided no direct muscular resistance against the knee's ensuing hyperextension deformity. Furthermore, the greater the hyperextension deformity, the longer the external moment arm

(EMA) available to body weight to perpetuate the deformity. Without bracing of the knee, the hyperextension deformity produced a vicious circle, allowing continuous stretching of the posterior structures of the knee, increased length of the external moment arm, greater extension external torque, and a continuous progression of the deformity.

A recurring theme in this chapter is the fact that the knee functions as the middle link of the lower limb, and it is therefore vulnerable to deforming loads from musculoskeletal pathology at either end of the lower extremity. This case report demonstrates how an excessive and fixed plantar flexed ankle can, over the years, predispose a person to genu recurvatum. As depicted in Figure 13-38, *B*, a relatively simple and inexpensive modification in footwear was used to treat the hyperextension deformity. Wearing tennis shoes with "built-up" heels provided excellent reduction in the severity of the genu recurvatum. The raised heel tilted the tibia and knee *anteriorly*, thereby significantly reducing the length of the deforming external moment arm at the knee. Body weight now produced less hyperextension torque at the knee, held in check by the anteriorly tilted tibia and the rigidity provided by the fused ankle joint.

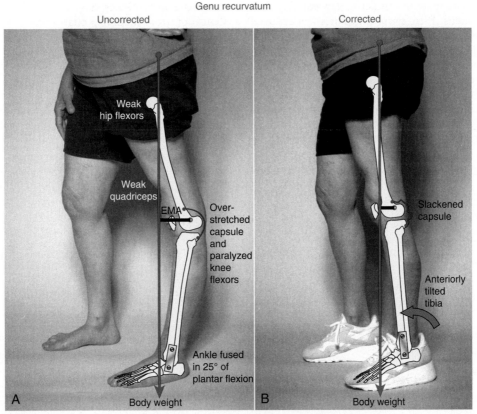

Genu recurvatum

FIGURE 13-38. Subject showing severe genu recurvatum of the left knee secondary to polio. In addition to sporadic muscle weakness throughout the left lower extremity, the left ankle was surgically fused in 25 degrees of plantar flexion. **A,** When the subject stands barefoot, the body weight acts with an abnormally large external moment arm *(EMA)* at the knee. The resulting large extensor torque amplifies the magnitude of the knee hyperextension deformity. **B,** Subject is able to reduce the severity of the recurvatum deformity by wearing tennis shoes with a built-up heel. The shoe tilts her tibia and knee forward (indicated by the green arrow), thereby reducing the length of the deforming external moment arm at the knee.

SYNOPSIS

The unique movements allowed at the knee can be observed during many activities that involve the lower limb as a whole. Consider, for example, a person jumping high into the air. During the preparatory phase of the jump, the body lowers as the hips and knees flex and the ankles dorsiflex. This action stretches the appropriate biarticular muscles as a way to augment their propulsive action as hip-and-knee extensors and ankle plantar flexors. When appropriately timed, these actions propel and functionally elongate the body, maximizing the distance of the jump. A person with limited motion, pain, or significant weakness of the hip, knee, or ankle muscles would naturally have great difficulty in performing this activity.

Although axial rotation of the knee is essential to a normal gait pattern, the full expression of this motion is most apparent during femoral-on-tibial activities, in which the femur (and the rest of the upper body) rotates relative to a fixed lower leg. This movement is fundamental to running and rapidly changing directions, as well as many sporting activities, including dance. This femoral-on-tibial motion is guided and stabilized by muscle activation, body weight, articular fit between the femoral condyles and the menisci, and tension in several ligaments, notably the ACL and collateral ligaments. As will be described in the next chapter, the tibia and talus typically also participate in this activity by rotating relative to a fixed calcaneus. Pain, muscle weakness, or reduced motion in any single joint in the lower limb will require some musculoskeletal compensation at one or several other joints. Such compensations often give important clues to the underlying cause of the origin of the pathomechanics.

In contrast to other joints of the lower limb, the stability of the knee is dependent less on its bony fit and more on the surrounding muscles and periarticular connective tissues. The lack of bony restraint to most knee motions enhances its range of motion, but at the expense of increasing the vulnerability of the knee to injury. The MCL, posterior-medial capsule, and ACL are particularly vulnerable to injury from large valgus and axial rotation forces that affect the lateral side of a weight-bearing lower limb, especially if the knee is in or near full extension. The extended knee, the joint's close-packed position, renders most tissues taut. Although this ligamentous pre-tension offers greater protection to the knee, the ligaments are closer to their mechanical failure point and therefore more vulnerable to injury when further strained.

Prevention of knee injuries is an important topic within sports medicine and demands continued attention and research. Although it may be possible to reduce the incidence of knee injuries during some noncontact sports, completely avoiding knee injury may be virtually impossible in certain high-velocity contact sports, such as American football or rugby. Protection may be maximized, however, by improving the athlete's ability to absorb or, when feasible, avoid the full effect of such an impact. This may be accomplished through better design of equipment and playing environment, and establishment of training programs that sufficiently strengthen and condition muscles, increase control and agility of the sport-specific movements, and improve the athlete's proprioception. Determining how and if these preventative approaches are successful requires systematic and controlled research performed by a wide range of health, physical education, and medical professionals.

As described previously in this chapter, biomechanics of the knee are strongly influenced by its central location between the hip and foot. During weight bearing, the position of the hip directly affects the position of the knee. This strong kinematic dependency has important clinical implications. Consider, for example, that contraction of the gluteus maximus can indirectly assist with knee extension provided that the foot is firmly planted on the ground. This concept is important when teaching a person with a transfemoral amputation to climb stairs while wearing an above-the-knee prosthesis. Many other clinical examples relate to the role of the hip abductor and external rotator muscles in controlling the frontal and horizontal plane alignment of the knee. This concept is heavily embedded within the treatment or prevention of ACL injury, abnormal tracking of the patella, or osteoarthritis of the knee. The next chapter will describe how the bones and joints of the ankle and foot influence the alignment of the lower leg, which also ultimately affects the tension within the structures of the knee.

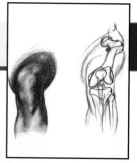

ADDITIONAL CLINICAL CONNECTIONS

CLINICAL CONNECTION 13-1
Further Biomechanical Considerations on the Function of the Patella

As described in the text, the patella displaces the tendon of the quadriceps anteriorly, thereby increasing the internal moment arm used by the knee extensor mechanism. In this way the patella can augment the torque potential of the quadriceps. Figure 13-39 shows an analogy between a mechanical crane and the human knee. Both use a "spacer" to increase the distance between the axis of rotation and the internal "supporting" force. The larger the internal moment arm, the greater the internal torque produced per level of force generated by the quadriceps muscle of the human knee (or transferred by the cable in the crane).

In cases of disease or trauma, the patella may need to be surgically removed. One study reported that the internal moment arm of a patellectomized knee reduced from 4.7 cm to 3.8 cm, when averaged across the full range of motion.[117] Depending on the patient, the clinician may consider the functional impact of this reduced moment arm (leverage) in one of two ways. First, the reduced leverage suggests that, in theory, the maximal knee extensor torque potential may be reduced by about 19%, although muscle hypertrophy or other neuromuscular adaptations may minimize this torque deficit. A second consideration, however, may be that without a patella a person would need to generate 23.5% *more force* to produce an equivalent pre-patellectomized extensor torque. The increased muscle force is required to compensate for the proportional loss in leverage. As a consequence, greater muscular-based compression force is generated on the tibiofemoral joint, creating greater wear on the articular cartilage (Figure 13-40). A subtle but important function of the patella, therefore, is to reduce the magnitude of the quadriceps force needed to perform ordinary submaximal efforts, such as ascending a step. This reduced demand indirectly lowers the compressive load across the articular cartilage and menisci at the knee. When considered over many years, this reduction would limit mechanical wear on the knee.

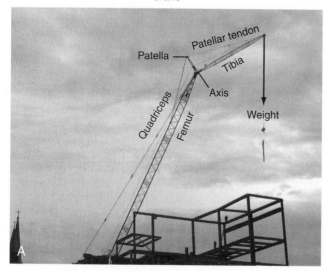

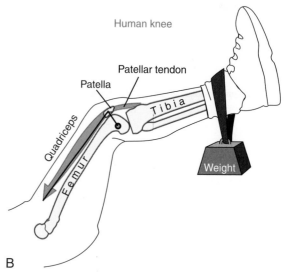

FIGURE 13-39. An analogy is made between a crane **(A)** and the human knee **(B).** In the crane, the moment arm is the distance between the axis and the tip of the metal piece that functions as a patella does.

Continued

ADDITIONAL CLINICAL CONNECTIONS

CLINICAL CONNECTION 13-1
Further Biomechanical Considerations on the Function of the Patella—cont'd

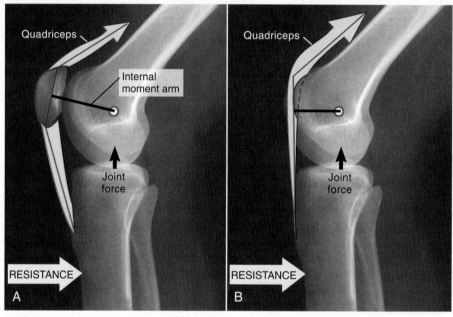

FIGURE 13-40. The quadriceps is shown contracting with a patella **(A)** and without a patella **(B).** In each case the quadriceps muscle maintains static rotary equilibrium at the knee by responding to an external resistance (torque). The magnitude of the external resistance (torque) is assumed to be equal in A and B. The moment arm *(black line)* is reduced in **B** because of the patellectomy. As a consequence, the quadriceps in **B** must produce a proportional greater force to match the external resistance. The greater force of the quadriceps creates a greater joint (reaction) force, which must cross the tibiofemoral joint.

ADDITIONAL CLINICAL CONNECTIONS

CLINICAL CONNECTION 13-2
Female Athletes at a Greater Risk for Anterior Cruciate Ligament Injury

Female athletes are at least three to five times more likely to experience an anterior cruciate ligament (ACL) injury compared with males playing at relatively similar levels of the same sport.[7,79,170,171,184] The risk is greatest in noncontact sports that involve jumping and landing combined with vigorous pivoting motions, such as basketball, soccer, and gymnastics.[171,179,246] The elevated risk of injury, combined with the ever-growing number of women participating in high-school and college sports, has led to an alarming increase in the number of ACL injuries in this relatively young population.

Considerable research has focused on the underlying causes for the gender bias in ACL injuries. Understanding why females are at an elevated risk for injury is an essential step in developing effective preventative measures. Research has focused on factors such as *anatomy* (including, for example, bone and joint alignment, strength of the ACL, overall ligamentous laxity, body mass index, size of the femoral intercondylar notch), *hormonal fluctuations, muscular strength* (including stiffness and fatigue), and *neuromuscular control.** Although some degree of actual or theoretic cause-and-effect relationships has been cited for each of these factors, a definitive and universal causal relationship is difficult to establish.

Risk factors possibly related to neuromuscular control have received considerable attention from the sports medicine community.[73] In particular, researchers have identified specific differences in the manner in which females and males land from a jump.[30,31,91] Several studies have demonstrated that females typically land with their knees in greater valgus alignment than males.[30,60,121,128] This landing was previously highlighted in Figure 13-21. Landing in this manner, particularly if unexpected and unprotected by specific muscular activation, can place large and potentially damaging tensile loads on the ACL, as well as the medial collateral ligament.[91,281] This potentially deleterious knee posture may arise from reduced control or strength of the knee musculature (i.e., different components within the quadriceps and

*References 30, 72, 80, 103, 182, 249.

hamstrings), or, more likely, from reduced control or strength of the hip abductor and external rotators muscles. As indicated in Figure 13-21, weakness or poor control of the hip abductors and external rotators allows the hip (femur) to assume a relative adducted and internally rotated position—kinematics that strongly contribute to valgus and excessive external rotation of the knee.

Furthermore, most research has shown that females land from a jump with hips and knees in slightly greater *extension* than males—frequently referred to as a "stiffer" landing.[30] Electromyographic (EMG) studies have also consistently shown that females display a greater quadriceps-to-hamstrings activation ratio compared with males at or immediately after the landing.[60,105,154,272] It has been theorized that the purported greater quadriceps activation in females increases the anterior translation of the tibia and thereby increases the strain on the ACL, especially when the subject lands with the knee closer to full extension. Combining this scenario with a large and unexpected valgus-and-axial rotation load on the knee is a potentially dangerous situation.

Partially in response to the research in this area, specific prevention programs have been developed that aim to reduce ACL injury in female athletes, most commonly for the sport of soccer. In addition to the traditional focus on improving strength, flexibility, aerobic conditioning, and sport-specific skills, most programs incorporate proprioceptive and "neuromuscular" coordination components within the training and warm-up activities.[68] These components include more complex and rigorous agility and plyometric training, in addition to educating the athletes about safer landing techniques. The hope is that the athletes can establish a prelanding muscular activation pattern that effectively stabilizes against a catastrophic valgus collapse of the knee.[30]

Most ACL prevention programs for female athletes have reported a decrease in the rate of injuries[73,89,155] Although the results are very promising, more rigorous research is needed to better understand the neuromuscular and biomechanical mechanisms behind the intervention. This should lead to further improvement of the prevention strategies and hopefully allow them to be directed toward a broader group of athletes.

ADDITIONAL CLINICAL CONNECTIONS

CLINICAL CONNECTION 13-3
Some Biomechanical Considerations When Performing Knee Exercises after Surgical Reconstruction of the Anterior Cruciate Ligament

Because a completely torn anterior cruciate ligament (ACL) does not heal of its own accord, surgical reconstruction is often recommended.[15,228] Surgical repair is often justified based on the overall functional importance of the ACL and on the fact that ACL-deficient knees frequently show premature signs of degeneration.[14]

Physical rehabilitation is an essential component of a successful ACL repair, and volumes of material have been published on differing physical rehabilitation protocols. Topics that have received considerable attention in the research literature are listed in the box.[15] One universal goal of treatment in postsurgical rehabilitation is to increase the strength, control, and normal activation pattern of the muscles of the knee. In theory, accomplishing these goals increases muscular stability around the knee, which helps safeguard the grafted material, improve gait kinematics, protect against reinjury, and limit joint deterioration.

Selected Topics of Interest in the Postsurgical ACL Rehabilitation Literature
- Immediate versus delayed motion
- Immediate versus delayed weight bearing
- Closed versus open kinematic chain exercises
- Bracing
- Home- versus clinic-based rehabilitation
- Neuromuscular electrical stimulation versus voluntary muscle contraction
- Specificity of exercise intensity and type
- Duration of rehabilitation

Considerable research has focused on the change in knee muscle function after ACL injury and reconstruction.[271] One issue is the relatively frequent persistent inhibition, atrophy, and weakness of the quadriceps, potentially negatively affecting the kinematics of the knee. Addressing persistent quadriceps weakness is therefore an important element of postsurgical rehabilitation.

Clinicians must be able to design strengthening exercises that offer significant resistance to cause hypertrophy of the quadriceps musculature without simultaneously damaging or straining the surgically grafted material. Excessive strain could result in permanent deformation of the graft or disruption of the graft fixation to the bone, thereby affecting the stability of the knee and the effectiveness of the surgery. In general, the concern after some ACL reconstructions is to avoid exercise situations in which a strong contraction of the quadriceps muscle would create excessive anterior translation of the tibia (or posterior translation of the femur). This concern is usually most relevant during the early phase of rehabilitation, when the grafted ACL material is most vulnerable to injury or being overstretched. Although this issue is always a concern, the degree of the concern will vary depending on the patient's history, time since surgery, type of graft or surgery, and training and philosophy of the orthopedic surgeon physical therapist, or athletic trainer.

The following two-part principle serves as the basis for understanding how activated knee muscle affects the strain (and therefore tension) in the ACL or grafted surrogate material: (1) *ACL strain increases as the line of force of the quadriceps more closely opposes the primary action of the ligament*, and (2) *the amount of ACL strain is proportional to the magnitude of the muscle activation.* As will be described, a muscle's line of force and the primary action of the ACL both change as a function of knee flexion angle.

For reasons described previously, strengthening of the quadriceps muscle is an important component of postsurgical rehabilitation of the ACL. With the knee in full extension, Herzog and Read reported that the line of force of the quadriceps (patellar tendon) is approximately 20 degrees relative to the long axis of the tibia (Figure 13-41, *A*). In theory, 34% of the force produced by the quadriceps (sine of 20 degrees) would pull the tibia anteriorly, directly opposing the primary action of the ACL. A mathematic-based computerized model using different data expands this concept across 80 degrees of flexion by plotting the tension in the ACL caused by forces generated by isolated, submaximal contraction of the quadriceps, and by the combined coactivation of both the quadriceps and hamstring muscles (Figure 13-42).[168] Note in this computerized model how sharply ACL tension increases during an isolated contraction of the quadriceps between 30 to 40 degrees of flexion and full knee extension. Tension in the ACL is greatest during quadriceps contraction with the knee in full extension because the extended knee creates the greatest angle-of-insertion of the patellar tendon into the tibial tuberosity (shown as 20 degrees in Figure 13-41, *A*). Although not shown in the graph associated with Figure 13-42, it should be clear that the tension in the ACL would increase proportionally to the increase in *magnitude* of the force in the quadriceps muscle. Theoretically, in the absence of quadriceps activity, regardless of knee angle, the ACL would not be subjected to a significant tensile load.

It is important to note in Figure 13-42 that coactivation of both the quadriceps and hamstring muscles in the last 20 to 30 degrees of extension reduces but does not eliminate the anterior translation force generated by the quadriceps. At these knee joint angles, the line of pull of the hamstrings has a relatively strong vertical bias, which reduces their ability to completely offset the strong anterior pull of the quadriceps on the ACL.

ADDITIONAL CLINICAL CONNECTIONS

CLINICAL CONNECTION 13-3
Some Biomechanical Considerations When Performing Knee Exercises after Surgical Reconstruction of the Anterior Cruciate Ligament—cont'd

The concepts described in the preceding paragraphs provide credence to the advice given to some patients to avoid exercises in the very early phases of post-ACL reconstruction rehabilitation that involve strong and isolated contraction of the quadriceps, specifically in the last 30 to 40 degrees of extension. For example, it is typically advised to avoid tibia-on-femoral full (knee) extension (via an open kinematic chain) while sitting on the edge of a mat. Not only does this exercise require *isolated* contraction of the quadriceps, but the external torque demands imposed on the quadriceps are greatest in full knee extension. As the knee approaches and reaches full extension, the quadriceps muscle must generate a relatively high force at a knee angle at which the muscle force maximally antagonizes (stretches) the ACL. This type of exercise, especially if performed with significant external load placed near the foot, would generate relatively high strain levels within the ACL. Although this exercise may be well tolerated in the late phase of the rehabilitation, it should nevertheless be performed with caution and with full knowledge of the potential effect on the ACL.

The biomechanics described earlier regarding quadriceps-based tension in the ACL change considerably when analyzed in greater knee flexion. With the knee flexed to 80 degrees, for example, the line of force of the quadriceps is approximately parallel with the long axis of the tibia (see Figure 13-41, *B*). Virtually *all* force generated by the quadriceps would pull the tibia superiorly against the femur; none of it would pull the tibia anteriorly against the ACL. As noted in Figure 13-42, ACL tension resulting from isolated quadriceps contraction is near zero at knee angles greater than 70 degrees of flexion. Of importance, *cocontraction* of both the quadriceps and hamstrings theoretically produces zero tension in the ACL at knee angles greater than 30 degrees of flexion. Hamstring activation generally unloads the ACL, most notably as the knee is flexed. The reason for this is very apparent in the 80 degree flexed knee depicted in Figure 13-41, *B*. The line of force of the hamstring muscles at 80 degrees of knee flexion is approximately 80 degrees to the long axis of the tibia. At this amount of flexion, 98% of the force in the hamstrings (based on the sine of 80 degrees) would pull the tibia posteriorly, very effectively unloading (and slackening) the ACL.

Exercises that involve femoral-on-tibial (closed kinematic chain) exercises in moderate degrees of knee flexion therefore place relatively low and usually acceptable levels of strain on the ACL.[12,16,27] In addition to their functional nature, these types of exercises are well ingrained into ACL rehabilitation protocols because they require quadriceps activation in a more flexed knee position, and they naturally require coactivation of the quadriceps and hamstrings muscles. (The hamstring muscles are essential to

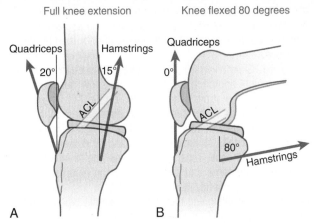

FIGURE 13-41. Lines of force of the quadriceps and hamstring muscles relative to the anterior cruciate ligament (ACL) for a knee in full extension **(A)** and in 80 degrees of flexion **(B).** Drawing based on mean data from five cadavers, based on the work of Herzog and Read.[88] Note that the change in joint angle significantly alters the line of force of the muscles and the orientation of the ACL. Angles-of-insertion of the muscles are indicated relative to the long axis of the tibia. Angles are approximate, and vectors are not drawn to scale.

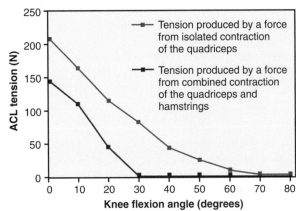

FIGURE 13-42. Relationship between the tension in the anterior cruciate ligament (ACL) and the knee joint angle during a submaximal force produced by (1) isolated contraction of the quadriceps and (2) a combined contraction from the quadriceps and hamstrings. The combined muscle force was designed to simulate cocontraction of the two sets of muscles. (Data based on work of Mesfar and Shirazi-Adl, using a three-dimensional finite element model of the entire knee joint, including muscles and ligaments.[168])

Continued

ADDITIONAL CLINICAL CONNECTIONS

CLINICAL CONNECTION 13-3
Some Biomechanical Considerations When Performing Knee Exercises after Surgical Reconstruction of the Anterior Cruciate Ligament—cont'd

the control of hip motion during the squat activity, for example.) As stated above, tension in the ACL remains at zero when the muscles are coactivated at knee angles greater than 30 degrees of flexion.

Closing Comments: This Clinical Connection describes a biomechanical approach to understanding how quadriceps activation affects the strain in and tension on the ACL. In summary, strain in the ACL can be *minimized* by exercises or activities that (1) coactivate the quadriceps and hamstrings in knee flexion angles greater than about 30 degrees and (2) demand low forces from the quadriceps, regardless of knee angle. Although these summary statements and data presented in Figures 13-41 and 13-42 are very useful, clinicians must take into account other variables when designing the most appropriate type of exercises for a given patient. These variables include the specific charac-

teristics of the patient (occupation, age, health, activity level, etc) and the time since surgery and type of surgical reconstruction. No one approach to the design of quadriceps strengthening exercises after ACL reconstruction is best for all patients and all clinical scenarios.[81,177,202,261,279] Although the theme of this feature has been on understanding *how* to limit the muscular-based tension in the ACL, it did not address equally important issues as far as *when* and the *extent to which* the tension should be limited. At some point in the rehabilitation process, tension in the ACL (or grafted material) likely facilitates healing and is actually considered therapeutic.[265] The clinician must continually be challenged to adjust exercise protocols for postsurgical ACL rehabilitation as new research on biomechanics, surgery, and material properties of the ACL and replacement materials continues to emerge.

ADDITIONAL CLINICAL CONNECTIONS

CLINICAL CONNECTION 13-4
Synergy among Monoarticular and Biarticular Muscles of the Hip and Knee

TYPICAL MOVEMENT COMBINATIONS: HIP-AND-KNEE EXTENSION OR HIP-AND-KNEE FLEXION:
Many movements performed by the lower extremities involve the cyclic actions of hip-and-knee extension or hip-and-knee flexion. These patterns of movement are fundamental components of walking, running, jumping, and climbing. Hip-and-knee extension propels the body forward or upward. Conversely, hip-and-knee flexion advances or swings the lower limb or is used to slowly lower the body toward the ground. These movements are controlled, in part, through a synergy among monoarticular and polyarticular muscles, many of which cross the hip and knee.

Figure 13-43 shows an interaction of muscles during the hip-and-knee extension phase of running. The vastus group and gluteus maximus—two monoarticular muscles—are active synergistically, along with the biarticular semitendinosus and rectus femoris muscles. The vastus group of the quadriceps and the semitendinosus are both electrically active, yet their net torque at the knee favors *extension*. This occurs because the contracting vastus muscles overpower the contraction efforts of the semitendinosus. As a consequence, the tension stored in the forced lengthening of the semitendinosus across the knee is used to assist with active extension at the hip. In the combined movement of hip-and-knee extension, therefore, the semitendinosus muscle (when considered as a whole) extends the hip but actually contracts or shortens a relatively short distance. Because the contraction excursion is low, so is the contraction velocity when considered over a similar time span.

The action of the semitendinosus muscle as described favors relatively high force production per level of neural drive or effort. The physiologic basis for this efficient muscular action rests on the force-velocity and length-tension relationships of muscle (see Chapter 3). Consider first the effect of muscle velocity on muscle force production. Muscle force per level of effort increases sharply as the contraction velocity is reduced. As an example, a muscle contracting at 6.3% of its maximum shortening velocity produces a force of about 75% of its maximum. Slowing the contraction velocity to only 2.2% of maximal (i.e., very near isometric) raises force output to 90% of maximum.[75] In the movement of hip-and-knee extension, the vastus muscles, by extending the knee, indirectly augment hip extension force by reducing the contraction velocity of the semitendinosus.

Consider next the effect of muscle length on the passive force produced within a biarticular muscle. Based on a muscle's passive length-tension relationship, the internal resistance or force within a muscle, such as the semitendinosus, increases as it is stretched. The passive force created within the stretched semitendinosus across the extending knee, in this particular example, is "recycled" and used to help extend the hip. In this manner the semitendinosus—as well as all biarticular hamstrings—functions as a "transducer" by transferring force ultimately produced by the contracting vastus muscles to the extending hip.

During active hip-and-knee extension, the gluteus maximus and rectus femoris have a relationship similar to that described between the vastus muscles and the semitendinosus. In essence,

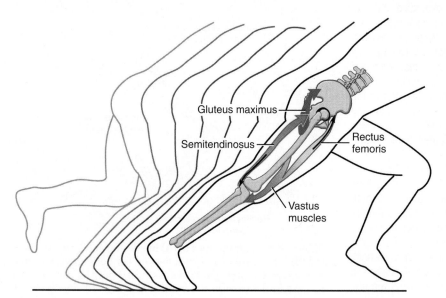

FIGURE 13-43. The action of several monoarticular and biarticular muscles are depicted during the hip-and-knee extension phase of running. Observe that the vastus muscles extend the knee, which then stretches the distal end of the semitendinosus. The gluteus maximus extends the hip, which stretches the proximal end of the rectus femoris. The stretched biarticular muscles are depicted by thin black arrows. The stretch placed on the active biarticular muscles reduces the rate and amount of their overall contraction. (See text for further details.)

Continued

ADDITIONAL CLINICAL CONNECTIONS

CLINICAL CONNECTION 13-4
Synergy among Monoarticular and Biarticular Muscles of the Hip and Knee—cont'd

TABLE 13-7. Examples of Muscle Synergies at the Hip and Knee

	Monoarticular Muscle(s)	Action	Biarticular Transducer(s)	Action Augmented
Active hip and knee extension	Vasti	Knee *extension*	Two-joint hamstrings	Hip *extension*
	Gluteus maximus	Hip *extension*	Rectus femoris	Knee *extension*
Active hip and knee flexion	Iliopsoas	Hip *flexion*	Two-joint hamstrings	Knee *flexion*
	Biceps femoris (short head), popliteus	Knee *flexion*	Rectus femoris	Hip *flexion*

Modified from Leiber RL: *Skeletal muscle: structure and function*, Baltimore, 1992, Williams & Wilkins.

the monoarticular gluteus maximus augments knee extension force by its dominating influence over hip extension. This dominance, in turn, stretches the activated rectus femoris. In this example the rectus femoris is the biarticular transducer, transferring force from the gluteus maximus to knee extension. A summary of these and other muscular interactions used during hip-and-knee flexion are listed in Table 13-7.

The functional interdependence among the hip-and-knee extensor muscles and among the hip-and-knee flexor muscles should be considered in evaluation of functional activities that require these active movement combinations. Consider, for example, the combined movements of hip-and-knee extension required to stand from a seated position. Weakness of the vastus muscles could indirectly cause difficulty in extending the hip, whereas weakness of the gluteus maximus could indirectly cause difficulty in extending the knee. Strengthening programs may benefit by designing resistive challenges that incorporate this natural synergy between these muscles. Consider also someone with patellofemoral joint pain during active contraction of the quadriceps. Encouraging this person to activate his or her hip extensor muscles to assist with knee extension may reduce the active demands placed on the quadriceps, thereby potentially lowering the compression forces placed on the patellofemoral joint.

ATYPICAL MOVEMENT COMBINATIONS: HIP FLEXION AND KNEE EXTENSION, OR HIP EXTENSION AND KNEE FLEXION:
Consider active movement patterns of the hip and knee that are "out of phase" with the more typical movement patterns described earlier. Hip flexion can occur with knee extension (Figure 13-44, *A*), or hip extension can occur with knee flexion (Figure 13-44, *B*). The physiologic consequences of these movements are very different from those described in Figure 13-43. In Figure 13-44, *A*, the biarticular rectus femoris must shorten a great distance, and with relatively high velocity, in

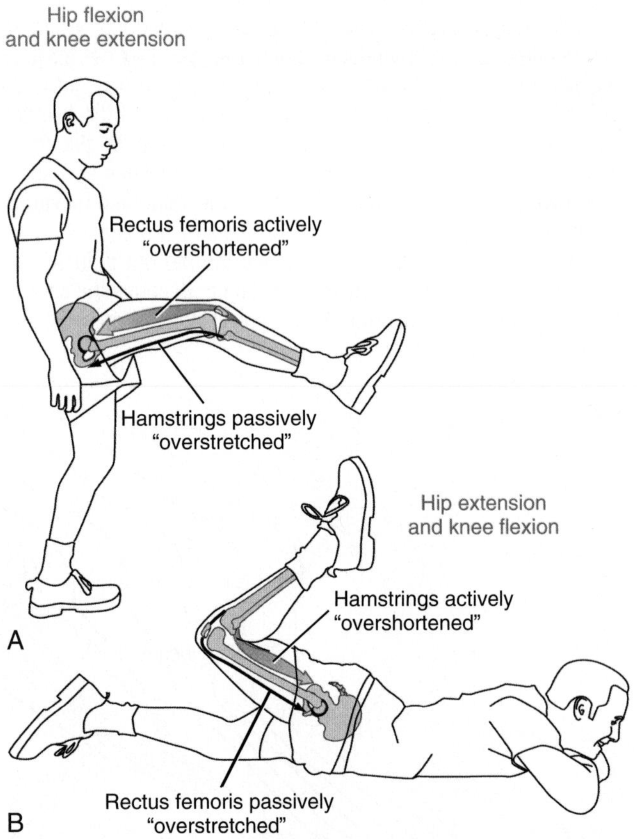

Hip flexion and knee extension

Rectus femoris actively "overshortened"

Hamstrings passively "overstretched"

Hip extension and knee flexion

Hamstrings actively "overshortened"

Rectus femoris passively "overstretched"

FIGURE 13-44. The motions of **(A)** hip flexion and knee extension and **(B)** hip extension and knee flexion. For both movements the near-maximal contraction of the biarticular muscles *(red)* causes a near-maximal stretch in the biarticular antagonist muscles *(black arrows)*.

ADDITIONAL CLINICAL CONNECTIONS

CLINICAL CONNECTION 13-4
Synergy among Monoarticular and Biarticular Muscles of the Hip and Knee—cont'd

order to simultaneously flex the hip and extend the knee. Even with maximal effort, active knee extension is usually limited during this action. Based on the length-tension and force-velocity relationships of muscle, the rectus femoris is not able to develop maximal knee extensor force. The biarticular hamstrings are also overstretched across both the hip and knee, thereby passively resisting knee extension.

The situation described in Figure 13-44, *A* also applies to the movement depicted in Figure 13-44, *B*. The biarticular hamstrings must contract to a very short length—a movement that is often accompanied by cramping. Furthermore, the biarticular rectus femoris is overstretched across both the hip and knee, thereby passively resisting knee flexion. For both reasons, knee flexion force and range of motion are usually limited by the out-of-phase movement.

The atypical movements depicted in Figure 13-44 may have a useful purpose. Consider the action of kicking a ball. Elastic energy is stored in the stretched rectus femoris by the preparatory movement of combined hip extension and knee flexion. The action of kicking the ball involves a rapid and near-full contraction of the rectus femoris to simultaneously flex the hip and extend the knee. The goal of this action is to dissipate *all* force in the rectus femoris as quickly as possible. In contrast, activities such as walking, jogging, or cycling use biarticular muscles in a manner that forces are developed more slowly and in a repetitive or cyclic fashion. In these examples, the length changes in the rectus femoris and semitendinosus, for instance, are relatively small throughout much of the activation cycle (as shown in Figure 13-43). In this way, muscles avoid repetitive cycles of storing and immediately releasing relatively large amounts of energy. More moderate levels of active and passive forces are cooperatively shared between muscles, thereby optimizing the metabolic efficiency of the movement.

REFERENCES

1. Amis AA: Current concepts on anatomy and biomechanics of patellar stability, *Sports Med Arthrosc Rev* 15:48-56, 2007.
2. Amis AA, Bull AM, Gupte CM, et al: Biomechanics of the PCL and related structures: posterolateral, posteromedial and meniscofemoral ligaments, *Knee Surg Sports Traumatol Arthrosc* 11:271-281, 2003.
3. Amis AA, Firer P, Mountney J, et al: Anatomy and biomechanics of the medial patellofemoral ligament, *Knee* 10:215-220, 2003.
4. Amis AA, Senavongse W, Bull AM: Patellofemoral kinematics during knee flexion-extension: an in vitro study, *J Orthop Res* 24:2201-2211, 2006.
5. Andrade JR, Grant C, Dixon AS: Joint distension and reflex muscle inhibition in the knee, *J Bone Joint Surg Am* 47:313-322, 1965.
6. Andriacchi TP, Birac D: Functional testing in the anterior cruciate ligament–deficient knee, *Clin Orthop Relat Res* 288:40-47, 1993.
7. Arendt E, Dick R: Knee injury patterns among men and women in collegiate basketball and soccer. NCAA data and review of literature, *Am J Sports Med* 23:694-701, 1995.
8. Armour T, Forwell L, Litchfield R, et al: Isokinetic evaluation of internal/external tibial rotation strength after the use of hamstring tendons for anterior cruciate ligament reconstruction, *Am J Sports Med* 32:1639-1643, 2004.
9. Arneja S, McConkey MO, Mulpuri K, et al: Graft tensioning in anterior cruciate ligament reconstruction: a systematic review of randomized controlled trials, *Arthroscopy* 25:200-207, 2009.
10. Besier TF, Draper CE, Gold GE, et al: Patellofemoral joint contact area increases with knee flexion and weight-bearing, *J Orthop Res* 23:345-350, 2005.
11. Besier TF, Gold GE, Beaupré GS, Delp SL: A modeling framework to estimate patellofemoral joint cartilage stress in vivo, *Med Sci Sports Exerc* 37:1924-1930, 2005.
12. Beynnon BD, Fleming BC: Anterior cruciate ligament strain in-vivo: a review of previous work, *J Biomech* 31:519-525, 1998.
13. Beynnon BD, Fleming BC, Johnson RJ, et al: Anterior cruciate ligament strain behavior during rehabilitation exercises in vivo, *Am J Sports Med* 23:24-34, 1995.
14. Beynnon BD, Johnson RJ, Abate JA, et al: Treatment of anterior cruciate ligament injuries, part 1, *Am J Sports Med* 33:1579-1602, 2005.
15. Beynnon BD, Johnson RJ, Abate JA, et al: Treatment of anterior cruciate ligament injuries, part 2, *Am J Sports Med* 33:1751-1767, 2005.
16. Beynnon BD, Johnson RJ, Fleming BC, et al: The strain behavior of the anterior cruciate ligament during squatting and active flexion-extension. A comparison of an open and a closed kinetic chain exercise, *Am J Sports Med* 25:823-829, 1997.
17. Bicos J, Fulkerson JP, Amis A: Current concepts review: the medial patellofemoral ligament, *Am J Sports Med* 35:484-492, 2007.
18. Bizzini M, Childs JD, Piva SR, Delitto A: Systematic review of the quality of randomized controlled trials for patellofemoral pain syndrome, *J Orthop Sports Phys Ther* 33:4-20, 2003.
19. Boden BP, Dean GS, Feagin JA Jr, Garrett WE Jr: Mechanisms of anterior cruciate ligament injury, *Orthopedics* 23:573-578, 2000.
20. Bohannon RW, Gajdosik RL, LeVeau BF: Isokinetic knee flexion and extension torque in the upright sitting and semireclined sitting positions, *Phys Ther* 66:1083-1086, 1986.
21. Boling MC, Bolgla LA, Mattacola CG, et al: Outcomes of a weight-bearing rehabilitation program for patients diagnosed with patellofemoral pain syndrome, *Arch Phys Med Rehabil* 87:1428-1435, 2006.
22. Boynton MD, Tietjens BR: Long-term followup of the untreated isolated posterior cruciate ligament–deficient knee, *Am J Sports Med* 24:306-310, 1996.
23. Bruce WD, Stevens PM: Surgical correction of miserable malalignment syndrome, *J Pediatr Orthop* 24:392-396, 2004.
24. Buford WL Jr, Ivey FM Jr, Malone JD, et al: Muscle balance at the knee–moment arms for the normal knee and the ACL-minus knee, *IEEE Trans Rehabil Eng* 5:367-379, 1997.
25. Buford WL Jr, Ivey FM Jr, Nakamura T, et al: Internal/external rotation moment arms of muscles at the knee: moment arms for the normal knee and the ACL-deficient knee, *Knee* 8:293-303, 2001.
26. Butler DL, Noyes FR, Grood ES: Ligamentous restraints to anterior-posterior drawer in the human knee. A biomechanical study, *J Bone Joint Surg Am* 62:259-270, 1980.
27. Bynum EB, Barrack RL, Alexander AH: Open versus closed chain kinetic exercises after anterior cruciate ligament reconstruction. A prospective randomized study, *Am J Sports Med* 23:401-406, 1995.
28. Calmels PM, Nellen M, van dB, I, et al: Concentric and eccentric isokinetic assessment of flexor-extensor torque ratios at the hip, knee, and ankle in a sample population of healthy subjects, *Arch Phys Med Rehabil* 78:1224-1230, 1997.
29. Campbell SE, Sanders TG, Morrison WB: MR imaging of meniscal cysts: incidence, location, and clinical significance, *AJR Am J Roentgenol* 177:409-413, 2001.
30. Chappell JD, Creighton RA, Giuliani C, et al: Kinematics and electromyography of landing preparation in vertical stop-jump: risks for non-contact anterior cruciate ligament injury, *Am J Sports Med* 35:235-241, 2007.
31. Chappell JD, Yu B, Kirkendall DT, Garrett WE: A comparison of knee kinetics between male and female recreational athletes in stop-jump tasks, *Am J Sports Med* 30:261-267, 2002.
32. Chhabra A, Starman JS, Ferretti M, et al: Anatomic, radiographic, biomechanical, and kinematic evaluation of the anterior cruciate ligament and its two functional bundles, *J Bone Joint Surg Am* 88(Suppl 4):2-10, 2006.
33. Clancy WG Jr, Sutherland TB: Combined posterior cruciate ligament injuries, *Clin Sports Med* 13:629-647, 1994.
34. Cochrane JL, Lloyd DG, Buttfield A, et al: Characteristics of anterior cruciate ligament injuries in Australian football, *J Sci Med Sport* 10:96-104, 2007.
35. Cole BJ, Dennis MG, Lee SJ, et al: Prospective evaluation of allograft meniscus transplantation: a minimum 2-year follow-up, *Am J Sports Med* 34:919-927, 2006.
36. Coqueiro KR, Bevilaqua-Grossi D, Bérzin F, et al: Analysis on the activation of the VMO and VLL muscles during semisquat exercises with and without hip adduction in individuals with patellofemoral pain syndrome, *J Electromyogr Kinesiol* 15:596-603, 2005.
37. Covey DC, Sapega AA, Riffenburgh RH: The effects of sequential sectioning of defined posterior cruciate ligament fiber regions on translational knee motion, *Am J Sports Med* 36:480-486, 2008.
38. Crenshaw SJ, Pollo FE, Calton EF: Effects of lateral-wedged insoles on kinetics at the knee, *Clin Orthop Relat Res* 375:185-192, 2000.
39. Crossley K, Bennell K, Green S, et al: Physical therapy for patellofemoral pain: a randomized, double-blinded, placebo-controlled trial, *Am J Sports Med* 30:857-865, 2002.
40. Crossley K, Bennell K, Green S, McConnell J: A systematic review of physical interventions for patellofemoral pain syndrome, *Clin J Sport Med* 11:103-110, 2001.
41. Csintalan RP, Schulz MM, Woo J, et al: Gender differences in patellofemoral joint biomechanics, *Clin Orthop Relat Res* 402:260-269, 2002.
42. deAndrade JR, Grant C, Dixon ASJ: Joint distension and reflex muscle inhibition in the knee, *J Bone Joint Surg Am* 47:313-322, 1965.
43. DeFrate LE, Gill TJ, Li G: In vivo function of the posterior cruciate ligament during weightbearing knee flexion, *Am J Sports Med* 32:1923-1928, 2004.
44. DeHaven KE, Lintner DM: Athletic injuries: comparison by age, sport, and gender, *Am J Sports Med* 14:218-224, 1986.
45. DeMorat G, Weinhold P, Blackburn T, et al: Aggressive quadriceps loading can induce noncontact anterior cruciate ligament injury, *Am J Sports Med* 32:477-483, 2004.
46. Dupont JY: Synovial plicae of the knee. Controversies and review, *Clin Sports Med* 16:87-122, 1997.
47. Eckstein F, Wirth W, Hudelmaier M, et al: Patterns of femorotibial cartilage loss in knees with neutral, varus, and valgus alignment, *Arthritis Rheum* 59:1563-1570, 2008.
48. Edwards A, Bull AM, Amis AA: The attachments of the anteromedial and posterolateral fibre bundles of the anterior cruciate ligament: Part 1: tibial attachment, *Knee Surg Sports Traumatol Arthrosc* 15:1414-1421, 2007.
49. Edwards A, Bull AM, Amis AA: The attachments of the anteromedial and posterolateral fibre bundles of the anterior cruciate ligament. Part 2: femoral attachment, *Knee Surg Sports Traumatol Arthrosc* 16:29-36, 2008.
50. Elias JJ, Kilambi S, Goerke DR, Cosgarea AJ: Improving vastus medialis obliquus function reduces pressure applied to lateral patellofemoral cartilage, *J Orthop Res* 27:578-583, 2009.
51. Englund M, Guermazi A, Roemer FW, et al: Meniscal tear in knees without surgery and the development of radiographic osteoarthritis among middle-aged and elderly persons: The Multicenter Osteoarthritis Study, *Arthritis Rheum* 60:831-839, 2009.
52. Englund M, Roos EM, Lohmander LS: Impact of type of meniscal tear on radiographic and symptomatic knee osteoarthritis: a sixteen-year

followup of meniscectomy with matched controls, *Arthritis Rheum* 48:2178-2187, 2003.

53. Escamilla RF, Fleisig GS, Zheng N, et al: Biomechanics of the knee during closed kinetic chain and open kinetic chain exercises, *Med Sci Sports Exerc* 30:556-569, 1998.

54. Feipel V, Simonnet ML, Rooze M: The proximal attachments of the popliteus muscle: a quantitative study and clinical significance, *Surg Radiol Anat* 25:58-63, 2003.

55. Feller JA, Amis AA, Andrish JT, et al: Surgical biomechanics of the patellofemoral joint, *Arthroscopy* 23:542-553, 2007.

56. Ferretti M, Levicoff EA, Macpherson TA, et al: The fetal anterior cruciate ligament: an anatomic and histologic study, *Arthroscopy* 23:278-283, 2007.

57. Fithian DC, Paxton EW, Stone ML, et al: Epidemiology and natural history of acute patellar dislocation, *Am J Sports Med* 32:1114-1121, 2004.

58. Fleming BC, Ohlén G, Renström PA, et al: The effects of compressive load and knee joint torque on peak anterior cruciate ligament strains, *Am J Sports Med* 31:701-707, 2003.

59. Fleming BC, Renstrom PA, Beynnon BD, et al: The effect of weight-bearing and external loading on anterior cruciate ligament strain, *J Biomech* 34:163-170, 2001.

60. Ford KR, Myer GD, Hewett TE: Valgus knee motion during landing in high school female and male basketball players, *Med Sci Sports Exerc* 35:1745-1750, 2003.

61. Franz JR, Dicharry J, Riley PO, et al: The influence of arch supports on knee torques relevant to knee osteoarthritis, *Med Sci Sports Exerc* 40:913-917, 2008.

62. Fredericson M, Yoon K: Physical examination and patellofemoral pain syndrome, *Am J Phys Med Rehabil* 85:234-243, 2006.

63. Fukuda Y, Woo SL, Loh JC, et al: A quantitative analysis of valgus torque on the ACL: a human cadaveric study, *J Orthop Res* 21:1107-1112, 2003.

64. Fulkerson JP: Diagnosis and treatment of patients with patellofemoral pain, *Am J Sports Med* 30:447-456, 2002.

65. Fulkerson JP, Hungerford DS: *Disorders of the patellofemoral joint*, 2nd ed, Baltimore, 1990, Williams & Wilkins.

66. Fulkerson JP, Tennant R, Jaivin JS, Grunnet M: Histologic evidence of retinacular nerve injury associated with patellofemoral malalignment, *Clin Orthop Relat Res* 197:196-205, 1985.

67. Gehring D, Melnyk M, Gollhofer A: Gender and fatigue have influence on knee joint control strategies during landing, *Clin Biomech (Bristol, Avon)* 24:82-87, 2009.

68. Gilchrist J, Mandelbaum BR, Melancon H, et al: A randomized controlled trial to prevent noncontact anterior cruciate ligament injury in female collegiate soccer players, *Am J Sports Med* 36:1476-1483, 2008.

69. Gill TJ, DeFrate LE, Wang C, et al: The biomechanical effect of posterior cruciate ligament reconstruction on knee joint function. Kinematic response to simulated muscle loads, *Am J Sports Med* 31:530-536, 2003.

70. Goodfellow J, Hungerford DS, Zindel M: Patello-femoral joint mechanics and pathology. 1. Functional anatomy of the patello-femoral joint, *J Bone Joint Surg Br* 58:287-290, 1976.

71. Grace TG, Sweetser ER, Nelson MA, et al: Isokinetic muscle imbalance and knee-joint injuries. A prospective blind study, *J Bone Joint Surg Am* 66:734-740, 1984.

72. Griffin LY, Agel J, Albohm MJ, et al: Noncontact anterior cruciate ligament injuries: risk factors and prevention strategies, *J Am Acad Orthop Surg* 8:141-150, 2000.

73. Griffin LY, Albohm MJ, Arendt EA, et al: Understanding and preventing noncontact anterior cruciate ligament injuries: a review of the Hunt Valley II meeting, January 2005, *Am J Sports Med* 34:1512-1532, 2006.

74. Griffith CJ, Wijdicks CA, LaPrade RF, et al: Force measurements on the posterior oblique ligament and superficial medial collateral ligament proximal and distal divisions to applied loads, *Am J Sports Med* 37:140-148, 2009.

75. Gross MT, Foxworth JL: The role of foot orthoses as an intervention for patellofemoral pain, *J Orthop Sports Phys Ther* 33:661-670, 2003.

76. Gupte CM, Bull AM, Thomas RD, Amis AA: A review of the function and biomechanics of the meniscofemoral ligaments, *Arthroscopy* 19:161-171, 2003.

77. Gupte CM, Smith A, Jamieson N, et al: Meniscofemoral ligaments—structural and material properties, *J Biomech* 35:1623-1629, 2002.

78. Gupte CM, Smith A, McDermott ID, et al: Meniscofemoral ligaments revisited. Anatomical study, age correlation and clinical implications, *J Bone Joint Surg Br* 84:846-851, 2002.

79. Gwinn DE, Wilckens JH, McDevitt ER, et al: The relative incidence of anterior cruciate ligament injury in men and women at the United States Naval Academy, *Am J Sports Med* 28:98-102, 2000.

80. Hashemi J, Chandrashekar N, Mansouri H, et al: The human anterior cruciate ligament: sex differences in ultrastructure and correlation with biomechanical properties, *J Orthop Res* 26:945-950, 2008.

81. Heijne A, Fleming BC, Renstrom PA, et al: Strain on the anterior cruciate ligament during closed kinetic chain exercises, *Med Sci Sports Exerc* 36:935-941, 2004.

82. Heino BJ, Powers CM: Patellofemoral stress during walking in persons with and without patellofemoral pain, *Med Sci Sports Exerc* 34:1582-1593, 2002.

83. Hemmerich A, Brown H, Smith S, et al: Hip, knee, and ankle kinematics of high range of motion activities of daily living, *J Orthop Res* 24:770-781, 2006.

84. Herrington L: The difference in a clinical measure of patella lateral position between individuals with patellofemoral pain and matched controls, *J Orthop Sports Phys Ther* 38:59-62, 2008.

85. Herrington L, Al-Sherhi A: A controlled trial of weight-bearing versus non-weight-bearing exercises for patellofemoral pain, *J Orthop Sports Phys Ther* 37:155-160, 2007.

86. Herrington L, Malloy S, Richards J: The effect of patella taping on vastus medialis oblique and vastus lateralis EMG activity and knee kinematic variables during stair descent, *J Electromyogr Kinesiol* 15:604-607, 2005.

87. Herrington L, Nester C: Q-angle undervalued? The relationship between Q-angle and medio-lateral position of the patella, *Clin Biomech (Bristol, Avon)* 19:1070-1073, 2004.

88. Herzog W, Read LJ: Lines of action and moment arms of the major force-carrying structures crossing the human knee joint, *J Anat* 182:213-230, 1993.

89. Hewett TE, Ford KR, Myer GD: Anterior cruciate ligament injuries in female athletes: Part 2, a meta-analysis of neuromuscular interventions aimed at injury prevention, *Am J Sports Med* 34:490-498, 2006.

90. Hewett TE, Myer GD, Ford KR: Anterior cruciate ligament injuries in female athletes: Part 1, mechanisms and risk factors, *Am J Sports Med* 34:299-311, 2006.

91. Hewett TE, Myer GD, Ford KR, et al: Biomechanical measures of neuromuscular control and valgus loading of the knee predict anterior cruciate ligament injury risk in female athletes: a prospective study, *Am J Sports Med* 33:492-501, 2005.

92. Hewett TE, Zazulak BT, Myer GD, Ford KR: A review of electromyographic activation levels, timing differences, and increased anterior cruciate ligament injury incidence in female athletes, *Br J Sports Med* 39:347-350, 2005.

93. Hinman RS, Bennell KL, Metcalf BR, Crossley KM: Temporal activity of vastus medialis obliquus and vastus lateralis in symptomatic knee osteoarthritis, *Am J Phys Med Rehabil* 81:684-690, 2002.

94. Hinman RS, Payne C, Metcalf BR, et al: Lateral wedges in knee osteoarthritis: what are their immediate clinical and biomechanical effects and can these predict a three-month clinical outcome? *Arthritis Rheum* 59:408-415, 2008.

95. Höher J, Harner CD, Vogrin TM, et al: In situ forces in the posterolateral structures of the knee under posterior tibial loading in the intact and posterior cruciate ligament–deficient knee, *J Orthop Res* 16:675-681, 1998.

96. Höher J, Vogrin TM, Woo SL, et al: In situ forces in the human posterior cruciate ligament in response to muscle loads: a cadaveric study, *J Orthop Res* 17:763-768, 1999.

97. Hollister AM, Jatana S, Singh AK, et al: The axes of rotation of the knee, *Clin Orthop Relat Res* 290:259-268, 1993.

98. Hollman JH, Ginos BE, Kozuchowski J, et al: Relationships between knee valgus, hip-muscle strength, and hip-muscle recruitment during a single-limb step-down, *J Sport Rehabil* 18:104-117, 2009.

99. Hootman JM, Dick R, Agel J: Epidemiology of collegiate injuries for 15 sports: summary and recommendations for injury prevention initiatives, *J Athl Train* 42:311-319, 2007.

100. Horton MG, Hall TL: Quadriceps femoris muscle angle: normal values and relationships with gender and selected skeletal measures, *Phys Ther* 69:897-901, 1989.

101. Hoy MG, Zajac FE, Gordon ME: A musculoskeletal model of the human lower extremity: the effect of muscle, tendon, and moment arm on the moment-angle relationship of musculotendon actuators at the hip, knee, and ankle, *J Biomech* 23:157-169, 1990.

102. Huberti HH, Hayes WC: Patellofemoral contact pressures. The influence of Q-angle and tendofemoral contact, *J Bone Joint Surg Am* 66:715-724, 1984.

103. Hughes G, Watkins J: A risk-factor model for anterior cruciate ligament injury, *Sports Med* 36:411-428, 2006.

104. Hunt MA, Birmingham TB, Giffin JR, Jenkyn TR: Associations among knee adduction moment, frontal plane ground reaction force, and lever arm during walking in patients with knee osteoarthritis, *J Biomech* 39:2213-2220, 2006.

105. Huston LJ, Greenfield ML, Wojtys EM: Anterior cruciate ligament injuries in the female athlete. Potential risk factors, *Clin Orthop Relat Res* 372:50-63, 2000.

106. Inman VT, Saunders JB: Referred pain from skeletal structures, *J Nerv Ment Dis* 99:660-667, 1944.

107. Ireland ML, Willson JD, Ballantyne BT, Davis IM: Hip strength in females with and without patellofemoral pain, *J Orthop Sports Phys Ther* 33:671-676, 2003.

108. Isaac DL, Beard DJ, Price AJ, et al: In-vivo sagittal plane knee kinematics: ACL intact, deficient and reconstructed knees, *Knee* 12:25-31, 2005.

109. Ishii Y, Terajima K, Terashima S, Koga Y: Three-dimensional kinematics of the human knee with intracortical pin fixation, *Clin Orthop Relat Res* 343:144-150, 1997.

110. Janousek AT, Jones DG, Clatworthy M, et al: Posterior cruciate ligament injuries of the knee joint, *Sports Med* 28:429-441, 1999.

111. Johnson F, Leitl S, Waugh W: The distribution of load across the knee. A comparison of static and dynamic measurements, *J Bone Joint Surg Br* 62:346-349, 1980.

112. Johnston LB, Gross MT: Effects of foot orthoses on quality of life for individuals with patellofemoral pain syndrome, *J Orthop Sports Phys Ther* 34:440-448, 2004.

113. Jordaan G, Schwellnus MP: The incidence of overuse injuries in military recruits during basic military training, *Mil Med* 159:421-426, 1994.

114. Jordan SS, DeFrate LE, Nha KW, et al: The in vivo kinematics of the anteromedial and posterolateral bundles of the anterior cruciate ligament during weightbearing knee flexion, *Am J Sports Med* 35:547-554, 2007.

115. Kan JH, Heemskerk AM, Ding Z, et al: DTI-based muscle fiber tracking of the quadriceps mechanism in lateral patellar dislocation, *J Magn Reson Imaging* 29:663-670, 2009.

116. Katchburian MV, Bull AM, Shih YF, et al: Measurement of patellar tracking: assessment and analysis of the literature, *Clin Orthop Relat Res* 412:241-259, 2003.

117. Kaufer H: Mechanical function of the patella, *J Bone Joint Surg Am* 53:1551-1560, 1971.

118. Kellis E, Baltzopoulos V: In vivo determination of the patella tendon and hamstrings moment arms in adult males using videofluoroscopy during submaximal knee extension and flexion, *Clin Biomech (Bristol, Avon)* 14:118-124, 1999.

119. Kennedy JC, Alexander IJ, Hayes KC: Nerve supply of the human knee and its functional importance, *Am J Sports Med* 10:329-335, 1982.

120. Kernozek TW, Ragan RJ: Estimation of anterior cruciate ligament tension from inverse dynamics data and electromyography in females during drop landing, *Clin Biomech (Bristol, Avon)* 23:1279-1286, 2008.

121. Kernozek TW, Torry MR, Iwasaki M: Gender differences in lower extremity landing mechanics caused by neuromuscular fatigue, *Am J Sports Med* 36:554-565, 2008.

122. Kerrigan DC, Lelas JL, Goggins J, et al: Effectiveness of a lateral-wedge insole on knee varus torque in patients with knee osteoarthritis, *Arch Phys Med Rehabil* 83:889-893, 2002.

123. Kessler MA, Glaser C, Tittel S, et al: Volume changes in the menisci and articular cartilage of runners: an in vivo investigation based on 3-D magnetic resonance imaging, *Am J Sports Med* 34:832-836, 2006.

124. Kim YC, Yoo WK, Chung IH, et al: Tendinous insertion of semimembranosus muscle into the lateral meniscus, *Surg Radiol Anat* 19:365-369, 1997.

125. Kiriyama S, Sato H, Takahira N: Gender differences in rotation of the shank during single-legged drop landing and its relation to rotational muscle strength of the knee, *Am J Sports Med* 37:168-174, 2009.

126. Koh TJ, Grabiner MD, De Swart RJ: In vivo tracking of the human patella, *J Biomech* 25:637-643, 1992.

127. Krevolin JL, Pandy MG, Pearce JC: Moment arm of the patellar tendon in the human knee, *J Biomech* 37:785-788, 2004.

128. Krosshaug T, Nakamae A, Boden BP, et al: Mechanisms of anterior cruciate ligament injury in basketball: video analysis of 39 cases, *Am J Sports Med* 35:359-367, 2007.

129. Kubo K, Ohgo K, Takeishi R, et al: Effects of series elasticity on the human knee extension torque-angle relationship in vivo, *Res Q Exerc Sport* 77:408-416, 2006.

130. Kulig K, Andrews JG, Hay JG: Human strength curves, *Exert Sport Sci Rev* 12:417-466, 1984.

131. Kumagai M, Mizuno Y, Mattessich SM, et al: Posterior cruciate ligament rupture alters in vitro knee kinematics, *Clin Orthop Relat Res* 395:241-248, 2002.

132. Kuroda R, Kambic H, Valdevit A, Andrish JT: Articular cartilage contact pressure after tibial tuberosity transfer. A cadaveric study, *Am J Sports Med* 29:403-409, 2001.

133. Lafortune MA, Cavanagh PR, Sommer HJ 3rd, Kalenak A: Three-dimensional kinematics of the human knee during walking, *J Biomech* 25:347-357, 1992.

134. Laprade J, Lee R: Real-time measurement of patellofemoral kinematics in asymptomatic subjects, *Knee* 12:63-72, 2005.

135. LaPrade RF, Tso A, Wentorf FA: Force measurements on the fibular collateral ligament, popliteofibular ligament, and popliteus tendon to applied loads, *Am J Sports Med* 32:1695-1701, 2004.

136. Lautamies R, Harilainen A, Kettunen J, et al: Isokinetic quadriceps and hamstring muscle strength and knee function 5 years after anterior cruciate ligament reconstruction: comparison between bone-patellar, tendon-bone, and hamstring tendon autografts, *Knee Surg Sports Traumatol Arthrosc* 16:1009-1016, 2008.

137. Lee SJ, Aadalen KJ, Malaviya P, et al: Tibiofemoral contact mechanics after serial medial meniscectomies in the human cadaveric knee, *Am J Sports Med* 34:1334-1344, 2006.

138. Lee TQ, Anzel SH, Bennett KA, et al: The influence of fixed rotational deformities of the femur on the patellofemoral contact pressures in human cadaver knees, *Clin Orthop Relat Res* 302:69-74, 1994.

139. Lee TQ, Morris G, Csintalan RP: The influence of tibial and femoral rotation on patellofemoral contact area and pressure, *J Orthop Sports Phys Ther* 33:686-693, 2003.

140. Lesher JD, Sutlive TG, Miller GA, et al: Development of a clinical prediction rule for classifying patients with patellofemoral pain syndrome who respond to patellar taping, *J Orthop Sports Phys Ther* 36:854-866, 2006.

141. Li G, Most E, DeFrate LE, et al: Effect of the posterior cruciate ligament on posterior stability of the knee in high flexion, *J Biomech* 37:779-783, 2004.

142. Li G, Rudy TW, Sakane M, et al: The importance of quadriceps and hamstring muscle loading on knee kinematics and in-situ forces in the ACL, *J Biomech* 32:395-400, 1999.

143. Li G, Zayontz S, Most E, et al: In situ forces of the anterior and posterior cruciate ligaments in high knee flexion: an in vitro investigation, *J Orthop Res* 22:293-297, 2004.

144. Lieb FJ, Perry J: Quadriceps function. An anatomical and mechanical study using amputated limbs, *J Bone Joint Surg Am* 50:1535-1548, 1968.

145. Lohmander LS, Englund PM, Dahl LL, Roos EM: The long-term consequence of anterior cruciate ligament and meniscus injuries: osteoarthritis, *Am J Sports Med* 35:1756-1769, 2007.

146. Lowry CD, Cleland JA, Dyke K: Management of patients with patellofemoral pain syndrome using a multimodal approach: a case series, *J Orthop Sports Phys Ther* 38:691-702, 2008.

147. Lu TW, O'Connor JJ: Lines of action and moment arms of the major force-bearing structures crossing the human knee joint: comparison between theory and experiment, *J Anat* 189:575-585, 1996.

148. Luyckx T, Didden K, Vandenneucker H, et al: Is there a biomechanical explanation for anterior knee pain in patients with patella alta? Influence of patellar height on patellofemoral contact force, contact area and contact pressure, *J Bone Joint Surg Br* 91:344-350, 2009.

149. Lyu SR: Relationship of medial plica and medial femoral condyle during flexion, *Clin Biomech (Bristol, Avon)* 22:1013-1016, 2007.

150. MacIntyre NJ, Hill NA, Fellows RA, et al: Patellofemoral joint kinematics in individuals with and without patellofemoral pain syndrome, *J Bone Joint Surg Am* 88:2596-2605, 2006.

151. MacIntyre NJ, McKnight EK, Day A, Wilson DR: Consistency of patellar spin, tilt and lateral translation side-to-side and over a 1 year period in healthy young males, *J Biomech* 41:3094-3096, 2008.

152. Maffulli N, Binfield PM, King JB, Good CJ: Acute haemarthrosis of the knee in athletes. A prospective study of 106 cases, *J Bone Joint Surg Br* 75:945-949, 1993.

153. Malghem J, Maldague B: Depth insufficiency of the proximal trochlear groove on lateral radiographs of the knee: relation to patellar dislocation, *Radiology* 170:507-510, 1989.

154. Malinzak RA, Colby SM, Kirkendall DT, et al: A comparison of knee joint motion patterns between men and women in selected athletic tasks, *Clin Biomech (Bristol, Avon)* 16:438-445, 2001.

155. Mandelbaum BR, Silvers HJ, Watanabe DS, et al: Effectiveness of a neuromuscular and proprioceptive training program in preventing anterior cruciate ligament injuries in female athletes: 2-year follow-up, *Am J Sports Med* 33:1003-1010, 2005.

156. Margheritini F, Rihn J, Musahl V, et al: Posterior cruciate ligament injuries in the athlete: an anatomical, biomechanical and clinical review, *Sports Med* 32:393-408, 2002.

157. Markolf KL, Burchfield DM, Shapiro MM, et al: Combined knee loading states that generate high anterior cruciate ligament forces, *J Orthop Res* 13:930-935, 1995.

158. Markolf KL, Feeley BT, Jackson SR, et al: Biomechanical studies of double-bundle posterior cruciate ligament reconstructions, *J Bone Joint Surg Am* 88:1788-1794, 2006.

159. Markolf KL, Graff-Radford A, Amstutz HC: In vivo knee stability. A quantitative assessment using an instrumented clinical testing apparatus, *J Bone Joint Surg Am* 60:664-674, 1978.

160. Markolf KL, O'Neill G, Jackson SR, McAllister DR: Effects of applied quadriceps and hamstrings muscle loads on forces in the anterior and posterior cruciate ligaments, *Am J Sports Med* 32:1144-1149, 2004.

161. Marzo JM, Gurske-DePerio J: Effects of medial meniscus posterior horn avulsion and repair on tibiofemoral contact area and peak contact pressure with clinical implications, *Am J Sports Med* 37:124-129, 2009.

162. Mascal CL, Landel R, Powers C: Management of patellofemoral pain targeting hip, pelvis, and trunk muscle function: 2 case reports, *J Orthop Sports Phys Ther* 33:647-660, 2003.

163. McDermott ID, Amis AA: The consequences of meniscectomy, *J Bone Joint Surg Br* 88:1549-1556, 2006.

164. McLean SG, Walker KB, Van Den Bogert AJ: Effect of gender on lower extremity kinematics during rapid direction changes: an integrated analysis of three sports movements, *J Sci Med Sport* 8:411-422, 2005.

165. McNair PJ, Marshall RN, Maguire K: Swelling of the knee joint: effects of exercise on quadriceps muscle strength, *Arch Phys Med Rehabil* 77:896-899, 1996.

166. Mesfar W, Shirazi-Adl A: Biomechanics of changes in ACL and PCL material properties or prestrains in flexion under muscle force-implications in ligament reconstruction, *Comput Methods Biomech Biomed Engin* 9:201-209, 2006.

167. Mesfar W, Shirazi-Adl A: Biomechanics of the knee joint in flexion under various quadriceps forces, *Knee* 12:424-434, 2005.

168. Mesfar W, Shirazi-Adl A: Knee joint mechanics under quadriceps–hamstrings muscle forces are influenced by tibial restraint, *Clin Biomech (Bristol, Avon)* 21:841-848, 2006.

169. Messier SP, Davis SE, Curl WW, et al: Etiologic factors associated with patellofemoral pain in runners, *Med Sci Sports Exerc* 23:1008-1015, 1991.

170. Messina DF, Farney WC, DeLee JC: The incidence of injury in Texas high school basketball. A prospective study among male and female athletes, *Am J Sports Med* 27:294-299, 1999.

171. Mihata LC, Beutler AI, Boden BP: Comparing the incidence of anterior cruciate ligament injury in collegiate lacrosse, soccer, and basketball players: implications for anterior cruciate ligament mechanism and prevention, *Am J Sports Med* 34:899-904, 2006.

172. Miyazaki T, Wada M, Kawahara H, et al: Dynamic load at baseline can predict radiographic disease progression in medial compartment knee osteoarthritis, *Ann Rheum Dis* 61:617-622, 2002.

173. Mizuno Y, Kumagai M, Mattessich SM, et al: Q-angle influences tibiofemoral and patellofemoral kinematics, *J Orthop Res* 19:834-840, 2001.

174. Mochizuki T, Akita K, Muneta T, Sato T: Pes anserinus: layered supportive structure on the medial side of the knee, *Clin Anat* 17:50-54, 2004.

175. Moran CJ, Poynton AR, Moran R, Brien MO: Analysis of meniscofemoral ligament tension during knee motion, *Arthroscopy* 22:362-366, 2006.

176. Morrison JB: The mechanics of the knee joint in relation to normal walking, *J Biomech* 3:51-61, 1970.

177. Morrissey MC, Drechsler WI, Morrissey D, et al: Effects of distally fixated versus nondistally fixated leg extensor resistance training on knee pain in the early period after anterior cruciate ligament reconstruction, *Physical Therapy* 82:35-43, 2002.

178. Mossber KA, Smith LK: Axial rotation of the knee in women, *J Orthop Sports Phys Ther* 4:236-240, 1983.

179. Mountcastle SB, Posner M, Kragh JF Jr, Taylor DC: Gender differences in anterior cruciate ligament injury vary with activity: epidemiology of anterior cruciate ligament injuries in a young, athletic population, *Am J Sports Med* 35:1635-1642, 2007.

180. Mundermann A, Dyrby CO, Hurwitz DE, et al: Potential strategies to reduce medial compartment loading in patients with knee osteoarthritis of varying severity: reduced walking speed, *Arthritis Rheum* 50:1172-1178, 2004.

181. Muneta T, Yamamoto H, Sakai H, et al: Relationship between changes in length and force in in vitro reconstructed anterior cruciate ligament, *Am J Sports Med* 21:299-304, 1993.

182. Myer GD, Ford KR, Paterno MV, et al: The effects of generalized joint laxity on risk of anterior cruciate ligament injury in young female athletes, *Am J Sports Med* 36:1073-1080, 2008.

183. Myklebust G, Bahr R: Return to play guidelines after anterior cruciate ligament surgery, *Br J Sports Med* 39:127-131, 2005.

184. Myklebust G, Engebretsen L, Braekken IH, et al: Prevention of anterior cruciate ligament injuries in female team handball players: a prospective intervention study over three seasons, *Clin J Sport Med* 13:71-78, 2003.

185. Nebelung W, Wuschech H: Thirty-five years of follow-up of anterior cruciate ligament-deficient knees in high-level athletes, *Arthroscopy* 21:696-702, 2005.

186. Nha KW, Papannagari R, Gill TJ, et al: In vivo patellar tracking: clinical motions and patellofemoral indices, *J Orthop Res* 26:1067-1074, 2008.

187. Nielsen AB, Yde J: Epidemiology of acute knee injuries: a prospective hospital investigation, *J Trauma* 31:1644-1648, 1991.

188. Noyes FR, Bassett RW, Grood ES, Butler DL: Arthroscopy in acute traumatic hemarthrosis of the knee. Incidence of anterior cruciate tears and other injuries, *J Bone Joint Surg Am* 62:687-695, 1980.

189. Ostermeier S, Holst M, Hurschler C, et al: Dynamic measurement of patellofemoral kinematics and contact pressure after lateral retinacular release: an in vitro study, *Knee Surg Sports Traumatol Arthrosc* 15:547-554, 2007.

190. Osternig LR, Bates BT, James SL: Patterns of tibial rotary torque in knees of healthy subjects, *Med Sci Sports Exerc* 12:195-199, 1980.

191. Pal S, Langenderfer JE, Stowe JQ, et al: Probabilistic modeling of knee muscle moment arms: effects of methods, origin-insertion, and kinematic variability, *Ann Biomed Eng* 35:1632-1642, 2007.

192. Paletta GA Jr, Manning T, Snell E, et al: The effect of allograft meniscal replacement on intraarticular contact area and pressures in the human knee. A biomechanical study, *Am J Sports Med* 25:692-698, 1997.

193. Palmieri-Smith RM, Kreinbrink J, Ashton-Miller JA, Wojtys EM: Quadriceps inhibition induced by an experimental knee joint effusion affects knee joint mechanics during a single-legged drop landing, *Am J Sports Med* 35:1269-1275, 2007.

194. Pandy MG, Shelburne KB: Dependence of cruciate-ligament loading on muscle forces and external load, *J Biomech* 30:1015-1024, 1997.

195. Pantano KJ, White SC, Gilchrist LA, Leddy J: Differences in peak knee valgus angles between individuals with high and low Q-angles during a single limb squat, *Clin Biomech (Bristol, Avon)* 20:966-972, 2005.

196. Papannagari R, DeFrate LE, Nha KW, et al: Function of posterior cruciate ligament bundles during in vivo knee flexion, *Am J Sports Med* 35:1507-1512, 2007.

197. Park SE, DeFrate LE, Suggs JF, et al: The change in length of the medial and lateral collateral ligaments during in vivo knee flexion, *Knee* 12:377-382, 2005.

198. Parolie JM, Bergfeld JA: Long-term results of nonoperative treatment of isolated posterior cruciate ligament injuries in the athlete, *Am J Sports Med* 14:35-38, 1986.

199. Patel D: Arthroscopy of the plicae–synovial folds and their significance, *Am J Sports Med* 6:217-225, 1978.

200. Patel VV, Hall K, Ries M, et al: A three-dimensional MRI analysis of knee kinematics, *J Orthop Res* 22:283-292, 2004.

201. Peeler J, Anderson JE: Structural parameters of the vastus medialis muscle and its relationship to patellofemoral joint deterioration, *Clin Anat* 20:307-314, 2007.

202. Perry MC, Morrissey MC, King JB, et al: Effects of closed versus open kinetic chain knee extensor resistance training on knee laxity and leg function in patients during the 8- to 14-week post-operative period after anterior cruciate ligament reconstruction, *Knee Surg Sports Traumatol Arthrosc* 13:357-369, 2005.

203. Petersen W, Loerch S, Schanz S, et al: The role of the posterior oblique ligament in controlling posterior tibial translation in the posterior cruciate ligament-deficient knee, *Am J Sports Med* 36:495-501, 2008.

204. Petrigliano FA, McAllister DR: Isolated posterior cruciate ligament injuries of the knee, *Sports Med Arthrosc Rev* 14:206-212, 2006.

205. Pincivero DM, Salfetnikov Y, Campy RM, Coelho AJ: Angle- and gender-specific quadriceps femoris muscle recruitment and knee extensor torque, *J Biomech* 37:1689-1697, 2004.

206. Pinskerova V, Johal P, Nakagawa S, et al: Does the femur roll-back with flexion? *J Bone Joint Surg Br* 86:925-931, 2004.

207. Pombo MW, Shen W, Fu FH: Anatomic double-bundle anterior cruciate ligament reconstruction: where are we today? *Arthroscopy* 24:1168-1177, 2008.

208. Powers CM: Patellar kinematics, part I: the influence of vastus muscle activity in subjects with and without patellofemoral pain, *Phys Ther* 80:956-964, 2000.

209. Powers CM: Patellar kinematics, part II: the influence of the depth of the trochlear groove in subjects with and without patellofemoral pain, *Phys Ther* 80:965-978, 2000.

210. Powers CM: Rehabilitation of patellofemoral joint disorders: a critical review, *J Orthop Sports Phys Ther* 28:345-354, 1998.

211. Powers CM: The influence of altered lower-extremity kinematics on patellofemoral joint dysfunction: a theoretical perspective, *J Orthop Sports Phys Ther* 33:639-646, 2003.

212. Powers CM, Chen PY, Reischl SF, Perry J: Comparison of foot pronation and lower extremity rotation in persons with and without patellofemoral pain, *Foot Ankle Int* 23:634-640, 2002.

213. Powers CM, Landel R, Perry J: Timing and intensity of vastus muscle activity during functional activities in subjects with and without patellofemoral pain, *Phys Ther* 76:946-955, 1996.

214. Powers CM, Ward SR, Chen YJ, et al: The effect of bracing on patellofemoral joint stress during free and fast walking, *Am J Sports Med* 32:224-231, 2004.

215. Powers CM, Ward SR, Fredericson M, et al: Patellofemoral kinematics during weight-bearing and non-weight-bearing knee extension in persons with lateral subluxation of the patella: a preliminary study, *J Orthop Sports Phys Ther* 33:677-685, 2003.

216. Pujol N, Blanchi MP, Chambat P: The incidence of anterior cruciate ligament injuries among competitive Alpine skiers: a 25-year investigation, *Am J Sports Med* 35:1070-1074, 2007.

217. Race A, Amis AA: Loading of the two bundles of the posterior cruciate ligament: an analysis of bundle function in a-P drawer, *J Biomech* 29:873-879, 1996.

218. Raimondo RA, Ahmad CS, Blankevoort L, et al: Patellar stabilization: a quantitative evaluation of the vastus medialis obliquus muscle, *Orthopedics* 21:791-795, 1998.

219. Rajala GM, Neumann DA, Foster C: Quadriceps muscle performance in male speed skaters, *J Strength Cond Res* 8:48-52, 1994.

220. Ramappa AJ, Apreleva M, Harrold FR, et al: The effects of medialization and anteromedialization of the tibial tubercle on patellofemoral mechanics and kinematics, *Am J Sports Med* 34:749-756, 2006.

221. Reilly DT, Martens M: Experimental analysis of the quadriceps muscle force and patello-femoral joint reaction force for various activities, *Acta Orthop Scand* 43:126-137, 1972.

222. Reischl SF, Powers CM, Rao S, Perry J: Relationship between foot pronation and rotation of the tibia and femur during walking, *Foot Ankle Int* 20:513-520, 1999.

223. Richter M, Kiefer H, Hehl G, Kinzl L: Primary repair for posterior cruciate ligament injuries. An eight-year followup of fifty-three patients, *Am J Sports Med* 24:298-305, 1996.

224. Roach KE, Miles TP: Normal hip and knee active range of motion: the relationship to age, *Phys Ther* 71:656-665, 1991.

225. Robinson JR, Bull AM, Thomas RR, Amis AA: The role of the medial collateral ligament and posteromedial capsule in controlling knee laxity, *Am J Sports Med* 34:1815-1823, 2006.

226. Robinson JR, Sanchez-Ballester J, Bull AM, et al: The posteromedial corner revisited. An anatomical description of the passive restraining structures of the medial aspect of the human knee, *J Bone Joint Surg Br* 86:674-681, 2004.

227. Robinson RL, Nee RJ: Analysis of hip strength in females seeking physical therapy treatment for unilateral patellofemoral pain syndrome, *J Orthop Sports Phys Ther* 37:232-238, 2007.

228. Roe J, Pinczewski LA, Russell VJ, et al: A 7-year follow-up of patellar tendon and hamstring tendon grafts for arthroscopic anterior cruciate ligament reconstruction: differences and similarities, *Am J Sports Med* 33:1337-1345, 2005.

229. Rue JP, Yanke AB, Busam ML, et al: Prospective evaluation of concurrent meniscus transplantation and articular cartilage repair: minimum 2-year follow-up, *Am J Sports Med* 36:1770-1778, 2008.

230. Salsich GB, Brechter JH, Farwell D, Powers CM: The effects of patellar taping on knee kinetics, kinematics, and vastus lateralis muscle activity during stair ambulation in individuals with patellofemoral pain, *J Orthop Sports Phys Ther* 32:3-10, 2002.

231. Salsich GB, Perman WH: Patellofemoral joint contact area is influenced by tibiofemoral rotation alignment in individuals who have patellofemoral pain, *J Orthop Sports Phys Ther* 37:521-528, 2007.

232. Sanchez AR 2nd, Sugalski MT, LaPrade RF: Anatomy and biomechanics of the lateral side of the knee, *Sports Med Arthrosc* 14:2-11, 2006.

233. Schöttle PB, Fucentese SF, Pfirrmann C, et al: Trochleaplasty for patellar instability due to trochlear dysplasia: a minimum 2-year clinical and radiological follow-up of 19 knees, *Acta Orthop* 76:693-698, 2005.

234. Schultz RA, Miller DC, Kerr CS, Micheli L: Mechanoreceptors in human cruciate ligaments. A histological study, *J Bone Joint Surg Am* 66:1072-1076, 1984.

235. Schulz MS, Russe K, Weiler A, et al: Epidemiology of posterior cruciate ligament injuries, *Arch Orthop Trauma Surg* 123:186-191, 2003.

236. Schutte MJ, Dabezies EJ, Zimny ML, Happel LT: Neural anatomy of the human anterior cruciate ligament, *J Bone Joint Surg Am* 69:243-247, 1987.

237. Seering WP, Piziali RL, Nagel DA, Schurman DJ: The function of the primary ligaments of the knee in varus-valgus and axial rotation, *J Biomech* 13:785-794, 1980.

238. Senavongse W, Amis AA: The effects of articular, retinacular, or muscular deficiencies on patellofemoral joint stability, *J Bone Joint Surg Br* 87:577-582, 2005.

239. Sharma L, Song J, Felson DT, et al: The role of knee alignment in disease progression and functional decline in knee osteoarthritis, *JAMA* 286:188-195, 2001.

240. Shelbourne KD, Davis TJ, Patel DV: The natural history of acute, isolated, nonoperatively treated posterior cruciate ligament injuries. A prospective study, *Am J Sports Med* 27:276-283, 1999.

241. Shelburne KB, Pandy MG, Anderson FC, et al: Pattern of anterior cruciate ligament force in normal walking, *J Biomech* 37:797-805, 2004.

242. Shelburne KB, Pandy MG, Torry MR: Comparison of shear forces and ligament loading in the healthy and ACL-deficient knee during gait, *J Biomech* 37:313-319, 2004.

243. Shelburne KB, Torry MR, Pandy MG: Muscle, ligament, and joint-contact forces at the knee during walking, *Med Sci Sports Exerc* 37:1948-1956, 2005.

244. Shelburne KB, Torry MR, Steadman JR, Pandy MG: Effects of foot orthoses and valgus bracing on the knee adduction moment and medial joint load during gait, *Clin Biomech (Bristol, Avon)* 23:814-821, 2008.

245. Shetty VD, Vowler SL, Krishnamurthy S, Halliday AE: Clinical diagnosis of medial plica syndrome of the knee: a prospective study, *J Knee Surg* 20:277-280, 2007.

246. Shimokochi Y, Shultz SJ: Mechanisms of noncontact anterior cruciate ligament injury, *J Athl Train* 43:396-408, 2008.

247. Shin CS, Chaudhari AM, Andriacchi TP: The influence of deceleration forces on ACL strain during single-leg landing: a simulation study, *J Biomech* 40:1145-1152, 2007.

248. Shrive NG, O'Connor JJ, Goodfellow JW: Load-bearing in the knee joint, *Clin Orthop Relat Res* 131:279-287, 1978.

249. Slauterbeck JR, Hickox JR, Beynnon B, Hardy DM: Anterior cruciate ligament biology and its relationship to injury forces, *Orthop Clin North Am* 37:585-591, 2006.

250. Slocum DB, Larson RL: Rotatory instability of the knee: its pathogenesis and a clinical test to demonstrate its presence. 1968, *Clin Orthop Relat Res* 454:5-13, 2007.

251. Smidt GL: Biomechanical analysis of knee flexion and extension, *J Biomech* 6:79-92, 1973.

252. Smith TO, Walker J, Russell N: Outcomes of medial patellofemoral ligament reconstruction for patellar instability: a systematic review, *Knee Surg Sports Traumatol Arthrosc* 15:1301-1314, 2007.

253. Solomonow M, Baratta R, Zhou BH, et al: The synergistic action of the anterior cruciate ligament and thigh muscles in maintaining joint stability, *Am J Sports Med* 15:207-213, 1987.

254. Song CY, Lin YF, Wei TC, et al: Surplus value of hip adduction in leg-press exercise in patients with patellofemoral pain syndrome: a randomized controlled trial, *Phys Ther* 89:409-418, 2009.

255. Souza RB, Powers CM: Differences in hip kinematics, muscle strength, and muscle activation between subjects with and without patellofemoral pain, *J Orthop Sports Phys Ther* 39:12-19, 2009.

256. Speer KP, Spritzer CE, Bassett FH 3rd, et al: Osseous injury associated with acute tears of the anterior cruciate ligament, *Am J Sports Med* 20:382-389, 1992.

257. Spoor CW, van Leeuwen JL: Knee muscle moment arms from MRI and from tendon travel, *J Biomech* 25:201-206, 1992.

258. Standring S: *Gray's anatomy: the anatomical basis of clinical practice*, ed 40, St Louis, 2009, Elsevier.

259. Steinkamp LA, Dillingham MF, Markel MD, et al: Biomechanical considerations in patellofemoral joint rehabilitation, *Am J Sports Med* 21:438-444, 1993.

260. Stensdotter AK, Hodges P, Ohberg F, Häger-Ross C: Quadriceps EMG in open and closed kinetic chain tasks in women with patellofemoral pain, *J Mot Behav* 39:194-202, 2007.

261. Tagesson S, Oberg B, Good L, Kvist J: A comprehensive rehabilitation program with quadriceps strengthening in closed versus open kinetic chain exercise in patients with anterior cruciate ligament deficiency: a randomized clinical trial evaluating dynamic tibial translation and muscle function, *Am J Sports Med* 36:298-307, 2008.

262. Tashman S, Kolowich P, Collon D, et al: Dynamic function of the ACL-reconstructed knee during running, *Clin Orthop Relat Res* 454:66-73, 2007.

263. Taunton JE, Ryan MB, Clement DB, et al: A retrospective case-control analysis of 2002 running injuries, *Br J Sports Med* 36:95-101, 2002.

264. Thomeé R, Renström P, Karlsson J, Grimby G: Patellofemoral pain syndrome in young women. II. Muscle function in patients and healthy controls, *Scand J Med Sci Sports* 5:245-251, 1995.

265. Tipton CM, Vailas AC, Matthes RD: Experimental studies on the influences of physical activity on ligaments, tendons and joints: a brief review, *Acta Med Scand Suppl* 711:157-168, 1986.

266. Tsuda E, Okamura Y, Otsuka H, et al: Direct evidence of the anterior cruciate ligament-hamstring reflex arc in humans, *Am J Sports Med* 29:83-87, 2001.

267. Uhorchak JM, Scoville CR, Williams GN, et al: Risk factors associated with noncontact injury of the anterior cruciate ligament: a prospective four-year evaluation of 859 West Point cadets, *Am J Sports Med* 31:831-842, 2003.

268. Van de Velde SK, DeFrate LE, Gill TJ, et al: The effect of anterior cruciate ligament deficiency on the in vivo elongation of the medial and lateral collateral ligaments, *Am J Sports Med* 35:294-300, 2007.

269. Van de Velde SK, Gill TJ, Li G: Evaluation of kinematics of anterior cruciate ligament-deficient knees with use of advanced imaging techniques, three-dimensional modeling techniques, and robotics, *J Bone Joint Surg Am* 91(Suppl 1):108-114, 2009.

270. Wang CJ, Walker PS: The effects of flexion and rotation on the length patterns of the ligaments of the knee, *J Biomech* 6:587-596, 1973.

271. Wexler G, Hurwitz DE, Bush-Joseph CA, et al: Functional gait adaptations in patients with anterior cruciate ligament deficiency over time, *Clin Orthop Relat Res* 348:166-175, 1998.

272. White KK, Lee SS, Cutuk A, et al: EMG power spectra of intercollegiate athletes and anterior cruciate ligament injury risk in females, *Med Sci Sports Exerc* 35:371-376, 2003.

273. Wilk KE, Davies GJ, Mangine RE, Malone TR: Patellofemoral disorders: a classification system and clinical guidelines for nonoperative rehabilitation, *J Orthop Sports Phys Ther* 28:307-322, 1998.

274. Williams GN, Snyder-Mackler L, Barrance PJ, et al: Muscle and tendon morphology after reconstruction of the anterior cruciate ligament with autologous semitendinosus-gracilis graft, *J Bone Joint Surg Am* 86:1936-1946, 2004.

275. Willson JD, Davis IS: Lower extremity strength and mechanics during jumping in women with patellofemoral pain, *J Sport Rehabil* 18:76-90, 2009.

276. Wilson NA, Press JM, Koh JL, et al: In vivo noninvasive evaluation of abnormal patellar tracking during squatting in patients with patellofemoral pain, *J Bone Joint Surg Am* 91:558-566, 2009.

277. Winter DA: *Biomechanics and motor control of human movement*, Hoboken, New Jersey, 2005, John Wiley & Sons.

278. Withrow TJ, Huston LJ, Wojtys EM, Ashton-Miller JA: The effect of an impulsive knee valgus moment on in vitro relative ACL strain during a simulated jump landing, *Clin Biomech (Bristol, Avon)* 21:977-983, 2006.

279. Witvrouw E, Danneels L, Van TD, et al: Open versus closed kinetic chain exercises in patellofemoral pain: a 5-year prospective randomized study, *Am J Sports Med* 32:1122-1130, 2004.

280. Wood L, Ferrell WR, Baxendale RH: Pressures in normal and acutely distended human knee joints and effects on quadriceps maximal voluntary contractions, *Q J Exp Physiol* 73:305-314, 1988.

281. Yu B, Lin CF, Garrett WE: Lower extremity biomechanics during the landing of a stop-jump task, *Clin Biomech (Bristol, Avon)* 21:297-305, 2006.

282. Zakaria D, Harburn KL, Kramer JF: Preferential activation of the vastus medialis oblique, vastus lateralis, and hip adductor muscles during isometric exercises in females, *J Orthop Sports Phys Ther* 26:23-28, 1997.

283. Zhao D, Banks SA, Mitchell KH, et al: Correlation between the knee adduction torque and medial contact force for a variety of gait patterns, *J Orthop Res* 25:789-797, 2007.

284. Zimny ML, Albright DJ, Dabezies E: Mechanoreceptors in the human medial meniscus, *Acta Anat (Basel)* 133:35-40, 1988.

STUDY QUESTIONS

1 As described in this chapter, the maximum-effort torques produced by the internal and external rotator muscles of the knee (when tested at 90 degrees of flexion) are of about equal magnitudes. How can this fact be justified given the disparity in the number of internal and external rotator muscles?

2 How can severe hyperextension of the knee while in a weight bearing position cause injury to *both* the ACL and the PCL?

3 Explain why the patellofemoral joint is least stable in the last 20 to 30 degrees of knee extension.

4 Why do most persons have slightly greater active knee flexion range of motion with the hip fully flexed as compared to fully extended?

5 List muscles and ligaments capable of resisting external rotation of the knee. Why would this function be especially important from a femoral-on-tibial (weight-bearing) perspective?

6 What is the primary mechanism by which the menisci reduce pressure across the articular surfaces of the knee?

7 Which of the following activities create greater compression stress (pressure) on the surfaces of the patellofemoral joint: (a) holding a partial squat with knees flexed to 10 to 20 degrees, or (b) holding a deep squat with knees flexed to 60 to 90 degrees? Why?

8 Why do the medial collateral ligament and the medial meniscus often become traumatized by a similar mechanism of injury?

9 Describe how contraction of the quadriceps muscle could elongate (strain) the anterior cruciate ligament? How is the strain on the ligament affected by (a) the knee joint angle and (b) the coactivation of quadriceps and hamstring muscle?

10 Describe the type of muscular activity of the quadriceps muscle during the early part of the stance phase of gait.

11 At about what arc of knee motion does the quadriceps muscle produce its largest internal torque? What factor(s) most likely account for this?

12 Justify (a) why the popliteus is called the "key to the knee," and (b) how the popliteus can provide both medial *and* lateral stability to the knee.

13 Describe the type of quadriceps and hamstring muscle activation (i.e., eccentric, concentric, etc) that occurs across the hip and knee while one *slowly* sits into a chair.

14 Polio affecting the L^2-L^4 spinal nerve roots would theoretically cause paralysis of what muscle group of the knee? (Hint: Consult Appendix IV, Part A.)

15 List three factors that could limit full knee extension.

Answers to the study questions can be found on the Evolve website.

Ankle and Foot

DONALD A. NEUMANN, PT, PhD, FAPTA

Walking and running require the foot to be sufficiently pliable to absorb stress and to conform to the countless spatial configurations between it and the ground. In addition, walking and running require the foot to be relatively rigid in order to withstand potentially large propulsive forces. The healthy foot satisfies the seemingly paradoxical requirements of shock absorption, pliability, and strength through a complex functional and structural interaction among its joints, connective tissues, and muscles. Although not emphasized enough in this chapter, the normal sensation of the healthy foot also provides important measures of protection and feedback to the muscles of the lower extremity.

This chapter sets forth a firm basis for an understanding of the evaluation and treatment of several disorders that affect the ankle and foot, many of which are kinesiologically related to the movement of the entire lower extremity. Several of the kinesiologic issues addressed in this chapter are related specifically to the process of walking, or gait, a topic covered in

detail in Chapter 15. Figure 15-12 should be consulted as a reference to the terminology used throughout Chapter 14 to describe the different phases of the gait cycle.

OSTEOLOGY

Basic Terms and Concepts

NAMING THE JOINTS AND REGIONS

Figure 14-1 depicts an overview of the terminology that describes the regions of the ankle and foot. The term *ankle* refers primarily to the talocrural joint: the articulation among the tibia, fibula, and talus. The term *foot* refers to all the tarsal bones, and the joints distal to the ankle. Within the foot are three regions, each consisting of a set of bones and one or more joints. The *rearfoot* (hindfoot) consists of the talus, calcaneus, and subtalar joint; the *midfoot* consists of the

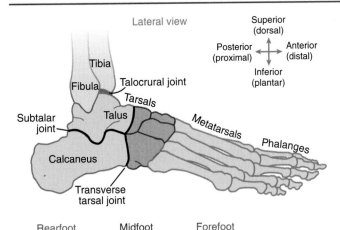

FIGURE 14-1. Overall organization of the bones, major joints, and regions of the foot and ankle.

remaining tarsal bones, including the transverse tarsal joint and the smaller distal intertarsal joints; and the *forefoot* consists of the metatarsals and phalanges, including all joints distal to and including the tarsometatarsal joints. Table 14-1 provides a summary of the organization of the bones and joints of the ankle and foot.

The terms *anterior* and *posterior* have their conventional meanings with reference to the tibia and fibula (i.e., the leg). When describing the ankle and foot, however, these terms are often used interchangeably with *distal* and *proximal*, respectively. The terms *dorsal* and *plantar* describe the superior (top) and inferior aspects of the foot, respectively.

OSTEOLOGIC SIMILARITIES BETWEEN THE DISTAL LEG AND THE DISTAL ARM

The ankle and foot have several features that are structurally similar to the wrist and hand. The radius in the forearm and

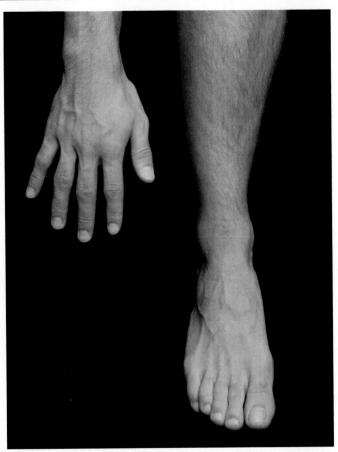

FIGURE 14-2. Topographic similarities between a pronated forearm and the ankle and foot. Note that the thumb and great toe are both located on the medial side of their respective extremity.

the tibia in the leg each articulates with a set of small bones—the carpus and tarsus, respectively. When the pisiform of the wrist is considered as a sesamoid (in contrast to a separate carpal bone), the carpus and tarsus have seven bones each. The general plan of the metatarsus and metacarpus, as well as the more distal phalanges, is very similar. A notable exception is that the first (great) toe in the foot is not as functionally developed as the thumb in the hand.

As described in Chapter 12, the entire lower extremity progressively internally or medially rotates during embryologic development. As a result, the great toe is positioned on the medial side of the foot, and the top of the foot is actually its dorsal surface. This orientation is similar to that of the hand when the forearm is fully pronated (Figure 14-2). This plantigrade position of the foot is necessary for walking and standing. With the forearm pronated, flexion and extension of the wrist are similar to plantar flexion and dorsiflexion of the ankle, respectively.

Individual Bones

FIBULA

The long and thin fibula is located lateral and parallel to the tibia (Figure 13-3). The fibular *head* can be palpated just lateral to the lateral condyle of the tibia. The slender shaft of the fibula transfers only about 10% of body weight through the

TABLE 14-1. Structural Organization of the Bones and Joints of the Ankle and Foot

	Ankle	Foot
Bones	Tibia Fibula Talus	*Rearfoot:* Calcaneus and talus* *Midfoot:* Navicular, cuboid, and cuneiforms *Forefoot:* Metatarsals and phalanges
Joints	Talocrural joint Proximal tibiofibular joint Distal tibiofibular joint	*Rearfoot:* Subtalar joint *Midfoot:* Transverse tarsal joint: talonavicular and calcaneocuboid; distal intertarsal joint: cuneonavicular, cuboideonavicular, and intercuneiform and cuneocuboid complex *Forefoot:* Tarsometatarsal, intermetatarsal, metatarsophalangeal, interphalangeal joints

*Talus is included as a bone of the ankle and of the foot.

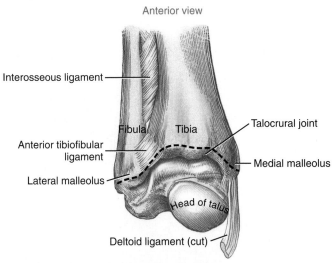

Anterior view

Interosseous ligament

Fibula   Tibia

Anterior tibiofibular ligament

Lateral malleolus

Head of talus

Talocrural joint

Medial malleolus

Deltoid ligament (cut)

FIGURE 14-3. An anterior view of the distal end of the right tibia and fibula, and the talus. The articulation of the three bones forms the talocrural (ankle) joint. The dashed line shows the proximal attachment of the capsule of the ankle joint.

leg; most of the weight is transferred through the thicker tibia. The shaft of the fibula continues distally to form the sharp and easily palpable *lateral malleolus* (from the Latin root *malleus,* hammer). The lateral malleolus functions as a pulley for the tendons of the fibularis (peroneus) longus and brevis. On the medial surface of the lateral malleolus is the *articular facet for the talus* (see ahead Figure 14-11). In the articulated ankle, this facet forms part of the talocrural joint (Figure 14-3).

DISTAL TIBIA

The distal end of the tibia expands to accommodate loads transferred across the ankle. On its medial side is the prominent *medial malleolus*. On the lateral surface of the medial malleolus is the *articular facet for the talus* (see ahead Figure 14-11). In the articulated ankle, this facet forms a small part of the talocrural joint. On the lateral side of the distal tibia is the *fibular notch,* a triangular concavity that accepts the distal end of the fibula at the distal tibiofibular joint (see ahead Figure 14-11).

In the adult the distal end of the tibia is twisted externally around its long axis approximately 20 or 30 degrees relative to its proximal end.[141] This natural torsion is evidenced by the slight externally rotated position of the foot during standing. This twist of the lower leg is referred to as *lateral tibial torsion,* based on the orientation of the bone's distal end relative to its proximal end.

Osteologic Features of the Fibula and Distal Tibia

Fibula
- Head
- Lateral malleolus
- Articular facet (for the talus)

Distal Tibia
- Medial malleolus
- Articular facet (for the talus)
- Fibular notch

TARSAL BONES

The seven tarsal bones are shown in four different perspectives in Figures 14-4 through 14-7.

Osteologic Features of the Tarsal Bones

Talus
- Trochlear surface
- Head
- Neck
- Anterior, middle, and posterior facets
- Talar sulcus
- Lateral and medial tubercles

Calcaneus
- Tuberosity
- Lateral and medial processes
- Anterior, middle, and posterior facets
- Calcaneal sulcus
- Sustentaculum talus

Navicular
- Proximal concave (articular) surface
- Tuberosity

Medial, Intermediate, and Lateral Cuneiforms
- Transverse arch

Cuboid
- Groove (for the tendon of the fibularis longus)

Talus

The talus is the most superiorly located bone of the foot. Its dorsal or *trochlear surface* is a rounded dome: convex anterior-posteriorly and slightly concave medial-laterally (see Figures 14-4 and 14-6). Cartilage covers the trochlear surface and its adjacent sides, providing smooth articular surfaces for the talocrural joint.[120] The prominent *head* of the talus projects forward and slightly medially toward the navicular. In the adult the long axis of the *neck* of the talus positions the head of this bone about 30 degrees medial to the sagittal plane. In small children the head is projected medially about 40 to 50 degrees, partially accounting for the often inverted appearance of their feet.

Figure 14-8 shows three articular facets on the plantar (inferior) surface of the talus. The *anterior* and *middle facets* are slightly curved and often continuous with each other. The articular cartilage that covers these facets also covers part of the adjacent head of the talus. The oval, concave *posterior facet* is the largest facet. As a functional set, the three facets articulate with the three facets on the dorsal (superior) surface of the calcaneus, forming the subtalar joint. The *talar sulcus* is an obliquely running groove between the anterior-middle and posterior facets.

Lateral and *medial tubercles* are located on the posterior-medial surface of the talus (see Figure 14-4). A groove formed between these tubercles serves as a pulley for the tendon of the flexor hallucis longus (see ahead Figure 14-12).

Calcaneus

The calcaneus, the largest of the tarsal bones, is well suited to accept the impact of the heel striking the ground during walking. The large and rough calcaneal *tuberosity* receives the attachment of the Achilles tendon. The plantar surface of the

Superior view

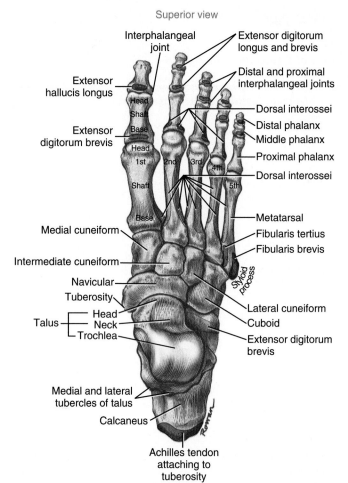

FIGURE 14-4. A superior (dorsal) view of the bones of the right foot. Proximal attachments of muscles are indicated in red, distal attachments in gray.

Inferior view

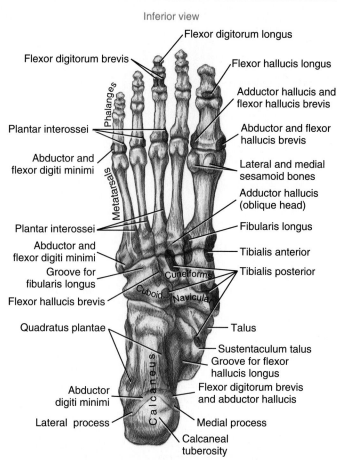

FIGURE 14-5. An inferior (plantar) view of the bones of the right foot. Proximal attachments of muscles are indicated in red, distal attachments in gray.

Medial view

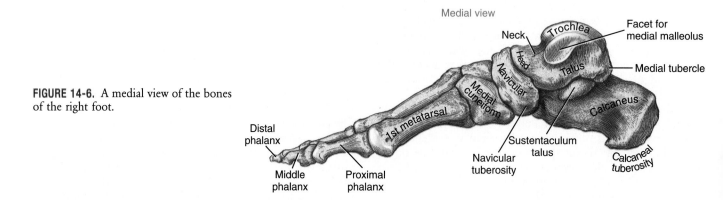

FIGURE 14-6. A medial view of the bones of the right foot.

tuberosity has *lateral* and *medial processes* that serve as attachments for many of the intrinsic muscles and the deep plantar fascia of the foot (see Figure 14-5).

The calcaneus articulates with other tarsal bones on its anterior and dorsal surfaces. The relatively small, curved anterior surface of the calcaneus joins the cuboid at the calcaneocuboid joint (see Figure 14-7). The more extensive dorsal surface contains three facets that join the matching facets on the talus (see Figure 14-8). The *anterior* and *middle facets* are relatively small and nearly flat. The *posterior facet* is large and convex, conforming to the concave shape of the equally large posterior facet on the talus. Between the posterior and medial facets is a wide oblique groove called the *calcaneal sulcus.* Located within this sulcus are the attachments of several strong ligaments that bind the subtalar joint. With the subtalar joint articulated, the sulci of the calcaneus and talus form a canal within the subtalar joint, known as the *tarsal sinus* (see Figure 14-7).

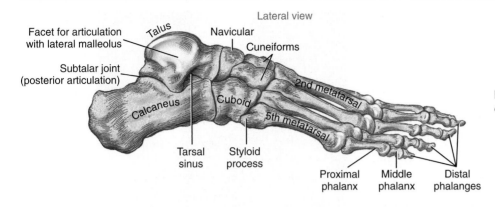

Lateral view

Facet for articulation
with lateral malleolus
Talus
Navicular
Cuneiforms
Subtalar joint
(posterior articulation)
Calcaneus
Cuboid
2nd metatarsal
5th metatarsal
Tarsal
sinus
Styloid
process
Proximal
phalanx
Middle
phalanx
Distal
phalanges

FIGURE 14-7. A lateral view of the bones of the right foot.

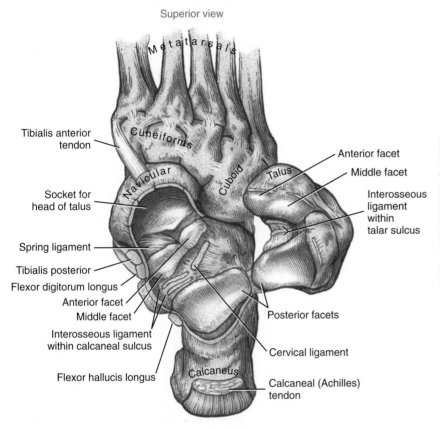

Superior view

Metatarsals
Tibialis anterior
tendon
Cuneiforms
Navicular
Cuboid
Talus
Anterior facet
Middle facet
Interosseous
ligament
within
talar sulcus
Socket for
head of talus
Spring ligament
Tibialis posterior
Flexor digitorum longus
Anterior facet
Middle facet
Interosseous ligament
within calcaneal sulcus
Posterior facets
Flexor hallucis longus
Calcaneus
Cervical ligament
Calcaneal (Achilles)
tendon

FIGURE 14-8. A superior view of the talus flipped laterally to reveal its plantar surface as well as the dorsal surface of the calcaneus. With the talus moved, it is possible to observe the three articular facets located on the talus and on the calcaneus. Note also the deep, continuous concavity formed by the proximal side of the navicular and the spring ligament. This concavity accepts the head of the talus, forming the talonavicular joint. (The interosseous and cervical ligaments and multiple tendons have been cut.)

The *sustentaculum talus* projects medially as a horizontal shelf from the dorsal surface of the calcaneus (see Figure 14-6). The sustentaculum talus lies under and supports the middle facet of the talus. (Sustentaculum talus literally means a "shelf for the talus.")

Navicular

The navicular is named for its resemblance to a ship (i.e., referring to "navy"). Its *proximal (concave) surface* accepts the head of the talus at the talonavicular joint (see Figure 14-4). The distal surface of the navicular bone contains three relatively flat facets that articulate with the three cuneiform bones.

The medial surface of the navicular has a prominent *tuberosity,* palpable in the adult at about 2.5 cm inferior and distal

(anterior) to the tip of the medial malleolus (see Figure 14-6). This tuberosity serves as one of several distal attachments of the tibialis posterior muscle.

Medial, Intermediate, and Lateral Cuneiforms

The cuneiform bones (from the Latin root meaning "wedge") act as a spacer between the navicular and bases of the three medial metatarsal bones (see Figure 14-4). The cuneiforms contribute to the *transverse arch* of the foot, accounting, in part, for the transverse convexity of the dorsal aspect of the midfoot.

Cuboid

As its name indicates, the cuboid has six surfaces, three of which articulate with adjacent tarsal bones (see Figures 14-4,

14-5, and 14-7). The distal surface articulates with the bases of both the fourth and fifth metatarsals. The cuboid is therefore homologous to the hamate bone in the wrist.

The entire, curved proximal surface of the cuboid articulates with the calcaneus (see Figure 14-4). The medial surface has an oval facet for articulation with the lateral cuneiform and a small facet for articulation with the navicular. A distinct *groove* runs across the plantar surface of the cuboid, which in life is occupied by the tendon of the fibularis longus muscle (see Figure 14-5).

RAYS OF THE FOOT

A *ray* of the forefoot is functionally defined as one metatarsal and its associated set of phalanges.

Metatarsals

The five metatarsal bones link the distal row of tarsal bones with the proximal phalanges (see Figure 14-4). Metatarsals are numbered 1 through 5, starting on the medial side. The first metatarsal is the shortest and thickest, and the second is usually the longest. The second and usually the third metatarsals are the most rigidly attached to the distal row of tarsal bones. These morphologic characteristics generally reflect the larger forces that pass through this region of the forefoot during the push off phase of gait. Each metatarsal has a *base* at its proximal end, a *shaft,* and a convex *head* at its distal end (see Figure 14-4, first metatarsal). The bases of the metatarsals have small *articular facets* that mark the site of articulation with the bases of the adjacent metatarsals.

Longitudinally, the shafts of the metatarsals are slightly concave on their plantar side (see Figure 14-6). This arched shape enhances the load-supporting ability of the metatarsals, and provides space for muscles and tendons. The plantar surface of the first metatarsal head has two small facets for articulation with two *sesamoid bones* that are imbedded within the tendon of the flexor hallucis brevis (see Figure 14-5). The fifth metatarsal has a prominent *styloid process* just lateral to its base, marking the attachment of the fibularis brevis muscle (see Figure 14-7).

Osteologic Features of a Metatarsal
- Base (with articular facets for articulation with the bases of adjacent metatarsals)
- Shaft
- Head
- Styloid process (on the fifth metatarsal only)

Phalanges

As in the hand, the foot has 14 phalanges. Each of the four lateral toes contains a proximal, middle, and distal phalanx (see Figure 14-4). The first toe—more commonly called the *great toe* or *hallux*—has two phalanges, designated as proximal and distal. In general, each phalanx has a concave *base* at its proximal end, a *shaft,* and a convex *head* at its distal end.

Osteologic Features of a Phalanx
- Base
- Shaft
- Head

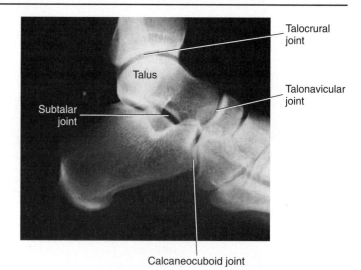

FIGURE 14-9. A radiograph from a healthy person showing the major joints of the ankle and foot: talocrural, subtalar, talonavicular, and calcaneocuboid. The talonavicular and calcaneocuboid joints are part of the larger transverse tarsal joint. Note the central location of the talus.

ARTHROLOGY

The major joints of the ankle and foot are the *talocrural, subtalar,* and *transverse tarsal joints* (Figure 14-9). As will be described, the talus is mechanically involved with all three of these joints. The multiple articulations made by the talus help to explain the bone's complex shape, with nearly 70% of its surface covered with articular cartilage. *An understanding of the shape of the talus is crucial to an understanding of the kinesiology of the ankle and foot.*

Terminology Used to Describe Movements

The terminology used to describe movements of the ankle and foot incorporates two sets of definitions: a fundamental set and an applied set. The *fundamental terminology* defines movement of the foot or ankle as occurring at right angles to the three standard axes of rotation (Figure 14-10, *A*). *Dorsiflexion* (extension) and *plantar flexion* describe motion that is parallel to the sagittal plane, around a medial-lateral axis of rotation. *Eversion* and *inversion* describe motion that is parallel to the frontal plane, around an anterior-posterior axis of rotation. *Abduction* and *adduction* describe motion that is parallel to the horizontal (transverse) plane, around a vertical (superior-inferior) axis of rotation. For at least the three major joints of the ankle and foot, these fundamental definitions are inadequate because most movements at these joints occur about an *oblique* axis rather than about the three standard, orthogonal axes of rotation depicted in Figure 14-10, *A*.

A second and more *applied terminology* has therefore evolved in the attempt to define the movements that occur perpendicular to the prevailing oblique axes of rotation at the ankle and foot (see Figure 14-10, *B*). *Pronation* is defined as a motion that has elements of eversion, abduction, and dorsiflexion. *Supination,* in contrast, is defined as a motion that has elements of inversion, adduction, and plantar flexion. The orientation of the oblique axis of rotation depicted in Figure 14-10, *B* varies across the major joints but, in general, has a pitch that

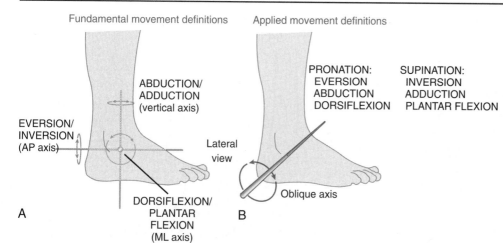

FIGURE 14-10. A, *Fundamental movement definitions* are based on the movement of any part of the ankle or foot in a plane perpendicular to the three standard axes of rotation: vertical, anterior-posterior *(AP),* and medial-lateral *(ML).* **B,** *Applied movement definitions* are based on the movements that occur at right angles to one of several oblique axes of rotation within the foot and ankle. The two main movements are defined as either pronation or supination.

TABLE 14-2. Terms That Describe Movements and Deformities of the Ankle and Foot

Motion	Axis of Rotation	Plane of Motion	Example of Fixed Deformity or Abnormal Posture
Plantar flexion Dorsiflexion	Medial-lateral	Sagittal	Pes equinus Pes calcaneus
Inversion Eversion	Anterior-posterior	Frontal	Varus Valgus
Abduction Adduction	Vertical	Horizontal	Abductus Adductus
Supination Pronation	Oblique (varies by joint)	Varying elements of inversion, adduction, and plantar flexion Varying elements of eversion, abduction, and dorsiflexion	Inconsistent terminology—usually implies one or more of the components of supination Inconsistent terminology—usually implies one or more of the components of pronation

is similar to that illustrated. The exact pitch of each major joint's axis of rotation is described in subsequent sections.

Pronation and supination motions have been called "triplanar" motions. Unfortunately, this description is misleading. The term *triplanar* implies only that the movements "cut through" each of the three cardinal planes, not that the joint exhibiting this movement possesses three degrees of freedom. *Pronation and supination occur in one plane.* Table 14-2 summarizes the terminology used to describe the movements of the ankle and foot, including the terminology that describes abnormal posture or deformity.

Structure and Function of the Joints Associated with the Ankle

From an anatomic perspective, the ankle includes one articulation: the *talocrural joint.* An important structural component of this joint is the articulation formed between the tibia and fibula—an articulation reinforced by the *proximal* and *distal tibiofibular joints* and the *interosseous membrane* of the leg (see Figure 13-3). Because of this functional association, the proximal and distal tibiofibular joints are included under the topic of the "ankle."

PROXIMAL TIBIOFIBULAR JOINT

The proximal tibiofibular joint is a synovial joint located lateral to and immediately inferior to the knee. The joint is

formed between the head of the fibula and the posterior-lateral aspect of the lateral condyle of the tibia (see Figure 13-4). The joint surfaces are generally flat or slightly oval, covered by articular cartilage.[120]

A capsule strengthened by anterior and posterior ligaments encloses the proximal tibiofibular joint (see Figures 13-7 and 13-9). The tendon of the popliteus muscle provides additional stabilization as it crosses the joint posteriorly. Very little gliding motion occurs at this joint; a firm articulation is needed to ensure that forces within the biceps femoris and lateral collateral ligament of the knee are transferred effectively from the fibula to the tibia.

DISTAL TIBIOFIBULAR JOINT

The distal tibiofibular joint is formed by the articulation between the medial surface of the distal fibula and the fibular notch of the tibia (Figure 14-11).[6] Anatomists frequently refer to the distal tibiofibular joint as a *syndesmosis,* which is a type of fibrous synarthrodial joint that is closely bound by an interosseous membrane.[120] Relatively little movement is permitted between the distal tibia and distal fibula.

The *interosseous ligament* provides the strongest bond between the distal end of the tibia and fibula (see Figure 14-3).[120] This ligament is an extension of the *interosseous membrane* between the tibia and fibula. The *anterior* and *posterior (distal) tibiofibular ligaments* also stabilize the joint (Figures 14-11 and 14-12). A stable union between the distal tibia and

Anterior-lateral view

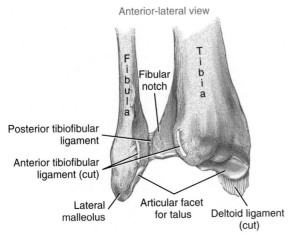

FIGURE 14-11. An anterior-lateral view of the right distal tibiofibular joint with the fibula reflected to show the articular surfaces.

Posterior view

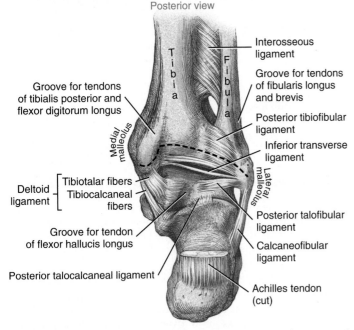

FIGURE 14-12. Posterior view of the right ankle region shows several ligaments of the distal tibiofibular, talocrural, and subtalar joints. The dashed line indicates the proximal attachments of the capsule of the talocrural (ankle) joint.

fibula is essential to the stability and function of the talocrural joint.

Ligaments of the Distal Tibiofibular Joint
- Interosseous ligament
- Anterior tibiofibular ligament
- Posterior tibiofibular ligament

TALOCRURAL JOINT

Articular Structure

The talocrural joint is the articulation of the trochlea (dome) and sides of the talus with the rectangular cavity formed by

The shape of the
talocrural joint

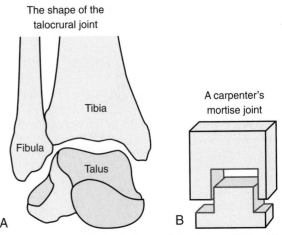

FIGURE 14-13. The similarity in shape of the talocrural joint **(A)** and a carpenter's mortise joint **(B)** is demonstrated. Note the extensive area of the talus that is lined with articular cartilage *(blue)*.

the distal end of the tibia and both malleoli (see Figures 14-3 and 14-9). The talocrural joint is often referred to as the "mortise," owing to its resemblance to the wood joint used by carpenters (Figure 14-13). The concave shape of the proximal side of the mortise is maintained by connective tissues that bind the tibia with the fibula. The confining shape of the talocrural joint provides a major source of natural stability to the ankle.[128]

The structure of the mortise must be sufficiently stable to accept the forces that pass between the leg and foot. Although variable, approximately 90% to 95% of the compressive forces pass through the talus and tibia; the remaining 5% to 10% pass through the lateral region of the talus and the fibula.[18] The talocrural joint is lined with about 3 mm of articular cartilage, which can be compressed by 30% to 40% in response to peak physiologic loads.[135] This load-absorption mechanism protects the subchondral bone from damaging stress.

Ligaments

A thin *capsule* surrounds the talocrural joint. Externally, the capsule is reinforced by collateral ligaments that help maintain the stability between the talus and the rectangular "socket" of the mortise.

The medial collateral ligament of the talocrural joint is called the *deltoid ligament,* based on its triangular shape. This ligament is broad and expansive (Figure 14-14). Its apex is attached to the medial malleolus, with its base fanning into three sets of superficial fibers (see box). Deeper tibiotalar fibers blend with and strengthen the medial capsule of the talocrural joint.

Distal Attachments of the Three Superficial Sets of Fibers within the Deltoid Ligament
- *Tibionavicular* fibers attach to the navicular, near its tuberosity.
- *Tibiocalcaneal* fibers attach to the sustentaculum talus.
- *Tibiotalar* fibers attach to the medial tubercle and adjacent part of the talus.

The primary function of the deltoid ligament is to limit eversion across the talocrural, subtalar, and talonavicular joints. Sprains of the deltoid ligament are relatively uncommon, in part because of the ligament's strength and because the lateral malleolus serves as a bony block against excessive eversion.

The *lateral collateral ligaments* of the ankle include the anterior and posterior talofibular and the calcaneofibular ligaments. Because of the relative inability of the medial malleolus to block the medial side of the mortise, the overwhelming majority of ankle sprains involve excessive inversion, often involving injury to the lateral collateral ligaments.[8]

The *anterior talofibular ligament* attaches to the anterior aspect of the lateral malleolus, then courses anteriorly and medially to the neck of the talus (Figure 14-15). This ligament is the most frequently injured of the lateral ligaments. Injury is often caused by excessive inversion or (horizontal plane) adduction of the ankle, especially when combined with plantar flexion—for example, when inadvertently stepping into a hole or onto someone's foot while landing from a jump.[115] The *calcaneofibular ligament* courses inferiorly and posteriorly from the apex of the lateral malleolus to the lateral surface of the calcaneus (see Figure 14-15). This ligament resists inversion across the talocrural joint (especially when fully dorsiflexed) and the subtalar joint. As a pair, the calcaneofibular and anterior talofibular ligaments limit inversion throughout most of the range of ankle dorsiflexion and plantar flexion.[21] About two thirds of all lateral ankle ligament injuries involve both of these ligaments.[36,54]

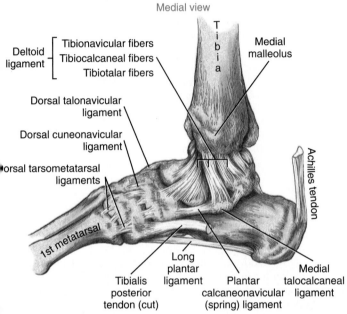

FIGURE 14-14. Medial view of the right ankle region highlights the medial collateral (deltoid) ligament.

> **Three Major Components of the Lateral Collateral Ligaments of the Ankle**
> * Anterior talofibular ligament
> * Calcaneofibular ligament
> * Posterior talofibular ligament

The *posterior talofibular ligament* originates on the posterior-medial side of the lateral malleolus and attaches to the lateral tubercle of the talus (see Figures 14-12 and 14-15). Its fibers run horizontally across the posterior side of the talocrural joint, in an oblique anterior-lateral to posterior-medial direction (Figure 14-16). The primary function of the posterior talofibular ligament is to stabilize the talus within the mortise.

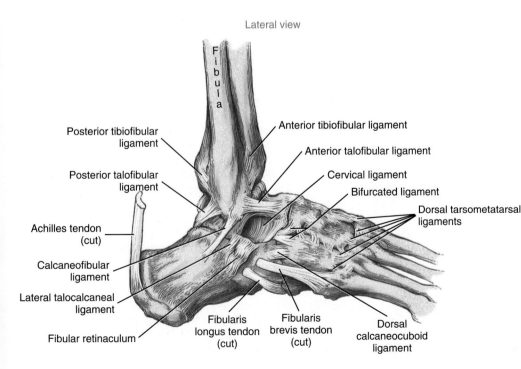

FIGURE 14-15. Lateral view of the right ankle region highlights the lateral collateral ligaments.

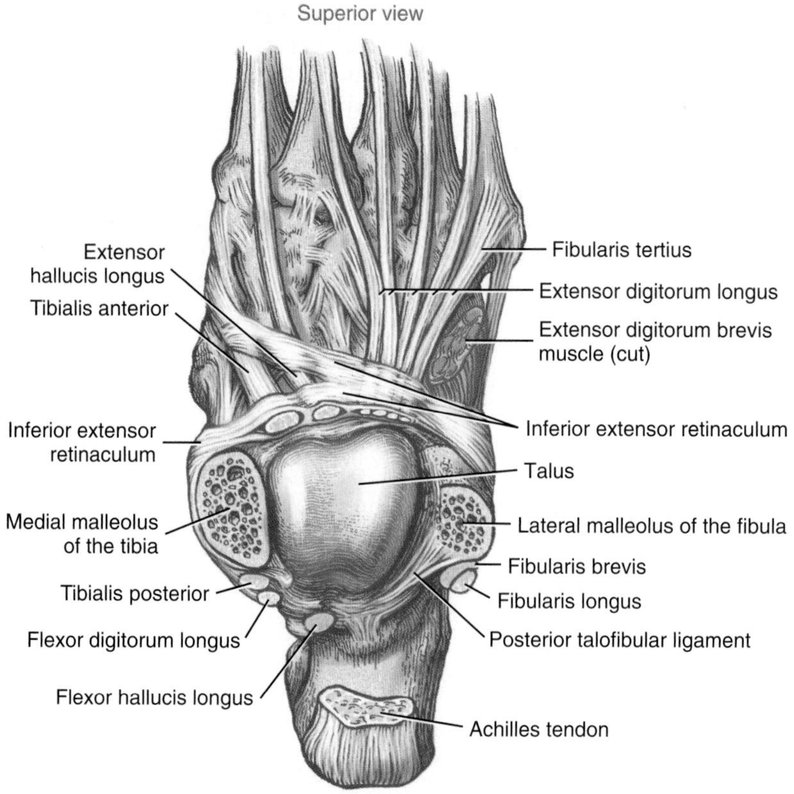
Superior view
Extensor hallucis longus
Tibialis anterior
Inferior extensor retinaculum
Medial malleolus of the tibia
Tibialis posterior
Flexor digitorum longus
Flexor hallucis longus
Fibularis tertius
Extensor digitorum longus
Extensor digitorum brevis muscle (cut)
Inferior extensor retinaculum
Talus
Lateral malleolus of the fibula
Fibularis brevis
Fibularis longus
Posterior talofibular ligament
Achilles tendon

FIGURE 14-16. A superior view displays a cross-section through the right talocrural joint. The talus remains, but the lateral and medial malleolus and all the tendons are cut.

In particular, it limits excessive abduction of the talus, especially when the ankle is fully dorsiflexed.[21]

The *inferior transverse ligament* is a small thick strand of fibers considered part of the posterior talofibular ligament (see Figure 14-12). The fibers continue medially to the posterior aspect of the medial malleolus, forming part of the posterior wall of the talocrural joint.

In summary, the medial and lateral collateral ligaments of the ankle limit excessive eversion and inversion, respectively, at every joint that the fibers cross. Because most of the ligaments course, to varying degrees, from anterior to posterior, they also limit anterior-to-posterior translation of the talus within the mortise. As described in the section on arthrokinematics, the movements of plantar flexion and dorsiflexion are kinematically linked to anterior and posterior translation of the talus, respectively. For these reasons, several of the collateral ligaments are stretched at the extremes of dorsiflexion or plantar flexion of the talocrural joint.

Several of the major ligaments that cross the talocrural joint also cross other joints of the foot, such as the subtalar and talonavicular joints. These ligaments therefore provide stability across multiple joints. Table 14-3 provides a summary of the movements that stretch the major ligaments of the ankle. This information helps explain the mechanisms that frequently injure these ligaments, as well as the rationale behind the manual stress tests performed to evaluate the structural integrity of the ligaments after injury.

Osteokinematics

The talocrural joint possesses one degree of freedom. Motion occurs around an axis of rotation that passes through the body of the talus and through the tips of both malleoli. Because the lateral malleolus is inferior and posterior to the medial malleolus (which should be verified by palpation), the axis of rotation departs slightly from a pure medial-lateral axis. As depicted in Figure 14-17, *A* and *B*, the axis of rotation (in red) is inclined slightly superiorly and anteriorly as it passes laterally to medially through the talus and both malleoli.[78] The axis deviates from a pure medial-lateral axis about 10 degrees in the frontal plane (see Figure 14-17, *A*) and 6 degrees in the horizontal plane (see Figure 14-17, *B*). Because of the pitch of the axis of rotation, dorsiflexion is associated with slight abduction and eversion, and plantar flexion with slight adduction and inversion.[118] By definition, therefore, the talocrural joint produces a movement of pronation and supination. Because the axis of rotation deviates only minimally from the pure medial-lateral axis, the main components of pronation and supination at the talocrural joint are overwhelmingly *dorsiflexion* and *plantar flexion* (see Figure 14-17, *D* and *E*).[76,119] The horizontal and frontal plane components of pronation and supination are indeed small,[88] and usually ignored in most clinical situations.

The 0-degree (neutral) position at the talocrural joint is defined by the foot held at 90 degrees to the leg. From this position, the talocrural joint permits about 15 to 25 degrees of dorsiflexion and 40 to 55 degrees of plantar flexion, although reported values differ considerably based on type and method of measurement.[10,40,118] Accessory movements at the nearby subtalar joint may contribute to about 20% of the total reported range of motion.[40] Dorsiflexion and plantar flexion at the talocrural joint need to be visualized when the foot is off the ground and free to rotate, and when the foot is fixed to the ground as the leg rotates forward, such as during the stance phase of gait.

TABLE 14-3. Movements That Stretch and Elongate the Major Ligaments of the Ankle*

Ligaments	Crossed Joints	Movements That Stretch or Elongate Ligaments
Deltoid ligament (tibiotalar fibers)	Talocrural joint	Eversion, dorsiflexion with associated posterior slide of talus within the mortise
Deltoid ligament (tibionavicular fibers)	Talocrural joint	Eversion, plantar flexion with associated anterior slide of talus within the mortise
	Talonavicular joint	Eversion, abduction
Deltoid ligament (tibiocalcaneal fibers)	Talocrural joint and subtalar joint	Eversion
Anterior talofibular ligament	Talocrural joint	Plantar flexion with associated anterior slide of talus within the mortise, inversion, adduction
Calcaneofibular ligament	Talocrural joint	Dorsiflexion with associated posterior slide of talus within the mortise, inversion
	Subtalar joint	Inversion
Posterior talofibular ligament	Talocrural joint	Dorsiflexion with associated posterior slide of talus within the mortise, abduction, inversion

*The information is based on movements of the unloaded foot relative to a stationary leg.

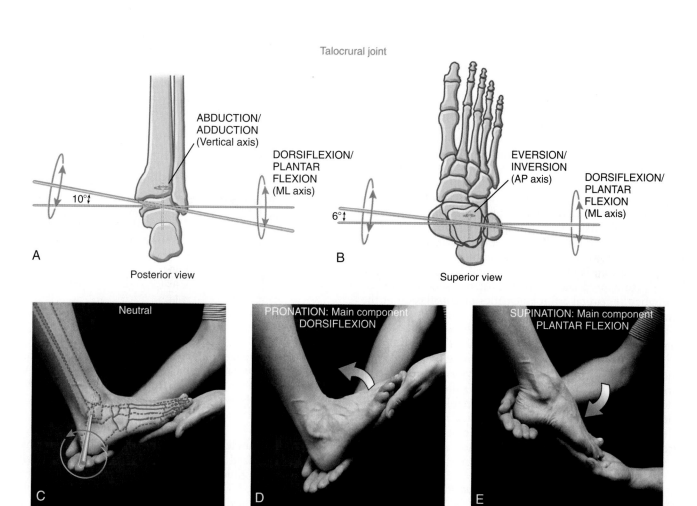

FIGURE 14-17. The axis of rotation and osteokinematics at the talocrural joint. The slightly oblique axis of rotation *(red)* is shown from behind **(A)** and from above **(B)**; this axis is shown again in **C.** The component axes and associated osteokinematics are also depicted in **A** and **B.** Note that, although subtle, dorsiflexion **(D)** is combined with slight abduction and eversion, which are components of pronation; plantar flexion **(E)** is combined with slight adduction and inversion, which are components of supination.

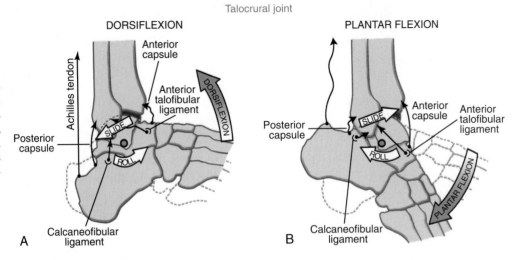

FIGURE 14-18. A lateral view depicts the arthrokinematics at the talocrural joint during passive dorsiflexion **(A)** and plantar flexion **(B)**. Stretched (taut) structures are shown as thin elongated arrows; slackened structures are shown as wavy arrows.

Arthrokinematics

The following discussion assumes that the foot is unloaded and free to rotate. During *dorsiflexion,* the talus rolls forward relative to the leg as it simultaneously slides *posteriorly* (Figure 14-18, *A*). The simultaneous posterior slide allows the talus to rotate forward with only limited anterior translation.[22,134] Figure 14-18, *A* shows the calcaneofibular ligament becoming taut in response to the posterior sliding tendency of the talus-calcaneal segment. Generally, *any collateral ligament that becomes increasingly taut on posterior translation of the talus also becomes increasingly taut during dorsiflexion.* Maximal dorsiflexion elongates the posterior capsule and all tissues capable of transmitting plantar flexion torque, such as the Achilles tendon.

Full dorsiflexion of the ankle is often limited after a sprain of the lateral ankle. One therapeutic approach aimed at increasing dorsiflexion involves passive joint mobilization of the talocrural joint. Specifically, the clinician applies a posterior-directed translation of the talus and foot relative to the leg.[38,134] An appropriately applied posterior slide is designed to mimic the natural arthrokinematics of dorsiflexion at the talocrural joint.

During plantar flexion, the talus rolls posteriorly as the bone simultaneously slides anteriorly (see Figure 14-18, *B*). Generally, *any collateral ligament that becomes increasingly taut on anterior translation of the talus also becomes increasingly taut during plantar flexion.* As depicted in Figure 14-18, *B*, the anterior talofibular ligament is stretched in full plantar flexion. (Although not depicted, the tibionavicular fibers of the deltoid ligament would also become taut at full plantar flexion [review Table 14-3]). Plantar flexion also stretches the dorsiflexor muscles and the anterior capsule of the joint.

Progressive Stabilization of the Talocrural Joint throughout the Stance Phase of Gait

At initial heel contact during walking, the ankle rapidly plantar flexes in order to lower the foot to the ground (Figure 14-19; from 0% to 5% of the gait cycle). As soon as the foot flat phase of gait is reached, the leg starts to rotate forward (dorsiflex) over the grounded foot.[68] Dorsiflexion continues until after just after heel off phase. At this point in the gait cycle, the ankle becomes increasing stable owing to the increased tension in many stretched collateral ligaments and

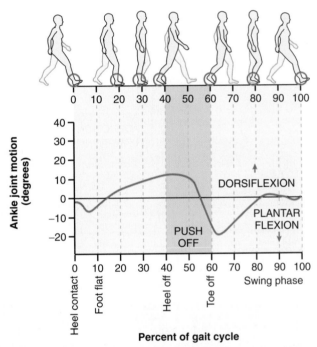

FIGURE 14-19. The range of motion of the right ankle (talocrural) joint is depicted during the major phases of the gait cycle. The push off (propulsion) phase (about 40% to 60% of the gait cycle) is indicated in the darker shade of green.

plantar flexor muscles (Figure 14-20, *A*). The dorsiflexed ankle is further stabilized as the wider anterior part of the talus wedges into the tibiofibular component of the mortise (see Figure 14-20, *B*).[18] The wedging effect causes the distal tibia and fibula to spread apart slightly. This action is resisted by tension in the distal tibiofibular ligaments and interosseous membrane.[6] At the initiation of the push off phase of walking (just after about 40% of the gait cycle; see Figure 14-19), the fully dorsiflexed talocrural joint is well stabilized to accept compression forces that may reach over four times body weight.[121] This inherent stability may partially account for the relatively low frequency of idiopathic osteoarthritis at the talocrural joint.[18,81] Posttraumatic arthritis at the talocrural

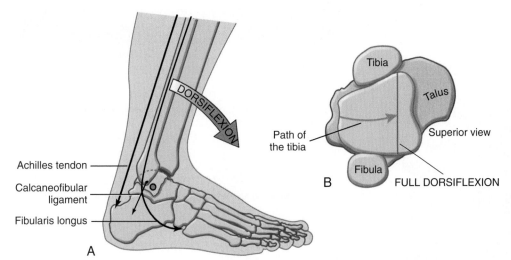

FIGURE 14-20. Factors that increase the mechanical stability of the fully dorsiflexed talocrural joint are shown. **A,** The increased passive tension in several connective tissues and muscles is demonstrated. **B,** The trochlear surface of the talus is wider anteriorly than posteriorly (see red line). The path of dorsiflexion places the concave tibiofibular segment of the mortise in contact with the wider anterior dimension of the talus, thereby causing a wedging effect within the talocrural joint.

joint is, however, relatively common. Residual incongruity within the mortise after trauma can increase intra-articular stress to damaging levels.

The slight natural spreading of the mortise at maximal dorsiflexion causes slight translation of the fibula.[13] The line of force of the stretched anterior and posterior (distal) tibiofibular ligaments and interosseous membrane produces a slight superior translation of the fibula that is transferred proximally to the proximal tibiofibular joint. For this reason, the proximal tibiofibular joint is related more functionally to the ankle (talocrural joint) than to the knee.

Structure and Function of the Joints Associated with the Foot

SUBTALAR JOINT

The subtalar joint, as its name indicates, resides under the talus (see Figure 14-9). To appreciate the extent of subtalar joint motion, one need only firmly grasp the unloaded calcaneus and twist it in a side-to-side and rotary fashion. During this motion, the talus remains essentially stationary within the tight-fitting talocrural joint. Pronation and supination during non–weight-bearing activities occur as the calcaneus moves relative to the fixed talus. In weight bearing such as during the stance phase of walking, for example, pronation and supination occur as the calcaneus remains relatively stationary. This situation requires complex kinematics involving the leg and talus (as a common unit) rotating *over* the stable calcaneus. This mobility at the subtalar joint allows the foot to assume positions that are independent of the orientation of the superimposed ankle and leg. This function is essential to activities such as walking across a steep hill, standing with feet held wide apart, quickly changing directions while walking or running, and keeping one's balance on a rocking boat.

Articular Structure

The large, complex subtalar joint consists of three articulations formed between the posterior, middle, and anterior facets of the calcaneus and the talus. These articulations are depicted in yellow in Figure 14-21.

Ankle Injury Resulting from the Extremes of Dorsiflexion or Plantar Flexion

The proximal and distal tibiofibular joints and interosseous membrane are functionally and structurally related to the talocrural joint. This relationship is apparent after an injury related to extreme dorsiflexion—for example, landing from a jump. An extreme and violent dorsiflexion of the ankle (leg over the foot) can cause the mortise to "explode" outward, injuring many of the collateral ligaments. The traumatic widening of the mortise can also injure the ligaments that support the distal tibiofibular joint and interosseous membrane—the so-called *high ankle or syndesmotic sprain*.[6] This type of injury occurs less frequently than the common inversion ankle sprain but usually requires a more prolonged recovery time.[12]

Full plantar flexion—the loose-packed position of the talocrural joint—slackens most collateral ligaments of the ankle and all plantar flexor muscles. In addition, plantar flexion places the narrower width of the talus between the malleoli, thereby releasing tension within the mortise. As a consequence, full plantar flexion causes the distal tibia and fibula to "loosen their grip" on the talus. Bearing body weight over a fully plantar flexed ankle, therefore, places the talocrural joint in a relatively unstable position. Wearing high heels or landing from a jump in a plantar flexed (and usually inverted) position increases the likelihood of destabilizing the mortis and potentially injuring the lateral ligaments of the ankle.[35]

The prominent *posterior articulation* of the subtalar joint occupies about 70% of the total articular surface area. (Some anatomy texts limit the description of the subtalar joint to the prominent posterior facets only, referring to it as the *talocalcaneal joint*.[120]) The concave posterior facet of the talus rests on the convex posterior facet of the calcaneus. The articulation is held tightly opposed by its interlocking shape, ligaments, body weight, and activated muscle. The closely aligned *anterior* and *middle articulations* consist of smaller,

Superior view

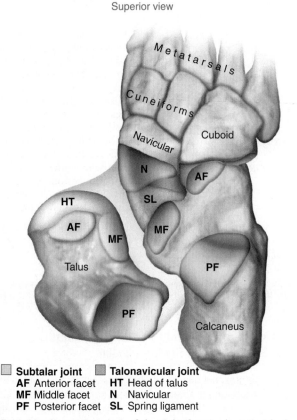

Subtalar joint   **Talonavicular joint**
AF Anterior facet   **HT** Head of talus
MF Middle facet   **N** Navicular
PF Posterior facet   **SL** Spring ligament

FIGURE 14-21. A superior view of the right foot is shown with the talus flipped medially, exposing most of its plantar surface. The articular surfaces of the *subtalar joint* are shown in yellow; the nearby articular surfaces of *talonavicular joint* are shown in light purple. Replacing the talus to its natural position joins the three sets of articular facets within the subtalar joint–anterior facet *(AF)*, middle facet *(MF)*, and posterior facet *(PF)*. Replacing the talus also rearticulates the talonavicular joint by joining the head of the talus *(HT)* within the concavity formed by the concave surfaces of the navicular *(N)* and the spring ligament *(SL)*.

TABLE 14-4. **Primary Functions of the Prominent Ligaments of the Subtalar Joint**	
Ligament	**Primary Function at the Subtalar joint**
Calcaneofibular	Limits excessive inversion
Tibiocalcaneal fibers of the deltoid ligament	Limits excessive eversion
Interosseous (talocalcaneal) Cervical	Both ligaments bind the talus with the calcaneus; limit the extremes of all motions, especially inversion

nearly flat joint surfaces. Although all three articulations contribute to movement at the subtalar joint, clinicians typically focus on the more prominent posterior articulation when performing mobilization techniques to increase the flexibility of the rearfoot.

Ligaments

The posterior and anterior-middle articulations within the subtalar joint are each enclosed by a separate capsule. The larger, posterior capsule is reinforced by three slender thickenings: *medial, posterior,* and *lateral talocalcaneal ligaments* (see Figures 14-12, 14-14, and 14-15). These ligaments are often indistinguishable from the capsule and serve as secondary stabilizers of the joint. Other more prominent ligaments provide the primary source of stabilization to the joint as a whole (Table 14-4). The *calcaneofibular ligament* limits excessive inversion, and the *deltoid ligament (tibiocalcaneal fibers)* limit excessive eversion. (The anatomy of these ligaments was described previously with the talocrural joint.)

The interosseous (talocalcaneal) and cervical ligaments attach directly between the talus and calcaneus[120] and therefore provide the greatest nonmuscular stability to the subtalar joint.

These broad and flat ligaments cross obliquely within the tarsal sinus and therefore are difficult to view unless the joint is disarticulated, as depicted previously in Figure 14-8. The *interosseous (talocalcaneal) ligament* has two distinct, flattened, anterior and posterior bands. These bands arise from the calcaneal sulcus and course superiorly to attach within the talar sulcus and adjacent regions. The larger *cervical ligament* has an oblique fiber arrangement similar to the interosseous ligament but attaches more laterally within the calcaneal sulcus. From this attachment the cervical ligament courses superiorly and medially to attach primarily to the inferior-lateral surface of the neck of the talus (hence the name "cervical") (see Figure 14-15). The interosseous and cervical ligaments limit the extremes of all motions–most notably inversion.[61,120,127]

Although the ligaments within the tarsal sinus are recognized as primary stabilizers at the subtalar joint, a precise anatomic description and a full understanding of their function are unclear.[53,127] This lack of knowledge has limited the development of standard clinical "stress tests" to aid in the diagnosis of ligamentous injury. Cadaveric study suggest that a lateral-to-medial translational force applied to the calcaneus specifically stresses the interosseous ligament.[127] This finding is consistent with the ligament's proposed function of resisting inversion at the subtalar joint.

Kinematics

The arthrokinematics at the subtalar joint involve a sliding motion among the three sets of facets, yielding a curvilinear arc of movement between the calcaneus and the talus. Although considerable variation exists from one person to another,[71] the axis of rotation is typically described as a line that pierces the lateral-posterior heel and courses through the subtalar joint in anterior, medial, and superior directions (Figure 14-22, *A* to *C*, red).[51,80,103] The axis of rotation is positioned 42 degrees from the horizontal plane (see Figure 14-22, *A*) and 16 degrees from the sagittal plane (see Figure 14-22, *B*).[80]

Pronation and supination of the subtalar joint occur as the calcaneus moves relative to the talus (or vice versa when the foot is planted) in an arc that is perpendicular to the axis of rotation (see the red circular arrows in Figure 14-22, *A* to *C*). Given the general pitch to the axis, only two of the three main components of pronation and supination are strongly evident: inversion and eversion, and abduction and adduction (see Figure 14-22, *A* and *B*). *Pronation,* therefore, has main components of *eversion* and *abduction* (see Figure 14-22,

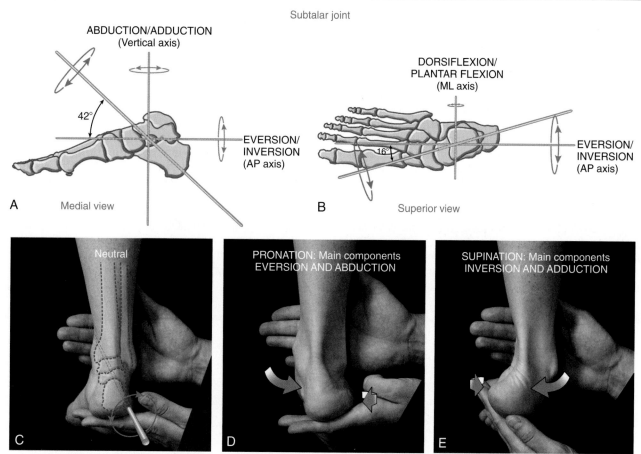

FIGURE 14-22. The axis of rotation and osteokinematics at the subtalar joint. The axis of rotation *(red)* is shown from the side **(A)** and above **(B);** this axis is shown again in **C.** The component axes and associated osteokinematics are also depicted in **A** and **B.** The movement of pronation, with the main components of eversion and abduction, is demonstrated in **D.** The movement of supination, with the main components of inversion and adduction, is demonstrated in **E.** In **D** and **E,** blue arrows indicate abduction and adduction, and purple arrows indicate eversion and inversion.

D); supination has main components of *inversion* and *adduction* (see Figure 14-22, *E*). The calcaneus does dorsiflex and plantar flex slightly relative to the talus; however, this motion is small and usually ignored clinically. Overall, the kinematic pattern expressed at the subtalar joint is much greater than at the talocrural joint.[76]

For simplicity, the osteokinematics of the subtalar joint have been pictorially demonstrated by the calcaneus moving relative to a fixed and essentially immobile talus. During walking, however, when the calcaneus is relatively immobile because of the load of body weight, a significant portion of pronation and supination occur by *horizontal plane rotation of the talus and leg.* Because of the inherent stability and fit provided by the mortise, the majority of the horizontal plane rotation of the talus is mechanically coupled to the rotation of the leg. Small horizontal plane accessory motions within the talocrural joint absorb a small component of this rotation.[96]

Range of Motion

Grimston and colleagues reported active range of inversion and eversion motions at the subtalar joint across 120 healthy subjects (aged 9 through 79 years).[40] Results showed that inversion exceeds eversion by nearly double: inversion, 22.6 degrees; eversion, 12.5 degrees. Although these data include accessory rotations at the talocrural joint, the much greater ratio of inver-

sion to eversion is typical of that reported for the subtalar joint alone.[5,125] Studies that measure *passive* range of motion usually report greater magnitudes of motion, with inversion-to-eversion ratios approaching 3:1.[142] Regardless of active or passive motion, the distally projecting lateral malleolus and the relatively thick deltoid ligament naturally limit eversion.

TRANSVERSE TARSAL JOINT (TALONAVICULAR AND CALCANEOCUBOID JOINTS)

The transverse tarsal joint, also known as the *midtarsal joint,* consists of two anatomically distinct articulations: the *talonavicular joint* and the *calcaneocuboid joint.* These joints connect the rearfoot with the midfoot (see organization of joints illustrated in Figure 14-23).

At this particular point in this chapter, it may be instructive to consider the functional characteristics of the transverse tarsal joint within the context of the other major joints of the ankle and foot. As described earlier, the talocrural (ankle) joint permits motion primarily in the sagittal plane: dorsiflexion and plantar flexion. The subtalar joint, however, permits a more oblique path of motion consisting of two primary components: inversion-eversion and abduction-adduction. This section now describes how the transverse tarsal joint, the most versatile joint of the foot, moves through a more oblique

SPECIAL FOCUS 14-2

Standard Clinical Measurements of Subtalar Joint Range of Motion

Accurately measuring the extent of pronation and supination at the subtalar joint through standard goniometry is very difficult. Measurement error reflects the inability of a standard, rigid goniometer to follow the oblique arc of pronation and supination, compounded by simultaneous movements in surrounding joints. As a method of improving the usefulness of this measurement, clinicians often report subtalar joint motion as a more simple frontal plane motion of inversion and eversion of the rearfoot (calcaneus).

The rather strict terminology described for subtalar motion is not always adhered to in clinical and research settings. "Shortcuts" in terminology have evolved that, unfortunately, limit the ability to effectively communicate the precise details of foot and ankle kinesiology. Pronation and supination at the subtalar joint

are often referred to simply as *eversion* and *inversion* of the calcaneus, respectively. Eversion, for example, is only a component of, rather than a synonym of, pronation. Comparisons of range-of-motion data among studies are often difficult, unless the motions are explicitly defined.

Clinically, the expression "subtalar joint neutral" is often used to establish a baseline or reference for evaluating a foot before fabrication of an orthotic device.[47] The neutral position of the subtalar joint is attained by placing the subject's calcaneus in a position that allows both lateral and medial sides of the talus to be equally exposed for palpation within the mortise. In this "neutral" position, the joint is typically one third the distance from full eversion and two thirds the distance from full inversion.

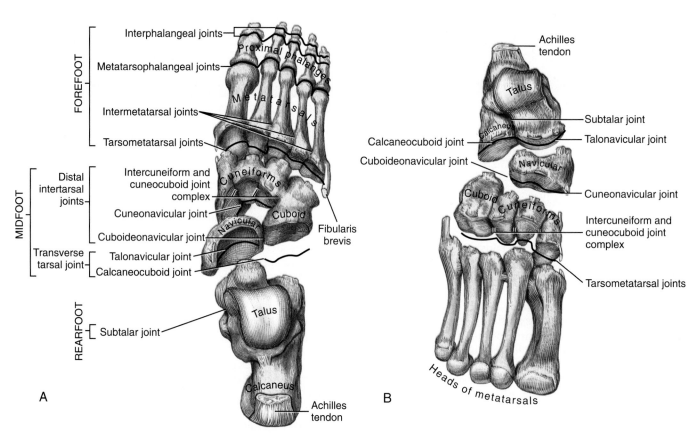

FIGURE 14-23. A, The bones and disarticulated joints of the right foot are shown from two perspectives: superior-posterior **(A)** and superior-anterior **(B).** The overall organization of the joints is highlighted in **A.**

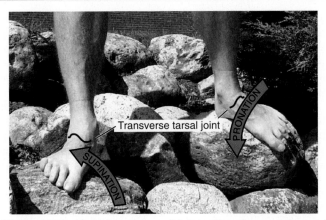

FIGURE 14-24. The transverse tarsal joints allow for pronation and supination of the midfoot while one stands on uneven surfaces.

path of motion, cutting nearly *equally through all three cardinal planes*. Among other important functions, the path of pronation and supination at the transverse tarsal joint allows the weight-bearing foot to adapt to a variety of surface contours (Figure 14-24).

The transverse tarsal joint has a strong functional relationship with the subtalar joint. As will be described, these two joints function cooperatively to control most of the pronation and supination posturing of the entire foot.

Articular Structure and Ligamentous Support

Talonavicular Joint

The talonavicular joint (the medial compartment of the transverse tarsal joint) resembles a ball-and-socket joint, providing substantial mobility to the medial (longitudinal) column of the foot. Much of this mobility is expressed as a twisting (inverting and everting) of the midfoot relative to the rearfoot.[74] The talonavicular joint consists of the articulation between the convex head of the talus and the continuous, deep concavity formed by the proximal side of the navicular bone and "spring" ligament (see Figure 14-8). The convex-concave relationship of the talonavicular joint is evident in Figure 14-21. The *spring ligament* (labeled as SL in Figure 14-21) is a thick and wide band of collagenous connective tissue, spanning the gap between the sustentaculum talus of the calcaneus and the medial-plantar surface of the navicular bone.[87] By directly supporting the medial and plantar convexity of the head of the talus, the spring ligament forms the structural "floor and medial wall" of the talonavicular joint. Considerable support is required in this region during standing because body weight tends to depress the head of the talus in plantar and medial directions—toward the earth. The surface of the spring ligament that directly contacts the head of the talus is lined with smooth fibrocartilage.[120] (The more formal and precise name of the spring ligament is the *plantar calcaneonavicular ligament*. The term "spring" is actually a misnomer because it has little, if any, elasticity; its highly collagenous nature offers considerable strength and resistance to elongation. Nevertheless, the term *spring* remains well established in the clinical and research literature.[87])

An irregularly shaped capsule surrounds the talonavicular joint. The ligaments reinforcing this capsule are summarized in the box.

> **Summary of Ligaments That Reinforce the Talonavicular Joint**
> - Interosseous ligament (of the subtalar joint) reinforces the capsule *posteriorly* (see Figure 14-8).
> - Dorsal talonavicular ligament reinforces the capsule *dorsally* (see Figure 14-14).
> - Bifurcated ligament (calcaneonavicular fibers) reinforces the capsule *laterally* (see Figure 14-15).
> - Anterior (tibionavicular) fibers of the deltoid ligament reinforce the capsule *medially* (see Figure 14-14).

Calcaneocuboid Joint

The calcaneocuboid joint is the lateral component of the transverse tarsal joint, formed by the junction of the anterior (distal) surface of the calcaneus with the proximal surface of the cuboid (see Figure 14-23). Each articular surface has a concave and convex curvature. The joint surfaces form an interlocking wedge that resists sliding. The calcaneocuboid joint allows less motion than the talonavicular joint, especially in the frontal and horizontal planes.[76] The relative inflexibility of the calcaneocuboid joint provides stability to the lateral (longitudinal) column of the foot.

The dorsal and lateral parts of the capsule of the calcaneocuboid joint are thickened by the *dorsal calcaneocuboid ligament* (see Figure 14-15).[102] Three additional ligaments further stabilize the joint. The *bifurcated ligament* is a Y-shaped band of tissue with its stem attached to the calcaneus, just proximal to the dorsal surface of the calcaneocuboid joint. The stem of the ligament flares into lateral and medial fiber bundles. The aforementioned medial (calcaneonavicular) fibers reinforce the lateral side of the talonavicular joint. The lateral (calcaneocuboid) fibers cross the dorsal side of the calcaneocuboid joint, forming the primary bond between the two bones.[120]

The long and short plantar ligaments reinforce the plantar side of the calcaneocuboid joint (Figure 14-25). The *long*

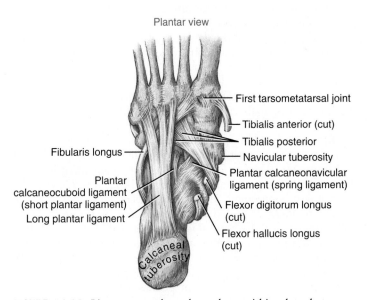

FIGURE 14-25. Ligaments and tendons deep within the plantar aspect of the right foot. Note the course of the tendons of the fibularis longus and tibialis posterior.

plantar ligament, the longest ligament in the foot, arises from the plantar surface of the calcaneus, just anterior to the calcaneal tuberosity. The ligament inserts on the plantar surface of the bases of the lateral three or four metatarsal bones. The *short plantar ligament*, also called the *plantar calcaneocuboid ligament*, arises just anterior and deep to the long plantar ligament and inserts on the plantar surface of the cuboid bone. By passing perpendicularly to the calcaneocuboid joint, the plantar ligaments provide excellent structural stability to the lateral column of the foot.[70]

Summary of Ligaments That Reinforce the Calcaneocuboid Joint

- Dorsal calcaneocuboid ligament reinforces the capsule *dorsal-laterally* (see Figure 14-15).
- Bifurcated ligament (calcaneocuboid fibers) reinforces the calcaneocuboid joint *dorsally* (see Figure 14-15).
- Long and short plantar ligaments (see Figure 14-25) reinforce the *plantar side* of the calcaneocuboid joint.

Kinematics

The transverse tarsal joint rarely moves without associated movements at nearby joints, especially the subtalar joint. To appreciate the mobility that occurs primarily at the transverse tarsal joint, hold the calcaneus firmly while maximally pronating and supinating the midfoot (Figure 14-26, *A* and *C*, respectively). During these motions the navicular spins within the talonavicular joint.[74] Combining motions across *both* the subtalar and transverse tarsal joints accounts for most of the pronation and supination throughout the foot (see Figure 14-26, *B* and *D,* respectively). As evident throughout Figure 14-26, mobility of the forefoot contributes to the pronation and supination of the entire foot.

Three noteworthy points should be made before the detailed kinematics of the transverse tarsal joint are addressed. *First,* two separate axes of rotation have been identified. *Second,* the amplitude and direction of movement is typically different during weight-bearing as compared with non–weight-bearing activities. *Third,* the ability of the transverse tarsal joint to stabilize the midfoot depends strongly on the position of the subtalar joint. The upcoming sections discuss each of these factors.

Axes of Rotation and Corresponding Movements

Manter originally described two axes of rotation for movement at the transverse tarsal joint: *longitudinal* and *oblique.*[80] Movement at this joint therefore occurs naturally in two unique planes, each oriented perpendicular to a specific axis of rotation. The *longitudinal axis* is nearly coincident with the straight anterior-posterior axis (Figure 14-27, *A* to *C*), with the primary component motions of *eversion* and *inversion* (see Figure 14-27, *D* and *E*). The *oblique axis,* in contrast, has a strong vertical *and* medial-lateral pitch (see Figure 14-27, *F* to *H*). Motion around this axis, therefore, occurs freely as a combination of *abduction and dorsiflexion* (Figure 14-27, *I*), and *adduction and plantar flexion* (see Figure 14-27, *J*).

The transverse tarsal joint possesses two separate axes of rotation, with each axis producing a unique kinematic pattern. Although this may be technically correct, the functional kinematics associated with most weight-bearing activities occur as

a blending of movements across *both* axes—a blend that yields the purest form of pronation and supination (i.e., movement that maximally expresses components of *all three* cardinal planes).[76,95] Pronation and supination at the transverse tarsal joint allow the midfoot (and ultimately the forefoot) to adapt to many varied shapes and contours.

Range of motion at the transverse tarsal joint is difficult to measure and isolate from adjacent joints. By visual and manual inspection, however, it is evident that the midfoot allows about twice as much supination as pronation. The amount of pure inversion and eversion of the midfoot occurs in a pattern similar to that observed at the subtalar joint: about 20 to 25 degrees of inversion and 10 to 15 degrees of eversion.

Arthrokinematics

The arthrokinematics at the transverse tarsal joint are best described in context with motion across both the rearfoot and midfoot. Consider the movement of active *supination* of the unloaded foot in Figure 14-26, *D.* The tibialis posterior muscle, with its multiple attachments, is the prime supinator of the foot.[64] Because of the relatively rigid calcaneocuboid joint, an inverting and adducting calcaneus draws the lateral column of the foot "under" the medial column of the foot. The important pivot point for this motion is the talonavicular joint. The pull of the tibialis posterior contributes to the spin of the navicular, and to the raising of the medial longitudinal

---

SPECIAL FOCUS 14-3

Position of the Subtalar Joint Affecting Stability of the Transverse Tarsal Joint

In addition to controlling the position of the rearfoot, the subtalar joint also indirectly controls the stability of the more distal joints, especially the transverse tarsal joint. Although the relevance of this concept is discussed later in this chapter, *full supination at the subtalar joint restricts the overall flexibility of the midfoot.* A loosely articulated skeletal model helps to demonstrate this principle. With one hand stabilizing the talus, maximally "swing" the calcaneus into full inversion and note that the lateral aspect of the midfoot "drops" relative to the medial aspect. As a result, the talonavicular and calcaneocuboid joints (components of the transverse tarsal joint) become twisted longitudinally, thereby increasing the rigidity of the midfoot. *Full pronation of the subtalar joint, in contrast, increases the overall flexibility of the midfoot.* Again, returning to a loosely articulated skeleton model, maximal eversion of the calcaneus untwists the medial and lateral aspects of the midfoot, placing them in a nearly parallel position. As a result, the talonavicular and calcaneocuboid joints untwist longitudinally, thereby increasing the flexibility of the midfoot. Make the effort to "feel" on a partner the increased multi-planar flexibility of the midfoot (and forefoot) as the calcaneus is gradually taken from a maximal inversion to a maximal eversion position.[9] As described in subsequent sections, the ability of the midfoot to change its flexibility has important mechanical implications during the stance phase of gait.

PRONATION of the foot (dorsal-medial view)

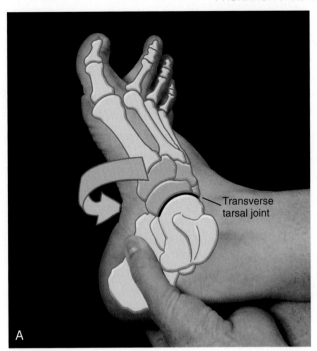

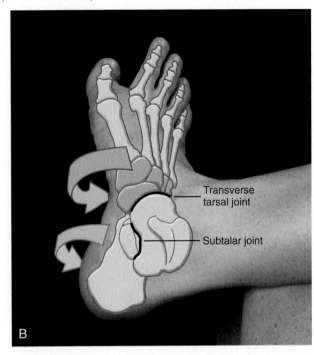

SUPINATION of the foot (plantar-medial view)

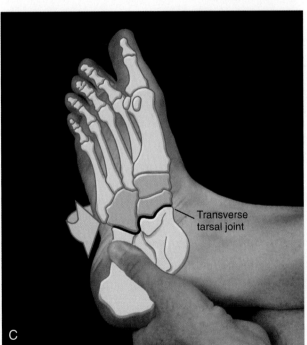

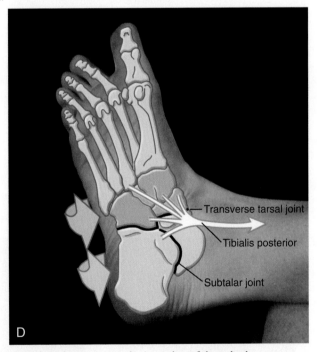

FIGURE 14-26. Pronation and supination of the unloaded right foot demonstrates the interplay of the subtalar and transverse tarsal joints. With the calcaneus held fixed, pronation and supination occur primarily at the midfoot (**A** and **C**). When the calcaneus is free, pronation and supination occur as a summation across both the rearfoot and midfoot (**B** and **D**). Rearfoot movement is indicated by pink arrows; midfoot movement is indicated by blue arrows. The pull of the tibialis posterior muscle is shown in **D** as it directs active supination over both the rearfoot and midfoot.

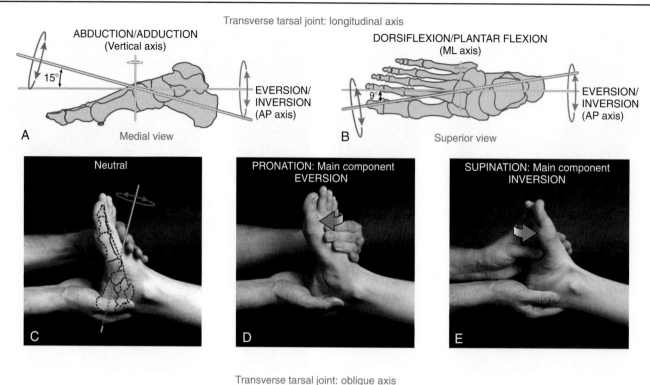

Transverse tarsal joint: longitudinal axis

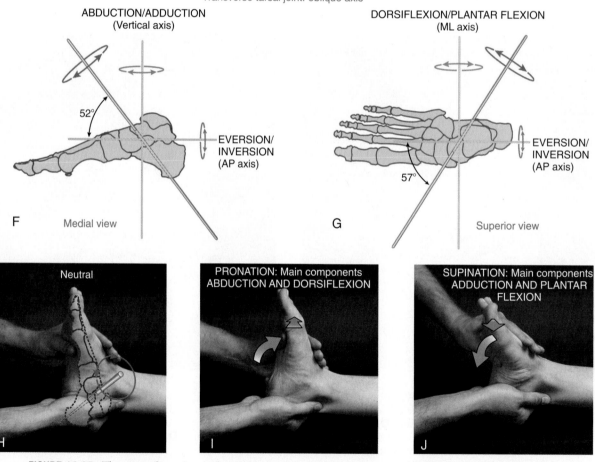

Transverse tarsal joint: oblique axis

FIGURE 14-27. The axes of rotation and osteokinematics at the transverse tarsal joint. The *longitudinal axis* of rotation is shown in red from the side (**A** and **C**) and from above (**B**). (The component axes and associated osteokinematics are also depicted in **A** and **B**.) Movements that occur around the longitudinal axis are (**D**) *pronation* (with the main component of eversion) and (**E**) *supination* (with the main component of inversion). The *oblique axis* of rotation is shown in red from the side (**F** and **H**) and from above (**G**). (The component axes and associated osteokinematics are also depicted in **F** and **G**.) Movements that occur around the oblique axis are (**I**) *pronation* (with main components of abduction and dorsiflexion) and (**J**) *supination* (with main components of adduction and plantar flexion). In **I** and **J**, blue arrows indicate abduction and adduction, and green arrows indicate dorsiflexion and plantar flexion.

arch (instep) of the foot. During this motion, the concave proximal surface of the navicular and the spring ligament both spin around the convex head of the talus.

Pronation of the unloaded foot occurs by similar but reverse kinematics as those described. The pull of the fibularis longus helps lower the medial side and raise the lateral side of the foot.

The previously described arthrokinematics of supination and pronation assume that the foot is unloaded, or off the ground. The challenge is to understand these arthrokinematics when the foot is *on* the ground, typically during the walking process. This topic is addressed later in this chapter.

Medial Longitudinal Arch of the Foot

Figure 14-28 shows the locations of the medial longitudinal and transverse arches of the foot. Both arches lend very important elements of stability and resiliency to the loaded foot. The talonavicular joint serves as the keystone to the medial longitudinal arch. For this reason, the structure and function of the medial longitudinal arch is addressed in this section. The transverse arch is described later during the study of the distal intertarsal joints.

The *medial longitudinal arch* is evident as the characteristic concave "instep" of the medial side of the foot. This arch is the primary load-bearing and shock-absorbing structure of the foot.[129] The bones that form the medial arch are the calcaneus, talus, navicular, cuneiforms, and associated three medial metatarsals. Without this arched configuration, the large and rapidly produced forces applied against the foot during running, for example, would likely exceed the physiologic weight-bearing capacity of the bones. Additional structures that assist the arch in absorbing loads are the plantar fat pads, sesamoid bones located at the plantar base of the great toe, and superficial plantar fascia (which attaches primarily to the overlying thick dermis, functioning primarily to reduce shear forces.) As will be described, the medial longitudinal arch and associated connective tissues are usually adequate to support the foot during relatively low-stress or near-static conditions—for example, standing at ease. Active muscular forces, however, assist the arch when the stresses and loads on the foot are larger and more dynamic, such as during standing on tiptoes, walking, jumping, or running. The following section describes the passive support mechanism provided by the medial longitudinal arch. The role of muscles in providing active support is described later, in the study of muscles of the ankle and foot.

Passive Support Mechanism of the Medial Longitudinal Arch

The talonavicular joint and associated connective tissues form the *keystone* of the medial longitudinal arch. Additional nonmuscular structures responsible for maintaining the height and general shape of this arch are the plantar fascia, spring ligament, and first tarsometatarsal joint. The *plantar fascia of the foot* provides the primary passive support to the medial longitudinal arch.[26,48] This extremely strong fascia consists of a series of thick, longitudinal and transverse bands of collagen-rich tissue.[59] The plantar fascia covers the sole and sides of the foot and is organized into superficial and deep fibers. The superficial fibers, introduced above, attach primarily to the overlying thick dermis. The more extensive deep plantar fascia attaches posteriorly to the medial process of the calcaneal tuberosity. From this origin, lateral, medial, and central

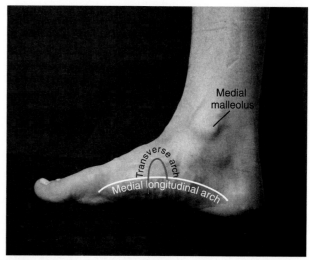

FIGURE 14-28. The medial side of a normal foot shows the medial longitudinal arch *(white)* and the transverse arch *(red)*.

sets of fibers course anteriorly, blending with and covering the first layer of the intrinsic muscles of the foot. The main, larger, central set of fibers extends toward the metatarsal heads, where the fibers attach to the plantar plates (ligaments) of the metatarsophalangeal joints and fibrous sheaths of the adjacent flexor tendons of the digits. Active toe extension therefore stretches the central band of deep fascia, adding tension to the medial longitudinal arch. This mechanism is useful because it increases tension in the arch when one stands on tiptoes, or during the push off phase of gait.

When one stands normally, the weight of the body falls through the foot near the region of talonavicular joint. This load is distributed anteriorly and posteriorly throughout the medial longitudinal arch, ultimately passing to the fat pads and the thick dermis over the heel and ball (metatarsal head region) of the foot (Figure 14-29, *A*). Normally the rearfoot receives about twice the compressive load as the forefoot.[20] The mean pressure under the forefoot is usually greatest in the region of the heads of the second and third metatarsal bones.

During standing, body weight tends to depress the talus inferiorly and flatten the medial longitudinal arch. This action increases the distance between the calcaneus and metatarsal heads. Tension in stretched connective tissues, especially the deep plantar fascia, acts as a semi-elastic tie-rod that "gives" slightly under load, allowing only a marginal drop in the arch (see stretched spring in Figure 14-29, *A*). Acting like a truss, the tie-rod supports and absorbs body weight. Experiments on cadaveric specimens indicate that the deep plantar fascia is the major structure that maintains the height of the medial longitudinal arch; cutting the fascia decreased arch stiffness by 25%.[48]

As the arch is depressed, the rearfoot normally pronates a few degrees. This is most evident from a posterior view as the calcaneus everts slightly relative to the tibia. As the foot is unloaded, such as through the shifting of body weight to the other leg during walking, the naturally elastic and flexible arch returns to its preloaded raised height. The calcaneus inverts slightly back to its neutral position, allowing the mechanism to repeat its shock absorption function once again.

Normal arch

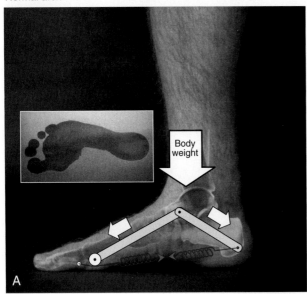

Dropped arch

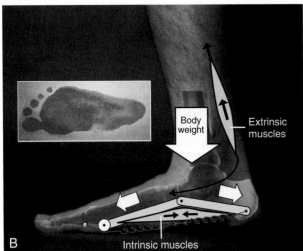

FIGURE 14-29. Models of the foot show a mechanism of accepting body weight during standing. **A,** With a normal medial longitudinal arch, body weight is accepted and dissipated primarily through elongation of the plantar fascia, depicted as a red spring. The footprint illustrates the concavity of the normal arch. **B,** With an abnormally dropped medial longitudinal arch, the overstretched and weakened plantar fascia, depicted as an overstretched red spring, cannot adequately accept or dissipate body weight. As a consequence, various extrinsic and intrinsic muscles are active as a secondary source of support to the arch. The footprint illustrates the dropped arch and loss of a characteristic instep.

Standing at ease on healthy feet typically produces very little activity from the intrinsic or extrinsic muscles of the foot.[4] The height and shape of the medial longitudinal arch is controlled primarily by passive restraints from the connective tissues depicted by the spring in Figure 14-29, *A*. Active muscle support during standing is usually required only as a "secondary line of support"–for example, when a heavy load

is held, or when the arch lacks inherent support because of overstretched connective tissues.[126]

Pes Planus—"Abnormally Dropped" Medial Longitudinal Arch
Pes planus or "flatfoot" describes a chronically dropped or abnormally low medial longitudinal arch.[58,144] This condition is often the result of joint laxity within the midfoot or proximal forefoot regions, typically combined with an overstretched or weakened plantar fascia, spring ligament, and tibialis posterior tendon.[97,129] During the stance phase of walking, the subtalar joint subsequently pronates excessively as the rearfoot assumes an exaggerated valgus posture (calcaneus excessively everted away from the midline).[129] The depressed talus and navicular bones often cause a callus on the adjacent skin.

Figure 14-29, *B* shows the foot of a person with pes planus. The abnormally wide midfoot region evident in the footprint is indicative of excessive laxity within the joints that normally support the arch.[55] A person with moderate or severe pes planus typically has a compromised ability to dissipate loads optimally throughout the foot. Active forces from intrinsic and extrinsic muscles are often required to compensate for the lack of tension produced in overstretched or weakened connective tissues. Increased muscular activity may be needed even during quiet standing, which may contribute to fatigue and various overuse symptoms, including pain, "shin splints," bone spurs, and a thickened and inflamed plantar fascia.[136]

Pes planus is often described as being either a rigid or a flexible deformity. The foot with *rigid pes planus* (as shown in Figure 14-29, *B*) demonstrates a dropped arch even in non–weight-bearing positions. This deformity is often congenital, secondary to bony or joint malformation, such as tarsal coalition (i.e., partial fusion of the calcaneus with the talus fixed in eversion). Pes planus may also occur from spastic paralysis and the resultant overpull from certain muscles. Because of the fixed nature and potential for producing painful symptoms, rigid pes planus may require surgical correction during childhood.

Flexible pes planus is the more common form of a dropped arch. The medial longitudinal arch appears essentially normal when unloaded but drops excessively on weight bearing. Acquired flexible pes planus is often associated with tendinopathy or generalized dysfunction of the tibialis posterior muscle, increased laxity of local connective tissues, or structural anomalies and/or compensatory mechanisms that cause excessive pronation of the foot. Surgical intervention is rarely indicated for flexible pes planus. Treatment is usually in the form of orthosis, specialized footwear, and exercise.[31,64,66]

COMBINED ACTION OF THE SUBTALAR AND TRANSVERSE TARSAL JOINTS

When the foot is *unloaded* (i.e., not bearing weight), pronation twists the sole of the foot outward, whereas supination twists the sole of the foot inward. While the foot is under load during the stance phase of walking, however, pronation and supination permit the leg and talus to rotate in all three planes relative to a relatively fixed calcaneus. This important mechanism is orchestrated primarily through an interaction among the subtalar joint, transverse tarsal joint, and medial longitudinal arch. Much remains to be learned about this complex topic.[68,76,82]

Pes Cavus—Abnormally Raised Medial Longitudinal Arch

In its least complicated form, *pes cavus* describes an abnormally *raised* medial longitudinal arch, typically associated with excessive rearfoot varus (inversion) (Figure 14-30). Excessive forefoot valgus (eversion) may also be present, often as a compensation mechanism used to keep the medial forefoot firmly in contact with the ground.

Pes cavus may be fixed or progressive and may manifest in early childhood or later in life. An abnormally raised medial longitudinal arch receives far less clinical attention than an abnormally dropped or low arch (pes planus).[79] Several factors can cause or are associated with pes cavus. Many relatively mild forms of pes cavus are considered *idiopathic* with a strong genetic predisposition, such as the subject depicted in Figure 14-30. Functional limitations associated with mild or subtle pes cavus vary from nonexistent to marked; often the disorder goes undiagnosed. Regardless of severity, a chronically high arch alters the biomechanics of walking and running. As clearly depicted in Figure

14-30, the abnormally high arch places the metatarsal bones at a greater angle with the ground. As a result, contact pressures can increase in the region of the metatarsal heads, often causing callus formation and metatarsalgia. Furthermore, a foot with a chronically raised (and relatively rigid) arch cannot optimally absorb the repeated impacts of running.[138] A person with pes cavus is therefore more vulnerable to stress-related injury, not only in the foot but also throughout the lower limb. This clinically held premise has received mixed support by several studies of military recruits during their basic training.[25,27,56,69,89]

More severe cases of pes cavus also exist—many of which are associated with a known cause. Pes cavus may be *posttraumatic*, caused by, for example, severe fracture, crush injury, or burn. An unresolved *"clubfoot"* in childhood may persist later in life as pes cavus. Perhaps the most involved cases of pes cavus have a *neurologic* origin, such as Charcot-Marie-Tooth disease, poliomyelitis, cerebral palsy, peripheral nerve injury, and various motor and sensory neuropathies. Although usually for different reasons, these disorders often cause marked force imbalances within the muscles that act on the foot. Over time, a persistent force imbalance ultimately causes the pes cavus deformity. For example, spastic or otherwise overpowering tibialis posterior and fibularis longus muscles combined with a weakened or paralyzed tibialis anterior muscle eventually favor development of a rearfoot varus and forefoot valgus deformity. The weakened tibialis anterior muscle may also allow the fibularis longus to overpull the first metatarsal into excessive plantar flexion. A combined rearfoot varus, forefoot valgus, and excessively plantar flexed first metatarsal are often the more prominent features of pes cavus.

Treatment of pes cavus varies depending on severity or progressive nature of the underlying cause. Conservative management may include stretching of tight muscles (including the typically tight gastrocnemius and soleus) and the use of specialized footware or orthotic devices.[79] Braces may be helpful for joint alignment or support in cases of muscle paralysis. In more severe or involved cases, surgery may be indicated, including osteotomy, tendon transfer, or Achilles tendon and other soft-tissue lengthening procedures.[143]

Pes cavus

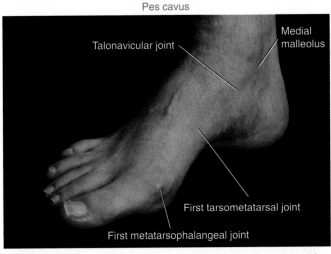

FIGURE 14-30. A photograph of a right foot of a man with idiopathic pes cavus. Several key joints and bony landmarks are indicated.

In the healthy foot the medial longitudinal arch rises and lowers cyclically throughout the gait cycle. During most of the stance phase, the arch lowers slightly in response to the progressive loading of body weight (Figure 14-31, *A*).[19,50] Structures that resist the lowering of the arch help to absorb local stress as the foot is progressively compressed by body weight. Although not always verifiable through controlled research, this load attenuation mechanism likely protects the foot and lower limb against stress-related injury.[27,56,86,138]

During the first 30% to 35% of the gait cycle, the subtalar joint pronates (everts), adding an element of flexibility to the midfoot (see Figure 14-31, *B*).[24] By late stance, the arch rises as the supinated subtalar joint adds rigidity to the midfoot. The rigidity prepares the foot to support the large loads produced at the push off phase of gait. The ability of the

foot to repeatedly transform from a flexible and shock-absorbent structure to a more rigid lever during each gait cycle is one of the most important and clinically relevant actions of the foot. As subsequently described, the subtalar joint is the principal joint that directs the pronation and supination kinematics of the foot.

Early to Mid-Stance Phase of Gait:
Kinematics of Pronation at the Subtalar Joint

Immediately after the heel contact phase of gait, the dorsi-flexed talocrural joint and slightly supinated subtalar joint rapidly plantar flex and pronate, respectively (compare Figures 14-19 and 14-31, *B*). Although the data plotted in Figure 14-31, *B* show only 2 degrees of average maximum eversion (beyond the resting posture),[24] other researchers

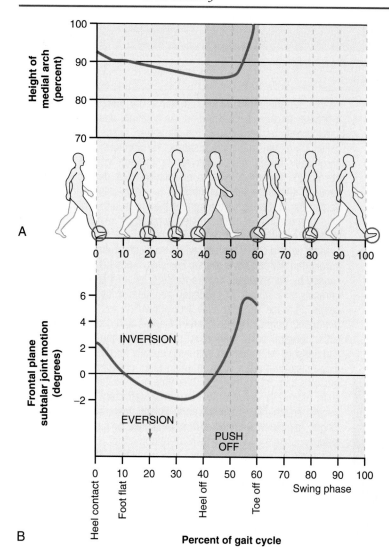

FIGURE 14-31. A, The percent change in height of the medial longitudinal arch throughout the stance phase (0% to 60%) of the gait cycle. On the vertical axis, the 100% value is the height of the arch when the foot is unloaded during the swing phase. **B,** Plot of frontal plane range of motion at the subtalar joint (i.e., inversion and eversion of the calcaneus) throughout the stance phase.[24] The 0-degree reference for frontal plane motions is defined as the position of the calcaneus (observed posteriorly) while a subject stands at rest. The push off phase of walking is indicated by the darker shade of purple.

using asymptomatic subjects report higher values, in the range of 5 to 9 degrees.[50,129,142] Differences in defining the 0-degree position of the subtalar joint, dissimilar sample sizes, and the varying measurement techniques account for much of this inconsistency within the literature.[142] For this reason, it is often difficult to define what constitutes "abnormal" eversion (pronation) during walking.

The pronation (eversion) at the subtalar joint during stance occurs primarily by two mechanisms. *First,* the calcaneus tips into slight eversion in response to the ground reaction force passing upward and just lateral to the midpoint of the posterior calcaneus. The simultaneous impact of heel contact also pushes the head of the talus medially in the horizontal plane and inferiorly in the sagittal plane. Relative to the calcaneus, this motion of the talus abducts and (slightly) dorsiflexes the subtalar joint. These motions are consistent with the formal definition of pronation. A loosely articulated skeletal model aids in the visualization of this motion. *Second,* during the early stance phase, the tibia and fibula, and to a lesser extent the femur, internally rotate after initial heel contact.[51,105] Because of the embracing configuration of the talocrural joint, *the internally rotating lower leg steers the subtalar joint into further pronation.* The argument is often raised that

with the calcaneus in contact with the ground, pronation at the subtalar joint causes, rather than follows, internal rotation of the leg; either perspective is valid.

The amplitude of pronation at the subtalar joint during early to mid-stance phase of walking is indeed relatively small–about 5 degrees on average–occurring for only one quarter of a second during average-speed walking. The amount and the speed of the pronation nevertheless influence the kinematics of the more proximal joints of the lower extremity. These effects can be readily appreciated by exaggerating and dramatically slowing the pronation action of the rearfoot during the initial loading phase of gait. Consider the demonstration depicted in Figure 14-32. While standing over a loaded and fixed foot, forcefully but slowly internally rotate the lower limb and observe the associated pronation at the rearfoot (subtalar joint) and simultaneous lowering of the medial longitudinal arch.[95] If sufficiently forceful, this action also tends to internally rotate, slightly flex, and adduct the hip and create a valgus stress on the knee (Table 14-5). These mechanical events are indeed exaggerated and do not all occur to this degree and pattern during walking at normal speed. Nevertheless, because of the linkages throughout the lower limb, excessive or uncontrolled pronation of the

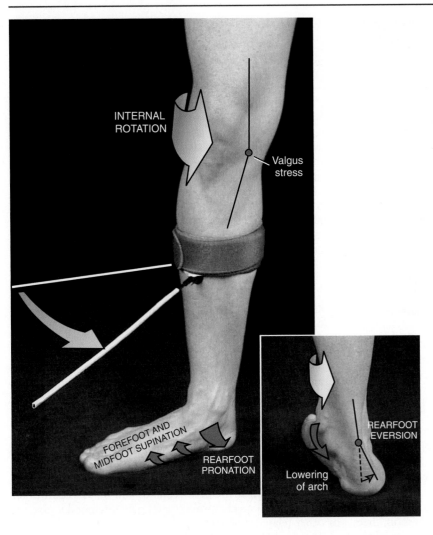

FIGURE 14-32. With the foot fixed, full internal rotation of the lower limb is mechanically associated with rearfoot pronation (eversion), lowering of the medial longitudinal arch, and valgus stress at the knee. Note that as the rearfoot pronates, the floor "pushes" the forefoot and midfoot into a relatively supinated position.

TABLE 14-5. Selected Actions that may be Associated with Exaggerated Pronation of the Subtalar Joint during Weight Bearing	
Joint or Region	**Action**
Hip	Internal rotation, flexion, and adduction
Knee	Increased valgus stress
Rearfoot	Pronation (eversion) with a lowering of medial longitudinal arch
Midfoot and forefoot	Supination (inversion)

rearfoot could exaggerate one or more of these mechanically related joint actions.[57] Clinically, a person who excessively pronates during early stance may complain of medial knee pain, possibly from excessive valgus stress placed on the knee and subsequent overstretching of the medial collateral ligament. Whether the overpronation causes excessive strain on the medial collateral ligament or vice versa is not always obvious.

Although widely accepted, a predictable kinematic relationship between the magnitude and timing of excessive pronation and excessive internal rotation throughout the lower limb has not been established conclusively.[105] Precise measurements of these kinematic relationships while a subject is walking are technically difficult. The kinematics themselves are highly variable and poorly defined. Some studies report the kinematics as a rotation of a single bone, and others report relative rotations between bones. Additional studies are needed in this area before definite cause-and-effect relationships are known. These relationships are important, as they serve as the basis for many exercises and for the use of orthotics to reduce painful conditions related to excessive or poorly controlled pronation.

Biomechanical Benefits of Limiting Pronation during the Stance Phase

Controlled pronation of the subtalar joint through the mid-stance phase of walking has several useful biomechanical effects. Pronation at the subtalar joint permits the talus and entire lower extremity to rotate internally slightly *after* the calcaneus has contacted the ground. The strong horizontal orientation of the facets at the subtalar joint certainly facilitates this action. Without such a joint mechanism, the plantar surface of the calcaneus would otherwise "spin" like a child's top against the walking surface, along with the internally rotating leg. Eccentric activation of supinator muscles, such as the tibialis posterior, can help to decelerate the pronation

Example of the Kinematic Versatility of the Foot

Earlier in this section, the point was made that pronation of the unloaded foot occurs primarily as a summation of the pronation at both the subtalar and transverse tarsal joints (review Figure 14-26, *B*). This summation of motion does not necessarily occur, however, when the foot is under the load of body weight. With the foot loaded or otherwise fixed to the ground, pronating the rearfoot may cause the midfoot and forefoot regions, which are receiving firm upward counterforce from the floor, to twist into relative *supination* (see Figure 14-32).[96] This reciprocal kinematic relationship between the rearfoot and more anterior regions of the foot demonstrates the versatility of the foot, either amplifying the other region's action when the foot is unloaded (see Figure 14-26, *B*), or counteracting the other region's action when the foot is loaded (see Figure 14-32).

The Use of a Foot Orthosis

Clinicians generally agree that some form of foot orthosis or specialized footwear can provide therapeutic benefits in persons with pes planus or other conditions that cause excessive pronation during walking or running.[32,64,92,98,108] In general, a foot orthosis is a device inserted into the shoe in order to modify the foot's mechanics. Often a wedge is placed on the medial aspect of the orthosis, effectively "bringing the floor up to the foot." This modification theoretically helps to control the rate, amount, and temporal sequencing of pronation at the subtalar joint. The precise mechanisms of how orthotics affect the kinematics and kinetics of the foot and lower limb are not completely understood.[29,32,77]

As an adjunct to orthosis, some clinicians also stress the need to improve the "eccentric control" of the muscles that decelerate pronation and other associated motions mechanically linked to pronation (such as those listed in Table 14-5). These muscle groups include the supinators of the foot (notably the tibialis posterior) and the more proximal external rotators and abductors of the hip. This therapeutic approach strives to reduce the rate of pronation as well as the rate of loading on the foot.

and resist the lowering of the medial longitudinal arch. Controlled pronation of the subtalar joint favors relative flexibility of the midfoot, allowing the foot to accommodate to the varied shapes and contours of walking surfaces.

Biomechanical Consequences of Abnormal Pronation during the Stance Phase

Innumerable examples exist on how malalignment within the foot affects the kinematics of walking. One common scenario results from excessive, prolonged, or poorly controlled pronation at the subtalar joint during the stance phase. This disorder can have multiple causes, including weakness of muscles throughout the lower extremity, laxity or weakness in the mechanisms that normally support and control the medial longitudinal arch, or abnormal shape or mobility of the tarsal bones. Regardless of cause, the rearfoot falls into excessive valgus (eversion) after heel contact.[83] Excessive subtalar joint pronation may be a compensation for excessive or restricted motion throughout the lower extremity, particularly in the frontal and horizontal planes.

Paradoxically, one of the most common structural deformities within an overpronated foot is a relatively fixed *rearfoot varus.* (Varus describes a segment of the foot that is *inverted* toward the midline.) As a response to rearfoot varus, the subtalar joint often overcompensates by excessively pronating, in speed and/or magnitude, to ensure that the medial aspect of the forefoot contacts the ground during stance phase.[15,85] Similar compensations may occur with a *forefoot varus* deformity. Whether the forefoot varus deformity causes or results from excessive pronation of the rearfoot is not always clear.

As described previously, excessive rearfoot pronation is typically associated with excessive (horizontal plane) internal rotation of the talus and leg during walking. Such a movement may create a "chain reaction" of kinematic disturbances and compensations throughout the entire limb, such as those depicted in Figure 14-32. As described in Chapter 13, the abnormal kinematic sequence between the tibia and femur may alter the contact area at the patellofemoral joint, potentially increasing stress at this joint. Furthermore, excessive

rearfoot eversion may create an increased valgus stress on the medial side of the knee.[104] These situations may predispose a person to patellofemoral joint pain syndrome or instability. For these reasons, clinicians often note the position of the subtalar joint while the patient stands and walks as part of an evaluation for a mechanical cause of patellofemoral joint pain or other related dysfunction.[137]

The underlying pathomechanics of an excessively pronated foot are complex and not fully understood. The pathomechanics can involve many kinematic relationships, both within the joints of the foot and between the foot and the rest of the lower limb. The origin of the pathomechanics may be related to interactions between the hip and knee (described in Chapter 13) and expressed distally as impairments at the subtalar joint. Even if the pathomechanics are obviously located within the foot, abnormal motion in the forefoot may be compensated for by abnormal motion in the rearfoot and vice versa. Furthermore, extrinsic factors, such as footwear, orthotics, terrain, and speed of walking or running, alter the kinematic relationships within the foot and lower extremity. An understanding of the complex kinesiology of the entire lower extremity is a definite prerequisite for the effective treatment of the painful or misaligned foot.

Mid-to-Late Stance Phase of Gait: Kinematics of Supination at the Subtalar Joint

At about 15% to 20% into the gait cycle, the entire stance limb reverses its horizontal plane motion from internal to external rotation.[52,105] External rotation of the leg while the foot remains planted coincides roughly with the beginning of the swing phase of the contralateral lower extremity. With the stance foot securely planted, external rotation of the femur, followed by the tibia, gradually reverses the horizontal plane direction of the talus from internal to external rotation. As a

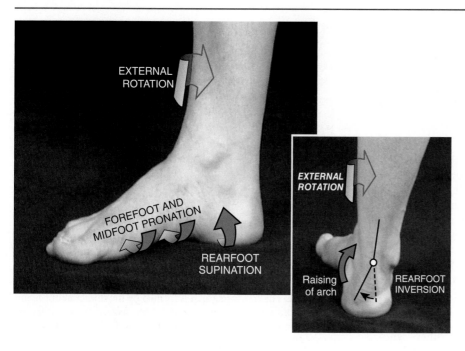

FIGURE 14-33. With the foot fixed to the ground, full *external rotation* of the lower limb is mechanically associated with: rearfoot supination (inversion) and raising of the medial longitudinal arch. Note that as the rearfoot supinates, the forefoot and midfoot pronate to maintain contact with the ground.

result, at about 30% to 35% into the gait cycle, the pronated (everted) subtalar joint starts to move sharply toward supination (inversion) (see Figure 14-31, *B*). As demonstrated in Figure 14-33, with the rearfoot supinating, the midfoot and forefoot must simultaneously twist into relative pronation in order for the foot to remain in full contact with the ground.[75,96] By late stance, the supinated subtalar joint and the elevated and tensed medial longitudinal arch convert the midfoot (and ultimately the forefoot) into a more rigid lever.[50,68] Muscles such as the gastrocnemius and soleus use this stability to transfer forces from the Achilles tendon, through the midfoot, to the metatarsal heads during the push off phase of walking or running.

A person who, for whatever reason, remains relatively pronated late into stance phase often has difficulty stabilizing the midfoot at a time when it is naturally required. Consequently, excessive activity may be required from extrinsic and intrinsic muscles of the foot to reinforce the medial longitudinal arch. Over time, hyperactivity may lead to generalized muscle fatigue and painful "overuse" syndromes throughout the lower limb and foot.

DISTAL INTERTARSAL JOINTS

The distal intertarsal joints are a collection of three joints or joint complexes, each occupying a part of the midfoot (review organization of joints of the foot; see Figure 14-23). The articular surfaces of the distal intertarsal joints are exposed and color-coded in Figure 14-34.

Collection of Articulations within the Distal Intertarsal Joints

- Cuneonavicular joint
- Cuboideonavicular joint
- Intercuneiform and cuneocuboid joint complex

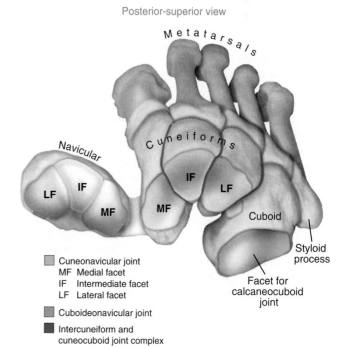

FIGURE 14-34. A posterior-superior view of the right foot is shown with the talus and calcaneus removed. The navicular bone has been flipped medially, exposing its anterior surface and the many articulations within the *distal intertarsal joints*. Articular surfaces have been colored-coded as follows: *cuneonavicular joint in light purple;* the small *cuboideonavicular joint in green;* and the *intercuneiform and cuneocuboid joint complex in blue.* Replacing the navicular to its natural position would join the three sets of articular facets within the cuneonavicular joint—medial facet *(MF)*, intermediate facet *(IF)*, and lateral facet *(LF)*. Replacing the navicular would also rearticulate the cuboideonavicular joint *(green)*.

Basic Structure and Function

As a group, the distal intertarsal joints (1) assist the transverse tarsal joint in pronating and supinating the midfoot, and (2) provide stability across the midfoot by forming the transverse arch of the foot. Motions in these joints are small and typically not formally described.

Cuneonavicular Joint

Three articulations are formed between the anterior side of the navicular and the posterior surfaces of the three cuneiform bones (see Figure 14-34, purple). Surrounding these articulations are plantar and dorsal ligaments. The slightly concave facets (lateral, intermediate, and medial) on each of the three cuneiforms fit into one of three slightly convex facets on the anterior side of the navicular. The major function of the cuneonavicular joint is to help transfer components of pronation and supination distally toward the forefoot.[74]

Cuboideonavicular Joint

The small synarthrodial (fibrous) or sometimes synovial cuboideonavicular joint is located between the lateral side of the navicular and a proximal region of the medial side of the cuboid (see Figure 14-34, green).[120] This joint provides a relatively smooth contact point between the lateral and medial longitudinal columns of the foot. Observations on cadaver specimens show that the articular surfaces slide slightly against each other during most movements of the midfoot, most notably during inversion and eversion.

Intercuneiform and Cuneocuboid Joint Complex

The intercuneiform and cuneocuboid joint complex consists of three articulations: two between the set of three cuneiforms, and one between the lateral cuneiform and medial surface of the cuboid (see Figure 14-34, blue). Articular surfaces are essentially flat and aligned nearly parallel with the long axis of the metatarsals. Plantar, dorsal, and interosseous ligaments strengthen this set of articulations.

The intercuneiform and cuneocuboid joint complex forms the *transverse arch* of the foot (Figure 14-35, *A*). This arch provides transverse stability to the midfoot. Under the load of body weight, the transverse arch depresses slightly, allowing body weight to be shared across all five metatarsal heads. The transverse arch receives support from intrinsic muscles; extrinsic muscles, such as the tibialis posterior and fibularis longus; connective tissues; and the keystone of the transverse arch: the intermediate (IF) cuneiform (see Figure 14-34).

TARSOMETATARSAL JOINTS

Anatomic Considerations

The tarsometatarsal joints are frequently called *Lisfranc's joints*, after Jacques Lisfranc, a French field surgeon in Napoleon's army who described an amputation in this region of the foot. As a group, the five tarsometatarsal joints separate the midfoot from the forefoot (review organization of joints in Figure 14-23). The joints consist of the articulation between the bases of the metatarsals and the distal surfaces of the three cuneiforms and cuboid. Specifically, the first (most medial) metatarsal articulates with the medial cuneiform, the second

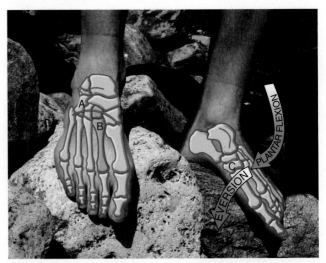

FIGURE 14-35. Structural and functional features of the midfoot and forefoot. **A,** The transverse arch is formed by the intercuneiform and cuneocuboid joint complex. **B,** The stable second ray is reinforced by the recessed second tarsometatarsal joint. **C,** Combined plantar flexion and eversion of the left tarsometatarsal joint of the first ray allow the forefoot to better conform to the surface of the rock.

with the intermediate cuneiform, and the third with the lateral cuneiform. The bases of the fourth and fifth metatarsals both articulate with the distal surface of the cuboid.

The articular surfaces of the tarsometatarsal joints are generally flat, although the medial two show slight, irregular curvatures. Dorsal, plantar, and interosseous ligaments add stability to these articulations. Only the first tarsometatarsal joint has a well-developed capsule.[120]

Kinematic Considerations

The tarsometatarsal joints serve as the base joints of the forefoot. Mobility is least at the second and third tarsometatarsal joints, in part because of strong ligaments and the wedged position of the base of the second ray between the medial and lateral cuneiforms (see Figure 14-35, *B*). Consequently, the second and third rays produce an element of longitudinal stability throughout the foot, similar to the second and third rays in the hand.[67] This stability is useful in late stance as the forefoot prepares for the dynamics of push off.

Mobility is greatest in the first, fourth, and fifth tarsometatarsal joints, most notably in the first (most medial) joint.[34] During walking, the first tarsometatarsal joint normally expresses about 10 degrees of sagittal plane movement; mobility in other planes is usually slight.[23]

During the early to mid-stance phase of walking, the first tarsometatarsal joint gradually *dorsiflexes* about 5 degrees. This motion occurs as body weight depresses the cuneiform region downward as the ground simultaneously pushes the distal end of the first ray upward. This movement is associated with a gradual lowering of the medial longitudinal arch[37]—a mechanism that helps absorb the stress of body weight acting on the foot. At late stance (push off) phase of gait, however, the first tarsometatarsal joint rapidly *plantar flexes* about 5 degrees.[23] The plantar flexion of the first ray, controlled in part by pull of the fibularis longus, effectively "shortens" the medial column of the foot slightly, thereby helping to raise the medial longitudinal arch. This mechanism increases the stability of the arch (and medial column of the foot) at a time in the gait cycle when the midfoot and forefoot are under higher loads.

Although the descriptions are dated and still partially unresolved, most literature describes a natural mechanical coupling of the kinematics at the first tarsometatarsal joint: specifically, plantar flexion occurs with slight eversion, and dorsiflexion with slight inversion.[37,45,68] Such passive mobility does indeed appear to occur naturally when assessed in a non–weight-bearing condition (Figure 14-36). These movement combinations are atypical, however, because they do not fit the standard definitions of pronation or supination. Nevertheless, the unique mobility at the first tarsometatarsal joint may provide useful functions. Combining plantar flexion and eversion, for example, allows the medial side of the foot to better conform around irregular surfaces on the ground (see Figure 14-35, *C*). (This motion of the first metatarsal is generally similar to the movement of the thumb metacarpal as the pronated hand attempts to grasp a large spherical object.) Exactly how these atypical movement combinations relate functionally to the overall kinematics of the foot during walking remains uncertain.

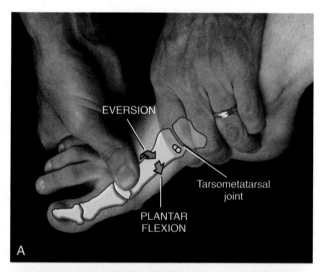

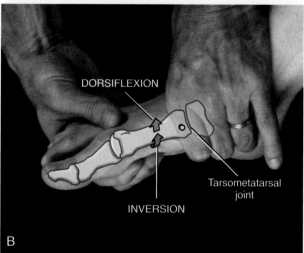

FIGURE 14-36. The osteokinematics of the first tarsometatarsal joint. Plantar flexion occurs with slight eversion **(A)**, and dorsiflexion occurs with slight inversion **(B)**.

INTERMETATARSAL JOINTS

Structure and Function

Plantar, dorsal, and interosseous ligaments interconnect the bases of the four lateral metatarsals. These points of contact form three small intermetatarsal synovial joints. Although interconnected by ligaments, a true joint does not typically form between the bases of the first and second metatarsals. This lack of articulation increases the relative movement of the first ray, in a manner similar to the hand. Unlike in the hand, however, the deep transverse metatarsal ligaments interconnect the distal end of all five metatarsals. Slight motion at the intermetatarsal joints augments the flexibility at the tarsometatarsal joints.

METATARSOPHALANGEAL JOINTS

Anatomic Considerations

Five metatarsophalangeal joints are formed between the convex head of each metatarsal and the shallow concavity of the proximal end of each proximal phalanx (see Figure 14-23). These joints are located about 2.5 cm proximal to the "web spaces" of the toes. With the joints flexed, the prominent heads of the metatarsals are easily palpable on the dorsum of the distal foot.

Articular cartilage covers the distal end of each metatarsal head (Figure 14-37). A pair of *collateral ligaments* spans each metatarsophalangeal joint, blending with and reinforcing the capsule. As in the hand, each collateral ligament courses obliquely from a dorsal-proximal to a plantar-distal direction, forming a thick cord portion and a fanlike accessory portion.

The accessory portion attaches to the thick, dense *plantar plate*, located on the plantar side of the joint. The plate, or ligament, is grooved for the passage of flexor tendons. Fibers from the deep plantar fascia attach to the plantar plates and sheaths of the flexor tendons. Two *sesamoid bones* located within the tendon of the flexor hallucis brevis rest against the plantar plate of the first metatarsophalangeal joint (Figure 14-38). Although not depicted in Figure 14-38, four deep *transverse metatarsal ligaments* blend with and join the adjacent plantar plates of all five metatarsophalangeal joints. By interconnecting all five plates, the transverse metatarsal ligaments help maintain the first ray in a similar plane as the lesser rays, thereby adapting the foot for propulsion and weight bearing

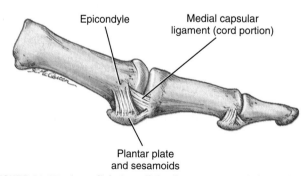

FIGURE 14-37. A medial view of the first metatarsophalangeal joint showing the cord and accessory portions of the medial (collateral) capsular ligament. The accessory portion attaches to the plantar plate and sesamoid bones. (Redrawn from Haines R, McDougall A: Anatomy of hallux valgus, *J Bone Joint Surg Br* 36:272, 1954.)

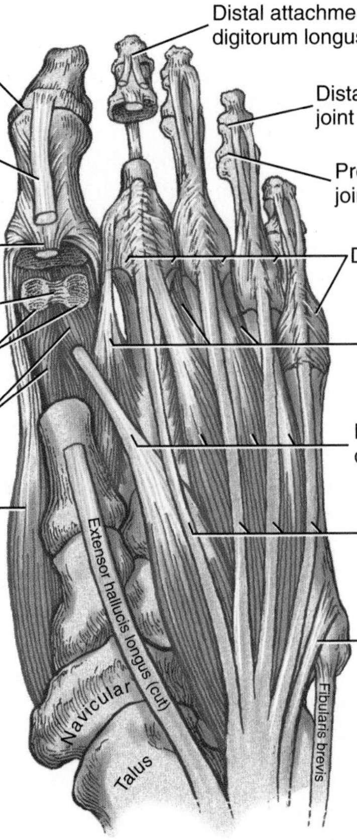

Superior view

Interphalangeal joint

Extensor hallucis longus (cut)

Extensor digitorum brevis (cut)

Plantar plate

Sesamoid bones

Flexor hallucis brevis

Abductor hallucis

Distal attachment of extensor digitorum longus and brevis (cut)

Distal interphalangeal joint

Proximal interphalangeal joint

Dorsal digital expansion

Dorsal interossei

Extensor digitorum brevis

Extensor digitorum longus

Fibularis tertius

Extensor hallucis longus (cut)

Navicular

Talus

Fibularis brevis

FIGURE 14-38. Muscles and joints of the dorsal surface of the right forefoot. The distal half of the first metatarsal is removed to expose the concave surface of the first metatarsophalangeal joint. A pair of sesamoid bones is located deep within the first metatarsophalangeal joint. The proximal phalanx of the second toe is removed to expose the concave side of the proximal interphalangeal joint.

rather than manipulation. In the hand, the deep transverse metacarpal ligament connects only the fingers, freeing the thumb for opposition.

A *fibrous capsule* encloses each metatarsophalangeal joint and blends with the collateral ligaments and plantar plates. A poorly defined *dorsal digital expansion* covers the dorsal side of each metatarsophalangeal joint. This structure (analogous to the extensor mechanism in the digits of the hand) consists of a thin layer of connective tissue that is essentially inseparable from the dorsal capsule and extensor tendons.

Kinematic Considerations

Movement at the metatarsophalangeal joints occurs in two degrees of freedom. *Extension* (dorsiflexion) and *flexion* (plantar flexion) occur approximately in the sagittal plane about a medial-lateral axis; *abduction* and *adduction* occur in the horizontal plane about a vertical axis. The second digit serves as the reference digit for naming the movements of abduction and adduction of the toes. (The reference digit for naming abduction and adduction in the hand is the third or middle digit.) The axes of rotation for all volitional movements of the metatarsophalangeal joints are through the center of each metatarsal head.

Most people demonstrate limited dexterity in active movements at the metatarsophalangeal joints, especially in abduction and adduction. From a neutral position, the toes can be passively extended about 65 degrees and flexed about 30 to 40 degrees. The great toe typically allows greater extension, to near 85 degrees.[131] This magnitude of extension is readily apparent as one stands up on "tiptoes."

Deformities or Trauma Involving the Metatarsophalangeal Joint of the Great Toe

Hallux Limitus

Hallux limitus, or "rigidus" in its less severe form, is primarily a posttraumatic condition characterized by gradual marked limitation of motion, articular degeneration, and pain at the metatarsophalangeal joint of the great toe. Although any trauma or sprain of the great toe can progress to hallux limitus, the mechanism of injury frequently involves forceful *hyperextension* of the metatarsophalangeal joint. More severe injuries may involve complete or incomplete tears of the plantar ligaments, capsule, and associated tendons, as well as fracture of the sesamoid bones.[14]

Injury caused by forced hyperextension of the great toe is often called "turf toe" and occurs relatively frequently in American football players. Historically, the term *turf toe* originated from the increase in this injury after the replacement of natural grass with artificial turf and the use of lighter-weight shoes.[11] Regardless of the initiating trauma, a diagnosis of hallux limitus is often made if pain persists along with reduced range of extension, usually to less than 55 degrees.[131] In some cases the condition will evolve to osteoarthritis; excessive osteophyte formation may then limit motion in all directions.

The impairments associated with hallux limitus can have significant impact on walking.[131] Normally, walking requires about 65 degrees of extension at the first metatarsophalangeal joint as the heel rises at late stance phase. A person with hallux limitus may attempt to avoid extending the painful great toe during the late stance phase of walking. Often this

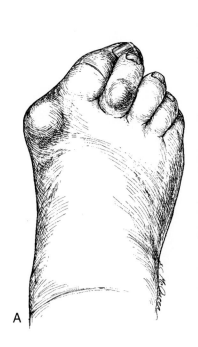

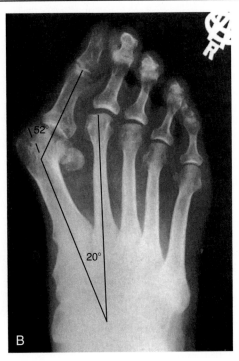

FIGURE 14-39. Hallux valgus. **A,** Multiple features of hallux valgus (bunion) and associated deformities. **B,** Radiograph shows the following pathomechanics often associated with hallux valgus: (1) adduction of the first metatarsal (toward the midline of the body), evidenced by the increased angle between the first and second metatarsal bones; (2) lateral deviation of the proximal phalanx with dislocation or subluxation of the first metatarsophalangeal joint; (3) displacement of the lateral sesamoid; (4) rotation (eversion) of the phalanges of the great toe; and (5) exposed first metatarsal head, forming the so-called "bunion." (From Richardson EG: Disorders of the hallux. In Canale ST, ed: *Campbell's operative orthopaedics,* vol 4, ed 9, St Louis, 1998, Mosby.)

is accomplished by walking on the outer surface of the affected foot, or by walking with the foot pointed outward and "rolling over" the medial arch of the foot.

Those affected may be advised to wear stiff-soled shoes (or stiff inserts placed within the shoes) and to avoid inclines or declines. Physical therapy has been shown to be effective in restoring range of motion and reducing pain.[117] Surgery is often recommended in more severe cases.

Hallux Valgus

The central feature of *hallux valgus* (or bunion) is a progressive lateral deviation of the great toe relative to the midline of the body. Although the deformity appears to involve primarily the metatarsophalangeal joint, the pathomechanics of hallux valgus typically involve the entire first ray (Figure 14-39, *A* and *B*). As depicted in the radiograph, hallux valgus is typically associated with excessive *adduction* of the first metatarsal (defined in this case relative to the body and not the second digit) about its tarsometatarsal joint.[30] The adducted position of the first metatarsal can eventually lead to lateral dislocation of the metatarsophalangeal joint, thereby completely exposing the metatarsal head as a lump or "bunion." The deformed metatarsophalangeal joint often becomes inflamed and painful. If the proximal phalanx laterally deviates in excess of about 30 degrees, the proximal phalanx often begins to evert about its long axis. The bunion deformity is also referred to as "hallux abducto-valgus" in order to account for the deviations in both horizontal and frontal planes.

The progressive axial rotation of the laterally deviated proximal phalanx of the hallux creates a muscular imbalance in the forces that normally align the metatarsophalangeal joint.[2] The abductor hallucis muscle (normally located *medial* to the first metatarsophalangeal joint) may gradually shift toward the plantar side of the joint. The subsequent unopposed pull of the adductor hallucis and lateral head of

the flexor hallucis brevis progressively increases the lateral deviation posture of the proximal phalanx. In time, the overstretched medial collateral ligament and capsule may weaken or rupture, removing an important source of reinforcement to the medial side of the joint. Persons with marked hallux valgus may avoid bearing weight over the first metatarsophalangeal joint, causing the lateral metatarsal bones to accept a greater proportion of the load. The pathomechanics of marked hallux valgus involve a zigzag-like collapse of the first ray, similar to the "ulnar drift" of the metacarpophalangeal joint in the hand with rheumatoid arthritis (see Chapter 8).

Although the cause of hallux valgus is not totally clear, genetics, incorrect footwear, pronated feet that cause valgus strain at the hallux, and asymmetry of the bones and joints can all contribute to the condition. The full spectrum of severe hallux valgus often includes dislocation and osteoarthritis of the metatarsophalangeal joint, metatarsus varus, valgus (lateral deviation) of the great toe, bunion formation (and bursitis) over the medial metatarsopophalangeal joint, hammer toe of the second digit, calluses, and metatarsalgia. Surgical intervention is often indicated in cases of marked deformity and dysfunction.

INTERPHALANGEAL JOINTS

As in the fingers, each toe has a *proximal interphalangeal* and a *distal interphalangeal joint.* The great toe, or hallux, being analogous to the thumb, has only one *interphalangeal joint.*

All interphalangeal joints of the foot possess similar anatomic features. The joint consists of the convex head of the more proximal phalanx articulating with the concave base of the more distal phalanx. The proximal phalanx of the second toe is removed in Figure 14-38 to expose the concave side of the proximal interphalangeal joint. The structure and function of the connective tissues at the interphalangeal joints are generally similar to those described for the metatarsophalangeal joints. Collateral ligaments, plantar plates, and capsules are present but smaller and less defined.

Mobility at the interphalangeal joints is limited primarily to flexion and extension. The amplitude of flexion generally exceeds extension, and motion tends to be greater at the proximal than the distal joints. Extension is limited primarily by passive tension in the toe flexor muscles and plantar ligaments.

ACTION OF THE JOINTS WITHIN THE FOREFOOT DURING THE LATE STANCE PHASE OF GAIT

The joints of the forefoot include the articulations associated with each ray, from the tarsometatarsal joint to the distal interphalangeal joints of the toe. Depending on the phase of gait, these joints provide an element of flexibility or stability to the forefoot.

During the end of the stance phase, the midfoot and forefoot must become relatively stable to accept the stress associated with push off. In addition to activation of local intrinsic and extrinsic muscles, a rising of the medial longitudinal arch further stabilizes the foot. Although the rise of the arch is highly variable, it averages 6 mm during the push off phase.[114] The primary mechanism used to lift the arch has been historically described as the "windlass effect," which is demonstrated by standing on tiptoes (Figure 14-40, *A*). Because of the attachments of the deep plantar fascia to the proximal phalanges, full extension of the metatarsophalangeal joints increases the tension throughout the medial longitudinal arch. In theory, the increased tension raises and stabilizes the arch. As the heel and most of the foot are lifted, body weight shifts anteriorly toward the more medial metatarsal heads. Local fat pads reduce potentially damaging stress to the bone, and the sesamoid bones protect the long flexor tendon of the great toe. Once stabilized by the stretched plantar fascia and a reinforced arch, the second and third rays act as rigid levers capable of withstanding the potentially large bending moments created by the contracting gastrocnemius and soleus muscles. The tensile force within the stretched plantar fascia during very late stance phase has been estimated to be near 100% of body weight.[26] Failure of the plantar fascia to transmit this force from the calcaneus to the base of the toes would limit the effectiveness of the windlass mechanism in raising the arch. This, indeed, is often observed by noting the guarded or ineffective manner of "push off" in a person who has had a plantar fasciotomy or is experiencing painful plantar fasciitis.

In contrast to the healthy foot, consider the pathomechanics involved as a person with an unstable "flat foot" (pes planus) attempts to rise up on tiptoes (see Figure 14-40, *B*). Although the individual has no neuromuscular pathology, there is significant loss in the lift of the heel, even on maximal muscular effort. Without an effective medial longitudinal arch, the unstable, unlocked midfoot and forefoot sag under body weight. This typically causes a movement toward *dorsiflexion* of the tarsometatarsal joints (in contrast to normal slight plantar flexion). This kinematic response may stretch the extrinsic toe flexor muscles and, if significant, limit toe extension. Regardless of the specific cause-and-effect relationship, the reduced extension of the metatarsophalangeal joints

Normal foot

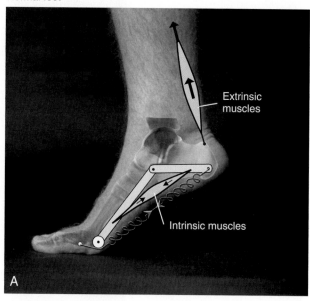

Extrinsic muscles

Intrinsic muscles

A

Foot with pes planus

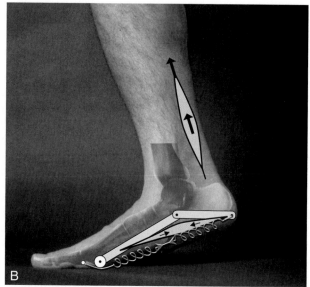

B

FIGURE 14-40. The "windlass effect" of the plantar fascia is demonstrated while a subject stands on tiptoes. (A windlass is a hauling or lifting device consisting of a rope wound around a cylinder that is turned by a crank. The rope is analogous to the plantar fascia, and the cylinder is analogous to the metatarsophalangeal joint.) **A,** In the normal foot, contraction of the extrinsic plantar flexor muscles lifts the calcaneus, thereby transferring body weight forward over the metatarsal heads. The resulting extension of the metatarsophalangeal joints (shown collectively as the white disk) stretches (or winds up) the plantar fascia within the medial longitudinal arch (red spring). The increased tension from the stretch raises the arch and strengthens the midfoot and forefoot. Contraction of the intrinsic muscles provides additional reinforcement to the arch. **B,** The foot with pes planus (flat foot) typically has a poorly supported medial longitudinal arch. During an attempt to stand up on tiptoes, the forefoot sags under the load of body weight. The reduced extension of the metatarsophalangeal joints limits the usefulness of the windlass effect. Even with strong activation of the intrinsic muscles, the arch remains flattened and the midfoot and forefoot unstable.

TABLE 14-6. Major Actions at Regions of the Ankle and Foot during the Stance Phase of Walking*

Region	Representative Joint	Early Stance		Mid to Late Stance	
		Action	**Desired Function**	**Action**	**Desired Function**
Ankle	Talocrural	Plantar flexion	Allows rapid foot contact with the ground	Dorsiflexion followed by rapid plantar flexion	Produces a stable joint to accept body weight, followed by thrust needed for push off
Rearfoot	Subtalar	Pronation and lowering of the medial longitudinal arch	Permits internal rotation of lower limb Allows the foot to function as a shock absorber Produces a pliable midfoot	Continued pronation changing to supination, followed by a raising of the medial longitudinal arch	Permits external rotation of lower limb Converts the midfoot to a rigid lever for push off
Midfoot	Transverse tarsal	Relative inversion as a response to counterforce from the ground	Allows full extent of subtalar joint pronation	Relative eversion	Allows the midfoot and forefoot to maintain firm contact with the ground
Forefoot	Metatarsophalangeal	Insignificant	–	Extension	Through the windlass effect, raises the medial longitudinal arch and stabilizes the midfoot and forefoot for push off

*Each region of the foot is represented by only one joint.

reduces the effectiveness of the windlass effect for stabilizing the foot.

The final section on kinematics closes with Table 14-6, which summarizes the important functions of the ankle and foot during the entire stance phase of walking.

MUSCLE AND JOINT INTERACTION

Innervation of Muscles and Joints

INNERVATION OF MUSCLES

Extrinsic muscles of the ankle and foot have their proximal attachments in the leg, and a few extend as far proximal as the femur. Intrinsic muscles, in contrast, have both their proximal and distal attachments within the foot.

The extrinsic muscles are arranged in three compartments of the leg: anterior, lateral, and posterior. A different motor nerve innervates the muscles within each compartment (see cross-sections in Figures 14-41 and 14-42). Each motor nerve is a branch of the sciatic nerve, formed from the L^4-S^3 spinal nerve roots of the sacral plexus.

Lateral to the head of the fibula, the common fibular (peroneal) nerve (L^4-S^2) divides into a deep and superficial branch (see Figure 14-41). The *deep branch of the fibular nerve* innervates the muscles within the *anterior compartment*: the tibialis anterior, extensor digitorum longus, extensor hallucis

longus, and fibularis (peroneus) tertius. The deep branch continues distally to innervate the extensor digitorum brevis (an intrinsic muscle located within the dorsum of the foot). It also supplies sensory innervation to a triangular area of skin in the web space between the first and second toes. The *superficial branch of the fibular nerve* innervates the fibularis longus and fibularis brevis within the *lateral compartment*. The nerve then continues distally as a sensory nerve to much of the skin on the dorsal and lateral aspects of the leg and foot.

The *tibial nerve* (L^4-S^3) and its terminal branches innervate the remainder of the extrinsic and intrinsic muscles of the foot and ankle (see Figure 14-42). The muscles within the *posterior compartment* are divided into superficial and deep sets. The *superficial* set includes the calf muscles: the gastrocnemius and soleus (together known as the *triceps surae*) and the small plantaris. The *deep* set includes the tibialis posterior, flexor hallucis longus, and flexor digitorum longus. As the tibial nerve approaches the medial side of the ankle, it sends a sensory branch to the skin over the heel.

Just posterior to the medial malleolus, the tibial nerve bifurcates into the *medial plantar nerve* (L^4-S^2) and *lateral plantar nerve* (L^5-S^3). The plantar nerves supply sensation to the skin on most of the plantar surface of the foot and motor innervation to all intrinsic muscles, except the extensor digitorum brevis. The general organization of the innervation of the intrinsic muscles of the foot is similar to that in the hand. The medial plantar nerve is analogous to the median

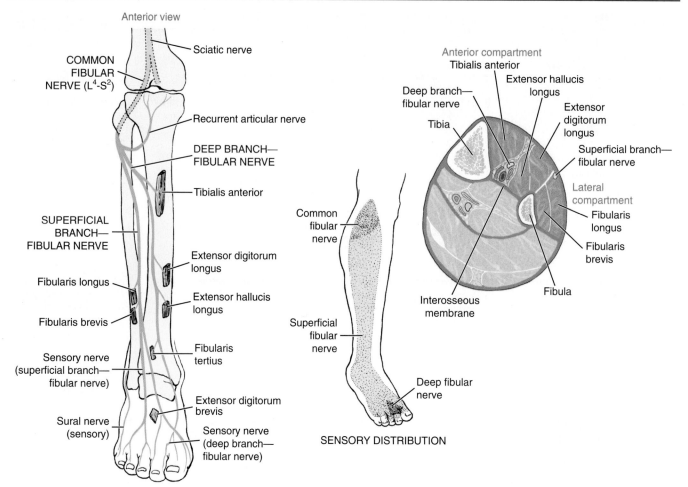

FIGURE 14-41. The path and general proximal-to-distal order of muscle innervation for the deep and superficial branches of the *common fibular (peroneal) nerve*. The primary spinal nerve roots are in parentheses. The general sensory distribution of this nerve (and its branches) is highlighted along the dorsal-lateral aspect of the leg and foot. The dorsal "web space" of the foot is innervated solely by sensory branches of the deep branch of the fibular nerve. The cross-section highlights the muscles and nerves located within the *anterior* and *lateral compartments* of the leg. (Modified with permission from deGroot J: *Correlative neuroanatomy,* ed 21, Norwalk, 1991, Appleton & Lange.)

nerve, whereas the lateral plantar nerve is analogous to the ulnar nerve.

The spinal nerve roots that supply the muscles of the lower extremity are listed in Appendix IV, Part A. Part B of this appendix lists key muscles typically used to test the functional status of the L^2-S^3 spinal nerve roots. Part C shows a dermatome map of the lower extremity.

SENSORY INNERVATION OF THE JOINTS

The *talocrural joint* receives sensory innervation from the deep branch of the fibular nerve. In general, the sensory innervation to the other joints of the foot is supplied by nerve branches that cross the region. Each major joint receives multiple sources of sensory innervation, traveling to the spinal cord primarily through S^1 and S^2 nerve roots.[120]

Anatomy and Function of the Muscles

The muscles of the ankle and foot not only control the specific actions of the underlying joints, but also provide the stability, thrust, and shock absorption necessary for locomotion. Both intrinsic and extrinsic muscles perform these functions. Additional discussion of the muscular interactions during walking follows in Chapter 15.

Because all extrinsic muscles cross multiple joints, they possess multiple actions. Many of these actions are evident by noting where the tendons cross the axes of rotation at the talocrural and subtalar joints (Figure 14-43). Although Figure 14-43 is oversimplified (by lacking the transverse tarsal joint as well as other components of pronation and supination of the foot), it can nevertheless serve as a useful guide to understanding many of the actions of the extrinsic muscles.

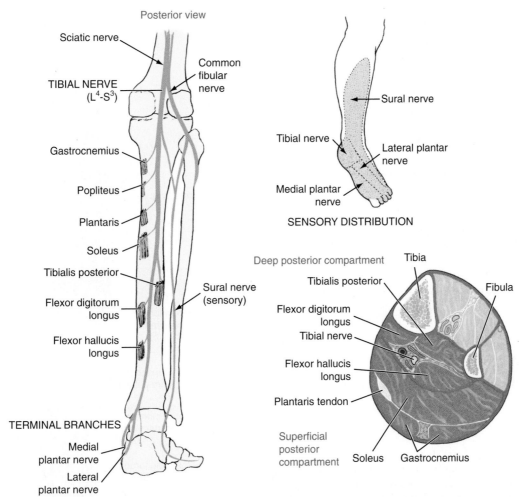

FIGURE 14-42. The path and general proximal-to-distal order of muscle innervation for the *tibial nerve* and its branches. The primary spinal nerve roots are in parentheses. The general sensory distribution of this nerve is highlighted along the lateral and plantar aspects of the leg and foot. The cross-section highlights the muscles and nerves located within the *deep* and *superficial parts of the posterior compartment* of the leg. (Modified with permission from deGroot J: *Correlative neuroanatomy,* ed 21, Norwalk, 1991, Appleton & Lange.)

EXTRINSIC MUSCLES

Anterior Compartment Muscles
Anatomy

The four muscles of the anterior compartment are listed in the box. As a group, these "pretibial" muscles have their proximal attachments on the anterior and lateral aspects of the proximal half of the tibia, the adjacent fibula, and the interosseous membrane (Figure 14-44). The tendons of these muscles cross the dorsal side of the ankle, restrained by a synovial-lined *superior* and *inferior extensor retinaculum.* Located most medially is the prominent tendon of the *tibialis anterior,* coursing distally to attach to the medial-plantar surface of the first tarsometatarsal joint (Figure 14-45). The tendon of the *extensor hallucis longus* passes just lateral to the tendon of the tibialis anterior as it courses toward the dorsal surface of the great toe (see Figure 14-44). Progressing laterally across the dorsum of the ankle are the tendons of the extensor digitorum longus and the fibularis tertius (or "third" fibularis

muscle). The four tendons of the *extensor digitorum longus* attach to the dorsal surface of the middle and distal phalanges via the dorsal digital expansion. The *fibularis tertius* is part of the extensor digitorum longus muscle and may be considered as this muscle's fifth tendon. The fibularis tertius attaches to the base of the fifth metatarsal bone.[140]

Muscles of the Anterior Compartment of the Leg (Pretibial "Dorsiflexors")

Muscles
- Tibialis anterior
- Extensor digitorum longus
- Extensor hallucis longus
- Fibularis tertius

Innervation
- Deep branch of the fibular nerve

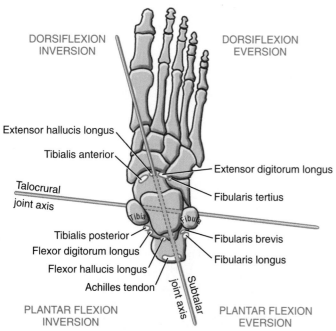

FIGURE 14-43. The multiple actions of muscles that cross the talocrural and subtalar joints, as viewed from above. The actions of each muscle are based on its position relative to the axes of rotation at the joints. Note that the muscles have multiple actions.

Joint Action

All four pretibial muscles are dorsiflexors because they cross anterior to the axis of rotation at the talocrural joint (see Figure 14-43). From the anatomic position, the *tibialis anterior* also inverts the subtalar joint by passing just medial to the axis of rotation. The tibialis anterior inverts and adducts the talonavicular joint, as well as providing secondary support to the medial longitudinal arch.

The primary actions of the *extensor hallucis longus* are dorsiflexion at the talocrural joint and extension of the great toe. Inversion at the subtalar joint is negligible because of its small moment arm, at least when analyzed from the anatomic position. In addition to dorsiflexion of the ankle, the *extensor digitorum longus* and *fibularis tertius* evert the foot.

The pretibial muscles are most active during the early stance phase and again throughout the entire swing phase of gait (see Figure 15-29, tibialis anterior). During early stance, the muscles are eccentrically active to control the rate of plantar flexion (i.e., the period between heel contact and foot flat; see Figure 14-19). Controlled plantar flexion is necessary for a soft landing of the foot. Through similar eccentric activation, the tibialis anterior helps to decelerate the lowering of the medial longitudinal arch and therefore indirectly helps to control pronation (eversion) of the rearfoot (review Figure 14-31). During the swing phase, the pretibial muscles actively dorsiflex the ankle and extend the toes to ensure that the foot clears the ground.

The ability to actively dorsiflex the foot in the near-sagittal plane requires a rather exacting balance of forces from the pretibial muscles. The eversion and/or abduction influence of the extensor digitorum longus and fibularis tertius must counterbalance the inversion and adduction influence of the tibialis anterior. With isolated paralysis of the tibialis anterior

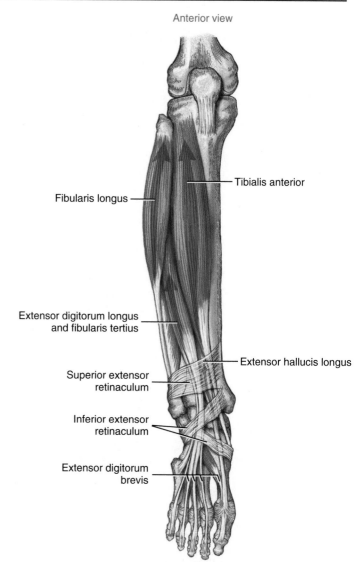

FIGURE 14-44. The pretibial muscles of the leg: tibialis anterior, extensor digitorum longus, extensor hallucis longus, and fibularis tertius. All four muscles dorsiflex the ankle.

muscle, the ankle can still actively dorsiflex, but would do so with an eversion-and-abduction bias.

Lateral Compartment Muscles
Anatomy

The fibularis longus and the fibularis brevis muscles (formerly called the *peroneus longus* and *peroneus brevis,* respectively) occupy the lateral compartment of the leg muscles (Figure 14-46). Both muscles attach proximally along the lateral fibula. The tendon of the *fibularis longus,* the more superficial of the two, courses distally a remarkable distance. After wrapping around the posterior side of the lateral malleolus, the tendon enters the plantar side of the foot through a groove in the cuboid bone. The tendon then travels between the long and short plantar ligaments to its final distal attachment on the plantar-lateral aspect of the first tarsometatarsal joint (see Figure 14-45). It is noteworthy that the fibularis longus and tibialis anterior attach on either side of the plantar surface first tarsometatarsal joint. This pair of muscles therefore provides kinetic stability to the base of the first ray.

Plantar view

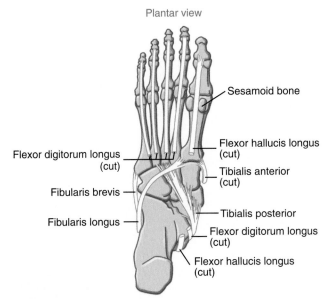

Sesamoid bone

Flexor hallucis longus (cut)

Tibialis anterior (cut)

Flexor digitorum longus (cut)

Fibularis brevis

Tibialis posterior

Fibularis longus

Flexor digitorum longus (cut)

Flexor hallucis longus (cut)

FIGURE 14-45. A plantar view of the right foot shows the distal course of the tendons of the fibularis longus, fibularis brevis, and tibialis posterior. The tendons of the tibialis anterior, flexor digitorum longus, and flexor hallucis longus are cut.

Lateral Compartment of the Leg ("Evertors")

Muscles
- Fibularis longus
- Fibularis brevis

Innervation
- Superficial branch of the fibular nerve

The tendon of the *fibularis brevis* travels posterior to the lateral malleolus alongside the fibularis longus. Both fibular tendons occupy the same synovial sheath as they pass under the *fibular retinaculum* (see Figure 14-46). Just distal to the retinaculum, the tendon of the fibularis brevis separates from the fibularis longus tendon and courses toward its distal attachment on the styloid process of the fifth metatarsal. Frequently observed in dancers, the styloid process may experience an avulsion fracture after a very strong contraction of the fibularis brevis, often in response to a sudden and extreme inversion movement of the ankle or foot.

Joint Action

The *fibularis longus* and *fibularis brevis* muscles are the primary evertors of the foot (see Figure 14-43). These muscles provide the main source of active stability to the lateral side of the ankle. For this reason, strengthening, conditioning, and coordination exercises involving these muscles are often designed for persons who may be vulnerable to inversion sprains of the ankle, such as athletes playing basketball or volleyball. Of interest, although these lateral muscles are very effective at resisting inversion, a purely reflexive muscular contraction in response to an unexpected inversion movement is typically too slow to prevent injury.[62] Other, more complex neuromuscular mechanisms are required for this protection, likely those involving feed-forward or anticipatory responses to an impending inversion injury.

Lateral view

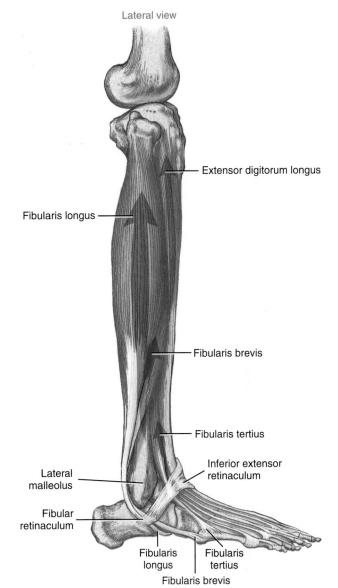

Extensor digitorum longus

Fibularis longus

Fibularis brevis

Fibularis tertius

Inferior extensor retinaculum

Lateral malleolus

Fibular retinaculum

Fibularis longus

Fibularis tertius

Fibularis brevis

FIGURE 14-46. A lateral view of the muscles of the leg is shown. Note how both the fibularis longus and fibularis brevis (primary evertors) use the lateral malleolus as a pulley to change direction of muscular pull across the ankle.

The fibularis longus and brevis have substantial moment arms for eversion across the subtalar joint—over 2 cm.[60] The lateral malleolus, serving as a fixed pulley, routes the fibular tendons posterior to the axis of rotation at the talocrural joint.[60] Both muscles therefore are also plantar flexors of the talocrural joint. Although not evident in Figure 14-43, the fibularis longus and brevis also abduct the subtalar and transverse tarsal joints.

The distal attachment of the fibularis longus generates eversion torque as far anterior as the forefoot. This is evident as the base of the first ray everts and depresses (plantar flexes) slightly during maximal-effort pronation of the unloaded foot. In addition, the fibularis longus stabilizes the first tarsometatarsal joint against the potent medial pull of the tibialis anterior. Without this stability, the first ray may migrate medially, predisposing a person to a hallux valgus deformity.[30]

The fibularis longus and brevis are most active throughout the middle and late stance phases of walking.[111,123] During most of this time, the subtalar joint is supinating (inverting) as the dorsiflexing talocrural joint rapidly changes its direction to plantar flexion (review Figures 14-19 and 14-31). An important function of the fibularis muscles during this phase of walking is to decelerate, and thus control, the rate and extent of the supinating subtalar joint. Furthermore, the active force within the fibularis longus helps to fixate the first ray securely to the ground, an action demonstrated by the forefoot in Figure 14-33. With weakness, paralysis, or inhibition of the fibularis longus, the potent supination pull of the tibialis posterior on the forefoot is unopposed. As a result, the forefoot follows the rearfoot into supination, causing the person to walk on the lateral border of the foot, possibly increasing the likelihood of an inversion sprain.

At very late stance phase, during push off, the fibularis longus and brevis muscles assist other muscles with plantar flexion at the talocrural joint. The lateral position of the fibularis muscles helps neutralize the strong inversion (supination) bias of the remaining active plantar flexors, including the tibialis posterior, and, to a limited degree, the gastrocnemius. The necessity for balance of these muscle forces is shown as a subject stands on tiptoes in Figure 14-47. As the heel rises, the strongly activated fibularis longus and tibialis posterior muscles neutralize each other as they form a functional "sling" that supports the transverse and medial longitudinal arches. The net effect of this muscle interaction slightly supinates the unloaded rearfoot, which provides further stability to the medial longitudinal arch and more distal regions of the foot. This stability ensures that the plantar flexion torque required to stand on tiptoes (or propel the body upward and forward) is effectively transferred distally through the foot, toward the metatarsal heads.

Furthermore, as the heel is raised during the push off phase of walking, contraction of the fibularis muscles, especially the longus, helps transfer body weight from the lateral to the medial side of the forefoot. This action shifts body weight toward the opposite foot, which has just entered its early stance phase of gait.

Posterior Compartment Muscles
Anatomy

The muscles of the posterior compartment are divided into two groups. The *superficial group* includes the gastrocnemius, soleus (together known as the *triceps surae*), and plantaris (Figure 14-48). The *deep group* includes the tibialis posterior, flexor digitorum longus, and flexor hallucis longus (Figure 14-49).

Muscles of the Posterior Compartment of the Leg

Superficial Group ("Plantar Flexors")
- Gastrocnemius
- Soleus
- Plantaris

Deep Group ("Invertors")
- Tibialis posterior
- Flexor digitorum longus
- Flexor hallucis longus

Innervation
- Tibial nerve

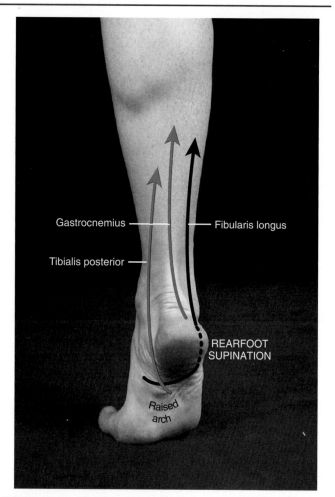

FIGURE 14-47. The line of force of several plantar flexor muscles while a subject rises on tiptoes. Note that the fibularis longus and tibialis posterior form a sling that supports the transverse and medial longitudinal arches. The pull of the gastrocnemius and tibialis posterior muscles causes a slight supination of the rearfoot, which adds further stability to the foot. (Invertor muscles are indicated by the red arrows; evertor muscle by the black arrow.)

Superficial Group. The *gastrocnemius* muscle forms the prominent belly of the calf. This two-headed muscle attaches by separate heads from the posterior side of the medial and lateral femoral condyles. The larger, medial head joins the lateral head midway down the leg to form a tendinous expansion that, after insertion of the tendon from the soleus muscle, forms the *Achilles tendon.* The broad flat *soleus* muscle lies deep to the gastrocnemius, arising primarily from the posterior side of the proximal fibula and middle tibia. Like the gastrocnemius, the soleus blends with the Achilles tendon for its distal attachment to the calcaneal tuberosity. The soleus is a very thick muscle, approximately twice the cross-sectional area as the overlying gastrocnemius.[139] The gastrocnemius crosses the knee but the soleus does not.

The *plantaris* muscle arises from the lateral supracondylar line of the femur. The fusiform muscle belly is only 7 to 10 cm long,[120] unusually small compared with the other muscles in the area. The plantaris has a very long, slender tendon that courses between the gastrocnemius and soleus, eventually fusing with the medial margin of the Achilles tendon.

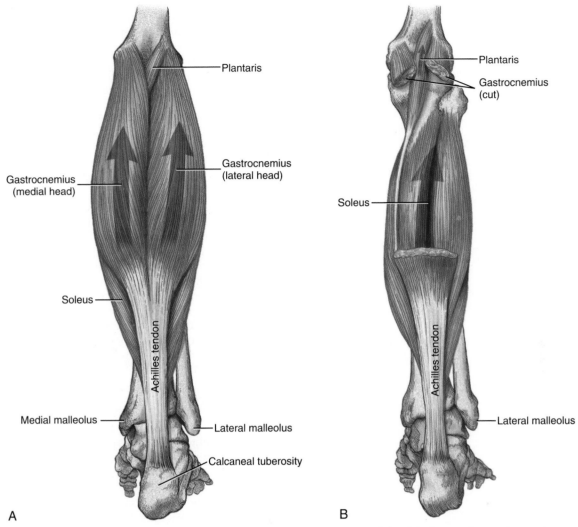

FIGURE 14-48. The superficial muscles of the posterior compartment of the right leg are shown: **A,** gastrocnemius; **B,** soleus and plantaris.

Deep Group. The tibialis posterior, flexor hallucis longus, and flexor digitorum longus muscles are located deep to the soleus muscle (see Figure 14-49). As a group, these muscles arise from the posterior side of the tibia, fibula, and interosseous membrane. The more centrally located tibialis posterior muscle is framed and partially covered by the flexor hallucis longus laterally and the flexor digitorum longus medially. At their distal musculotendinous junctions, all three muscles enter the plantar aspect of the foot from its medial side (see Figure 14-45). The position of the tendons as they cross the ankle and foot explains the strong supination (inversion) component of these muscles, most notably the tibialis posterior (see Figure 14-43).[60] The tibialis posterior, flexor digitorum longus, and tibial neurovascular bundle course through the *tarsal tunnel,* located just deep to the flexor retinaculum (Figure 14-50). The tarsal tunnel is analogous to the carpal tunnel in the wrist. "Tarsal tunnel syndrome" (analogous to carpal tunnel syndrome) is characterized by entrapment of the tibial nerve beneath the flexor retinaculum and subsequent paresthesia over the plantar aspect of the foot.

The tendon of the *flexor hallucis longus* courses distally through the ankle in a groove formed between the tubercles

of the talus and the inferior edge of the sustentaculum talus (see Figure 14-12). Fibrous bands convert this groove into a synovial-lined canal, anchoring the position of the tendon. The deeper (lateral) position of the tendon relative to the tibialis posterior and flexor digitorum longus explains why the flexor hallucis longus is *not* a structure within the tarsal tunnel. Once in the plantar aspect of the foot, the tendon of the flexor hallucis longus courses between the two sesamoid bones of the first metatarsophalangeal joint, finally attaching to the plantar side of the base of the distal phalanx of the great toe (see Figure 14-45).

The tendon of the *flexor digitorum longus* courses distally across the ankle posterior to the medial malleolus. At about the level of the base of the metatarsals, the main tendon of the flexor digitorum longus divides into four smaller tendons, each attaching to the base of the distal phalanx of the lesser toes (see Figure 14-45).

The tendon of the *tibialis posterior* muscle lies just anterior to the tendon of the flexor digitorum longus in a shared groove on the posterior side of the medial malleolus (see Figure 14-50). The tendon of the tibialis posterior continues distally and passes deep to the flexor retinaculum but

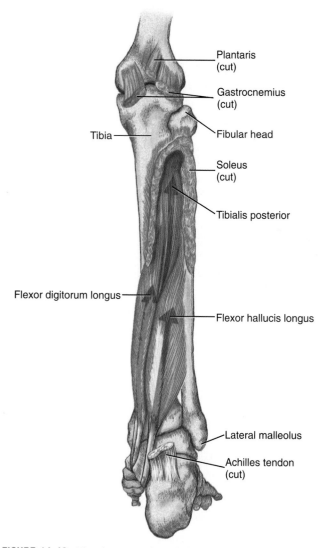

Plantaris
(cut)

Gastrocnemius
(cut)

Fibular head

Tibia

Soleus
(cut)

Tibialis posterior

Flexor digitorum longus

Flexor hallucis longus

Lateral malleolus

Achilles tendon
(cut)

FIGURE 14-49. The deep muscles of the posterior compartment of the right leg: the tibialis posterior, flexor digitorum longus, and flexor hallucis longus.

superficial to the deltoid ligament. At this point the tendon divides into superficial and deep parts, establishing attachments to *every tarsal bone, except the talus,* and to the bases of several of the more central metatarsals (see Figure 14-45). The most prominent distal attachment of the tibialis posterior is on the navicular tuberosity. The tendon is usually palpable for several centimeters just proximal to the navicular tuberosity during resisted adduction and inversion of the foot.

The main tendon of the tibialis posterior provides direct mechanical support to the adjacent spring ligament, thereby adding significant stability to the medial longitudinal arch.[87] A ruptured or overstretched tibialis posterior tendon typically results in the collapse of the medial longitudinal arch, with an associated drop in the height of the talus.[64,129]

The tendons of both the tibialis posterior and the flexor digitorum longus use the medial malleolus as a fixed pulley to direct their force posterior to the axis of rotation at the talocrural joint.[60] An analogous pulley exists for the fibularis longus and brevis tendons, as these structures pass posterior to the lateral malleolus (see Figure 14-46). Tendons of the tibialis posterior and flexor digitorum longus are positioned posterior to the medial malleolus by the flexor retinaculum. The flexor hallucis longus uses a different plantar flexion pulley system, formed proximally by the medial and lateral tubercles of the talus and distally by the sustentaculum talus of the calcaneus.

Joint Action

With the exception of the fibularis longus and brevis, all muscles that plantar flex the talocrural joint also supinate (invert) the subtalar or transverse tarsal joints. This strong inversion bias is evidenced by the position of all muscles within the posterior compartment of the leg relative to the subtalar joint (see Figure 14-43). From the anatomic position, even the triceps surae inverts slightly, as the force of the Achilles tendon passes just medial to the subtalar joint's axis of rotation.[60]

The tibialis posterior, flexor hallucis longus, and flexor digitorum longus are the primary supinators of the foot. The tibialis posterior likely produces the greatest supination

FIGURE 14-50. A medial view of the flexor retinaculum that covers the tendons of the tibialis posterior, flexor digitorum longus, and tibial neurovascular bundle. (From Richardson EG: Neurogenic disorders. In Canale ST, ed: *Campbell's operative orthopaedics,* vol 4, ed 9, St Louis, 1998, Mosby.)

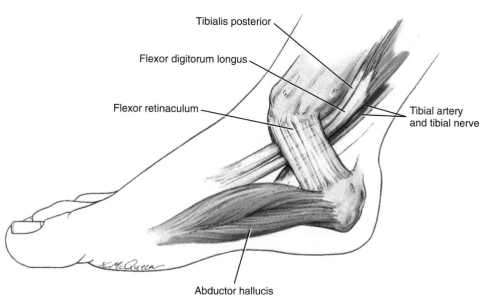

Tibialis posterior

Flexor digitorum longus

Flexor retinaculum

Tibial artery
and tibial nerve

Abductor hallucis

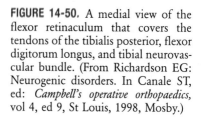

torque (especially in the direction of adduction) across the subtalar and transverse tarsal joints.[31,60,65] The muscle's extensive distal attachments, especially to the navicular, provide an effective inversion "twist" of the midfoot (see Figure 14-26, *D*). In addition to plantar flexion and supination, the flexor digitorum longus and flexor hallucis longus have additional actions at the more distal joints of the foot, especially at the metatarsophalangeal and interphalangeal joints.

Activation of the Plantar Flexor and Supinator Muscles during Walking. The plantar flexor and supinator muscles are active throughout most of the stance phase of gait, particularly between foot flat and toe off phases (see activation of the gastrocnemius and soleus, for example, in Figure 15-29).[123,124] These muscles become active immediately after the dorsiflexor muscles relax. From foot flat to just before heel off, the plantar flexors act eccentrically to decelerate the forward rotation (dorsiflexion) of the leg over the fixed talus.[50,93] Between the heel off and toe off phases, however, the muscles switch to a concentric activation to assist with the necessary thrust for push off and early swing phase. Furthermore, active forces in the flexor hallucis longus, flexor digitorum longus, and intrinsic foot muscles (lumbricals and interossei) hold the plantar surface of the extending toes firmly against the ground. This action expands the weight-bearing surfaces of the toes, thereby minimizing contact pressures.

The tibialis posterior, flexor hallucis longus, and flexor digitorum longus muscles are all capable of resisting pronation and assisting with supination during the stance phase of walking. Of the three muscles, however, the tibialis posterior is most designed for this function.[4,31,64] EMG studies show that the tibialis posterior is active during the stance phase longer than any other supinator muscle, from just before foot flat through heel off phase.[123] As the entire foot contacts the ground, the tibialis posterior decelerates the pronating rearfoot, which assists with a gradual and controlled lowering of the medial longitudinal arch (review Figure 14-31). Through this eccentric action, the tibialis posterior absorbs some of the impact of loading. Persons who excessively and/or rapidly pronate during the stance phase may place excessive braking (decelerating) demands on the tibialis posterior, possibly leading to tendinopathy, muscle fatigue, or stress-related anterior leg pain (more generically known as "shin splints").[110] It is not always certain whether excessive pronation causes or results from tibialis posterior dysfunction.[64,129] In either scenario, reduced function of the tibialis posterior limits an important shock absorption mechanism of the foot.

Throughout mid to late stance, contraction of the tibialis posterior helps guide the rearfoot *toward* supination. This same muscular force may assist with the concurrent external rotation of the lower leg and talus, as well as reestablishing the height of the medial longitudinal arch.

Plantar Flexion Torque Generated for Propulsion. At the very end of stance phase, the muscles within the posterior compartment concentrically contract to plantar flex the talocrural joint. The fibularis longus and brevis (within the lateral compartment) also contribute to this torque. The amount of muscular activity produced by the plantar flexor muscles during push off depends strongly on the speed and vigor

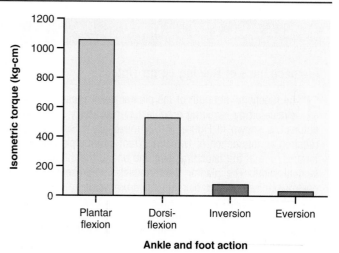

FIGURE 14-51. The magnitude of maximal-effort isometric torque is shown for four actions of the ankle and foot. (N = 86 healthy men and women.)[116]

of walking. Although these muscles provide the primary propulsive force for walking, secondary energy sources may include the ipsilateral hip extensors (generated at early stance) and the ipsilateral hip flexors (generated at very late stance).[16,106]

In healthy persons, maximal isometric plantar flexion torque exceeds the torque potential of all other movements about the ankle and foot combined (Figure 14-51).[41,100,116] Such a large plantar flexion torque reserve is needed to rapidly accelerate the body up and forward during brisk walking, running, jumping, and climbing. Plantar flexion torque is greatest when the ankle approaches full dorsiflexion (i.e., when plantar flexor muscles are elongated) and is least when the ankle is fully plantar flexed.[99] The ankle is typically dorsiflexed as one prepares to sprint or jump. Of interest, as the ankle vigorously plantar flexes at the "take off" of a sprint or jump, the contracting gastrocnemius is simultaneously elongated by the action of the extending knee. This biarticular arrangement prevents the gastrocnemius from overshortening, allowing greater torques throughout a larger range of ankle motion.[52] Because the soleus muscle does not cross the knee, its length-tension relationship is unaffected by the position of the knee. The relative slow-twitch muscle characteristics of the soleus are more suited to control the slow and subtle postural sway movements of the leg over the talus during standing. The faster-twitch characteristics of the gastrocnemius, on the other hand, are apparently better suited for providing a propulsive plantar flexion torque for activities that also involve dynamic knee extension, such as jumping and sprinting.

Of all the plantar flexor muscles, the gastrocnemius and soleus are by far the most powerful, theoretically capable of producing about 80% of the total plantar flexion torque at the ankle.[93] The large torque potential of the triceps surae results in part from the muscles' large cross-sectional area and relatively long moment arm. The protruding calcaneal tuberosity provides the triceps surae with a moment arm of about 5.3 cm from the talocrural joint, nearly twice the average moment arm of the other plantar flexor muscles.[60]

SPECIAL FOCUS 14-7

Biomechanics of Raising up on Tiptoes

The functional strength of the plantar flexor muscles is often evaluated by requiring a subject to repeatedly stand up on tiptoes. As shown in Figure 14-52, maximally raising the body requires an interaction of two concurrent internal plantar flexion torques, one at the talocrural joint and one at the metatarsophalangeal joints. The plantar flexor muscles, represented by the gastrocnemius, plantar flex the *talocrural joint* by rotating the calcaneus and talus within the mortise. The primary torque used to raise the body, however, occurs through extension across the *metatarsophalangeal joints.* Acting about the medial-lateral axes of rotation at the toes, the gastrocnemius has an internal moment arm that greatly exceeds the external moment arm of body weight (compare *B* and *C* in Figure 14-52). Such a large mechanical advantage is rare in the musculoskeletal system. Acting as a second-class lever with the pivot point at the metatarsophalangeal joints, the gastrocnemius lifts the body using mechanics similar to those of a person lifting a large load with a wheelbarrow. If, for instance, the gastrocnemius functions with a mechanical advantage of 3:1 (i.e., ratio of the internal-to-external moment arms, or *B/C* in the Figure 14-52), the muscle needs to produce a lifting force of only one third, or 33%, of body weight to support the plantar flexed position. Rarely in the body does a muscle produce a force less than the load it is supporting. As a biomechanical tradeoff, however, the gastrocnemius, in theory, needs to shorten a distance three times *greater* than the vertical displacement of the body's center of mass (see Chapter 1). (A more precise estimate of the vertical displacement requires knowledge of the average angle of pennation of all the plantar flexor muscles.) Nevertheless, the nature of this mechanical tradeoff allows one to stand up on tiptoes with relative ease.

Figure 14-52 shows the importance of ample extension range of motion at the metatarsophalangeal joints. Not only do the plantar flexor muscles use these joints to augment their internal moment arm, but, as described earlier, full extension of these joints pulls the plantar fascia taut via the windlass effect. This action helps the intrinsic muscles support the medial longitudinal arch and maintain a rigid forefoot, thereby allowing the foot to accept the load imposed by body weight.

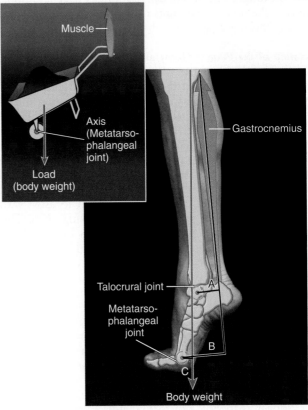

FIGURE 14-52. A mechanical model shows the biomechanics of standing on tiptoes. The force of a contracting gastrocnemius muscle acts with a relatively short internal moment arm from the talocrural joint *(A),* and a relatively long internal moment arm from the metatarsophalangeal joints *(B),* Once on tiptoes, the line of gravity from body weight falls just posterior to the axis of rotation at the metatarsophalangeal joints. As a result, body weight acts with a relatively small external moment arm *(C),* from the metatarsophalangeal joints.

MUSCULAR PARALYSIS AFTER INJURY TO THE FIBULAR OR TIBIAL NERVE

Injury to the Common Fibular Nerve and Its Branches

The *common fibular nerve* winds around the neck of the fibula, just deep to the fibularis longus. This nerve is injured relatively frequently from lacerations or trauma that involves a fractured proximal fibula. Injury to the *deep branch of the fibular nerve* can result in paralysis of *all* the dorsiflexor (pretibial) muscles (see Figure 14-41). With paralysis of the dorsiflexor muscles, the foot rapidly and uncontrollably plantar flexes immediately after the heel contact phase of walking. During the swing phase, the hip and knee must excessively flex to ensure that the toes clear the ground.

Paralysis of the dorsiflexor muscles dramatically increases the likelihood of developing a plantar flexion contracture at

the talocrural joint. This deformity is referred to as a *drop-foot* or *pes equinus.* In a surprisingly short period, a plantar flexed posture may lead to adaptive shortening and tightening of the Achilles tendon as well as several other collateral ligaments of the ankle. The relentless pull of gravity can also contribute to a plantar flexion contracture, often requiring an ankle-foot orthosis to maintain adequate dorsiflexion during walking.

An injury to the *superficial branch of the fibular nerve* may result in paralysis of the fibularis longus and fibularis brevis (see Figure 14-41). Over time, paralysis may lead to a supinated or inverted posture of the foot, a condition called *pes varus.* An injury to the *common fibular nerve* may involve both deep and superficial nerve branches. The resulting paralysis of all dorsiflexor *and* evertor muscles strongly predisposes a person to a deformity of combined plantar flexion of the

TABLE 14-7. Nerve Injury and Common Resulting Deformities or Abnormal Postures throughout the Ankle, Foot*, and Toes

Nerve Injury and Associated Muscle Paralysis	Possible Ensuing Deformity or Abnormal Posture	Common Clinical Name	Examples of Structures Likely to Experience Adaptive Shortening and Subsequent Tightness
Injury to the *deep branch of the fibular nerve* with paralysis of pretibial muscles	Plantar flexion of the talocrural joint	Drop-foot or pes equinus	Achilles tendon, posterior capsule of the talocrural joint
Injury to the *superficial branch of the fibular nerve* with paralysis of the fibularis longus and brevis	Inversion of the foot	Pes varus	Tibialis posterior, tibiocalcaneal fibers of the deltoid ligament and adjacent capsule of the subtalar joint
Injury to the *common fibular nerve* with paralysis of all dorsiflexor and evertor muscles	Plantar flexion of the talocrural joint and inversion of the foot	Pes equinovarus	Achilles tendon, tibialis posterior muscle
Injury to the *proximal portion of the tibial nerve* with paralysis of *all* plantar flexor and supinator muscles	Dorsiflexion† of the talocrural joint and eversion of the foot	Pes calcaneovalgus	Dorsiflexor and evertor muscles, anterior talofibular ligament and adjacent capsule of the subtalar joint
Injury to the *middle portion of the tibial nerve* with paralysis of supinator muscles	Eversion of the foot	Pes valgus	Fibularis muscles
Injury involving the *medial and lateral plantar nerves*	Hyperextension of the metatarsophalangeal joints, and flexion of the interphalangeal joints	Clawing of the toes	Extensor digitorum longus and brevis

*The *foot* refers primarily to the subtalar and transverse tarsal joints.
†Severity depends on the influence of gravity.

ankle and supination of the foot, a condition referred to as *pes equinovarus*.

Injury to the Tibial Nerve and Its Branches

Injury to the tibial nerve may cause varying levels of weakness or paralysis in the muscles of the posterior compartment (see Figure 14-42). Isolated paralysis of the gastrocnemius and soleus because of tibial nerve injury is rare. Nevertheless, regardless of underlying pathology, paralysis of these muscles results in profound loss of plantar flexion torque. Over time, a fixed dorsiflexion posture may result at the talocrural joint, a condition known as *pes calcaneus*. The term *calcaneus* is used to describe the often prominent heel pad that forms in response to the heel of the chronically dorsiflexed ankle sharply striking the ground at the initiation of the stance phase.

Paralysis involving primarily the supinator muscles of the foot may result in a fixed pronated deformity, primarily the result of the unopposed action of the fibularis longus and brevis muscles. The term *pes valgus* typically describes both eversion and abduction components of the pronation deformity. Paralysis involving *all* the muscles of the posterior compartment increases the potential for a fixed deformity called *pes calcaneovalgus*.

Injury to the tibial nerve within the leg typically involves the more distal *medial* and *lateral* plantar nerves (see Figure 14-42). Paralysis of the intrinsic muscles within the foot often results in a "clawing" of the toes: hyperextension of the metatarsophalangeal joints with flexion of the interphalangeal

joints. This deformity results primarily from an unopposed pull of the extrinsic toe extensor muscles across the metatarsophalangeal joints. The pathomechanics of clawing caused by weakness of the intrinsic muscles of the foot are similar to those of clawing of the fingers after a combined ulnar and median nerve injury (see Chapter 8).

The common fixed deformities or abnormal postures of the ankle, foot, and toes are summarized according to nerve injury in Table 14-7.

INTRINSIC MUSCLES

Anatomic and Functional Considerations

Intrinsic muscles are those that originate and insert within the foot. The following discussion highlights the primary attachments and actions of the intrinsic muscles. More detailed attachments of these muscles is presented in Appendix IV, Part D.

The dorsum of the foot has one intrinsic muscle, the extensor digitorum brevis, which is innervated by the deep branch of the fibular nerve. The *extensor digitorum brevis* originates on the dorsal-lateral surface of the calcaneus, just proximal to the calcaneocuboid articulation. The muscle belly sends four tendons: one to the dorsal surface of the great toe (often designated as the extensor hallucis brevis), and three that join the tendons of the extensor digitorum longus of the second through the fourth toes (see Figure 14-44). The extensor digitorum brevis assists the extensor hallucis longus and extensor digitorum longus in extension of the toes.

Intrinsic muscles of the foot

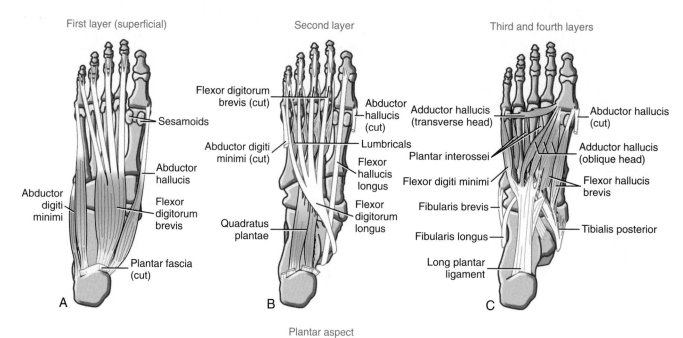

First layer (superficial)

Second layer

Third and fourth layers

Sesamoids

Flexor digitorum brevis (cut)

Abductor digiti minimi (cut)

Abductor hallucis (cut)

Lumbricals

Flexor hallucis longus

Flexor digitorum longus

Quadratus plantae

Abductor hallucis

Abductor digiti minimi

Flexor digitorum brevis

Plantar fascia (cut)

Adductor hallucis (transverse head)

Plantar interossei

Flexor digiti minimi

Fibularis brevis

Fibularis longus

Long plantar ligament

Abductor hallucis (cut)

Adductor hallucis (oblique head)

Flexor hallucis brevis

Tibialis posterior

A   B   C

Plantar aspect

FIGURE 14-53. The intrinsic muscles of the plantar aspect of the foot are organized into four layers.

The remaining intrinsic muscles originate and insert within the plantar aspect of the foot. These muscles are organized into *four layers* (Figure 14-53). The plantar fascia is located just superficial to the first layer of muscles.

Layer 1

The intrinsic muscles in the first layer of the foot are the flexor digitorum brevis, abductor hallucis, and abductor digiti minimi (see Figure 14-53, *A*). As a group, these muscles originate on the lateral and medial processes of the calcaneal tuberosity and nearby connective tissues. The *flexor digitorum brevis* attaches to both sides of the plantar aspect of the middle phalanges of the four lesser toes. Proximal to this distal attachment, each tendon divides to allow passage of the tendons of the flexor digitorum longus. (Note the similar relationship between the flexor digitorum superficialis and profundus of the hand.) The flexor digitorum brevis assists the flexor digitorum longus with flexing the toes. The *abductor hallucis* forms the medial border of the foot, providing a covered passage for the nerves that enter the plantar aspect of the foot. The abductor muscle attaches distally to the medial border of the proximal phalanx of the great toe, sharing an attachment with the medial head of the flexor hallucis brevis (see Figure 14-53, *C*). The *abductor digiti minimi* helps form the lateral-plantar margin of the foot, attaching distally to the lateral border of the base of the proximal phalanx of the fifth toe. Each muscle abducts and assists with flexion of its respective digit.

> **Intrinsic Muscles of the Foot, Layer 1**
> - Flexor digitorum brevis
> - Abductor hallucis
> - Abductor digiti minimi

Layer 2

The intrinsic muscles in the second layer are the quadratus plantae and the lumbricals (see Figure 14-53, *B*). Both muscles are anatomically related to the tendons of the flexor digitorum longus. The *quadratus plantae* (flexor digitorum accessorius) attaches by two heads to the plantar aspect of the calcaneus. Both heads attach distally to the lateral edge of the common tendon of the flexor digitorum longus. The quadratus plantae helps to stabilize the tendons of the flexor digitorum longus, preventing them from migrating medially.[72] The four *lumbricals* have their proximal attachment from the tendons of the flexor digitorum longus. These small fleshy muscles pass on the medial side of the lesser toes to attach into the extensor digital expansion. The lumbricals flex the metatarsophalangeal joints and extend the interphalangeal joints—actions that are functionally equivalent to the actions performed by the lumbricals of the hand.

> **Intrinsic Muscles of the Foot, Layer 2**
> - Quadratus plantae
> - Lumbricals

Layer 3

The intrinsic muscles in the third layer are the adductor hallucis, flexor hallucis brevis, and flexor digiti minimi (see Figure 14-53, *C*). As a group, these short muscles arise from the plantar aspect of the cuboid, cuneiforms, and bases of more central metatarsal bones, and from local connective tissues. Similar to the adductor pollicis in the hand, the *adductor hallucis* arises from two heads: oblique and transverse. Both heads attach to the lateral base of the proximal phalanx of the great toe and adjacent lateral sesamoid bone.[101] The muscle adducts and assists with flexion of the metatarsophalangeal joint of the great toe. The *flexor hallucis brevis* has two heads that attach distally to the medial and lateral sides of the base of the proximal phalanx of the great toe. Medial and lateral sesamoid bones are located within the two tendons of this muscle, providing greater leverage for the production of toe flexion torque.[1] The *flexor digiti minimi* attaches to the lateral base of the proximal phalanx of the fifth toe, sharing a common attachment with the abductor digiti minimi. Both short flexor muscles flex the metatarsophalangeal joint of their respective toes.

Intrinsic Muscles of the Foot, Layer 3
* Adductor hallucis
* Flexor hallucis brevis
* Flexor digiti minimi

Layer 4

The fourth layer of intrinsic muscles contains three plantar and four dorsal interossei muscles. The *plantar interossei* are shown in Figure 14-53, *C*, along with the muscles of the third layer. The dorsal interossei are illustrated in Figure 14-38. The overall plan of the interossei is nearly identical to that of the hand, except that the "reference digit" for abduction and adduction of the toes is the second instead of the third digit as in the hand.

Intrinsic Muscles of the Foot, Layer 4
* Plantar interossei (three)
* Dorsal interossei (four)

The *dorsal interossei* are two-headed, bipennate muscles. The second digit contains two dorsal interossei, whereas the third and fourth digits contain one each. All dorsal interossei insert on the base of the proximal phalanges; the first and second interossei insert on the medial and lateral side of the second digit, respectively, and the third and fourth dorsal interossei insert on the lateral side of the third and fourth digit (review attachments in Figure 14-4). Each dorsal interosseus muscle abducts the metatarsophalangeal joint. Each of the third, fourth, and fifth digits contains a *plantar interosseus* muscle. Each muscle consists of one head and inserts on the medial side of the base of the corresponding proximal phalanx (review attachments in Figure 14-5). These muscles adduct their respective metatarsophalangeal joint.

The actions assigned to each of the intrinsic muscles assume the foot is unloaded and the toes are free to move. Although these unique actions allow the clinician to test the strength and dexterity of these muscles, the actions are not very relevant functionally. The intrinsic muscles of the foot are used less for manual dexterity, such as in the hand, and more for assisting with standing and walking balance and, most notably, providing structural stability to the foot and the medial longitudinal arch during the push off phase of walking. These functions explain why most of the intrinsic muscles are maximally active during late stance, just as the heel is rising off the floor.[52]

Most of the intrinsic muscles of the foot are anatomically analogous to an intrinsic muscle of the hand. One exception, however, is that the foot does *not* contain muscles that perform opposition of the first and fifth digits. Understanding these analogies should help with learning the anatomy, innervation, and action of these muscles. Table 14-8 summarizes the relevant information on the intrinsic muscles of the foot.

SYNOPSIS

As an integrated complex, the ankle and foot function as the dynamic interface between the lower extremity and the earth's surface. This interface is amazingly adaptable: pliable enough to absorb repetitive loading and to accommodate to irregular ground surfaces, yet sufficiently rigid to support body weight and the muscular thrust of walking and running.

Twenty-eight individual muscles, acting across 32 joints or joint complexes, control the movement and posture of the ankle and foot. As a means to organize the anatomy, the ankle and foot are conveniently divided into three regions: the rearfoot, midfoot, and forefoot. Although movement can occur independently within these regions, this is generally not the case—especially during the stance phase of walking. Most often, the movements within each region are intended to amplify or accommodate to movements produced in other regions of the foot and lower limb, typically in response to active muscle and ground reaction forces.

The most effective way to summarize the kinesiology of the ankle and foot is to follow the main events of the stance phase of walking, starting as the heel contacts the ground. At *early stance* phase, the ankle rapidly plantar flexes as the rearfoot pronates (everts). During this so-called *load-acceptance phase of gait*, the dorsiflexor and supinator (invertor) muscles act eccentrically to decelerate the prevailing kinematics, as well as absorb the impact of the foot striking the ground.

As part of this load-acceptance and shock-absorption mechanism, the medial longitudinal arch depresses slowly in response to body weight. Several tissues help support as well as decelerate the lowering of the arch, including the spring ligament, capsule of the talonavicular joint, plantar fascia, and, if needed, muscles like the tibialis posterior. Tissues that slow the lowering of the arch absorb energy and therefore protect the foot. Failure to control the extent or rate of the combined rearfoot pronation and associated lowering of the medial longitudinal arch may, over time, lead to damaging stress and associated pain in local tissues. Treatment for this problem may involve orthotics or specialized shoes, taping, activity modification, and selected stretching, strengthening, and reeducation of lower extremity muscles that directly or indirectly control the ankle and foot.

During the *middle and late stance phases* of gait, the entire lower limb (which was previously internally rotating) sharply changes its rotation direction. The now externally rotating lower limb, although the movement is slight and barely perceptible, helps initiate the gradual transition from an everting to an inverting rearfoot. Mechanically coupled with an impending rising of the medial longitudinal arch, the foot, ideally, becomes increasingly rigid. The increased rigidity acts to stabilize the foot—both longitudinally and transversely—during the push off phase of walking. The rising of the arch during this latter part of the stance phase is driven primarily through concentric action of invertor muscles (notably the tibialis

TABLE 14-8. Summary of the Relevant Information on the Intrinsic Muscles of the Foot

Intrinsic Muscle	Location	Isolated Action	Innervation	Analogous Muscle in the Hand
Extensor digitorum brevis	Dorsum of the foot	Extension of the toes	Deep branch of the fibular nerve	None
Flexor digitorum brevis	Layer 1	Flexion of the proximal interphalangeal and metatarsophalangeal joints of the lesser toes	Medial plantar nerve	Flexor digitorum superficialis
Abductor hallucis	Layer 1	Abduction and (assistance with) flexion of the metatarsophalangeal joint of the great toe	Medial plantar nerve	Abductor pollicis brevis
Abductor digiti minimi	Layer 1	Abduction and (assistance with) flexion of the metatarsophalangeal joint of the fifth digit	Lateral plantar nerve	Abductor digiti minimi
Quadratus plantae	Layer 2	Provides medial stabilization to the common tendons of the flexor digitorum longus	Lateral plantar nerve	None
Lumbricals	Layer 2	Flexion of the metatarsophalangeal joints and extension of the interphalangeal joints of the lesser toes	*Second digit:* Medial plantar nerve *Third through fifth digits:* Lateral plantar nerve	Lumbricals
Adductor hallucis	Layer 3	Adduction and (assistance with) flexion of the metatarsophalangeal joint of the great toe	Lateral plantar nerve	Adductor pollicis
Flexor hallucis brevis	Layer 3	Flexion of the metatarsophalangeal joint of the great toe	Medial plantar nerve	Flexor pollicis brevis
Flexor digiti minimi	Layer 3	Flexion of the metatarsophalangeal joint of the fifth digit	Lateral plantar nerve	Flexor digiti minimi
Plantar interossei (three)	Layer 4	Adduction of the metatarsophalangeal joints of the third, fourth, and fifth digits (relative to a reference in line through the second digit)	Lateral plantar nerve	Palmar interossei
Dorsal interossei (four)	Layer 4	Abduction of the metatarsophalangeal joints of the second, third, and fourth digits (relative to a reference in line through the second digit)	Lateral plantar nerve	Dorsal interossei

posterior) and intrinsic muscles. As the heel rises, just before the toe off phase, body weight is transferred forward toward the metatarsal heads. The continued coactivation of intrinsic and extrinsic muscles, in conjunction with the windlass effect across the extending metatarsophalangeal joints, provides the final elements of stability to the propelling foot.

Impairments of the ankle and foot have multiple causes, including pathology affecting the connective tissues, muscles, peripheral nerves, or the central nervous system. The ankle and foot are also very vulnerable to direct mechanical trauma. Acute trauma may occur from an isolated event involving a relatively large damaging stress, such as an inversion sprain, fracture of the styloid process of the fifth metatarsal, or severe hyperextension of the great toe. Chronic trauma may result from an accumulation of lower magnitude stress over an extended time, leading to plantar fasciitis, displacement of the tendon of the fibularis longus relative to the fibula, tibialis

posterior tendinopathy, "heel spurs," or metatarsalgia. Often, stress caused by microtrauma is associated with abnormal alignment within the joints of the foot or in proximal parts of the lower extremity. Abnormal alignment may lead to excessive kinematic compensations that stress or induce fatigue in muscles and supporting connective tissues. Because of the frequency and regular necessity of using the foot, many stress-related conditions involve inflammation and associated pain.

Knowledge of the anatomy and kinesiology of the ankle and foot is a prerequisite to understanding the associated pathomechanics. Muscle and joint interactions must be understood both when the foot is unloaded and when the foot is fixed to the ground. Furthermore, the clinician must appreciate the mechanical interdependence between the kinematics of the ankle and foot and more proximal regions of the lower limb.

ADDITIONAL CLINICAL CONNECTIONS

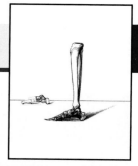

CLINICAL CONNECTION 14-1
Chronic Ankle Instability

Lateral ankle sprains are among the most common injuries in sports, particularly in basketball (most notably in females), volleyball, and lacrosse.[7] Most of these injuries involve excessive *inversion* of the ankle or foot, with subsequent injury to the lateral collateral ligaments and fibular (peroneal) muscle tendons.[122] The mechanism of injury varies but typically involves a strong and unexpected inversion torque to the weight-bearing ankle and foot, often in conjunction with external rotation of the lower limb.[62] Although estimates vary, 30% to 40% of persons who experience an isolated inversion sprain will later experience multiple ankle sprains to the same foot, typically associated with chronic pain and generalized instability.[63,133] Persons with *chronic ankle instability* (CAI) typically report that their ankle frequently "gives way" while they are involved in sporting events or even during relatively nonstressful activities. In addition to the loss of function, persons with CAI are likely at a greater risk for developing ankle osteoarthritis.[84]

Why certain persons develop CAI and others do not is not well understood.[42] A considerable amount of evidence suggests that the pathogenesis of CAI involves diminished sensation after repeated damage to the ligaments and embedded mechanoreceptors of the ankle.[33,43,62,130] Distorted sensory input reduces the body's ability to generate an effective and timely defensive response to protect the ankle, especially after an unexpected and rapid inversion perturbation. Indeed, subsequent research has shown that persons with CAI have altered ankle proprioception (positional awareness), increased postural unsteadiness or reduced balance (most notably while standing on one limb), reduced reaction times in local muscles (notably the fibularis longus and brevis), and altered recruitment patterns of muscles throughout the entire lower limb.* Gait analysis has revealed that persons with CAI enter the stance phase of gait with their subtalar joint *inverted 6 to 7 degrees greater* than in normal controls.[91] Authors of the study argue that the inversion bias just before and after heel strike may reflect the subjects' inability to correctly detect ankle position, or a delay in activation of the fibularis muscles, or a combination thereof. Both of these abnormal

---

*References 17, 28, 44, 73, 111, 130.

responses are believed to be the result of damage to the mechanoreceptors located within the injured ligaments.[91] Biomechanically, greater inversion at heel strike increases the likelihood that the upward-directed ground forces at heel strike would create a large and unexpected inversion torque. Furthermore, the authors reported that instead of normally controlling eversion during early stance phase through eccentric activation of invertor muscles, persons with CAI, on average, activated their evertor muscles in a *concentric* fashion. This mechanism of muscular control is not ideal for safely absorbing forces at and immediately after heel impact.

Hubbard and colleagues reported that persons with CAI, on average, have an abnormally anteriorly aligned position of the distal fibula.[49] The altered position of the fibula may have resulted from increased tension in the repeatedly stretched anterior talofibular ligament, or swelling around the mortise. The authors also suggested that the malaligned fibula is the result of increased "tone" in the fibularis muscles secondary to increased activity in the gamma motoneuron system. This increased neural activity may be a response to abnormal afferent impulses from the damaged mechanoreceptors embedded within the injured lateral ankle ligaments.[94] Regardless of cause, excessive anterior migration of the distal fibula will alter the kinematics and likely increase the stress within the talocrural joint.

In summary, the specific pathogenesis of CAI is unclear and likely involves several factors.[39,43,112] Research consistently implicates diminished proprioception about the ankle, which reduces overall postural steadiness as well as the body's dynamic response to protecting the ankle from injury.[107] It remains uncertain, however, whether the postural unsteadiness often associated with CAI is the *cause or the effect* of repeated ankle sprains.[28]

Evaluation and treatment of persons with CAI should address not only the instability at the ankle (through bracing, taping, and strengthening muscles),[107,113] but also balance and strength deficits within the body as a whole, especially while the person stands on one limb or progresses from double- to single-limb support. This use of "balance boards" or other dynamic challenges to the upright position has been shown to be effective in treatment of CAI.[42,44,90,109,132]

ADDITIONAL CLINICAL CONNECTIONS

ADDITIONAL CLINICAL CONNECTION 14-2
Palpation of Selected Anatomy of the Ankle and Foot

The ability to palpate and thus identify the bones and joints of the body is an essential clinical skill, routinely used in both evaluation and treatment of musculoskeletal disorders. Such a skill allows the clinician a "window" into the working anatomy (and ultimately the kinesiology) of the region. Skill with palpation (1) facilitates clinical communication and documentation, (2) improves the ability to identify specific key tissues, often for the purpose of diagnosing or monitoring a patient's condition, (3) improves the effectiveness of essentially any manually based treatment, and (4) helps in the assessment of normal and abnormal movement and posture.

The following section provides examples of bony regions of the ankle and foot that are routinely palpated as part of the assessment or treatment of common musculoskeletal disorders. These bony regions or joints are highlighted in medial and lateral perspectives using a radiograph and photograph of a healthy 23-year-old man (Figures 14-54 and 14-55). Each figure is associated with a table that describes (1) a method for palpating the structure, and (2) examples of why clinicians are interested in the region.

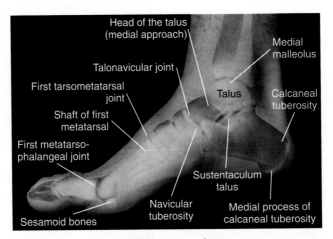

Medial perspective

Structure	Where to Palpate	Possible Reasons for Palpation

Medial malleolus	Extreme distal end of medial tibia	• Assess tenderness of the proximal attachment of the deltoid ligament
		• Assess leg length
		• Estimate medial-lateral axis of rotation at the talocrural joint
		• Anatomic reference for locating structures in the tarsal tunnel, such as:
		  o tendon of the tibialis posterior
		  o flexor digitorum longus
		  o tibial nerve and terminal branches (medial and lateral plantar nerves)

Calcaneal tuberosity	Posterior-plantar heel region	• Evaluate for Achilles tendinitis • Check for abnormal bone formation (possibly related to excessive stress placed on the Achilles tendon)
Medial process of calcaneal tuberosity	Plantar-medial heel region	• Evaluate for plantar fasciitis, heel spurs, or inflamed proximal attachment of many intrinsic muscles of the foot
Sustentaculum talus	Approximately 2-3 cm inferior to the tip of the medial malleolus	• Anatomic reference for locating medial surface of the subtalar joint • Evaluate tenderness of (a) distal attachment of tibiocalcaneal fibers of the deltoid ligament, (b) proximal attachment of the "spring" ligament

ADDITIONAL CLINICAL CONNECTIONS

ADDITIONAL CLINICAL CONNECTION 14-2
Palpation of Selected Anatomy of the Ankle and Foot—cont'd

Structure	Where to Palpate	Possible Reasons for Palpation
Navicular tuberosity	As a relatively sharp projection, located approximately 4 cm inferior-and-anterior to the tip of the medial malleolus	• General reference for locating the navicular bone, including the nearby talonavicular and first cuneonavicular joints. • Assess height of medial longitudinal arch • Assess tibialis posterior tendinopathy
Sesamoid bones	Plantar aspect of metatarsophalangeal joint of great toe (typically difficult to distinguish from flexor tendons crossing the joint)	• Evaluate for tenderness associated with sesamoiditis or fracture (common in dancers)
First metatarsophalangeal joint	Dorsal or medially; immediately distal to the head of the first metatarsal bone	• Evaluate severity of hallux valgus ("bunion") or hallux rigidus ("turf toe")
Shaft of the first metatarsal	Dorsal or medial aspect of forefoot	• Assess alignment (e.g., valgus or varus) and overall flexibility of the forefoot • Evaluate plantar flexed first ray, such as that often associated with pes cavus, or increased tension in the fibularis longus
Tarsometatarsal joint	Immediately proximal to the base of the metatarsal	• Evaluate laxity or alignment of the joint of the first digit • Assess Lisfranc's dislocation (typically second digit)
Talonavicular joint	Immediately posterior (and slightly superior) to the navicular tuberosity	• Evaluate for sprain, tenderness, and general mobility of the medial component of the transverse tarsal joint • Check stability of the keystone of the medial longitudinal arch
Head of the talus	Medial approach: About midway between the anterior-distal edge of the medial malleolus and the navicular tuberosity	• Assess height of medial longitudinal arch

FIGURE 14-54. Medial perspective using a radiograph and photograph of a healthy 23-year-old man.

Continued

ADDITIONAL CLINICAL CONNECTIONS

ADDITIONAL CLINICAL CONNECTION 14-2
Palpation of Selected Anatomy of the Ankle and Foot—cont'd

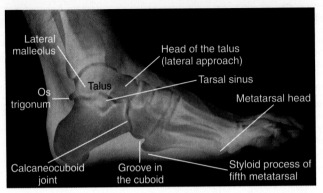

Lateral perspective

Structure	Where to Palpate	Possible Reasons for Palpation
Lateral malleolus	Extreme distal end of fibula	• Estimate medial-lateral axis of rotation at the talocrural joint • Reference for locating the tendons (and sheaths) of the fibularis longus and brevis • Testing the stability or alignment of the distal tibiofibular joint
Tarsal sinus	As a slight depression, just anterior to the extreme distal aspect of the lateral malleolus. This sinus (or canal) courses obliquely through the subtalar joint	• Assess tenderness in the anterior talofibular ligament. • Evaluate swelling possibly from injury to the cervical (talocalcaneal) ligament, located within the tarsal sinus
Head of the talus	Lateral approach: Immediately superior to the tarsal sinus	• In conjunction with a medial palpation approach, used to determine "subtalar neutral position."
Metatarsal head	Plantar aspect of the distal end of the metatarsal bone	• Assess severity of metatarsalgia (frequently on second or third digits)
Styloid process of fifth metatarsal	As a sharp projection, located at the approximate midpoint of the lateral side of the foot	• Assess possible avulsion fracture and tear of the fibularis brevis tendon.
Groove in the cuboid	Immediately proximal to the styloid process of the fifth metatarsal	• Assess tenderness of the tendon of the fibularis longus.
Calcaneocuboid joint	About 2 cm proximal to the styloid process of the fifth metatarsal	• Evaluate subluxation or other trauma associated with the cuboid
Os trigonum (infrequent appearance of an accessory bone, usually located posterior-lateral to the talus)	On the posterior aspect of the ankle, posterior to the lateral malleolus; depending on its size, however, this structure may not be readily palpable.	• Evaluate possible impingement of the os trigonum within the talocrural joint, usually at the extremes of plantar flexion.

FIGURE 14-55. Lateral perspective using a radiograph and photograph of a healthy 23-year-old man.

ADDITIONAL CLINICAL CONNECTIONS

CLINICAL CONNECTION 14-3
Plantar Flexor Muscles Indirectly Extending the Knee

An important function of the plantar flexor muscles is to stabilize the knee in extension.[93] This function becomes evident during observation of the gait of a person with weakened or subactivated plantar flexor muscles. Normally the plantar flexor muscles "brake" or decelerate ankle dorsiflexion (leg moving forward on foot) during the mid-to-late stance phase of gait. Excessive dorsiflexion at this time in the gait cycle can contribute to knee instability. Figure 14-56, *A* shows a hypothetic case of a person with a weakened soleus muscle unable to control forward rotation of the leg. The excessively dorsiflexed ankle shifts the force of body weight well *posterior* to the medial-lateral axis of rotation at the knee. This shift can create a sudden and often unexpected knee flexion torque. The dorsiflexed ankle, in this case, biases flexion of the knee. Normally the soleus muscle is able to resist excessive forward rotation of the leg, thereby maintaining body weight closer to the knee's medial-lateral axis of rotation.

With the foot fixed to the ground, active contraction of the plantar flexion muscles can actually assist in extending the knee (see Figure 14-56, *B*).[46] In this example, contraction of the soleus muscle rotates the leg posteriorly about the talocrural joint's axis of rotation. Although any plantar flexor muscle is theoretically capable of this action, the soleus is particularly well suited to stabilize the knee in extension. As a predominately slow-twitch muscle, the soleus can produce relatively low forces over a relatively long duration before fatiguing. Marked spasticity in the soleus muscle can exert a potent and chronic knee extension bias that, over time, can contribute to genu recurvatum deformity.

The ability of the plantar flexor muscles to assist indirectly with knee extension is a potentially important clinical phenomenon. Equally important in this regard is the ability of the *hip extensor muscles* to assist indirectly with knee extension. With the foot planted to the ground, strong activation of a hip extensor (such as that depicted in Figure 14-56, *B)* can pull the femur posteriorly.[3] If the femur is pulled into full hip extension, body weight can help mechanically lock the knee into extension. A hip or knee flexion contracture would reduce the effectiveness of this mechanical locking.

By far, the most direct and effective knee extensor muscle is the quadriceps. In cases of quadriceps weakness, however, it is clinically very useful to know how other muscles can assist (even if slightly) with knee extension. Even persons with strong quadriceps can benefit from recruiting hip extensor and plantar flexor muscles as indirect extensors of the knee. Reducing local demands on the quadriceps can minimize forces at the patellofemoral joint, which is often a desired strategy (at least in the short term) for someone with pain, instability, or arthritis at this joint.

FIGURE 14-56. Two examples of how the ankle affects the position and stability of the knee during standing. **A,** The weakened soleus muscle is unable to decelerate ankle dorsiflexion. With the foot fixed to the ground, ankle dorsiflexion occurs as a forward rotation of the leg over the talus. The forward position of the leg shifts the force of body weight well posterior to the knee, causing it to "buckle" into flexion. **B,** Normal strength and control of the soleus muscle can cause the ankle to plantar flex. With the foot fixed to the ground, plantar flexion rotates the leg posteriorly, bringing the knee toward extension. The contraction of a hip extensor muscle (such as the gluteus maximus) is also shown helping to extend the knee by pulling the femur posteriorly. (Note: The downward-directed body weight vectors could be considered as acting upward as ground reaction forces; either assumption is valid.)

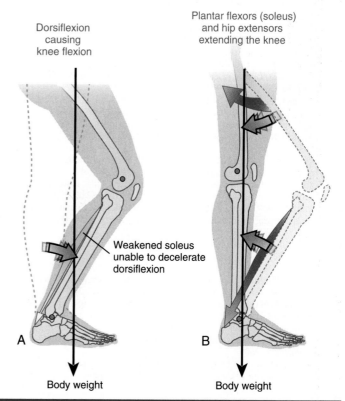

Dorsiflexion causing knee flexion

Plantar flexors (soleus) and hip extensors extending the knee

Weakened soleus unable to decelerate dorsiflexion

A

B

Body weight

Body weight

REFERENCES

1. Aper RL, Saltzman CL, Brown TD: The effect of hallux sesamoid excision on the flexor hallucis longus moment arm, *Clin Orthop Relat Res* 325:209-217, 1996.
2. Arinci Incel N, Genc H, Erdem HR, Yorgancioglu ZR: Muscle imbalance in hallux valgus: an electromyographic study, *Am J Phys Med Rehabil* 82:345-349, 2003.
3. Arnold AS, Anderson FC, Pandy MG, Delp SL: Muscular contributions to hip and knee extension during the single limb stance phase of normal gait: a framework for investigating the causes of crouch gait, *J Biomech* 38:2181-2189, 2005.
4. Basmajian JV, Stecko G: The role of muscles in arch support of the foot, *J Bone Joint Surg Am* 45:1184-1190, 1963.
5. Beimers L, Tuijthof GJ, Blankevoort L, et al: In-vivo range of motion of the subtalar joint using computed tomography, *J Biomech* 41:1390-1397, 2008.
6. Beumer A, van Hemert WL, Swierstra BA, et al: A biomechanical evaluation of the tibiofibular and tibiotalar ligaments of the ankle, *Foot Ankle Int* 24:426-429, 2003.
7. Beynnon BD, Vacek PM, Murphy D, et al: First-time inversion ankle ligament trauma: the effects of sex, level of competition, and sport on the incidence of injury, *Am J Sports Med* 33:1485-1491, 2005.
8. Jones MH, Amendola AS: Acute treatment of inversion ankle sprains: immobilization versus functional treatment. *Clin Orthop Relat Res* 455:169-172, 2007.
9. Blackwood CB, Yuen TJ, Sangeorzan BJ, Ledoux WR: The midtarsal joint locking mechanism, *Foot Ankle Int* 26:1074-1080, 2005.
10. Boone DC, Azen SP: Normal range of motion of joints in male subjects, *J Bone Joint Surg Am* 61:756-759, 1979.
11. Bowers KD Jr, Martin RB: Turf-toe: a shoe-surface related football injury, *Med Sci Sports* 8:81-83, 1976.
12. Boytim MJ, Fischer DA, Neumann L: Syndesmotic ankle sprains, *Am J Sports Med* 19:294-298, 1991.
13. Bozkurt M, Tonuk E, Elhan A, et al: Axial rotation and mediolateral translation of the fibula during passive plantarflexion, *Foot Ankle Int* 29:502-507, 2008.
14. Bronner S, Novella T, Becica L: Management of a delayed-union sesamoid fracture in a dancer, *J Orthop Sports Phys Ther* 37:529-540, 2007.
15. Buchanan KR, Davis I: The relationship between forefoot, midfoot, and rearfoot static alignment in pain-free individuals, *J Orthop Sports Phys Ther* 35:559-566, 2005.
16. Buczek FL, Cooney KM, Walker MR, et al: Performance of an inverted pendulum model directly applied to normal human gait, *Clin Biomech (Bristol, Avon)* 21:288-296, 2006.
17. Bullock-Saxton JE: Local sensation changes and altered hip muscle function following severe ankle sprain, *Phys Ther* 74:17-28, 1994.
18. Calhoun JH, Li F, Ledbetter BR, Viegas SF: A comprehensive study of pressure distribution in the ankle joint with inversion and eversion, *Foot Ankle Int* 15:125-133, 1994.
19. Cashmere T, Smith R, Hunt A: Medial longitudinal arch of the foot: stationary versus walking measures, *Foot Ankle Int* 20:112-118, 1999.
20. Cavanagh PR, Rodgers MM, Iiboshi A: Pressure distribution under symptom-free feet during barefoot standing, *Foot Ankle* 7:262-276, 1987.
21. Colville MR, Marder RA, Boyle JJ, Zarins B: Strain measurement in lateral ankle ligaments, *Am J Sports Med* 18:196-200, 1990.
22. Corazza F, Stagni R, Castelli VP, Leardini A: Articular contact at the tibiotalar joint in passive flexion, *J Biomech* 38:1205-1212, 2005.
23. Cornwall MW, McPoil TG: Motion of the calcaneus, navicular, and first metatarsal during the stance phase of walking, *J Am Podiatr Med Assoc* 92:67-76, 2002.
24. Cornwall MW, McPoil TG: Three-dimensional movement of the foot during the stance phase of walking, *J Am Podiatr Med Assoc* 89:56-66, 1999.
25. Cowan DN, Jones BH, Robinson JR: Foot morphologic characteristics and risk of exercise-related injury, *Arch Fam Med* 2:773-777, 1993.
26. Erdemir A, Hamel AJ, Fauth AR, et al: Dynamic loading of the plantar aponeurosis in walking, *J Bone Joint Surg Am* 86:546-552, 2004.
27. Esterman A, Pilotto L: Foot shape and its effect on functioning in Royal Australian Air Force recruits. Part 1: prospective cohort study, *Mil Med* 170:623-628, 2005.
28. Evans T, Hertel J, Sebastianelli W: Bilateral deficits in postural control following lateral ankle sprain, *Foot Ankle Int* 25:833-839, 2004.
29. Ferber R, Davis IM, Williams DS III: Effect of foot orthotics on rearfoot and tibia joint coupling patterns and variability, *J Biomech* 38:477-483, 2005.
30. Ferrari J, Malone-Lee J: A radiographic study of the relationship between metatarsus adductus and hallux valgus, *J Foot Ankle Surg* 42:9-14, 2003.
31. Flemister AS, Neville CG, Houck J: The relationship between ankle, hindfoot, and forefoot position and posterior tibial muscle excursion, *Foot Ankle Int* 28:448-455, 2007.
32. Franettovich M, Chapman A, Blanch P, Vicenzino B: A physiological and psychological basis for anti-pronation taping from a critical review of the literature, *Sports Med* 38:617-631, 2008.
33. Freeman MA, Dean MR, Hanham IW: The etiology and prevention of functional instability of the foot, *J Bone Joint Surg Br* 47:678-685, 1965.
34. Fritz GR, Prieskorn D: First metatarsocuneiform motion: a radiographic and statistical analysis, *Foot Ankle Int* 16:117-123, 1995.
35. Fujii T, Kitaoka HB, Luo ZP, et al: Analysis of ankle-hindfoot stability in multiple planes: an in vitro study, *Foot Ankle Int* 26:633-637, 2005.
36. Fujii T, Luo ZP, Kitaoka HB, An KN: The manual stress test may not be sufficient to differentiate ankle ligament injuries, *Clin Biomech (Bristol, Avon)* 15:619-623, 2000.
37. Glasoe WM, Yack HJ, Saltzman CL: Anatomy and biomechanics of the first ray, *Phys Ther* 79:854-859, 1999.
38. Green T, Refshauge K, Crosbie J, Adams R: A randomized controlled trial of a passive accessory joint mobilization on acute ankle inversion sprains, *Phys Ther* 81:984-994, 2001.
39. Gribble PA, Hertel J, Denegar CR: Chronic ankle instability and fatigue create proximal joint alterations during performance of the Star Excursion Balance Test, *Int J Sports Med* 28:236-242, 2007.
40. Grimston SK, Nigg BM, Hanley DA, Engsberg JR: Differences in ankle joint complex range of motion as a function of age, *Foot Ankle* 14:215-222, 1993.
41. Guette M, Gondin J, Martin A, et al: Plantar flexion torque as a function of time of day, *Int J Sports Med* 27:171-177, 2006.
42. Hale SA, Hertel J, Olmsted-Kramer LC: The effect of a 4-week comprehensive rehabilitation program on postural control and lower extremity function in individuals with chronic ankle instability, *J Orthop Sports Phys Ther* 37:303-311, 2007.
43. Hertel J: Functional instability following lateral ankle sprain, *Sports Med* 29:361-371, 2000.
44. Hertel J, Olmsted-Kramer LC: Deficits in time-to-boundary measures of postural control with chronic ankle instability, *Gait Posture* 25:33-39, 2007.
45. Hicks JH: The mechanics of the foot. I. The joints, *J Anat* 87:345-357, 1953.
46. Higginson JS, Zajac FE, Neptune RR, et al: Effect of equinus foot placement and intrinsic muscle response on knee extension during stance, *Gait Posture* 23:32-36, 2006.
47. Holmes CF, Wilcox D, Fletcher JP: Effect of a modified, low-dye medial longitudinal arch taping procedure on the subtalar joint neutral position before and after light exercise, *J Orthop Sports Phys Ther* 32:194-201, 2002.
48. Huang CK, Kitaoka HB, An KN, Chao EY: Biomechanical evaluation of longitudinal arch stability, *Foot Ankle* 14:353-357, 1993.
49. Hubbard TJ, Hertel J, Sherbondy P: Fibular position in individuals with self-reported chronic ankle instability, *J Orthop Sports Phys Ther* 36:3-9, 2006.
50. Hunt AE, Smith RM: Mechanics and control of the flat versus normal foot during the stance phase of walking, *Clin Biomech (Bristol, Avon)* 19:391-397, 2004.
51. Inman VT: *The joints of the ankle*, Baltimore, 1976, Williams & Wilkins.
52. Inman VT, Ralston HJ, Todd F: *Human walking*, Baltimore, 1981, Williams & Wilkins.
53. Jotoku T, Kinoshita M, Okuda R, Abe M: Anatomy of ligamentous structures in the tarsal sinus and canal, *Foot Ankle Int* 27:533-538, 2006.
54. Kaikkonen A, Hyppänen E, Kannus P, Järvinen M: Long-term functional outcome after primary repair of the lateral ligaments of the ankle, *Am J Sports Med* 25:150-155, 1997.
55. Kanatli U, Gözil R, Besli K, et al: The relationship between the hindfoot angle and the medial longitudinal arch of the foot, *Foot Ankle Int* 27:623-627, 2006.
56. Kaufman KR, Brodine SK, Shaffer RA, et al: The effect of foot structure and range of motion on musculoskeletal overuse injuries, *Am J Sports Med* 27:585-593, 1999.

57. Khamis S, Yizhar Z: Effect of feet hyperpronation on pelvic alignment in a standing position, *Gait Posture* 25:127-134, 2007.

58. Kitaoka HB, Luo ZP, An KN: Three-dimensional analysis of flatfoot deformity: cadaver study, *Foot Ankle Int* 19:447-451, 1998.

59. Kitaoka HB, Luo ZP, Growney ES, et al: Material properties of the plantar aponeurosis, *Foot Ankle Int* 15:557-560, 1994.

60. Klein P, Mattys S, Rooze M: Moment arm length variations of selected muscles acting on talocrural and subtalar joints during movement: an in vitro study, *J Biomech* 29:21-30, 1996.

61. Knudson GA, Kitaoka HB, Lu CL, et al: Subtalar joint stability. Talocalcaneal interosseous ligament function studied in cadaver specimens, *Acta Orthop Scand* 68:442-446, 1997.

62. Konradsen L: Sensori-motor control of the uninjured and injured human ankle, *J Electromyogr Kinesiol* 12:199-203, 2002.

63. Konradsen L, Bech L, Ehrenbjerg M, Nickelsen T: Seven years follow-up after ankle inversion trauma, *Scand J Med Sci Sports* 12:129-135, 2002.

64. Kulig K, Burnfield JM, Reischl S, et al: Effect of foot orthoses on tibialis posterior activation in persons with pes planus, *Med Sci Sports Exerc* 37:24-29, 2005.

65. Kulig K, Burnfield JM, Requejo SM, et al: Selective activation of tibialis posterior: evaluation by magnetic resonance imaging, *Med Sci Sports Exerc* 36:862-867, 2004.

66. Kulig K, Reischl SF, Pomrantz AB, et al: Nonsurgical management of posterior tibial tendon dysfunction with orthoses and resistive exercise: a randomized controlled trial, *Phys Ther* 89:26-37, 2009.

67. Lakin RC, DeGnore LT, Pienkowski D: Contact mechanics of normal tarsometatarsal joints, *J Bone Joint Surg Am* 83:520-528, 2001.

68. Leardini A, Benedetti MG, Berti L, et al: Rear-foot, mid-foot and fore-foot motion during the stance phase of gait, *Gait Posture* 25:453-462, 2007.

69. Lees A, Lake M, Klenerman L: Shock absorption during forefoot running and its relationship to medial longitudinal arch height, *Foot Ankle Int* 26:1081-1088, 2005.

70. Leland RH, Marymont JV, Trevino SG, et al: Calcaneocuboid stability: a clinical and anatomic study, *Foot Ankle Int* 22:880-884, 2001.

71. Lewis GS, Kirby KA, Piazza SJ: Determination of subtalar joint axis location by restriction of talocrural joint motion, *Gait Posture* 25:63-69, 2007.

72. Lewis OJ: The comparative morphology of M. flexor accessorius and the associated long flexor tendons, *J Anat* 96:321-333, 1962.

73. Löfvenberg R, Kärrholm J, Sundelin G, Ahlgren O: Prolonged reaction time in patients with chronic lateral instability of the ankle, *Am J Sports Med* 23:414-417, 1995.

74. Lundberg A, Svensson OK, Bylund C, et al: Kinematics of the ankle/foot complex—Part 2: pronation and supination, *Foot Ankle* 9:248-253, 1989.

75. Lundberg A, Svensson OK, Bylund C, et al: Kinematics of the ankle/foot complex—Part 3: influence of leg rotation, *Foot Ankle* 9:304-309, 1989.

76. Lundgren P, Nester C, Liu A, et al: Invasive in vivo measurement of rear-, mid- and forefoot motion during walking, *Gait Posture.* 28:93-100, 2008.

77. MacLean C, Davis IM, Hamill J: Influence of a custom foot orthotic intervention on lower extremity dynamics in healthy runners, *Clin Biomech (Bristol, Avon)* 21:623-630, 2006.

78. Mann RA: Biomechanics of the foot. In: *American academy of orthopedic surgeons*, editors: Atlas of orthotics: biomechanical principles and application, St Louis, 1975, Mosby.

79. Manoli A, Graham B: The subtle cavus foot, "the underpronator" [Review], *Foot Ankle Int* 26:256-263, 2005.

80. Manter JT: Movements of the subtalar joint and transverse tarsal joint, *Anat Rec* 80:397-410, 1941.

81. Martin RL, Stewart GW, Conti SF: Posttraumatic ankle arthritis: an update on conservative and surgical management, *J Orthop Sports Phys Ther* 37:253-259, 2007.

82. Mattingly B, Talwalkar V, Tylkowski C, et al: Three-dimensional in vivo motion of adult hind foot bones, *J Biomech* 39:726-733, 2006.

83. McCulloch MU, Brunt D, Vander LD: The effect of foot orthotics and gait velocity on lower limb kinematics and temporal events of stance, *J Orthop Sports Phys Ther* 17:2-10, 1993.

84. McKinley TO, Rudert MJ, Koos DC, Brown TD: Incongruity versus instability in the etiology of posttraumatic arthritis, *Clin Orthop Relat Res* 423:44-51, 2004.

85. McPoil TG, Knecht HG, Schuit D: A survey of foot types in normal females between ages of 18 and 30 years, *J Orthop Sports Phys Ther* 9:406-409, 1988.

86. Mei-Dan O, Kahn G, Zeev A, et al: The medial longitudinal arch as a possible risk factor for ankle sprains: a prospective study in 83 female infantry recruits, *Foot Ankle Int* 26:180-183, 2005.

87. Mengiardi B, Zanetti M, Schöttle PB, et al: Spring ligament complex: MR imaging–anatomic correlation and findings in asymptomatic subjects, *Radiology* 237:242-249, 2005.

88. Michelson JD, Helgemo SL Jr: Kinematics of the axially loaded ankle, *Foot Ankle Int* 16:577-582, 1995.

89. Milgrom C, Giladi M, Kashtan H, et al: A prospective study of the effect of a shock-absorbing orthotic device on the incidence of stress fractures in military recruits, *Foot Ankle* 6:101-104, 1985.

90. Mohammadi F: Comparison of 3 preventive methods to reduce the recurrence of ankle inversion sprains in male soccer players, *Am J Sports Med* 35:922-926, 2007.

91. Monaghan K, Delahunt E, Caulfield B: Ankle function during gait in patients with chronic ankle instability compared to controls, *Clin Biomech (Bristol, Avon)* 21:168-174, 2006.

92. Mundermann A, Nigg BM, Neil HR, Stefanyshyn DJ: Foot orthotics affect lower extremity kinematics and kinetics during running, *Clin Biomech (Bristol, Avon)* 18:254-262, 2003.

93. Murray MP, Guten GN, Sepic SB, et al: Function of the triceps surae during gait. Compensatory mechanisms for unilateral loss, *J Bone Joint Surg Am* 60:473-476, 1978.

94. Myers JB, Riemann BL, Hwang JH, et al: Effect of peripheral afferent alteration of the lateral ankle ligaments on dynamic stability, *Am J Sports Med* 31:498-506, 2003.

95. Nester C, Bowker P, Bowden P: Kinematics of the midtarsal joint during standing leg rotation, *J Am Podiatr Med Assoc* 92:77-81, 2002.

96. Nester CJ, Findlow AF, Bowker P, Bowden PD: Transverse plane motion at the ankle joint, *Foot Ankle Int* 24:164-168, 2003.

97. Neville C, Flemister A, Tome J, Houck J: Comparison of changes in posterior tibialis muscle length between subjects with posterior tibial tendon dysfunction and healthy controls during walking, *J Orthop Sports Phys Ther* 37:661-669, 2007.

98. Nigg BM, Khan A, Fisher V, Stefanyshyn D: Effect of shoe insert construction on foot and leg movement, *Med Sci Sports Exerc* 30:550-555, 1998.

99. Nistor L, Markhede G, Grimby G: A technique for measurements of plantar flexion torque with the Cybex II dynamometer, *Scand J Rehabil Med* 14:163-166, 1982.

100. Ordway NR, Hand N, Briggs G, et al: Reliability of knee and ankle strength measures in an older adult population, *J Strength Cond Res* 20:82-87, 2006.

101. Owens S, Thordarson DB: The adductor hallucis revisited, *Foot Ankle Int* 22:186-191, 2001.

102. Patil V, Ebraheim N, Wagner R, Owens C: Morphometric dimensions of the dorsal calcaneocuboid ligament, *Foot Ankle Int* 29:508-512, 2008.

103. Piazza SJ: Mechanics of the subtalar joint and its function during walking, *Foot Ankle Clin* 10:425-442, 2005.

104. Powers CM, Maffucci R, Hampton S: Rearfoot posture in subjects with patellofemoral pain, *J Orthop Sports Phys Ther* 22:155-160, 1995.

105. Reischl SF, Powers CM, Rao S, Perry J: Relationship between foot pronation and rotation of the tibia and femur during walking, *Foot Ankle Int* 20:513-520, 1999.

106. Requião LF, Nadeau S, Milot MH, et al: Quantification of level of effort at the plantarflexors and hip extensors and flexor muscles in healthy subjects walking at different cadences, *J Electromyogr Kinesiol* 15:393-405, 2005.

107. Richie DH Jr: Effects of foot orthoses on patients with chronic ankle instability, *J Am Podiatr Med Assoc* 97:19-30, 2007.

108. Root ML: Development of the functional orthosis, *Clin Podiatr Med Surg* 11:183-210, 1994.

109. Rotem-Lehrer N, Laufer Y: Effect of focus of attention on transfer of a postural control task following an ankle sprain, *J Orthop Sports Phys Ther* 37:564-569, 2007.

110. Ruohola JP, Kiuru MJ, Pihlajamaki HK: Fatigue bone injuries causing anterior lower leg pain, *Clin Orthop Relat Res* 444:216-223, 2006.

111. Santilli V, Frascarelli MA, Paoloni M, et al: Peroneus longus muscle activation pattern during gait cycle in athletes affected by functional ankle instability: a surface electromyographic study, *Am J Sports Med* 33:1183-1187, 2005.

112. Santos MJ, Liu W: Possible factors related to functional ankle instability, *J Orthop Sports Phys Ther* 38:150-157, 2008.
113. Sawkins K, Refshauge K, Kilbreath S, Raymond J: The placebo effect of ankle taping in ankle instability, *Med Sci Sports Exerc* 39:781-787, 2007.
114. Scott SH, Winter DA: Biomechanical model of the human foot: kinematics and kinetics during the stance phase of walking, *J Biomech* 26:1091-1104, 1993.
115. Self BP, Harris S, Greenwald RM: Ankle biomechanics during impact landings on uneven surfaces, *Foot Ankle Int* 21:138-144, 2000.
116. Sepic SB, Murray MP, Mollinger LA, et al: Strength and range of motion in the ankle in two age groups of men and women, *Am J Phys Med* 65:75-84, 1986.
117. Shamus J, Shamus E, Gugel RN, et al: The effect of sesamoid mobilization, flexor hallucis strengthening, and gait training on reducing pain and restoring function in individuals with hallux limitus: a clinical trial, *J Orthop Sports Phys Ther* 34:368-376, 2004.
118. Sheehan FT, Seisler AR, Siegel KL: In vivo talocrural and subtalar kinematics: a non-invasive 3D dynamic MRI study, *Foot Ankle Int* 28:323-335, 2007.
119. Siegler S, Chen J, Schneck CD: The three-dimensional kinematics and flexibility characteristics of the human ankle and subtalar joints—Part I: kinematics, *J Biomech Eng* 110:364-373, 1988.
120. Standring S: *Gray's anatomy: the anatomical basis of clinical practice*, ed 40, St Louis, 2009, Elsevier.
121. Stauffer RN, Chao EY, Brewster RC: Force and motion analysis of the normal, diseased, and prosthetic ankle joint, *Clin Orthop Relat Res* 127:189-196, 1977.
122. Strauss JE, Forsberg JA, Lippert FG III: Chronic lateral ankle instability and associated conditions: a rationale for treatment, *Foot Ankle Int* 28:1041-1044, 2007.
123. Sutherland DH: An electromyographic study of the plantar flexors of the ankle in normal walking on the level, *J Bone Joint Surg Am* 48:66-71, 1966.
124. Sutherland DH: The evolution of clinical gait analysis. Part l: kinesiological EMG, *Gait Posture* 14:61-70, 2001.
125. Taylor KF, Bojescul JA, Howard RS, et al: Measurement of isolated subtalar range of motion: a cadaver study, *Foot Ankle Int* 22:426-432, 2001.
126. Thordarson DB, Schmotzer H, Chon J, Peters J: Dynamic support of the human longitudinal arch. A biomechanical evaluation, *Clin Orthop Relat Res* 316:165-172, 1995.
127. Tochigi Y, Amendola A, Rudert MJ, et al: The role of the interosseous talocalcaneal ligament in subtalar joint stability, *Foot Ankle Int* 25:588-596, 2004.
128. Tochigi Y, Rudert MJ, Saltzman CL, et al: Contribution of articular surface geometry to ankle stabilization, *J Bone Joint Surg Am* 88:2704-2713, 2006.
129. Tome J, Nawoczenski DA, Flemister A, Houck J: Comparison of foot kinematics between subjects with posterior tibialis tendon dysfunction and healthy controls, *J Orthop Sports Phys Ther* 36:635-644, 2006.
130. Van Deun S, Staes FF, Stappaerts KH, et al: Relationship of chronic ankle instability to muscle activation patterns during the transition from double-leg to single-leg stance, *Am J Sports Med* 35:274-281, 2007.
131. Van Gheluwe B, Dananberg HJ, Hagman F, Vanstaen K: Effects of hallux limitus on plantar foot pressure and foot kinematics during walking, *J Am Podiatr Med Assoc* 96:428-436, 2006.
132. Verhagen E, van der Beek A, Twisk J, et al: The effect of a proprioceptive balance board training program for the prevention of ankle sprains: a prospective controlled trial, *Am J Sports Med* 32:1385-1393, 2004.
133. Verhagen RA, de Keizer G, van Dijk CN: Long-term follow-up of inversion trauma of the ankle, *Arch Orthop Trauma Surg* 114:92-96, 1995.
134. Vicenzino B, Branjerdporn M, Teys P, Jordan K: Initial changes in posterior talar glide and dorsiflexion of the ankle after mobilization with movement in individuals with recurrent ankle sprain, *J Orthop Sports Phys Ther* 36:464-471, 2006.
135. Wan L, de Asla RJ, Rubash HE, Li G: In vivo cartilage contact deformation of human ankle joints under full body weight, *J Orthop Res* 26:1081-1089, 2008.
136. Wearing SC, Smeathers JE, Sullivan PM, et al: Plantar fasciitis: are pain and fascial thickness associated with arch shape and loading? *Phys Ther* 87:1002-1008, 2007.
137. Whittingham M, Palmer S, Macmillan F: Effects of taping on pain and function in patellofemoral pain syndrome: a randomized controlled trial, *J Orthop Sports Phys Ther* 34:504-510, 2004.
138. Williams DS III, McClay IS, Hamill J: Arch structure and injury patterns in runners, *Clin Biomech (Bristol, Avon)* 16:341-347, 2001.
139. Winter DA: *Biomechanics and motor control of human movement*, New Jersey, 2005, John Wiley & Sons.
140. Witvrouw E, Borre KV, Willems TM, et al: The significance of peroneus tertius muscle in ankle injuries: a prospective study, *Am J Sports Med* 34:1159-1163, 2006.
141. Yoshioka Y, Siu DW, Scudamore RA, Cooke TD: Tibial anatomy and functional axes, *J Orthop Res* 7:132-137, 1989.
142. Youberg LD, Cornwall MW, McPoil TG, Hannon PR: The amount of rearfoot motion used during the stance phase of walking, *J Am Podiatr Med Assoc* 95:376-382, 2005.
143. Younger AS, Hansen ST Jr: Adult cavovarus foot, *J Am Acad Orthop Surg* 13:302-315, 2005.
144. Younger AS, Sawatzky B, Dryden P: Radiographic assessment of adult flatfoot, *Foot Ankle Int* 26:820-825, 2005.

STUDY QUESTIONS

1 List the bones that make up (a) the ankle and (b) the rearfoot. Which bone is common to both regions?

2 Explain how excessive tibial torsion could mask the functional expression of excessive femoral anteversion.

3 Describe the path of the tendon of the flexor hallucis longus, from its belly to its insertion on the great toe.

4 Describe the primary arthrokinematics of inversion and eversion at the talonavicular joint.

5 Describe how the first tarsometatarsal joint is frequently involved with the development of hallux valgus (bunion).

6 Using Figure 14-43 as a reference, contrast the inversion torque potential of the tibialis anterior and the extensor hallucis longus.

7 Explain why a person with a weak calf muscle may complain of "buckling" of the knee prior to the push off phase of walking.

8 Compare the distal attachments of the fibularis brevis and fibularis tertius. Justify how these muscles have different actions within the sagittal plane but similar actions in the frontal plane.

9 Which structures (joints and connective tissues) bind the fibula to the tibia?

10 Describe the roll-and-slide arthrokinematics of dorsiflexion at the talocrural joint with the foot free (Figure 14-18, *A*) and with the foot fixed (Figure 14-20, *A*).

11 Which part of the gait cycle requires greater dorsiflexion at the talocrural joint: the stance phase or the swing phase?

12 What factors contribute to the stability of the talocrural joint in full dorsiflexion?

13 Which muscle is considered the most *direct antagonist* to the fibularis longus?

14 Propose a mechanism that could explain why active plantar flexion torque at the ankle is about 20% to 30% greater with the knee extended than when flexed.

15 Which deformity would most likely develop after weakness of the invertor muscles? Which muscles would you stretch? Which muscles would you attempt to strengthen?

⊖ *Answers to the study questions can be found on the Evolve website.*

Kinesiology of Walking

GUY G. SIMONEAU, PhD, PT

Walking (ambulation) serves an individual's basic need to move from place to place and is therefore one of the most common activities that people do on a daily basis. Ideally, walking is performed both efficiently, to minimize fatigue, and safely, to prevent falls and associated injuries.[188] Years of practice provide a healthy person with the control needed to ambulate while carrying on a conversation, looking in various directions, and even handling obstacles and other destabilizing forces with minimal effort.

Although a healthy person makes walking seem effortless, the challenge of ambulation can be recognized by looking at individuals at both ends of the lifespan (Figure 15-1). Early in life, the young child needs 11 to 15 months to learn how to stand and walk.[67,180] Once on their feet, children will refine their gait so that it visually resembles a mature adult walking pattern by 4 to 5 years of age,[26,172,178,179,180] with further refinement taking place over possibly several more years.* Late in life, walking often becomes an increasingly greater challenge. Because of decreased strength, decreased balance, or disease, the elderly may require a cane or walker to ambulate safely.

---

*References 26, 27, 48, 66, 75, 77, 80.

Walking child   **Walking adult**   **Walking elder**

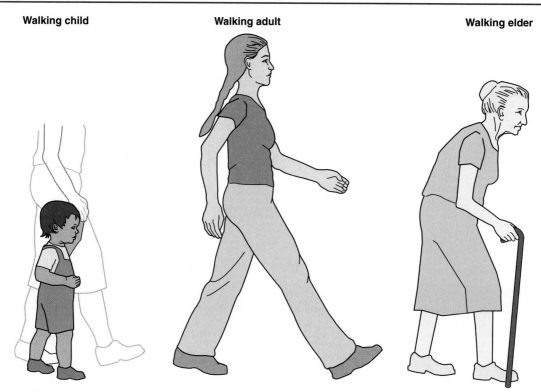

FIGURE 15-1. Walking at various stages in life.

Patla[144] eloquently expressed the importance of ambulation in our lives: "Nothing epitomizes a level of independence and our perception of a good quality of life more than the ability to travel independently under our own power from one place to another. We celebrate the development of this ability in children and try to nurture and sustain it throughout the lifespan."

This chapter provides a description of the fundamental kinesiologic characteristics of walking. Unless indicated otherwise, the information provided refers to individuals with a normal and mature gait pattern, walking on level surfaces at a steady average speed. Although this chapter provides enough details to be read independently of the rest of this book, reading Chapters 12 to 14 will facilitate an even greater understanding of walking.

Major Topics
- Spatial and temporal descriptors
- Control of the body's center of mass
- Joint kinematics
- Energy expenditure
- Muscle activity
- Walking kinetics
- Gait dysfunctions

The observation of walking, which is the focus of this chapter, provides information on the outcome of a complex set of "behind the scenes" interactions between sensory and motor functions. For a person to walk, the central nervous system must generate appropriate motor actions from the integration of visual, proprioceptive, and vestibular sensory inputs. Although this chapter covers the intricacy of limb and muscular actions performed during walking, it does not cover

the concept of motor control. To gain a greater understanding of the complexity of the motor control of walking, the reader is advised to examine other sources on the topic.*

HISTORICAL PERSPECTIVE OF GAIT ANALYSIS

"If a man were to walk on the ground alongside a wall with a reed dipped in ink attached to his head the line traced by the reed would not be straight but zig-zag, because it goes lower when he bends and higher when he stands upright and raises himself."[6] This early written record by Aristotle (384-322 BC) of observation of walking and numerous earlier paintings and sculptures of individuals engaged in the process of walking are testament that both the casual and detailed observation of ambulation has been of interest throughout history.

Despite this earlier interest, it was not until 1836 that the Weber brothers[200] published the first notable scientific work on gait, having benefited from the advances in science provided by individuals such as Galileo Galilei (1564-1642), Giovanni Borelli (1608-1679), and Isaac Newton (1642-1727), to name only a few. Willhelm, a physicist and electrician, and Eduard, an anatomist and physiologist, using instruments such as a stopwatch, a tape measure, and a telescope, described and measured elements of walking, such as step length, cadence, foot-to-ground clearance, and vertical excursion of the body. They also defined basic elements of the gait cycle, such as swing phase, stance phase, and double-limb support periods. Many of the terms they introduced remain in use today. The Webers hypothesized that the basic principle of walking is one of least muscular effort—a concept known to be true today, although the exact methods by which the body

---

*References 85, 107, 139, 142, 165, 212.

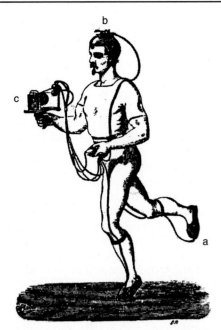

FIGURE 15-2. Marey's instrumented shoes used for the measurement of gait. (From Marey EJ: *La machine animal*, Paris, 1873, Librairie Germer Baillière.)

minimizes energy expenditure are still being studied.[137,209,210] An extensive account of the Weber brothers' work was published in 1894 and translated in 1992.[198,199]

In the nineteenth century, other researchers, such as Marey, Carlet, and Vierordt, made use of ingenious technology to expand our knowledge of gait. Most often cited among Marey and Carlet's many novel methods of measurement are shoes that had air chambers attached to a recorder to indicate the swing and stance phase of gait (Figure 15-2).[112,113,114] Another clever idea, by Vierordt, was the use of ink in small spray nozzles attached to the shoes and limbs.[189] The ink sprayed on the floor and wall as the individual walked, providing a permanent record of movement.

Concurrently, advances in the field of cinematography created a powerful medium to study and record the kinematic patterns of humans and animals walking. Muybridge may be the most recognized individual of his time to use cinematography to document sequence of movements. Muybridge is most famous for settling an old controversy regarding a trotting horse. In 1872, using sequence photography, he showed that all four feet of a trotting horse are indeed simultaneously off the ground for very brief periods of time. Muybridge created an impressive collection of photographs on human and animal gait, which was initially published in 1887 and assembled and reproduced in 1979.[133,134]

Initially, the description of gait was limited to planar analyses; the motion was typically recorded in the sagittal plane and less frequently in the frontal plane. Braune and Fisher[15,16] are credited as being the first, from 1895 to 1904, to perform a comprehensive three-dimensional analysis of a walking individual. By using four cameras (two pairs of cameras recording motion for each side of the body) and a number of light tubes attached to various body segments, they documented joint kinematics in three dimensions. They were also the first to use the principles of mechanics to measure dynamic quantities such as segmental acceleration, segmental inertial properties, and intersegmental loads (e.g., joint torques and forces). Their

analysis of joint torques, limited to the swing phase of gait, refutes the earlier concept, suggested by Weber and Weber in 1836, that lower extremity motion during the swing phase of gait could be explained solely by a passive pendulum theory.[201]

Throughout the twentieth century, the understanding of walking was greatly enhanced by many scientific advances. Instrumentation to document kinematics evolved from simple video cameras, with film that required painstaking analysis with a ruler and protractor, to highly sophisticated infrared systems, with real-time coordinate data of limb segments. Notable researchers who contributed to the description of the kinematics of gait using a variety of imaging techniques include Eberhart,[49] Murray,[125,127] Inman,[83] Winter,[204] and Perry.[147] Noteworthy is the work by Murray, a physical therapist and researcher, who published several papers in the 1960s, 1970s, and 1980s describing the kinematics of many aspects of normal and abnormal gait (Figure 15-3).[126-128,130,131,176] Among other accomplishments, data from her research—on the kinematics of walking in individuals with disabilities—influenced the design of artificial joints and lower extremity prosthetic limbs.

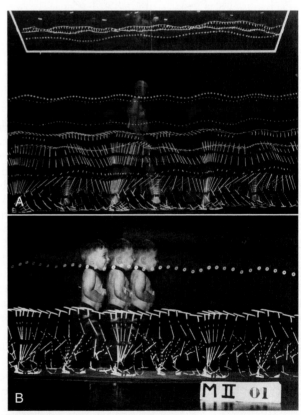

FIGURE 15-3. A sample of the technology used by Murray to record the basic kinematics of gait. An older man **(A)** and a young boy **(B)** wear reflective targets while walking in a semidark hallway. A camera was used with the shutter opened, and light was flashed 20 times per second to track the location of the markers. An additional brighter flash of light was used to photograph the man or boy while he was walking. This early technique allowed the visualization of an entire gait cycle with a single photograph. A ceiling-mounted mirror was also employed to observe horizontal plane motion. (**A,** From Murray MP, Gore DR: Gait of patients with hip pain or loss of hip joint motion. In Black J, Dumbleton JH, eds: *Clinical biomechanics: a case history approach*, New York, 1981, Churchill Livingstone. **B,** From Stratham L, Murray MP: Early walking patterns of normal children, *Clin Orthop Relat Res* 79:8, 1971.)

Gait analysis laboratory

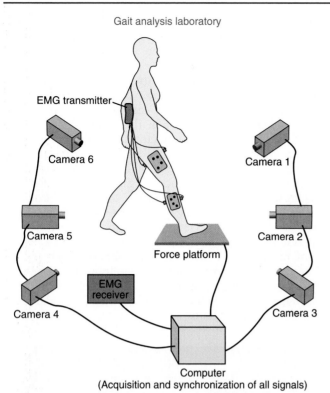

FIGURE 15-4. Instrumentation used in a typical gait laboratory to study walking.

Similarly, a more extensive understanding of the kinetics of gait was made possible through the development of devices to measure the forces taking place at the foot-ground interface. Amar,[2] Elftman,[52] Bresler and Frankel,[17] and Cunningham and Brown[38] all made significant contributions to this field. With the ability to measure the forces between the foot and the ground came computational methods to calculate the forces and torques taking place at the joints of the lower extremities during the stance phase of ambulation.[145,166,206]

The development of surface and intramuscular electrodes provided the opportunity to record the electrical activity of muscles during gait.[62,181] When this information is integrated with the kinematics of walking, the role that each muscle plays during gait can be better appreciated and more objectively described. Many researchers, including Sutherland,[179] Perry,[147] Inman,[83] and Winter,[204] have made notable contributions to the study of electromyography (EMG) during walking.

Today, gait analysis is routinely performed in specialized biomechanics laboratories (Figure 15-4). Three-dimensional

kinematic data are obtained by using two or more synchronized high-speed cameras. Ground reaction forces are measured using force platforms embedded in the floor. Muscle activity patterns are recorded by multichannel, often telemetered, electromyographic systems. Ultimately, lower extremity joint forces, torques, and powers are calculated with a combination of kinematic data, ground reaction forces, and anthropometric characteristics of the individual (Figure 15-5). These data are then used to describe and study normal and abnormal gait.

Patients with a variety of pathologies can potentially benefit from instrumented gait analyses. Currently the primary beneficiaries of this technology, however, are children with cerebral palsy. In this population, instrumented gait analysis is often used before surgery to help determine the proper intervention. It is employed again after surgery to objectively evaluate the outcome.[64] More comprehensive descriptions of the history, tools, and methods used for gait analysis can be found in other sources.[7,93,181-183,188,202]

Sophisticated technology, such as that described earlier, provides detailed information that can enhance the ability to describe and understand walking. Because such technology is rarely available in the typical clinical setting, clinicians must routinely rely on direct visual observation to evaluate the walking characteristics of their patients.[140] Such observational analysis requires a thorough knowledge and understanding of normal gait. Learning about walking, as presented here, is a more dynamic and rewarding experience if the study of this chapter is combined with the observations of gait patterns of relatives, friends, neighbors, and patients in the clinical setting.

SPATIAL AND TEMPORAL DESCRIPTORS

This section describes measurements of distance and time as related to walking.

Gait Cycle

Walking is the result of a cyclic series of movements. As such, it can be conveniently characterized by a detailed description of its most fundamental unit: a *gait cycle* (Figure 15-6). The gait cycle is initiated as soon as the foot contacts the ground. Because foot contact is normally made with the heel, the 0% point or beginning of the gait cycle is often referred to as *heel contact* or *heel strike*. The 100% point or completion of the gait cycle occurs as soon as the same foot once again makes contact with the ground. *Initial contact* is often used as a substitute term for heel contact when an individual makes first

FIGURE 15-5. Typical approach used for the analysis of human motion. Variables in the colored ovals can be precisely measured. Computational methods, in the rectangles, are used to calculate the variables in the green circles.

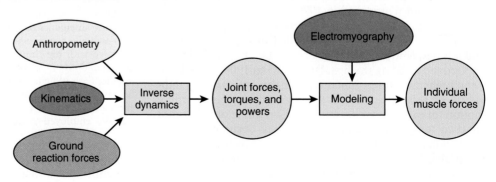

The gait cycle

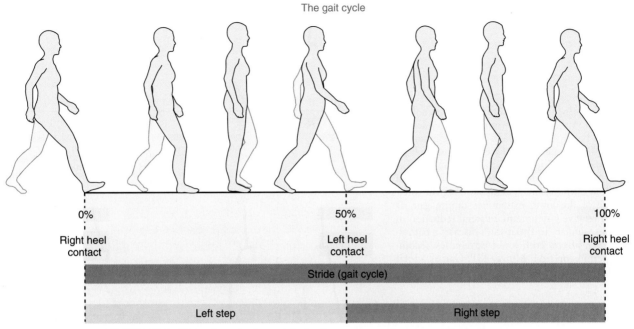

FIGURE 15-6. The gait cycle from right heel contact to subsequent right heel contact.

contact with the ground with a part of the foot other than the heel, but for the purpose of this chapter, focusing on normal walking, the term *heel contact* will be used.

A *stride* (synonymous with a gait cycle) is the sequence of events taking place between successive heel contacts of the same foot. In comparison, a *step* is the sequence of events that occurs within successive heel contacts of opposite feet, for example, between right and left heel contacts. A gait cycle, therefore, has two steps—a left step and a right step.

The most basic spatial descriptors of gait include the length of a stride and the length of a step (Figure 15-7). *Stride length* is the distance between two successive heel contacts of the same foot. *Step length*, in contrast, is the distance between successive heel contacts of the two different feet. Comparing right with left step lengths can help to evaluate the symmetry of gait between the lower extremities (Figure 15-8). *Step width* is the lateral distance between the heel centers of two consecutive foot contacts and is on average around 8 to 10 cm (see Figure 15-7).[73,111,117,118] *Foot angle,* the amount of "toe-out," is the angle between the line of progression of the body and the long axis of the foot. About 5 to 7 degrees is considered average.[118] Although the stated norms are for adults, a noteworthy publication[80] of data collected from 360 children 7 to 12 years of age documents a normal step width and foot angle

of 8 to 10 cm and 2.5 to 6 degrees, respectively—values relatively similar to those in healthy young adults.

Spatial Descriptors of Gait	
• Stride length	• Step width
• Step length	• Foot angle

The most basic temporal descriptor of gait is *cadence,* the number of steps per minute, which is also called *step rate.* Other temporal descriptors of gait are *stride time* (the time for a full gait cycle) and *step time* (the time for the completion of a right or a left step). Note that with symmetric gait, step time can be derived from cadence (i.e., step time is the reciprocal of cadence).

Temporal Descriptors of Gait
• Cadence
• Stride time
• Step time
Spatial-Temporal Descriptor
• Walking speed

Spatial descriptors of gait

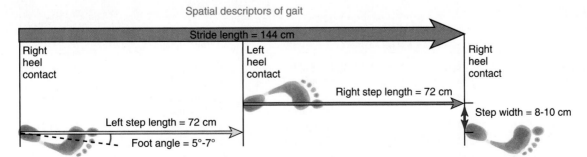

FIGURE 15-7. Spatial descriptors of gait and their typical values for a right gait cycle.

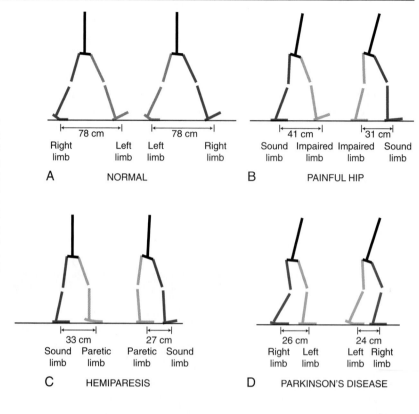

FIGURE 15-8. Influence of impairment and pathology on step length. **A** illustrates the symmetric step length expected in a healthy individual. **B** and **C** are examples of step length asymmetry often seen in those with an impairment or pathology that affects a single lower extremity. Note the bilateral shortening of the normal step length in both instances, demonstrating the interdependence of the lower extremities during gait. **D** illustrates a relatively symmetric bilateral reduction in step length secondary to Parkinson's disease, a pathology that often affects both lower extremities. (Modified with permission from Murray MP: Gait as a total pattern of movement, *Am J Phys Med* 46:290, 1967.)

Walking speed combines both spatial and temporal measurements by providing information on the distance covered in a given amount of time. The units of measure are typically meters per second (m/sec) or miles per hour (mph). Speed can be calculated by measuring the time it takes to cover a given distance, or the distance covered in a given amount of time, or by multiplying the step rate by the step length. Walking speed varies considerably among individuals based on factors such as age and physical characteristics (e.g., height and weight).[36,93] Of all spatial and temporal measurements of gait, speed may be the best and most functional measure of an individual's walking ability.

For healthy adults, a gait cycle (i.e., two consecutive steps) takes slightly more than 1 second and covers approximately 1.44 m (4.5 feet), resulting in a walking speed of 1.37 m/sec. Data in Table 15-1 indicate that, at a freely chosen walking speed, women exhibit a slower walking speed, shorter step length, and faster cadence than men. These differences are likely in part reflective of anthropometric disparities between genders. Even when anthropometrically matched with men,

though, women still demonstrate a higher cadence and shorter step length than men when walking at the same speed.[56,129]

> **Normal Values for Walking Based on Data from Table 15-1**
> - Walking speed: 1.37 m/sec (3 mph)
> - Step rate: 1.87 steps/sec (110 steps/min)
> - Step length: 72 cm (28 inches)

The classic data in Table 15-1 were derived from more than 2300 pedestrians walking outdoors in a large city and who were unaware that their gait characteristics were being measured. Table 15-2 provides data from a select number of studies,* including a smaller number of subjects who walked indoors on an instrumented walkway used to precisely and reliably measure spatial and temporal characteristics of gait. Unlike the pedestrians in the studies in Table 15-1, these

*References 13, 73, 79, 111, 118, 208.

TABLE 15-1. **Normative Data for Walking Speed, Step Rate, and Step Length**				
	Drillis (1961)[47] (New York City)	**Molen (1973)[122] (Amsterdam)**	**Finley and Cody (1970)[55] (Philadelphia)**	**Average over Gender and City**
Walking speed (m/sec)	1.46*	1.39 (males) 1.27 (females)	1.37 (males) 1.24 (females)	1.37
Step rate (steps/sec)	1.9*	1.79 (males) 1.88 (females)	1.84 (males) 1.94 (females)	1.87
Step length (m)	0.76*	0.77 (males) 0.67 (females)	0.74 (males) 0.63 (females)	0.72

Data obtained from more than 2300 pedestrians unaware of being observed as they walked.
*Males and females are averaged together for these data.

TABLE 15-2. Selected Data for Temporal and Spatial Gait Parameters Derived from Individuals Walking in a Laboratory Setting on an Instrumented Walkway[*]

	Walking Speed (m/sec)	Cadence[†] (steps/min)	Stride Length[‡] (m)	Step Width (cm)	Foot Angle (degrees)
Marchetti et al (2008)[111]	1.43 (1.35-1.51)	119.1 (115.1-123.1)	70.7 (67.8-74.2) 72.6 (69.1-76.1)	8.1 (7.0-9.2)	
Hollman et al (2007)[79]	1.48 ± 0.15				
Youdas et al (2006)[208]	1.40 ± 0.13	119.6 ± 7.6	1.42 ± 0.13		
Menz et al (2004)[118]	1.43 ± 0.14	110.8 ± 6.9	0.77 ± 0.06	8.6 ± 3.2	6.7 ± 5.0
Bilney et al (2003)[13]	1.46 ± 0.16	114.7 ± 6.4	1.53 ± 0.14		
Grabiner et al (2001)[73§]				10.8 ± 2.7 8.7 ± 2.3	

[*]Data are means ± standard deviations, with the exception of Marchetti and colleagues, for whom data are means and 95% confidence intervals. All data are for healthy adults, and all groups include both males and females.
[†]Divide cadence by 60 to obtain step rate in steps per second.
[‡]The data by Marchetti and colleagues are for left and right step length, and the data by Menz and colleagues are for step length.
[§]Data for two different groups of subjects.

subjects were aware that their walking characteristics were being measured, which may account in part for the small differences noted between the data in the two tables.

The data in Tables 15-1 and 15-2 were collected from individuals walking at their freely chosen speed, which may not always be fast enough to reach a destination in the desired amount of time. When an increase in walking speed is needed, two strategies are available: increasing the stride, or step length, and increasing the cadence (Figure 15-9). Typically an individual combines both strategies until the longest reasonable step length is reached. From that point on, a further increase in walking speed is solely related to an increase in cadence. *It must be reemphasized, therefore, that all values (spatial, temporal, kinematic, and kinetic variables) obtained from the measurements of walking vary based on walking speed.* For proper reference and interpretation, reports of gait characteristics should always include the walking speed at which the data were collected.

Stance and Swing Phases

To help describe events taking place during the gait cycle, it is customary to subdivide the gait cycle from 0% to 100%. As stated earlier, heel or foot contact with the ground is considered the start of the gait cycle (0%), and the next ground contact made by the same foot is considered the end of the gait cycle (100%). Throughout this chapter, gait is described using the right lower extremity as a reference. A full gait cycle for the right lower extremity can be divided into two major phases: stance and swing (Figure 15-10). *Stance phase* (from right heel contact to right toe off) occurs as the right foot is on the ground, supporting the body's weight. *Swing phase* (from right toe off to the next right heel contact) occurs as the right foot is in the air, being advanced forward for the next contact with the ground. At normal walking speed, the stance phase occupies approximately 60% of the gait cycle, and the swing phase occupies the remaining 40%.

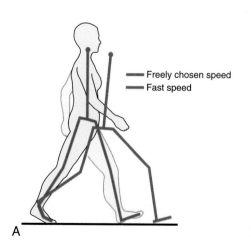
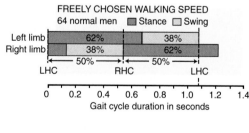
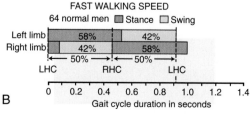

FIGURE 15-9. Methods to increase walking speed. **A** illustrates the longer step length used to increase walking speed. **B** illustrates the shorter gait cycle duration (faster walking cadence) used to increase walking speed. It also illustrates that at the faster walking speed, a smaller percentage of the gait cycle is spent in double-limb support (16% at fast speed compared with 24% at free speed walking). (Data from Murray MP, Kory RC, Clarkson BH, Sepic SB: Comparison of free and fast speed walking patterns of normal men, *Am J Phys Med* 45:8, 1966.)

SPECIAL FOCUS 15-1

Simple Clinical Measurements of Walking

Sophisticated instrumentation, such as walkways and foot switches, exists to make spatial and temporal measurements of foot placement during gait.* For most clinical applications, this information can, however, be measured with readily available tools and a little imagination. Average walking speed can be measured using a stopwatch and a known distance. Step length and step width can be measured by the use of ink marks made by shoes or feet on a roll of paper covering the floor. This technique works especially well to document abnormal gait patterns, including asymmetry in step length.

Clinically, simple measurements of walking speed and distance can be helpful in monitoring functional progress or documenting functional limitations. Results obtained from a patient can be compared with normal values provided in Tables 15-1 and 15-2 or with minimum standards required to perform a specific task, such as crossing a street within the time allowed by the stoplights.[†] The following are two proposed minimum standards, based on community-living activities: the ability to walk 300 m (1000 feet) in less than 11.5 minutes (walking speed of 0.45 m/sec or 1 mph); the ability to walk at a speed of 1.3 m/sec (3 mph) for 13 to 27 m (42 to 85 feet) to cross a street safely.

---

*References 13, 73, 80, 111, 118, 190, 208.
†References 55, 57, 103, 153, 194, 195.

Gait Cycle
- Stance phase = 60% of gait cycle
- Swing phase = 40% of gait cycle

Within a gait cycle, the body experiences two periods of *double-limb support* (when both feet are in contact with the ground simultaneously) and two periods of *single-limb support* (when only one foot is on the ground) (see Figure 15-10). We observe the first period of double-limb support at 0% to 10% of the gait cycle. During that time period, the body's weight is being transferred from the left to the right lower extremity. The right lower extremity is then in single-limb support until 50% of the gait cycle has been reached. During that time, the left lower extremity is in its swing phase, being advanced forward. The second period of double-limb support takes place at 50% to 60% of the gait cycle and serves the purpose of transferring the weight of the body from the right to the left lower extremity. Finally, at 60% to 100% of the gait cycle the body is again in single-limb support, this time on the left lower extremity. This period of left single-limb support corresponds to the swing phase of the right lower extremity.

As gait speed increases, the percentage of the gait cycle spent in periods of double-limb support becomes shorter (see Figure 15-9). Race walkers aim to walk as fast as possible while always keeping one foot in contact with the ground. For these athletes, greater speeds are achieved by increasing cadence and stride length and by minimizing periods of double-limb support to the point at which stance and swing phase times are about equal. Whereas maximum walking speed in adults 20 to 50 years of age is approximately 2.4 to 2.5 m/sec (5.5 to 5.7 mph),[14] walking speed during race walking can be in excess of 3.3 m/sec (7.5 mph).[129,169]

During running, the periods of double-limb support disappear altogether to be replaced by periods when both feet are off the ground simultaneously. The transition from walking to running normally takes place at a step rate of approximately 180 steps/min or at a speed of approximately 2.1 to 2.2 m/sec (4.8 to 5.0 mph).[43,163] Above that speed it is more energy efficient to run than to walk.

Conversely, at a slow walking speed, the periods of double-limb support occupy an increasingly greater percentage of the

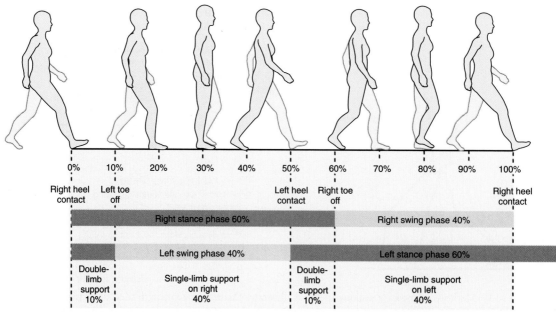

FIGURE 15-10. Subdivision of the gait cycle illustrating the phases of stance and swing and periods of single- and double-limb support.

gait cycle. A slower gait provides greater stability because both feet are on the ground simultaneously for a greater percentage of the cycle. In fact, the reduced speed, shorter step length, and slower cadence commonly seen in the elderly with fear of falling or strength deficits serve to improve gait stability and prevent falls.[96]

SUBDIVISION OF STANCE AND SWING PHASES

Five specific events are typically described during stance phase: heel contact, foot flat, mid stance, heel off (or heel rise), and toe off (Figure 15-11 and Table 15-3). *Heel contact* is defined as the instant the heel comes in contact with the ground, at 0% of the gait cycle. *Foot flat* corresponds to the instant the entire plantar surface of the foot comes in contact with the ground. This event occurs at approximately 8% of the gait cycle. *Mid stance* is most often defined as the point at which the body's weight passes directly over the supporting lower extremity. It is also defined as the time when the foot of the lower extremity in the swing phase passes the lower extremity in the stance phase (i.e., the feet are side by side). A third definition of mid stance is the time when the greater trochanter of the femur is vertically above the midpoint of the supporting foot in the sagittal plane. In reality, these three definitions all correspond to about 30% of the gait cycle or 50% of the stance phase. *Heel off*, the timing of which varies appreciably among individuals, occurs at somewhere between 30% and 40% of the gait cycle. It corresponds to the instant the heel comes off the ground. *Toe off*, which occurs at 60% of the gait cycle, is defined as the instant the toes come off the ground.

A period referred to as *push off* is also often used. This period roughly corresponds to the movement of ankle plantar flexion at 40% to 60% of the gait cycle.

Although there is a significant amount of variation in the description of the swing phase of gait, this phase is traditionally subdivided into three sections: early, mid, and late swing (see Figure 15-11). *Early swing* is the period from the time of toe off to mid swing (60% to 75% of the gait cycle). *Mid swing* corresponds to the time from slightly before to slightly after the mid stance event of the opposite lower extremity, when the foot of the swing limb passes next to the foot of the stance limb (75% to 85% of the gait cycle). *Late swing* is the period from the end of mid swing to foot contact with the ground (85% to 100% of the gait cycle).

TABLE 15-3. Common Terminology Defining the Subdivisions of the Gait Cycle

Phases	Events	Percentage of Cycle	Events of Opposite Limb
Stance	Heel contact	0	
	Foot flat	8	
		10	Toe off
	Mid stance	30	Mid swing (25%-35%)
	Heel off	30-40	
		50	Heel contact
	Toe off	60	
Swing	Early swing	60-75	
	Mid swing	75-85	Mid stance (80%)
	Late swing	85-100	
		90	Heel off (80%-90%)
	Heel contact	100	

SPECIAL FOCUS 15-2

Take Time to Develop Your Observation Skills

The events of the gait cycle can be observed by watching people walking in normal surroundings (streets, malls, airports). Like any clinical skill, observational gait analysis improves with practice. Repeated observation of individuals with normal gait patterns sharpens the ability to recognize normal gait variations and identify abnormal gait deviations. Opportunities to practice this skill with a person already trained in observational gait analysis further sharpen these skills.

An alternate and relatively more recent terminology, proposed by Perry,[147] consists of eight events that divide the gait cycle into seven periods (Figure 15-12). The events are *initial contact, opposite toe off, heel rise, opposite initial contact, toe off, feet adjacent, tibia vertical,* and *initial contact* for the next stride. The four time periods during stance are *loading response, mid stance,*

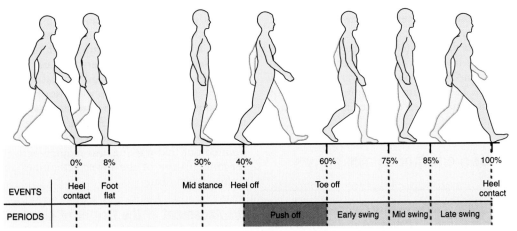

FIGURE 15-11. Traditional subdivisions of the gait cycle.

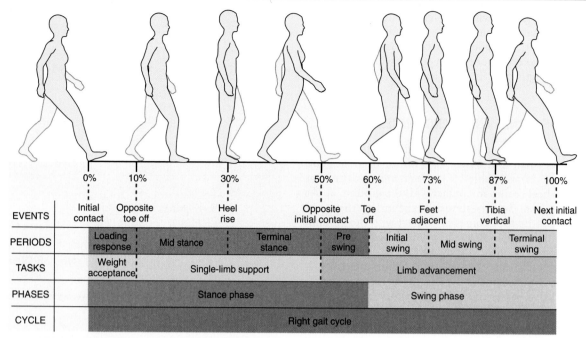

EVENTS	0% Initial contact	10% Opposite toe off		30% Heel rise		50% Opposite initial contact	60% Toe off	73% Feet adjacent		87% Tibia vertical	100% Next initial contact
PERIODS	Loading response	Mid stance		Terminal stance		Pre swing	Initial swing	Mid swing		Terminal swing	
TASKS	Weight acceptance	Single-limb support					Limb advancement				
PHASES	Stance phase						Swing phase				
CYCLE	Right gait cycle										

FIGURE 15-12. Terminology to describe the events of the gait cycle. *Initial contact* corresponds to the beginning of stance when the foot first contacts the ground at 0% of gait cycle. *Opposite toe off* occurs when the contralateral foot leaves the ground at 10% of gait cycle. *Heel rise* corresponds to the heel lifting from the ground and occurs at approximately 30% of gait cycle. *Opposite initial contact* corresponds to the foot contact of the opposite limb, typically at 50% of gait cycle. *Toe off* occurs when the foot leaves the ground at 60% of gait cycle. *Feet adjacent* takes place when the foot of the swing limb is next to the foot of the stance limb at 73% of gait cycle. *Tibia vertical* corresponds to the tibia of the swing limb being oriented in the vertical direction at 87% of gait cycle. The final event is, again, initial contact, which in fact is the start of the next gait cycle.

These eight events divide the gait cycle into seven periods. *Loading response,* between initial contact and opposite toe off, corresponds to the time when the weight is accepted by the lower extremity initiating contact with the ground. *Mid stance* is from opposite toe off to heel rise (10% to 30% of gait cycle). *Terminal stance* begins when the heel rises and ends when the contralateral lower extremity touches the ground, from 30% to 50% of gait cycle. *Pre-swing* takes place from foot contact of the contralateral limb to toe off of the ipsilateral foot, which is the time corresponding to the second double-limb support of the gait cycle (50% to 60% of gait cycle). *Initial swing* is from toe off to feet adjacent, when the foot of the swing limb is next to the foot of the stance limb (60% to 73% of gait cycle). *Mid swing* is from feet adjacent to when the tibia of the swing limb is vertical (73% to 87% of gait cycle). *Terminal swing* is from a vertical position of the tibia to immediately before heel contact (87% to 100% of gait cycle). The first 10% of the gait cycle corresponds to a task of weight acceptance—when body mass is transferred from one lower extremity to the other. Single-limb support, from 10% to 50% of the gait cycle, serves to support the weight of the body as the opposite limb swings forward. The last 10% of stance phase and the entire swing phase serve to advance the limb forward to a new location.

terminal stance, and *pre swing.* Swing phase has three time periods: *initial swing, mid swing,* and *terminal swing.* With a few exceptions, this terminology is in general agreement with the earlier description of gait.

The existence of two different terminologies can be confusing, especially when many use them interchangeably. In this chapter, the terminology proposed by Perry in 1992 is used predominantly.[147] To eliminate confusion, the timing of the events during gait is most often described as a percentage of the gait cycle.

DISPLACEMENT AND CONTROL OF THE BODY'S CENTER OF MASS

Walking can be defined as a series of losses and recoveries of balance. Ambulation is initiated by allowing the body to lean forward. For a fall to be prevented, momentary recovery of balance is achieved by moving either foot forward to a new location. Once gait is initiated, the body's forward momentum carries the center of mass (CoM) of the body beyond the foot's new location, necessitating a step forward with the other foot. Forward progression is then achieved by the successive and alternate relocations of the feet. The smooth, controlled transition between loss and recovery of balance continues as long as forward displacement of the body is desired. Ambulation stops when foot placement stops the forward momentum of the body and balance is regained over the static base of support. Although this description provides a useful and relatively accurate explanation of gait, it must be pointed out that walking also requires active participation of the musculature of the lower extremities and consequently energy expenditure.

Displacement of the Center of Mass

The body's CoM is located just anterior to the second sacral vertebra, but the best visualization of the movement of the

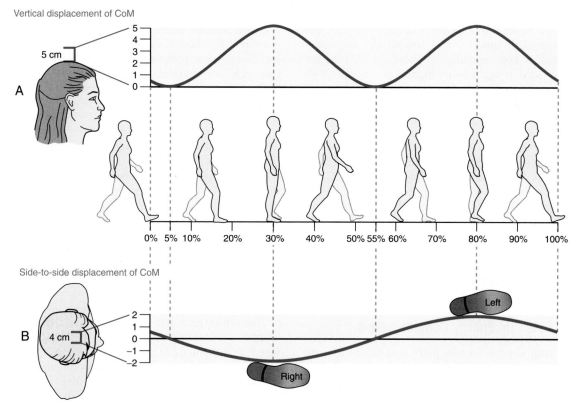

FIGURE 15-13. Center of mass (CoM) displacement during gait. The vertical and the side-to-side displacements of the CoM are illustrated in **A** and **B,** respectively. The CoM is at its lowest and most central position, in the side-to-side direction, in the middle of double-limb support (5% and 55% of the gait cycle)–a position of relative stability with both feet on the ground. Conversely, the CoM is at its highest and most lateral position at mid stance (30% and 80% of the gait cycle)–a position of relative instability. During single-limb support, the trajectory of the CoM is never directly over the base of support. This fact is illustrated in **B,** with the vertical projection of the CoM always located between the footprints.

CoM is by tracking the displacement of the head or torso. Clearly, the most notable displacement of the body during gait is in the forward direction (Figure 15-13). Superimposed on this forward displacement, however, are two sinusoidal patterns of movement that correspond to the movement of the CoM in the vertical and side-to-side directions.

In the vertical direction, the CoM oscillates up and down to describe two full sine waves per gait cycle (see Figure 15-13, *A*). This movement of the CoM is best understood by looking at the individual from the side. Minimum height of the CoM occurs at the midpoint of both periods of double-limb support (5% and 55% of the gait cycle). Maximum height of the CoM occurs at the midpoint of both periods of single-limb support (30% and 80% of the gait cycle). A total vertical displacement of approximately 5 cm is noted at the average walking speed in the adult male.

Displacement of the Center of Mass
- Total vertical displacement: 5 cm
- Total side-to-side displacement: 4 cm

During ambulation the CoM is also alternately shifted from the right to the left lower extremity, creating a single side-to-side (right-to-left) sinusoidal pattern per gait cycle (see Figure 15-13, *B*). Maximum position of the CoM to the right occurs at the midpoint of the stance phase on the right lower

extremity (30% of the gait cycle), and maximum position of the CoM to the left occurs at the midpoint of the stance phase on the left lower extremity (80% of the gait cycle). A total side-to-side displacement of approximately 4 cm occurs during normal ambulation.[83] The amount of displacement increases when the individual has a wider base of support during gait (i.e., walking with the feet wider apart) and decreases with a narrower base of support (i.e., walking with the feet closer together).

Next consider the total pattern of motion of the CoM during a full gait cycle (see Figure 15-13). Starting shortly after right heel contact, the CoM is moving forward, upward, and toward the right foot. This general direction of movement continues for the first 30% of the gait cycle–the body is essentially "climbing and shifting its mass" over the supporting lower extremity. At right mid stance, the CoM reaches its highest and most lateral position toward the right. Just after right mid stance, the CoM continues forward but starts moving in a downward direction and toward the left side of the body–the body is essentially "falling away" from the supporting lower extremity. This is a critical moment in the gait cycle. With the left limb in its swing phase, the body depends on the left lower extremity to make secure contact with the ground to accept the weight transfer and to prevent a fall. Shortly after left heel contact, during the double-limb support phase, the CoM is located midway between the feet and reaches its lowest position as it continues to move forward and toward the left lower extremity. From right toe off to mid stance on the left lower extremity (80% of the gait cycle), the CoM moves forward, upward, and toward the left lower extremity, which is now providing support. At 80% of the gait cycle, the CoM is again at its highest point, but in its most lateral position to the left. Shortly after left mid stance, the movement of the CoM shifts downward and toward the right side of the body. The gait cycle is completed, and the process repeated, when the right heel contacts the ground.

Noteworthy is the fact that the body's CoM is never directly located over the body's base of support during single-limb support (see Figure 15-13, *B*). This fact illustrates the relative imbalance of the body during gait, especially during single-limb support, when the foot must be positioned just slightly lateral to the vertical projection of the body's CoM to control its side-to-side movement. Proper location of the foot by hip motion in the frontal plane (i.e., hip abduction and adduction) is crucial considering the limited ability of the muscles of the subtalar joint to control the side-to-side motion of the CoM.[203]

Kinetic and Potential Energy Considerations

Although walking appears to take place at a steady forward speed, the body actually speeds up and slows down slightly with each step. When the supporting lower extremity is in front of the body's CoM, the body slows down. Conversely, when the supporting lower extremity is behind the body's CoM, the body speeds up. The body reaches its lowest velocity, therefore, at mid stance, once it has "climbed" on the supporting lower extremity, and its highest velocity during double-limb support, once it has "fallen away" from the sup-

porting lower extremity and before "climbing" on the opposite limb. Because kinetic energy of the body during ambulation is a direct function of its velocity (Equation 15-1), minimum kinetic energy is present at mid stance (30% and 80% of the gait cycle) and maximum kinetic energy is reached at double-limb support (5% and 55% of the gait cycle) (Figure 15-14).

$$\text{Kinetic energy} = 0.5\ mv^2 \qquad \textbf{(Equation 15.1)}$$

where *m* is the mass of the body, and *v* is the velocity of the body's CoM.

Kinetic energy is complemented by potential energy (see Figure 15-14). Potential energy is a function of the mass of the body, the gravitational field acting on the body, and the height of the body's CoM (Equation 15-2). During gait, maximum potential energy is achieved when the CoM reaches its highest points (30% and 80% of the gait cycle). Minimum potential energy of the body occurs at double-limb support (5% and 55% of the gait cycle), when the body's CoM is at its lowest points.

$$\text{Potential energy} = mgh \qquad \textbf{(Equation 15.2)}$$

where *m* is the mass of the body, *g* is the potential downward acceleration of the body resulting from gravity, and *h* is the height of the body's CoM.

In a graphic representation of the changes in kinetic and potential energy during gait, a relationship between the curves is readily observed (see Figure 15-14). The times of maximum potential energy correspond to the times of minimum kinetic energy and vice versa. As potential energy is lost from mid stance to double-limb support (the CoM of the body going

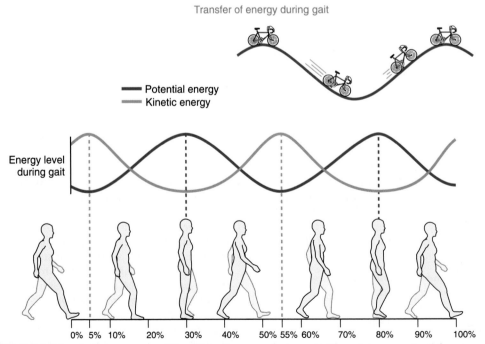

FIGURE 15-14. Transfer between potential and kinetic energy during gait. The minimum potential energy exists when the center of mass (CoM) is at its lowest points (5% and 55% of the gait cycle). The maximum potential energy occurs when the CoM is at its highest points (30% and 80% of the gait cycle). The reverse occurs for kinetic energy. This transfer between potential and kinetic energy is analogous to riding a bicycle that gains speed while going down a hill and loses speed while climbing up the next hill.

from its highest to its lowest location), kinetic energy is gained (the CoM of the body going from its minimum to maximum speed). Conversely, as kinetic energy is lost from double-limb support to mid stance, potential energy is gained. Therefore the body, acting to a great extent as an inverted pendulum, appears to use an optimal magnitude of vertical oscillation to most effectively transfer mechanical energy between its potential and kinetic forms. Deviation from this optimal vertical oscillation, by adoption of either a "bouncy" or a "flat" gait, has been demonstrated to increase energy expenditure.[1,115,141]

In closing, it must be noted that although the cyclic transfer between kinetic and potential energy minimizes the metabolic cost of walking, this process alone is not sufficient to sustain steady-speed ambulation.[19] Consequently, unlike the movement of a perfect pendulum, walking is dependent on the energy generated by muscles. Muscles of the lower extremity must generate forces to assist with forward propulsion of the body during stance phase and help with the advancement of the lower limb during the swing phase.[201]

JOINT KINEMATICS

During gait, the body's CoM is displaced linearly as a result of the summation of the angular rotation of the joints of the lower extremities, which is not unlike a car moving forward owing to the rotation of its tires. Movements at the joints of the lower extremities therefore are described as a function of angular rotation. Although joint angular rotation occurs primarily in the sagittal plane, important motion, although of smaller magnitude, also occurs in the frontal and horizontal planes.

Most often throughout this chapter, the angular rotation that takes place at the joint itself is described (i.e., the relative motion of one bone compared with another). In some instances (e.g., for the sagittal plane motion of the pelvis), the movement of the bones in space is described *without* regard to movement at the joint. The reader must therefore be careful to recognize when a discussion pertains to joint kinematics and when it pertains to bone kinematics.

Sagittal Plane Kinematics

Sagittal plane movement of the pelvis is small and is described here as movement of the bony structure itself. Conversely, the sagittal plane kinematics of the hip, knee, ankle, tarsometatarsal, and first metatarsophalangeal joints are of larger magnitude and are described as joint motion. In this section, as in the entire chapter, the gait cycle is described from right heel contact to subsequent right heel contact.

PELVIS

Movement of the pelvis in the sagittal plane is described as short-arc rotations in anterior and posterior directions about a medial-lateral axis through the hip joints (see Chapter 12). (The direction of the pelvic tilt is based on movement of the iliac crests.) The neutral position (0 degrees of pelvic tilt) is defined as the orientation of the pelvis in relaxed stance. Because the pelvis is a relatively rigid structure, both iliac crests are considered as moving together. During gait at normal speed, the amount of anterior and posterior pelvic tilt is small (i.e., a total of approximately 2 to 4 degrees). Although the

movement of the pelvis is described as movement of an independent "detached" structure, the kinematics actually take place primarily at the hip joints (through pelvic-on-femoral flexion and extension) and, to a lesser degree, at the lumbosacral joints (through pelvic-on-lumbar flexion and extension).

The pattern of motion of the pelvis over the full gait cycle resembles a sine wave with two full cycles (Figure 15-15, *A*). At right heel contact, the pelvis is in a near neutral position. From 0% to 10% of the gait cycle, a period of double-limb support, a small amount of posterior pelvic tilt occurs. The pelvis then begins tilting anteriorly during the period of single-limb support, reaching a slight anterior pelvic tilted position just after mid stance (30% of the gait cycle). In the second half of the stance phase, the pelvis tilts posteriorly until just after toe off. During initial and mid swing (60% to 87% of gait), the pelvis again tilts anteriorly before starting to tilt in the posterior direction in terminal swing.

In general, pelvic tilting increases with the speed of ambulation.[83] Significant variability in the amount, timing, and direction of tilt, however, has been noted across walking speed and among individuals. The generally noted greater magnitude of pelvic tilt with faster walking speed serves to increase functional limb length, which in turn serves to increase step length.

The sagittal plane tilt of the pelvis during walking is caused by the sum of the passive and active forces produced by the hip joint capsule and the hip flexor and extensor muscles. In pathologic situations, persons with marked hip flexion contractures show an exaggerated anterior tilt of the pelvis in the second half of the stance phase (i.e., at 30% to 60% of the gait cycle). This is attributed to increased passive tension in the shortened anterior hip structures, creating an anterior tilting tendency of the pelvis as full hip extension is attempted. An excessive anterior pelvic tilt can, to a degree, compensate for the lack of passive hip extension in the latter part of stance and is typically associated with increased lumbar lordosis.

HIP

At a typical walking speed the hip is flexed approximately 30 degrees at heel contact (see Figure 15-15, *B*). As the body moves forward over the fixed foot, the hip extends. Maximum hip extension of approximately 10 degrees is achieved before toe off. Flexion of the hip is initiated during pre-swing, and the hip is at about 0 degrees of flexion by toe off (60% of gait). During the swing phase, the hip further flexes to bring the lower extremity forward for the next foot placement. Maximum flexion (slightly more than 30 degrees) is achieved just before heel contact. Note that at heel contact the hip has already started to extend in preparation for weight acceptance. Overall, approximately 30 degrees of flexion and 10 degrees of extension (from the anatomic neutral position) are needed at the hip for normal walking.[65,159] As for all of the joints of the lower extremities, the magnitude of hip movement is proportional to walking speed.

Individuals with limited sagittal plane hip mobility may appear to walk without a gait deviation as the movement of the pelvis and lumbar spine, compensating for reduced hip motion, may be initially unnoticed. Apparent hip extension, detectable with good visual observational skills, can be achieved through an anterior pelvic tilt and associated increase in lumbar lordosis. Conversely, a posterior pelvic tilt accompanied by a flattening of the lumbar spine provides apparent hip flexion. To

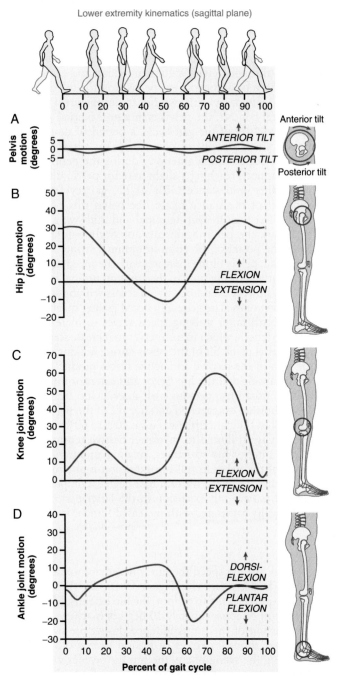

FIGURE 15-15. Sagittal plane angular rotation of the pelvis **(A)**, hip **(B)**, knee **(C)**, and ankle **(D)** during a gait cycle.

ambulate, individuals with a fused (i.e., ankylosed) hip use an exaggerated posterior and anterior pelvic tilt as a means to compensate for the absence of sagittal plane hip mobility (Figure 15-16).[71,185] Because the pelvis and lumbar spine motions are mechanically linked at the sacroiliac joint, exaggerated pelvic tilting during walking may increase the stress at the lumbar spine. These stresses could eventually irritate the structures within this region, resulting in low back pain.

KNEE

The kinematic pattern of the knee is slightly more complex than that of the hip (see Figure 15-15, *C*).[65,159] At heel contact the knee is flexed approximately 5 degrees, and it continues

to flex an additional 10 to 15 degrees during the initial 15% of the gait cycle. This slight knee flexion, controlled by eccentric action of the quadriceps, serves the purpose of shock absorption and weight acceptance as body weight is progressively transferred to this lower extremity. Following initial flexion, the knee approaches near full extension until about heel off (occurring at 30% to 40% of the gait cycle). At this point the knee starts flexing, reaching approximately 35 degrees of flexion by the time of toe off (60% of gait cycle). Maximum knee flexion of approximately 60 degrees is assumed by the beginning of mid swing (73% of gait cycle). Knee flexion during initial swing serves to shorten the length of the lower limb, facilitating toe clearance. In mid and terminal swing, the knee extends to just short of full extension before starting to flex slightly in preparation for heel contact.

Normal function of the knee during gait on a level surface requires range of motion from nearly full extension to approximately 60 degrees of flexion. A limitation of knee extension (i.e., knee flexion contracture) results in a functionally shorter limb, affecting the kinematics of both the stance limb and the swing limb. The stance limb, lacking full knee extension, must assume a partially "crouched" position, involving the hip, knee, and ankle, and the normal swing limb needs greater knee and possibly hip flexion to clear the toes from the ground. The uneven functional limb length also leads to excessive trunk and CoM movement, increasing the metabolic demands of walking. A flexed knee posture during gait also increases the muscular demand on the knee extensors, resulting in further metabolic costs.

A lack of sufficient knee flexion during the swing phase of gait interferes with toe clearance as the foot moves forward. To compensate, the hip must flex excessively. If the knee is immobilized in full extension with an orthosis or a cast, more noticeable compensations, such as hip "hiking" and hip circumduction, are required.

ANKLE (TALOCRURAL JOINT)

At the ankle, heel contact occurs with the talocrural joint in a slightly plantar flexed position (between 0 and 5 degrees) (see Figure 15-15, *D*). Shortly after heel contact (the first 8% of the gait cycle), the foot is positioned flat on the ground by a movement of plantar flexion controlled eccentrically by the ankle dorsiflexors. Then, during stance, up to 10 degrees of ankle dorsiflexion occurs as the tibia moves forward over the foot, which is in firm contact with the ground (from 8% to 45% of the gait cycle). Shortly after heel off (occurring at 30% to 40% of the gait cycle), the ankle begins to plantar flex, reaching a maximum of 15 to 20 degrees of plantar flexion just after toe off. During the swing phase the ankle is again dorsiflexed to a neutral position to allow the toes to clear the ground.[65,159]

Average speed of ambulation requires approximately 10 degrees of dorsiflexion and 20 degrees of plantar flexion. It is of note that greater dorsiflexion is needed during the stance phase than during the swing phase of gait. As at the knee and the hip, limitation of motion at the ankle leads to an abnormal gait pattern. For example, limited ankle plantar flexion may result in a decreased push off, possibly leading to a shorter step length.

Conversely, a lack of adequate dorsiflexion mobility during stance, for example from a "tight" Achilles tendon, may cause a premature heel off, resulting in a "bouncing" type of gait pattern. Alternatively, a "toeing-out" gait pattern

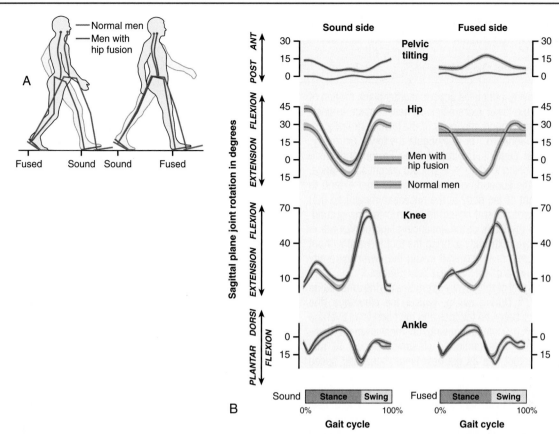

FIGURE 15-16. Body diagram **(A)** and average sagittal plane kinematic patterns **(B)** of men with unilateral hip fusion *(red lines)* compared with men with normal hip motion *(green lines)*. The lack of mobility of one hip drastically affects motion of the pelvis, the ipsilateral knee, and the contralateral hip. Less significant effects are noted at the contralateral knee and at both ankles. This figure illustrates how impairment (i.e., reduced mobility of the hip) that affects a single joint will affect motion of the other joints. (Modified from Gore DR, Murray MP, Sepic SB, Gardner GM: Walking patterns of men with unilateral surgical hip fusion, *J Bone Joint Surg Am* 57:759, 1975.)

is often employed to partially compensate for limited ankle dorsiflexion. With excessive toeing-out of the foot, the individual rolls off the medial aspect of the foot in the second half of stance phase. Another commonly accepted compensation for lack of ankle dorsiflexion is increased foot pronation. With or without toeing-out, excessive foot pronation can lead to greater stresses applied to the supporting soft-tissue structures of the plantar aspect of the foot.

In extreme cases in which there is a pes equinus deformity (i.e., fixed plantar flexion of the ankle), the individual may walk on the forefoot (metatarsal heads) with extended toes, with the heel never coming in contact with the ground. This condition is most commonly observed in individuals with cerebral palsy.

Limited ankle dorsiflexion also interferes with clearing the toes during swing phase. To compensate, increased knee and/or hip flexion of the swing limb is needed. Limited dorsiflexion in swing may result from plantar flexor tightness, calf spasticity, or ankle dorsiflexor weakness.

FIRST TARSOMETATARSAL JOINT

The first tarsometatarsal joint, the function of which is described in Chapter 14, has a slight amount of plantar flexion and dorsiflexion that helps adjust the flexibility and stability of the foot's medial longitudinal arch during gait.[8,68]

FIRST METATARSOPHALANGEAL JOINT

The metatarsophalangeal (MTP) joint of the hallux (great toe) is crucial to normal gait. At heel contact, the MTP joint is slightly extended. From shortly after heel contact to heel off, the MTP joint is in a relatively neutral position. Between heel off to just before toe off, the MTP joint extends approximately 45 to 55 degrees beyond neutral position. (This is the angle measured between the long axis of the first metatarsal and the proximal phalanx of the hallux.[83]) During the late part of stance phase and initial swing, the joint flexes and returns to a near neutral position.

Limited MTP joint extension because of a soft-tissue injury, such as a joint sprain (turf toe) or degeneration of the joint (hallux rigidus), typically results in an exaggerated toeing-out gait. One consequence of this abnormal gait pattern is a less efficient push off. Toeing-out also creates increased stress to the medial structures of the knee and foot, including the hallux, as mentioned earlier.

Frontal Plane Kinematics

Joint rotations within the frontal plane are of smaller amplitude compared with those in the sagittal plane. These rotations are important, however, especially at the hip and subtalar joints.

SPECIAL FOCUS 15-3

SPECIAL FOCUS 15-3

Summary of Sagittal Plane Kinematics

Several underlying principles govern sagittal plane motion of the joints of the lower extremities. At heel contact, to position the foot on the ground, the joints of the lower extremity are aligned to "reach forward," or to elongate the lower extremity. Shortly after heel contact, controlled knee flexion and ankle plantar flexion cushion loading for a smooth weight acceptance. All the joints of the supporting lower extremity then extend to support the weight of the body at the necessary height so that the foot of the contralateral swing limb can clear the ground. During swing, all the joints of the advancing limb participate in shortening the lower extremity to bring the foot forward without tripping on the ground. In terminal swing the lower extremity again "reaches forward" for the next heel contact.

The level of control of the lower extremities during ambulation is remarkable.[12,204] During swing, typical toe clearance (the minimum distance between the toes and the floor) is on average between 1.2 and 1.9 cm depending on measurement techniques.[10,117,120,123,171] This minimum clearance occurs at mid swing, when the foot has its greatest linear horizontal speed (4.5 m/sec). The transition from the swing to the stance phase is also amazingly well controlled. To provide smooth contact with the ground, vertical heel speed slows just before heel contact to only 0.05 m/sec. This level of control is the basis of the argument against using the term heel "strike" to describe the typically well-controlled heel contact with the ground. Further evidence of the fine control taking place during walking is expressed by the small clearance observed between the edge of steps and the foot during stair descent.[167]

PELVIS

Frontal plane motion of the pelvis during walking is best observed from either in front of or behind the individual, watching the iliac crests rise and fall in relationship to the horizontal plane. The pelvis rotates through a total excursion of about 10 to 15 degrees as a result of pelvic-on-femoral (hip) adduction and abduction on the stance limb. During weight acceptance on the right lower extremity (i.e., the first 15% to 20% of the gait cycle), the left iliac crest drops slightly below the height of the right iliac crest (Figure 15-17, *A*); this drop of the left iliac crest reflects pelvic-on-femoral adduction of the right stance hip (see Figure 15-17, *B*).[143] This initial downward motion of the left side of the pelvis is the result of gravity acting on the trunk and is controlled to a great extent by eccentric activation of the right hip abductors. From 20% to 60% of the gait cycle, the left iliac crest is elevated by concentric activation of the right hip abductors, assisted by a slight shift of the CoM of the trunk toward the right side. This shift brings the mass of the trunk over the right hip, thereby reducing the external torque demands on the right hip abductors. The elevation of the left iliac crest (on the swing limb) effectively produces abduction of the right stance hip. Throughout the swing phase on the right, a similar pattern occurs of initial controlled lowering of the right iliac crest followed by its progressive elevation.[31,161]

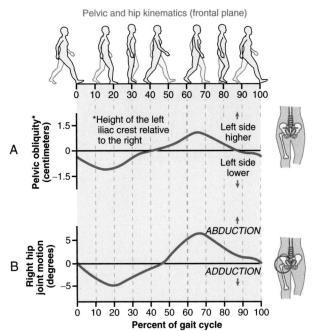

FIGURE 15-17. Frontal plane pelvis and hip motion for a full gait cycle starting with right heel contact. **A** illustrates the alignment of the pelvis itself considering the height of the left iliac crest in relationship to the right iliac crest. During right stance phase, the left iliac crest initially drops slightly before progressively moving upward. This movement is controlled by a strong activation, initially eccentric then concentric, of the right hip abductors. Therefore a small drop of the contralateral pelvis during early stance is considered normal. In the second half of the gait cycle, the relatively higher left iliac crest during the initial part of right swing phase reflects the controlled lowering of the right iliac crest by the left hip abductors when a person initially stands on the left lower extremity. **B** illustrates frontal plane hip motion. When considering the movement of the pelvis (described earlier) in relationship to the femur, in the early part of stance on the right, the drop of the left iliac crest contributes to right hip adduction. As the left iliac crest is elevated in the latter section of the right stance phase and the right iliac crest is lowered in the early part of the right swing phase, right hip abduction is created. (Data from Ounpuu S: Clinical gait analysis. In Spivack BS, ed: *Evaluation and management of gait disorders*, New York, 1995, Marcel Dekker.)

HIP

The pattern of elevation and depression of the iliac crests reflects the frontal plane motion of the hips (see Figure 15-17, *B*). During the stance phase this frontal plane motion occurs primarily from pelvic-on-femoral kinematics (see Chapter 12). A much smaller and variable amount of frontal plane motion likely occurs during stance by way of femoral-on-pelvic kinematics. During the swing phase, the motion of the pelvis (about the stance limb) combines with motion of the advancing femur to return the hip to its neutral frontal plane position.[31,159]

KNEE

Because of its articular geometry and strong collateral ligaments, the knee is relatively stable in the frontal plane, allowing only a very small amount of angular movement.[11,99,159] Benoit and colleagues[11] studied the kinematics at the tibiofemoral joints of six healthy subjects by recording the move-

SPECIAL FOCUS 15-4

Possible Causes for Excessive Hip Frontal Plane Motion during Walking

Excessive frontal plane movement of the stance hip is quite common, causing exaggerated medial-lateral shifts in the center of mass (CoM). There are at least three reasons why excessive movement of the pelvis and hip in the frontal plane may be observed: weakness of the hip abductors, reduced "shortening" of the swing limb, and a discrepancy in limb length.

The drop of the contralateral iliac crest (i.e., hip adduction) during early to mid stance is normally controlled by an eccentric activation of the hip abductor muscles of the stance limb. Inadequate abduction torque from these muscles often leads to excessive frontal plane motion during stance.[138] While standing on one limb, a person with moderate hip abductor weakness demonstrates an excessive drop of the pelvis to the side of the lifted lower extremity (Figure 15-18).[21] This action is referred to as a *positive Trendelenburg sign.* Typically, however, a person with weakened hip abductors, especially if severe, compensates by leaning the trunk to the *same side* as the weakened muscle during any single-limb support activities, whether standing or walking. During walking, this is called a "compensated" Trendelenburg gait or gluteus medius limp. Leaning of the trunk to the side of weakness minimizes the external torque demands resulting from body weight on the abductor muscles of the stance limb.

Another deviation that is observed by looking at the movement of the pelvis in the frontal plane is called hip "hiking." Hip hiking on the side of the swing lower extremity compensates for the inability of the knee and/or ankle of the lower extremity to sufficiently shorten the limb for clearance of the foot. The classic example is walking with a knee orthosis, keeping the knee in full extension. Hip hiking is more accurately described as the excessive elevation of the iliac crest on the side of the swing limb. Elevation results from pelvic-on-femoral abduction of the stance limb. Muscles involved in this movement include the primary abductors of the stance limb, the quadratus lumborum of the swing limb, and possibly the abdominals and back extensors on the side of the swing limb.

A significant limb length difference also affects movement of the pelvis in the frontal plane. Limb length discrepancy can be severe, secondary to a fracture of the femur or a unilateral coxa vara or valga, or it can be slight (<0.5 cm) owing to natural variability. During periods of double-limb support, the iliac crest of the longer lower extremity is positioned higher than the iliac crest of the shorter lower extremity. This pelvic obliquity, which is occurring for every gait cycle, results in increased cyclic side bending of the lumbar spine.

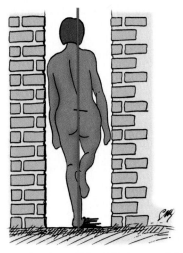

FIGURE 15-18. Excessive drop of the right (non–weight-bearing side) iliac crest resulting from a weak gluteus medius on the weight-bearing side. (Modified from Calvé J, Galland M, De Cagny R: Pathogenesis of the limp due to coxalgia: the antalgic gait, *J Bone Joint Surg Am* 21:12, 1939.)

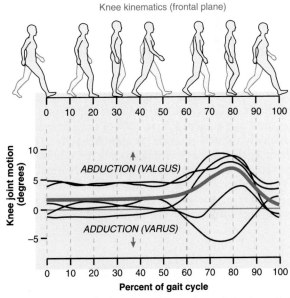

FIGURE 15-19. Frontal plane angular motion of the knee is illustrated. The purple line is the average of four of the five subjects. The smaller black lines are each subject's individual data. (Data from Lafortune MA, Cavanagh PR, Sommer HJ III, Kalenak A: Three-dimensional kinematics of the human knee during walking, *J Biomech* 25:347, 1992.)

ment of reflective markers attached to the pins inserted in the cortexes of each subject's femur and tibia. As subjects walked at a self-selected speed, the movements were measured in three-dimensions through the use of four infrared cameras. Overall, the authors found a minimal and inconsistent pattern of abduction-adduction movement (less than 3 degrees) at the knee during the first 80% of stance phase. In the last 20% of stance, just before toe off, approximately 5 degrees of knee adduction took place in most subjects. Benoit and colleagues'

data are generally consistent with those of a previously published study by Lafortune and co-workers who used similar invasive methods on five subjects walking at 1.2 m/sec.[99] Lafortune and colleagues reported the knee to be in an average of 1.2 degrees of abduction (valgus) at the time of heel contact (Figure 15-19). This alignment remained unchanged throughout the stance phase.

Lafortune and colleagues also reported data for the swing phase of gait, indicating that the knee typically abducted an additional 5 degrees during initial swing phase. Maximum abduction occurred when the knee was near its maximum flexion angle. The knee returned to its slightly abducted position before the next heel contact. The data from both studies provide a unique contribution to the literature. Most other published data on these kinematics are from studies using skin-mounted markers, which generally are associated with greater error.

ANKLE (TALOCRURAL JOINT)

The primary motion of the talocrural joint is dorsiflexion–plantar flexion. Although, as described in Chapter 14, the ankle everts and abducts slightly with dorsiflexion, and inverts and adducts slightly with plantar flexion, these secondary frontal and horizontal plane motions are very small and are not discussed in this chapter.

FOOT AND SUBTALAR JOINT

The triplanar motions of pronation and supination occur through interaction of the subtalar and transverse tarsal joints. Pronation combines components of eversion, abduction, and dorsiflexion; supination combines inversion, adduction, and plantar flexion. This chapter considers the frontal plane motions of eversion and inversion at the subtalar joint to represent the more global motions of foot pronation and supination, respectively. Subtalar joint motions are typically measured as the angle made between the posterior aspect of the calcaneus and the posterior aspect of the lower leg (Figure 15-20).

The subtalar joint is inverted approximately 2 to 3 degrees at the time of heel contact (Figure 15-21). Immediately after heel contact, rapid eversion of the calcaneus begins and continues until mid stance (30% to 35% of the gait cycle), where a maximally everted position of approximately 2 degrees is reached. At that time, the subtalar joint reverses its direction of movement and starts toward inversion. Normally, a relatively neutral position of the calcaneus is reached at about 40% to 45% of the gait cycle, at approximately heel off. Between heel off and toe off, calcaneal inversion continues

until it reaches a value of approximately 6 degrees of inversion.[35] During swing, the calcaneus returns to a slightly inverted position in preparation for the next heel contact. This pattern of motion is generally agreed on in the literature; however, the reported amount of foot pronation during gait varies based on the techniques and preferences for measurement. Reischl and co-workers,[150] using a three-dimensional model of the foot, report a mean peak pronation of 10.5 ± 3.4 degrees, occurring at 26.8% ± 8.7% of the gait cycle.

The movement of foot pronation or supination during walking is accompanied by changes in height of the foot's medial longitudinal arch.[8,68] A detailed review of this associated kinesiology is provided in Chapter 14.

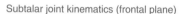

Subtalar joint kinematics (frontal plane)

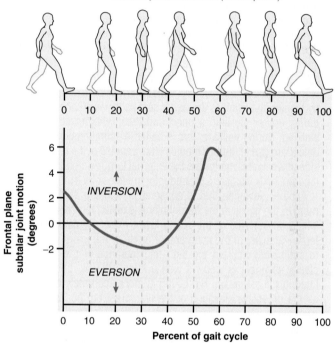

FIGURE 15-21. Frontal plane inversion and eversion of the calcaneus as an indicator of subtalar joint motion during walking. (Data from Cornwall MW, McPoil TG: Three-dimensional movement of the foot during the stance phase of walking, *J Am Podiatr Med Assoc* 89:56, 1999.)

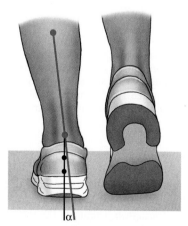

α = Frontal plane
Subtalar joint angle

FIGURE 15-20. Method to measure rear foot (subtalar joint) motion. The inversion or eversion angle, made by the lines bisecting the lower leg *(purple line)* and the calcaneus *(black line)*, is measured as a simplified indicator of the amount of foot pronation or supination. This measurement can be made at a single point or throughout the gait cycle by the analysis of individual images recorded using a video system.

⬢ **SPECIAL FOCUS 15-5**

Summary of Frontal Plane Kinematics

The best location from which to observe frontal plane kinematics of the joints of the lower extremities is behind the individual. Hip motion plays an important role in reducing the vertical displacement of the body's center of mass (CoM). The rapid pronation (calcaneal eversion) of the foot after heel contact participates in the process of weight acceptance and provides a flexible and adaptable foot structure for making contact with the ground. Later in the stance phase, between heel off and toe off, the inversion of the calcaneus associated with supination of the foot provides a more rigid foot structure, which helps propel the body forward.

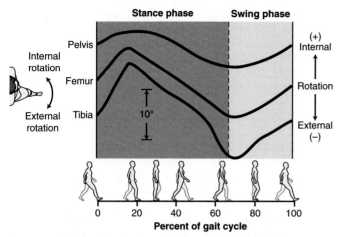

FIGURE 15-22. Pattern of horizontal plane motion of the pelvis, femur, and tibia as viewed from above. The pattern of motion is similar for the three bony structures, with progressively larger amplitude of movement for the more distal structures. View from above, for the right lower extremity, internal rotation of the pelvis corresponds with a counterclockwise motion. (From Mann RA: Biomechanics of the foot. In American Academy of Orthopedic Surgeons, ed: *Atlas of orthotics: biomechanical principles and application,* St Louis, 1975, Mosby, 1975.)

Horizontal Plane Kinematics

Information currently available about lower extremity kinematics in the horizontal plane during walking is provided by only a limited number of studies. To improve the accuracy of these measurements, some investigators fixed rigid metal pins in the pelvis, femur, and tibia of their subjects. Attached to these metal pins were markers that allowed video cameras to track bone movement. In some studies only the movement of the bony structures in space was observed; reports from other studies described the relative motion that took place at the joint itself.[82,99]

The following section cites data on movement of the bones as well as movement of the joints. Although the number of studies describing horizontal plane kinematics has increased in recent years, this area of study is not well understood and results are difficult to generalize across the population. The lack of understanding is associated with the technical difficulty of trying to measure a relatively small amount of movement, in combination with the natural high variability of this motion among subjects.

PELVIS

During walking, the pelvis rotates in the horizontal plane around a vertical axis of rotation through the hip joint of the stance limb. The following description of pelvic rotation is based on a *top view for a right gait cycle.* At right heel contact the right anterior-superior iliac spine (ASIS) is forward compared with the left ASIS. For the initial 15% to 20% of the gait cycle, the pelvis rotates in an internal (counterclockwise) rotation, as viewed from above in Figure 15-22. Throughout the rest of stance on the right lower extremity, an external (clockwise) rotation of the pelvis occurs as the left ASIS progressively moves forward along with the advancing left swing limb. At right toe off, the right ASIS is now behind the left. During swing of the right lower extremity, the right ASIS

progressively moves forward. Throughout the gait cycle, the pelvis rotates 3 to 4 degrees in each direction. A greater amount of rotation of the pelvis occurs with increasing walking speed to increase step length.

FEMUR

After heel contact, the femur rotates internally for the first 15% to 20% of the gait cycle (see Figure 15-22). At about 20% of the gait cycle, the femur reverses its direction and rotates externally until shortly after toe off. Internal rotation of the femur takes place throughout most of the swing phase. Overall, the femur rotates approximately 6 to 7 degrees in each direction during gait.[25]

TIBIA

The pattern of movement of the tibia is very similar to the movement described for the femur (see Figure 15-22). The magnitude of the rotation is about 8 to 9 degrees in each direction.

HIP

Both the femur and the pelvis rotate simultaneously. At right heel contact, the right hip is in slight external rotation based on the relative posterior position of the contralateral (left) ASIS (Figure 15-23). A net internal rotation movement of the right hip occurs during most of stance on the right lower extremity, as the contralateral (left) ASIS is brought forward. A maximum internally rotated position is achieved by 50% of gait. External rotation of the right hip occurs from 50% of gait until mid swing, as the right lower extremity is advanced forward. From mid swing to right heel contact, a slight amount of right hip internal rotation takes place.[31,159,179]

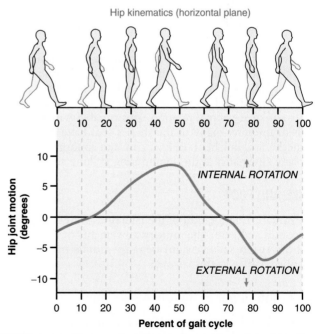

FIGURE 15-23. Horizontal plane angular motion of the hip. (Data from Sutherland DH, Kaufman KR, Moitoza JR: Kinematics of normal human walking. In Rose J, Gamble JG, eds: *Human walking,* ed 2, Philadelphia, 1994, Williams & Wilkins.)

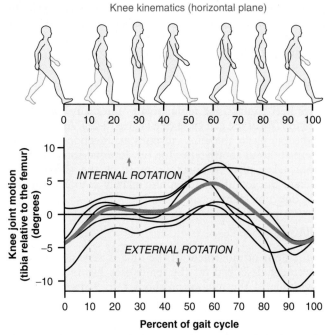

Knee kinematics (horizontal plane)

FIGURE 15-24. Horizontal plane angular motion of the knee. The blue line is the average of the five subjects. The smaller black lines are each subject's individual data. (Data from Lafortune MA, Cavanagh PR, Sommer III HJ, Kalenak A: Three-dimensional kinematics of the human knee during walking, *J Biomech* 25:347, 1992.)

KNEE

There are two studies of particular interest that used intracortical pins attached to the femur and tibia as a means to precisely document horizontal plane rotation of the knee during ambulation.[11,99] Figure 15-24 illustrates data from a study by Lafortune and colleagues for each subject, along with the group average.[99] Clearly, and consistent with data from Benoit and co-workers,[11] the amount and direction of the horizontal plane rotation of the knee is highly variable. Much of this variability is masked by the process of averaging the data across individuals, as performed in Figure 15-24 and in many descriptive and research reports. In fact, although Figure 15-24 shows an overall trend toward internal rotation during the stance phase, data by Benoit and colleagues[11] indicate an average overall pattern of knee external rotation. This variability makes it difficult to interpret many of the studies that have proposed a biomechanical link between knee pain and abnormal horizontal plane kinematics at this joint during walking and running.

ANKLE AND FOOT

Horizontal plane rotation of the talocrural joint is slight and not considered here. The primary movements of the subtalar joint (inversion and eversion) are in the frontal plane and are described earlier in this chapter.

Trunk and Upper Extremity Kinematics

The trunk and upper extremities play an important role in maintaining balance and minimizing energy expenditure during gait. In addition, small intricate spinal movements and muscular actions at the trunk serve to dampen the gait-related oscillations and accelerations produced by the movement of the lower extremities.[86,119] As a result, accelerations of the head segment are 10% to 40% less than those of the lower portion of the trunk. This dampening effect, keeping the head more stable, serves an important role in optimizing visual and vestibular function during gait.

TRUNK

During ambulation, translation of the CoM follows the general pattern of translation of the head and trunk (see Figure 15-13). In addition, the trunk rotates in the horizontal plane around its vertical axis. The shoulder girdle rotates in the opposite direction as the pelvis. The average total rotational excursion of the shoulder girdle is approximately 7 to 9 degrees.[18,132] This pattern of movement of the trunk makes a small contribution to the overall efficiency of gait.[18] Restriction of trunk motion increases energy expenditure during walking by as much as 10%.[149]

Although the preceding paragraph briefly describes the horizontal plane motion of the trunk, Rozumalski and colleagues[155] in 2008 published data on segmental motion throughout the lumbar spine during ambulation. The uniqueness of this study is related to the methods of data collection, which included three-dimensional video analysis of markers rigidly fixed to the spinous processes of all lumbar segments using surgically inserted Kirshner wires. The data indicate complex intervertebral lumbar motion of up to 3 to 5 degrees in each direction, in all three planes.[155] These kinematics, although modest, are likely necessary to allow the previously described small triplanar pelvic motions to occur while the trunk is kept in a relatively erect posture.

SHOULDER

In the sagittal plane the shoulder exhibits a sinusoidal pattern of movement that is out of phase with hip flexion and extension. As the hip (femur) moves toward extension, the ipsilateral shoulder (humerus) moves toward flexion, and vice versa.[174] At heel contact, the shoulder is in its maximally extended position of approximately 25 degrees beyond the neutral position. The shoulder then progressively rotates forward to reach a maximum of 10 degrees of flexion by 50% of the gait cycle. In the second half of the gait cycle, as the ipsilateral hip moves forward toward flexion, the shoulder extends to return to 25 degrees of extension by the next heel contact.

The pattern of movement of the shoulder is consistent across individuals, although the magnitude of movement varies greatly. In general, the amplitude of shoulder movement increases with greater speed. Arm swing is partly active, rather than fully passive, especially for the movement of shoulder extension that requires some activation of the posterior deltoid muscle.[197] The major function of arm swing is to balance the rotational forces in the trunk.[51] Restriction of arm motion has not been shown to have a significant effect on the energy cost of ambulation.[149,207]

ELBOW

The elbow is normally in approximately 20 degrees of flexion at heel contact. As the shoulder flexes in the first 50% of the gait cycle, the elbow also flexes to a maximum of approximately 45 degrees. In the second half of the gait cycle, as the shoulder extends, the elbow extends to return to 20 degrees of flexion.[132]

Summary of Horizontal Plane Kinematics

Figure 15-25 summarizes the direction of horizontal plane rotation of the major bones of the lower extremity and subtalar joint during walking, using different sets of data.[35,71,110] The pelvis, femur, and tibia rotate internally, well after heel contact (i.e., through about 15% to 20% of the gait cycle). This mass internal rotation is accompanied by subtalar joint eversion. As described in Chapter 14, an everting subtalar joint tends to increase the pliability of the midfoot region, including the transverse tarsal joint. A pliable midfoot serves to cushion the impact of limb loading. After about 15% to 20% of the gait cycle, the pelvis, femur, and tibia all begin to externally rotate until toe off. Simultaneously to this external rotation of the pelvis, femur, and tibia the subtalar joint begins moving toward inversion, which tends to increase the stability of the midfoot region. This stability enables the midfoot to serve as a rigid lever in terminal stance and pre-swing, allowing the plantar flexors to lift the calcaneus without the midfoot collapsing under the body's weight. Further investigation, such as that performed by Reischl and colleagues,[150] is needed to clearly elucidate the exact relationship that exists between the timing and magnitude of pronation of the foot and rotation of the tibia and femur.

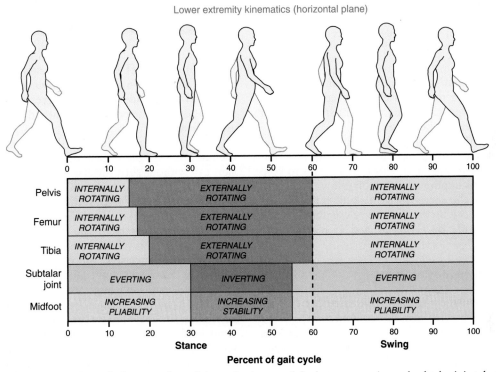

FIGURE 15-25. Horizontal plane rotation of the major bones of the lower extremity and subtalar joint during walking. The graph shows the direction of rotation, which is not necessarily the same as the absolute joint position.

ENERGY EXPENDITURE

Energy expenditure during gait is measured by the amount of energy used in calories per meter walked per kilogram of body weight. Typically, energy expenditure is measured indirectly by quantifying oxygen consumption.[154] When walking, the body strives to minimize energy cost. Conservation of energy is achieved by optimizing the excursion of the CoM, controlling the body momentum, and taking advantage of intersegmental transfers of energy.[201]

The metabolic efficiency of walking is greatest at a walking speed of approximately 1.33 m/sec (3 mph).[154] Not surprisingly, this walking speed roughly corresponds to that freely adopted by individuals ambulating on the street (see Table 15-1). Walking faster or slower than that optimal speed increases the energy cost of ambulation (Figure 15-26).

Walking speed is equal to the product of step length and cadence (step rate). Maximum energy efficiency of walking is achieved by the body's innate ability to adopt an ideal combination of step length and step rate. This combination is demonstrated across all walking speeds. Although the energy cost of ambulation increases with walking speed, the efficiency of walking is greatest at the maintained step length–

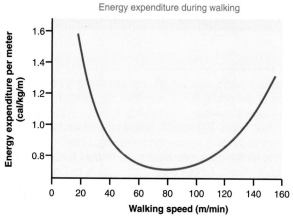

FIGURE 15-26. Energy expenditure as a function of walking speed. The lowest energy expenditure per meter walked is at a speed of approximately 1.33 m/sec (80 m/min). (Data from Ralston HJ: Effects of immobilization of various body segments on energy cost of human locomotion, *Ergon Suppl* 53, 1965.)

step rate ratio of 0.0072 m/steps/min for men and 0.0064 m/steps/min for women across all walking speeds.[211] At any given walking speed, imposition of a different step length or step rate increases energy expenditure.

With abnormal gait the energy cost of ambulation increases (Table 15-4).[39,135] As a consequence, individuals with abnormal gait patterns tend to walk more slowly as a means to keep the rate of energy consumption at a comfortable aerobic level. Further discussion of the energetics of walking in individuals with pathologic gaits can be found in Perry's textbook[147] and reviews of the literature by Gonzalez and Corcoran[69] and Waters and Mulroy.[196]

Energy-Saving Strategies of Walking

During gait, five kinematic strategies serve to reduce the displacement of the CoM which, in turn, has long been believed to decrease energy cost. Vertical displacement of the CoM is reduced by the combined actions of the first four strategies. The fifth strategy serves to reduce the side-to-side displace-

TABLE 15-4. Increased Energy Cost of Walking Associated with Specific Conditions

Conditions	Increased Energy Cost (%)*
Immobilization of one ankle[149,192]	3-6
Immobilization of one knee in full extension[92,193]	23-33
Immobilization of one knee at 45 degrees of flexion[149]	37
Immobilization of one hip, arthrodesis[192]	32
Unilateral transtibial amputation, walking with prosthesis[60]	20-38
Unilateral transfemoral amputation, walking with prosthesis[60]	20-60
Postcerebrovascular accident, moderate-to-severe residual deficits[34]	55

*Percentage increase based on energy cost of normal gait.

TABLE 15-5. Kinematic Strategies to Optimize Energy Expenditure during Gait

Direction of Action	Name of Strategy	Action
Vertical	Horizontal plane pelvic rotation	Reduces the downward displacement of the center of mass (CoM)
Vertical	Sagittal plane ankle rotation	Reduces the downward displacement of the CoM
Vertical	Stance phase knee flexion	Reduces the upward displacement of the CoM
Vertical	Frontal plane pelvic rotation	Reduces the upward displacement of the CoM
Side to side	Frontal plane hip rotation (step width)	Reduces the side-to-side excursion of the CoM

ment of the CoM (Table 15-5). The strategies detailed in this chapter are based on the *six determinants* of gait originally described by Saunders and colleagues in 1953.[158] A detailed account of these determinants is found in the work of Inman and colleagues.[82,83]

To appreciate the effects of the four kinematic strategies used to optimize the vertical displacement of the CoM, envision gait without such mechanisms. This can be achieved by using two pencils connected at the eraser ends (Figure 15-27, *A*). During walking, a large vertical oscillation of the eraser end of the pencils (representing the pelvis and therefore the body's CoM) is readily observed. The eraser end is highest when the pencils are side by side in a vertically oriented position (i.e., mid stance). Conversely, the eraser end is lowest when the pencils are maximally angled (i.e., double-limb support). This gait pattern results in a large displacement of the CoM.

Saunders and colleagues[158] in their classic manuscript, suggested that the goal of these strategies is to reduce the displacement of the CoM so as to decrease the energy expenditure related to the muscular effort needed to cyclically lift the body. This view has since been challenged in favor of a model in which the vertical displacement of the body acts more like an inverted pendulum, taking advantage of the transfer between potential and kinetic energy.[97] More recent data actually suggest that an optimal amount of vertical oscillation of the CoM exists, one that is neither too "flat" or too "bouncy," which minimizes energy cost.[1,70,97,115,141] These data provide a new perspective on the interpretation of the goal of the original *determinants* of gait, possibly from "minimizing" to "optimizing" the CoM displacement. Additional work is needed to better understand the relationship among lower extremity kinematics, CoM excursion, and energy cost of ambulation.

VERTICAL DISPLACEMENT OF THE CENTER OF MASS

Reducing the downward displacement of the CoM is achieved by horizontal plane pelvic rotation and sagittal plane ankle rotation. Horizontal plane rotation of the pelvis advances the entire swing limb forward, thereby minimizing the amount of hip flexion and extension needed for a given step length (compare Figure 15-27, *A* with Figure 15-27, *B*). As a consequence of the lower extremities remaining closer to a vertical orientation throughout the gait cycle, the lowest points of the CoM trajectory are raised, which reduces the downward displacement of the CoM. Sagittal plane ankle rotation makes use of the configuration of the ankle-foot complex (Figure 15-27, *C*). At heel contact the alignment of the ankle places the large protruding calcaneus in contact with the ground, functionally elongating the lower extremity. Near the end of stance, as the hip extends and the knee begins to flex, the lower extremity is elongated by plantar flexion of the ankle (i.e., heel rise). This functional elongation of the lower extremity at both ends of stance phase further reduces the downward displacement of the CoM (compare Figure 15-27, *B* with Figure 15-27, *C*).[41,90,91]

Limiting the upward displacement of the CoM is partially achieved by stance phase knee flexion, when the lower extremity is in its most vertical orientation (see Figure 15-27, *D*). Frontal plane pelvic rotation further assists in reducing upward displacement of the CoM (see Figure 15-27, *E*). During stance phase, the contralateral iliac crest falls as the ipsilateral iliac crest rises. Throughout a complete gait cycle, therefore, the iliac crests alternately rise and fall like the ends of a seesaw, but the point just anterior to the second sacral vertebra (i.e., the point representing the body's CoM) remains relatively stationary, as would the pivot point of a seesaw.[41,91]

As shown in Figure 15-28, the combination of the four aforementioned strategies reduces the total net vertical displacement of the CoM. The downward displacement of the CoM is reduced by horizontal plane pelvic rotation and sagittal plane ankle rotation. The upward displacement of the CoM is reduced by stance phase knee flexion and frontal plane pelvic rotation. Although still debated, the work by Della Croce and colleagues[41] suggests that sagittal plane ankle rotation has the largest influence on CoM vertical displacement, followed by pelvic obliquity, stance phase knee flexion, and frontal plane pelvic rotation.

SIDE-TO-SIDE DISPLACEMENT OF THE CENTER OF MASS

While a person walks, his or her CoM shifts side-to-side and remains within the dynamic base of support provided by the feet (see Figure 15-13). The amplitude of this lateral displacement, partially reflected by step width, is largely a function of frontal plane hip motion (i.e., hip abduction and adduction). The normally adopted 8- to 10-cm step width during ambulation reduces side-to-side displacement of the body, primarily as a strategy to reduce energy expenditure.[46,135] Because, however, this step width also decreases the potential size of the dynamic base of support, it likely represents a mechanical compromise between energy conservation and stability of the body as a whole. Theoretically a step width greater than 8 to 10 cm provides greater stability at a cost of increased energy expenditure. Persons with balance disorders, for example, often choose to walk with a wider base of support as a means to improve their stability. Although this strategy increases the energy cost of walking, the tradeoff is likely worthwhile, considering the often negative consequences of falling.

But, as discussed earlier with regard to vertical displacement of the CoM, the normally adopted step width of 8 to 10 cm seems to reflect the inherent ability of the body to naturally use kinematic strategies that are optimal to minimize energy expenditure. It has been demonstrated that ambulation with either a lesser or a larger step width increases energy cost of ambulation in young healthy individuals.[46]

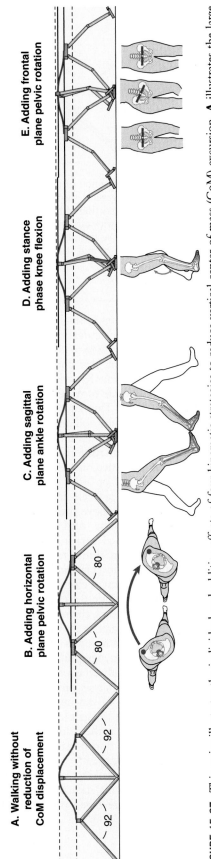

FIGURE 15-27. This series illustrates the individual and additive effects of four kinematic strategies to reduce vertical center of mass (CoM) excursion. **A** illustrates the large vertical oscillation of the CoM while a person walks *without* the strategies. **B** illustrates that rotation of the pelvis in the horizontal plane functionally lengthens the lower extremities and reduces the magnitude of the hip flexion-extension angle required for a given step length, thereby reducing the downward displacement of the CoM. **C** illustrates that further reduction of the downward displacement of the CoM is achieved by rotation of the ankle in the sagittal plane. **D** illustrates that the small amount of knee flexion present during stance reduces the functional length of the lower extremity and therefore the upward displacement of the CoM. **E** shows that the contralateral pelvic drop during stance also reduces the net overall elevation of the CoM. The angle values in **A** and **B** are for illustrative purposes only and do not represent the actual hip angles during walking.

A. Walking without reduction of CoM displacement

B. Adding horizontal plane pelvic rotation

C. Adding sagittal plane ankle rotation

D. Adding stance phase knee flexion

E. Adding frontal plane pelvic rotation

A. Walking without reduction of CoM displacement

B. Walking with reduction of CoM displacement

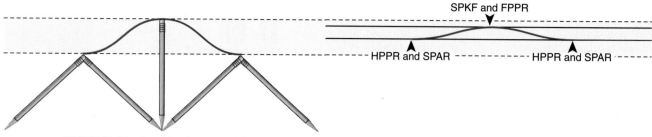

FIGURE 15-28. Combined action of the four kinematic strategies to reduce vertical CoM excursion. Without these strategies, a large vertical displacement of the body's CoM *(red)* would occur during walking **(A)**. **B** illustrates the combined action of horizontal plane pelvic rotation *(HPPR)* and sagittal plane ankle rotation *(SPAR)* to reduce the downward displacement of the CoM during double-limb support. It also shows the action of stance phase knee flexion *(SPKF)* and frontal plane pelvic rotation *(FPPR)* to reduce the upward displacement of the CoM at mid stance.

MUSCLE ACTIVITY

During a gait cycle, virtually all muscles of the lower extremities exhibit one or two short bursts of electrical activity, lasting from generally 100 to 400 msec (about 10% to 40% of the gait cycle). Like all other elements of gait, this phasic muscular activation is repeated during each stride. Knowledge of when muscles are active during the gait cycle provides insight into their specific kinesiologic function. This knowledge allows gait deviations to be more easily understood and treated.

Activity of the lower extremity and trunk musculature has been studied extensively using EMG. In its simplest interpretation, muscular activity can be determined on a temporal basis; the muscle is simply considered "on" or "off." The muscle is considered "on" when the amplitude of its electromyographic signal reaches a predetermined value above the resting level. Otherwise, the muscle is considered to be "off," or electrically silent. As examples, the red horizontal bars in Figure 15-29 illustrate when selected muscles are "on" during the gait cycle.[94]

Another method of reporting muscular activity during walking is to express the relative amount of electromyographic signal compared with a reference standard (review topic of EMG in Chapter 3). In many gait studies, the reference is the maximum signal recorded during a gait cycle for that same muscle, which explains why there are no units on the Y axis in Figure 15-29 and why the electromyographic signal representation for each muscle takes full advantage of the graph's vertical dimension.[204] This type of analysis provides insight into the relative level of activation of the muscle (i.e., an index of muscular effort) throughout the gait cycle.

Finally, the reader is reminded that the timing and especially relative activation of muscles during gait vary based on parameters such as walking velocity,[4,22,42,78,187] additional loading,[187] and inclination[101] of the walking surface. Unless otherwise stated, the electromyographic data presented and discussed throughout this chapter are based on an average walking velocity of approximately 1.37 m/sec.

Trunk

Only the actions of the erector spinae and the rectus abdominis are discussed here. It is noteworthy that these muscles show simultaneous activation on the right and the left sides of the body.

ERECTOR SPINAE

The erector spinae, at the level of the lumbar region, show two well-defined periods of activity. The first period is from slightly before heel contact to about 20% of the gait cycle. The second period is from 45% to 70% of the gait cycle, which corresponds to opposite heel contact.[3,22,28,100] These two bursts of activity, from both the right and left erector spinae, control the forward angular momentum of the trunk relative to the hips shortly after heel contact for each step.

RECTUS ABDOMINIS

This muscle has very low and variable activity throughout the gait cycle.[3,37,195] Nevertheless, increased activity occurs at between 20% and 40% and again at between 70% and 90% of the gait cycle. This small increase in activity coincides with the time the hip flexors are actively flexing the hip. Increased activity of the rectus abdominis bilaterally therefore stabilizes the pelvis and lumbar spine and provides a stable fixation point for the hip flexor muscles, principally the iliopsoas and rectus femoris.

Hip

Three muscle groups at the hip have been extensively studied during normal ambulation: the hip extensors, such as the gluteus maximus and the hamstrings; the hip flexors, such as the iliacus and the psoas; and the hip abductors, such as the gluteus medius and minimus.[4,22,78,101,187] Less well documented is the role of the hip adductors and rotators.[22,78]

HIP EXTENSORS

Activation of the gluteus maximus begins at terminal swing and serves two purposes—initiating hip extension and preparing the musculature for weight acceptance at the beginning of stance (review Figure 15-15). At heel contact the gluteus maximus is therefore already activated to extend the hip and prevent forward "jackknifing," or uncontrolled trunk flexion, over the femur. This "jackknifing" would occur if the forward displacement of the trunk were to continue at a steady velocity while the forward translation of the pelvis normally slightly but suddenly slowed at heel contact. The gluteus maximus

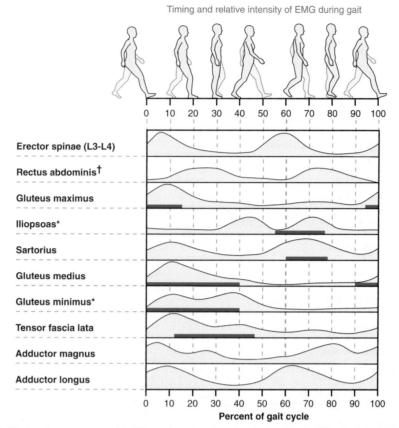

Timing and relative intensity of EMG during gait

FIGURE 15-29. **A, B,** An electromyographic illustration showing the timing *(dark red bars)* and relative intensity *(light brown shading)* of muscle activation during walking. (Muscle timing data from Knutson and Soderberg, 1995[94]; relative intensity of muscle activation data from Winter, 1991[204]; Bechtol,* 1975[9]; Carlsoo,† 1972.[23]) These general patterns of muscle activations are consistent with data reported in several other studies.[22,42,78,101,187] Although the Y axis is not labeled, it does nevertheless depict the relative intensity of muscle activation for each muscle as a function of the maximum value obtained during the gait cycle. The reader should be alerted to the fact that although all muscles fill the full vertical dimension of their graph, some muscles, such as the rectus abdominis, are in fact only minimally active during gait. For other muscles, such as the gluteus medius, their peak in activation represents a more significant effort.

remains active from heel contact to mid stance (i.e., first 30% of the gait cycle) to support the weight of the body and produce hip extension. Strong activation of the gluteus maximus when the foot is firmly planted also assists indirectly with knee extension. During the swing phase, the gluteus maximus is largely inactive until terminal swing, when a modest activation is needed to first decelerate the flexing hip and then initiate its extension.

The hamstring muscles are active during the first 10% of the gait cycle, likely for similar reasons as the gluteus maximus (see Figure 15-29, *B*).

HIP FLEXORS

Electromyographic data on the hip flexors is relatively sparse in the literature, likely reflecting the need to use intramuscular electrodes for data collection. Available data indicate that the iliopsoas becomes active well before toe off and remains so through initial swing.[4] The activation at between 30% and 50% of the gait cycle is likely initially eccentric, as the hip is extending at that time, followed by a concentric action to initiate hip flexion just before toe off. Despite the continued hip flexion into terminal swing, the hip flexor muscles are active only in the first 50% of the swing phase. Hip flexion

in the second half of the swing phase is a result of the forward momentum that the thigh gains in initial swing. The rectus femoris also acts as a hip flexor and therefore assists with the aforementioned actions.[4,136] The key roles of the hip flexors are to advance the lower extremity forward during swing in preparation for the next step and to lift the lower extremity to allow for toe clearance during swing.

The sartorius, another anterior muscle of the hip, is also active as a hip flexor from toe off until mid swing. The activation during early stance phase, as illustrated in Figure 15-29, *A*, has not been consistently reported by other studies, especially those using intramuscular electromyographic electrodes.[4] Studies reporting activation of this muscle in early stance typically used surface electromyographic electrodes, which raises the possibility that the increase in electromyographic signal is the result of "cross-talk" (see discussion of EMG in Chapter 3), the electromyographic signal effectively originating from the underlying vasti muscles.

HIP ABDUCTORS

Whereas hip flexors and extensors have their primary role in the sagittal plane, the hip abductors—gluteus medius, gluteus minimus, and tensor fascia lata—stabilize the pelvis in the

Timing and relative intensity of EMG during gait

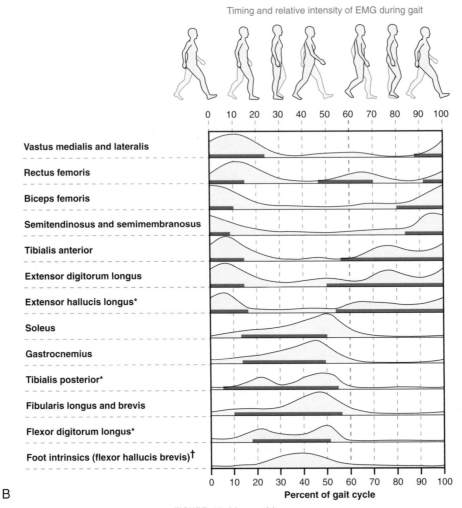

FIGURE 15-29, cont'd.

frontal plane. The gluteus medius is active toward the very end of the swing phase in preparation for heel contact. The gluteus medius and minimus, the two primary hip abductors, are most active during the first 40% of the gait cycle, especially during single-limb support. The primary function of the abductors is to control the slight lowering of the contralateral pelvis on the side of the swing limb (review Figure 15-17). After this eccentric action, these muscles act concentrically to initiate the relative abduction of the hip that occurs in later stance. As described earlier in this chapter and extensively in Chapter 12, adequate frontal plane torque from the hip abductor muscles is crucial for frontal plane stability during gait. A cane used in the hand contralateral to the weak hip abductors is an effective way to reduce the demands placed on the weakened abductors, thereby reducing excessive frontal plane movement of the pelvis resulting from body weight (see Chapter 12).

The hip abductors also control the alignment of the femur in the frontal plane. Inadequate muscular activation may result in excessive adduction of the femur, causing poor alignment of the lower extremity and excessive valgus torque at the knee during the stance phase. Other accessory roles of the gluteus medius include assisting with hip flexion and internal rotation, using anterior fibers, and assisting with hip extension and external rotation, using posterior fibers.

HIP ADDUCTORS AND HIP ROTATORS

The hip adductors show two bursts of activity during gait.[204] The first burst occurs at heel contact and the second just after toe off. The initial burst of activity serves to stabilize the hip through coactivation with the hip extensors and hip abductors. It is probable that the adductor magnus and other adductors assist with hip extension at this time in the gait cycle. The second burst of activity, after toe off, likely assists with initiating hip flexion. As illustrated in Figure 12-34, the adductors have a moment arm to extend the hip when it is flexed (i.e., the hip position at heel contact) and a moment arm to flex the hip when it is in extension (i.e., the hip position at toe off).

The hip internal rotators (tensor fascia lata, gluteus minimus, and anterior fibers of the gluteus medius) are active throughout much of the stance phase. During this time, these internal rotators move the contralateral side of the pelvis forward in the horizontal plane, thereby assisting with advancement of the swing limb (see Figure 12-36).

The hip external rotators, consisting of the six short external rotators, the posterior fibers of the gluteus medius, and the gluteus maximus, are most active during early stance. These muscles, in conjunction with the hip internal rotators, control the alignment of the hip in the horizontal plane. In particular, they control pelvic rotation while the lower limb is fixed to the ground. Consider the important action of these rotators in the rapid change of direction during walking or running.

Eccentric activation of the external rotators may be especially important to the control of the internal rotation of the lower limb in early stance (review Figure 15-25). Inadequate strength or control of the external rotators may result in excessive internal rotation of the femur, often seen in conjunction with excessive foot pronation.

Knee

Two muscle groups play a critical role at the knee during ambulation: the knee extensors and knee flexors.[22,42,78,101,187]

KNEE EXTENSORS

As a group, the quadriceps is active in the very late stage of the swing phase in preparation for heel contact (see Figure 15-29, *B*). The major burst of activity, however, occurs shortly after heel contact. The function of the quadriceps at this time is to control the knee flexion that takes place in the first 10% of the gait cycle. Eccentric activation serves to cushion the rate of weight acceptance on the lower extremity (i.e., shock absorption) and to prevent excessive knee flexion. The quadriceps then acts concentrically to extend the knee and support the weight of the body during mid stance.

Nene and colleagues critically compared the EMG activity of the rectus femoris and vasti components of the quadriceps during walking.[136] They established that the rectus femoris was *not* active at heel contact as traditionally thought, but only before and after toe off. The function of the rectus femoris at toe off is likely aimed at controlling the extent of knee flexion. By using both surface and intramuscular electrodes in this study, Nene and co-workers concluded that the burst of rectus femoris electromyographic signal typically reported at heel contact in the literature (and shown in Figure 15-29, *B*) is a result of cross-talk from the underlying vastus intermedius muscle.[136]

In summary, it appears that the muscular components within the quadriceps have different functions during gait, at least as expressed during normal walking speed. Being active at heel contact, the vasti function primarily as shock absorbers. According to Andersson and colleagues,[4] the rectus femoris may assist with this action during walking at speeds that exceed 2 m/sec and during running. The primary function of the rectus femoris in gait occurs in the transition from stance to swing phase and appears directed at assisting with initiating hip flexion as well as controlling knee flexion.

KNEE FLEXORS

The hamstrings are most active from a period just before to just after heel contact. Before heel contact, the hamstrings decelerate knee extension in preparation for the placement of the foot on the ground. During the initial 10% of stance, the hamstrings are active to assist with hip extension and to provide stability to the knee through coactivation. The short head of the biceps femoris may also assist with knee flexion during the swing phase. Most of the knee flexion during pre-swing and the swing phase of gait is performed passively as a result of the flexing hip and a small gastrocnemius activation.[164,204]

Ankle and Foot

At the ankle and foot, several muscles play a crucial role in normal gait: the tibialis anterior, extensor digitorum, extensor hallucis longus, gastrocnemius, soleus, tibialis posterior, and fibularis longus and brevis.[*]

TIBIALIS ANTERIOR

The tibialis anterior has two periods of activity. At heel contact, a strong eccentric activation is present to decelerate the passive plantar flexion of the ankle caused by the weight of the body being applied on the most posterior section of the calcaneus. If unopposed by the eccentric activation of the tibialis anterior and other ankle dorsiflexors, this large, passive plantar flexion torque results in the gait deviation referred to as "foot slap." This term is derived from the characteristic sound made by the foot slapping the ground just after heel contact. From heel contact to foot flat, the tibialis anterior may also assist with decelerating foot pronation, also through eccentric activation. The poor mechanical advantage of the muscle to invert the foot, however, raises some doubt with regard to the effectiveness of the tibialis anterior in strongly controlling foot pronation.

The second period of activation of the tibialis anterior occurs during the swing phase. The purpose of this activation is to produce sufficient dorsiflexion of the ankle to clear the toes from the ground. Extreme weakness of the tibialis anterior and the other ankle dorsiflexors typically results in a "drop foot" during the swing phase. As a mechanism of compensation, the individual typically excessively flexes the knee and hip during swing. Other compensatory maneuvers, such as vaulting, hip circumduction, and hip hiking (illustrated later in this chapter), may also be adopted to clear the toes from the ground. A common remedy for a drop-foot is a posterior ankle-foot orthosis that passively maintains ankle dorsiflexion during swing.

EXTENSOR DIGITORUM AND EXTENSOR HALLUCIS LONGUS

Similar to the tibialis anterior, the extensor digitorum longus and extensor hallucis longus decelerate plantar flexion of the ankle at heel contact. These muscles, however, lack the line of force to decelerate foot pronation during loading response and mid stance. During the swing phase, the toe extensors assist with dorsiflexion of the ankle and extend the toes to ensure that the toes clear the ground. Minor activity of the extensor digitorum longus and extensor hallucis longus during push off may provide stability to the ankle through coactivation with the ankle plantar flexors.[204]

ANKLE PLANTAR FLEXORS

The soleus and gastrocnemius (triceps surae) are active throughout most of the stance phase, with the notable exception of the first 10% of the gait cycle. During this period, plantar flexion of the foot is controlled by an eccentric action of the ankle dorsiflexors. From about 10% of the gait cycle to heel off (approximately 30% to 40% of the gait cycle), the ankle plantar flexors are active eccentrically to control the

---

*References 22, 42, 61, 78, 101, 124, 187, 191.

Role of Triceps Surae

Work by Stewart and colleagues[175] provides some interesting additional insight into the functional role of the triceps surae in the stance phase of walking. In a healthy group of subjects, electrical stimulation of the soleus during the stance phase led to a reduced amount of knee flexion during this part of the gait cycle. In contrast, electrical stimulation of the biarticular gastrocnemius during the stance phase produced greater than normal knee flexion, as well as an increased ankle dorsiflexion. These findings suggest a complex biomechanical link between the sagittal plane control of the knee and ankle during the stance phase. Such a disruption in control of these two joints is often seen in individuals with certain neuromuscular diseases.

forward movement of the tibia and fibula relative to the talus (i.e., ankle dorsiflexion). Excessive or uncontrolled forward movement of the leg results in exaggerated ankle dorsiflexion and possibly uncontrolled knee flexion.

The major burst of activity of the ankle plantar flexors occurs near heel off and decreases rapidly to near zero at toe off. During this brief period, shortening of the muscles creates an ankle plantar flexion torque that participates in the forward propulsion of the body. This action is referred to as *push off.*

The gastrocnemius also generates low-level muscular activity in initial swing, presumably to help with knee flexion. Note that because the rectus femoris is also active during initial swing, a small amount of coactivation of the knee flexors and extensors is taking place.[204]

The other plantar flexors of the ankle (tibialis posterior, flexor hallucis longus, flexor digitorum longus, and peroneals) assist the gastrocnemius-soleus group in the previously described actions. Some additional actions of these muscles are noteworthy.

TIBIALIS POSTERIOR

The tibialis posterior, a potent supinator muscle of the foot, is active from 5% to 55% of the gait cycle. Tibialis posterior decelerates pronation of the foot at between 5% and about 35% of the cycle and supinates the foot at between 35% and 55% (mid stance to toe off) of the cycle.[87] The tibialis posterior muscle acts on both the foot and the tibia throughout mid and late stance phase of gait. Based on its line of pull, shortening of this muscle could supinate the rearfoot (and raise the arch of the foot) as it simultaneously externally rotates the lower leg relative to the foot. Indeed, both of these coupled kinematics occur as the tibialis posterior is active. Although speculation, it is interesting to consider how dorsiflexion of the talocrural joint (which occurs through 50% of the gait

"Bottom-up" or "Top-down" Control of the Global "Pronation" of the Lower Extremity during Early Stance

As described earlier in the chapter and textbook, an important kinesiologic component of the loading response period of the gait cycle is a global internal rotation of the lower extremity in conjunction with pronation of the foot. This motion is often loosely described clinically as global "pronation" of the entire lower extremity. Such motion, when controlled, provides at least two useful biomechanical functions. First, the pronation at the subtalar joint (in particular its horizontal component) allows for dissipation of the residual internal rotation of the lower limb after heel contact. Second, pronation at the subtalar joint acts in concert with a controlled lowering of the medial longitudinal arch—both movements designed to help absorb some of the impact of loading. To be most effective, the overall "pronation response" of the lower limb must be performed within limited amplitude and prescribed duration. In worst-case scenarios, excessive lower limb pronation, especially during participation in sports that involve running and jumping, may result in a "medial collapse" of the knee, potentially leading to a variety of lower extremity pathologies, including patellofemoral pain syndrome[148] and noncontact injury of the anterior cruciate ligament.[40]

A fundamental clinically relevant question relates to the source of the initiation and control of the global pronation of the lower extremity during the early part of the stance phase of walking and running.[74,148] Because of the weight-bearing nature of the stance phase, it has long been presumed that internal rotation of the lower extremity occurs *in response* to the overall pronation pattern of the foot. Pronation of the foot causes internal rotation of the tibia, which in turn leads to internal rotation of the femur. This view suggests a "bottom-up" kinesiologic control of global pronation of the lower extremity and is the basis for prescribing specialized footwear and foot orthoses for persons who demonstrate excessive (and pain-producing) global pronation of the entire lower extremity.[74]

Conversely, a more recent view advocating a "top-down" control of global lower limb pronation has been proposed. Based on this perspective, excessive pronation of the entire lower extremity primarily results from too much internal rotation and adduction of the femur secondary to inadequate activation or strength of the hip external rotator and abductor muscles throughout but especially during early stance.[121,170] This poorly controlled femoral motion would lead to excessive internal rotation of the tibia and ultimately excessive pronation of the foot. Proponents of this top-down perspective infer that correction of excessive pronation of the lower limb and the associated "medial collapse" of the knee is best achieved through therapeutic efforts that improve the control and strength of the musculature of the hip.

It is likely that both the bottom-up and top-down kinesiologic perspectives are complementary as opposed to exclusionary. Continued clinical and biomechanical research is required to further refine diagnostic and treatment approaches for individuals with lower extremity pathologies related to excessive or poorly controlled global pronation of the lower extremity.

cycle) may serve to stretch this muscle at a time when it may be overshortening during its coupled external rotation-supination action on the lower leg and foot. Maintaining adequate length (and tension) in this muscle at this time may assist in raising the medial longitudinal arch and adding the necessary rigidity to the foot to prepare for its impending push off.

There is evidence in the literature that individuals with excessively pronated (flat) feet exhibit greater activation of supinator muscles such as the tibialis posterior, tibialis anterior, and flexor hallucis longus.[124] Active individuals with overly pronated feet may develop overuse and subsequent strain of the supinator muscles as they attempt to control the excessive pronation bias of the foot during early stance.

The tibialis posterior receives special attention in the treatment of people with cerebral palsy. The often hyperactive tibialis posterior, along with the soleus muscle, may cause an equinovarus deformity of the foot and ankle, resulting in the individual's walking on a foot that is plantar flexed and supinated.

FIBULARIS MUSCLES

The fibularis brevis and longus are active from about 10% of the gait cycle to just before toe off. In addition to their function as plantar flexors, these pronator (evertor) muscles help counteract the strong inversion effect caused by activation of the tibialis posterior and other deep posterior muscles. The fibularis longus also assists in the kinematics of the foot by holding the first ray rigidly to the ground, which provides a firm base of support for the action of the foot as a rigid lever during the terminal stance and pre-swing phases of gait.

INTRINSIC MUSCLES OF THE FOOT

The intrinsic muscles of the foot are typically active from mid stance to toe off (30% to 60% of the gait cycle). These muscles stabilize the forefoot and raise the medial longitudinal arch, thereby providing a rigid lever for ankle plantar flexion in terminal stance and pre-swing. They also likely help with controlling toe extension between heel off and toe off.

KINETICS

Understanding the forces that are responsible for movement during gait plays a critical role in understanding normal and pathologic movement. Although the kinetics (study of forces) of walking are not visually observable, they are ultimately responsible for the observed kinematics.

Ground Reaction Forces

During ambulation, forces are applied under the surface of the foot every time a person takes a step. The forces applied to the ground by the foot are called *foot forces*. Conversely, the forces applied to the foot by the ground are called *ground* (or *floor*) *reaction forces*. These forces are of equal magnitude but opposite direction. (Newton's Third Law—the law of action and reaction—states that forces are always present in pairs, equal in magnitude and opposite in direction.) This chapter focuses primarily on ground reaction forces because of the impact they potentially have on the body.

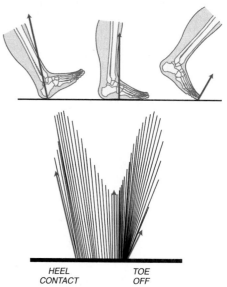

FIGURE 15-30. The bottom portion of the figure illustrates the classic "butterfly" representation of the ground reaction forces for a step. Each line represents the resultant force from the vector addition of the vertical and anterior-posterior forces at regular time intervals (i.e., every 10 msec in this case). The top portion of the figure represents how the successive lines from the "butterfly" reflect the progression of force application under the foot from heel contact to toe off. The vectors in red indicate heel contact, mid stance, and toe off. (Data from Whittle M: *Gait analysis: an introduction,* ed 4, Oxford, 2007, Butterworth-Heinemann.)

The description of the ground reaction forces follows a Cartesian coordinate system, with the forces being expressed along three orthogonal axes: vertical, anterior-posterior, and medial-lateral. The vector summation of the three forces gives a single resultant force vector between the foot and the ground. Such vector summation performed for the vertical and anterior-posterior components of the ground reaction forces leads to the classic "butterfly" representation of the ground reaction forces for a single step (Figure 15-30).

Peak Ground Reaction Forces
(as a Percent of Body Weight)
- Vertical: 120% body weight (BW)
- Anterior-posterior: 20% BW
- Medial-lateral: 5% BW

VERTICAL FORCES

The vertical forces are those directed perpendicular to the supporting surface. These vertical ground reaction forces peak twice in a given gait cycle. Forces are slightly greater than body weight at the time of the loading response and again at the time of terminal stance (see Figure 15-31, *A* and *C*). During mid stance, the ground reaction forces are slightly less than body weight. This fluctuation in force is a result of the vertical acceleration of the body's CoM. (Force is a function of mass and acceleration: $F = ma$.) At the time of loading response, the body's CoM is moving downward (review Figure 15-13). A vertical ground reaction force greater than one's body weight, therefore, is needed to initially decelerate the downward movement of the body and then accelerate it

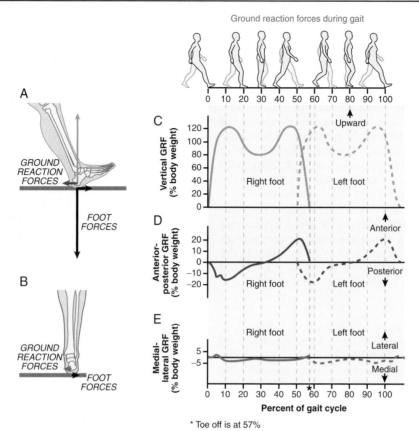

FIGURE 15-31. Ground reaction forces (GRFs) during gait. **A** illustrates the vertical *(orange arrows)* and anterior-posterior GRFs *(red arrows)* and foot forces *(black arrows)* at 10% of gait cycle. **B** illustrates the medial-lateral forces at 10% of gait cycle. **C, D,** and **E** show the GRFs for a gait cycle. Dashed lines are data for the stance phase on the left foot.

upward. (This is similar to jumping on a bathroom scale and briefly reading a weight that is higher than static body weight.) At mid stance, the vertical ground reaction forces are less than body weight as a result of a relative "unweighting" caused by the upward momentum of the body gained during the early part of stance. The higher ground reaction force at terminal stance reflects the combined push provided by the plantar flexors and the need to reverse the downward movement of the body that occurs in terminal stance through pre-swing.

ANTERIOR-POSTERIOR FORCES

In the anterior-posterior direction, shear forces are applied parallel to the supporting surface. At heel contact the ground reaction force is in the posterior direction (i.e., the foot applies an anteriorly directed force to the ground) (see Figure 15-31, *D*). At that time, sufficient friction is required between the foot and the ground to prevent the foot from slipping forward (picture the classic cartoon of a person falling to the ground after slipping on a banana peel). As the magnitude of the ground reaction force in the horizontal direction increases with longer steps and a faster walking speed, requirements for friction between the foot and the ground to prevent the foot from slipping increase.[33,76,106] Accordingly, the required coefficient of friction for ambulation is calculated as the ratio of the resultant shear force (which is the vector addition of the combined horizontal forces in the anterior-posterior and medial-lateral directions) divided by the vertical force applied under the foot.[20,33] Strategies to prevent slipping are minimiz-

ing the distance between foot location and the CoM of the body and reducing walking speed. This is why people often take shorter and narrower steps when walking on an icy surface–they are decreasing the demand for friction by keeping the feet nearly directly under the CoM.

During terminal stance and pre-swing, the ground reaction force is directed anteriorly, with the foot applying a posteriorly directed force to the ground to propel the body forward. The magnitude of the propulsive force depends on walking speed and, especially, attempts to accelerate. Inadequate friction between the foot and the ground at this time often causes the foot to slide backward without propelling the body forward. This explains the difficulty experienced when one accelerates quickly while walking on a slippery surface.

The peak anterior-posterior ground reaction force is typically equal to about 20% of body weight. These shear forces are in large part the result of the CoM of the body being either posterior (at heel contact) or anterior (at terminal stance and pre-swing) to the foot. The larger the step length, the greater the shear forces because of the greater angle between the lower extremity and the floor. Inertial properties of the body, such as momentum, also contribute to anterior-posterior ground reaction forces.

The posteriorly directed ground reaction force at heel contact momentarily slows the forward progression of the body. Conversely, the body is momentarily accelerated forward at toe off as a result of an anteriorly directed ground reaction force. Note that the propulsive force of one limb is applied simultaneously with the braking force of the opposite limb during the times of double-limb support (see Figure 15-31, *D*). When one walks at a constant velocity, the propulsive force occurring late in stance balances the braking force occurring early in stance. Because these forces are of relatively equal magnitude but of opposite direction, they provide balance to the body when the weight is transferred from one lower extremity to the other at the time of double-limb support. Slowing down requires a greater braking force than propulsive force, and speeding up requires the opposite.

MEDIAL-LATERAL FORCES

The magnitude of the ground reaction force in the medial-lateral direction is relatively small (i.e., less than 5% of body weight) and more variable across individuals (see Figure 15-31, *B* and *E*). As with anterior-posterior shear force, the magnitude and direction of this shear force depends mostly on the relationship between the position of the body's CoM and the location of the foot. During the initial 5% or so of the gait cycle, a small, laterally directed ground reaction shear force is produced to stop the small lateral-to-medial velocity of the foot that is typically present at the time of heel contact. During the rest of stance phase, however, the CoM of the body is medial to the foot (review Figure 15-13), causing a laterally directed force to be applied to the ground by the foot and therefore a medially directed ground reaction force. These medially directed ground reaction forces throughout stance initially decelerate the lateral movement of the CoM. Then, these ground reaction forces accelerate the CoM medially toward the contralateral lower extremity, which is swinging forward and preparing to make the next foot contact with the ground.

Although the action of the medial-lateral ground reaction forces may not be easily felt during normal gait, they can be readily felt during walking while taking very large steps or when jumping from side to side. In fact, greater peak values in medial-lateral ground reaction forces are often seen in individuals with wider step widths. The need for friction can again be appreciated by observing someone walking on ice. Individuals walking on icy surfaces reduce their step widths almost as if they were walking on a tightrope. This learned adaptation is intended to keep the body's CoM directly over the feet to minimize the medial-lateral ground reaction forces and therefore the need for friction. Ice skaters make use of these medial-lateral ground reaction forces to propel their bodies forward. This is achieved by using a blade that digs into the ice, providing an adequate resistance for propulsion.

Path of the Center of Pressure

The path of the center of pressure (CoP) under the foot throughout stance follows a relatively reproducible pattern (Figure 15-32). (The term *pressure* is used to describe the ground reaction force related to its specific area of application.) At heel contact, the CoP is located just lateral to the midpoint of the heel. It then moves progressively to the lateral midfoot region at mid stance, and to the medial forefoot region (under the first or second metatarsal head) during heel off to toe off. The location of the CoP helps to explain the tendency for the ankle and foot to plantar flex and evert, respectively, at heel contact (Figure 15-33). Both tendencies are partially controlled by eccentric activation of ankle muscles, namely the ankle dorsiflexors, including the tibialis anterior.

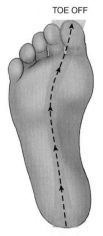

Path of the center of pressure on the plantar surface of the foot

FIGURE 15-32. Path of the center of pressure (CoP) under the foot from heel contact to toe off. The shaded area is representative of individual variability of the path of the CoP.

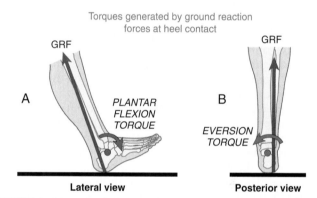

FIGURE 15-33. At heel contact, the point and direction of application of the ground reaction force *(GRF)* on the calcaneus falls posterior to the axis of rotation of the talocrural joint *(green circle),* thereby creating a plantar flexion torque at the ankle **(A).** This external torque requires the generation of an opposing dorsiflexion internal torque by the ankle dorsiflexors. In **B,** the lateral location of the ground reaction force on the calcaneus (relative to its near midpoint depicted as a purple circle) produces an eversion torque at the subtalar joint. This tendency is partially controlled by action of the tibialis anterior.

Joint Torques and Powers

During gait, the ground reaction forces applied under the foot generate an *external torque* on the joints of the lower extremities. This fact is illustrated in Figure 15-34. During the loading response on the right limb, the line of action of the ground reaction force is located behind the ankle and knee but anterior to the hip. As a consequence, the ground reaction forces at heel contact produce ankle plantar flexion, knee flexion, and hip flexion. To prevent collapse of the lower extremity, these external torques are resisted by *internal torques* created by the activation of the ankle dorsiflexors, the knee extensors, and the hip extensors.

A simplified analysis of the magnitude of the internal (muscular) torques, as could be derived from a body diagram similar to Figure 15-34, assumes a condition of static equilibrium. A more accurate calculation, however, requires the use of the inverse dynamic approach, which takes into account

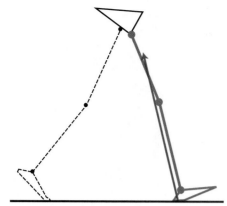

FIGURE 15-34. During the loading response the line of action of the ground reaction forces (posterior to the ankle, posterior to the knee, and anterior to the hip) promotes ankle plantar flexion, knee flexion, and hip flexion. (Modified from Whittle M: *Gait analysis: an introduction,* ed 4, Oxford, 2007, Butterworth-Heinemann.)

the dynamic nature of the action.[5] This approach requires the knowledge of the anthropometric characteristics of the individual's segment masses, location of the segments' CoM, segments' mass center inertia matrix, precise magnitude of body position and motion (each segment's linear and angular velocity), and ground reaction forces during the gait cycle (review Figure 15-5). In this chapter, much of the data on internal torques during walking are based on the inverse dynamic approach.

As stated previously, the activation of muscles creates most of the internal torques that control joint motion, especially in midrange positions. This internal torque is associated with concentric muscle activation when the joint moves in the direction of the muscle's action; in contrast, internal torque is associated with eccentric muscle activation when the joint moves in the direction opposite the muscle's action. In either case, the magnitude of the internal torque reasonably matches the description of muscular activation provided earlier in this chapter.

Internal torques can also be created by passive forces generated by the deformation and recoil of connective tissues, such as the capsule, tendons, and ligaments. It is not always possible to state with certainty the relative contribution of active and passive forces to the prevailing internal torque across a joint. In some cases, however, such as in the middle of the range of motion, it may be a fairly simple deductive process to identify the structures responsible (likely active muscles), but in other cases, such as near the end of the range of motion, contributions of both active and passive structures may need to be considered.[201] Many gait deviations associated with muscle weakness rely heavily on passive tensions created at the end range of a joint's position for the internal torques required for ambulation.

The literature often uses the term *net* internal joint torque in attempts to account for coactivation of agonist-antagonist muscle groups. For example, the flexion torque produced by the hip flexor muscles during the swing phase may be associated with slight (eccentric) activation of muscles that extend the hip. In theory, this extensor torque subtracts from the hip flexion torque, thereby yielding a net flexion torque. Although during walking this antagonistic torque is likely small, it is something to consider, especially in pathology such as stroke

or Parkinson's disease. This chapter does not consistently use the modifying term *net*, although it is implied.

The concept of internal torque provides valuable insight into the role of particular muscles and connective tissues in controlling a joint during walking. Internal torque does not, however, describe the *rate* of work performed by the muscles or passive deformation of connective tissues; this requires knowledge of power. Joint power is the product of the net internal joint torque and the joint angular velocity. Joint power reflects the net rate of generating or absorbing energy by all muscles and other connective tissues crossing a joint. A positive value indicates power *generation*, which reflects concentric muscle activation and a release of energy from previously stretched connective tissues. A negative value, in contrast, indicates power *absorption*, which reflects eccentric muscle activation and the stretching of passive connective tissues.[201] The concept of power generation and absorption may be better understood with the example of performing a jump. During the initial squatting movement preceding a jump, most muscles of the lower extremities work eccentrically, absorbing energy. This energy is then released by a concentric muscle activation and release of energy from stretched connective tissues during the upward movement of the body. Application of this concept in the field of strength building is known as *plyometric training.*

It must be reemphasized that power generation and absorption are based on the *product* of angular velocity and internal torque. Consider, for example, that even a large internal torque may create only a small amount of power if the angular velocity is very low. Alternatively, the same torque creates a very large power if the angular velocity is large. This concept is important to consider when interpreting the data provided in Figures 15-35, 15-36, 15-38, and 15-42.[9,204,205]

The following sections highlight the primary torques and powers generated during walking. These sections also provide figures that summarize the kinematics and kinetics of the hip, knee, and ankle in the sagittal plane, and the hip in the frontal plane. Careful study of these figures should provide an increased understanding of the relationships among joint motion, torque, power, and muscle activation during gait. There is overall strong agreement in the literature on the pattern and magnitude of the torque and power data in the sagittal plane during ambulation. But as with the kinematic data, as torque and power are partially derived from the kinematic data, there is more variation in the literature for frontal and especially horizontal plane torque and power data.[54,72,104,116,159]

Analysis of joint torques and powers gives a more complete picture of the biomechanics of gait.[44,65,102,152,201] These variables help establish the relative contribution of various joints and muscle groups to provide support and propulsion of the body.[19,89,105] The understanding and treatment of pathologic gait benefit from this type of information.

HIP

In the early part of stance phase, in the *sagittal plane,* the hip musculature generates a hip extension torque that serves to accept the weight of the body, control the forward momentum of the trunk, and extend the hip (Figure 15-35, *A* and *B*). In the second half of stance, a flexion torque is generated to initially decelerate hip extension and then initiate hip flexion before toe off. This hip flexion torque is the result of a combination of passive forces from structures anterior to the hip joint, including the joint capsule, and activity of the hip flexors.[201] In initial swing, a small hip flexion torque, corresponding to the concentric activation of the hip flexors, further assists hip flexion. In the second half of swing (at about 80% of the gait cycle), an extensor torque is needed to initially decelerate the movement of hip flexion, then initiate hip extension.

Figure 15-35, *C* shows the power curve for the hip in the sagittal plane. In the first 35% of the gait cycle, power is generated to support the body, raise the CoM, control the trunk, and propel the body forward.[205] Power is then absorbed until approximately 50% of the gait cycle is reached, reflecting the deceleration of hip extension secondary to resistance provided by the anterior hip structures and the eccentric activation of the hip flexors. In pre-swing and initial swing, power is generated to flex the hip.[201] A small amount of energy fluctuation takes place during the second half of swing, reflecting the combination of change in hip angular velocity and torque needed to first decelerate hip flexion then to initiate hip extension.

To complete the description of sagittal plane hip movement during gait, Figure 15-35, *D* illustrates the relative intensity and type of muscle activation of two primary antagonistic muscles of the hip. The areas of the electromyographic curve are coded to represent the muscles' presumed eccentric activation (shaded area) and concentric activation (hatched area), based on the direction of hip angular motion. In general, the muscular activations correlate with power absorption (eccentric action) and power generation (concentric action).

In the *frontal plane,* a large abduction torque occurs throughout the stance phase to support the mass of the body that is located medial to the hip joint (Figure 15-36, *A* and *B*). Power absorption occurs in the early part of stance (see Figure 15-36, *C*) as the opposite side of the pelvis is initially lowered (see Figure 15-36, *A*). These kinematics are controlled through eccentric activation of the hip abductors (see Figure 15-36, *D*). Two bursts of power generation are seen at approximately 20% and 50% of the gait cycle, as the contralateral pelvis is raised (see Figure 15-36, *C*).

In the *horizontal plane,* an external rotation torque is used to decelerate the internal rotation of the femur in the first 20% of the gait cycle (Figure 15-37, *A*). This torque is followed by an internal rotation torque that advances the contralateral side of the pelvis forward during the remainder of stance. Note the small magnitude of these torques, approximately 15% of those in the sagittal and frontal planes. The eccentric activation of the hip external rotators in the initial 20% of the gait cycle accounts for the power absorption noted at that time in Figure 15-37, *B*. However, as stated earlier, variability exists in the reporting of these horizontal plane data for the hip, partially attributed to their smaller magnitude, the difficulties in making accurate kinematic measurements in the horizontal plane, and various methods of data processing.[104,152,159,160]

KNEE

In the *sagittal plane,* at heel contact, a very brief (first 4% of the gait cycle) initial flexion torque presumably ensures that the knee is flexed to provide an adequate knee alignment for shock absorption (Figure 15-38, *A* and *B*). A large extension torque needed for the loading response quickly follows this brief flexion torque. This extensor torque continues until 20% of

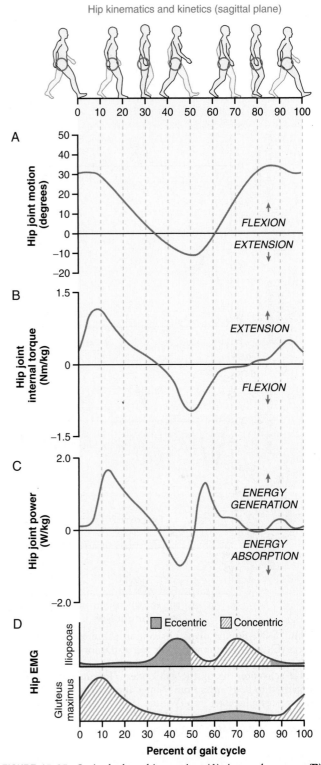

FIGURE 15-35. Sagittal plane hip motion **(A),** internal torques **(B),** powers **(C),** and electromyographic signal **(D)** for a gait cycle. The electromyographic curves represent the relative intensity of the muscle activation during the gait cycle. (Torque and power data normalized to body mass from Winter and colleagues, 1996,[205] and electromyographic data from Winter, 1991,[204] and Bechtol, 1975.[9]) As in Figure 15-29, note that electromyographic signal amplitude is illustrated so that its maximum value during the gait cycle fills the vertical dimension of the graphs. The signal is therefore normalized to the maximum value obtained during the gait cycle, not to its maximum capability to generate force.

Hip kinematics and kinetics (frontal plane)

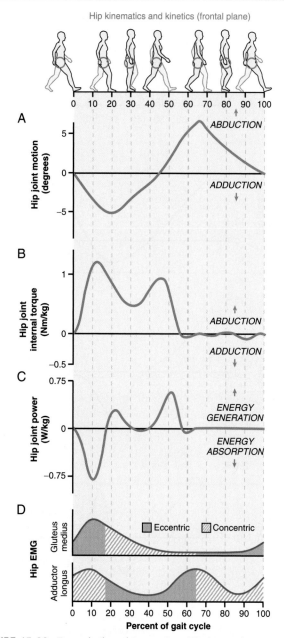

FIGURE 15-36. Frontal plane hip motion **(A)**, internal torques **(B)**, powers **(C)**, and electromyographic signal **(D)** for a gait cycle. The electromyographic curves represent the relative intensity of the muscle activation during the gait cycle. (Torque and power data normalized to body mass from Winter and colleagues, 1996,[205] and electromyographic data from Winter, 1991.[204]) See legend in Figure 15-35 for additional comments on the normalization of the electromyographic data. *EMG,* electromyography.

Hip kinetics (horizontal plane)

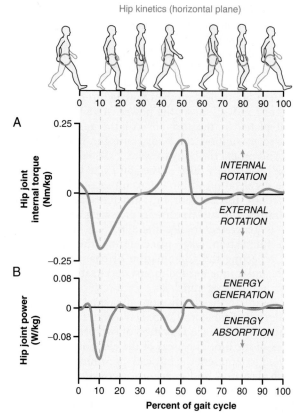

FIGURE 15-37. Horizontal plane internal torques **(A)** and powers **(B)** for the hip. (Data normalized to body mass from Winter DA, Eng JJ, Ishac M: Three-dimensional moments, powers and work in normal gait: implications for clinical assessments. In Harris GF, Smith PA, eds: *Human motion analysis: current applications and future directions,* New York, 1996, IEEE Press.)

control knee flexion. In terminal swing, an internal flexion torque is generated to decelerate knee extension.

The power curve for the sagittal plane reflects the action of the musculature surrounding the knee (see Figure 15-38, *C* and *D*). The short-duration power generation at early stance shows that the knee flexion torque creates flexion of the knee. Then power absorption momentarily takes place, reflecting the eccentric action of the quadriceps at 5% to 15% of the gait cycle). This is followed by another brief instant of power generation, indicating the start of knee extension produced by the continued knee extension torque. Just before toe off, at 50% to 60% of the gait cycle, power is absorbed by the knee extensors to control knee flexion. In the second half of the swing phase, the hamstrings absorb energy as the swing limb is decelerated (see Figure 15-38, *C* and *D*), until initiating knee flexion just before the next heel contact.

In the *frontal plane* (Figure 15-39, *A*), during stance, an internal abduction torque at the knee counters the external adduction (varus) torque created by the resultant ground reaction force passing medial to the knee (Figure 15-40). The internal abduction torque is created by a combination of active and passive structures, including the iliotibial band, the tensor fascia lata, and the lateral ligaments of the knee. Despite the large torques (see Figure 15-39, *A*), power values in this plane are very low because of the very small amount of knee movement and hence low angular velocity during stance (see Figure 15-39, *B*). Nevertheless, the pattern of

gait has been reached, initially to control knee flexion, then to extend the knee. From 20% to 50% of the gait cycle, an internal flexion torque is present at the knee despite the knee extending at 20% to 40% of the gait cycle. Because little activity of the hamstrings is present at that time, the internal flexion torque likely results from passive tension in the posterior knee structures, including the capsule, that are being elongated. Knee flexion, in preparation for the swing phase, starts at 40% of the gait cycle, which matches the direction of the internal flexion torque at the knee at 40% to 50% of the gait cycle. Just before toe off, however, a small internal extension torque occurs to

Knee kinematics and kinetics (sagittal plane)

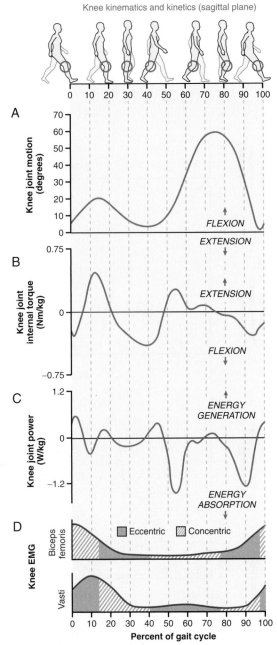

FIGURE 15-38. Sagittal plane knee motion **(A),** internal torques **(B),** powers **(C),** and electromyographic signal **(D)** for a gait cycle. The electromyographic curves represent the relative intensity of the muscle activation during the gait cycle. (Torque and power data normalized to body mass from Winter and colleagues, 1996,[205] and electromyographic data from Winter, 1991.[204]) See legend in Figure 15-35 for additional comments on normalization of the electromyographic data. *EMG,* electromyography.

Knee kinetics (frontal plane)

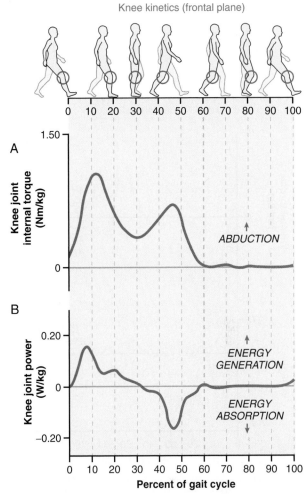

FIGURE 15-39. Frontal plane internal torques **(A)** and powers **(B)** for the knee. (Data normalized to body mass from Winter DA, Eng JJ, Ishac M: Three-dimensional moments, powers and work in normal gait: implications for clinical assessments. In Harris GF, Smith PA, eds: *Human motion analysis: current applications and future directions,* New York, 1996, IEEE Press.)

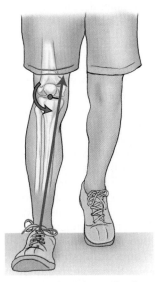

FIGURE 15-40. The instant of weight application on the foot during gait creates a varus torque at the knee.

initial energy generation followed by energy absorption suggests a small movement of knee abduction (valgus) initially followed by a small amount of knee adduction (varus).

In the *horizontal plane* the joint torques at the knee are similar to those at the hip, with an external rotation torque in the first half of stance and an internal rotation torque in the second half (Figure 15-41, *A*). These torques are likely passive, being generated by knee ligaments in response to the active hip torques created in the horizontal plane.[53] During loading response, a small amount of power is absorbed as the

Knee kinetics (horizontal plane)

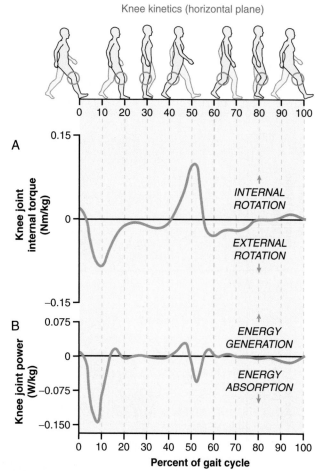

FIGURE 15-41. Horizontal plane internal torques **(A)** and powers **(B)** for the knee. (Data normalized to body mass from Winter DA, Eng JJ, Ishac M: Three-dimensional moments, powers and work in normal gait: implications for clinical assessments. In Harris GF, Smith PA, eds: *Human motion analysis: current applications and future directions,* New York, 1996, IEEE Press.)

knee's capsular and ligamentous structures resist the internal rotation motion of the femur on the tibia (or external rotation of the knee) (see Figure 15-41, *B*). Again, these torque and power values are of small magnitude in contrast to those in the sagittal and frontal planes.

ANKLE

In the *sagittal plane* a small dorsiflexion torque is generated at the ankle immediately after heel contact (Figure 15-42, *A* and *B*). This torque serves to control the movement of plantar flexion generated by the application of body weight on the calcaneus (review Figure 15-33). A plantar flexion torque prevails throughout the rest of stance, initially to control the tibia advancing over the foot, then to plantar flex the ankle at push off. A very small dorsiflexion torque is present during swing to keep the ankle dorsiflexed to clear the toes from the ground.

In the sagittal plane, power is absorbed just after heel contact as a result of the muscular deceleration of ankle plantar flexion (see Figure 15-42, *C*). Then some energy absorption occurs until push off, reflecting the eccentric activation of the plantar flexors at 10% to 40% of the gait cycle (see Figure 15-42, *D*), as the tibia is slowly advanced over the

Ankle kinematics and kinetics (sagittal plane)

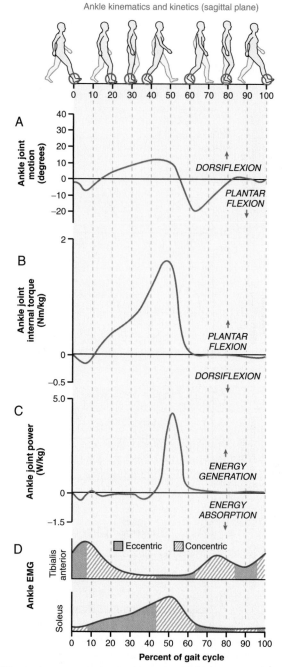

FIGURE 15-42. Sagittal plane ankle motion **(A)**, internal torques **(B)**, powers **(C)**, and electromyographic signal **(D)** for a gait cycle. The electromyographic curves represent the relative intensity of the muscle activation during the gait cycle. (Torque and power data normalized to body mass from Winter and colleagues, 1996,[205] and electromyographic data from Winter, 1991.[204]) See legend in Figure 15-35 for additional comments on normalization of the electromyographic data. *EMG,* electromyography.

foot. The relatively slow ankle angular displacement (and assumed velocity) at 10% to 40% of the gait cycle explains the small power values (see Figure 15-42, *C*). A large generation of energy occurs at push off (from 40% to 60% of the gait cycle) primarily as a result of a concentric action of the ankle plantar flexors, but with some contribution (approximately 10% to 15% of the power burst) from a return of the

Ankle kinetics (frontal plane)

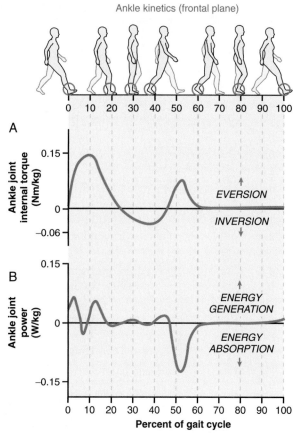

FIGURE 15-43. Frontal plane internal torques **(A)** and powers **(B)** for the ankle. (Data normalized to body mass from Winter DA, Eng JJ, Ishac M: Three-dimensional moments, powers and work in normal gait: implications for clinical assessments. In Harris GF, Smith PA, eds: *Human motion analysis: current applications and future directions,* New York, 1996, IEEE Press.)

Ankle kinetics (horizontal plane)

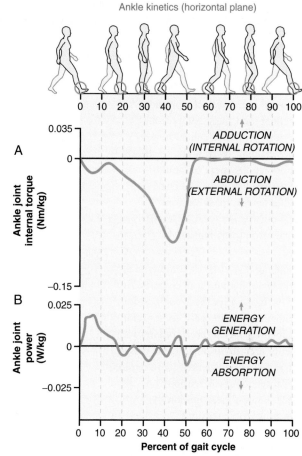

FIGURE 15-44. Horizontal plane internal torques **(A)** and powers **(B)** for the ankle. (Data normalized to body mass from Winter DA, Eng JJ, Ishac M: Three-dimensional moments, powers and work in normal gait: implications for clinical assessments. In Harris GF, Smith PA, eds: *Human motion analysis: current applications and future directions,* New York, 1996, IEEE Press.)

energy absorbed through stretching of the ankle plantar flexors before heel off. This power generation noted at push off is considered by many (although not all) to be the primary contributor to the forward propulsion of the body during normal gait, with gravity and the hip extensors also likely playing significant roles.[19,89,151]

The torques and especially the power values in the *frontal* and *horizontal planes* at the ankle are very small and exhibit large variation among people (Figures 15-43 and 15-44). In the frontal plane, stance phase is characterized by a small initial eversion torque (from 0% to 20% of gait) followed by an inversion torque (from 20% to 45% of gait) and a smaller eversion torque just before toe off.[205] In the horizontal plane an external rotation torque is present during the stance phase. This external rotation torque should in fact be called an *abduction torque* based on the description of ankle and foot movements provided in Chapter 14.

Joint and Tendon Forces

Joint surfaces, ligaments, and tendons are all subjected to large tensile, compressive, or shear forces during walking. Knowledge of the magnitude of these forces is of interest, especially to the clinician, orthopedic surgeon, and bioengineer. The design of surgical joint implants, in particular, requires these

types of data. Direct measurements in men and women are obviously not readily obtainable; therefore these forces are typically calculated indirectly through biomechanical analysis including modeling and optimization techniques.

Forces applied to various structures of the lower extremities during ambulation are presented in Table 15-6. These forces can be surprisingly large. Consider, for example, that the compressive force at the hip during ambulation at 1.4 m/ sec has been measured at 6.4 times body weight.[168]

GAIT DYSFUNCTIONS

Most of us take for granted our ability to walk. The fact is, unless we have personally experienced an injury or a physical impairment, we do not think of walking as a difficult task. The information provided thus far in this chapter, however, reminds us of the complexity of walking. Many actions must occur simultaneously at each part of the gait cycle for ambulation to take place with maximum efficiency.

Normal gait requires sufficient range of motion and strength at each participating joint. Walking also requires

TABLE 15-6. Magnitude of Forces (in Multitude of Body Weight) Applied to the Lower Extremity Structures during Ambulation at Various Speeds

Structures (Types of Force)	Magnitude (BW)	Speed*
Ankle		
Talocrural joint (peak compression)[168]	4.2	1.4 m/sec
Talocrural joint (peak compression)[32]	4.8	114 steps/min
Talocrural joint (peak compression)[162]	12.0	4.2 m/sec (running)
Talocrural joint (peak anterior shear†)[173]	0.6	116 steps/min
Talocrural joint (peak posterior shear†)[173]	0.3	116 steps/min
Achilles tendon (peak tension)[58]	2.0	1.5 m/sec
Achilles tendon (peak tension)[59]	4.0	1.7 m/sec
Achilles tendon (peak tension)[162]	7.0	4.2 m/sec (running)
Ankle dorsiflexors (peak tension)[32]	1.0	114 steps/min
Plantar fascia (peak tension)[162]	2.1	4.2 m/sec (running)
Knee		
Tibiofemoral joint (peak compression)[168]	4.6	1.4 m/sec
Patellofemoral joint (peak compression)[95]	0.3	1.0 m/sec
Patellofemoral joint (peak compression)[98]	1.5	1.5 m/sec
Patellofemoral joint (peak compression)[184]	0.8	1.0 m/sec
Patellofemoral joint (peak compression)[162]	9.0	4.2 m/sec (running)
Anterior cruciate ligament (peak tension)[32]	1.5	114 steps/min
Posterior cruciate ligament (peak tension)[32]	0.4	114 steps/min
Patellar tendon (peak tension)[59]	3.0	1.7 m/sec
Patellar tendon (peak tension)[162]	5.8	4.2 m/sec (running)
Hamstrings (peak tension)[32]	1.1	114 steps/min
Hip		
Hip (peak compression)[168]	6.4	1.4 m/sec
Hip (peak compression)[146]	3.1	0.9 m/sec
Adductor magnus (peak tension)[146]	0.3	0.9 m/sec
Gluteus medius (peak tension)[146]	0.5	0.9 m/sec

*m/sec, Meters per second.
†Direction of shear of tibia on talus.

sophisticated control of movement through the central nervous system. The complexity of walking creates many opportunities for the normal gait pattern to be affected by impairment. The adaptability of the system, however, creates many opportunities to modify the gait pattern to preserve "walking," despite even severe impairments. In these cases a normal gait pattern is sacrificed for the ability to move from one location to another independently. We have all used this ability to adapt gait, even if only for a painful blister under the foot or for walking on hot sand at the beach. In essence, an abnormal or a pathologic gait pattern reflects an effort to preserve ambulation through adaptation. The cost of gait deviation is, typically, increased energy expenditure and application of abnormal stresses to the body.

Three common causes of pathologic gait patterns are listed in the box. Each includes many specific and general pathologies. The observed deviations may be the direct reflection of the specific impairment, or they may be a biomechanical compensation for some aspect of the impairment. The features of pathologic gait therefore depend on the nature of the impairment as well as the ability of the individual to compensate for that impairment.

Causes of Pathologic Gait Patterns
- Pain
- Central nervous system disorders
- Musculoskeletal system impairments

Pain can cause an abnormal gait pattern that is often referred to as an *antalgic gait.* The pattern of weight avoidance on the painful limb often leads to characteristic features. The primary findings are a shorter step length, in conjunction with decreased stance time on the painful side. If the pain is related to hip joint compression from hip abductor muscle activation, lateral displacement of the head and trunk toward the painful weight-bearing lower extremity occurs (see Chapter 12). If the source of pain is other than the hip, the trunk may lean slightly toward the swing limb in an attempt to alleviate weight bearing on the injured stance limb.

Many neurologic disorders, such as cerebrovascular accidents (CVAs), Parkinson's disease, and cerebral palsy, can cause abnormal gait patterns.[39,45,177] Spasticity of muscles, defined as increased tone and resistance to stretch, results in inappropriate muscle activity and increased stiffness. It often affects the extensor musculature of individuals with cerebral palsy and CVA, resulting in a gait pattern that appears stiff-legged, accompanied by a tendency to circumduct and scuff the toes. Hyperactive hip adductors may contribute to a scissoring gait pattern. Parkinson's disease is associated with a lack of arm swing, flexed trunk, and short accelerating steps, also called *festinating gait*. Cerebellar lesions are associated with an ataxic gait pattern characterized by unsteady uncoordinated steps and a wide base of support. Apraxia, defined as a disorder of voluntary movement, occurs in some disease processes affecting the elderly. Gait apraxia may result in an ambulation pattern characterized by a wide base of support, short stride, and shuffling. Individuals with impaired sensory function and balance may show an unsteady gait pattern.[165] With neurologic disorders, the primary cause of gait dysfunction is an inability to generate and control appropriate levels of muscle force.

Deficits in the musculoskeletal system, such as excessive or limited joint range of motion and/or limited muscle strength, can cause a wide variety of gait deviations. Abnormal joint range of motion may occur secondary to injury, tightness, or contracture of connective tissues and muscles; abnormal joint structure; joint instability; or congenital connective tissue laxity. In most cases, abnormal range of motion in one joint leads to some form of compensation in one or more surrounding joints. Muscular weakness may result from disuse atrophy after an injury or a limited neural drive secondary to a peripheral neural injury. Whatever the cause, weakness ultimately leads to modification of the gait pattern. Tables 15-7 through 15-12 and Figures 15-45 through 15-50 present some of the most common gait deviations observed in the general population.

Text continued on page 671.

TABLE 15-7. Gait Deviations at the Ankle and Foot Secondary to Specific Ankle and Foot Impairments*

Observed Gait Deviation at the Ankle or Foot	Likely Impairment	Selected Pathologic Precursors	Mechanical Rationale and/or Associated Compensations
"Foot slap": rapid ankle plantar flexion occurs after **heel contact.**[†] The name *foot slap* is derived from the characteristic noise made by the forefoot hitting the ground.	Mild weakness of ankle dorsiflexors	Common peroneal nerve palsy and distal peripheral neuropathy	Ankle dorsiflexors have sufficient strength to dorsiflex the ankle during swing but not enough to control ankle plantar flexion after heel contact. No other gait deviations.
"Foot flat": Entire plantar aspect of the foot touches the ground at **initial contact,**[‡] followed by normal, passive ankle dorsiflexion during the rest of stance.	Marked weakness of ankle dorsiflexors	Common peroneal nerve palsy and distal peripheral neuropathy	Sufficient strength of the dorsiflexors to partially, but not completely, dorsiflex the ankle during swing. Normal dorsiflexion occurs during stance as long as the ankle has normal range of motion. No other gait deviations.
Initial contact with the ground is made by the forefoot followed by the heel region. Normal passive ankle dorsiflexion occurs during stance.	Severe weakness of ankle dorsiflexors	Common peroneal nerve palsy and distal peripheral neuropathy	No active ankle dorsiflexion is possible during swing. Normal dorsiflexion occurs during stance as long as the ankle has normal range of motion. Likely requires excessive knee and hip flexion during swing to avoid catching the toes on the ground.
Initial contact is made with the forefoot, but the heel never makes contact with the ground during stance.	Heel pain Plantar flexion contracture (pes equinus deformity) or spasticity of ankle plantar flexors	Calcaneal fracture, plantar fasciitis Upper motor neuron lesion, cerebral palsy, cerebrovascular accident (CVA)	Purposeful strategy to avoid weight bearing on the heel. To maintain the weight over the forefoot, the knee and hip are kept in flexion throughout stance, leading to a "crouched gait." Requires short steps.
Initial contact is made with the forefoot, and the heel is brought to the ground by a posterior displacement of the tibia at midstance (see Figure 15-45).	Plantar flexion contracture (pes equinus deformity) or spasticity of ankle plantar flexors	Upper motor neuron lesion (cerebral palsy, CVA) Ankle fusion in a plantar flexed position	Knee hyperextension occurs during stance owing to the inability of the tibia to move forward over the foot. Hip flexion and excessive forward trunk lean during terminal stance occur to shift the weight of the body over the foot.
Premature elevation of the heel in **mid or terminal stance.**	Lack of ankle dorsiflexion	Congenital or acquired muscular tightness of ankle plantar flexors	Characteristic bouncing gait pattern.

Continued

TABLE 15-7. Gait Deviations at the Ankle and Foot Secondary to Specific Ankle and Foot Impairments—cont'd

Observed Gait Deviation at the Ankle or Foot	Likely Impairment	Selected Pathologic Precursors	Mechanical Rationale and/or Associated Compensations
Heel remains in contact with the ground late in **terminal stance.**	Weakness or flaccid paralysis of plantar flexors with or without a fixed dorsiflexed position of the ankle (pes calcaneus deformity)	Peripheral or central nervous system disorders Excessive surgical lengthening of the Achilles tendon	Excessive ankle dorsiflexion results in prolonged heel contact, reduced push off, and a shorter step length.
Supinated foot position and weight bearing on the lateral aspect of the foot during **stance.**	Pes cavus deformity	Congenital structural deformity	A high medial longitudinal arch is noted with reduced midfoot mobility throughout swing and stance
Excessive foot pronation occurs during **stance,** with failure of the foot to supinate in mid stance. Normal medial longitudinal arch noted during swing.	Rearfoot varus and/or forefoot varus	Congenital or acquired structural deformity	Excessive foot pronation and associated flattening of the medial longitudinal arch may be accompanied by a general internal rotation of the lower extremity during stance.
Excessive foot pronation with weight bearing on the medial portion of the foot during **stance.** The medial longitudinal arch remains absent during **swing.**	Weakness (paralysis) of ankle invertors Pes planus deformity	Upper motor neuron lesion Congenital structural deformity	An overall excessive internal rotation of the lower extremity during stance is possible.
Excessive inversion and plantar flexion of the foot and ankle occur during **swing** and at **initial contact.**	Pes equinovarus deformity caused by spasticity of the plantar flexors and invertors	Upper motor neuron lesion (cerebral palsy, CVA)	Contact with the ground is made with the lateral border of the forefoot. Weight bearing on the lateral border of the foot during stance.
Ankle remains plantar flexed during **swing** and can be associated with dragging of the toes, typically called *drop foot* (see Figure 15-46).	Weakness of dorsiflexors and/or pes equinus deformity	Common peroneal nerve palsy	Hip hiking, hip circumduction, or excessive hip and knee flexion of the swing lower extremity or vaulting of the stance limb may be noted to lift the toes off the ground and prevent the toes from dragging during swing.

*Within this context, an impairment is a loss or an abnormality in physiologic or anatomic structure or function.

†The terms in bold indicate when in the gait cycle the gait deviation is expressed.

‡*Initial contact* is often used instead of *heel contact* to reflect the fact that with many gait deviations the heel is not the section of the foot that makes initial contact with the ground.

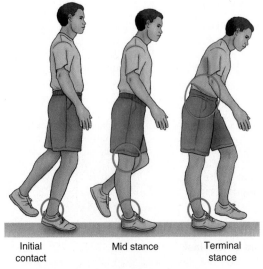

FIGURE 15-45. Individuals with an ankle plantar flexion contracture will make initial contact with the ground with the forefoot region. At mid stance, bringing the heel to the ground will result in knee hyperextension. Forward lean of the trunk occurs in terminal stance as a strategy to maintain forward progression of the center of mass.

Initial contact   Mid stance   Terminal stance

○ Impairment: ankle plantar flexion contracture
○ Compensations: knee hyperextension (mid stance); forward trunk lean (terminal stance)

TABLE 15-8. Gait Deviations Seen at the Ankle and Foot as a Compensation for an Impairment of the Ipsilateral Knee, Ipsilateral Hip, or Contralateral Lower Extremity

Observed Gait Deviation at the Ankle or Foot	Likely Impairment	Mechanical Rationale
Vaulting: compensatory mechanism demonstrated by exaggerated ankle plantar flexion during **mid stance**;* leads to excessive vertical movement of the body (see Figure 15-47).	Any impairment of the contralateral lower extremity that reduces hip flexion, knee flexion, or ankle dorsiflexion during swing	Strategy used to allow the foot of a functionally long contralateral lower extremity to clear the ground during swing.
Excessive foot angle during **stance** that is called *toeing-out*	Retroversion of the neck of the femur or tight hip external rotators	Foot is in excessive toeing-out because of excessive external rotation of the lower extremity.
Reduction of the normal foot angle during **stance** that is called *toeing-in*	Excessive femoral anteversion or spasticity of the hip adductors and/or hip internal rotators	General internal rotation of the lower extremity.

*The terms in bold indicate when in the gait cycle the gait deviation is expressed.

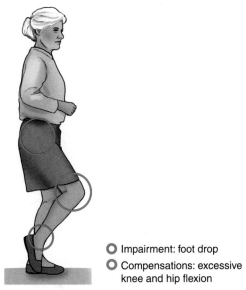

○ Impairment: foot drop
○ Compensations: excessive knee and hip flexion

FIGURE 15-46. Weak ankle dorsiflexors may result in a foot drop during swing phase, requiring excessive hip and knee flexion for the toes to clear the ground as the limb is advanced forward during swing.

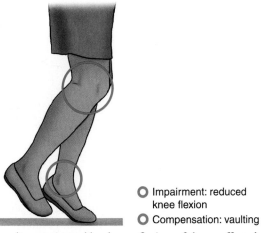

○ Impairment: reduced knee flexion
○ Compensation: vaulting

FIGURE 15-47. Vaulting through excessive ankle plantar flexion of the unaffected stance limb is used to compensate for limited functional shortening of the affected swing limb.

TABLE 15-9. Gait Deviations at the Knee Secondary to Specific Knee Impairments

Observed Gait Deviation at the Knee	Likely Impairment	Selected Pathologic Precursors	Mechanical Rationale and/or Associated Compensations
Rapid extension of the knee (knee extensor thrust) after **initial contact***	Spasticity of the quadriceps	Upper motor neuron lesion	Depending on the status of the posterior structures of the knee, may occur with or without knee hyperextension.
Knee remains extended during the **loading response,** but there is no extensor thrust	Weak quadriceps	Femoral nerve palsy, L^3-L^4 compression neuropathy	Knee remains fully extended throughout stance. An associated anterior trunk lean in the early part of stance moves the line of gravity of the trunk slightly anterior to the axis of rotation of the knee (see Figure 15-48). This keeps the knee extended without action of the knee extensors. This gait deviation may lead to an excessive stretching of the posterior capsule of the knee and eventual knee hyperextension (genu recurvatum) during stance.
	Knee pain	Arthritis	Knee is kept in extension to reduce the need for quadriceps activity and associated compressive forces. It may be accompanied by an antalgic gait pattern characterized by a reduced stance time and shorter step length.
Genu recurvatum during **stance**	Knee extensor weakness	Poliomyelitis	Secondary to progressive stretching of the posterior capsule of the knee.
Varus thrust during **stance**	Laxity of the posterior and lateral ligamentous joint structures of the knee	Traumatic injury or progressive laxity	Rapid varus deviation of the knee during mid stance, typically accompanied by knee hyperextension.
Flexed position of the knee during **stance** (see Figure 15-49) and lack of knee extension in **terminal swing**	Knee flexion contracture >10 degrees (genu flexum), hamstring overactivity (spasticity)	Upper motor neuron lesion	Associated increase in hip flexion and ankle dorsiflexion during stance.
	Knee pain and joint effusion	Trauma or arthritis	Knee is kept in flexion because this is the position of lowest intraarticular pressure.
Reduced or absent knee flexion during **swing**	Spasticity of knee extensors	Upper motor neuron lesion	Compensatory hip hiking and/or hip circumduction could be noted.
	Knee extension contracture	Immobilization or surgical fusion	

*The terms in bold indicate when in the gait cycle the gait deviation is expressed.

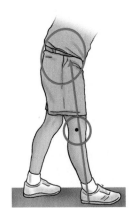

○ Impairment: weak quadriceps
○ Compensation: forward trunk lean

FIGURE 15-48. Weak quadriceps leading to anterior trunk lean to move the center of mass of the body anterior to the axis of rotation of the knee.

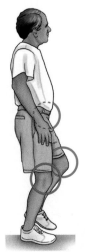

○ Impairment: knee flexion contracture
○ Compensations: exaggerated knee and hip flexion

FIGURE 15-49. Knee flexion contracture resulting in a crouched gait of the stance limb. To clear the toes during swing, the unaffected contralateral side must compensate with exaggerated knee and hip flexion.

TABLE 15-10. Gait Deviations Seen at the Knee as a Compensation for an Impairment of the Ipsilateral Ankle, Ipsilateral Hip, or Contralateral Lower Extremity

Observed Gait Deviation at the Knee	Likely Impairment	Mechanical Rationale
Knee is kept in flexion during **stance*** despite the knee having normal range of motion on examination	Impairments at the ankle or the hip including a pes calcaneus deformity, plantar flexor weakness, and hip flexion contracture	Exaggerated ankle dorsiflexion or hip flexion during stance forces the knee in a flexed position. The contralateral (healthy) swing limb shows exaggerated hip and knee flexion to clear the toes owing to the functionally shorter stance limb.
Hyperextension of the knee (genu recurvatum) from **initial contact to pre-swing**	Ankle plantar flexion contracture (pes equinus deformity) or spasticity of ankle plantar flexors	Knee must hyperextend to compensate for the lack of forward displacement of the tibia during mid stance (see Figure 15-45).
Antalgic gait	Painful stance lower extremity	Characterized by a shorter step length and stance time on the side of the painful lower extremity; it may be accompanied by ipsilateral trunk lean with hip pain or a contralateral trunk lean with knee and foot pain.
Excessive knee flexion in **swing**	Lack of ankle dorsiflexion of the swing limb or a short stance limb	Strategy to increase toe clearance of the swing limb; is typically accompanied by increased hip flexion.

*The terms in bold indicate when in the gait cycle the gait deviation is expressed.

TABLE 15-11. Gait Deviations at the Hip, Pelvis, and Trunk Secondary to Specific Hip, Pelvis, or Trunk Impairments

Observed Gait Deviation at the Hip, Pelvis, or Trunk	Likely Impairment	Selected Pathologic Precursors	Mechanical Rationale and/or Associated Compensations
Backward trunk lean during **loading response.***	Weak hip extensors	Poliomyelitis	This action moves the line of gravity of the trunk behind the hip and reduces the need for hip extension torque.
Lateral trunk lean toward the **stance** lower extremity; because this movement compensates for a weakness, it is often called *compensated Trendelenburg gait* and is referred to as a *waddling gait* if bilateral.	Marked weakness of the hip abductors	Guillain-Barré or poliomyelitis	Shifting the trunk over the supporting limb reduces the demand on the hip abductors.
	Hip pain	Arthritis	Shifting the trunk over the supporting lower extremity reduces compressive joint forces associated with the action of hip abductors (see Figure 15-18).
Excessive downward drop of the contralateral pelvis during **stance.** (Referred to as *positive Trendelenburg sign* if present during single-limb standing.)	Mild weakness of the gluteus medius of the stance limb	Guillain-Barré or poliomyelitis	Although the Trendelenburg sign may be seen in single-limb standing, a compensated Trendelenburg gait is often seen in severe weakness of the hip abductors.
Forward bending of the trunk during **mid** and **terminal stance,** as the hip is moved over the foot.	Hip flexion contracture	Hip osteoarthritis	Forward trunk lean is used to compensate for lack of hip extension. An alternative adaptation could be excessive lumbar lordosis.
	Hip pain	Hip osteoarthritis	Keeping the hip at 30 degrees of flexion minimizes intraarticular pressure.
Excessive lumbar lordosis in **terminal stance.**	Hip flexion contracture	Arthritis	Lack of hip extension in terminal stance is compensated for by increased lordosis.
Trunk lurches backward and toward the unaffected stance limb from **heel off** to **mid swing.**	Hip flexor weakness	L^2-L^3 nerve compression	Hip flexion is passively generated by a backward movement of the trunk.
Posterior tilt of the pelvis during **initial swing.**	Hip flexor weakness	L^2-L^3 nerve compression	Abdominals are used during initial swing to advance the swing lower extremity.
Hip circumduction: semicircle movement of the hip during **swing** (see Figure 15-50).	Hip flexor weakness	L^2-L^3 nerve compression	Semicircle movement combining hip flexion, hip abduction, and forward rotation of the pelvis.

*The terms in bold indicate when in the gait cycle the gait deviation is expressed.

TABLE 15-12. Gait Deviations Seen at the Hip, Pelvis, and Trunk as a Compensation for an Impairment of the Ipsilateral Ankle, Ipsilateral Knee, or Contralateral Lower Extremity

Observed Gait Deviation at the Hip, Pelvis, or Trunk	Likely Impairment	Mechanical Rationale
Forward bending of the trunk during the **loading response***	Weak quadriceps	Trunk is brought forward to move the line of gravity anterior to the axis of rotation of the knee, thereby reducing the need for knee extensors (see Figure 15-48).
Forward bending of the trunk during **mid** and **terminal stance**	Pes equinus deformity	Lack of ankle dorsiflexion during stance results in knee hyperextension at mid stance and forward trunk lean during terminal stance to move the weight of the body over the stance foot (see Figure 15-45).
Excessive hip and knee flexion during **swing** (see Figure 15-46)	Often caused by lack of ankle dorsiflexion of the swing limb; may also be caused by a functionally or anatomically short contralateral stance lower extremity	Used to clear the toes of the swing limb
Hip circumduction during **swing** (see Figure 15-50)	Lack of shortening of the swing limb secondary to reduced hip flexion, reduced knee flexion, and/or lack of ankle dorsiflexion	Used to lift the foot of the swing limb off the ground and provide toe clearance
Hip hiking (elevation of the ipsilateral pelvis during **swing**)	Lack of shortening of the swing limb secondary to reduced hip flexion, reduced knee flexion, and/or lack of ankle dorsiflexion Functionally or anatomically short stance limb	Used to lift the foot of the swing lower extremity off the ground and provide toe clearance.
Excessive backward horizontal rotation of the pelvis on the side of the stance lower extremity in terminal stance	Ankle plantar flexor weakness	Ankle plantar flexor weakness leads to prolonged heel contact and lack of push off. An increased pelvic horizontal rotation is used to lengthen the limb and maintain adequate step length.

*The terms in bold indicate when in the gait cycle the gait deviation is expressed.

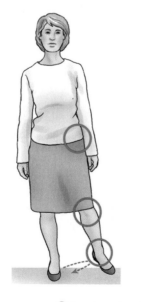
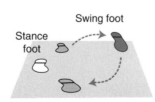

○ Impairment: reduced knee flexion and/or lack of ankle dorsiflexion

○ Compensation: hip circumduction

FIGURE 15-50. Hip circumduction during swing is used to compensate for the inability to shorten the swing limb because of inadequate knee flexion or ankle dorsiflexion.

SYNOPSIS

Walking integrates the functions of all regions of the lower extremities. To fully understand the kinesiology of locomotion, the reader must consider the near simultaneous and relatively rapid musculoskeletal interactions that occur among multiple joints and planes, across both lower limbs and, to some extent, the trunk and upper extremities. In addition, the internal and external forces that act on each lower limb must be considered as it is freely moving as well as when it is fixed to the ground.

For a foundation to be set forth for study of this complex human activity so fundamental to everyday life, terms and conventions must initially be defined. One of the first conventions discussed in this chapter is the description of walking based on a single gait cycle. The gait cycle consists of all events that occur between consecutive heel contacts of the same limb; ambulation at steady walking velocity is simply a repetition of that gait cycle. In its simplest subdivision, a gait cycle consists of a stance phase (heel contact to toe off) that encompasses approximately the first 60% of the gait cycle, and a swing phase that encompasses the remainder of the cycle (toe off to the next heel contact).

Throughout the gait cycle, the major joints of the lower limb rotate as a way to advance the body while also providing support against the external torques imposed by gravity. As the body is propelled forward, its CoM is also displaced slightly in both the medial-lateral and vertical directions. The natural cyclic displacement of the body gives walking the quality of an inverted pendulum, allowing a cyclic and smooth transfer of potential and kinetic mechanical energy. Such a mechanism is advantageous to minimize energy cost.

In this chapter the biomechanics associated with the forward translation of the body as a whole are focused on the rotation of the joints of the lower limbs—most specifically the hip, knee, ankle, and foot. The greatest range of joint motion occurs within the sagittal plane, which reflects the primary forward direction of movement of the body. Less obvious but equally important are the frontal and horizontal plane rotations of the joints of the lower limbs. In addition to their modest contribution to the forward progression of the body, these extra-sagittal plane motions help optimize the vertical and medial-lateral displacements of the body's CoM.

During walking, a limitation of motion at any one joint can have a profound effect on the quality and efficiency of movement of the body as a whole. Consider, for example, the disrupted walking pattern after the isolated loss of the last 15 degrees of knee extension. Walking is still possible, but only with significant kinematic compensations made by other joints, at a cost of an increased expenditure of energy.

Based on information provided in Appendix IV of this textbook, 50 muscles operate each lower extremity. No muscle has identical actions, and all are active to varying degrees at one time or another during the gait cycle. Many of these muscles express their specific actions in multiple ways: eccentrically, concentrically, or isometrically; across one or multiple joints; or as movers of either the distal or proximal segment of a joint, or a combination thereof. Consider the tibialis posterior muscle, for example. Before mid stance, the muscle is active eccentrically as it controls the lowering of the medial longitudinal arch. After mid stance, the same muscle is active concentrically as it lifts the arch and assists with external rotation of the tibia. This concentric action continues as it contributes to the ankle plantar flexion torque generated during push off. Inhibition of this muscle action as a result of weakness or tendinopathy could significantly interfere with the natural transformation of the foot from a pliable platform at loading response to a more rigid lever at push off. Understanding this level of detail of each muscle's action is essential to recognizing as well as treating associated underlying pathomechanics.

A noticeable gait deviation will likely result if a muscle or muscle group fails to activate at an appropriate time and magnitude of effort. The deviation can often be minimized through biomechanical compensations naturally learned by the individual. Often, however, it is the role of the clinician to devise strategies that can either compensate for or eliminate the gait deviation. These strategies typically include exercises that aim to increase the control, strength, or flexibility of targeted muscles. In addition, strategies often include patient education, endurance and gait retraining activities, and the use of bracing, orthoses, electrical stimulators, biofeedback, or other assistive devices such as a cane.

Walking may be considered the ultimate kinesiologic expression of the neuromuscular and musculoskeletal interactions of the lower body. Although the kinesiology of walking is complex, a thorough understanding of the subject serves as the direct or indirect basis for the evaluation and treatment of most disorders involving the lower limb. These disorders vary considerably and include local muscle injury or overuse, painful or replaced joints, neurologic trauma or disease, reduced endurance after bed rest or surgery, and the actual amputation, paralysis, or loss of control of a lower limb. The kinesiology presented in this chapter is intended to be a starting point for a study that lasts a lifetime.

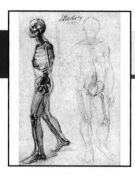

ADDITIONAL CLINICAL CONNECTIONS

CLINICAL CONNECTION 15-1
Eccentric, Isometric, or Concentric Muscle Activation: Is It Really Always Known for Certain?

Much attention has been paid in this chapter to the type of activation of a muscle or muscle group during the different parts of the gait cycle. In a broad sense, isometric activation occurs when an activated muscle does not change length. Concentric activation occurs as the activated muscle is actually shortening (contracting), whereas eccentric activation occurs as the activated muscle is being elongated by some other more dominant force. As described in Chapter 3, the force output of a muscle is dependent on its type of activation, given a constant effort. This issue is therefore very relevant to the study of gait.

In most clinical or laboratory settings, the specific type of activation of a muscle can be estimated only by comparing its established action against the rotation direction of the joint that the muscle is crossing. For example, the tibialis anterior is assumed to experience an eccentric activation after heel contact based on the fact that the ankle is plantar flexing at the time this primary dorsiflexor muscle is active. This clinical connection considers variables that may interfere with the logic of this practical method of analysis.

First, consider an activated pluri-articular muscle of the lower extremity. It is not unusual for such a muscle to contract across one joint while at the same time being elongated across a more proximal or distal joint. The joint kinematics illustrated in Figure 15-15 provide an opportunity to consider such a situation for pluri-articular muscles acting principally in the sagittal plane. For example, it may not be possible to determine with absolute certainty the net change in length of the activated rectus femoris as it is being elongated through hip extension and simultaneously shortened as a result of knee extension at 15% to 40% of the gait cycle. Similarly, the actual net change in length of the gastrocnemius may be quite challenging to determine when one considers the combination of ankle and knee movements during gait.[63,84]

To add to the complexity of the process of estimating the type of activation a muscle is experiencing during walking is the fact that net change in length of the muscle is affected by *both* the change in length of the activated muscle fibers and the stretch in its related tendon. Based on its stiffness, a tendon may elongate a significant amount when under load. The Achilles tendon, for example, elongates up to 8% of its resting length after a maximal contraction of the calf muscles.[108] The magnitude of elongation is dependent on the specific architecture of the muscle-tendon unit, but also on the amount and rate of the application of the force.

This physiologic property of a tendon may obscure the actual length change in the entire muscle-tendon unit during activation. It is possible that in some kinematic conditions, depending on the muscle, the overall contraction of the muscle fibers may be offset by a similar elongation of the tendon. In this example, an activation previously thought to be isometric for the entire muscle-tendon unit (based on no change in joint angle) may, in fact, be slightly concentric at the level of the muscle fibers.

Real-time ultrasonography now provides the ability to make direct measurements of the lengths of muscle fibers during dynamic movement.[29,30,109] This technique was used to study the specific function of the vastus lateralis during gait shortly after heel contact, a time when this muscle is known to be strongly activated and assumed to be active eccentrically. Despite the knee moving toward flexion, the length of the muscle fibers actually remained relatively constant—the load placed on the muscle caused significant lengthening of the tendon of the vastus lateralis. The authors of the same study also observed similar results when analyzing the muscle fibers of the tibialis anterior immediately after heel contact—a time when the muscle is strongly activated while the ankle moves toward plantar flexion. In both scenarios, an activation previously thought to be eccentric for the entire muscle-tendon unit was observed to be essentially isometric in nature at the level of the muscle fibers. The lengthening of the tendon is likely being used to dampen the impact on the overall muscle and for storage of elastic energy.[29]

These data expose the oversimplification of interpreting a muscle's type of action based on electromyographic and kinematic data alone. In some muscles, especially during short-arc movements as those described earlier, the compliance within the tendon (and other connective tissue) may account for some or all of the changes in joint motion. It is interesting to consider that the two factors highlighted in this clinical connection—pluri-articular muscles and tendon compliance—may minimize muscle fiber length changes during movement and thereby help maintain the muscle in a more optimal portion of its length-tension curve.

This clinical connection is not intended to negate the standard empiric method for inferring if a muscle is active isometrically, concentrically, or eccentrically, but rather highlights the potential limitation of this method in assessment of all muscles over a wide range of function.

ADDITIONAL CLINICAL CONNECTIONS

CLINICAL CONNECTION 15-2
Walking and Running—a Kinesiologic Continuum

Running, a natural progression of bipedal locomotion when we need to move faster, shares many of the same fundamental kinesiologic principles as walking. However, notable differences need to be considered to provide optimal assessment and interventions for those seeking care for running-related injuries. It is not uncommon for individuals with impairments in the lower limbs to complain of pain when running and not while walking.

Similar to walking, running is a cyclic action that can be summarized through the description of a full cycle—from foot contact of one limb to the next foot contact of the same limb. Also as with walking, although a general pattern of movement can be described for running, joint kinematics and kinetics, as well as the intensity and timing of muscle activation, differ substantially across the spectrum of running velocity, from slow jogging to sprinting. This speed-dependent kinesiology of running is often implicated in running-related injuries, as running faster typically requires greater movement amplitude, movement velocity, and generation of forces. A lack of progressive accommodations to these greater demands on the musculoskeletal system of the lower extremities has the potential to lead to injuries such as tendinitis and stress fractures.[81,186] In general, the description of running provided here will be kept in general terms and give typical values that apply to running at a moderate jogging speed.

An individual transitions from walking to running not because of the inability to walk faster, but because of the greater energy efficiency of running compared with walking when a walking speed of approximately 2.1 to 2.2 m/sec is reached.[43,157,163] By definition, running occurs when the two periods of double-limb support during walking are replaced by two "flight" periods—when both feet are off the ground at the same time. When transitioning from walking to running, the duration of stance phase for each limb drops suddenly from 60% to 40% of the cycle. The faster the running velocity, the shorter the duration of the running cycle and the lower the percentage of the stance phase in the total running cycle (Figure 15-51). Mechanically, when switching from walking to running, the body has transitioned from a mode of locomotion resembling an inverted pendulum to one resembling a "spring."[22,156] The cyclic transfer of potential and kinetic energy taking place over a relatively extended stance limb during walking has been replaced by a strategy taking advantage of elastic energy initially stored and then released by muscles, tendons, and other connective tissues on a relatively flexed stance limb during running (Figure 15-52).

Through visual observation, it should be readily apparent that the movements of the joints of the lower extremities occur much more rapidly during running compared with walking. This is primarily because of the shorter duration of the gait cycle but also, although to a lesser extent, the greater magnitude of joint move-

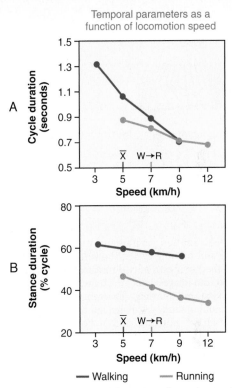

Temporal parameters as a function of locomotion speed

FIGURE 15-51. Time-duration of a gait and running cycle over a range of walking and running speeds **(A).** Stance phase duration over a range of walking and running speeds **(B).** Note: 5 km/hr (1.3 m/sec) is reflective of an average walking velocity (indicated by X̄), and 7 km/hr (2 m/sec) is reflective of the speed when individuals transition from walking to running (indicated by W→R). (Data from Cappellini G, Ivanenko YP, Poppele RE, Lacquaniti F: Motor patterns in human walking and running, *J Neurophysiol* 95:3426, 2006.)

ment used for running.[24] At the hip, in the sagittal plane, the pattern of movement during running is very similar to that during walking, with the exception of a larger amount of hip flexion at initial foot contact and slightly more hip extension at toe off. The pattern of sagittal plane motion at the knee during running is also similar to that during walking, with the notable exception of a greater amount of knee flexion throughout the full cycle. During running the knee is flexed to as much as 20 to 30 degrees at initial contact, before flexing a few additional degrees in the early part of stance. This is followed by a small amount of knee extension, returning the knee back to the flexion angle at initial contact, before starting to flex again just before toe off to initiate swing

Continued

ADDITIONAL CLINICAL CONNECTIONS

CLINICAL CONNECTION 15-2
Walking and Running—a Kinesiologic Continuum—cont'd

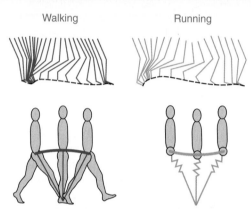

FIGURE 15-52. Top images illustrate stick diagrams representing the walking and running cycles, showing the slightly more flexed attitude of the lower extremity during stance and swing phases of running. Bottom images depict the trajectory of the center of mass during walking and running. The center of mass resembles an inverted pendulum during walking, indicating the transfer between the "out-of-phase" potential and kinetic energy (compare with Figure 15-14). This is in contrast to running, which takes advantage of a transfer between "in-phase" potential and kinetic energy of the body and elastic energy from the muscles, tendons, and other connective tissues of the lower extremities. (Data from Cappellini G, Ivanenko YP, Poppele RE, Lacquaniti F: Motor patterns in human walking and running, *J Neurophysiol* 95:3426, 2006.)

phase. Given this relatively flexed attitude of the stance limb and the need to move the swing limb more quickly, maximum knee flexion during swing is 80 to 110 degrees—again, specific angles varying with running velocity.

At slow running speed, similar to walking, most runners make initial contact with the ground with the heel region. These runners are often referred to as *rearfoot strikers*. Those who instead make initial ground contact with the entire undersurface of the foot or the forefoot region are called *midfoot* and *forefoot strikers,* respectively. As running speed increases, most runners will progressively change the region of initial contact to the forefoot. Regardless of the foot contact pattern, in general, the ankle is near a neutral position at initial foot contact. Initial contact is immediately followed by a dorsiflexion movement of the ankle. This dorsiflexion movement results in part from the greater knee flexion that is present during running, requiring eccentric control from the ankle plantar flexors. This is in sharp contrast to the small amount of ankle plantar flexion, controlled by an eccentric action from the dorsiflexors to generate a dorsiflexion internal torque (Figure

15-53), occurring immediately after heel contact during walking. The movement of dorsiflexion occurring in the early part of stance, up to approximately 20 degrees, is followed by rapid plantar flexion (up to approximately 30 degrees) later in stance, before toe off. As with walking, the ankle is then brought back toward dorsiflexion during swing.

In the frontal and transverse planes the overall kinematic patterns taking place at the hip (combined internal rotation and adduction followed by external rotation and abduction), knee, and foot (pronation followed by supination) during the stance phase of running are overall similar to those observed during walking. The notable differences are that joint motions occur at much greater angular velocity and are typically of a few degrees greater magnitude. These movements, either of excessive amplitude, poorly controlled, or both, are often believed to contribute to acute and chronic injuries of the lower limb. Clinically, observation and quantification of these movements is difficult but nevertheless of utmost importance in determining optimal intervention approaches (see Special Focus 15-8).[50,121,170]

As would be suspected, Figure 15-53 shows that the vertical ground reaction forces during running are of greater magnitude than those measured during walking. In this illustration the smooth single peak shape of the curve is characteristic of a runner making initial contact with the forefoot—the ankle plantar flexors readily and smoothly transferring impact loading into propulsive forces. The vertical ground reaction force profile of a rearfoot striker would exhibit an additional, highly characteristic, initial impact peak within the first 10% of the stance phase. Vertical ground reaction forces during running can be as high as three to four times body weight, being progressively larger as running speed increases. In the anterior-posterior direction, similar to what occurs during walking, both rearfoot and forefoot strikers show an initial breaking force in the first half of stance, followed by a propulsive force in the second half of stance. The speed-dependent magnitude of these forces ranges from 0.3 to 0.6 times body weight, which is two to four times the magnitude of those measured during walking.[24,88]

The larger ground reaction forces combined with the often larger joint angular movements during running are associated with larger internal joint torques. Figure 15-53 compares the internal joint torque curves for walking and running for the hip, knee, and ankle. The shapes of the curves for the hip and the knee are generally similar for walking and running, but the internal joint torques are of greater magnitude during running. At the ankle the joint torque profile for running is notably different from that during walking, with the absence of the initial dorsiflexion torque. This is reflective of the kinematics at the ankle, with initial

ADDITIONAL CLINICAL CONNECTIONS

CLINICAL CONNECTION 15-2
Walking and Running—a Kinesiologic Continuum—cont'd

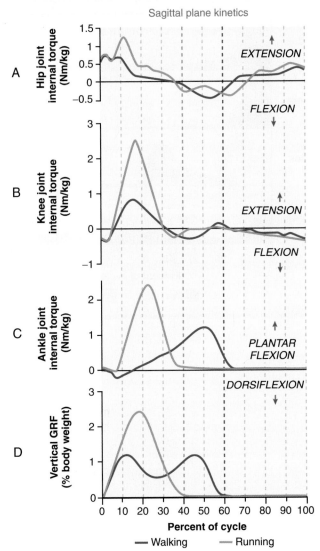

FIGURE 15-53. Sagittal plane internal torques for the hip **(A),** knee **(B),** and ankle **(C),** and vertical ground reaction forces *(GRF)* **(D)** for a walking (5.4 km/hr) and running (9.4 km/hr) cycle for one individual. Vertical dashed blue and orange lines indicate transition between stance and swing phases. (Data from Cappellini G, Ivanenko YP, Poppele RE, Lacquaniti F: Motor patterns in human walking and running, *J Neurophysiol* 95:3426, 2006.)

contact being immediately followed by a (leg-on-foot) dorsiflexion movement. The pattern and magnitude of the joint torque at the ankle vary appreciably based on running speed and across runners according to the manner with which the foot makes initial contact with the ground. In comparison with those who make initial ground contact with the heel, forefoot strikers rely much more heavily on the ankle plantar flexors to cushion the initial loading on the lower extremity. Determining the pattern of foot contact with the ground is part of a comprehensive evaluation of runners with lower extremity injuries, especially injuries to the foot, ankle, and lower leg.

As described in this chapter, the power across a joint is the product of torque and angular velocity. It is therefore not surprising that the power generated or absorbed across the joints of the lower extremity during running is several times the magnitude of that experienced during walking. The presence of greater power and torque is expressed through the significant increase in muscular activation measured during running compared with walking. Figure 15-54 displays the magnitude and pattern of activation of four representative muscles, comparing walking at 5 km/hr (an average walking speed) and running at 9 km/hr (a slow jogging speed). The vastus medialis and gluteus medius are reflective of the more proximal musculature, showing a relatively similar activation pattern during walking and running. Conversely, consistent with the changes in ankle kinematics and kinetics, the activation patterns of the ankle musculature, the tibialis anterior and gastrocnemius, are notably different between walking and running. For all muscles, progressively larger muscle activation is noted during running, and this difference is amplified as running speed increases. (See Cappellini and colleagues[22] for the muscle activation profiles of 32 muscles across a spectrum of walking and running speeds.)

From an injury and prevention perspective, one of the most important differences between walking and running is the magnitude of the forces applied to the musculoskeletal system (see Table 15-6). The magnitude and repetitive nature of these forces require adequate strength and endurance of the lower extremity musculature as well as progressive tissue adaptation over time. Furthermore, it is important to consider the influence of factors such as running speed and surface incline, which modify the running kinematics and kinetics and the demands on the system in a manner that potentially lead to injuries. Clinically, "training errors," leading to injuries during running, are more readily identified and understood with a better knowledge of how kinematics and kinetics change over a continuum of walking and running velocities.

Continued

ADDITIONAL CLINICAL CONNECTIONS

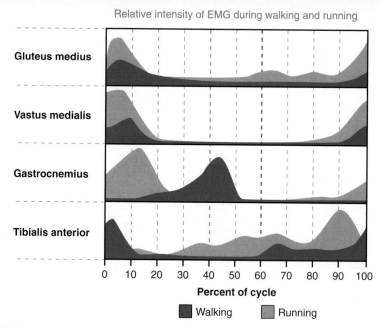

FIGURE 15-54. Relative intensity and profile of activation of four selected muscles during walking (5 km/hr) and running (9 km/hr). Vertical dashed blue and orange lines indicate transition between stance and swing phases. (Data from Cappellini G, Ivanenko YP, Poppele RE, Lacquaniti F: Motor patterns in human walking and running, *J Neurophysiol* 95:3426, 2006.)

REFERENCES

1. Alexander RM: Flat and bouncy walking, *J Physiol* 582(2):474, 2007.
2. Amar J: Trottoir dynamographique, *Comptes rendus hebdomadaires des séances de l'Académie des Sciences* 163:130-133, 1916.
3. Anders C, Wagner H, Puta C, et al: Trunk muscle activation patterns during walking at different speeds, *J Electromyogr Kinesiol* 17:245-252, 2007.
4. Andersson EA, Nilsson J, Thorstensson A: Intramuscular EMG from the hip flexor muscles during human locomotion, *Acta Physiol Scand* 161:361-370, 1997.
5. Andrews JG: Euler's and Lagrange's equations for linked rigid-body models of three-dimensional human motion. In Allard P, Stokes IAF, Blanchi JP, editors: *Three-dimensional analysis of human movement*, Champaign, Ill, 1995, Human Kinetics.
6. Aristotle: parts of animals. *Movement of animals, Progression of animals.* Translated by Peck AL and Forster ES, Cambridge, Mass, 1968, Harvard University Press.
7. Baker R: The history of gait analysis before the advent of modern computers, *Gait Posture* 26:331-342, 2007.
8. Bandholm T, Bousen L, Haugaard S, et al: Foot medial longitudinal-arch deformation during quiet standing and gait in subjects with medial tibial stress syndrome, *J Foot Ankle Surg* 47(2):89-95, 2008.
9. Bechtol CO: Normal human gait. In Bowker JH, Hall CB, editors: *Atlas of orthotics: American academy of orthopaedic surgeons*, St Louis, 1975, Mosby.
10. Begg R, Best R, Dell'Oro L, Taylor S: Minimum foot clearance during walking: strategies for the minimization of trip-related falls, *Gait Posture* 25:191-198, 2007.
11. Benoit DL, Ramsey DK, Lamontagne M, et al: In vivo knee kinematics during gait reveals new rotation profiles and smaller translations, *Clin Orthop Relat Res* 454:81-88, 2007.
12. Best R, Begg R: A method for calculating the probability of tripping while walking, *J Biomech* 41(5):1147-1151, 2008.
13. Bilney B, Morris M, Webster K: Concurrent related validity of the GAITRite walkway system for quantification of the spatial and temporal parameters of gait, *Gait Posture* 17:68-74, 2003.
14. Bohannon RW: Comfortable and maximum walking speed of adults aged 20-79 years: reference values and determinants, *Age Ageing* 26:15-19, 1997.
15. Braune W, Fisher O: Der Gang des Menschen [The human gait]. Leipzig, Germany, *BG Teubner*, 1895-1904.
16. Braune W, Fisher O: *The human gait (translation by Maquet P, Furlong R)*, Berlin, 1987, Springer-Verlag. (Original work published 1895-1904.).
17. Bresler B, Frankel JP: Forces and moments in the leg during walking, *Am Soc Mech Eng Trans* 72:27, 1950.
18. Bruijn SM, Meijer OG, van Dieen JH, et al: Coordination of leg swing, thorax rotations, and pelvis rotations during gait: the organization of total body angular momentum, *Gait Posture* 27:455-462, 2008.
19. Buczek FL, Cooney KM, Walker MR, et al: Performance of an inverted pendulum model directly applied to normal human gait, *Clin Biomech (Bristol, Avon)* 21:288-296, 2006.
20. Burnfield JM, Powers CM: The role of center of mass kinematics in predicting peak utilized coefficient of friction during walking, *J Forensic Sci* 52:1328-1333, 2007.
21. Calvé J, Galland M, De Cagny R: Pathogenesis of the limp due to coxalgia: the antalgic gait, *J Bone Joint Surg* 21:12, 1939.
22. Cappellini G, Ivanenko YP, Poppele RE, Lacquaniti F: Motor patterns in human walking and running, *J Neurophysiol* 95:3426-3437, 2006.
23. Carlsoo S: *How man moves: kinesiological methods and studies*, New York, 1972, Crane, Russak & Company.
24. Cavanagh PR: The biomechanics of lower extremity action in distance running, *Foot Ankle* 7:197-217, 1987.
25. Chan CW, Rudins A: Foot biomechanics during walking and running, *Mayo Clin Proc* 69:448, 1994.
26. Chester VL, Tingley M, Biden EN: A comparison of kinetic gait parameters for 3-13 year olds, *Clin Biomech* 21:726-732, 2006.
27. Chester VL, Wrigley AT: The identification of age-related differences in kinetic gait parameters using principal component analysis, *Clin Biomech (Bristol, Avon)* 23:212-220, 2008.
28. Chevutschi A, Lensel G, Vaast D, Thevenon A: An electromyographic study of human gait both in water and on dry ground, *J Physiol Anthropol* 26:467-473, 2007.
29. Chleboun GS, Busic AB, Graham KK, Stuckey HA: Fascicle length change of the human tibialis anterior and vastus lateralis during walking, *J Orthop Sports Phys Ther* 37:372-379, 2007.
30. Chleboun GS, Harrigal ST, Odenthal JZ, et al: Vastus lateralis fascicle length changes during stair ascent and descent, *J Orthop Sports Phys Ther* 38:624-631, 2008.
31. Chumanov ES, Wall-Scheffler C, Heiderscheit BC: Gender differences in walking and running on level and inclined surfaces, *Clin Biomech (Bristol, Avon)* 23:1260-1268, 2008.
32. Collins JJ: The redundant nature of locomotor optimization laws, *J Biomech* 28:251, 1995.
33. Cooper RC, Prebeau-Menezes LM, Butcher MT, Bertram JEA: Step length and required friction in walking, *Gait Posture* 27:547-551, 2008.
34. Corcoran PJ, Jebsen RH, Brengelman GL, Simons BC: Effects of plastic and metal leg braces on speed and energy cost of hemiparetic ambulation, *Arch Phys Med Rehabil* 51:69, 1970.
35. Cornwall MW, McPoil TG: Three-dimensional movement of the foot during the stance phase of walking, *J Am Podiatr Med Assoc* 89:56, 1999.
36. Craik RL, Dutterer L: Spatial and temporal characteristics of foot fall patterns. In Craik RL, Oatis CA, editors: *Gait analysis: theory and application*, St Louis, 1995, Mosby.
37. Cromwell RL, Aadland-Monahan TK, Nelson AT, et al: Sagittal plane analysis of head, neck, and trunk kinematics and electromyographic activity during locomotion, *J Orthop Sports Phys Ther* 31:255-262, 2001.
38. Cunningham D, Brown G: Two devices for measuring the forces acting on the human body during walking, *Exp Stress Anal* 75-90, 1952.
39. D'Angelo MG, Berti M, Piccinini L, et al: Gait pattern in Duchenne muscular dystrophy, *Gait Posture* 29:36-41, 2009.
40. Davis I, Ireland ML, Hanaki S: ACL injuries–the gender bias, *J Orthop Sports Phys Ther* 37:A1-A32, 2007.
41. Della Croce U, Riley PO, Lelas JL, Kerrigan DC: A refined view of the determinants of gait, *Gait Posture* 14:79-84, 2001.
42. Den Otter AR, Geurts ACH, Mulder T, Duysens J: Speed related changes in muscle activity from normal to very slow walking speeds, *Gait Posture* 19:270-278, 2004.
43. De Smet K, Segers V, Lenoir M, De Clercq D: Spatiotemporal characteristics of spontaneous overground walk-to-run transition, *Gait Posture* 29:54-59, 2009.
44. DeVita P, Helseth J, Hortobagyi T: Muscles do more positive than negative work in human locomotion, *J Exp Biol* 210:3361-3373, 2007.
45. Don R, Serrao M, Vinci P, et al: Foot drop and plantar flexion failure determine different gait strategies in Charcot-Marie-Tooth patients, *Clin Biomech (Bristol, Avon)* 22:905-916, 2007.
46. Donelan JM, Kram R, Kuo AD: Mechanical and metabolic determinants of the preferred step width in human walking, *Proc Biol Sci.* 268:1985-1992, 2001.
47. Drillis R: The influence of aging on the kinematics of gait. In *Geriatric Amputee (NAS-NRC Pub. No. 919)*, Washington, DC, 1961, NAS-NRC.
48. Dusing SC, Thorpe DE: A normative sample of temporal and spatial gait parameters in children using the GAITRite electronic walkway, *Gait Posture* 25:135-139, 2007.
49. Eberhart H: *Fundamental studies of human locomotion and other information relating to design of artificial limbs*, Report to U.S. Veterans' Association. Berkeley, 1947, University of California.
50. Ekegren CL, Miller WC, Celebrini RG, et al: Reliability and validity of observational risk screening in evaluating dynamic knee valgus, *J Orthop Sports Phys Ther* 39(9), 2009 (in press).
51. Elftman H: The function of the arms in walking, *Hum Biol* 11:529, 1939.
52. Elftman H: The measurement of the external force in walking, *Science* 88:152-153, 1938.
53. Eng JJ, Winter DA: Kinetic analysis of the lower limbs during walking: what information can be gained from a three-dimensional model? *J Biomech* 28:753, 1995.
54. Ferrari A, Benedetti MG, Pavan E, et al: Quantitative comparison of five current protocols in gait analysis, *Gait Posture* 28:207-216, 2008.
55. Finley F, Cody K: Locomotive characteristics of urban pedestrians, *Arch Phys Med Rehabil* 51:423, 1970.
56. Finley F, Cody K, Finizie R: Locomotion patterns in elderly women, *Arch Phys Med Rehabil* 50:140, 1969.
57. Finley FR, Cody KA, Sepic SB: Walking patterns of normal women, *Arch Phys Med Rehabil* 51:637, 1970.
58. Finni T, Komi PV, Lukkariniemi J: Achilles tendon loading during walking: application of a novel optic fiber technique, *Eur J Appl Physiol* 77:289, 1998.
59. Finni T, Lepola V, Komi PV: Tendomuscular loading in normal locomotion conditions. In Kyrolainen H, Avela J, Takala T, editors: *Limiting*

factors of human neuromuscular performance, Jyvaskyla, Finland, 1999, University of Jyvaskyla.

60. Fisher SV, Gullickson G: Energy cost of ambulation in health and disability: a literature review, *Arch Phys Med Rehabil* 59:124, 1978.

61. Franettovich M, Chapman A, Vicenzino B: Tape that increases medial longitudinal arch height also reduces leg muscle activity: a preliminary study, *Med Sci Sports Exerc* 40(4):593-600, 2008.

62. Frigo C, Crenna P: Multichannel SEMG in clinical gait analysis: a review and state-of-the-art, *Clin Biomech (Bristol, Avon)* 24:236-245, 2009.

63. Fukunaga T, Kubo K, Kawakami Y, et al: In vivo behaviour of human muscle tendon during walking, *Proc Biol Sci* 268:229-233, 2001.

64. Gage JR: Gait analysis in cerebral palsy. In *Clinic in developmental medicine*, London, 1991, Mac Keith Press.

65. Ganley JK, Powers CM: Gait kinematics and kinetics of 7-year-old children: a comparison to adults using age-specific anthropometric data, *Gait Posture* 21:141-145, 2005.

66. Ganley JK, Powers CM: Intersegmental dynamics during the swing phase of gait: a comparison of knee kinetics between 7 year-old children and adults, *Gait Posture* 23:499-504, 2006.

67. Garrett M, McElroy AM, Staines A: Locomotor milestones and baby-walkers: cross sectional study, *BMJ* 324:1494, 2002.

68. Glasoe WM, Yack HJ, Saltzman CL: Anatomy and biomechanics of the first ray, *Phys Ther* 79:854, 1999.

69. Gonzalez EG, Corcoran PJ: Energy expenditure during ambulation. In Downey JA, Myers SJ, Gonzalez EG, Lieberman JS: *The physiological basis of rehabilitation medicine*, ed 2, Boston, 1994, Butterworth-Heinemann.

70. Gordon KE, Ferris DP, Kuo AD: Metabolic and mechanical costs of reducing vertical center of mass movement during gait, *Arch Phys Med Rehabil* 90:136-144, 2009.

71. Gore DR, Murray MP, Sepic SB, Gardner GM: Walking patterns of men with unilateral surgical hip fusion, *J Bone Joint Surg Am* 57:759, 1975.

72. Gorton GE, Hebert DA, Gannotti ME: Assessment of the kinematic variability among 12 motion analysis laboratories, *Gait Posture* 29:398-402, 2009.

73. Grabiner PC, Biswas T, Grabiner MD: Age-related changes in spatial and temporal gait variables, *Arch Phys Med Rehabil* 82:31-35, 2001.

74. Gross MT, Foxworth JL: The role of foot orthoses as an intervention for patellofemoral pain, *J Orthop Sports Phys Ther* 33:661-670, 2003.

75. Hausdorff JM, Zemany L, Peng CK, Goldberger AL: Maturation of gait dynamics: stride-to-stride variability and its temporal organization in children, *J Appl Physiol* 86:1040-1047, 1999.

76. Heiden TL, Sanderson DJ, Inglis JT, Siegmund GP: Adaptations to normal human gait on potentially slippery surfaces: the effects of awareness and prior slip experience, *Gait Posture* 24:237-246, 2006.

77. Hillman SJ, Stansfield BW, Richardson AM, Robb JE: Development of temporal and distance parameters of gait in normal children, *Gait Posture* 29:81-85, 2009.

78. Hof AL, Elzinga H, Grimmius W, Halbertsma JPK: Detection of non-standard EMG profiles in walking, *Gait Posture* 21:171-177, 2005.

79. Hollman JH, Kovash FM, Kubik JJ, Linbo RA: Age-related differences in spatiotemporal markers of gait stability during dual task walking, *Gait Posture* 26:113-119, 2007.

80. Holm I, Tveter AT, Fredriksen PM, Vollestad N: A normative sample of gait and hopping on one leg parameters in children 7-12 years of age, *Gait Posture* 29:317-321, 2009.

81. Hreljac A: Impact and overuse injuries in runners, *Med Sci Sports Exerc* 36:845-849, 2004.

82. Inman VT, Ralston HJ, Todd F: Human locomotion. In Rose J, Gamble JG, editors: *Human walking*, ed 2, Philadelphia, 1994, Williams & Wilkins.

83. Inman VT, Ralston HJ, Todd F: *Human walking*, Baltimore, 1981, Williams & Wilkins.

84. Ishikawa M, Pakaslahti J, Komi PV: Medial gastrocnemius muscle behavior during human running and walking, *Gait Posture* 25:380-384, 2007.

85. Ivanenko YP, Poppele RE, Lacquaniti F: Motor control programs and walking, *Neuroscientist* 12:339-348, 2006.

86. Kavanagh JJ, Morrison S, Barrett RS: Lumbar and cervical erector spinae fatigue elicit compensatory postural responses to assist in maintaining head stability during walking, *J Appl Physiol* 101:1118-1126, 2006.

87. Kaye RA, Jahss MH: Tibialis posterior: a review of anatomy and biomechanics in relation to support of the medial longitudinal arch, *Foot Ankle* 11:244, 1991.

88. Keller TS, Weisberger AM, Ray JL, et al: Relationship between vertical ground reaction force and speed during walking, slow jogging, and running, *Clin Biomech (Bristol, Avon)* 11:253-259, 1996.

89. Kepple TM, Siegel KL, Stanhope SJ: Relative contributions of the lower extremity joint moments to forward progression and support during gait, *Gait Posture* 6:1, 1997.

90. Kerrigan DC, Croce UD, Marciello M, Riley PO: A refined view of the determinants of gait: significance of heel rise, *Arch Phys Med Rehabil* 81:1077, 2000.

91. Kerrigan DC, Riley PO, Lelas JL, Della Croce U: Quantification of pelvic rotation as a determinant of gait, *Arch Phys Med Rehabil* 82:217-220, 2001.

92. Kerrigan DC, Viramontes BE, Corcoran PJ, LaRaia PJ: Measured versus predicted vertical displacement of the sacrum during gait as a tool to measure biomechanical gait performance, *Am J Phys Med Rehabil* 74:3, 1995.

93. Kirtley C: *Clinical gait analysis: theory and practice*, Philadelphia, 2006, Churchill Livingstone.

94. Knutson LM, Soderberg GL: EMG: use and interpretation in gait. In Craik RL, Oatis CA, editors: *Gait analysis: theory and application*, St Louis, 1995, Mosby.

95. Komistek RD, Stiehl JB, Dennis DA, et al: Mathematical model of the lower extremity joint reaction forces using Kane's method of dynamics, *J Biomech* 31:185, 1998.

96. Kressig RW, Gregor RJ, Oliver A, et al: Temporal and spatial features of gait in older adults transitioning to frailty, *Gait Posture* 20:30-35, 2004.

97. Kuo AD: The six determinants of gait and the inverted pendulum analogy: a dynamic walking perspective, *Hum Mov Sci* 26:617-656, 2007.

98. Kuster M, Wood GA, Sakurai S, Blatter G: Stress on the femoropatellar joint in downhill walking—a biomechanical study, *Z Unfallchir Versicherungsmed* 86:178, 1993.

99. Lafortune MA, Cavanagh PR, Sommer III HJ, Kalenak A: Three-dimensional kinematics of the human knee during walking, *J Biomech* 25:347, 1992.

100. Lamoth CJC, Meijer OG, Daffertshofer A, et al: Effects of chronic low back pain on trunk coordination and back muscle activity during walking: changes in motor control, *Eur Spine J* 15:23-40, 2006.

101. Lay AN, Hass CJ, Nichols TR, Gregor RJ: The effect of sloped surfaces on locomotion: an electromyographic analysis, *J Biomech* 40:1276-1285, 2007.

102. Lee JL, Hidler J: Biomechanics of overground vs. treadmill walking in healthy individuals, *J Appl Physiol* 104:747-755, 2008.

103. Lerner-Frankiel MB, Vargas S, Brown MB, et al: Functional community ambulation: What are your criteria? *Clin Manage* 6:12, 1990.

104. Liu J, Lockhart TE: Comparison of 3D joint moments using local and global inverse dynamic approaches among three different age groups, *Gait Posture* 23:480-485, 2006.

105. Liu MQ, Anderson FC, Schwartz MH, Delp SL: Muscle contributions to support and progression over a range of walking speeds, *J Biomech* 41:3243-3252, 2008.

106. Lockart TE, Spaulding JM, Park SH: Age-related slip avoidance strategy while walking over a known slippery surface, *Gait Posture* 26:142-149, 2007.

107. Mackay-Lyons M: Central pattern generation of locomotion: a review of the evidence, *Phys Ther* 82:69-83, 2002.

108. Magnusson SP, Hansen P, Aagaard P, et al: Differential strain patterns of the human gastrocnemius aponeurosis and free tendon, in vivo, *Acta Physiol Scand* 177:185-195, 2003.

109. Magnusson SP, Narici MV, Maganaris CN, Kjaer M: Human tendon behavior and adaptation, in vivo, *J Physiol* 586:71-81, 2008.

110. Mann RA: Biomechanics of the foot. In American Academy of Orthopaedic Surgeons, editors: *Atlas of Orthotics: Biomechanical Principles and Application*, St Louis, 1975, Mosby.

111. Marchetti GF, Whitney SL, Blatt PJ, et al: Temporal and spatial characteristics of gait during performance of the dynamic gait index in people with and people without balance or vestibular disorders, *Phys Ther* 88:640-651, 2008.

112. Marey EJ: De la measure dans les different acts de la locomotion, *Comptes rendus de l'Academie des Sciences de Paris* 97:820-825, 1883.

113. Marey EJ: *La machine animal*, Paris, 1873, Librairie Germer Baillière.

114. Marey EJ: *Movement*, London, 1895, W. Heinemann.

115. Massaad F, Lejeune TM, Detrembleur C: The up and down bobbing of human walking: a compromise between muscle work and efficiency, *J Physiol* 582(2):789-799, 2007.

116. McGinley JL, Baker R, Wolfe R, Morris ME: The reliability of the three-dimensional kinematic gait measurements: a systematic review, *Gait Posture* 29:360-369, 2009.

117. Menant JC, Steele JR, Menz HB, et al: Effects of walking surfaces and footwear on temporo-spatial gait parameters in young and older people, *Gait Posture* 29:392-397, 2009.

118. Menz HB, Latt MD, Tiedemann A, et al: Reliability of the GAITRite walkway system for the quantification of temporo-spatial parameters of gait in young and older people, *Gait Posture* 20:20-25, 2004.

119. Menz HB, Lord SR, Fitzpatrick RC: Acceleration patterns of the head and pelvis when walking on level and irregular surfaces, *Gait Posture* 18:35-46, 2003.

120. Mills PM, Barrett RS, Morrison S: Toe clearance variability during walking in young and elderly men, *Gait Posture* 28:101-107, 2008.

121. Mizner RL, Kawaguchi JK, Chmieleski TL: Muscle strength in the lower extremity does not predict postinstruction improvements in the landing patterns of female athletes, *J Orthop Sports Phys Ther* 38:353-361, 2008.

122. Molen HH: *Problems on the evaluation of gait*, Amsterdam, 1973, Free University.

123. Moosabhoy MA, Gard SA: Methodology for determining the sensitivity of swing leg toe clearance and leg length to swing leg joint angles during gait, *Gait Posture* 24:493-501, 2006.

124. Murley GS, Landorf KB, Menz HB, Bird AR: Effect of foot posture, foot orthoses and footwear on lower limb muscle activity during walking and running: a systematic review, *Gait Posture* 29:172-187, 2009.

125. Murray MP: Gait as a total pattern of movement, *Am J Phys Med* 46:290, 1967.

126. Murray MP, Gore DR: Gait of patients with hip pain or loss of hip joint motion. In Black J, Dumbleton JH, editors: *Clinical biomechanics: a case history approach*, New York, 1981, Churchill Livingstone.

127. Murray MP, Gore DR, Clarkson BH: Walking patterns of patients with unilateral hip pain due to osteoarthritis and avascular necrosis, *J Bone Joint Surg Am* 53:259, 1971.

128. Murray MP, Gore DR, Sepic SB, Mollinger LA: Antalgic maneuvers during walking in men with unilateral knee disability, *Clin Orthop Relat Res* 199:192, 1985.

129. Murray MP, Guten GN, Mollinger LA, Gardner GM: Kinematic and electromyographic patterns of Olympic race walkers, *Am J Sports Med* 11:68, 1983.

130. Murray MP, Kory RC, Clarkson BH, Sepic SB: Comparison of free and fast speed walking patterns of normal men, *Am J Phys Med* 45:8, 1966.

131. Murray MP, Kory R, Sepic S: Walking patterns of normal women, *Arch Phys Med Rehabil* 51:637, 1979.

132. Murray MP, Sepic SB, Barnard EJ: Patterns of sagittal rotation of the upper limbs in walking: study of normal men during free and fast speed walking, *Phys Ther* 47:272, 1967.

133. Muybridge E: *Animal locomotion*, Philadelphia, 1887, University of Pennsylvania Press.

134. Muybridge E: *Human and animal locomotion*, New York, 1979, Dover.

135. Nankaku M, Tsuboyama T, Kakinoki R, et al: Gait analysis of patients in early stages after total hip arthroplasty: effect of lateral trunk displacement on walking efficiency, *J Orthop Sci* 12:550-554, 2007.

136. Nene A, Byrne C, Hermens H: Is rectus femoris really a part of quadriceps? Assessment of rectus femoris function during gait in able-bodied adults, *Gait Posture* 20:1-13, 2004.

137. Neptune RR, Sasaki K, Kautz SA: The effect of walking speed on muscle function and mechanical energetics, *Gait Posture* 28:135-143, 2008.

138. Neumann DA: Biomechanical analysis of selected principles of hip joint protection, *Arthritis Care Res* 2:146, 1989.

139. Nielsen JB: How we walk: central control of muscle activity during human walking, *Neuroscientist* 9:195-204, 2003.

140. Norkin CC: Examination of gait. In O'Sullivan SB, Schmitz TJ: *Physical rehabilitation*, ed 5, Philadelphia, 2007, FA Davis.

141. Ortega JD, Farley CT: Minimizing center of mass vertical movement increases metabolic cost in walking, *J Applied Physiol* 99:2099-2107, 2005.

142. O'Sullivan SB, Schmitz TJ: *Physical rehabilitation*, ed 5, Philadelphia, 2007, FA Davis.

143. Ounpuu S: Clinical gait analysis. In Spivack BS, editor: *Evaluation and management of gait disorders*, New York, 1995, Marcel Dekker.

144. Patla A: A framework for understanding mobility problems in the elderly. In Craik RL, Oatis CA, editors: *Gait analysis: theory and application*, St Louis, 1995, Mosby.

145. Paul JP: Forces transmitted by joints in the human body, *Proc Inst Mech Eng* 181:8, 1966.

146. Pederson DR, Brand RA, Davy DT: Pelvic muscle and acetabular contact forces during gait, *J Biomech* 30:959, 1997.

147. Perry J: *Gait analysis: normal and pathological function*, Thorofare, NJ, 1992, Slack.

148. Powers CM: The influence of altered lower-extremity kinematics on patellofemoral joint dysfunction: a theoretical perspective, *J Orthop Sports Phys Ther* 33:639-646, 2003.

149. Ralston HJ: Effects of immobilization of various body segments on energy cost of human locomotion, *Ergon Suppl* 53, 1965.

150. Reischl SF, Powers CM, Rao S, Perry J: Relationship between foot pronation and rotation of the tibia and femur during walking, *Foot Ankle Int* 20:513, 1999.

151. Requiao LF, Nadeau S, Milot MH, et al: Quantification of level of effort at the plantarflexors and hip extensors and flexor muscles in healthy subjects walking at different cadences, *J Electromyogr Kinesiol* 15:393-405, 2005.

152. Riley PO, Paolini G, Della Croce U, et al: A kinematic and kinetic comparison of overground and treadmill walking in healthy subjects, *Gait Posture* 26:17-24, 2007.

153. Robinett CS, Vondran MA: Functional ambulation velocity and distance requirements in rural and urban communities, *Phys Ther* 68:1371, 1988.

154. Rose J, Ralston HJ, Gamble JG: Energetics of walking. In Rose J, Gamble JG, editors: *Human walking*, ed 2, Philadelphia, 1994, Williams & Wilkins.

155. Rozumalski A, Schwartz MH, Wervey R, et al: The in vivo three-dimensional motion of the human lumbar spine during gait, *Gait Posture* 25:378-384, 2008.

156. Saibene F, Minetti AE: Biomechanical and physiological aspects of legged locomotion in humans, *Eur J Appl Physiol* 88:297-316, 2003.

157. Sasaki K, Neptune RR: Muscle mechanical work and elastic energy utilization during walking and running near the preferred gait transition speed, *Gait Posture* 23:383-390, 2006.

158. Saunders JB, Inman VT, Eberhart HD: The major determinants in normal and pathological gait, *J Bone Joint Surg Am* 35:543, 1953.

159. Schache AG, Baker R: On the expression of joint moments during gait, *Gait Posture* 25:440-452, 2007.

160. Schache AG, Baker R, Vaughan CL: Differences in lower limb transverse plane joint moments during gait when expressed in two alternative reference frames, *J Biomech* 40:9-19, 2007.

161. Schnall BL, Baum BS, Andrews AM: Gait characteristics of a soldier with a traumatic hip disarticulation, *Phys Ther* 88:1568-1577, 2008.

162. Scott SH, Winter DA: Internal forces of chronic running injury sites, *Med Sci Sports Exerc* 22:357, 1990.

163. Segers V, Aerts P, Lenoir M, De Clercq D: Spatiotemporal characteristics of the walk-to-run and run-to-walk transition when gradually changing speed, *Gait Posture* 24:247-254, 2006.

164. Shiavi R: Electromyographic patterns in adult locomotion: a comprehensive review, *J Rehabil* 22:85, 1985.

165. Shumway-Cook A, Woollacott MH: *Motor control: translating research into clinical practice*, Philadelphia, 2006, Lippincott, Williams & Wilkins.

166. Siegler S, Liu W: Inverse dynamics in human locomotion. In Allard P, Cappozzo A, Lundberg A, Vaughan CL, editors: *Three-dimensional analysis of human locomotion*, New York, 1997, John Wiley & Sons.

167. Simoneau GG, Cavanagh PR, Ulbrecht JS, et al: The influence of visual factors on fall-related kinematic variables during stair descent by older women, *J Gerontol Med Sci* 46:M188, 1991.

168. Simonsen EB, Dyhre-Poulsen P, Voigt M, et al: Bone-on-bone forces during loaded and unloaded walking, *Acta Anat (Basel)* 152:133, 1995.

169. Smidt GL: Rudiments of gait. In Smidt GL, editor: *Gait in rehabilitation*, New York, 1990, Churchill Livingstone.

170. Souza RB, Powers CM: Differences in hip kinematics, muscle strength, and muscle activation between subjects with and without patellofemoral pain, *J Orthop Sports Phys Ther* 39:12-19, 2009.

171. Sparrow WA, Begg RK, Parker S: Variability in the foot-ground clearance and step timing of young and older men during single-task and dual-task treadmill walking, *Gait Posture* 28:563-567, 2008.

172. Stansfield BW, Hillman SJ, Hazlewood ME, et al: Normalisation of gait data in children, *Gait Posture* 17:81-87, 2003.

173. Stauffer RN, Chao EYS, Brewster RC: Force and motion analysis of the normal, diseased and prosthetic ankle joint, *Clin Orthop Relat Res* 127:189, 1977.

174. Stephenson JL, Lamontagne A, De Serres S: The coordination of upper and lower limb movements during gait in healthy and stroke individuals, *Gait Posture* 29:11-16, 2009.

175. Stewart C, Postans N, Schwartz MH et al: An exploration of the function of the triceps surae during normal gait using functional electrical stimulation, *Gait Posture* 26:482-488, 2007.

176. Stratham L, Murray MP: Early walking patterns of normal children, *Clin Orthop Relat Res* 79:8, 1971.

177. Sudarsky L: An overview of neurological diseases causing gait disorder. In Spivack BS, editor: *Evaluation and management of gait disorders*, New York, 1995, Marcel Dekker.

178. Sutherland D: Dimensionless gait measurements and gait maturity, *Gait Posture* 4:209-211, 1996.

179. Sutherland DH, Kaufman KR, Moitoza JR: Kinematics of normal human walking. In Rose J, Gamble JG, editors: *Human walking*, ed 2, Philadelphia, 1994, Williams & Wilkins.

180. Sutherland DH, Olshen RA, Cooper L, Woo SL: The development of mature gait, *J Bone Joint Surg Am* 62A:336-353, 1980.

181. Sutherland DH: The evolution of clinical gait analysis. Part I: kinesiological EMG, *Gait Posture* 14:61-70, 2001.

182. Sutherland DH: The evolution of clinical gait analysis. Part II: kinematics, *Gait Posture* 16:159-179, 2002.

183. Sutherland DH: The evolution of clinical gait analysis. Part III: kinetics and energy assessment, *Gait Posture* 21:447-461, 2005.

184. Taylor SJ, Walker PS, Perry JS, et al: The forces in the distal femur and the knee during walking and other activities measured by telemetry, *J Arthroplasty* 13:428, 1998.

185. Thambyah A, Hee HT, Das S, Lee SM: Gait adaptations in patients with longstanding hip fusion, *J Orthop Surg* 11:154-158, 2003.

186. van Gent RN, Siem D, van Middelkoop M, et al: Incidence and determinants of lower extremity running injuries in long distance runners: a systematic review, *Br J Sports Med* 41:469-480, 2007.

187. van Hedel HJA, Tomatis L, Muller R: Modulating of leg muscle activity and gait kinematics by walking speed and bodyweight unloading, *Gait Posture* 24:35-45, 2006.

188. Vaughan CL: Theories of bipedal walking: an odyssey, *J Biomech* 36:513-523, 2003.

189. Vierordt KH: *Das gehen des menschen in gesunden und kranken zuständen nach selbstregistrirenden methoden dargestellt*, Tubingen, Germany, 1881, Laupp.

190. Walsh JP: Foot fall measurement technology. In Craik RL, Oatis CA, editors: *Gait analysis: theory and application*, St Louis, 1995, Mosby.

191. Warren GL, Maher RM, Higbie EJ: Temporal patterns of plantar pressures and lower-leg muscle activity during walking: effect of speed, *Gait Posture* 19:91-100, 2004.

192. Waters RL, Barnes G, Husserel T, et al: Comparable energy expenditure after arthrodesis of the hip and ankle, *J Bone Joint Surg Am* 70:1032, 1988.

193. Waters RL, Campbell J, Thomas L, et al: Energy costs of walking in lower-extremity plaster casts, *J Bone Joint Surg Am* 64:896, 1982.

194. Waters RL, Lunsford BR, Perry J, Byrd R: Energy-speed relationship of walking: standard tables, *J Orthop Res* 6:215, 1988.

195. Waters RL, Morris JM: Electrical activity of muscles of the trunk during walking, *J Anat* 111:2, 191-199, 1972.

196. Waters RL, Mulroy S: The energy expenditure of normal and pathologic gait, *Gait Posture* 9:207, 1999.

197. Webb D, Tuttle RH, Baksh M: Pendular activity of human upper limbs during slow and normal walking, *Am J Phys Anthropol* 93:477, 1993.

198. Weber W, Weber E: *Mechanik der menschlichen gewerkzeuge. [Mechanics of the human walking apparatus]*. Berlin, Germany, 1894, Springer-Verlag.

199. Weber W, Weber E: *Mechanics of the human walking apparatus*, (Translation by Maquet P, Furlong R.) Berlin, Germany, 1991, Springer-Verlag. (Original work published in 1894.).

200. Weber W, Weber E: *The mechanics of human motion*, Gottingen, Germany, 1836, Dieterischen Buchhandlung.

201. Whittington B, Silder A, Heiderscheit B, Thelen DG: The contribution of passive-elastic mechanisms to lower extremity joint kinetics during human walking, *Gait Posture* 27:628-634, 2008.

202. Whittle M: *Gait analysis: an introduction*, ed 4, Oxford, UK, 2007, Butterworth-Heinemann.

203. Winter DA: *Anatomy, biomechanics and control of balance during standing and walking*, Waterloo, Ontario, Canada, 1995, Waterloo Biomechanics.

204. Winter DA: *The biomechanics and motor control of human gait: normal, elderly and pathological*, ed 2, Waterloo, Canada, 1991, University of Waterloo Press.

205. Winter DA, Eng JJ, Ishac M: Three-dimensional moments, powers and work in normal gait: implications for clinical assessments. In Harris GF, Smith PA, editors: *Human motion analysis: current applications and future directions*, New York, 1996, IEEE Press.

206. Winter DA, Eng JJ, Ishac MG: A review of kinetic parameters in human walking. In Craik RL, Oatis CA, editors: *Gait analysis: theory and application*, St Louis, 1995, Mosby.

207. Yizhar Z, Boulos S, Inbar O, Carmeli E: The effect of restricted arm swing on energy expenditure in healthy men, *Int J Rehabil Res* Dec 5, 2008 [Epub ahead of print].

208. Youdas JW, Hollman JH, Aalbers MJ, et al: Agreement between the GAITRite walkway system and a stopwatch-footfall count method for measurement of temporal and spatial gait parameters, *Arch Phys Med Rehabil* 87:1648-1652, 2006.

209. Zajac FE, Neptune RR, Kautz SA: Biomechanics and muscle coordination of human walking part I: introduction to concepts, power transfer, dynamics and simulations, *Gait Posture* 16:215-232, 2002.

210. Zajac FE, Neptune RR, Kautz SA: Biomechanics and muscle coordination of human walking part II: lessons from dynamical simulations and clinical implications, *Gait Posture* 17:1-17, 2003.

211. Zarrugh MY, Todd FN, Ralston HJ: Optimization of energy expenditure during level walking, *Eur J Appl Physiol* 33:293, 1974.

212. Zehr EP, Duysens J: Regulation of arm and leg movement during human locomotion, *Neuroscientist* 10:347-361, 2004.

STUDY QUESTIONS

1 At what point(s) in the gait (walking) cycle is the potential energy (A) greatest, and (B) least?

2 At 10% into the gait cycle, describe the position and direction of rotation of the hip, knee, and ankle with respect to the sagittal plane.

3 A, Describe the rotation at the ankle at between 5% and 40% of the gait cycle with respect to the sagittal plane. B, Describe the type of muscle activation (eccentric, isometric, concentric) of the ankle plantar flexor and dorsiflexor muscles within the context of the kinematics described in part A.

4 Between mid and late stance (about 30% to 50% of the gait cycle), a person with a tight or short heel cord (Achilles tendon) often makes kinematic compensations within the foot as a way to allow continued forward rotation of the leg relative to the ground. Describe a kinematic compensation that may allow this, including the specific joint(s) where it may occur.

5 At what point(s) in the gait (walking) cycle are the vertical ground reaction forces (A) greatest and (B) least?

6 A, For 0% to about 50% of the gait cycle, describe the kinematics of the hip joint in the horizontal plane. B, Using Figure 15-29, A as a guide, discuss a possible role of the gluteus minimus and the gluteus medius muscles during these kinematics.

7 Describe kinematic strategies typically used to optimize the vertical and medial-lateral displacements of the center of mass of the body during walking.

8 For about 5% to 20% of the gait cycle, correlate the functional association between the frontal plane kinematics at the stance hip with the type of muscle activation of the gluteus medius.

9 What are the two basic kinematic mechanisms used to increase walking speed?

10 Describe the primary differences in the kinematics, kinetics, and muscular activations at the ankle during walking and running. (Assume for running that the person is a "heel striker.")

11 A, For mid and terminal stance (about 30% and 50% of the gait cycle), describe the likely position and direction of movement of the subtalar joint in the frontal plane. Use frontal plane movements of inversion and eversion (of the calcaneus) as a reference for your description. B, Using Figure 15-29, B as a guide, explain the most likely role of the tibialis posterior muscle in controlling these kinematics.

12 What is one likely role of the adductor longus muscle at 60% to 75% of the gait cycle?

13 Describe the changes that typically occur in gait in aged persons. What natural protection may these changes provide?

14 At what point in the gait (walking) cycle are the following two muscles most likely at their greatest length? A, semitendinosus; B, gastrocnemius.

15 Figure 15-40 shows the primary mechanics associated with the production of a varus torque at the knee at the instant of heel contact. Which tissues at the knee are capable of limiting this torque?

⊖ *Answers to the study questions can be found on the Evolve website.*

IV

Reference Materials for Muscle Attachments and Innervation of the Lower Extremity

Part A:
Spinal Nerve Root Innervations of the Muscles of the Lower Extremity

Part B:
Key Muscles for Testing the Function of Spinal Nerve Roots (L^2 to S^3)

Part C:
Dermatomes of the Lower Extremity

Part D:
Attachments and Innervation of the Muscles of the Lower Extremity

Part A: Spinal Nerve Root Innervations of the Muscles of the Lower Extremity

Muscle	Spinal Nerve Root							
	Lumbar					Sacral		
	L¹	L²	L³	L⁴	L⁵	S¹	S²	S³
Psoas minor	**X**							
Psoas major	*X*	**X**	**X**	*X*				
Iliacus		**X**	**X**	*X*				
Pectineus		**X**	**X**	*X*				
Sartorius		**X**	**X**					
Quadriceps		*X*	**X**	*X*				
Adductor brevis		**X**	**X**	*X*				
Adductor longus		**X**	**X**	*X*				
Gracilis		**X**	**X**	*X*				
Obturator externus			**X**	**X**				
Adductor magnus		*X*	**X**	**X**	**X**	*X*		
Gluteus medius				**X**	**X**	**X**		
Gluteus minimus				**X**	**X**	**X**		
Tensor fasciae latae				**X**	**X**	**X**		
Gluteus maximus					**X**	**X**	*X*	
Piriformis						**X**	**X**	
Gemellus superior					**X**	**X**	**X**	
Obturator internus					**X**	**X**	**X**	
Gemellus inferior				**X**	**X**	**X**		
Quadratus femoris				**X**	**X**	**X**		
Biceps (long head)					*X*	**X**	**X**	
Semitendinosus				*X*	**X**	**X**	**X**	
Semimembranosus				*X*	**X**	**X**	*X*	
Biceps (short head)					**X**	**X**	*X*	
Tibialis anterior				**X**	**X**			
Extensor hallucis longus				*X*	**X**	**X**		
Extensor digitorum longus				*X*	**X**	**X**		
Fibularis tertius				*X*	**X**	**X**		
Extensor digitorum brevis				*X*	**X**	**X**		
Fibularis longus				*X*	**X**	**X**		
Fibularis brevis				*X*	**X**	**X**		
Plantaris				*X*	**X**	**X**		
Gastrocnemius						**X**	**X**	
Popliteus				**X**	**X**	**X**		
Soleus					*X*	**X**	**X**	
Tibialis posterior				*X*	**X**	*X*		
Flexor digitorum longus					**X**	**X**	**X**	
Flexor hallucis longus					*X*	**X**	**X**	
Flexor digitorum brevis					*X*	**X**	**X**	
Abductor hallucis					*X*	**X**	**X**	
Flexor hallucis brevis					*X*	**X**	**X**	
Lumbrical I					*X*	**X**	**X**	
Abductor digiti minimi						*X*	**X**	**X**
Quadratus plantae						*X*	**X**	**X**
Flexor digiti minimi						*X*	**X**	**X**
Abductor digiti minimi						*X*	**X**	**X**
Adductor hallucis						*X*	**X**	**X**
Plantar interossei							**X**	**X**
Dorsal interossei							**X**	**X**
Lumbricals II, III, IV						*X*	**X**	**X**

Data based on two primary references: Standring S. *Gray's anatomy: the anatomical basis of clinical practice*, 40th ed, St Louis: Elsevier, 2009; Kendall FP, McCreary EK, Provance PG et al: *Muscles: testing and function with posture and pain*, ed 5, Philadelphia, 2005, Lippincott Williams & Wilkins.
X, minor-to-moderate literature support; **X**, major distribution.

Part B: Key Muscles for Testing the Function of Spinal Nerve Roots (L^2 to S^3)

The table shows the key muscles typically used to test the function of individual spinal nerve roots of the lumbosacral plexus (L^2 to S^3). Reduced strength in a key muscle may indicate an injury to or pathologic process within the associated spinal nerve root. Significant overlap exists in muscle innervation.

Key Muscles	Primary Nerve Root	Sample Test Movements
Iliopsoas	L^2	Hip flexion
Adductor longus	L^2	Hip adduction
Quadriceps	L^3	Knee extension
Tibialis anterior	L^4	Ankle dorsiflexion
Extensor digitorum longus	L^5	Toe extension
Gluteus medius	L^5	Hip abduction
Gluteus maximus	S^1	Hip extension with knee flexed
Semitendinosus	S^1	Knee flexion and internal rotation
Gastrocnemius and soleus	S^2	Ankle plantar flexion
Flexor hallucis longus	S^2	Flexion of the great toe
Dorsal and plantar interossei	S^3	Abduction and adduction of the toes

Part C: Dermatomes of the Lower Extremity

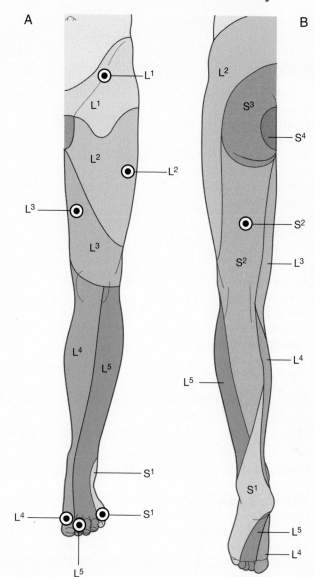

FIGURE IV-1.   Dermatomes of the lower extremity. **A,** Anterior. **B,** Posterior. Bold dots indicate regions often used clinically to test each dermatome. (*L^1*, first lumbar nerve root; *S^1*, first sacral nerve root; and so on.) (From Drake R, Vogl W, Mitchell A: *Gray's anatomy for students,* Philadelphia, 2005, Churchill Livingstone.)

Part D: Attachments and Innervation of the Muscles of the Lower Extremity

HIP AND KNEE MUSCULATURE

Adductor Brevis
Proximal attachment: anterior surface of the inferior pubic ramus
Distal attachment: proximal one third of the linea aspera of the femur
Innervation: obturator nerve

Adductor Longus
Proximal attachment: anterior surface of the body of the pubis
Distal attachment: middle one third of the linea aspera of the femur
Innervation: obturator nerve

Adductor Magnus
Anterior Head
Proximal attachment: ischial ramus
Distal attachment (horizontal fibers): extreme proximal end of linea aspera of femur
Distal attachment (oblique fibers): entire linea aspera of the femur
Innervation: obturator nerve

Posterior (Extensor) Head
Proximal attachment: ischial tuberosity
Distal attachment: adductor tubercle of the femur
Innervation: tibial portion of sciatic nerve

Articularis Genu
Proximal attachment: anterior surface of the distal femoral shaft
Distal attachments: proximal capsule and synovial membrane of the knee
Innervation: femoral nerve

Biceps Femoris
Long Head
Proximal attachments: from a common tendon with the semitendinosus; originating from a medial impression on the posterior surface of the ischial tuberosity and part of the sacrotuberous ligament
Distal attachment: head of the fibula
Innervation: tibial portion of the sciatic nerve

Short Head
Proximal attachment: lateral lip of the linea aspera below the gluteal tuberosity
Distal attachment: head of the fibula
Innervation: common fibular (peroneal) portion of the sciatic nerve

Gemellus Inferior
Proximal attachment: upper part of the ischial tuberosity
Distal attachment: blends with the tendon of the obturator internus
Innervation: nerve to the quadratus femoris and gemellus inferior

Gemellus Superior
Proximal attachment: dorsal surface of the ischial spine
Distal attachment: blends with the tendon of the obturator internus
Innervation: nerve to the obturator internus and gemellus superior

Gluteus Maximus
Proximal attachments: outer ilium, posterior gluteal line, thoracolumbar fascia, posterior side of sacrum and coccyx, and part of sacrotuberous and posterior sacroiliac ligaments
Distal attachments: gluteal tuberosity and iliotibial band
Innervation: inferior gluteal nerve

Gluteus Medius
Proximal attachment: outer surface of the ilium, above the anterior gluteal line
Distal attachment: lateral surface of the greater trochanter
Innervation: superior gluteal nerve

Gluteus Minimus
Proximal attachment: outer surface of the ilium between the anterior and inferior gluteal lines, as far posterior as the greater sciatic notch
Distal attachments: anterior-lateral aspect of the greater trochanter and portion of superior capsule of the joint
Innervation: superior gluteal nerve

Gracilis
Proximal attachments: anterior aspect of lower body of pubis and inferior ramus of pubis
Distal attachment: proximal medial surface of the tibia just posterior to the upper end of the attachment of the sartorius
Innervation: obturator nerve

Iliopsoas
Psoas Major
Proximal attachments: transverse processes and lateral bodies of the last thoracic and all lumbar vertebrae including the intervertebral discs
Distal attachment: lesser trochanter of the femur

Iliacus
Proximal attachments: superior two thirds of the iliac fossa, inner lip of the iliac crest, and small region of the sacrum across the sacroiliac joint
Distal attachment: lesser trochanter of the femur via the lateral side of psoas major tendon
Innervation of Iliopsoas: femoral nerve (Psoas major also receives branches from L^1)

Obturator Externus
Proximal attachments: external surface of the obturator membrane and surrounding external surfaces of the inferior pubic ramus and ischial ramus
Distal attachment: medial surface of the greater trochanter at the trochanteric fossa
Innervation: obturator nerve

Obturator Internus
Proximal attachments: internal side of the obturator membrane and immediately surrounding surfaces of the inferior pubic

ramus and ischial ramus; bony attachments extend superiorly within the pelvis to the greater sciatic notch

Distal attachment: medial surface of the greater trochanter just anterior and superior to the trochanteric fossa

Innervation: nerve to the obturator internus and gemellus superior

Pectineus

Proximal attachment: pectineal line on superior pubic ramus

Distal attachment: pectineal (spiral) line on the posterior surface of the femur

Innervation: femoral nerve and occasionally a branch from the obturator nerve

Piriformis

Proximal attachment: anterior side of the sacrum between the sacral foramina; blends partially with the capsule of the sacroiliac joint

Distal attachment: apex of the greater trochanter

Innervation: nerve to the piriformis

Popliteus

Proximal attachment: by an intracapsular tendon that attaches to the lateral aspect of the lateral femoral condyle

Distal attachments: posterior surface of the proximal tibia above the soleal line; also attaches to lateral meniscus

Innervation: tibial nerve

Psoas Minor

Proximal attachments: transverse processes and lateral bodies of the last thoracic and the first lumbar vertebra including the intervertebral disc

Distal attachment: pubis near the pectineal line

Innervation: branches from L^1

Quadratus Femoris

Proximal attachment: lateral surface of the ischial tuberosity just anterior to the attachments of the semimembranosus

Distal attachment: quadrate tubercle (middle of intertrochanteric crest)

Innervation: nerve to the quadratus femoris and gemellus inferior

Rectus Femoris

Proximal attachments: straight tendon–anterior-inferior iliac spine; reflected tendon–groove around the superior rim of the acetabulum and into the capsule of the hip

Distal attachment: base of the patella and, via the patellar tendon, the tibial tuberosity

Innervation: femoral nerve

Sartorius

Proximal attachment: anterior-superior iliac spine

Distal attachment: along a line on the proximal medial surface of the tibia

Innervation: femoral nerve

Semimembranosus

Proximal attachment: lateral impression on the posterior surface of the ischial tuberosity

Distal attachments: posterior aspect of the medial condyle of the tibia; additional attachments include the medial collateral ligament, oblique popliteal ligament, popliteus muscle, and medial meniscus

Innervation: tibial portion of the sciatic nerve

Semitendinosus

Proximal attachments: from a common tendon with the long head of the biceps femoris originating from a medial impression on the posterior surface of the ischial tuberosity and part of the sacrotuberous ligament

Distal attachment: proximal medial surface of the tibia, just posterior to the lower end of the attachment of the sartorius

Innervation: tibial portion of the sciatic nerve

Tensor Fasciae Latae

Proximal attachment: outer surface of the iliac crest just posterior to the anterior-superior iliac spine

Distal attachment: proximal one third of the iliotibial band of the fascia lata

Innervation: superior gluteal nerve

Vastus Intermedius

Proximal attachment: anterior-lateral regions of the upper two thirds of the femoral shaft

Distal attachments: lateral base of the patella, and, via the patellar tendon, the tibial tuberosity

Innervation: femoral nerve

Vastus Lateralis

Proximal attachments: upper region of intertrochanteric line, anterior and inferior border of the greater trochanter, lateral region of the gluteal tuberosity, lateral lip of the linea aspera

Distal attachments: lateral capsule of the knee, base of the patella, and, via the patellar tendon, the tibial tuberosity

Innervation: femoral nerve

Vastus Medialis

Proximal attachments: lower region of intertrochanteric line, medial lip of linea aspera, proximal medial supracondylar line, fibers from adductor magnus

Distal attachments: medial capsule of the knee, base of the patella, and, via the patellar tendon, the tibial tuberosity

Innervation: femoral nerve

ANKLE AND FOOT MUSCULATURE

Extensor Digitorum Longus

Proximal attachments: lateral condyle of tibia, proximal two thirds of the medial surface of the fibula, and adjacent interosseous membrane

Distal attachments: by four tendons that attach to the proximal base of the dorsal surface of the middle and distal phalanges via the dorsal digital expansion

Innervation: deep branch of the fibular (peroneal) nerve

Extensor Hallucis Longus

Proximal attachments: middle section of the medial surface of the fibula and adjacent interosseous membrane

Distal attachments: dorsal base of the distal phalanx of the great toe

Innervation: deep branch of the fibular nerve

Fibularis (Peroneus) Brevis
Proximal attachment: distal two thirds of the lateral surface of the fibula
Distal attachment: styloid process of the fifth metatarsal
Innervation: superficial branch of the fibular nerve

Fibularis (Peroneus) Longus
Proximal attachments: lateral condyle of tibia, head, and proximal two thirds of the lateral surface of the fibula
Distal attachment: lateral surface of the medial cuneiform and lateral side of the base of first metatarsal bone
Innervation: superficial branch of the fibular nerve

Fibularis (Peroneus) Tertius
Proximal attachments: distal one third of the medial surface of the fibula and adjacent interosseous membrane
Distal attachment: dorsal surface of the base of the fifth metatarsal
Innervation: deep branch of the fibular nerve

Flexor Digitorum Longus
Proximal attachments: posterior surface of the middle one third of the tibia just medial to the proximal attachment of the tibialis posterior
Distal attachments: by four separate tendons to the base of the distal phalanx of the four lesser toes
Innervation: tibial nerve

Flexor Hallucis Longus
Proximal attachment: distal two thirds of most of the posterior surface of the fibula
Distal attachment: plantar surface of the base of the distal phalanx of the great toe
Innervation: tibial nerve

Gastrocnemius
Proximal attachments: by two separate heads from the posterior aspect of the lateral and medial femoral condyle
Distal attachment: calcaneal tuberosity via the Achilles tendon
Innervation: tibial nerve

Plantaris
Proximal attachments: most inferior part of lateral supracondylar line of the femur and oblique popliteal ligament of the knee
Distal attachment: joins the medial aspect of the Achilles tendon to insert on the calcaneal tuberosity
Innervation: tibial nerve

Soleus
Proximal attachments: posterior surface of the fibula head and proximal one third of its shaft and from the posterior side of the tibia near the soleal line
Distal attachment: calcaneal tuberosity via the Achilles tendon
Innervation: tibial nerve

Tibialis Anterior
Proximal attachments: lateral condyle and proximal two thirds of the lateral surface of the tibia and the interosseous membrane

Distal attachment: medial and plantar aspects of the medial cuneiform and the base of the first metatarsal
Innervation: deep branch of the fibular nerve

Tibialis Posterior
Proximal attachments: proximal two thirds of the posterior surface of the tibia and fibula and adjacent interosseous membrane
Distal attachments: tendon attaches to every tarsal bone but the talus, plus the bases of the second through the fourth metatarsal bones; main insertion is on the navicular tuberosity and the medial cuneiform bone
Innervation: tibial nerve

INTRINSIC MUSCLES OF THE FOOT

Extensor Digitorum Brevis
Proximal attachment: lateral-distal aspect of the calcaneus just proximal to the calcaneocuboid joint
Distal attachments: usually by four tendons: one to the dorsal surface of the great toe, and the other three join the tendons of the extensor digitorum longus of the second through the fourth toes
Innervation: deep branch of the fibular nerve

LAYER 1
Abductor Digiti Minimi
Proximal attachments: medial and lateral processes of the calcaneal tuberosity, plantar aponeurosis, and plantar surface of the base of the fifth metatarsal bone with flexor digiti minimi
Distal attachment: lateral side of the proximal phalanx of the fifth toe, sharing an attachment with the flexor digiti minimi
Innervation: lateral plantar nerve

Abductor Hallucis
Proximal attachments: flexor retinaculum, medial process of the calcaneus and plantar fascia
Distal attachment: medial side of the base of proximal phalanx of the hallux, sharing an attachment with the medial tendon of the flexor hallucis brevis
Innervation: medial plantar nerve

Flexor Digitorum Brevis
Proximal attachments: medial process of calcaneal tuberosity and central part of the plantar fascia
Distal attachments: each of four tendons splits and inserts on the sides of the plantar aspect of the base of the middle phalanx of the lesser toes
Innervation: medial plantar nerve

LAYER 2
Lumbricals
Proximal attachments: from the tendons of the flexor digitorum longus muscle
Distal attachments: each muscle crosses the medial side of each metatarsophalangeal joint to insert into the dorsal digital expansion of the four lesser toes
Innervation: to second toe—medial plantar nerve; to third through fifth toes—lateral plantar nerve

Quadratus Plantae

Proximal attachments: by two heads from the medial and lateral aspect of the plantar surface of the calcaneus, distal to the calcaneal tuberosity

Distal attachment: lateral border of the flexor digitorum longus common tendon

Innervation: lateral plantar nerve

LAYER 3

Adductor Hallucis

Proximal Attachment

Oblique head: plantar aspect of the base of the second through fourth metatarsal and the fibrous sheath of the fibularis longus tendon

Transverse head: plantar aspect of the ligaments that support the metatarsophalangeal joints of the third through fifth toes

Distal attachments: both heads converge to insert on the lateral base of the proximal phalanx of the great toe along with the lateral tendon of the flexor hallucis brevis

Innervation: lateral plantar nerve

Flexor Digiti Minimi

Proximal attachments: plantar surface of the base of the fifth metatarsal bone and fibrous sheath covering the tendon of the fibularis longus

Distal attachment: lateral surface of the base of the proximal phalanx of the fifth toe blending with the tendon of the abductor digiti minimi

Innervation: lateral plantar nerve

Flexor Hallucis Brevis

Proximal attachments: plantar surface of the cuboid and lateral cuneiform bones, and on parts of the tendon of the tibialis posterior muscle

Distal attachments: by two tendons in which the lateral tendon attaches to the lateral base of the proximal phalanx of the great toe with the adductor hallucis, and the medial tendon attaches to the medial base of the proximal phalanx of the great toe with the abductor hallucis; a pair of sesamoid bones is located within the tendons of this muscle

Innervation: medial plantar nerve

LAYER 4

Dorsal Interossei

Proximal Attachments

First: adjacent sides of the first and second metatarsals

Second: adjacent sides of the second and third metatarsals

Third: adjacent sides of the third and fourth metatarsals

Fourth: adjacent sides of the fourth and fifth metatarsals

Distal Attachments*

First: medial side of the base of the proximal phalanx of the second toe

Second: lateral side of the base of the proximal phalanx of the second toe

Third: lateral side of the base of the proximal phalanx of the third toe

Fourth: lateral side of the base of the proximal phalanx of the fourth toe

Innervation: lateral plantar nerve

Plantar Interossei

Proximal Attachments

First: medial side of the third metatarsal

Second: medial side of the fourth metatarsal

Third: medial side of the fifth metatarsal

Distal Attachments*

First: medial side of the proximal phalanx of the third toe

Second: medial side of the proximal phalanx of the fourth toe

Third: medial side of the proximal phalanx of the fifth toe

Innervation: lateral plantar nerve

---

*Attaches into the dorsal digital expansion of the toes.

Index

Page numbers followed by *f* indicate figures; *t,* tables; *b,* boxes.